Organ
Transplantation
AND Replacement

ST BARTHOLOMEW'S AND THE ROYAL LONDON SCHOOL OF MEDICINE AND DENTISTRY

WHITECHAPEL LIBRARY, TURNER STREET, LONDON E1 2AD
020 7882 7110

4 WEEK LOAN
Books are to be returned on or before the last date below,
otherwise fines may be charged.

Organ
Transplantation
AND Replacement

G. JAMES CERILLI, M.D.

Professor of Surgery
Albany Medical College of Union University
Albany, New York

With 90 contributors

J. B. Lippincott Company PHILADELPHIA
LONDON MEXICO CITY NEW YORK ST. LOUIS SÃO PAULO SYDNEY

Acquisitions Editor: Lisette Bralow
Sponsoring Editor: Sanford J. Robinson
Manuscript Editor: Helen Ewan
Indexer: Betty Herr Hallinger
Designer: Susan Hess Blaker
Production Manager: Kathleen P. Dunn
Production Coordinator: Fred D. Wood IV
Compositor: Ruttle, Shaw & Wetherill, Inc.
Printer/Binder: Maple Press

1 3 5 6 4 2

Library of Congress Cataloging-in-Publication Data

Organ transplantation and replacement.

  Includes bibliographies and index.
  1. Transplantation of organs, tissues, etc.
I. Cerilli, G. James, 1933-   [DNLM: 1. Trans-
plantation. WO 660 0669]
RD120.7.0718   1987   617'.95   87-2839
ISBN 0-397-50732-1

Contributors

Linda Abress, B.A.
Graduate Research Assistant
Department of Sociology
University of Minnesota
Minneapolis, Minnesota

Guy P. J. Alexandre, M.D.
Professor of Surgery
Chief, Department of Renal Transplantation
Cliniques Universitaires St. Luc
Brussels, Belgium

Carol Anderson, B.A.
Graduate Research Assistant
Department of Sociology
University of Minnesota
Minneapolis, Minnesota

Nancy L. Ascher, M.D., Ph.D.
Assistant Professor of Surgery
Clinical Director of Liver Transplant Program
University of Minnesota Medical School—
    Minneapolis
Minneapolis, Minnesota

A. Bannett, M.D.
Professor of Surgery
Director of Transplantation
Albert Einstein Medical Center
Philadelphia, Pennsylvania

Clyde F. Barker, M.D., F.A.C.S.
John Rhea Barton Surgical Associates
Professor and Chairman
Director, Harrison Division of Surgical Research
University of Pennsylvania School of Medicine
Philadelphia, Pennsylvania

Glenn R. Barnhart, M.D.
Assistant Professor of Surgery
Virginia Commonwealth University
Medical College of Virginia School of Medicine
Richmond, Virginia

William H. Bay, M.D.
Associate Professor of Medicine
Department of Medicine
Director, Dialysis
University Hospitals
The Ohio State University
Columbus, Ohio

Folkert O. Belzer, M.D., F.A.C.S.
A.R. Curreri Professor of Surgery
Chairman of the Department of Surgery
University of Wisconsin Medical School
Madison, Wisconsin

Alan H. Bennett, M.D., F.A.C.S
Professor of Surgery (Urological)
Head, Division of Urological Surgery
Albany Medical College of Union University
Albany, New York

Alan I. Benvenisty, M.D.
Associate Professor of Medicine
Director of Emergency Services
Columbia University College of Physicians and
    Surgeons
New York, New York

Alan G. Birtch, M.D., F.A.C.S.
Professor of Surgery
Southern Illinois University School of Medicine
Assistant Chairman, Department of Surgery
Chairman, Division of General Surgery
Chief, Section of Transplantation
St. John's Hospital and Memorial Medical Center
Springfield, Illinois

Christopher R. Blagg, M.D., F.R.C.P.
Professor of Medicine
University of Washington School of Medicine
Executive Director
Northwest Kidney Center
Seattle, Washington

Lauren Brasile, B.S.
Research Associate
Department of Surgery
Albany Medical College of Union University
Albany, New York

William E. Braun, M.D.
Director of Histocompatibility and Immunogenetics
   Laboratory
Consultant in Transplantation
Cleveland Clinic Foundation
Cleveland, Ohio

Darrell A. Campbell, Jr., M.D.
Associate Professor of Surgery
Chief, General Surgery Division of Transplantation
University of Michigan Medical Center
Ann Arbor, Michigan

James Cicciarelli, Ph.D.
Adjunct Assistant Professor of Surgery
University of California, Los Angeles
UCLA School of Medicine
Los Angeles, California

Zane Cohen, M.D., F.R.C.S.(C), F.A.C.S.
Associate Professor of Surgery
Head, Colon and Rectal Residency Program
University of Toronto Faculty of Medicine
Toronto, Ontario

Geoffrey M. Collins, M.D.
Director, Transplant Division
Pacific Presbyterian Medical Center
San Francisco, California

Jack G. Copeland, M.D.
Professor of Surgery
Chief, Section of Cardiovascular and Thoracic
   Surgery
University of Arizona Health Sciences Center
Tucson, Arizona

Robert J. Corry, M.D.
Professor of Surgery
Chairman, Department of Surgery
University of Iowa College of Medicine
Iowa City, Iowa

P. William Curreri, M.D.
Professor and Chairman
Department of Surgery
University of South Alabama College of Medicine
Mobile, Alabama

Donald C. Dafoe, M.D.
Associate Professor of Surgery
University of Michigan Medical Center
Ann Arbor, Michigan

Steven V. Edelman, M.D.
Division of Endocrinology & Metabolism
University of California, San Diego,
School of Medicine
San Diego, California

Carlos O. Esquivel, M.D., Ph.D.
Assistant Professor of Surgery

University of Pittsburgh School of Medicine
Pittsburgh, Pennsylvania

Gary E. Friedlaender, M.D., F.A.C.S.
Professor and Chairman
Department of Orthopaedics and Rehabilitation
Yale University School of Medicine
Chief of Orthopaedics and Rehabilitation
Yale-New Haven Hospital
New Haven, Connecticut

William H. Frist, M.D.
Director, Heart–Lung Transplantation
Vanderbilt University Medical Center
Nashville, Tennessee

Robert D. Gordon, M.D.
Assistant Professor of Surgery
University of Pittsburgh School of Medicine
Pittsburgh, Pennsylvania

Carl E. Haisch, M.D.
Assistant Professor of Surgery
Director of Transplantation
University of Vermont College of Medicine
Burlington, Vermont

Mark A. Hardy, M.D.
Professor of Surgery
Director of Transplantation and Dialysis
Columbia University College of Physicians and
   Surgeons
New York, New York

Lee A. Hebert, M.D.
Professor of Medicine
Director, Division of Renal Diseases
Department of Medicine
Ohio State University College of Medicine
Columbus, Ohio

Debra A. Hullett, Ph.D.
Project Associate
University of Wisconsin
Madison, Wisconsin

Shunzaburo Iwatsuki, M.D.
Associate Professor of Surgery
University of Pittsburgh School of Medicine
Pittsburgh, Pennsylvania

Stuart W. Jamieson, M.B., F.R.C.S., F.A.C.S.
Professor and Head
Division of Cardiothoracic Surgery
University of Minnesota Hospital
Director, Minnesota Heart and Lung Institute
Minneapolis, Minnesota

Barry D. Kahan, Ph.D., M.D.
Professor of Surgery
Director, Division of Immunology and Organ
   Transplantation
University of Texas Medical School at Houston
Houston, Texas

Robert C. Kelch, M.D.
Professor of Pediatrics
University of Michigan Medical Center
Ann Arbor, Michigan

Ronald H. Kerman, Ph.D.
Professor of Surgery
Head, Histocompatibility and Immune Evaluation
 Laboratories
University of Texas Medical School at Houston
Houston, Texas

John W. Konnak, M.D.
Professor of Surgery
University of Michigan Medical Center
Ann Arbor, Michigan

Kevin J. Lafferty, Ph.D.
Research Director
Barbara Davis Center for Childhood Diabetes
Denver, Colorado

H. M. Lee, M.D., F.A.C.S.
Professor and Chairman
Division of Vascular Surgery
Director, Clinical Transplant Program
Virginia Commonwealth University
Medical College of Virginia School of Medicine
Richmond, Virginia

Neil Lempert, M.D.
Professor of Surgery
Director, Transplant Program
Albany Medical College of Union University
Albany, New York

Mark M. Levinson, M.D.
Assistant Professor
University of Arizona Health Sciences Center
Tucson, Arizona

Robert B. Love, M.D.
Fourth Year Resident
University of Wisconsin
Madison, Wisconsin

Richard R. Lower, M.D.
Professor of Surgery
Chairman, Division of Cardiothoracic Surgery
Virginia Commonwealth University
Medical College of Virginia School of Medicine
Richmond, Virginia

Arnold Luterman, M.D., F.R.C.S., F.A.C.S.
Professor of Surgery
Director, Burn Center
University of South Alabama College of Medicine
Mobile, Alabama

Leonard Makowka, M.D., Ph.D.
Assistant Professor of Surgery
University of Pittsburgh School of Medicine
Pittsburgh, Pennsylvania

Thomas L. Marchioro, M.D., F.A.C.S.
Professor of Surgery
Chief, Division of Transplantation
University of Washington School of Medicine
Seattle, Washington

James F. Markmann, B.A.
Medical Scientist Training Program Trainee
University of Pennsylvania School of Medicine
Philadelphia, Pennsylvania

Arthur J. Matas, M.D., F.A.C.S.
Associate Professor of Surgery
Montefiore Medical Center/Albert Einstein College
 of Medicine
New York, New York

Robert M. Merion, M.D.
Assistant Professor of Surgery
University of Michigan Medical Center
Ann Arbor, Michigan

Anthony P. Monaco, M.D.
Professor of Surgery
Harvard Medical School
Director of Division of Organ Transplantation
New England Deaconess Hospital
Boston, Massachusetts

Cheryl M. Montefusco, Ph.D.
Associate Professor of Surgery
Montefiore Medical Center/Albert Einstein College
 of Medicine
New York, New York

Francis D. Moore, M.D.
Moseley Professor of Surgery, Emeritus
Harvard Medical School
Surgeon-in-Chief, Emeritus
Peter Bent Brigham Hospital
Boston, Massachusetts

Kay C. Moudry, RNC
Pancreas Transplant Registry Coordinator
Department of Surgery
University of Minnesota
Minneapolis, Minnesota

John S. Najarian, M.D.
Regents' Professor and Chairman
Department of Surgery
University of Minnesota Hospitals & Clinics
Minneapolis, Minnesota

Ali Naji, M.D., Ph.D.
Assistant Professor of Surgery
University of Pennsylvania School of Medicine
Philadelphia, Pennsylvania

Thomas D. Overcast, J.D., Ph.D.
Partner, White, Overcast and Thomas
Consultant in Medicolegal Affairs
Seattle, Washington

Israel Penn, M.D., F.R.C.S.(Eng), F.R.C.S.(Can), F.A.C.S.
Professor of Surgery
University of Cincinnati Medical Center
Chief of Surgery
V.A. Medical Center
Cincinnati, Ohio

Stephen J. Prowse, Ph.D.
Assistant Professor of Microbiology and Immunology
The Barbara Davis Center for Childhood Diabetes
Denver, Colorado

Leslie L. Rocher, M.D.
Assistant Professor of Internal Medicine
University of Michigan Medical Center
Ann Arbor, Michigan

Robert H. Rubin, M.D.
Associate Professor of Medicine
Chief of Infectious Disease for Transplantation
Massachusetts General Hospital
Harvard Medical School
Boston, Massachusetts

Oscar Salvatierra, Jr., M.D.
Professor of Surgery and Urology
Chief, Transplant Service
University of California, San Francisco, School of Medicine
San Francisco, California

Mukund Sargur, M.D.
Senior Fellow
University of Washington School of Medicine
Seattle, Washington

James A. Schulak, M.D.
Associate Professor of Surgery
Case Western Reserve University School of Medicine
Director of Transplantation
University Hospitals of Cleveland
Cleveland, Ohio

Aileen B. Sedman, M.D.
Assistant Professor of Pediatrics
University of Michigan Medical Center
Ann Arbor, Michigan

Byers W. Shaw, Jr., M.D.
Associate Professor of Surgery
Chief of Transplantation Service
Department of Surgery
University of Nebraska Medical Center
Omaha, Nebraska

Richard K. Sibley, M.D.
Associate Professor of Pathology
Stanford University School of Medicine
Stanford, California

Richard Silverman, M.D.
Research Fellow
Division of General Surgery
Toronto General Hospital
Department of Surgery
University of Toronto Faculty of Medicine
Toronto, Ontario, Canada

Richard L. Simmons, M.D.
Professor of Surgery and Microbiology
Associate Director, Clinical Transplantation
University of Minnesota Medical School—Minneapolis
Minneapolis, Minnesota

Roberta G. Simmons, Ph.D.
Professor of Sociology and Psychiatry
University of Minnesota
Minneapolis, Minnesota

Richard S. Smith, M.D.
Professor and Chairman
Department of Ophthalmology
Albany Medical College of Union University
Albany, New York

Dale C. Snover, M.D.
Associate Professor
Associate Director of Anatomic Pathology
University of Minnesota Medical School—Minneapolis
Minneapolis, Minnesota

Hans W. Sollinger, M.D., Ph.D.
Associate Professor of Surgery and Pathology
Director, Histocompatibility Laboratory
University of Wisconsin Medical School
Madison, Wisconsin

James H. Southard, Ph.D.
Assistant Professor of Surgery
Department of Surgery
University of Wisconsin Medical School
Madison, Wisconsin

Jean-Paul Squifflet, M.D.
Associate, Chief of Clinics
Cliniques Universitaires St. Luc
Brussels, Belgium

Thomas E. Starzl, M.D.
Professor of Surgery
Chief of Transplantation
University of Pittsburgh School of Medicine
Pittsburgh, Pennsylvania

T. B. Strom, M.D.
Associate Professor of Medicine
Harvard Medical School
Boston, Massachusetts

David E. R. Sutherland, M.D., Ph.D.
Professor of Surgery

University of Minnesota Medical School—
   Minneapolis
Minneapolis, Minnesota

Vivian A. Tellis, M.D., F.A.C.S.
Associate Professor of Surgery
Co-Director of the Transplant Program
Montefiore Medical Center/Albert Einstein College
   of Medicine
New York, New York

Paul I. Terasaki, Ph.D.
Professor of Surgery
Division of UCLA Tissue Typing Laboratory
University of California, Los Angeles
UCLA School of Medicine
Los Angeles, California

E. Donnall Thomas, M.D.
Professor of Medicine
University of Washington School of Medicine
Associate Director for Clinical Research
Fred Hutchinson Cancer Research Center
Seattle, Washington

Nicholas L. Tilney, M.D., F.A.C.S., F.R.C.S.(Glas)
Professor of Surgery
Director, Surgical Research Laboratory
Harvard Medical School
Director, Transplant Service
Brigham & Women's Hospital
Boston, Massachusetts

Satoru Todo, M.D.
Visiting Assistant Professor of Surgery
University of Pittsburgh School of Medicine
Pittsburgh, Pennsylvania

Nina E. Tolkoff-Rubin, M.D., F.A.C.P.
Associate Professor of Medicine
Director, Hemodialysis Unit
Massachusetts General Hospital
Harvard Medical School
Boston, Massachusetts

Jeremiah G. Turcotte, M.D.
Professor of Surgery
Director, Organ Transplantation Center

Director, Transplant Policy Center
University of Michigan Medical Center
Ann Arbor, Michigan

Andreas G. Tzakis, M.D.
Assistant Professor of Surgery
University of Pittsburgh School of Medicine
Pittsburgh, Pennsylvania

Frank J. Veith, M.D., F.A.C.S.
Professor of Surgery
Director of the Transplant Program and Chief of
   Vascular Surgical Services
Montefiore Medical Center/Albert Einstein College
   of Medicine
New York, New York

Louis Vignati, M.D.
Instructor
Department of Medicine
Harvard Medical School
Boston, Massachusetts
Director, Diabetes Center
New England Sinai Hospital
Stoughton, Massachusetts

Ramses Wassef, M.D., MSc., F.R.C.S. (c)
Fellow
Medical Research Council of Canada
Division of General Surgery
Toronto General Hospital
Department of Surgery
University of Toronto Faculty of Medicine
Toronto, Ontario, Canada

G. Melville Williams, M.D.
Professor of Surgery
Chief, Division of Transplantation and Vascular
   Surgery
Johns Hopkins University School of Medicine
Baltimore, Maryland

R. Patrick Wood, M.D.
Assistant Professor of Surgery
Director of Student Education
Department of Surgery
University of Nebraska College of Medicine
Omaha, Nebraska

Preface

The successful transfer of tissue and organs from one individual to another has been one of the great achievements of modern medicine and surgery. The enormous progress made in transplantation in the 1960s was followed by a period of stability, with relatively few improvements in the 1970s. However, beginning in the late 1970s and in the 1980s, there has been a veritable explosion of new information both in basic transplant immunology and clinical transplantation. This information has been transferred into new methods of management for transplant patients, new organs being successfully transplanted, and a rising success rate. It was because of this extraordinary recent progress and the amount of information that has recently been accumulated that it became apparent that there was a need for a comprehensive textbook in transplantation that documented these accomplishments. Therefore, the objectives in compiling *Organ Transplantation and Replacement* are to:

1. Provide a summary of the pertinent science upon which transplantation is founded, namely, the fundamentals of transplant immunology.
2. Cover in detail the current practice and principles of renal transplantation, the transplant discipline about which most is known.
3. Describe the status of the science of *all* organs that are currently being transplanted.
4. Introduce the knowledge that is available on artificial organ replacement, particularly of the heart and pancreas, since replacement therapy complements organ transplantation and will do so increasingly in the future.

I decided that the optimal approach was to elicit the contributions of the experts in the field; therefore, this is a multi-author textbook. Thus the reader will find that in most instances, the chapters have been written by individuals who have been major contributors to the progress in transplantation.

There are several topics that are discussed, by design, in more than one section. This is appropriate for several reasons. Certain topics, for instance, the ethics of transplantation, relate to multiple aspects of transplantation (i.e., legality, the management of the transplant recipient, donor selection, and so forth). There are important programs that currently deserve emphasis, since they are on the frontier of transplantation, such as transplantation of the pancreas and pancreatic islets. Some topics are very extensive and even controversial. Thus more than one perspective is presented to aid in their comprehension.

If there is a general tone throughout the text, it is certainly one of optimism. Optimism for what has been accomplished and optimism for the future. However, we must also be realistic. While the successes of transplantation have been impressive, the successes have been incomplete. For example, current documented 15-year graft survival for cadaveric kidney allografts is approximately 20%. It is anticipated that this will increase with the introduction of cyclosporine and other current improvements, but even the most optimistic projections will increase graft survival to only 50% at 15 years. This is inadequate, and therefore kidney transplantation therapy is still palliative. Pancreatic islet transplantation has not been successful. While the results of whole-organ pancreas transplantation have improved, the technique is difficult and the successful transplantation of islets would broaden the application of this approach to the management of type 1 diabetes. Finally, we still depend on toxic drugs for immunosuppression and the management of rejection. The era of the biologic manipulation of the human recipient is just beginning. Biologic manipulation of the transplant recipient is the key to transplantation becoming safer and more successful. Lastly, mechanical organ replacement is still in its infancy. Progress has been exciting and substantial, and in the future it will not only complement transplantation, but will stand alone as a therapeutic modality. *Organ Transplantation and Replacement,* therefore, is designed not only to inform the reader of the current state of the art and science of transplantation and organ replacement, but hopefully to challenge, excite, and stimulate the audience to solve the problems that remain, such as those listed above. It is thus intended to be not only a compilation of past accomplishments, but also a catalyst for future developments.

I would like to acknowledge the encouragement and support provided in editing this text by Sharon Persbacker, Joann Stewart, and Mr. Brian Freed. Each of these individuals was extremely helpful in the enormous task of editing this major textbook. I also wish to acknowledge some of those who were instrumental in developing my transplantation career, particularly, Dr. Thomas Starzl, Dr. Thomas Marchioro, and Dr. William Waddell.

G. James Cerilli, M.D.

Foreword

For centuries surgeons have yearned for the day when they would be able to replace damaged or diseased tissues or organs by performing grafts from one human being to another and, perhaps more ambitiously, from lower animals to humans. More than 400 years ago Ambroise Paré listed "to supply the defects of nature" as one of the five things he considered to be "proper to the duties of a chirurgion." Happily this day is near at hand, thanks in part to a few pioneering studies dating back to the beginning of this century, but mainly to the burgeoning of interest and activity on the part of biologists and surgeons since the end of World War II.

This comprehensive and impressive volume is essentially an up-to-date, in-depth progress report on the attainment of this goal. No one can possibly know the whole of transplantation, for two main reasons. First, the intrusion of transplantation into and its considerable impact upon a variety of other disciplines, which include immunobiology, genetics, oncology, internal medicine, biochemistry, cellular and molecular biology, cryobiology, and jurisprudence has given the field enormous scope. Second, each tissue or organ is to some extent unique in its requirements for allotransplantation. These include, among other things, the development of some kind of adaptation of the recipient towards the graft and of the graft towards the recipient. Through necessity, therefore, this volume is an integrated symposium. Each of its various sections has been contributed by one or more international authorities who have been assigned generous amounts of space to cover their selected topics.

My own professional career as a transplantation biologist has been almost coeval with the explosive development of the field. I have witnessed periods of slow progress punctuated by periods of intense activity, in turn galvanized by the discovery (usually empirical) of new phenomena or by conceptual advances. Many of these have played important roles in the development of immunobiology. A few, after appropriate trials, have led to clinical application. These include anti-lymphocyte globulin; tissue typing, and especially matching for HLA-DR; "passenger cells"; the "transfusion effect" in renal transplantation; monoclonal antibodies; cyclosporine; total lymphoid irradiation; and pancreatic or islet transplantation.

We are now at that point where renal transplantation is firmly established as the preferred treatment of end-stage renal failure, and a considerable measure of success is attainable with cardiac and liver transplants. There are firm grounds for optimism about the future of pancreatic and lung graft. Obviously, these successes with organ grafts have required the solution of many challenging technical problems.

Although great progress has been made in understanding the host immune response and its effectuation—and in certain species we have learned how to manipulate it and even turn it off completely in an antigenically specific manner that does not require ongoing treatment with drugs or other agents—a relatively safe, specific means of abrogating the host response to allografts in humans has yet to be discovered. This remains a goal for the future.

Rupert E. Billingham

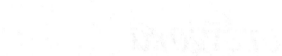

Contents

Organ
Transplantation
AND Replacement

PART ONE

Past, Present, Future

CHAPTER 1

The History of Transplantation—A Lesson for Our Time

Francis D. Moore

While the history of transplantation occupies a central focus in any text on transplantation, its importance far outweighs its inclusion as background because the history of transplantation is a paradigm of modern clinical advance. In it are to be found in full flower all the social and scientific forces involved in bioscience progress. Legislators, science policy advisors, sociologists, and scientists alike should study this history so that some components of success may be preserved.

Here we find the story of the work of a few pioneers, often unknown to their peers. It is a tale of a science whose application could not be clearly foreseen, a story of collaboration between clinician and scientist, with both sides contributing equally but at different times. Here is exemplified the bioengineering aspect of clinical work in general and of surgery in particular, improving as it goes without any clear "breakthroughs." Finally we see the widening social impact of a new procedure on public acceptance, government policy, and the emergence of a payment mechanism to make it generally available. In this brief account, there is room for only a few details of this fascinating story.

TRADING ORGANS— THE PRIMITIVE PERIOD

Moving Kidneys Around

A method of blood vessel anastomosis is required in order to move major vascularized organs such as the kidney from place to place in the same animal or from one animal to another. Alexis Carrel was the first to recognize this as a bioscientific problem that would yield to an engineering solution. His simple method of vascular anastomosis using fine needles and thread has been used ever since 1902, with but few modifications. It depends merely on careful dissection, exact identification of the several layers of the severed vessels to be joined, control of bleeding from both ends, and sewing them together in a manner that everts the intima.[9]

Having learned to perform this anastomosis, Carrel and Emerick Ullmann were amongst the first to study the transferring of organs in animals. The early cat kidney transplantations performed by Carrel were done "en masse," removing both kidneys, aorta, vena cava, and ureters with the kidneys, to give him sizeable vessels for anastomosis. He recognized that the transferred organs functioned normally, put out urine, and maintained life. He sensed that something was causing their loss, but he did not coin the term *rejection*. It did not seem to be infection or infarction. The concept of rejection was there, if not the modern term.[10]

Other workers, both in this country and abroad, were performing work of this type between 1900 and 1930. In almost all these experiments, kidneys were used because of their simple vascular supply; the presence of the ureter, which gives index of function within minutes; and the fact that it was a paired organ.

A New Process of Destruction

Along with this primitive work on trading organs came the realization that the loss of the grafted organ was due to a process quite distinct from infarction (i.e., loss of blood supply), avascular necrosis (i.e., loss of arterial supply), infection, or inflammation. The term *rejection* indicated a process by which the new host denied the organ a new place of residence. It was soon understood that this might have some relationship to the immunologic process by which an organism combats invading bacterial infection.

Early experiments with chickens, and with the understanding of the genetic implications of the freemartin phenomena, increased the immunogenetic background in this field.[8,15,23] Emile Holman, a surgeon of the Hopkins, Harvard, and Stanford, in the mid 1920s carried out in man an experiment whose repercussions are yet to be fully understood. He grafted the skin of a mother onto a badly burned child. When, some days later, he put more skin on the child, the child not only rejected the mother's skin quite rapidly (a foretaste of the "second set" phenomena) but, in addition, developed a severe necrotizing inflammation of his own skin. This suggested shared antigens and the development of an autoimmune disease as the cause of a necrotizing dermatitis. Holman clearly saw the remarkable implications of this experiment but was unable to pursue them further.[18]

The end of this period was marked by the experiments of David Hume, George Thorn, Gustave Dammin, and their group at the Peter Bent Brigham Hospital in Boston.[19] There, starting about 1951, kidneys were grafted from one subject to another, using the thigh as the recipient site. There had been one previous emergency experience based on using the arm as the site for a temporary kidney. With one exception, all these experiences showed that while the kidney was rejected, function was good for a time. One of the most important aspects of this Harvard/Brigham experience was that it was sophisticated collaborative scientific work involving medicine and surgery, pathology, radiology, and immunology, with mutual respect of all parties for the role that each played. There was no one department seeking to play a "prima donna" role and putting the others down as merely technical. It was a full-dress, fully academic collaboration, the results of which were published in detail in the literature. It was a forecast of the sort of group collaboration that was to mark the efforts of many leading institutions during the coming decades.

DIALYSIS, THE SECOND SET REACTION, AND THE TWINS—THE PERIOD OF PROMISE

World War II brought many severely injured young men together with many ingenious physicians and surgeons. Out of this experience came many aspects of medicine and surgery that we regard now as "modern," even though, 40 years later, we simply roll them up into the general history of the 20th century. This series of advances included antibiotics, plasma fractionation, massive blood transfusion, endotracheal positive pressure anesthesia, primary vascular anastomosis for arterial injury, dialysis, and the study of skin grafts. All of these contributed to advance in transplant science.

Dialysis

Willem Kolff, working in Holland during the War, made a dialysis machine using sausage casing and some tomato cans.[21] He had been inspired in this work by the previous studies of Abel, Rowntree, and Turner at Johns Hopkins[1] who showed that dialysis might indeed clear the blood of low–molecular weight substances that accumulate in renal failure. Kolff's own accounts of this early period deserve rereading. All his dialysis patients died. As he said, "It was a good thing the boss was away!" because he might have been fired! That commentary on the judgment of people in clinical authority over a new concept was to be repeated again on many occasions. One example was during the Korean War when a respected commander, reviewing the death of soldiers with renal failure after dialysis, said that we should "stop this business" because "nearly all of them" died. The index word in that sentence is "nearly." The commander did not realize that without dialysis, they all would have died. The patients' lives were severely threatened by their wounds; when even a few were saved by dialysis, it was immensely significant.

In any event, following World War II, Kolff generously gave his apparatus to several countries and institutions for further experimentation and work. It was George Thorn, Professor of Medicine at the Peter Bent Brigham Hospital and Harvard Medical School, working from 1947 to 1950 with a bioengineer/surgeon, Carl W. Walter (and with others later, including Benjamin Miller and John Merrill), who made dialysis a part of standard therapy in the United States.[28] Dialysis is an interesting example of the duality of priority seen so often in science. To Kolff (or to Abel) must go the credit for inventing this machine; he in turn acknowledged his gratitude to his predecessors. To Thorn and his group must go the credit for taking a visionary new device and incorporating it into standard practice by the application of clinical and engineering skill.

With dialysis came a renewed focus on the kidneys, which now could be understood better than before. Thus, by 1950, the stage was set for major advances in the study of renal disease.

The Early Clinical Experiences

During the early 1950s, several patients underwent renal transplantation in Paris and Boston; these all ultimately failed as immunosuppression was not used.[*]

In 1954, a physician in Boston telephoned Dr. John Merrill suggesting that a patient dying of chronic glomerulonephritis be dialyzed. Merrill was at first hesitant since dialysis was then used largely for treatment of acute reversible tubular necrosis, especially in post-obstetric or post-traumatic patients. The physician then indicated that the patient had an identical twin; both the referring physician and Merrill clearly understood the implications.

The patient was transferred to the hospital. There, with the collaboration of geneticists, surgeons, and scientists of a variety of backgrounds, it was demonstrated that the twins were in point of fact truly identical. The kidney transplant was carried out by Dr. Joseph Murray from healthy twin to sick twin. Function was excellent and there was prolonged survival.[27] At that time, it seemed unlikely that there would be many more experiences of this apparently unique type. But Murray's operation was soon to be repeated and now has reached many hundreds of twin pairs worldwide. There were many apprehensions about the twin grafts, particularly the concern that the twin kidney or the twin, might come down with the disease. While this fear has been realized in some instances, the salvage has been good. The general lesson still applies: While it is possible to foresee insuperable difficulties for almost any new concept, a cautious trial in an ethical setting, and with good scientific backup, is the only chance for success. One can never assume freedom from hazard. For our story here, the twin

experience told a very simple and clear lesson: With the immunogenetic barrier overcome, a transplanted kidney could give new life to a dying patient.

The Second Set Response

In World War II, with many aircraft pilots severely burned (especially around the face and neck), and these burns a burdensome challenge to the care of military casualties, the British Medical Research Council focused anew on the problem. Finding a brilliant young immunologist and biologist, Dr. Peter Medawar, they asked him to work with a plastic surgeon, Dr. Thomas Gibson, in Edinburgh. They were to attempt to perfect skin grafting in man and, if possible, to examine the use of skin from other donors.

In carrying out these experiments, Dr. Medawar soon observed that he could rely on one standard laboratory finding. If an initial skin graft was placed from Animal A on Animal B, it had a survival of about 7 days. Then, if a second set of skin was applied in exactly the same fashion between the same two animals, the second set of skin was rejected in about half that period of time. This was therefore called the *second set response*. Its historic importance in transplantation science, histocompatibility, and immunogenetics can scarcely be overemphasized.[25]

In all of science, there is nothing quite as precious as a reliable experimental model. Such things as Koch's postulates in infectious disease, for example, or the culture of malignant cells, the response of isolated hearts to glycosides, are all examples where a standard biologic model has been of immense importance in conceptualizing a field and standardizing a reliable experimental approach. In the study of tissue immunity, there had never been a standard model to provide this sort of conceptual and experimental focus until Dr. Medawar defined the second set response.

With his characteristic energy and imagination, Dr. Medawar then proceeded to unravel many aspects of tissue immunology using the second set response as endpoint. He soon moved on to a whole variety of new studies in immunology and histocompatibility, for which he was later given the Nobel Prize, and was knighted.[4] At about the same time (1943–1953), Dr. MacFarlane Burnet of Melbourne was working on the impact of immune responses on clones of immune cells. He evolved the theory of clonal selection, which meant that when one cell of a clone enjoyed a close fit of its antibody chemistry to a foreign antigen, it was at the same

---

[*] Voronoy, a Russian surgeon, performed five unsuccessful human renal allografts between 1936 and 1949. While he had little concept of tolerable ischemia time for codonesic grafts, he appreciated immunological process in graft loss.[17a]

time stimulated to reproduce.[5] Whatever the later fate of this theory, its importance lay in the fact that a theoretical construct was made to analyze the mechanism by which antigenic configurations interacted with living cells and their progeny.

1954 was an important milestone year in the history of transplantation. It was in that year that the first twin transplant was performed and when Peter Medawar gave the Dunham Lectures at Harvard, telling a huge and avid audience of his studies of tissue immunology. With the twins standing as witness to the success of transplantation, and with immunologic science given an entirely new insight into the response of tissues from different individuals (a little bit reminiscent of the blood groups, as both Holman[18] and Williamson[51] had predicted many years before), the explosion was clearly ready to take place. Few people noted a connection, but it was also in 1954 that Gibbon performed his first successful operation with an extracorporeal pump-oxygenator.[16]

6-MERCAPTOPURINE, AZOTHIOPRINE, IMMUNO-SUPPRESSION, TISSUE-TYPING, AND WORLDWIDE ACCEPTANCE— THE PERIOD OF PROMISE FULFILLED

Clinical Immunosuppression

Between 1954 and 1962, more identical twins were transplanted and a few desperate experiments were carried out with clinical transplantation under whole-body x-ray as immunosuppression. Then came chemical immunosuppression.

Since April 1962, all transplantation of tissues between unrelated individuals have been done with the patient under the influence of a chemical agent to suppress the immune response of the patient to the graft.

The birth of immunosuppressive chemotherapy, like so many other things in science, might have occurred in several places. Various investigators were studying whole-body irradiation as a means of immune suppression, irradiation of the graft itself, and the use of drugs such as nitrogen mustard. The breakthrough came when Schwartz and Dameshek of Tufts University made observations on the effect of 6-mercaptopurine on xenogeneic solute protein.[37] They used a laboratory model in which the antigen was bovine or human serum albumin given either to a rat or a hamster. By radioactive tagging of the albumin, it was possible to study its disappearance curve. Without immunosuppression, it

very rapidly disappeared from the circulation, removed by circulating antibody, but when they gave the animals 6-mercaptopurine, the foreign protein had a normal half-life in the body fluids of the recipient.

The story goes that Dr. Schwartz had talked with several drug companies in an effort to obtain cancer chemotherapeutic agents to study their effect on immunity. He got no response except from Dr. George Hitchings at the Burroughs-Wellcome Company, who sent some 6-mercaptopurine, still difficult to obtain, and quite precious. It was thought to act by making a false substitution for other purines in nucleic acids of the genome.

Their report of "induced immune tolerance" in *Nature* was observed by many investigators. Because of the prior work of Billingham, Brent, and Medawar on "natural tolerance" observable in the newborn or in the embryo,[4] these investigators used the term *induced tolerance* for what we would now call *immunosuppression.*

At that time, several investigators, including Dempster[38] in London and Küss[22] in Paris, had perfected a model in the dog for a kidney transplanted from another dog; the other native kidney could be removed if a survival endpoint was sought. It was a perfect biologic model for the study of drug immunosuppression.

Mr. Roy Calne was then a young surgeon doing postgraduate surgical research in London. Reading this report, he and Zukoski applied 6-mercaptopurine to the kidney graft model. Within weeks of these first trials, it was evident that an entirely new era of experimental kidney transplantation was begun. They soon could report dogs at 6 to 7 weeks after kidney grafting, with kidneys that functioned well. While the kidneys were not histologically normal, the massive lymphocytic infiltration (at that time the hallmark of tissue rejection) was largely absent.[6] Desiring to work on this further and achieve collaboration with other transplant researchers both on the chemical and biologic side, and with clinical experience, Mr. Calne set out for the United States.

He came to this country for two reasons. He wanted to work with Murray and his group at the Laboratories of Surgical Research at the Peter Bent Brigham Hospital and the Harvard Medical School. He likewise came to this country because he wanted to be near Dr. George Hitchings and the laboratories of Burroughs-Wellcome, Inc. They could supply him with additional new drugs. Upon first landing in this country, he went directly to see Dr. Hitchings, and then came to Boston.

Soon Calne and Murray were achieving the

same sort of laboratory success that Calne had experienced in London. Dr. Hitchings was anxious to produce a drug similar to 6-mercaptopurine, but one that might be longer acting and possibly less toxic. Within a few months, working with his collaborator, Dr. Gertrude Elion, he had struck on a derivative of 6-mercaptopurine, substituted at the sulfur atom. This was originally called "BW-322," then "azothioprine," and later, "Imuran." Dr. Hitchings tells the story that when he sent this drug to Mr. Calne to work with in Boston, he did not hear much for a while. And then he called Mr. Calne to see how things were going, and Calne replied (with "typical British reserve") that "BW-322 is not without promise." Dr. Hitchings took the signal, and his chemists went into production. Soon, the results in dogs were clearly better than those with 6-mercaptopurine, the toxicity was less marked, and prolonged kidney graft acceptance in the dog became the rule.

The fact that immunosuppression might work in man as well as in animals had been suggested by a prior successful transplant between two fraternal twins using a sublethal dose of whole-body irradiation as immunosuppression.[26] This key experience gave the group additional fortitude in proceeding to man with azothioprine after about 18 months experience in the dog. Amongst the first patients operated upon with immunosuppressive chemotherapy was a patient whose course after operation in April 1962 was singularly smooth and who survived for a long period of time.[30]

It was the operation in April 1962 and that particular patient that gave organ transplantation as we know it today, its first great boost.

Other experiments along similar lines were being carried out by Starzl,[41] Küss,[22] and Hamburger[17] in Paris and by other groups in this country. Starzl's work was particularly notable because of his early successes, also in 1962.

In medical history, it is a mistake to regard a breakthrough as unique and the only opportunity for the particular event to have occurred. Many advances in medicine in this century have this character: If they had not occurred at that particular historical moment, they would have occurred soon in someone else's hands. This in no way detracts from the significance of the skill and luck that marks the first success. This widespread concern and awareness accounts for the very widespread acceptance of certain remarkable advances. When many groups, institutions, hospitals, and research laboratories are "ready" for such a discovery. This was the case with immunosuppressive chemotherapy in transplant science.

The use of other immunosuppressive agents with Imuran was explored immediately by clinical research groups both in this country and abroad. These included low-dose whole-body irradiation, irradiation of the grafted kidney either before or after it was placed, the use of ACTH, and cortisone.

The fact that rejection was not an "all-or-none" phenomenon was critical to the progression of renal transplantation. Goodwin[16a] first noted the reversal of rejection in human renal transplants. The institution of combination therapy, that is, Imuran and routine steroids, which was associated with improved results, was another clinical milestone.[42]

Acceptances, as Well as Practice, Make Close to Perfect

In the early days of kidney transplantation under immunosuppressive chemotherapy, the morbidity and mortality were high. Increased sophistication in handling of the ureter, the management of sepsis, understanding of complications, and the use of cortisone of course helped. But the major reduction in morbidity and mortality from kidney transplantation came about with the widespread realization by the late 1960s that once kidney rejection was out of control, the best treatment was removal of the kidney. This simple and common sense step, alone, reduced the patient mortality manyfold; it must be emphasized that without dialysis such would be quite impossible.

Between 1965 and 1975, kidney transplantation became a widespread practice for the treatment of renal failure. Many surgical improvements and better tissue preservation acted as sort of a continuous bioengineering structure to improve results remarkably.[47]

Tissue-Typing

At the same time that these events were transpiring, between 1965 and 1975, two other events were to transpire that profoundly influenced the whole field of immunology, transplantation of kidneys and later of other organs.

First was the discovery of tissue types and tissue-typing. This discovery is traceable to the work of Professor Dausset in Paris[33]; it was brought to this country by Dr. Paul Terasaki of the University of California at Los Angeles.[46] Here is a discovery that arose directly from the reality of surgical transplantation of the kidney. Its implications have had far-reaching reverberations throughout the field of genetics and immunology.

Dausset showed that human lymphocytes had

characteristic antigens designated as HLA. Finding the tissue type of donor and recipient enabled us to understand how closely related two siblings or cousins, parent and child, really were, or how antigenically similar two unrelated individuals were. It was later shown that these tissue-typed antigens had specific locations on the genome. This led to gene mapping for histocompatibility antigens. It soon became apparent that the histocompatibility antigens were associated with immunologic capability and, in some cases, with the occurrence of specific diseases.

There is an analogy with the blood groups; like so many biologic analogies, it should not be taken too far. Genetic diversity leads to a very heterogeneous mix of HLA types in the population. It has been noted that random unrelated cadaver matches in certain small regions of Europe were much more likely to be similar than those in the United States. In some countries of Europe, essentially the same population has existed for many centuries in a small area or city with little genetic diversity. In the United States, by contrast, if there is any characteristic of the population, it is that of its genetic heterogeneity. Random cadaver grafts did better in Europe than in the United States.

At the same time that the histocompatibility antigens were being unravelled by Dausset and coworkers, there was increasing evidence that there were several ways of direct matching of potential donor and recipient. In each method, some tissue, fluid, or cell mixture from the potential donor was used as a challenge to the immune response of the recipient and the reaction observed either under the microscope or by bioassay (such as the mixed lymphocyte culture). These were much more sophisticated examples of the sort of matching attempted by the crossed skin grafts that had been done in the 1950s when judging whether or not two people were closely related and how reasonable it might be to expect them to accept grafts of tissue or organs. A registry of kidney transplantation was now set up in this country and later duplicated by one in Europe; the registry could report about 25,000 kidney transplantations carried out worldwide by about 1975. The total to 1987 is not known but is presumed over 100,000.

Clinical Progress

There were many problems. The choice between long-term dialysis and kidney transplantation was still to remain an urgent enigma for many patients, for many years. There were problems with loss of the kidney, surgical complications, difficulties in finding donors, and the hyperimmune sensitized recipient.

But events of the 1950s and 1960s had culminated, by 1970 to 1975, in worldwide acceptance of kidney transplantation as a viable alternative either to death from renal failure, on the one hand, or a lifetime of dialysis on the other hand. The promise visualized by a few visionary workers in the 1950s was fulfilled within 15 to 20 years.

THE LIVER, HEART, AND OTHER TISSUES; BIOENGINEERING AND SURGICAL RESULTS; DONOR RECRUITMENT; CYCLOSPORIN

The Liver

The application of modern surgical techniques and the modern concepts of transplantation to the liver was probably first explored by Welch, who experimented with ectopic transplants of the liver, that is, transplants of the liver that place the liver in a different site in the abdomen, giving it an arterial supply, a venous supply (sometimes not of portal origin), and a place for the bile to drain.[50]

This work did not seem to hold much promise. About 1957, Moore[29] in Boston and Starzl[41] in Chicago reported on animal experiments on orthotopic liver transplantation done simultaneously. The liver is nourished by a much more complicated blood supply than is the kidney, and transplantation or removal obviously involves interruption of the inferior vena cava, the main venous return to the heart. Without some sort of a venous shunting mechanism, the animal would die during the operation for lack of cardiac venous return, with pooling of blood in the lower extremities. Despite these difficulties, the work in Boston and Chicago progressed rapidly and, by 1958, short-term survival in the dog, limited by rejection, was reported.

When immunosuppressive chemotherapy became available, clinical transplantation of the liver was attempted. Calne, who had previously worked on the kidney experiments, as previously mentioned, had by now returned to England where he was Professor of Surgery at the University of Cambridge. While Moore and his group abandoned the operation after only four clinical transplants, Calne and Starzl continued to work very actively from 1965 onward.[7,43*] By 1975, transplantation of the liver could be reported from the two centers (Starzl

---

* The first clinical liver transplant was performed by Starzl in 1963 but was unsuccessful; prolonged survival was not achieved until 1967 by the same group.[40]

in Denver, Calne in Cambridge), numbering about 100 cases. Though survival was often distressingly short of ideal, there were a few long-term successes. A worthwhile horizon became dimly visible.

With the advent of cyclosporin (see below) and much more widespread adoption of the procedure based on the techniques of Starzl and some of the chemotherapeutic methods of Calne, the operation became much more widespread. By 1980, liver transplantation was being performed in approximately a dozen centers in this country and as many in Europe. Patients requiring the operation were usually those with advanced post-necrotic cirrhosis, children with biliary atresia, and certain cases of biliary neoplasm. As of this time (1986–1987), transplantation of the liver has only recently received acceptance as standard therapy in most countries of the world, and it stands about where kidney transplantation did in 1970, although over 250 liver transplants were performed by Starzl's group in 1985. It is my conviction, however, that the operation will never be as widely done as kidney transplantation; the liver is not a paired organ; cadaver donors must always be used. In addition, the operation itself is of extreme complexity and very demanding technically; there will always be only a very limited number of surgeons with the skill to complete these operations successfully (both in donor and recipient) in significant numbers of patients.

The Heart

Within a few years of the commencement of kidney transplantation on a clinical scale, Barnard, a surgeon of South Africa (1967), carried out cardiac transplantation operations. The latter attracted worldwide attention.[2] Although Dr. Barnard's patient did not survive for long, the perceived daring of the operation, the necessity of obtaining a heart from a person in whom the heart was still beating and in whom death had been declared on the basis of brain changes, combined with the universal sentiment that the heart is the seat of life, made the operation very spectacular for news media and the public throughout the world.

Within a few years, a large number of attempts had been made to transplant the heart, notably in Paris, London, and in this country, largely in Houston, Texas. In 1968, more than 20 cardiac transplantations were carried out with great technical expertise, but with a minimum of sophistication in chemical immunosuppression. The net result of all these early operations (following Barnard's lead) was catastrophic. Most of the patients died early; survival could not be ensured. It seemed the very prototype of the expenditure of skill and resources without commensurate benefit. The public, as well as cautious physicians, was disillusioned.

At the same time, a surgeon at Stanford University, Dr. Norman Shumway, was starting his work with cardiac transplantation. Within a few years he was to become preeminent in the world and remains so today.[39,44] Shumway's work was quietly pursued in a systematic way. He looked at various indices of cardiac rejection in the electrocardiographic tracings. He studied various histologic aspects of rejection and continued forward with the operation until, at a point in the middle 1970s, he had broken through what seemed to be a barrier. About 30 or 40 successful operations with quite a few long-term survivors stood as testimony to his work. Lower, in Richmond, Virginia, and a former student of Shumway, and several other surgeons began to report long-term survivors.[24] About 1980, the operation began to spread to other centers, and, at this time, there are, as with the liver, multiple centers carrying out cardiac transplantation systematically and with satisfactory results, both in this country and in Europe.

Unlike the liver, the vascular arrangements of the heart are reasonably simple and involve large vessels whose anastomosis does not present the challenge of small size. Open heart surgery had progressed in such spectacular fashion under the use of the pump-oxygenator that immunosuppressive methods learned from the kidney were entirely applicable to the heart.

Artificial Support of Organ Function

As previously mentioned, the artificial kidney had presented a model for which a duplicate has been sought in other organ failure systems. For the liver, this has taken the form of ex vivo liver perfusion or blood filtration in an attempt to repair the biochemical defect of liver failure, or to tide the patient over either a period of not having normal liver function preoperatively or rejection of the transplant. In the case of the liver, these efforts have not been productive and are rarely used.

In the case of the heart, an artificial pump that could take the place of the heart for days or weeks has been an obvious possibility ever since the success by Gibbon in using the pump-oxygenator for shorter periods. By 1980, various efforts to develop an artificial heart had been made, and, by 1982, the artificial heart could be used in a widely publicized patient in Salt Lake City,[13] under the general guidance of Dr. Kolff, the man who had developed the artificial kidney 40 years before.

At this time, the artificial heart has been extensively explored, and it is possible that its most important application will lie in temporary support pending either the availability of a transplant or, if a transplant fails, the availability of a second heart. Like the artificial kidney, the artificial heart does not suffer rejection. While it does not require immunosuppressive chemotherapy, it is associated with a high incidence of microembolic disease in the brain.

The artificial heart has usually been placed orthotopically in the chest. While such a device would seem both logical and potentially widely available, and thus in some ways appealing, there is at the present time no completely acceptable mechanical alternative to a transplant. Were a prolonged-support mechanical heart to become available outside the body such as the artificial kidney, and be free of embolic hazards, it might fill this need. If a suitable transplant is available, it remains preferable to the artificial heart from almost every point of view. Cerebral microembolism is an overriding fault in the mechanical heart. This balance between alternatives may change in the coming years as the balance between donor heart availability and artificial heart engineering changes.

Efforts in 1984 to 1985 to place the heart of a young baboon in the cardiac locus of a neonate, as a xenograft, failed. This was predictable on the basis of all known data on the biology of xenografting at this time; it appears to be another example of ill-founded biological optimism justified on the basis of desperate straits. A wait for a human heart might have been advisable.

Lung, Pancreas, Bone Marrow

There is not space here to detail the development of our current knowledge of transplantation of other tissues and organs. In each case, a very small group of persistent investigators has continued to work, often with inadequate funding. For each patient to which it was applied, it would be the only source of hope in an otherwise dismal prognosis.

Transplantation of the lung,[12] stimulated by the work of Veith, and of the heart and lung,[34] stimulated by the efforts of Jamieson, has been a natural outgrowth of experience with the heart. It became evident early in this work that transplantation of a single lung, by introducing a high-resistance arterial circuit in a low-pressure ventricular outflow tract, diverted all the blood to the other lung. Transplantation of both lungs appears to be surgically no less complex and physiologically more viable than transplantation of a single lung. For persons suffering from late-state pulmonary arterial disease or emphysema (particularly with cor pulmonale) such a transplant offers the potential of important salvage.

A major and continuing contributor to the field of lung transplant has been Veith, who has studied and advocated the use of single lung transplants rather than the heart–lung en bloc transplant. His initial work, reported in 1969,[48] demonstrated that a single lung could be transplanted without developing a fixed high vascular resistance; in other work and in some clinical cases, Veith has ligated the opposite pulmonary artery to promote perfusion of the transplanted lung. The opposite lung has remained viable and functional. More recently, Veith reported his clinical results with single lung transplantation.[49] Again, the emphasis has been on the maintenance of normal perfusion/ventilation relationships. Prolonged survival was not obtained. For the vast majority of patients having disease of heart and lungs, often etiologically and physiologically related, the en bloc transplant would appear essential.

Even though this chapter makes no effort to review the work of all centers currently active in transplantation, the work of Najarian[31] at the University of Minnesota deserves special mention. Najarian was a pioneer in the application of kidney transplants to the pediatric patient and later extended his work in treating certain complications of late diabetes by transplantation of healthy kidneys to the diabetic patient. Some of this work has been done in conjunction with his extensive exploration of the use of antilymphocyte globulin, a field in which his work is preeminent.

In addition, Najarian's department has carried forward the studies of pancreatic transplantation very aggressively, working both with islet cell and whole-organ transplants, and has reported some encouraging results.[45]

Transplantation of the pancreas would be particularly important for certain types of diabetics in whom disorders of vision and renal and central nervous system function are sequellae. While transplantation of pancreatic islets has been uniformly unsuccessful, transplantation of the whole pancreas has now been performed with reasonable success in a very few patients.[35] Their greatly lessened requirement for exogenous insulin or total freedom from such requirement is a clear indication of islet cell survival. The success rate of whole organ pancreatic grafts is rapidly increasing under the influence of several investigators, including Sutherland, Sollinger, Dubernad, and Russell.

Transplantation of the bone marrow was first studied in the early days of kidney transplantation when it was considered to be a possible means of infusing tolerant cells (i.e., from the same ultimate donor) for the kidney to come. Although this was unsuccessful, it became clear that transplantation of bone marrow was not a complicated procedure; simple aspiration and reinjection were often sufficient. Its utility was greatest in patients suffering from bone marrow destruction (as in certain forms of chemical toxicity and aplastic anemia), or where bone marrow destruction was an essential aspect of tumor chemotherapy, as in some of the leukemias. Since the marrow contains many immunologically competent cells, an obvious by-product is graft-versus-host disease, which can be of great severity. Attempting to achieve the precise balance between marrow restoration and avoidance of crippling graft-versus-host disease has been the central focus of modern research in bone marrow transplantation and has been successfully accomplished in many instances despite a continuing high mortality.[14] Transplantation of the spleen carries the same risk of severe graft-versus-host disease.

Surgical and Clinical Improvement— Where Does it Come From?

If medicine is applied human biology, surgery is its bioengineering handmaiden. There are three features of engineering of particular importance in surgical advance. They have been manifest repeatedly in the transplant field. First is *problem definition.* An able engineering approach defines problems after very careful study to indicate where the mechanical, technical, or operative difficulties lie. It then moves on to *problem solution,* often using methods of basic science. *Repeated performance* is the third aspect of clinical bioengineering. It is very subtle. In many examples in surgery, this repeated performance has been carried out by surgeons in large and small communities, as well as in universities. They initiate small improvements that collectively improve results.

In the case of transplantation, the wider dissemination of the operation has resulted in many technical improvements. The tendency for operations, when performed in several major centers, to be done with a lower morbidity and mortality and a lesser requirement of supportive therapy (transfusions, antibiotics) is very notable. The skills of many are applied to procedures often started by a single person. The declining patient mortality from kidney transplantation is in part due to this subtle aspect of surgical bioengineering. By contrast, the improved survival of the individual kidney as a functioning organ is to be traced only in part to widespread acceptance and bioengineering advance,

and more to a greater sophistication in immunosuppressive chemotherapy.

As time passes, this bioengineering improvement can be so great as to reduce risk to a level deemed quite impossible in the light of the first trials. While transplantation of kidney, liver, and heart are good examples of this phenomenon, open heart operations and coronary bypass surgery, the use of insulin, anesthetics, and other new drugs are also examples. It would be unfortunate if policy-making groups were to believe it possible, at the very outset of some new development in biomedicine, to predict its 3- to 5-year course, let alone its ultimate place. Those cannot be predicted on the basis of laboratory study or initial clinical application.

Donor Procurement

In the early days of kidney transplantation, sibling or other family-related donors appeared to be preferable. The results were and still are better than with cadaveric donors. It was not clear at that time whether the better results were because the donor was in the next operating room and the kidney was very fresh, or because the tissues were better matched on an immunologic basis. As tissue-typing and crossmatching became available, it became clear that family donors generally showed a closer genetic match.

The major operation of removing a kidney from a family donor is not without risk. While only a very few, there have been donor deaths. The injury of one person to help another is not new to medicine and surgery, as witness death in childbirth or the widespread use of blood transfusion. But to remove an organ from one person to help another was a new phenomenon. As this aspect came into focus about 1970, the use of living donors gradually fell out of favor at some centers, particularly in Europe. As previously mentioned, this latter situation may have been due to the fact that European cadaveric random-donor matches appear to be slightly closer than in the United States.

Whatever the rights and wrongs of this issue of living donors for kidney, there is no alternative with the heart and liver. Cadaver donors must be used.

The procurement of a suitable number of viable cadaver organs has been a problem for organ banks and regional exchanges in many regions of this country and in most of the countries of Europe. It has not attracted the public attention and support that it should. There is a need for better public understanding of the fact that traumatic deaths in young people (often the most shocking and upsetting to the family) are the very ones that offer the greatest hope of salvage for others. The matter of donor procurement constitutes a major bottleneck in transplantation of both the heart and the liver. Yet even with kidney, the waiting times are long. This is the one aspect of transplantation that most requires public support and understanding. Newspapers, magazines, radio, television, and advertising could help the public to understand their own key role in the distribution of scarce but precious human resources.

Recent development in organ procurement is a story in itself. Regional exchanges have been successful both in Europe and the United States. Through such methods a registry of potential recipients is maintained together with their tissue-typing information and, in many instances, blood or tissue samples for crossmatching. As cadaver donors become available, the tissue is procured by specially trained surgical teams. The most suitable recipient is selected; oftentimes, the tissue, cooled to a little above 0°C, is transported by helicopter. While these developments are a source of encouragement and satisfaction to those concerned with treating extremely ill patients, they have also been the source of controversy and potential abuse. The selection of the most suitable recipient can be confused by issues of financial resources for extra payment and the accusation of "buying and selling human organs." The maintenance of this activity in an atmosphere free of taint and corruption is clearly a job for major medical centers with strong supervision from within and constant peer review of open transactions.

Cyclosporin

About 1975 a new drug, based on a fungus extract, began to become available.[3,20] Several workers both in Europe and in this country began to experiment with the drug. While rather toxic, its renal damage is reversible, and oncogenesis is not more frequent than with Imuran. It can be used to support the transplantation of any organ. The impression soon became widespread that cyclosporin had revolutionized transplantation, particularly of heart and liver. The evidence is still not conclusive on that score. While cyclosporin may provide improved immunosuppression, there is another possibility to account for the improved results. The new drug arrived on the scene at the very time that heart and liver transplantations were ready to be spread to many centers. The spread and further bioengineering improvement of these procedures was coincident with the introduction and use of cyclosporin.

Toxicity and Oncogenesis

The toxicity of immunosuppressive drugs was anticipated from the start. The normal mammalian immune system is responsible for warding off the threat of infection from ordinary commensal bacteria and chance invasion by virulent pathogens. Clearly, the clinical acceptance of an immunosuppressive chemotherapeutic drug to be used for transplantation depends partly on achieving some degree of selectivity: The immune response to foreign tissue is to be abated somewhat but without a lethal loss of general immunity.

Despite such selectivity, global suppression of immunity has been a hazard in the organ recipient since the very earliest work with whole-body irradiation. Other effects such as skin, liver, and renal toxicity vary with the drug and combination of drugs being used, the genetics of the patient, and the particular circumstances of the case.

The observation of tumor formation during immunosuppressive chemotherapy came very early in the use of these drugs and has been noteworthy throughout this history.[32] The initial interpretation was that normal "immune surveillance" is responsible for the frequent or constant killing off of tumor cell lines within the body of any higher organism; with immune suppression, tumors form and grow. That there is some substance to such a surmise is given support by the remarkable case reported by Wilson and associates.[52] Here, a kidney was transplanted from a donor later found to be suffering from widespread subclinical carcinoma of the lung. The transplanted kidney soon became the site for growth of the ectopic lung cancer. Understanding the implication of this finding, the immunosuppressive drug (Imuran) was discontinued, whereat the patient rejected both the tumor and the kidney. A subsequent kidney transplant was successful.

In some instances with injectible immunosuppressive drugs, the tumor has been found to be in the precise site of injection, suggesting some local carcinogenic effect as well as loss of immune surveillance. In many instances, the tumors have been of a mesenchymal type (sarcomas and lymphomas)—less frequently, epithelial carcinomas. The exact chain of biological events leading to cancer in immunosuppressed patients has yet to be elucidated.

Fiscal Costs and Social Acceptance

At the time of the first successful twin transplantation in 1954, few would have predicted that only

30 years later there would be widespread political unrest and fiscal self-searching by states and governments, concerning the expenditure of large sums of money to support tissue transplantation for a relatively few patients.

One of the initial steps forcing this evaluation was the passage of legislation in 1972, amending the Social Security Act, to make available federal funds for the treatment of renal failure. This initially modest program had come to cost, by 1984, almost two billion dollars annually. It poses many ethical questions. Most pressing was the query as to what was so deserving about renal failure as to make federal support with tax dollars more available than for patients suffering from diabetes, multiple sclerosis, heart disease, or stroke. Clearly there is no answer to such a question. A major stimulus for the development of this legislation was the perception that large numbers of patients were being denied this sophisticated therapy because the facilities were not available. One might say that the United States was backing into a national health service by way of the urinary tract. As is so frequently the case with congressional legislation in health, something that appeared very prominent in the public eye at the time attracted major federal funding. The attractive components were of course the development of dialysis and transplantation and a general awareness of the widespread nature of chronic renal failure and its newly discovered treatability. But within this legislation were soon to be found huge expenses associated with dialysis and transplantation.

As cardiac transplantation became available, the cost per case appeared to be even greater. Public attention, as always, was riveted on the heart. For many people in the United States who casually read the public press, the word *transplantation* refers specifically to the heart—the average man-on-the-street being ignorant of the long prior experience with the kidney.

Little wonder then, that by 1983, federal panels were established to examine costs and benefits of transplantation. Various states gathered task forces to issue reports on the acceptability or nonacceptability of transplantation as "standard therapy" to be paid for by regular payment mechanisms.[11,36] The availability of widespread standard payment mechanisms, some of them tax supported (Medicare, Medicaid) and others by quasi public-interest third-party payors (Blue Cross, Blue Shield), further forced this decision-making process on the public.

Several philosophic issues arise here that may have been given inadequate attention. First is the fact that the expenditure of large amounts of re-sources on relatively few patients has been characteristic of medicine for many centuries and in all fields of medical care. In fact, in a report published in 1982, it was shown that about 13% of patients use about 50% of resources.[53] This asymmetry is quite obvious: Not everyone gets sick, and some people have long-term highly expensive illnesses. Others may die suddenly or suffer eminently treatable illnesses at little expense. Viewing this in perspective and understanding the immense cost of treatment of severe burns, certain forms of fractures, cancer, the long-term care of stroke patients, the analogous asymmetrical expense for transplant patients at least falls into place as a familiar social phenomenon, not something new.

Social costs in such a field as this must also be evaluated against the result achieved. This type of analysis is simply not an outcome of conventional cost/benefit calculation. The contrast between transplantation and treatment of recurrent cancer is appropriate. The treatment of recurrent cancer can at times be extremely prolonged and very expensive. With the exception of a tiny group of three or four cancers, late recurrent metastatic malignancy still remains 100% fatal. By contrast, transplantation is usually performed in young people who are otherwise reasonably healthy and who could have a reasonably normal life ahead of them if success were achieved.

Finally, the evaluation of medical costs in any social framework must be evaluated against costs of other activities of that society. Many expensive features of our society, including cosmetics, banker and brokerage fees, and breakfast foods, of dubious benefit to millions of purchasers, must be contrasted with the high-benefit potential to a few people involved in relatively expensive medical procedures such as transplantation.

While the political rhetoric and biased viewpoints that attend such discussions will inevitably continue, two or three social imperatives seem clear.

First, the costs of transplantation and any other medical procedure should be held to a minimum by thrifty, expert management. Such management can decrease costs, but the major cost savings will arise from improved immunosuppression, organ procurement, and clinical research.

Second, such treatment should be available to all segments of our society, regardless of ability to pay from private funds.

Third, while transplantation might appear to be "false technology" in the sense that it does not address the basic source of the disease (e.g., post-necrotic cirrhosis, cardiomyopathy, chronic glomerulonephritis), it is effective for individual patients: "Never underestimate the clinical effectiveness of false technology." This is an important aphorism when addressing the individual patient or the parent of a sick child. It is this ultimate physician/patient contact that has dictated the utilization of medical resources since Hippocrates. While this may appear sentimental to some, this sort of decision in transplantation in no way differs from other personal judgments in our society. The needs of the individual patient will therefore remain controlling in the further development of tissue transplantation as long as we enjoy a free society.

REFERENCES

1. Abel JJ, Rowntree LG, Turner BB: On the removal of diffusible substances from the circulating blood of living animals by dialysis. J Pharmacol Exp Ther 5:275–316, 1913–1914

2. Barnard CN: Human cardiac transplantation: An evaluation of the first two operations performed at the Groote Schuur Hospital, Cape Town. Am J Cardiol 22:584–596, 1968

3. Beveridge T. In White DJ (ed): Cyclosporine A, p 35. Amsterdam, Elsevier, 1982

4. Billingham RE, Brent L, Medawar PB: Actively acquired tolerance of foreign cells. Nature 172:603–606, 1953

5. Burnet FM: A modification of Jern's theory of antibody production using the concept of clonal selection. Aust J Sci 20:67–70, 1957

6. Calne RY: The rejection of renal homograft; inhibition in dogs by 6-mercaptopurine. Lancet 1:417–418, 1960

7. Calne RY, Williams R: Liver transplantation in man: I. Observations on technique and organization in five cases. Br Med J 4:535–548, 1968

8. Cannon JA, Longmire WP Jr: Studies of successful skin homografts in the chicken. Description of a method of grafting and its application as a technic of investigation. Ann Surg 135:60–68, 1952

9. Carrel A: La Technique operatoire des anastomoses vasculaires et la transplantation des visceres. Lyon Med 98:859–864, 1902

10. Carrel A: Results of the transplantation of blood vessels, organs, and limbs. JAMA 51:1662–1667, 1908

11. Report of the Massachusetts Task Force on Organ Transplantation. George J Annas, Chairman, Department of Public Health, Comm of MA, October 1984

12. Derom F, Barbier F, Ringoir S et al: A case of lung homotransplantation in man (preliminary report). Tijdschr Diergeneeskd 25:109–114, 1969

13. De Vries WC, Anderson JL, et al: The clinical use of the total artificial heart. N Engl J Med 310:273–278, 1984

14. Dirk WvB (ed): Bone Marrow Transplantation. New York, Dekker, 1985

15. Dunsford I, Bowley CC, Hutchison AM et al: A human blood-group chimera. Br Med J 2:81, 1953

16. Gibbon JH, Miller BJ, Fineberg C: An improved mechanical heart–lung apparatus. Med Clin North Am 37:1603, 1953

16a. Goodwin WE, Kaufman JJ, Mims MM et al: Human renal transplantation—I. Clinical experiences with six cases of renal homotransplantation. I Urol 89:13, 1963

17. Hamburger J, Dormont J: Functional and morphologic alterations in long-term kidney transplants. In Rapaport FT, Dausset J (eds): Human Transplantation, pp 201–214. New York, Grune & Stratton, 1968

17a. Hamilton DM, Reid WA: Voronoy and the first Kidney allograft. Surg Gynecol Obstet 159:289, 1984

18. Holman E: Protein sensitization in isoskingrafting. Is the latter of practical value? Surg Gynecol Obstet 38:100–106, 1924

19. Hume D, Merrill JP, Miller BF: Homologous transplantations of human kidneys. J Clin Invest 31:640, 1952

20. Kahan BD (ed): Cyclosporine A. Transplantation Proceedings Reprint of Supplement *1,XVII*. New York, Grune & Stratton, 1985

21. Kolff WJ, Berk HThJ: The artificial kidney: a dialyser with a great area. Acta Med Scand 117:121–134, 1944

22. Küss R, Legrain M, Mathe G et al: Homotransplantation renale chez l'homme hors de tout lien de parente. Survie jusqu'au dix-septieme mois. Rev Franc Etud Clin Biol 7:1048–1066, 1962

23. Lillie FR: The theory of the free-martin. Science 43:611–613, 1916

24. Lower RR, Dong E Jr, Shumway NE: Long-term survival of cardiac homografts. Surgery 58:110–119, 1965

25. Medawar PB: A second study of the behavior and fate of skin homografts in rabbits. (A report to the War Wounds Committee of the Medical Research Council). J Anat 79:157–176, 1945

26. Merrill JP, Murray JE, Harrison JH et al: Successful homotransplantation of the kidney between nonidentical twins. N Engl J Med 262:1251–1260, 1960

27. Merrill JP, Murray JE, Harrison JH et al: Successful homotransplantation of the human kidney between identical twins. JAMA 160:277–282, 1956

28. Merrill JP, Thorn GW, Walter CW et al: The use of an artificial kidney. I. Technique. J Clin Invest 29:412, 1950

29. Moore FD, Smith LL, Burnap TK et al: One-stage homotransplantation of the liver following total hepatectomy in dogs. Transplantation Bull 6:103–107, 1959

30. Murray JE, Merrill JP, Harrison JH et al: Prolonged survival of human-kidney homografts by immunosuppressive drug therapy. N Engl J Med 268:1315–1323, 1963

31. Najarian JS, Kjellstrand CM, Simmons RL et al: Renal transplantation for diabetic glomerulosclerosis. Ann Surg 178:477, 1973

32. Penn I, Hammond W, Brettschneider L et al: Malignant lymphomas in transplantation patients. Transplant Proc 1:106–112, 1969

33. Rapaport FT, Dausset J: Ranks of donor-recipient histocompatibility for human transplantation. Science 167:1260–1262, 1970

34. Reitz BA: Heart–lung transplantation: A review. Heart Transplantation 1:8, 1982

35. Reemstma K, Lucas JF Jr, Rogers RE et al: Islet cell function of the transplanted canine pancreas. Ann Surg 158:645–653, 1963

36. Roberts SD, Maswell DR, Gross TL: Cost-effective care of end-stage renal disease: A billion dollar question. Intern Med 92:243–248, 1980

37. Schwartz R, Stack J, Dameshek W: Effect of 6-mercaptopurine on primary and secondary immune responses. J Clin Invest 38:1394–1403, 1959

38. Shackman R, Dempster JW, Wrong OM: Kidney homotransplantation in the human. Br J Urol 35:222–255, 1963

39. Shumway NE: Cardiac replacement in perspective. Heart Transplantation III:3–5, 1983

40. Starzl TE, Groth CT, Brettschneider L et al: Orthotop homotransplantation of the human liver. Ann Surg 168:392, 1968

41. Starzl TE, Marchioro TL, Huntley RT et al: Experimental and clinical homotransplantation of the liver. Ann NY Acad Sci 120:739–765, 1964

42. Starzl TE, Marchioro TL, Waddell WR: The reversal of rejection in human renal homografts with subsequent development of homograft tolerance. Surg Gynecol Obstet 117:385–395, 1963

43. Starzl TE, Putnam CW: Experience in Hepatic Transplantation. Philadelphia, W.B. Saunders Company, 1969

44. Stinson EB, Dong E Jr, Schroeder JS et al: Cardiac transplantation in man. IV. Early results. Ann Surg 170:588–592, 1969

45. Sutherland ER, Goetz FC, Najarian JS: One hundred pancreas transplants at a single institution. Ann Surg 200:414–440, 1984

46. Terasaki PI: Antibody response to homografts. II. Preliminary studies of the time of appearance of lymphoagglutinins upon homografting. Am Surg 25:896–899, 1959

47. Tilney NL, Strom TB, Vineyard GC et al: Factors contributing to the declining mortality rate in renal transplantation. N Engl J Med 299:1321–1325, 1978

48. Veith FJ, Richards K: Mechanism and prevention of fixed high vascular resistance in autografted and allografted lungs. Science 163:699–701, 1969

49. Veith FJ, Spencer KK, Siegelman SS et al: Single lung transplantation in experimental and human emphysema. Ann Surg 178:463–476, 1973

50. Welch CS: A note on transplantation of the whole liver in dogs. Transplantation Bull 2:54, 1955

51. Williamson CS: Further studies on the tranplantation of the kidney. J Urol 16:231–253, 1926

52. Wilson RE, Hager EB, Hampers CL et al: Immunologic rejection of human cancer transplanted with renal allograft. N Engl J Med 278:479–483, 1968

53. Zook CJ, Moore FD: High-cost users of medical care. N Engl J Med 302:996–1002, 1980

CHAPTER 2

Highlights of Recent Progress in Transplantation

G. James Cerilli

During the mid-1970s, there was relatively little progress in transplantation, and the discipline of transplantation was in a clinical and an experimental doldrum. The clinical results in transplantation had not improved and, in fact, were deteriorating. There was little that offered much promise for improvement in clinical results. In contrast, a review of the very recent clinical and experimental progress in transplantation reveals a plethora of new information that offers great promise for not only helping to explain the pathogenesis of graft rejection but also further accelerating the progress that has been made in clinical transplantation during the past 2 to 3 years. This chapter will highlight *selected* subjects in transplantation in which either significant recent progress has been made or a fund of knowledge is accumulating that may lead to dramatic change in transplantation. It is obviously not possible to include all components of transplantation without writing an additional textbook. Rather, these are selected highlights of recent progress that the author hopes the reader will find of interest and possibly stimulate further reading and investigation.

MECHANISM OF GRAFT REJECTION

Any attempt to simplify the complex process of graft rejection into a single or even relatively few mechanisms is doomed to failure. Nevertheless, our understanding of graft rejection is essential if successful manipulation of the rejection process is to be achieved.

Cell Types Involved in Graft Rejection

The cell populations that are involved in graft rejection were recently reported by Bradley.[10] Infiltrating cells that are harvested from renal allografts that were either from recipients that were rejecting (untreated) or cyclosporine treated show similar levels of nonspecific cytotoxicity; only cells from grafts of untreated recipients show alloantigen-specific target cell lysis. Thus, it seems that specific cytotoxic T cells rather than nonspecific responses play the major and essential role in allograft rejection in the rat. Both T helper and T suppressor cells are important in allograft rejection. In the rat, cardiac allograft model T suppressor cells become activated during cardiac allograft rejection, but their inhibitory effect on rejection is totally negated by the interleukin 2 (IL-2)-driven helper/cytotoxic effector pathway.[82] Blocking this pathway by ART-18, which blocks IL-2 at the receptor level, eliminates the stimulation of effector cells by T helper cells. This suggests a role for the T helper cell in developing a very specific suppressor cell that may be independent of IL-2 and possibly is a mechanism for the development of allograft tolerance.

The pattern of the cellular infiltrate as well as the cell types involved are important variables in evaluating the severity of renal allograft rejection.[79] The total T subset infiltrate, regardless of its pattern, does not correlate with rejection. However, an intense infiltrate of LEU-2 cells in a diffuse cortical pattern is associated with eventual rejection, as is an intense manifestation of humoral vascular rejection. Thus, the greatest relative risk of irreversible rejection is an intense infiltration of LEU-2 cells in a diffuse cortical pattern. Thus, certain T cell subpopulations and specific distribution patterns correlate with eventual graft outcome. T cells are essential for allograft rejection as (1) they are invariably present in rejecting allografts, (2) rejection can be minimized by depriving the recipient of T cells, and (3) rejection capability can be transferred to immunoincompetent hosts by purified T cells.[88] However, it is conceivable that the relative roles of T cytotoxic/suppressor cells and Th (helper/inducer) cells is semantic because of the inconsistent correlation between T cell phenotypes and T cell function. Nevertheless, Th cells have an important role in allograft rejection because they are important providers of IL-2. Also, Th and inflammatory cells release factors that can contribute to microvascular lesions and graft necrosis. An understanding of the important T cell subsets participating in graft rejection is essential if highly specific monoclonal antibody immunotherapy is to be effective. Monoclonal antibody directed against Th subsets probably achieves its immunosuppressive effect by inhibiting the critical source of T cell help.

The normal rejection process involves the recognition of certain antigens by the host as foreign. Using a panel of monoclonal antibodies to a variety of T cell and Dr antigens, it was demonstrated in 20 rejected human liver transplants that following transplantation, but not before, bile duct epithelium as well as the portal and central vein and hepatic artery epithelium expressed Dr/Ia antigens.[23] These structures are known preferential targets of the rejection process. These studies suggest that the transplantation process induced and stimulated expression of Dr/Ia antigens on structures that appear to be a prime target for immune destruction; this may be an important mechanism in the pathogenesis of liver allograft rejection. These cell surface antigens can be evaluated using monoclonal antibodies, as summarized by Krensky and Clayberger1 in a paper entitled "Diagnostic and therapeutic implications of T cell surface antigens."[49] These monoclonal antibodies (M_{Ab}), which are useful for the definition of T cell antigens, can also affect the immune response in several ways: They (1) can bind directly to such antigens, thus removing a potential antigenic stimulus; (2) may destroy a critical T cell subset, illustrated by the use of OKT3 or anti-T12 in clinical transplantation; (3) may bind to lymphocyte receptors and block the interaction between lymphocyte reception and major histocompatibility complex (MHC) gene products, and (4) may inhibit self-recognition processes involved in the immune response.

The fact that IL-2 plays an essential role in the immune response and graft rejection has led to studies on the effect of anti-IL-2 receptor monoclonal antibody on allograft rejection.[45] If the IL-2 receptor could be selectively blocked, the interaction between IL-2 and the receptor would be inhibited, blocking the clonal expansion of T cells. This concept is plausible because the IL-2 receptor is not present on resting T cells. It is tested by evaluating the effect of a monoclonal antibody against the murine IL-2 receptor as to its ability to prolong allograft survival of heterotopic heart transplants. Treating the heart transplant recipients with the monoclonal antibody markedly prolonged heart graft survival, and, in one third of the animals, the graft survival appeared to be indefinite. These results further support the important role of the IL-2 receptor in graft rejection and provide intriguing evidence as to its suitability for immunomodulation.

Clearly, monoclonal antibodies can categorize lymphocytes and T cells into subunits. The molecular structure responsible for these subunits and T cell antigen receptors seems to be a surface complex constituting a clono-typic 90 KD Ti heterodimer and the invariant 20 and 25 KD T3 molecules.[77] There are several thousand T1 and T3 molecules on the surface of T-lymphocytes, and these glycoproteins are expressed during late thymic development. Thus, it may eventually be possible to target immunomodulating antibodies to very specific molecules of the T cell antigen receptor.

NORMAL IMMUNE RESPONSE

Effect of Graft Modulation

Dr. Lafferty has recently summarized the theory and practice of immunoregulation by tissue treatment prior to transplantation.[50] Two signals are required for lymphocyte activation. The first signal is provided by antigen adhering to the potentially responding lymphocyte; the second signal is provided by an inductive molecule that is believed to possess costimulator activity. This concept of the stimulator cell led to the concept of passenger leukocytes playing a central role in the immune response leading to graft rejection, that is, the removal of such cells can induce a marked reduction in the graft's immunogenicity. The concept of influencing graft immunogenicity by altering the antigenic structure of the graft was expanded by the studies of Matthys van der Rijn in a very unique experiment.[104] A cloned genomic DNA fragment coding for the HLA-A2 antigen was transferred into a human fibroblast that was negative for this HLA antigen. After such transfer, the fibroblast cells expressed molecules on their surface that were biochemically indistinguishable from the HLA-A2 antigen from the cell line from which the HLA-A2 gene was isolated. Cytolytic T cells that were cloned to have specific reactivity against the HLA-A2 antigen would recognize the human HLA-A2 fibroblast into which the HLA-A2 gene coding have been transferred. This remarkable experiment indicates that it may ultimately be possible to alter the immunologically important antigens on the surface of a cell so that the recipient no longer recognizes that it is foreign. While such observations are a long way from clinical application, nevertheless, they present directions for research that have the potential of significantly affecting the field of transplantation.

Modification of the Normal Immune Response

There are several unique nonbiological methods for modifying the normal immune response. Mice on a nucleotide-free diet have a decreased cell-mediated immunity and a prolonged survival of H-2 incompatible cardiac allografts.[103] Graft-versus-host disease in bone marrow allografted mice is significantly decreased, and the immunosuppressive efficacy of low-dose cyclosporine is markedly enhanced by a nucleotide-free diet. The mechanism for this decreased immunologic response is presumably based on the observation that nucleotide-deprived mice failed to exhibit normal levels of TH $1.2+$ and Lyt $-1+1$ lymphocytes and Il-2 production following immune stimulation. Thus, specific dietary manipulation can affect the normal immune response. The testis and the subarachnoid and intracerebral spaces are reconfirmed as an immunologically privileged site; thus, the anatomical location of transplanted tissue is relevant to the normal immune response.[39,102a] The prolonged survival of allografted rat parathyroid tissue when transplanted to the testis is not based upon the lower temperature within the testis or on the lack of cells bearing class II histocompatibility antigens, which are required for antigen processing. When allografts placed within the testis were pretreated with estrogen to suppress Leydig cell synthesis of testosterone, most testicular implanted grafts were rejected promptly, suggesting that local steroid secretion is important in the immune privileged site of the testis. Similarly the subarachnoid and intracerebral sites for allografted pancreatic islets produced very prolonged graft survival. The reconfirmation that these sites are immunologically privileged has the potential for clinical application, particularly with endocrine tissue.

Antigen-specific reactions between donor and recipient may involve other nonimmunologic mechanisms that lead to graft rejection. Monocyte procoagulant activity and plasminogen activator may play a role in human renal allograft rejection.[18] The secretion of coagulation proteins by monocytes and macrophages is part of the host immune response. A variety of antigens stimulate procoagulant activity, which in vitro is T cell dependent. Thus, lymphocytes may program macrophages to produce an antigen-specific response resulting in the expression of procoagulant activity; this links the immune and coagulation systems in rejection. Thus, monocyte procoagulant activity probably plays an important role in pathogenesis of rejection, possibly because of its ability to cause local hypercoagulability and therefore vascular thrombosis and necrosis.

HISTOCOMPATIBILITY

Clinical

The relevance of tissue-typing in transplantation, although still not completely defined, is becoming increasingly clarified. Matching, particularly for the combination of HLA-A, -B, and -Dr, does seem to correlate with graft success, particularly as time passes post-transplantation. In more than 8000 first cadaver transplants, very well-matched grafts for Dr and HLA-B (zero antigen incompatibility) had a 20% better graft survival than poorly matched grafts.[72] The major difference in graft survival with matching seems to be between those patients with no A, B, or Dr mismatches and those with any number of antigens mismatched. The difference in graft survival between two or six mismatched antigens appears relatively small. This conclusion is supported by a recent report in which there was a marked improvement in cadaver graft survival if there were no mismatched antigens at any of the three HLA loci (A, B, or Dr), that is, an 83% 1-year graft survival compared with a 64% graft survival in patients with a single mismatched antigen.[61] This difference is so large that it strongly supports efforts to expand the size of the donor pool so that a patient would have a greater likelihood of obtaining a kidney with a zero antigen mismatch. Statistical analysis indicates that an increase of the donor pool by a factor of 30 would result in about 50% of the patients being able to receive a kidney with no mismatched antigens. It is important to understand that without such a natural pool, the actual impact of matching on the overall graft survival of all patients transplanted is very small. For instance, in a more recent analysis of Terasaki,[98] only about 6% of patients in a multivariate analysis had a zero antigen mismatch kidney transplant. The 1-year graft survival in the remaining 94% of the patients (one to six antigens mismatched) was unaffected by the degree match if they were treated with cyclosporine.

The impact of cyclosporine on the role of matching was recently analyzed in 3000 patients.[97] This study indicates that zero A, B, Dr mismatched patients have only a 7% to 10% advantage over two to six A, B, Dr mismatched patients when treated with cyclosporine compared with a 17% to 21% advantage in the non-cyclosporine-treated patients. Similarly, the 1-year graft survival in a Southeast Organ Procurement Foundation study[47] was the same in well-matched versus poorly matched patients (72% vs. 73%) in patients treated with cyclosporine. Thus, improved immunosuppression may be gradually overcoming the adverse clinical effect of poor matching.

Relevance of Specific Antigens

The relevance to graft outcome of specific HLA or "non-HLA" antigens received continuing emphasis during the past year. First, Vanrenterghem,[106] supporting the observation by Van Rood, reported that the Drw6 antigen may be a gene influencing the intensity of the immune response, as positive Drw6 recipients had more rejection episodes than negative Drw6 recipients. Second, an antigen system on the vascular endothelial cells (VEC) and not on the lymphocyte (HLA) is important in the pathogenesis of rejection. Patients receiving HLA identical renal transplants who have rejected their grafts appear to be mismatched for at least one VEC–specific antigen.[17] In contrast, patients who have done well with HLA identical grafts appear identical for the six VEC antigens studied. This confirmed previous observations in that (1) there is an antigen system located on the VEC but not on the lymphocyte, (2) these VEC antigens have an important immunologic role in rejection, and (3) typing for this VEC antigen system may improve graft results. Third, private epitopes (e.g., HLA 2,3,4) can be grouped into public specifications based upon crossreactivity between some HLA antigens. Thus, several private specificities may be grouped into a single cross reaction group (CREG) because they share a backbone antigen. Screening highly sensitized patients on the basis of CREG groups and identifying the antibodies particularly to the high-frequency public epitopes simplifies the logistics of finding a negative crossmatch donor for a highly sensitized recipient by decreasing the number of sensitized patients that should be logically screened against any given donor.[70a] An analysis of the data from 4000 patients of the Southeast Organ Procurement Foundation revealed a similar correlation between graft outcome and matching, whether private or public antigen specificities were used.[81] Thus, the concept of public specificities may simplify the matching process and the process of obtaining a kidney for sensitized patients.

Sensitization

The incidence of hyperacute rejection in centers with a highly sensitive crossmatch test was recently compared to that in centers with a low-sensitivity crossmatch test.[80] An increased crossmatch sensitivity is associated with an improved graft survival because of a slightly lower (but not statistically significant) incidence of hyperacute rejection or primary nonfunction. The more sensitive crossmatch technique of immunofluorescent flow cytometry does seem capable of detecting a population of sensitized patients who are likely to have irreversible rejection.[99] However, the antiglobulin-augmented crossmatch, although a more sensitive method for the detection of antibody, did not correlate with first kidney graft survival and does not predict hyperacute or accelerated rejection.[44] Thus, some methods and not others, while being more sensitive detectors of low levels of antibody, may not correlate with clinical course, and great care must be exercised in choosing the proper screening method for defining sensitization to a specific donor.

The transplantation of highly sensitized patients might be more readily accomplished by a transient pretransplantation decrease in antibody levels of the recipient, similar to the approach used in transplanting AB O incompatible combinations. Unfortunately, attempts to remove preformed cytotoxic anti-HLA antibodies in highly sensitized patients using a combination of plasma exchange and immunosuppressive therapy prior to transplantation have had inconsistent results. The level of circulating antibodies in one study was not sufficiently reduced for the patients to obtain a successful kidney transplant.[40] However, recently the combination of plasma exchanges, prednisolone, and cyclophosphamide led to successful grafting in four of five highly cytotoxic patients.[25] Such efforts are critical if highly sensitized patients, who constitute an increasing percentage of patients awaiting transplantation, are to be successfully transplanted.

This brief discussion on histocompatibility has attempted to indicate recent trends occurring in the field of histocompatibility. The overall current practical impact of histocompatibility is still controversial, and the difficulty in establishing the true clinical impact of tissue-typing is reflected in the report of Tiwari,[100] in which transplant centers from the European Dialysis and Transplant Association were classified as giving either strong, moderate, minor, or no clinical importance to matching. There was no difference in graft survival among the centers; thus, in this particular analysis, overall clinical results were independent of the emphasis that a respective center placed upon matching in choosing a donor for a given recipient.

ORGAN PRESERVATION

Kidney preservation is reasonably adequate for the clinical needs of 1986. However, current methodology and success of kidney preservation is inadequate if two major problems are ultimately to be solved. First, the transplantation of sensitized patients will probably require the establishment of a much larger donor pool. This will require the ability to preserve kidneys for significantly longer periods of time. Current preservation techniques are also inadequate for another reason. The use of donor-specific transfusions (DST) in living donors modulates the recipient to be immunologically less reactive to donor-specific antigens. Currently, this protocol requires several weeks prior to the transplant. However, there is evidence that the time required for such immunologic modulation may be significantly shorter. If this is true, successful long-term preservation of cadaveric kidneys could be coupled with immunologic manipulation of a cadaveric kidney recipient. This would couple the optimal form of immunosuppression, that is, biological manipulation of the host, with the optimal form of organ donor, that is, cadaver, thus possibly achieving a graft survival with cadaveric grafts approximating that is now being achieved with related donors. Heart, pancreas, and liver preservation is currently not optimal for the most efficient transplantation of these organs.

The current methods, pump perfusion vs. cold storage or renal preservation, are reasonably comparable in terms of graft results. However, immediate graft function may be lower in patients treated with cyclosporine and preserved with cold storage compared with those treated with pulsatile perfusion ($p < 0.005$).[64] This suggests a need for conservative initial doses of cyclosporine with kidneys that are preserved by cold storage. Others, however, do not believe that cyclosporine decreases long-term graft survival of cold-stored kidneys.

There is currently great emphasis on the role of oxygen-derived free radicals that are toxic to cells and generated at the time of reperfusion of stored organs. Several investigators have recently shown that the utilization of scavengers of oxygen-derived free radicals can enhance the preservation of kidneys. The infusion of the free radical scavenger superoxide dismutase into an autotransplanted preserved kidney substantially ameliorates the reperfusion injury. Blocking the generation of superoxide radicals from xanthine oxidase with allopurinol provides equal protection.[46] Treating hypothermically perfused rat kidneys with superoxide dismutase or catalase, both of which are known to be free radical scavengers, provides a similar result.[4] Similarly, in the perfused rabbit lung model, lung edema following 5 hours of preservation is markedly decreased if the lung is treated with either catalase or superoxide dismutase.[90] Oxygen-derived free radical scavengers also protect the liver from ischemic damage.[3] However, the protection was not as great as with the kidney. While most of the emphasis is now on the use of oxygen-derived free radical scavengers in improving organ preservation, other approaches are improving organ preservation. Masaki[57] has obtained successful preservation of the canine kidney for 96 to 120 hours by simple surface cooling with a modified Collins' solution containing urokinase. The urokinase may exert its beneficial effect by inhibiting the deposition of fibrin formed inside the renal vessels during storage as well as inhibiting the formation of fibrin that occurs immediately following reperfusion of the organ. Similarly, Fujimura[26] was able to successfully preserve the canine lung for 24 hours using only a modified extracellular fluid.

The capability of preserving the liver, lung, kidney, and the heart differ but for unknown reasons. Ischemia leads to a fall in ATP in heart, liver, and kidney that is accompanied by increasing levels of ADP and AMP only in the kidney and liver.[78] Thus, reperfusion led ATP to be promptly regenerated from ADP and AMP only in the kidney and liver. Thus, these studies suggest that maintenance of ADP and AMP levels in the liver and kidney may account for their decreased susceptibility to preservation injury.

It has long been known that the "quality" of the organ at the beginning of the preservation period influences its susceptibility to deterioration during preservation and its immediate function. There is now evidence that hormonal depletion of the donor contributes to poor organ quality and that administration to the donor of a combination of insulin, cortisol, and T3 improves the function of transplanted hearts and kidneys.[69]

These new avenues of investigation hold promise for the long-term preservation of organs, thus improving the possibility of transplanting sensitized patients and increasing the feasibility of successful immunologic manipulation of recipients of cadaveric grafts.

CLINICAL RENAL TRANSPLANTATION

Risk Factors

It is increasingly possible to define risk factors in clinical renal transplantation, allowing more appropriate patient selection. The relationship between graft outcome and time on hemodialysis is becoming increasingly clear. In more than 3000 non-diabetic, first cadaver kidney transplants performed between 1978 and 1983 in 30 United Kingdom transplant centers, long periods on dialysis were associated with a reduced risk of graft failure, that is, the longer the duration on dialysis, the lower the risk of rejection ($p < 0.00001$).[30] This relationship was observed when other factors relating to graft survival, such as HLA matching, age, serum lymphocyte reactivity, and, most importantly, the number of transfusions were controlled. This improved graft survival may be secondary to the acquired deficiency in cell-mediated immunity associated with chronic hemodialysis. However, this concept is not universally accepted, as evidenced by a recent report of more than 300 patients in whom pretransplant dialysis did not influence graft survival.[62]

Increasingly, patients are being transplanted who have a positive crossmatch on historic sera but a negative crossmatch on current sera. The graft survivals in this group seem reasonably comparable to those who have negative crossmatches on all sera samples. Recent analysis of the risk factors in such patients indicates that if the patient is 40 years of age or older, there is increased risk of mortality. Also, the 1-year graft survival is significantly lower in patients who become sensitized by rejecting a graft (43%) compared with patients who are sensitized through other mechanisms (69%). Thus, sensitization secondary to previous graft failure seems to be a greater risk factor than sensitization induced by other causes.[16] In this analysis of 260 sensitized patients, those who received their first transplants had a graft survival of 65% compared with patients receiving second or subsequent transplants (48%) ($p < 0.05$). Graft function was independent of any of the following variables: (1) peak antibody titer; (2) current antibody titer; (3) decline in magnitude of the antibody from peak to current; or (4) surprisingly, time elapsed from the most recent positive crossmatch and the day of transplantation.[31] These important findings will help define the optimal clinical circumstances of transplanting sensitized patients.

The relative patient risks of dialysis versus transplantation have been controversial. The comparison has been difficult because of a rapidly evolving data base. However, when 85 variables were recently examined, age, duration of diabetes, left ventricular failure, and myocardial infarction all contributed to mortality.[41] When these variables were controlled, the patient survival post-therapy was the same for cadaver kidney transplantation and dialysis, but was approximately 10% to 12% better for patients receiving living-related donor transplantation. When these prognostic factors were not controlled, patient survival for those receiving a transplant was almost twice that of patients remaining on dialysis. It seems, however, that for the diabetic patient it is clearly advantageous (improved survival), to undergo transplantation rather than any form of dialysis. This is particularly true after 5 years of follow-up and in these patients with coronary artery disease.[44b] The quality of life, which has been shown to be much better following transplantation, tends to add to the advantages of transplantation.

Some histocompatibility antigens or combinations, such as the combination of Drw6 in the recipient but absent in the donor have been suggested as being associated with a higher risk of graft rejection. Now B8 and Dr3 seems to be associated with increased graft failure.[24] This increased incidence of graft failure ($p = 0.01$) suggests that this haplotype (A1-B8-Dr3) confers a hyperresponder state to the recipient. Nevertheless, the concept that certain haplotypes have more immunologic significance than others deserves further investigation because of its obvious clinical relevance.

Donor-Specific Transfusions

The utilization of donor-specific transfusions with living-related donors is one of the most important advances in clinical transplantation because it demonstrated for the first time that biological manipulation of the human adult was not only possible but could predictably improve graft survival. However, its application is limited because of the relatively small and decreasing role of living-related donors in transplantation. However, the application of this concept is broadened by the observation that successful renal transplantation is enhanced by the utilization of donor-specific transfusions with unrelated living donors.[9,86] Thus, successful immunologic manipulation of the unrelated, antigenically disparate, donor using donor-specific transfusions appears possible, yielding graft survival approximating HLA identical living-related donors. If DSTs are beneficial with unrelated donors, they should be applicable to cadaveric transplantation if the beneficial effect could be induced with transfusions given at or just before transplantation. In a recent report, the administration of donor-specific blood from a one haploidentical living-related donor to recipients the day before and the day of surgery yielded an improved graft survival over a nondonor specific transfusion group.[27] However, the graft survival with perioperative transfusions was not quite as good as with the standard DST protocol; the 1-year graft survival with the standard DST, perioperative DST, or without DST was 96%, 91%, and 78%, respectively. Nevertheless, the improved graft survival using donor-specific transfusions around the time of transplantation may make possible immunomodulation of recipients of cadaveric kidneys.

Repeated exposure to the same antigens may be an important factor in inducing this beneficial immunologic response of transfusions. Living-related donors who received three donor-specific transfusions but who ultimately received a cadaveric graft have a higher graft survival rate than patients who received repetitive random transfusions.[75] This effect is not dependent upon recipient mismatched antigens but may be related to the reinforcement of an immunologic response induced by repetitive exposure to the same antigens. Although the number of patients in this study was small, if confirmed, these observations coupled with the results of the previous paper offer promise for successful biological manipulation of the immune response in cadaveric graft recipients.

Graft Outcome

Several factors that influence the clinical course of patients following transplantation have recently been reported. Cyclosporine-treated patients who develop steroid-resistant rejection episodes will be less likely to respond to ALG than patients maintained on azathioprine.[59] Thus, these patients may be more difficult (50% success rate) to reverse by current antirejection protocols. Although there have been sporadic reports suggesting that immunosuppression can be successfully discontinued in a stable patient post-transplantation, most reports indicate that this is associated with ultimate graft loss. For example, a reduction of azathioprine therapy to less than 100 mg/day in stable patients (good renal function 5 + years post-transplantation) is associated with a higher graft failure rate ($p < 0.001$) than that seen in patients whose immunosuppression is maintained.[74] Thus, recipients with long-term stable function have not achieved permanent tolerance to donor antigens. However, it is possible that "partial" tolerance may sporadically occur following cadaveric transplantation.[93]

A cadaveric kidney recipient in whom all immunosuppression had been discontinued except for betamethasone, 0.5 mg once every 3 days, maintained good renal function for more than 1 year. Suppressor T cells specific for donor alloantigens, nonspecific suppressor T cells, as well as antibody suppressive to autologous lymphocytes that reacted with donor antigens in mixed leukocyte culture (MLC) all developed post-transplantation. Thus, partial tolerance may occur in some patients post-transplantation. Such tantalizing observations offer hope that exogenous immunosuppression may be discontinued following transplantation. However, any recipient/donor "tolerance" induced by immunosuppressive drugs appears quite fragile. For instance, the reduction in delayed hypersensitivity induced by azathioprine and prednisone can be completely reversed in mice with appropriate doses of cimetidine.[111] This illustrates the clinical important of drug–drug interactions and emphasizes the fragility of the immunologic effects of chemically induced immunosuppression.

Role of ABO Blood Group

A better understanding of the quantitative and qualitative aspects of the molecular structure of A,B blood group determinants could facilitate transplantation across the ABO barrier. For instance, the relative ease of transplanting A2 kidney donors into blood group O recipients is thought to be related to the different structure of the A2 determinate as compared with the A1; the A2 determinate more closely resembles the "O" antigen. Also, the anti-A sera titers and the reaction of antibodies with blood group A glycolipid structures have now been correlated with the clinical course of patients.[12]

Blood group O organs have been thought to be the "universal" donor. However, anti-recipient, anti-A or B antibody formation was observed in 5 of 26 A or B blood group patients who had received kidneys from O donors. A clinically significant hemolytic reaction from the autoantibodies was observed in 2 of these patients. This autoimmune hemolytic reaction was probably due to the transfer of passenger B-lymphocytes, which proliferate and produce antibody to recipient blood group antigens, with the kidney.[63] It is also possible that the blood group O determinate is itself immunogenic.

Data Analysis

Clinical transplantation generates enormous quantities of data that is used in patient management. The large number of factors that impact on graft survival and the appropriate analysis of such factors is conducive to computer analysis. A software program has been developed that provides rapid access to a large data base of transplantation case histories and a method for storing, retrieving, and regenerating actual survival curves with a computer.[21,43] This technology allows for more careful analysis as well as the storage of the enormous amounts of data currently being generated by the discipline of clinical transplantation.

OTHER ORGAN TRANSPLANTATION

Heart

The recent increase in the number of cardiac transplants has been paralleled by a marked improvement in the 1-year graft survival and the expansion of cardiac transplantation to successfully include older patients.[94] Although the results with cardiac transplantation have improved, hyperacute rejection occasionally occurs, despite a negative lymphocyte crossmatch with the donor. For example, three patients who experienced hyperacute rejection in the absence of any lymphocytotoxic antibody all had antivascular endothelial cell antibody present pretransplantation.[11] In one of these patients, antivascular endothelial cell antibody directed specifically against the vascular endothelial cells (VEC) of the donor heart was detected in the absence of any anti-donor lymphocytotoxic antibody. Such observations highlight the clinical importance of VEC antigens as a target of antibody leading to hyperacute rejection in cardiac transplantation. The relatively normal myocardium seen frequently in the presence of diffuse coronary artery "atherosclerosis" in patients undergoing chronic cardiac rejection also illustrates the importance of the VEC as an immunologic target during chronic rejection of heart allografts. However, cellularly mediated rejection as well as humeral antibody is important in cardiac rejection.[112] Lymphocyte cultures (11 of 14) obtained from biopsies of heart transplant recipients exhibited donor-specific alloactivity against both Class 1 and Class 2 HLA antigens. All lymphocyte cultures responded to IL-2, indicating that these lymphocyte cultures contained activated cells expressing the IL-2 receptors. Thus, both antibody-mediated and cellularly mediated mechanisms appear important in cardiac rejection. Histocompatibility matching appears to be relevant in cardiac transplantation (88% 1000-day survival for well matched, 66% for poorly matched).[109]

While the beneficial effect of third-party transfusions or donor-specific transfusions is well documented for renal allografts, their effect on cardiac allograft survival remains unknown. There is no benefit of either pretransplantation blood transfusions or perioperative donor-specific transfusions on baboon heterotopic cardiac graft survival.[20] In contrast, there is a significant prolongation of heart allograft survival in mice receiving either donor-specific or third-party massive perioperative blood transfusions.[81] When small amounts of blood are given to these mice, no prolongation in graft survival is obtained. Massive transfusions may initiate a transient nonspecific alteration of immune responsiveness. Thus, the effect of blood transfusions in human clinical cardiac transplantation currently remains undefined.

Liver

The results in liver transplantation have improved with the 4-year graft survival in pediatric liver transplant recipients approximating 75%. The major risk factors in hepatic transplantation are now better defined.[83] In adults, short-term survival is best with primary hepatic malignancies but is the worst at 3 years. At 1-year post-transplantation, adults with primary biliary cirrhosis have the best survival rate (70%); whereas patients with inborn errors of metabolisms have the worst survival rate. Patient age dramatically impacts upon survival in patients with cirrhosis, with a 67% survival rate in those under the age of 40 years and a 0% survival rate in those over the age of 40 years. These correlations improve recipient selection. Rejection of the liver, like the heart, involves cellular immune mechanisms. Activated T cells that demonstrate donor specificity have been found in 6 of 11 biopsies from hepatic transplants.[28] Thus, there is recent further understanding of the immunologic process of liver rejection and the risk factors associated with liver transplantation.

Pancreas

There has been significant recent progress in the transplantation of the whole pancreas, but relatively little improvement has been made in the transplantation of human pancreatic islets. The technique of implanting the pancreatic exocrine drainage into the bladder using a cuff of duodenum around the ampulla of Vater is a major technical improvement and has improved the survival rate of whole pancreatic grafts.[87] Autotransplants of the canine pancreas with the exocrine drainage into the urinary bladder maintain normal islet and exocrine structure and function 13 to 18 months after the initial surgery.[56] Urinary tract infection does not impair pancreatic graft function, and the bladder wall remains essentially normal. Thus, the clinical and laboratory results currently suggest that the pancreatic duct is best managed by drainage into the bladder. However, there are recent opposing views. Dr. Calne[14] suggests that the venous drainage of the graft into the systemic circulation is not physiologically advantageous and that maintaining its drainage into the portal circulation is preferable. However, most data indicate that venous drainage need not be portal in order to obtain adequate homeostasis. There is now evidence that pancreas transplantation may prevent the early diabetic nephropathy that develops following the transplantation of a normal kidney into a diabetic patient.[7]

The clinical transplantation of pancreatic islets has not recently improved but continues to attract attention because of its simplicity. Whether rejection, failure of implant, or other reasons may be the cause of the lack of success is unknown. However, the ability to consistently prevent the onset of diabetes by the injection (intrahepatic or splenic) of autologous islets in the monkey strongly suggests that the major problem is islet immunogenicity or susceptibility to immunosuppressive drugs.[34] The immunogenicity of transplanted islets can be decreased by treating the islets prior to transplantation with ultraviolet radiation.[37] Successful long-term function of ultraviolet irradiated islets was achieved both with allografts and xenografts. Ultraviolet irradiation may act by inducing a metabolic change in the dendritic cells of the islet grafts leading to defective antigen presentation. However, other observations that would support this concept are inconsistent. The pretreatment of donor islets with anti-IA antisera or antidendritic cell antibody does not always prolong islet cell function following islet transplantation to the renal subcapsular position.[33] Some data does not support, therefore, the hypothesis that the immunogenicity of islet allografts was reduced by eliminating IA+ cells from the graft. Thus, in some experimental models, particularly in the rodent, it is possible to prolong islet cell function

by altering islet immunogenicity; however, this effect is inconsistent and its mechanism is as yet unknown.

One of the problems in the transplantation of islets is the inability to obtain an adequate number of islets. The ability to preserve islets for prolonged periods of time would help to alleviate this obstacle, and successful autotransplantation of cryopreserved dispersed pancreatic grafts in dogs has been reported.[107] Although only a partial success was achieved by cryopreservation, this approach does offer promise for the preservation of islets. While cyclosporine is being used successfully with whole-organ transplantation of the pancreas, as well as pancreatic islets,[23b] it is suggested that it may be toxic to islet function.[29] Glucose regulation and insulin release are decreased immediately after intravenously infusing Cyclosporin A in a dog model. Cyclosporine may not act by direct toxicity, but possibly through other mechanisms, such as decreasing pancreatic blood flow. Thus, much remains to be learned regarding the interaction of pancreatic islets, pancreatic exocrine cells, pancreatic blood flow, immunosuppressive drugs, and, most importantly, the immunogenicity of an islet graft itself. If islets could be transplanted successfully, this would provide a simplified approach for the long-term management of diabetes.

Bone Marrow

High-dose chemotherapy or radiotherapy followed by autologous bone marrow transplantation has cured some patients with resistant lymphoma. However, not all patients have suitable autologous marrow. Peripheral blood monocytes have now been successfully used as stem cells in place of bone marrow to treat dogs with spontaneous lymphoma. This may widen the applicability of this approach in human patients.[2a]

CHEMICAL IMMUNOSUPPRESSION

General

Even though some progress has been made in the chemical manipulation of the immune response since the introduction of azathioprine and steroids, this approach is still very imperfect. The addition of cyclosporine to the therapeutic armamentarium has enhanced immunosuppressive flexibility. The optimal utilization of cyclosporine is still undetermined, but there is an increasing trend to utilize it as an adjuvant drug along with azathioprine and corticosteroids. Low-dose ALG, azathioprine, cyclosporine, and prednisone for cadaver grafts results in a patient and graft survival at least equal to the standard cyclosporine with prednisone and ALG or azathioprine and prednisone protocols but with lower serum creatinine levels and less cyclosporine toxicity.[15] The combination immunotherapy shows greater additive effects on the therapeutic side than toxic effects of the drug. Our experience at the Albany Medical Center with 119 patients during the last 30 months (up to 3/87) has been similar. Administration of low-dose azathioprine (less than 1 mg/kg), low-dose prednisone (starting at 30 mg/day, tapering to 10 mg/day by Day 45), and low-dose cyclosporine (3 mg/kg/day–5 mg/kg/day, maintaining blood levels of 250 ng/ml–350 ng/ml) has yielded a 1-year cadaveric graft survival of 81%, with nephrotoxicity being unusual. These clinical observations are supported by the finding that the combination of cyclosporine and azathioprine or total lymphoid irradiation (TLI) and azathioprine significantly prolonged canine renal graft survival compared with any single agent. Combination therapy also resulted in the highest percentage of long-term survivors (over 60 days) of any groups tested.[1] Because TLI is logistically difficult, this canine model supports the clinical observation that, at the present time, the combination of cyclosporine and azathioprine and corticosteroids may be the optimal immunosuppressive regimen.

The introduction of cyclosporine and combination immunotherapy will impact on the relevance of histocompatibility matching in transplantation.[38] It appears that the impact of mismatched antigens on graft survival is less in cyclosporine-treated patients than in azathioprine-treated patients.

Similarly, cyclosporine has influenced the rationale of organ sharing. Poorly matched kidneys used locally (short cold ischemic time) do as well as well-matched transplants that are shared (long cold ischemic time) if the patients are treated with cyclosporine.[2]

Cost as well as nephrotoxicity has stimulated the conversion of patients on cyclosporine to azathioprine. It is possible to successfully convert patients who have been stable for 6 months after transplantation using a gradual transition from Cyclosporin A to azathioprine oover approximately a 2-week period. Almost 90% of patients tolerate such conversion without difficulty, with many having an improved serum creatinine level. Those experiencing rejection episodes can be controlled with steroid therapy and returned to cyclosporine.[89] It must be understood that the long-term effect on graft survival of converting to Imuran from cyclosporine is not known.

Cyclosporine—Mechanism of Action

The active component of Cyclosporin A has been thought to reside in the parent molecule. However, the predominant metabolite, M17, is also a potent immunosuppressive.[76] M17 and, to a lesser extent, M1 and M21 inhibit the in vitro response of human mononuclear cells in the mixed lymphocyte culture (MLC) and in mitogen assays. Such observations may make possible the separation of the toxic effects of cyclosporine from its immunosuppressive effect. Cyclosporine's effectiveness may depend upon a relative sparing of specific suppressor cells early in the allogeneic response, ultimately leading to a state of tolerance as these suppressor cells mature. Patients who have had a combined renal, pancreatic, and splenic transplant have splenocytes that have alloantigen-specific cytotoxic T cell precursors.[32] Therefore, cyclosporine can prevent allograft rejection, but it does not necessarily prevent or ameliorate graft-versus-host disease, which was seen in those patients receiving splenic transplants. Furthermore, the cyclosporine clearly does not prevent in vitro T cell priming of alloantigen recognition. The primed cytotoxic precursors were present and could be expanded in the recipient in the presence of IL-2 to become fully active cytotoxic cells. While it is now well documented that cyclosporine inhibits T cell activation by blocking IL-2 production, it also inhibits the induction of IL-2 responsiveness. Not only is IL-2 production directly inhibited by cyclosporine, but when IL-2 is added to a MLC containing cyclosporine, the MLC will only partially recover in responsiveness despite the presence of adequate IL-2.[60,105]

Cyclosporine binds to a specific cell protein called *cyclophlin*.[36] The Cyclosporin A binding activity of cyclophlin is dependent upon sulfhydryl groups, as are many inhibitors of a MLC. Organs such as the kidney that are particularly sensitive to cyclosporine toxicity have a high concentration of cyclophlin. Cyclosporine can also modulate the expression of class I antigens[23a] and even prevent the induction of MHC class II antigen expression on endothelial cells. This strongly suggests that Cyclosporin A may, in part, achieve its immunosuppressant effect by impacting on the afferent limb of the immune response at the point of antigen recognition by the recipient.[35] The effectiveness of cyclosporine is influenced by the time of its administration in relation to transplantation and rejection episodes. Cyclosporine seems to be ineffective as an immunosuppressive if a population of cytotoxic T cells has been generated and therefore it cannot prevent the second set rejection.[102] However, it seems capable of reversing early skin rejection and of preventing rejection even when introduced several days after grafting. The clinical implications of this are obvious in that cyclosporine utilization is frequently delayed in clinical transplantation, awaiting the resolution of an acute tubular necrosis. Such studies would suggest that the delay in onset of utilization of cyclosporine may mitigate or eliminate its immunosuppressive effectiveness if a rejection episode has simultaneously occurred. Thus, as more knowledge is obtained about cyclosporine, its mechanism of action is becoming increasingly complex.

Cyclosporine Toxicity

Cyclosporine nephrotoxicity is currently avoided by frequent monitoring of cyclosporine blood levels that fluctuate widely and do not reflect tissue/drug interaction. Cyclosporine levels can now be determined directly in kidney tissue itself, which may more accurately reflect the likelihood of nephrotoxicity.[101] However, nephrotoxicity is not the only toxic effect of cyclosporine. Cyclosporine hepatotoxicity may have a 50% incidence if patients are carefully studied.[55] Also, cyclosporine has induced fetal toxicity in the rat.[58] There is a high incidence of rodent fetal mortality or runting with the high dose of 25 mg/kg. Cyclosporine crosses the human placenta, but fetal toxicity has not been noted in the few patients who have become pregnant while on cyclosporine; the dosage in such patients is smaller than that reported in this rat model.

The effects of other drugs on the nephrotoxicity and lethality of cyclosporine are currently receiving emphasis in an attempt to influence the risk/benefit ratio. Most efforts to minimize the toxicity of cyclosporine have been directed toward establishing and monitoring the appropriate dosage. Applying a different concept, verapamil and adenosine triphosphate–magnesium chloride (ATP-MgCl$_2$) pretreatment results in a reversal of the usual decrease in glomerular filtration and impaired tubular absorption induced by cyclosporine.[91] Similarly, prostaglandin E prevents a lethal nephrotoxicity without appearing to compromise the immunosuppressive ability of cyclosporine in the skin allograft model.[54] Thus, both prostaglandin E$_1$ and verapamil reduce cyclosporine-induced nephrotoxicity. Cyclosporine administration will decrease mouse survival in the cecal ligation/puncture peritonitis model. Copovithane is a synthetic immunostimulative polymer. This agent will significantly reverse the deleterious effect of cyclosporine in mice with fecal peritonitis without interfering with the immunosuppressive effect in this model.[65] The additional mortality induced by cyclosporine in the cecal ligation/puncture model can be eliminated by copovithane without adversely affecting skin allograft survival in these same animals. The potential application of this observation is great; in cyclosporine-treated patients with sepsis, it may be possible to use an immunostimulator without significantly inhibiting the effect of cyclosporine on allograft skin in cases of serious burns or in patients receiving a transplant. Further studies are necessary; the more prevalent concept is that it is difficult to differentiate the immunsuppressive properties of a drug from its toxic effects.

Other Immunosuppressive Drugs

Although, in the past year, most of the emphasis on the mechanism of action of immunosuppressive drugs has centered around cyclosporine, other drugs are also being investigated. The responsiveness of patients to corticosteroids varies greatly. On similar dosages, some patients become steroid toxic, whereas others do not. Some rejection episodes respond to steroid therapy, while other patients to not respond to a similar protocol. This latter phenomenon was recently studied. It was found that the response to mitogens of the peripheral blood lymphocytes from patients with good graft function was more inhibited by administered methylprednisolone than the response in patients who had poor graft function.[52] This correlation exists both prior to transplantation and after renal transplantation. Thus, individual patient's lymphocyte sensitivity to some drugs may relate to their immunosuppressive capability. It is becoming increasingly apparent that the route of administration and the actual timing of the drug administration may be critical to its efficacy. Direct infusion of prednisolone into an allografted renal artery is a more effective antirejection therapy than systemic infusion.[77a] In addition, administering cyclosporine at different stages of the circadian cycle changes its immunosuppressive effectiveness.[16a] Thus, much remains to be learned about optimal usage of immunosuppressive drugs.

A new immunosuppressive drug, FR 900506, which is a fermentation product, will inhibit IL-1 and IL-2 production and MLC reactivity and will significantly prolong renal, skin, and heart allograft survival.[70] This drug may be a new class of immunosuppressive agents. In addition, 15-deoxyspergualin shows great promise as a new class of immunosuppressive drug, since it significantly prolongs the survival of allografted heart, skin, islets, and kidneys. This agent appears to act via an effect on the mononuclear cells rather than the lymphocyte.[23c,107a]

These recent observations indicate that much remains to be learned about the toxic and immunosuppressive manifestations of drugs now used or under investigation in clinical transplantation. However, such studies offer enormous promise for enhancing the immunosuppressive capabilities of chemical immunosuppressants as well as preventing their toxic effects.

BIOLOGICAL MANIPULATION OF THE IMMUNE RESPONSE

The future of transplantation lies not in achieving permanent graft acceptance by the chronic administration of toxic immunosuppressant drugs but, it is hoped, by specifically inhibiting the immune response to the immunologically significant antigens present in the transplanted organ.

Transfusions

It has been my view that the improved graft survival obtained with donor-specific transfusions represents the most important advance in transplantation in many years. This concept offers increasing promise for successful immunologic manipulation of the recipient, leading to specific inhibition of the recipient's immune response to donor antigens. The current status of DSTs is discussed in detail elsewhere in this text, but very recent developments in this concept deserve to be highlighted. The incidence of sensitization induced by whole blood transfusions can be reduced by administering Imuran simultaneously with the whole blood. However, the ability to control sensitization by concordant administration of Imuran is not effective if the patient has had a prior transplant and a high lymphocyte panel activity (PRA) level or if the exchange involved a child to mother DST.[19] Thus, Imuran can decrease DST sensitization, but only in "low responders" or low-risk persons.

The specific component of whole blood that is responsible for the beneficial immunologic effect of DSTs is unknown. The buffy coat component is effective in improving graft survival for both living-related donors and for patients receiving cadaver grafts.[66] Similarly, purified platelets are as effective as whole blood in prolonging kidney grafts but do not appear to elicit the same degree of sensitization

in the rhesus monkey model.[5] In similar experiments, kidney transplants were performed in primates on unrelated, mismatched host/donor combinations following three transfusions of third-party or donor-specific platelets.[8] Platelet recipients of either donor-specific or third-party platelets had a mean graft survival three times that of normal controls; only the use of donor-specific platelets did not increase the incidence of positive crossmatches prior to transplantation. Thus, using specific components rather than whole blood may decrease sensitization while maintaining the beneficial effect of donor-specific transfusions.

Random transfusions may be as effective as donor-specific transfusions in living-related donors. In the Collaborative Transplant Study Group, there was a graft survival rate of 91% in patients receiving donor-specific transfusions, 75% in nontransfused recipients, and 90% in recipients receiving three or more random transfusions.[71] The induction of lymphocytotoxic antibodies against their potential related donor was rare with three to five random transfusions. These data suggest that there is no advantage to administering donor-specific transfusions to potential recipients of a one haplotype-HLA match in related kidney transplants. Similarly, third-party transfusions seem to be effective in HLA-identical related donor combination transplants.[68] Patients receiving an HLA-identical transplant had a marked decrease in the number and severity of rejection episodes if they received third-party transfusions prior to transplantation compared with patients not transfused. However, both of these studies suggest that third-party transfusions are beneficial in the immunologically optimal related donor combinations and may be as effective as donor-specific transfusions.

The role of random transfusions in cadaveric transplantation remains confusing and controversial. Most recent studies indicate improved graft survival in transfused recipients of cadaveric grafts. However, in a very recent report by Opelz[73] in a multicenter study, no long-term beneficial effects of transfusion were noted.

Mechanism of Action of Transfusions

The mechanism by which donor-specific transfusions enhance graft survival is still unknown, but it has been suggested that the beneficial effect of donor-specific transfusions is due to clonal deletion.[96] Multiple transfusions hyperimmunize patients, and, with transplantation, a vigorous anamnestic response may occur. This response occurs during the high-dose phase of immunosuppression, which is given during the early period post-transplantation. This high-dose immunosuppression kills or inactivates the clones of reactive cells that are targeted to donor antigens. These decloned patients may therefore undergo successful transplantation because those cells that are specifically targeted for donor antigen will have been removed by the high dose of immunosuppression. However, another explanation for the effectiveness of donor-specific transfusions is that the prolongation of kidney graft survival may be mediated by auto anti-idiotypic antibodies induced by donor-specific transfusions.[13] DST may induce an antibody that selectively inhibits the anti-donor antigen receptors of recipient T cells. Another possible mechanism by which blood transfusions may improve graft survival is by inducing prostaglandin synthesis, because the inhibition of prostaglandin synthesis by indomethacin has a detrimental effect on transfusion-induced immune suppression.[85]

The immunologic mechanism leading to improved graft survival induced by transfusions is indeed complex. Renal recipients who are Drw6 positive seem to be high responders, leading to a lower graft survival and higher incidence of leukocytotoxic antibodies after rejection. Drw6-positive recipients who received more than one transfusion had a very poor graft outlook compared with recipients in the other groups.[51] This suggests that Drw6-positive recipients require a different transfusion policy and should not be given more than one blood transfusion. If they do receive more than one blood transfusion, it is preferable that they receive an HLA-Dr identical kidney.

The beneficial effect of transfusions is not simply due to the identification of high responders, but transfusions most likely induce an immunologic change in the recipient. However, the beneficial immunologic process initiated is unknown. Prostaglandin E production increases following blood transfusions.[42] Prostaglandin E suppresses several immune responses through unknown mechanisms. The complexity of the interrelationship between donor organ, recipient, and transfusions is further illustrated by studies on the suppression of antibody response and prolongation of skin graft survival by multiple blood transfusions in the rat.[53] Rats receiving one to three blood transfusions produce high-titer cytotoxic antibodies, but additional blood transfusions lead to a decrease in the antibody titers. After 15 transfusions, the recipients have either no or very low titers of antibody. Multiple transfusions thus result in a humoral nonreactivity to the donor following an initial antibody response. Also multiple (> 15) transfusions lead to prolonged skin survival.

An active immunoregulatory process that inhibited antibody production appears to have been induced by repeated transfusions. If this phenomenon applied to man then continued, transfusions of patients sensitized from donor-specific transfusions might render them suitable recipients from their anticipated donor.

Monoclonal Antibody

Increasingly, monoclonal antibodies are being used to treat acute rejection episodes in renal transplantation. The monoclonal antibody OKT3 was highly effective in efficiently reversing acute cadaver kidney allograft rejection in a multicenter randomized study.[48] Similarly, in a single-center study, there was a 100% 1-year graft survival using OKT3 without cyclosporine with living-related donors, 83% among nondiabetic cadaver kidney recipients younger than 50 years of age, and 74% among cadaver and older recipients who did not develop the complications of OKT3.[67] Thus, OKT3 appears to be effective in reversing rejection in patients who are on cyclosporine, suggesting that OKT3 can also reverse steroid- or ALG-resistant rejection in cyclosporine-treated patients. OKT-3, used without other immunsuppressive drugs, is highly immunogenic, and its chemical effectiveness is very transient owing to antibody formation to the OKT-3. Based on current data, it should therefore be used in conjunction with other immunosuppressive agents.[106a]

Another monoclonal antibody, CBL,1, produced against the CEM lymphoblast line, has been used to treat allograft rejection in more than 50 patients receiving a renal transplant.[95] In this series, 11 of 11 patients with a living-related donor and persistent rejection responded to the antibody, and 4 of 8 patients with cadaveric donor and rejection were successfully treated. An antiblast antibody may react only against those cells that are actually reacting against the antigen of the transplanted organ. Also, monoclonal antibodies to the IL-2 receptor or to complement are being evaluated as antirejection therapy. The monoclonal antibody, C ampath-1, that fixes human complement, appears useful in very preliminary trials.[35a]

"Tolerance"

A form of spontaneous but incomplete tolerance may occur at random in allograft recipients. Efforts are being expanded to increase the regularity and predictability of recipient/donor long-term compatibility that is minimally dependent upon immunosuppression. One mechanism by which this may be achieved is the generation of large numbers of T suppressor cells specifically targeted toward donor antigens. Rats treated with KCL-extracted donor antigen preparation from buffy coat combined with a 3-day course of cyclosporine displayed prolonged graft survival ($p < 0.01$) compared with control subjects.[110] Adaptive transfer of spleen cells presumably containing suppressor cells into virgin secondary syngeneic hosts also led to prolonged graft survival. Thus, donor-specific graft prolongation can be achieved, presumably through the induction of large numbers of suppressor cells. Similarly, adult bone marrow cells as well as juvenile bone marrow cells (which had been used in almost all previous experiments) are capable of significantly prolonging graft survival in ALS-treated recipients.[22] Thus, antilymphocyte serum and bone marrow–derived antigen continue to be successful in producing prolonged allograft survivals in the rodent models. A limited success in the primate model with this approach does not seem to be reproducible in human trials even though specific unresponsiveness to donor antigen was obtained in two patients.

The exact class of antigens responsible for producing prolonged graft survival when coupled with immunosuppression has not been defined. A purified erythrocyte preparation (containing Class I but not Class II antigens) injected intravenously in the rat prior to transplantation is able to induce prolonged if not indefinite renal graft survival without producing sensitization.[108] This approach is not transferable to man because the human red cell does not contain Class 1 histocompatibility antigens. In a cardiac allograft model in mice, Class 1 antigens are also tolerogenic. When EL4 murine thymoma cells containing only Class 1 antigens are injected prior to transplantation in mice later receiving cardiac allografts, very significant graft prolongation is obtained, with 75% of the mice having very long-term (greater than 50 days) graft survival ($p < 0.0004$).[92] Thus, again, Class 1 antigens, in the absence of Class 2 antigens, are able to minimize allograft rejection, indicating significant tolerogenic

potential of Class 1 antigens in the rodent model. The exact mechanism by which the exogenous antigen leads to prolonged graft survival is unknown, but the increased number of suppressor T cells induced by the exogenous antigen may be relevant. A possible explanation for prolonged graft survival in the absence of specific tolerance is that the donor organ cells become replaced by recipient cells. This concept, however, is not supported by the finding that skin endothelial cells from long-term successful grafts have retained donor antigenicity.[6]

The passive transfer of sera from animals carrying long-term liver allografts to other animals has yielded very long-term acceptance with heart allografts in the sera recipients. Subsequently placed skin grafts from the same donor are permanently accepted, while third party grafts were rejected.[44a] Such observations are exciting and continue to tantalize transplant surgeons with the hope of a "magic potion" that will yield permanent graft survival without use of toxic drugs.

SUMMARY

There continues to be rapid expansion of information in basic immunology and clinical transplantation, which is improving current graft survival. Most importantly, an analysis of the very recent literature indicates that there are many clues that will even further improve the results in clinical transplantation and possibly lead to the "magic bullet" that will make it possible to produce permanent specific immunologic compatibility between the graft and the recipient in man. With the achievement of such an objective, the side effects and the complications of the immunosuppressive agents could be minimized, if not eliminated, opening the door for an even wider clinical application of transplantation. When this occurs, and it will occur, the applicability of transplantation will be limited only by the supply of organs and the willingness of society to pay for necessary costs of such technology.

REFERENCES

1. Aeder MI, Lewis WI, Sutherland DER, Najarian JS: Combination immunotherapy for prolongation of renal allograft survival. Transplant Proc 17:2675, 1985
2. Alexander JW, Vaughn W, Pfaff WW et al: Local use of kidneys with poor HLA matches is as good as shared use with good matches in the cyclosporine era. Abstract. American Society of Transplant Sur-

geons, p 25. May 1986 (to be published in Transplantation)
2a. Appelbaum FR, Deeg HJ, Storb R et al: Cure of malignant lymphoma in dogs with peripheral blood stem cell transplantation. Transplantation 42:19, 1986
3. Atalla SL, Toledo–Pereyra LH, MacKenzie GH, Cederna JP: Influence of oxyen-derived free radical

scavengers on ischemic livers. Transplantation 40:584, 1985

4. Bennett JF, Bry WI, Collins GC et al: Prevention of free radical damage in kidney preservation. Abstract. American Society of Transplant Surgeons, p 63. May 1985

5. Betuel H, Cantarovitch D, Robert F et al: Platelet transfusions preparative for kidney transplantation. Transplant Proc 17:2335, 1985

6. Bogman MJJT, de Waal RMW, Koene RAP: Persistent expression of donor-antigens in endothelium of long-standing skin allografts. Transplant Proc vol XIX, Feb 1987, Proceedings of XI International Congress of Transplantation Society

7. Bohman SO, Wilczek H, Tyden G et al: Recurrent diabetic nephropathy in renal transplants placed in diabetic patients and the protective effect of simultaneous pancreatic transplantation. Transplant Proc vol XIX, Feb 1987, Proceedings of XI International Congress of Transplantation Society

8. Borleffs JCC, Jonker M, Neuhaus P et al: Donor-specific platelet transfusions, cytotoxic antibodies, and kidney grafting in rhesus monkeys. Transplant Proc 17:2428, 1985

9. Bowen PA, House MA, Bairas D et al: Successful renal transplantation using distantly related or unrelated living donors with donor-specific blood transfusion. Transplantation 39:451, 1985

10. Bradley JA, Mason DW, Morris PJ: Evidence that rat renal allografts are rejected by cytotoxic T cells and not by nonspecific effectors. Transplantation 39:169, 1985

11. Brasile L, Zerbe T, Rabin B et al: Identification of the antibody to vascular endothelial cells in patients undergoing cardiac transplantation. Transplantation 40:672, 1985

12. Breimer ME, Brynger H, Rydberg L, Samuelsson BE: Transplantation of blood group A_2 kidneys to O recipients. Biochemical and immunological studies of blood group A antigens in human kidneys. Transplant Proc 17:2640, 1985

13. Burlingham WJ, Sparks–Mackety EMF, Wendel T et al: Beneficial effect of pretransplant donor-specific transfusions: Evidence for an idiotype network mechanism. Transplant Proc 17:2376, 1985

14. Calne RY: Paratopic segmental pancreas grafting: Technique with portal venous drainage. Lancet 1:595, 1984

15. Canafax DM, Sutherland DER, Simmons RL et al: Combination immunosuppression: Three drugs (azathioprine, cyclosporine, prednisone) for mismatched-related and four drugs (antilymphocyte globulin, azathioprine, cyclosporine, prednisone) for cadaver renal allograft recipients. Transplant Proc 17:2671, 1985

16. Cardella CJ, Falk JA, Halloran P et al: Risk factors in renal transplant recipients with a positive crossmatch on noncurrent sera. Transplant Proc 17:2446, 1985

16a. Cavallini M, Halberg F, Sutherland DER et al: Optimization by timing of oral cyclosporine to prevent acute kidney allograft rejection in dogs. Transplantation 41:654, 1986

17. Cerilli J, Brasile L, Lempert N et al: Overview of the vascular endothelial cell antigen system. Transplant Proc 17:2314, 1985

18. Cole EH, Cardella CJ, Schulman J, Levy GA: Monocyte procoagulant activity and plasminogen activator. Transplantation 40:363, 1985

19. Colombe B, Amend W, Vincenti F et al: Reduction in donor-specific transfusion by antibody responses to Imuran. Transplant Proc 17:2494, 1985

20. Cooper DKC, Rose AG, Toit ED et al: Failure of pretransplant third-party and preoperative donor-specific blood transfusion to improve heterotopic cardiac allograft survival in baboons. Transplantation 40:569, 1985

21. D'Amaro J, de Lange P, van Rood JJ: Storage, retrieval and regeneration of actuarial survival curves with a personal computer. Abstract. International Symposium on Relevant Immunological Factors in Clinical Kidney Transplantation, p 114. Heidelberg, June 1985

22. DeFazio SR, Hartner WC, Monaco AP, Gozzo JJ: Mouse skin graft prolongation with donor strain bone marrow and antilymphocyte serum. Transplantation 40:563, 1985

23. Demetris AJ, Lasky S, van Thiel DH et al: Induction of Dr/IA antigens in human liver allografts. Transplantation 40:504, 1985

23a. de Waal RMW, Bogman MJJT, Cornelissen IMHA et al: Expression of donor class I major histocompatibility antigens on the vascular endothelium of mouse skin allografts. Transplantation 42:178, 1986

23b. Dibelius A, Königsberger H, Walter P et al: Prolonged reversal of diabetes in the rat by transplantation of allogenic islets from a single donor and cyclosporine treatment. Transplantation 41:426, 1986

23c. Dickneite G, Schorlemmer HU, Walter P et al: The influence of $(\pm)$-15-dexoyspergualin on experimental transplantation and its immunopharmacological mode of action. Behring Inst Mitt 80:93, 1986

24. Dyer PA, Martin S, Kippax R et al: HLA-DR3 is a marker of graft failure in cadaveric renal transplantation. Transplant Proc 17:2248, 1985

25. Fauchald P, Leivestad T, Bratlie A et al: Plasma exchanges and immunosuppressive therapy prior to renal transplantation in highly sensitized patients. Transplant Proc vol XIX, Feb 1987, Proceedings of XI International Congress of Transplantation Society

26. Fujimura S, Kondo T, Handa M et al: Successful 24-hour preservation of canine lung transplants using modified extracellular fluid. Transplant Proc 17:1466, 1985

27. Fukuda Y, Dohi E, Ono H et al: Effect of donor-specific transfusion performed the day before and

during renal transplantation. Transplant Proc 17:2366, 1985

28. Fung, JJ, Iwatsuki S, Shaw B et al: Current status of immunologic monitoring in hepatic allograft recipients with acute rejection. Abstract. American Society of Transplant Surgeons, p 37. May 1985

29. Garvin PJ, Long S, Niehoff ML: Effect of cyclosporine on islet cell function. Surg Forum 36:328, 1985

30. Gilks WR, Bradley BA, Gore SM: The effect of duration of pretransplant dialysis on kidney graft survival. Transplant Proc 17:2801, 1985

31. Goeken NE: Outcome of renal transplantation following a positive crossmatch with historical sera: The second analysis of the ASHI survey. Transplant Proc 17:2443, 1985

32. Gonwa TA, Goeken NE, Schulak JA et al: Failure of cyclosporine to prevent in vivo T cell priming in man. Transplantation 40:299, 1985

33. Gores PF, Sutherland DER, Platt JL et al: Elimination of Ia-positive cells does not influence islet allograft survival in the renal subcapsular position. Surg Forum 36:326, 1985

34. Gray DWR, Warnock G, Sutton R et al: Successful autotransplantation of isolated islets of Langerhans in the cynomolgus monkey. Transplant Proc vol XIX, Feb 1987, Proceedings of the XI International Congress of the Transplantation Society

35. Groenewegen G, Buurman WA, Jeunhomme GMAA, van der Linden CJ: Effect of cyclosporine on MHC Class II antigen expression on arterial and venous endothelium in vitro. Transplantation 40:21, 1985

35a. Hale G, Waldmann H, Friend P et al: Pilot study of Campath-1, a rat monoclonal antibody that fixes human complement, as an immunosuppressant in organ transplantation. Transplantation 42:308, 1986

36. Handschumacher RE, Harding MW, Rice J et al: Cyclophlin: A specific cytosolic binding protein for Cyclosporin A. Science 226:544, 1984

37. Hardy MA, Lau H, Weber C, Reemtsma K: Pancreatic islet transplantation: Induction of graft acceptance by ultraviolet irradiation of donor tissue. Ann Surg 200:441, 1984

38. Harris KR et al: Azathioprine and cyclosporine: Different tissue matching criteria needed. Lancet 2:802, 1985

39. Head JR, Bilingham RE: Immune privilege in testis. Transplantation 40:269, 1985

40. Hillebrand G, Castro LA, Samtleben W et al: Removal of preformed cytotoxic antibodies in highly sensitized patients using plasma exchange and immunosuppressive therapy, azathioprine, or cyclosporine prior to renal transplantation. Transplant Proc 17:2501, 1985

41. Hutchinson TA, Duncan C, Thomas JC et al: Prognostically controlled comparison of dialysis and renal transplantation. Kidney Int 26:44, 1984

42. Jackson V, Tsakiris D, Tonner E et al: In vitro prostaglandin E production following multiple blood transfusions in dialysis patients. Transplant Proc 17:2386, 1985

43. Janssen R, Reuter R: Interactive analysis of (kidney) transplant data. Abstract. International Symposium on Relevant Immunological Factors in Clinical Kidney Transplantation, p 122. Heidelberg, June 1985

44. Johnson AH, Hallman J, Alijani MR et al: Clinical relevance of the antiglobulin-augmented crossmatch: Prospective study. Transplant Proc vol XIX, Feb 1987, Proceedings of the XI International Congress of the Transplantation Society

44a. Kamada N, Shinomiya T, Tamaki T et al: Immunosuppressive activity of serum from liver-grafted rats. Transplantation 42:581, 1986

44b. Khauli RB, Steinmuller DR, Novic AC et al: A critical look at survival of diabetics with end-stage renal disease: Transplantation versus dialysis therapy. Transplantation 41:598, 1986

45. Kirkman RL, Barrett LV, Gaulton GN et al: The effect of anti-interleukin-2 receptor monoclonal antibody on allograft rejection. Transplantation 40:719, 1986

46. Koyama I, Bulkley GB, Williams GM, Im MJ: The role of oxygen free radicals in mediating the reperfusion injury of cold-preserved ischemic kidneys. Transplantation 40:590, 1985

47. Kramer NC, Vaughn WK, Bollinger RR et al: Comparison of cyclosporine and conventional immunosuppressive therapy in renal transplantation: A prospective multicenter study. Transplant Proc 17:2196, 1985

48. Kreis H, Goldstein G: Monoclonal antibodies for the treatment of acute rejection episodes in renal transplantation. Transplant Proc 17:2751, 1985

49. Krensky AM, Claybergerl C: Diagnostic and therapeutic implications of T cell surface antigens. Transplantation 39:339, 1985

50. Lafferty KJ, Prowse SJ: Theory and practice of immunoregulation by tissue treatment prior to transplantation. World J Surg 8:187, 1984

51. Lagaaij EL, Persijn GG, Hendriks GFJ et al: HLA-DRw6-positive recipients should be given only a single pretransplant blood transfusion. Transplant Proc 17:2254, 1985

52. Langhoff E, Ladefoged J: In vivo and in vitro lymphocyte sensitivity in relation to glucocorticoids and renal graft prognosis. Transplant Proc 17:2635, 1985

53. Lenhard V, Renner D, Hansen B, Opelz G: Suppression of antibody response and prolongation of skin graft survival by multiple blood transfusions in the rat. Transplantation 39:424, 1985

54. Lopatin WB, Makowka L, Gilas T et al: A new role for prostaglandin E_1 (CL115,574) as a nephrocytoprotective agent for acute cyclosporine toxicosis. Surg Forum 36:341, 1985

55. Lorber MI, Van Buren CT, Flechner SM et al: Hepatobiliary complications of cyclosporine therapy in renal transplantation. Transplantation 43(1):35, 1987

56. MacAulay MA, Fraser RB, Morais A, MacDonald AS: Acinar structure and function in canine pancreatic autografts with duct drainage into the urinary bladder. Transplantation 39:490, 1985

57. Masaki Y, Uchida H, Osakabe T et al: Successful 96- and 120-hour preservation of the canine kidney by simple surface cooling with high units of urokinase and modified Collins' solution. Transplant Proc 17:1449, 1985

58. Mason RJ, Thomson AW, Whiting PH et al: Cyclosporine-induced fetotoxicity in the rat. Transplantation 39:9, 1985

59. Matas AJ, Tellis VA, Quinn T et al: Treatment of steroid-resistant rejection in patients receiving cyclosporine. Abstract. American Society of Transplant Surgeons, p 53. May 1985

60. Matsuura T, Kunikata S, Kanda H et al: Studies on the mode of action of cyclosporine. Transplant Proc 17:2712, 1985

61. Mickey MR, Carnahan B, Terasaki PI: Effectiveness of zero, A, B and DR mismatch for cadaver kidneys. Transplant Proc 17:2222, 1985

62. Migliori R, Fryd D, Payne W et al: Can renal transplantation be safely done without prior chronic dialysis therapy? Transplantation 43(1):51, 1987

63. Minakuchi J, Toma H, Takahashi K, Ota K: Auto-Anti-A or B antibody induced by ABO unmatched blood group kidney allograft. Abstract. International Symposium on Relevant Immunological Factors in Clinical Kidney Transplantation, p 124. Heidelberg, June 1985

64. Mittal VK, Toledo–Pereyra LH, Kaplan MP et al: Effect of preservation method on function in the cyclosporine era. Transplant Proc 17:2815, 1985

65. Moffat FL, Falk RE, Teodorczyk–Injeyan J et al: Reversal of cyclosporine-induced mortality with a synthetic polymeric immunostimulant in a murine model of fecal peritonitis. Transplantation 39:369, 1985

66. Norman DJ, Barry JM, Durr M, Wetzsteon P: A preliminary analysis of a randomized study of buffy coat transfusions in renal transplantation. Transplant Proc 17:2330, 1985

67. Norman DJ, Barry JM, Funnell B et al: OKT3 for treatment of acute and steroid- and ATG-resistant acute rejection in renal allograft transplantation. Transplant Proc 17:2744, 1985

68. Norman DJ, Wetzsteon P, Barry JM, Fischer S: Blood transfusions are beneficial in HLA-identical sibling kidney transplants. Transplant Proc 17:2347, 1985

69. Novitzky D, Cooper DKC, Reichart B: The value of hormonal therapy in improving organ viability in the transplant donor. Abstract. XI International Congress of the Transplantation Society, S32.1. August 1986 (to be published in Transplant Proc)

70. Ochiai T, Nakajima K, Nagata M et al: Effect of a new immunosuppressant, FR 900506,k on experimental organ transplantation. Transplant Proc vol XIX, Feb 1987, Proceedings of the XI International Congress of the Transplantation Society

70a. Oldfather JW, Anderson CB, Phelan DL et al: Prediction of crossmatch outcome in highly sensitized dialysis patients based on the identification of serum HLA antibodies. Transplantation 42:267, 1986

71. Opelz G: Comparison of random transfusions with donor-specific transfusions for pretreatment of HLA one-haplotype-matched related donor kidney transplant recipients. Transplant Proc 17:2357, 1985

72. Opelz G: Effect of HLA matching, blood transfusions, and presensitization in cyclosporine-treated kidney transplant recipients. Transplant Proc 17:2179, 1985

73. Opelz G: Pretransplant blood transfusions should be given to renal transplant recipients. Presented at the XI International Congress of the Transplantation Society, Plenary Session 4. Helsinki, Finland, August 7, 1986

74. Parfrey PS, Hutchinson TA, Lowry RP et al: The role of azathioprine reduction in late renal allograft failure. Transplantation 39:147, 1985

75. Rodey G, Cross D, Shield C: Influence of third-party, single-donor transfusion on cadaveric graft survival. Transplant Proc 17:2333, 1985

76. Rosano TG, Freed BM, Cerilli J, Lempert N: Immunosuppressive metabolites of cyclosporine in the blood of renal allograft recipients. Transplantation 42(3):262, 1987

77. Royer HD, Campen TJ, Ramarli D et al: Molecular aspects of human T lymphocyte antigen recognition. Transplantation 39:571, 1985

77a. Ruers TJM, Buurman WA, Smits JFM et al: Local treatment of renal allografts—a promising way to reduce the dose of immunosuppressive drugs: Comparison of various ways of administering prednisolone. Transplantation 41:156, 1986

78. St. Cyr JA, Bianco RW, Ascher NL, Koker JE: Consequences of ischemia on organ energy metabolism. Transplant Proc 17:1468, 1985

79. Sanfilippo F, Kolbeck PC, Vaughn WK, Bollinger RR: Renal allograft cell infiltrates associated with irreversible rejection. Transplantation 40:679, 1985

80. Sanfilippo F, MacQueen JM, LeFor WM et al: The influence of crossmatch test sensitivity on outcome in cadaver renal transplantation. Transplant Proc 17:2454, 1985

81. Sanfilipo F, Vaughn WK, Spees EK et al: Effect of HLA-A, -B matching on cadaver renal allograft rejection comparing public and private specificities. Transplantation 38:483, 1984

82. Schneider TM, Kupiec–Weglinski JM, Towpik E et al: Effects of lymphocytes and interleuken-2 receptor antibody on cardiac graft survival. Surg Forum 36:366, 1985

83. Shaw BW, Gordon RD, Iwatsuki S, Starzl TE: Defining major risk factors in hepatic transplantation. Abstract. American Society of Transplant Surgeons, p 33. May 1985

84. Shelby J, Fick J, Kolegraff RJ et al: Prolonged heart allograft survival induced by massive preoperative blood transfusions. Transplantation 40:334, 1985

85. Shelby J, Marushack MM, Nelson EW: Effect of prostaglandin inhibitors on transfusion-induced immune suppression. Transplantation 43(1):113, 1987

86. Sollinger HW, Kalayoglu M, Belzer FO: Use of the donor specific transfusion protocol in living unrelated donor–recipient combinations. Ann Surg 204(3):315, 1987

87. Sollinger HW, Kalayoglu M, Hoffman RM, Belzer FO: Results of segmental and pancreaticosplenic transplantation with pancreaticocystostomy. Transplant Proc 17:360, 1985

88. Steinmuller D: Which T cells mediate allograft rejection? Transplantation 40:229, 1985

89. Stuart FP, Haag BW, Jones K et al: Conversion from cyclosporine to azathioprine therapy six months after kidney transplantation. Transplant Proc 17:2681, 1985

90. Stuart RS, Baumgartner WA, Borkon AM et al: Five-hour hypothermic lung preservation with oxygen free–radical scavengers. Transplant Proc 17:1454, 1985

91. Sumpio BE, Chaudry IH, Baue AE: Alleviation of cyclosporine nephrotoxicity with verapamil and adenosine triphosphate-magnesium chloride treatment. Surg Forum 36:336, 1985

92. Superina RA, Wood KJ, Morris PJ: Class I major histocompatibility antigen pretreatment prolongs cardiac allograft survival in mice. Surg Forum 36:356, 1985

93. Suzuki S, Mizuochi I, Sada M, Amemiya H: Transplantation tolerance mediated by suppressor T cells and suppressive antibody in a recipient of a renal transplant. Transplantation 40:357, 1985

94. Szentpetery S, Morris JS, Hanrahan J et al: Cardiac transplantation in the sixth decade of life. Transplant Proc vol XIX, Feb 1987, Proceedings of the XI International Congress of the Transplantation Society

95. Takahashi H, Terasaki PI, Kinukawa T et al: Reversal of transplant rejection by monoclonal antiblast antibody. Lancet 2:1156, 1983

96. Terasaki PI: The beneficial transfusion effect on kidney graft survival attributed to clonal deletion. Transplantation 37:119, 1984

97. Terasaki PI, Cats S, Mickey MR et al: Impact of cyclosporine. Abstract. American Society of Transplant Surgeons Annual Meeting, p 45. May 1985

98. Terasaki PI, Mickey R, Cecka M et al: HLA-matching effects in the long term (5 years) and in the cyclosporine era. Abstract. American Society of Transplant Surgeons Annual Meeting, p 27. May 1986 (to be published in Transplantation)

99. Thistlethwaite JR, Buckingham M, Stuart JK et al: The T-cell immunofluorescence flow cytometric crossmatch: Correlation of results with rejection and graft loss in cadaveric donor renal transplant recipients. Transplant Proc vol XIX, Feb 1987, Proceedings of the XI International Congress of the Transplantation Society

100. Towari JL: Review: Kidney transplantation and HLA. In Terasaki PI (ed): Clinical Kidney Transplants 1985. Los Angeles,UCLA Tissue-Typing Laboratory, 1985

101. Totterman TH, Lindgren PG, Frodin L et al: Cyclosporine determinations in kidney needle biopsies: Method and clinical results. Transplant Proc 17:2730, 1985

102. Towpik E, Kupiec–Weglinski JW, Schneider TM et al: Cyclosporine and experimental skin allografts. Transplantation 40:714, 1985

102a. Tze WJ, Tai J: Intrathecal allotransplantation of pancreatic endocrine cells in diabetic rats. Transplantation 41:531, 1986

103. Van Buren CT, Kulkarni AD, Fanslow WC, Rudolph FB: Dietary nucleotides, a requirement for helper/inducer T-lymphocytes. Transplantation 40:694, 1985

104. van der Rijn M, Bernabeu C, Royer–Pokora B et al: Recognition of HLA-A2 by cytotoxic T lymphocytes after DNA transfer into human and murine cells. Science 226:1083, 1984

105. van Oers RHJ, Yong S, Schellekens PThA, Aarden LA: The mechanism of action of cyclosporine is not primarily at the level of the interleukin 2 system. Transplant Proc 17:2700, 1985

106. Vanrenterghem Y, Roels L, Dendievel J et al: Are cyclosporine-treated HLA-DRw6-positive cadaveric kidney allograft recipients high responders? Transplant Proc 17:2252, 1985

106a. Vigeral P, Chkoff H, chatenoud L et al: Prophylactic use of OKT-3 monoclonal antibody in cadaver kidney recipients: Utilization of OKT 3 as the sole immunosuppressive agent. Transplantation 41:730, 1986

107. Walsh TN, Alderson D, Farndon JR: Successful autotransplantation of cryopreserved dispersed pancreatic grafts in dogs. Transplantation 38:546, 1984

107a. Walter P, Thies J, Harbauer G et al: Allogeneic heart transplantation in the rat with a new antitumoral durg—15-Deoxyspergualin. Transplant Proc 18:1293, 1986

108. Wood KJ, Evins J, Morris PJ: Suppression of renal allograft rejection in the rat by Class I antigens on purified erythrocytes. Transplantation 39:56, 1985

109. Yacoub M, Festenstein H, Doyle P et al: The influence of HLA matching in cardiac allograft recipients receiving CyA and Imuran. Transplant Proc vol XIX, Feb 1987, Proceedings of the XI International Congress of the Transplantation Society

110. Yoshimura N, Kahan BD: Suppressor cell activity of cells infiltrating rat renal allografts prolonged by perioperative administration of extracted histocompatibility antigen and cyclosporine. Transplantation 40:708, 1985

111. Zapata–Sirvent RL, Narrod JA, Hansbrough JF: Restoration of delayed hypersensitivity in mice receiving immunosuppressive drugs by cimetidine. Transplantation 39:449, 1985

112. Zeevi A, Fung JJ, Griffith BP et al: Characterization of activated lymphocytes grown from heart biopsies from heart transplanted patients. Abstract. American Society of Transplant Surgery, p 41. May 1985

PART TWO

Immunologic Considerations in Transplantation

CHAPTER 3

The Normal Immune Response

Stephen J. Prowse   Kevin J. Lafferty

In mammals, the central lymphoid tissue contains stem cells that differentiate and populate peripheral lymphoid tissue. T cells mature in the thymus and are responsible for the cell-mediated arm of the immune response. B cells probably mature in the bone marrow and periphery and are responsible for the humoral arm of the immune response.

When foreign antigen enters the body, it first encounters phagocytic cells. These antigen-presenting cells are able to process antigen and display it on their surface. T cells with surface receptors for specific antigen are able to directly interact with antigen on the surface of the antigen-presenting cell. The T cell actually recognizes a complex made up of the antigen fragment and a major histocompatibility complex antigen. This interaction probably results in the release of the cytokine interleukin-1 from the antigen-pesenting cells. The interleukin-1 then interacts with the T cells, as a result of which they move to an activated state. Thus, T cell activation is a two-signal process, signal [1] being antigen, and signal [2] being interleukin-1. Once activated, the T cells can perform effector functions. Activated T cells secrete the lymphokine interleukin-2, leading to T cell clonal expansion and provide the signals required to activate B cells to produce antibody. B cells have immunoglobulin on their surface and are able to bind antigen. Upon binding antigen, they become activated, whereby they can present processed antigen fragments to antigen-specific activated T cells. The activated T cells then release factors that result in the proliferation and differentiation of the B cells into antibody-secreting cells.

Each T and B cell has the capability of recognizing only one antigen. Exposure to that antigen in the presence of the appropriate signals results in the expansion of clones of cells with specificity for that antigen. Activated B cells secrete antibody specific for the antigen to which they have been activated. Antibody is able to bind antigen, greatly enhancing phagocytosis and antigen elimination. Activated T cells can lyse cells and release a variety of lymphokines that affect many cells, including B cells, macrophages, and natural killer cells.

Both T and B cells contain genes that code for proteins capable of binding antigen. Since one cell recognizes only one antigen but a large number of antigens can be recognized by an individual organism, the diversity must be generated during cell differentiation. During antigen-independent differentiation, the DNA is rearranged such that one variable region gene is selected and brought adjacent to a constant region gene to form a complete gene coding for a receptor molecule.

Immune responses are regulated by molecules of the major histocompatibility complex (MHC). This complex is a cluster of genes coding for cell surface proteins, which are the major antigens involved in transplantation responses. There are two main types of major histocompatibility complex antigens: Class I antigens, which are present on most cells, and Class II antigens, which are present predominantly on lymphoid cells. The theory of allogeneic reactivity sees the MHC antigen as the control molecule of the immune system, which, of its very nature, must be the component responsible for the restriction of T cell specificity (MHC restriction). Minor antigens are any other cell surface components that do not express this function. The theory predicts that MHC antigen of itself is not the barrier to tissue grafting. The major barrier is provided by antigen presented on the surface of *active* antigen presenting cells (APCs).

For this reason, it is possible to reduce allograft immunogenicity by removal of passenger leucocytes from the tissue prior to grafting.

It is possible to manipulate the immune system in various ways so as to induce unresponsiveness or tolerance to a specific antigen. Tolerance to allogeneic tissues can be induced in both neonatal and adult animals. The mechanism of tolerance induction is not understood, but it is likely that both active (suppression) and passive (clonal deletion) mechanisms can play a role in the different forms of tolerance.

This chapter cannot hope to cover the entire immune system in minute detail. That is not our goal. We will attempt to provide the immunologic basis for the understanding of transplantation biology. Here we have a problem. In the past 5 to 10 years, transplantation biology has undergone a minor revolution; the notion that transplantation antigen alone is the barrier to grafting must be discarded. It is now possible, in animal systems, to successfully graft a number of different tissues that express major histocompatibility complex (MHC) antigens (both Class I and sometimes Class I and Class II MHC antigen) without immunosuppression of the host. This situation was considered impossible by classical transplantation theory. Medawar, one of the greatest transplantation biologists, told us that graft rejection resulted from antigen recognition by the immune system of the host. He concluded that it would be possible to transplant tissues only between persons with the same antigenic composition (such as identical twins) without recourse to immunologic intervention. However, in all other cases, the recipient would have to be manipulated to induce antigen-specific unresponsiveness (tolerance), or broad nonspecific immunosuppression would be required to allow acceptance of a graft from an unrelated member of the same species (allograft). Clearly, the classical concepts of transplantation biology do not provide an adequate explanation for the new experimental observations. One of our prime aims in this chapter is to develop a theoretical framework to explain these phenomena.

Within the chapter, we introduce the "Transplantation Paradox," which arises from the following observations. The allograft reaction, a most violent immune reaction, is mediated by antigen recognition; however, the antigens involved in this process are very weak immunogens, that is, the isolated transplantation antigens often cannot be used to induce allograft immunity. Instead, immunization with the isolated antigens can lead to enhanced allograft acceptance. Any attempt to understand the immunology of transplantation must provide an explanation of this paradox. The answer to the paradox comes from the new understanding of T cell biology. It is now clear that when we immunize an animal with exogenous antigen X, the thymus-derived lymphocytes (T cells) of the animal that respond to this antigen have a receptor specificity that is *not* anti-X, as would have been expected from our experience with B cell biology. If you immunize a person with tetanus toxin, he or she makes anti-tetanus toxin antibodies. T cells resulting from the immunization of an animal or a person with X are of specificity c.x (Fig. 3-1). When we write c.x, we mean that the specificity of the T cell receptor is defined by both c and x; the receptor reacts with neither c nor x alone. In this situation, c is one of the MHC antigens, and x is a derivative of X. This totally unexpected phenomenon has come to be known as MHC restriction of T cell specificity.

We have a solution for this central immunologic problem. The T cell is not immunized by X, it is immunized by a processed product of X, which we call x (see Fig. 3-1). Antigen processing is carried out by one of the phagocytic cells, which we call the antigen-presenting cell (APC). The APC, for reasons that will be discussed in detail later, must present this product x on its surface in some form of association with c, that is, in association with MHC antigen. So the *ligand*, the structure that binds to the T cell receptor, is not the immunizing antigen, X, but c.x (see Fig. 3-1). We now call X the *nominal antigen*, x is the processed product of X, and c.x is the ligand, which is presented to the T cell receptor.

In this chapter, we will discuss basic immunologic principles and explain why MHC antigens play such a dominant role in the regulation of T cell function. This approach provides an answer to the "Transplantation Paradox." This need to explain the new biology of T cells and its relevance to transplantation requires us to take a somewhat unconventional approach, which can make the reading difficult in the sense that preconceived notions of how the immune system works leave little room for new concepts. There is a need for new terminology; thus, we have included a glossary of terms at the end of this chapter. This chapter is written for the serious reader prepared to join the struggle to understand the immune system. This is no simple task.

CLASSICAL EXPECTATION

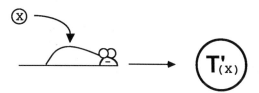

EXPERIMENTAL OBSERVATION

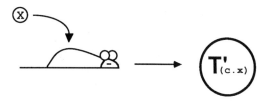

CELLULAR MECHANISM

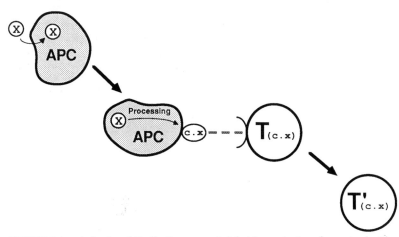

FIGURE 3-1.   *Activation of T cells. It was expected that immunization of an animal with antigen X results in activation of T cells displaying anti-X receptors, T'(X) (classical expectation). However, experiments showed that such T cells have receptors of specificity (c.x), where c is one of the major histocompatibility antigens and x is a derivative of X (experimental observation). The T cell is not immunized by X, but by a processed product of X. Antigen presenting cells (APC) internalize X, process it, and present this product x on their surface in association with c, the MHC antigens.*

THE IMMUNE SYSTEM

Among the vertebrates, the first line of defense against infection is nonspecific and nonadaptive. Skin acts as a barrier, preventing the entry of microorganisms into the body. By means of a second nonspecific mechanism, organisms that enter the body may be engulfed and digested by phagocytic cells. Such nonadaptive defense mechanisms have also been seen in invertebrates such as crayfish and snails. In many invertebrates, recognition is often aided by circulating molecules capable of specifically reacting with foreign particles.[53] The outstanding characteristic of the vertebrate immune system is its capacity to mount an adaptive response. For the immunologist, the term *adaptive* indicates a system with the capability of learning how to cope with the unknown. It is this adaptive nature of the mammalian immune system, its capacity to learn to respond to new environmental threats, that distinguishes it from the immune function expressed by most invertebrates. However, there is no sharp distinction between the immune systems of the invertebrates and the vertebrates, because some corals[24] and ascidians[16] are able to mount an adaptive response to foreign agents.

The vertebrate lymphoid system is a diffuse organ system distributed in aggregates throughout the body whose function is the provision of machinery for immune recognition and the mobilization of an adaptive response to the entry of foreign agents into the body. For this reason, these lymphoid aggregates are usually found close to the endothelial surfaces of the alimentary tract and along the path of lymphatics flowing from the extremities where the aggregates (lymph nodes) act as filters (Note: Most birds do not have lymph nodes monitoring lymph flow). The vertebrate immune system uses specifically reactive cells and specific antibodies in a combined attack on invading foreign agents. The *cellular* immune response is governed by thymus-derived cells and is responsible for defense against intracellular bacteria, recovery from viral infection, and graft rejection. (Antibodies can also play a part in the

process of graft rejection.) The *antibody* (humoral) response is primarily responsible for immunity to extracellular bacterial infections and the prevention of viral spread from one organ to another by way of the blood stream. The cell-mediated immune system also regulates the induction and expression of humoral immunity.

Structure of the Immune System

The lymphoid tissue is composed of central and peripheral components.[13] The central lymphoid tissue is the primary source of lymphopoiesis. It consists of bone marrow, which provides both a source of hemopoietic stem cells and a site where antibody-forming B cells can develop, and the thymus, the organ where bone marrow-derived stem cells differentiate into T cells. T cells from the thymus migrate to the periphery by way of the blood stream, where they function as regulators of B cell activity (helper T cells). Peripheral T cells also provide the antigen-specific component of cell-mediated immunity (CMI) (Fig. 3-2) and are thought to suppress certain immune responses. The existence and function of antigen-specific suppressor cells is a topic of considerable debate.

Peripheral lymphoid tissue is made up of lymph

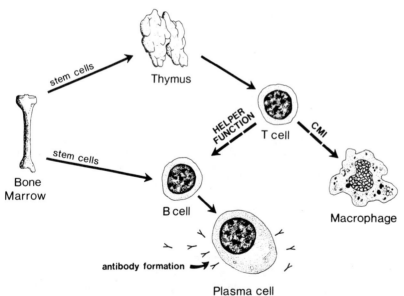

FIGURE 3-2. *Pathway of lymphocyte differentiation. The bone marrow and thymus constitute the central lymphoid tissue. Stem cells from the marrow migrate to the thymus where they differentiate along the T cell pathway. B cell development can occur in the bone marrow. B cell differentiation is also seen in peripheral lymphoid organs. After differentiation in the thymus, T cells migrate to the periphery where they can undergo further activation and clonal expansion and take part in T cell–mediated immune reactions such as acting as helper cells for B cell differentiation and interacting with macrophages in various aspects of the cell-mediated response.*

nodes, the spleen, and membrane-associated lymphoid tissue such as the gut-associated lymphoid tissue. Lymphocytes circulate through the body tissues. They constitute the cellular surveillance system, being ready to recognize and respond to foreign agents that have gained access to the tissues. Lymphocytes migrate into the lymphatic circulation either by passing directly across the post-capillary venules of the lymph node, the major pathway of lymphocyte migration from blood to lymph, or by passage into peripheral tissues and migration along afferent lymphatic channels. Dendritic cells (these cells play an important role in processing and presenting antigen to lymphocytes) are also found in lymph-draining organs and peripheral tissues. Peripheral lymph, containing these lymphocytes and dendritic cells, flows into the lymph node along with antigens and any other particulate matter that may have gained access to the body. An immune response is initiated in these draining nodes, and antigen-specific cells along with immunoglobulin are subsequently released into the efferent lymph. Several efferent lymphatic vessels eventually join to form the cervical (or right lymphatic duct) and the thoracic duct through which the lymph flows, finally reaching the blood stream by entry into the subclavian veins.

A typical lymph node has an outer layer known as the *cortex*, which is divided into B-lymphocyte areas (the primary follicles) surrounded by T-lymphocyte-containing tissue (Fig. 3-3). Primary follicles may contain germinal centers with dividing lymphocytes, which are the site of an ongoing immune response. A structural network called the *reticulum* supports macrophages and reticular dendritic cells, which probably have antigen-presenting functions through their ability to trap and process antigen into a form that can be presented to T cells. Activated T and B cells accumulate in the lymph node medulla, from which they can enter the efferent lymphatics. Antibody-forming B cells (plasma cells) usually remain in the medulla of the lymph node. Other antibody-secreting lymphocytes, which do not have the morphology of plasma cells, are found in lymph leaving the stimulated node. The spleen behaves like a large lymph node, trapping antigen from the blood rather than from lymphatics and initiating immune responses. A vigorous immune response may result in a dramatic increase in spleen size; lymph nodes also become enlarged following antigenic stimulation. This increase in size is partly due to cellular proliferation following antigenic challenge but is predominantly the result of a greatly increased rate of lymphocyte migration into these organs following antigenic stimulation. Membrane-associated lymphoid tissue consists of Peyer's patches, the vermiform appendix, and lymphoid tissue associated with the small intestine and the bron-

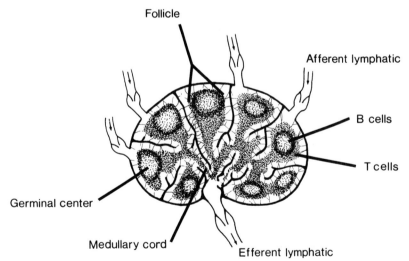

FIGURE 3-3. *Structure and function of the lymph node. Lymph nodes are situated along the pathway of lymphatic drainage from the periphery. Efferent lymphatics run into the outer cortical area of the node, filter through the node and leave by the efferent lymphatic along the pathway toward the major collecting lymphatic trunks. Lymphoid follicles in the cortex of the node are the site of B cell differentiation, with B cells primarily associated with the germinal center of the follicle and T cells in a layer surrounding the follicle and in the area of the corticomedullary junction. Mature antibody-secreting plasma cells accumulate in the medullary cords. Activated T cells and B cells leave the node via the efferent lymphatic.*

chi. This lymphoid tissue contains APCs, T cells, and predominantly IgA-secreting B cells.

Foreign antigen that has gained access to an animal is trapped by phagocytic cells where it is processed and prepared for presentation to the lymphocytes responsible for the initiation of specific immune responses, that is, the generation of antigen-specific T cells and the production of antibody. This process is discussed in detail later in this chapter. The most prominent characteristic of the immune system is its capacity to deal in an adaptive manner with novel agents that have gained access to the body.

Immunologic Theory

Modern immunologic theory developed with a shift away from the strict deterministic view of the chemists who thought that antibody folding occurred on the surface of antigen and, in this way, had a highly specific structure complementary to the antigenic determinant (*epitope*) that served as the template. This deterministic approach was very comfortable for chemists familiar with stoichiometric relationships between reactants of a chemical interaction. However, the concept had an aura of Lamarkian dogma about it: Were we looking at an example of the environment directing the behavior of body components (proteins) that should be under genetic control? The notion had little to offer in terms of understanding immunologic memory, the capacity of the immune system to respond more effectively to a second encounter with the same antigen. This adaptive capacity of the immune system is the characteristic that differentiates the immune system from many other systems in biology.

The next conceptual development was to move away from the notion of a chemical interaction between antigen and the raw immunoglobulin chain. Biologists working in this area, Jerne (1955), Talmage (1959), Burnet and Fenner (1949), were influenced by Darwinian ideas. They were driven by a need for biology to be consistent with a concept of adaptive development, derived from the random generation of change, followed by selection of the configuration appropriate for the particular situation.

The biologists concentrated on cells as the moving force for the immune system. Why couldn't such cells be governed by the same laws that regulate the behavior of individuals in a population? Populations adapt to environmental change by selection of the best suited to the environment, followed by reproductive expansion. Let us consider how the system would behave if antigen selected the cell with the appropriate immunologic receptor and then induced it to clonal expansion. Here was a Darwinian view

of the immune system, one that would explain the adaptive nature of immune responses.

Any model of this nature had to see receptor diversity generated by a totally random process independent of antigen (similar to mutation seen in biological systems). Burnet coined the term *somatic mutation* to explain the phenomenon, and these ideas culminated in the *clonal selection theory* of immune reactivity.

Recent developments in the biology of the immune system fit comfortably into this conceptual framework. We now know that the genes that control the primary structure of the specific receptors of the immune system, antibody and the T cell receptor, are structurally similar (Fig. 3-4). Each is composed of a number of parts, V (variable region), D (diversity segment), J (joining segment), and C (constant region), which specify different portions of the receptor molecule. These genetic components, each of which is present in a number of slightly different forms in the germ line, lie separated from one another in the genome. During the process of lymphocyte differentiation, these components are shuffled around and rearranged to form a particular VDJC combination (Fig. 3-4). This rearrangement appears to occur in a random fashion and provides the machinery for a process of somatic diversification. Further mutational events may also occur once the process of gene rearrangement has taken place.

Major Histocompatibility Complex (MHC) Antigens

MHC antigens were first defined in terms of graft rejection.[52] However, since their initial description, it has become clear that these molecules play a major regulatory role in the immune system. Snell studied tumor graft rejection and set about developing congeneic lines of animals that resisted tumor growth; these are the *congeneic-resistant* mouse lines.[52] The idea was to isolate the genetic elements responsible for resistance to tumor growth. Of some 38 congeneic-resistant lines developed, 30 were shown to differ from their partners at the H-2 locus. This dominant tumor resistance locus of the mouse was also known to be associated with skin graft rejection. It then became clear that resistance to tumor growth was also an expression of the allograft response. Thus, it appeared that there was a dominant genetic locus that controlled histocompatibility (at least for tumor grafts). In this way, the H-2 locus of the mouse came to be known as the MHC. Homologous structures have since been described in all vertebrate species studied in detail (e.g., HLA in man). Throughout this chapter, we will use the symbol c in a generic sense to designate the MHC of the species.

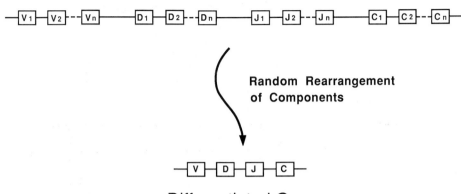

Differentiated Gene

FIGURE 3-4. *Structural rearrangement of antibody and T cell receptor genes. Genes that control the primary structure of the specific receptors of the immune system, antibody and the T cell receptor, are structurally similar. Each is made up of a number of parts, V (variable region), D (diversity segment), J (joining segment), and C (constant region), which specify different portions of the receptor molecule. These genetic components, each of which is present in a number of slightly different forms in the germ line, lie separated from one another in the genome. During lymphocyte differentiation, these components are rearranged to form a particular VDJC combination. This rearrangement is random and provides the machinery for the process of somatic diversification.*

MHC antigens can be identified both serologically and in terms of in vitro lymphocyte reactivity. MHC antigens carry a number of different epitopes, and those defined serologically are not necessarily the same as those defined by lymphocyte reactivity. Serum from a mouse strain A that has been immunized with alloantigens from a mouse of strain B will have antibody against several epitopes carried by strain B MHC antigens. Most of these epitopes will be common to a number of mouse strains, but several of them will be unique to strain B. These are referred to as public and private specificities, respectively. Such serologic definition of MHC antigens forms the basis of tissue-typing and MHC matching for clinical organ transplantation.

MHC antigens are divided into Class I and Class II antigens. Each class shows strong homologies both within and between species; however, there is much less homology between the Class I and Class II MHC antigens. The Class I molecule is a transmembrane glycoprotein noncovalently linked on the cell surface with β_2-microglobulin,[27] which is not a transmembrane protein. Synthesis of β_2-microglobulin is required for expression of the Class I antigen on the cell surface. The Class I MHC molecule has five distinct regions: three globular domains above the cell membrane, one transmembrane domain, and one region within the cytoplasm of the cell (Fig. 3-5). Carbohydrate residues are attached to the external domains. Class I MHC antigens are found on virtually every cell in the body, but the level of antigen expression may vary considerably from one cell to another, often increasing following exposure to lymphokine.[59]

The Class II MHC antigens consist of two polypeptide chains held together by noncovalent interactions (Fig. 3-5).[27] These molecules are also transmembrane globular glycoproteins with two external domains—one transmembrane domain, and one cytoplasmic region. Class II antigens are found primarily on bone marrow-derived lymphoreticular cells; however, some epithelial cells may acquire Class II antigen during inflammatory processes.[23] These MHC molecules show structural homology with the immunoglobulin receptor of the B cell, the T cell receptor, and the thy 1 molecule expressed on the surface of mouse T cells (Fig. 3-5). The reason for this homology is not clear at the present time. One speculation is that these structures represent a set of membrane molecules that sense and transport information across the membrane. In terms of the theoretical development used in this chapter, the symbol c, which represents the MHC, includes both Class I and Class II MHC antigens.

SIGNALING IN THE IMMUNE SYSTEM

For early theorists, antigen recognition and immune induction were seen as parts of the same process. As Medawar put it in 1963, "antigen like the em-

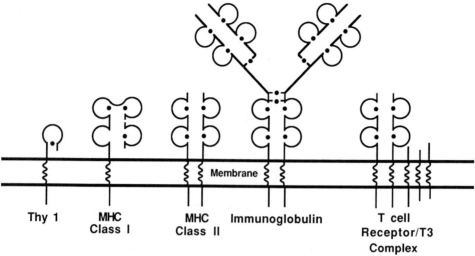

FIGURE 3-5. *The immunoglobulin gene superfamily. The products of these genes comprise a group of cell surface proteins with strong structural homology. Some and possibly all of these molecules have a signaling function, passing information from the exterior to the interior of the cell. The gene superfamily includes Thy 1, classes I and II MHC molecules, immunoglobulin, and the T cell receptor. Thy 1 has a molecular weight of ~25–28 kilodaltons (kD) and is found on mouse T cells. Class I MHC antigen (~43kD) is expressed on the cell surface in a noncovalent association with β_2-microglobulin. Class II MHC antigen consists of two noncovalently bonded subunits of ~34–36kD (α chain) and ~24–28 kD (β chain). Immunoglobulin is comprised of disulfide-bonded heavy and light chains. Immunoglobulin light chains have a molecular weight of ~22 kD; their heavy chains vary in molecular size (~53 kD) according to the nature of their constant region. The T cell receptor is considered to be a molecular complex consisting of a disulfide-bonded heterodimer made up of an α chain (~49 kD) and a β chain (~43 kD), and the three polypeptides (δ, γ, and ϵ) of the T3 molecule.*

bryonic inducer drives the process of lymphocyte differentiation."[43] To these immunologists, one signal provided by ligand engagement of the lymphocyte receptor was seen to be sufficient to initiate the differentiation process. We now know this to be an oversimplification. The signal provided by ligand binding alone is not sufficient to drive the activation process. Activation occurs only when this signal is provided in conjunction with the second signal, which is a hormone-like activity provided by one of the interleukins. This signal will be referred to as signal [2]. Provision of either signal [1] or signal [2] alone is not sufficient for lymphocyte activation. The realization that there was a need for a two-signal model to explain lymphocyte activation came with the recognition that lymphocytes, which constitute the animal's system of immunocytes, were composed of two major classes. T- and B-lymphocytes, and with the further demonstration that B cell activity was often, if not always, T cell dependent. Bretcher and Cohn[9] suggested that two signals were required for B cell induction. Signal one was provided, as in the classical sense, by antigen engagement of the lymphocyte receptor. However, induction occurred only when this signal was delivered

in conjunction with the second signal provided by the helper T cell. In this case, the second signal would be a lymphokine.

Our own studies of alloreactivity lead to the proposition that the first step in the chain of antigen-specific immune reactions was the activation of the T cell and that this was also a two-signal process (Fig. 3-6). According to this notion, an APC was required for T cell activation. The function of this cell is, first, to process antigen and present it in the form of a ligand that is recognizable by the T cell receptor and, second, to provide the inductive molecule that provides the second signal for T cell activation. In this case, the second signal would be a monokine. In our theoretical analysis, we used the term *costimulator activity (CoS)* in a generic sense to describe the function of the second signal for both T cells and B cells. Experimental analysis has shown that both IL-1 and IL-2 express costimulator activity; however, we must not conclude, at this stage of our knowledge, that these are the only molecules with costimulator activity. This model for immune induction sees the APC as playing an active role in the process of T cell activation. The production of CoS activity by the APC is an active function of this

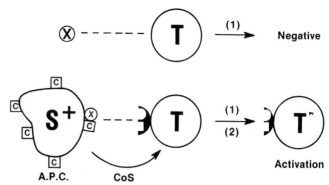

FIGURE 3-6. *The two-signal (stimulator cell) model for T cell activation. Engagement of the T cell receptor by antigen X, provides signal (1) for the mature T cell. This signal alone is not sufficient to activate the process of T cell priming. T cell activation (priming) occurs when the T cell receives signal (1) in conjunction with signal (2) provided by an inductive molecule that comes from the stimulator cell; stimulator cells express the S⁺ pheno-type. The model postulates that a* control structure *(shown as the black squares) on the surface of the S⁺ cell regulates the release of costimulator (CoS) activity. Engagement of the control molecule by the T cell receptor provides the signal that triggers release of CoS from the S⁺ cell. Syngeneic T cells do not carry a receptor for self control molecules (C), since such a molecule is part of the set of self antigens: reactivity to these antigens is eliminated during lymphocyte differentiation in the thymus. However, if exogenous antigen, X, is processed by the APC and presented in associa-tion with c, such that c.x ≠ c, then the T cell with the receptor for this altered self structure can signal the S⁺ cell and so trigger the release of costimulator activity leading to the activation of the T cell.*

MHC Regulation of Immune Function

A major conceptual problem in modern immuno-biology is explaining why antigens that regulate graft rejection (MHC antigens) play such an essen-tial role in the control of immune function. The simple answer to this question is that a molecular structure that functions as a control molecule in the immune system must, of its very nature, constitute the MHC antigens of the species. Although this statement is true, it is not immediately obvious. In the theoretical section that follows, we will attempt to derive this conclusion from first principles.

The essential elements of the two-signal theory for T cell activation are shown in Figure 3-6. This model is based upon the finding that T cell activa-tion is a two-signal process[37] and the *assumption* that a control molecule, designated c in Figure 3-6, reg-ulates the release of CoS activity from the S⁺ cell; cells with the capacity to produce costimulator ac-tivity express the S⁺ phenotype. Engagement of c by the T cell receptor is required to trigger the pro-cess of CoS release from the S⁺ cell. In this sense,

the control structure is operating as a switching mechanism. We also assume that the surface mol-ecule can act as an antigen and that this antigenic property is distinct from its signal transduction func-tion on the surface of the S⁺ cell. The purpose of our theoretical approach is to derive the known properties of the immune system from the logical implications of this assumption concerning the ex-istence and function of the control molecule, c. If the derivations fit with experimental findings, the two-signal theory provides a useful model that de-scribes the biology of the immune system.

Figure 3-6 shows the initial steps in the re-sponse of T cells to exogenous antigen X. The direct interaction of X with the T cell does not lead to activation; interaction with the T cell receptor pro-vides signal [1], and, in the absence of signal [2], no activation occurs. However, if X can be processed by the APC (S⁺) and presented on the surface of this cell in association with c, T cells with receptor specificity c.x can interact with this ligand on the APC. Binding of the T cell receptor provides signal [1], and engagement of c by the receptor triggers the production of signal [2], and, as a result, the T cell is activated.

It can be seen from Figure 3-6 that T cells

activated this way are not specific for X, the exogenous antigen, but for c.x, the complex of x, the degraded product of X, and the control molecule; that is, when T cells respond to exogenous antigen (X), the specificity of T cells is defined both by X and by c. The question that now arises is: What is the nature of c?

A theoretical analysis of alloreactivity allows us to define control structure c. Consider the interaction between stimulator cells of c genotype, ^cSc, and allogeneic T cells of c1 genotype, which can express a receptor for c because it is not a self-antigen, $^{c1}T(c)$. When discussing alloreactivity, we must symbolically designate the genotype of the interacting cells. In the same way that we use ABO both to define blood group antigens (as particular structures) as well as to describe the genotype of persons who express these particular antigens, we use c to describe the control structure molecule *as well as* the genotype of the cell that expresses this antigen. The superscript on the left side of the symbol for the particular cell defines the genotype of that cell.

This reaction has the form,

$$^cSc\ +\ ^{c1}T(c)\ \frac{(1)}{(2)}{\longrightarrow}\ ^{c1}T'(c) \qquad\text{(a)}$$

This allogeneic interaction will lead to efficient T cell activation, and, in this case, the T cell response will not be restricted by the genotype of the responding T cell. Experimental observation reveals that we see reactions of the type described by (a) when c and c1 are allogeneic at the MHC locus. Thus, MHC structures can act as control molecules. Since the T cell response to exogenous antigen is of specificity (c.x), we see why the T cell response is often MHC-restricted; that is, the phenomenon of MHC restriction results from the requirement for T cell activation. The Mls locus can also behave as a control molecule defined by reaction (a). However, thus far, these structures have not been shown experimentally to influence T cell reactivity to antigen.

The two-signal model for T cell activation implies that MHC restriction is not an intrinsic property of the T cell receptor, rather it is something imposed on the T cell by its activation requirements. That is, MHC restriction is the result of an influence extrinsic to the T cell and, in fact, is not always observed. There are other examples of situations in which T cells appear to have unrestricted specificities.[33,48]

Definition of T Cell Subsets

Early in the development of T cell biology, classification was based on function—always a dangerous procedure in the developmental phase of a scientific discipline when such function is often poorly defined. The T cell was no exception to this rule, and the subject is now painfully attempting to extract itself from a confusing morass of functional definition.

Functional definition of T cell subsets arose when these cells were first recognized and described as a distinct class of lymphocytes. T cells were thymus-derived lymphocytes required for full expression of B cell function.[15,44] These cells were therefore termed *helper T cells.* As the biology of the T cell unravelled, helper T cells had to be distinguished from the cytotoxic subset that had the capacity to specifically kill target cells—clearly a different function than that of the helper cells. T cells were found to be responsible for delayed-type hypersensitivity (DTH) reactions; suppressor T cells, which depress the immune response, were also described. Thus, T cell subsets came to be defined in terms of function. While there is no argument that T cells can express different functional activities, there is considerable debate as to whether these functional differences result from physiologic differences in the properties of distinct T cell subsets.[37]

A better way to define these subsets is in terms of the antigenic markers they carry. In the case of human T cells, monoclonal antibodies have been used to define two distinct antigenic markers, which are expressed, mutually exclusively, on the surface of mature T cells; immature T cells may express both sets of markers. These antibodies have been defined as CD4 and CD8, where CD represents cluster of differentiation.[60] In this chapter, we use CD4 and CD8 to describe the two major T cell subsets.

At this stage of our understanding, we can say that, as a general rule—although like all rules, this one has some exceptions—CD8 T cells are reactive to or restricted by Class I MHC antigens. CD4 T cells, on the other hand, are usually reactive to or restricted by Class II MHC antigens. At present, we cannot make any general statements relating T cell function exclusively to one or the other of these major T cell subsets.

T CELL BIOLOGY

In the preceding section, we discussed the signal requirements for T cell activation. Both CD4 and CD8 subsets have the same signal requirements.[37] T cell priming requires two signals: Signal [1] is provided by engagement of the T cell receptor, and signal [2] is provided by CoS activity. Experimental evidence suggests that both IL-1 and IL-2 express CoS activity [1]. However, it would be unwise to conclude that these two interleukins are the only molecules that can express CoS activity.

T Cell Triggering

The primed T cell, T', can be induced to produce lymphokine (lk) when triggered by antigen.[38] In this case, triggering of the primed T cell requires only the delivery of signal [1]. Currently, available evidence suggests that lymphokines (IL-2, gamma interferon [γ-IF] IL-3, B cell growth factor [BCGF], and B cell differentiation factor [BCDF]) are produced concordantly when T' cell populations are triggered by antigen. Both CD4 and CD8 cells can produce lymphokine.[2] However, whether all T' cells in a given population produce all lymphokines is currently a subject of debate and experimental investigation. What is significant for the understanding of T cell biology is the fact that cells of either subset have the capacity to both express cytotoxic activity and produce lymphokine.

Cytotoxic Activity

Activated T cells (T') can interact with and kill target cells that they recognize. This is a prominant characteristic of the CD8 population but is not an exclusive property of these Class I MHC antigen-reactive cells. Cytotoxic activity is usually seen in vitro, and we assume that this T cell function is also expressed in vivo. At present, we have no direct evidence for the expression of cytotoxic activity in vivo. In fact, we have situations where simple expression of cytotoxic activity will not explain the biological behavior of CD8 cells in the living animal. An important goal for future immunologic research is the in vivo validation of phenomena that have been described so elegantly in vitro.

Clonal Expansion

T' cells express receptors for T cell growth factors (TCGF). IL-2 is a TCGF, and it is becoming apparent that other lymphokines may also express TCGF activity. Thus, T cells, since they can be triggered to produce IL-2, can cooperate with one another in the process of clonal expansion, resulting in increased numbers of primed T cells.

T Cell Function

The function of T cells is determined to a large extent by their receptor specificity. As previously indicated, T cell specificities are set by their activation requirements, that is, the interaction with a metabolically active APC with the capacity to produce CoS activity. T cell specificity is predominately ^{c}T(c.x) or ^{c1}T(c). Thus, T cells can only interact with antigen presented on the surface of another cell in the form c.x or with allogeneic MHC antigen. T cells are, therefore, confined to taking part in cellular interactions. It follows that T cells can interact only with cells that have the capacity to present antigen in the form of c.x or with cells that carry allogeneic MHC antigen. In terms of syngeneic cellular interactions—the interactions that occur within any one animal—T cells can only interact directly with macrophages, dendritic cells, and B cells. T cells cannot interact directly with other T cells because T cells in general cannot process and present antigen.

If we make the assumption that T cells must recognize and interact with the cells that they regulate (there is experimental evidence to support this proposition), T cells can directly influence only the behavior of macrophages with B cells; direct T/T interactions cannot occur. Since this is a somewhat controversial viewpoint, let us see how these ideas fit within the framework of known T cell function.

The T cell receptor has a similar basic structure to the immunoglobulin molecule (see Fig. 3-5). In the cell membrane, the specific receptor is associated in a noncovalent linkage with the T3 component of the receptor system. The T3 component is possibly involved in signal transmission across the cell membrane. T3 is highly conserved among mammals, and T cells of differing specificity appear to carry the same T3 molecule. Antibody to T3 can trigger T cells in a nonspecific manner. Also, binding of T3 antibody can result in opsonization of the T cell and its removal from the circulation by the phagocytic system.

Cell-Mediated Immunity (CMI)

CMI results from the triggering of lymphokine release from previously sensitized T' cells. Antigen (X) is processed by macrophages at, or close to, the site of antigen's entry into the body and is displayed on the surface of these cells in the form c.x. Binding of antigen to the primed T cell of specificity (c.x), ^{c}T (c.x), results in triggering of lymphokine release.

Whereas the interaction of the sensitized T cell with its ligand is highly specific, the function of the lymphokines released is generally nonspecific. Many lymphokines are released following triggering of the primed T cell, only some of which are well characterized and are listed in Table 3-1. IL-2, which was previously discussed, maintains the growth of T cells and is responsible for clonal expansion. Interleukin-3 (IL-3) is a lymphokine that stimulates the growth and differentiation of granulocytes from bone marrow stem cells. Migration inhibition factor (MIF) and macrophage chemotactic factor (MCF) are lymphokines secreted by T cells that are involved in the inflammatory processes.

TABLE 3-1   *Lymphokines Produced by Activated T Cells*

LYMPHOKINE		FUNCTION
ACT ON LYMPHOCYTES		
Interleukin-2	IL-2	Maintains the growth of activated T cells
B cell growth factor	BCGF	Maintains B cell growth
B cell differentiation factor	BCDF	Induces B cell differentiation
Suppressor factors	—	Suppresses T and B cell functions, not well characterized
ACT ON MACROPHAGES		
Macrophage activating factor	MAF	Activates macrophages, may be same as gamma-IFN
Migration inhibition factor	MIF	Prevents macrophage mobility
Macrophage chemotactic factor	MCF	Attracts macrophages
Procoagulant induction	—	An activation activity, affects coagulation
Fc receptor induction	—	Induces elevated number of Fc receptors
ACT ON BONE MARROW		
Interleukin-3	IL-3	Promotes the growth and differentiation of stem cells
Colony stimulating factor	CSF	As above, may include IL-3
ACT ON PMN		
Eosinophol chemotactic factor	ECF	Attracts eosinophils
Eosinophil stimulators	—	Induces eosinophilia
Chemotactic factors	—	Attracts PMN
OTHER FUNCTIONS		
Gamma-interferon	IFN	Induces elevated MHC expression and has antiviral activity, may be the same as MAF
Osteoclast activating factor	OAF	Activates osteoclasts, may be the same as MAF
Lymphotoxins	LT	May be involved in cell damage mediated by LC

MIF inhibits the migration of macrophages from the site of T cell–ligand interaction, and MCF attracts other mononuclear cells to form an inflammatory focus. Macrophage activating factor (MAF) is a lymphokine that activates macrophages and enables them to kill gram-negative bacilli and tumor cells; tissue macrophages are unable to perform these functions unless they have been exposed to lymphokine. MAF may be the same molecule as γ-IFN. This lymphokine can also modulate the expression of MHC antigen on the cell surface, trigger the activation of natural killer (NK) cells, and arrest viral replication.

Activated macrophages kill bacteria much more efficiently than resting phagocytic cells. This is not a specific process; cells activated in response to infection with one organism are often able to kill a second unrelated organism with equal efficiency. Macrophage activation is associated with an in-

crease in hydrolytic enzymes within the cell and an increase in the number of cell surface receptors for immunoglobulin and complement components. The activated cells have increased motility and enhanced phagocytic capacity, and they generate oxygen-derived free radicals, which can be bactericidal. Such radical formation may also be associated with tissue damage seen at the site of the DTH reaction. Cell-mediated immunity of this type plays an important role in the elimination of infectious agents from the body and may contribute to the pathogenesis of autoimmune disease.[8] The processing of nominal antigen by macrophages results in the formation of a ligand made up of the MHC and the processed antigen (c.x). However, both Class I and Class II MHC antigens can act as control molecules.[37] In the case of processed antigen, the ligand is formed from an interaction of x with the Class II antigen of the MHC. Processed antigen is presented in association with Class I MHC antigen only when x is the product of a virus that is multiplying within the cell. Some fusion viruses can bypass this need for active growth by directly fusing with the cell membrane. We use the symbol K as a generic representation of Class I MHC antigen and Ia as a generic representation of Class II MHC antigen. Thus, processed exogenous antigen is presented in the form Ia.x. Since CD4 T cells are reactive to Class II MHC-restricted antigen, it is the CD4 T cell population that plays the most prominent role in the regulation of this form of immunity.

The cytotoxic potential of T′ cells has been thought to play a role in the expression of CMI, particularly, in the elimination of infectious virus from an animal. However, this interpretation is still open to question.[49] In the case of viruses, infection of cells that lack Class II MHC antigen—the majority of tissue parenchymal cells—results in the presentation of viral antigen on the cell surface in association with Class I MHC antigen, that is, in the form of the ligand K.x. Primed T cells specific for this ligand, T′(K.x), are usually of the CD8 type and can express cytotoxic activity. Such cells have been shown to be responsible for the elimination of infectious virus from the lungs of influenza-infected mice.[49] However, primed CD8 cells also have the capacity to produce and secrete lymphokine, and the capacity of these cells to eliminate virus has now been shown to be CsA sensitive.[49] Since CsA does not affect the cytotoxic activity of T′ cells, it would appear that the in vivo function of these primed CD8 cells is a lymphokine-dependent process; that is, inflammatory mechanisms or γ-IFN production rather than a direct cytotoxic effect could be playing an important role in the elimination of infectious virus. This question requires further investigation.

Natural Killer (NK) Cells

Cytotoxic T-lymphocytes (CTL) interact with their target cell by way of the ligand-specific receptor. During the testing of CTL against various tumor targets, it became apparent that lymphoid cells from normal animals could be highly cytotoxic against certain specified target cells.[46] This activity showed no evidence of target cell specificity or memory and was attributed to the activity of NK cells. NK cells are nonadherent, nonphagocytic and have no surface immunoglobulin, nor do they show any MHC preference in their killing activity. Essentially any stimulation of an animal's immune system results in an increase in NK activity, an effect probably mediated by one of the lymphokines (γ-IFN). Since NK cells will only lyse a limited range of target cells, their in vivo significance is still unclear.

Suppression

Experiments in many laboratories have led to the development of complex networks of induction and suppression of immune activity.[6,57] It should be noted that there are many ways of suppressing immune responses. For example, the presence of antibody will inhibit the expression of a DTH reaction in a sensitized animal. The rapid removal of antigen will also diminish the response to antigen. Animals with a highly active reticuloendothelial system tend to mount lower responses to antigen because of the rapid degradation and removal of antigen.

Suppression has been studied in many different types of systems, including suppression of antibody and mitogen responses, responses against alloantigens, GVHD, and contact sensitivity. In many of the suppressor systems studied, the suppressive activity can be abolished by pretreatment of the putative suppressor cells with anti-T cell antibody and complement prior to testing, identifying them as T cells. The precise mode of action of suppressor cells is still unclear. They may act by preventing proliferation of T and/or B cells or by preventing stimulation by APC. In some systems, suppression seems to be antigen specific, suggesting that suppressor cells are capable of specific antigen recognition. Nonspecific suppression is seen in systems involving mitogen-activated suppressor cells. These activated T cells may act by absorbing factors required for cell growth such as IL-2. Some suppressor cells seem to act by releasing suppressive factors, the mode of action of which is unclear. Further investigation should provide information on the relationship of suppressor cells in various systems and their importance in regulating immune responses.

Cyclosporin A (CsA) and T Cell Function

Cyclosporin A (CsA) has provided a tool for the analysis of T cell function in vivo.[7] CsA, a fungal metabolite, is a cyclic peptide comprised of 11 amino acids. The agent has a relatively specific effect on lymphocyte function without inhibiting the T cell-independent activity of the phagocytic system. It is this cellular specificity that makes the agent so useful clinically. This agent's capacity to spare the phagocytic system while inhibiting lymphocyte activity allows the nonspecific immune system to cope with some bacterial infections even though the T cell component of the immune system has been incapacitated. However, the phagocytic system is less efficient in the absence of T cell modulation.

CsA has a relatively specific site of action, and its effect on T cell biology is now relatively well understood.[7]

The priming reaction (conversion of T to T' by signals [1] and [2]) is relatively CsA insensitive. Thus, IL-2 receptor expression is observed in the presence of CsA (1 µg/ml), and there is now strong evidence for T cell priming in vivo in the presence of this agent.[7] Clonal expansion (e.g., increased number of T' by IL-2) is also insensitive to CsA.

However, the triggering reaction (the release of lymphokines from T' by antigen, that is, signal [1]) is extremely sensitive to CsA, being significantly inhibited at concentrations as low as 10 ng/ml. Lymphokine production by constitutive producers, such as certain tumor lines, is not inhibited by CsA at 1 ng/ml, nor is lymphokine production inhibited when CsA is added to T cells that have mRNA for lymphokine synthesis in their cytoplasm.[21] Thus, we can conclude that CsA prevents lymphokine production by interfering with the transmission of signal [1] to the T cell nucleus. This event is required to functionally activate the set of lymphokine genes, resulting in DNA transcription followed by synthesis and secretion of their molecular products. Once transcription has occurred, the cell is insensitive to CsA. CsA does not interfere with the expression of cytotoxic activity by T'cells.[7]

B CELL BIOLOGY

B cells differentiate from stem cells in the bone marrow. These marrow-derived stem cells also migrate to peripheral lymphoid tissue where they can develop into B cells and antibody-forming plasma cells. As pre-B cells mature, genomic components of the immunoglobulin genes are rearranged to produce a particular combination (see Fig. 3-4); this is a random process contributing to the somatic diversification of antibody specificity. Further maturation of the B cell results in the expression of membrane bound forms of IgM and IgD on the cell surface. Following antigenic stimulation, IgD is lost and the IgM molecule is secreted.

Immunoglobulin Structure

Early observations from the studies of infectious disease showed that human serum contained a substanced called antibody, which could neutralize toxins and destroy bacteria. As techniques improved it became possible to purify antibody and study its structure. A typical antibody molecule (Fig. 3-7) consists of two heavy and two light chains joined by disulfide bonds.[30] Enzymatic cleavage of the immunoglobulin molecule gives rise to a number of fragments that have biological activity. Fc fragments consist of the CH_2 and CH_3 domains joined by disulfide bonds. This fragment binds to cells with Fc receptors that play a major role on the phagocytosis of antigen–antibody complexes. $F(ab)_2$ fragments consist of two heavy–light chain complexes joined by a disulfide bond. These fragments contain the antigen combining sites and bind antigen with a valency of two, as does the whole antibody molecule. Each chain of the molecule consists of constant regions and variable regions giving rise to antibody diversity. The molecule has intrachain disulfide bonds, which give the molecule a globular structure (see Fig. 3-7).

Isotypes

In both humans and in rodents, there are a number of classes or isotypes of immunoglobulins that have different properties and can mediate different functions. For example, in humans, there are four IgG isotypes: IgG_1, IgG_2, IgG_3, and IgG_4. Of these, only types 1, 2, and 3 can fix complement. IgA_1 and IgA_2 are usually found in mucous secretions and exist as a dimer with the two molecules being joined by a joining chain (J chain). The dimer also has a secretory piece attached as a possible protection against proteolysis by gastric enzymes. IgA does not fix complement. IgM exists as a pentamer and is the first antibody to appear in an immune response. Since complement activation requires a complex of two antibody molecules, pentameric IgM is very efficient at fixing complement. IgE exists in minute quantities in normal serum and is the antibody associated with allergic reactions. The antibody binds to the surface of mast cells and, upon interaction with antigen, triggers the release of inflammatory mediators and initiates immediate-type hypersensitivity (ITH) reactions. IgD is an immunoglobulin found on the surface of lymphocytes during their differentiation.

Allotypes

Genetic analysis of antibody genes has been carried out in mice, rabbits, and humans using serologic procedures to follow the inheritance of distinctive antigenic markers on immunoglobulin molecules. These markers are known as allotypes and are antigenic determinants that characterize immunoglobulin chains from different forms of the same gene (alleles).[21] Allotypic differences are localized to the constant regions and have been used in mapping constant region genes. Allotypic markers are inherited in a mendelian fashion.

Idiotypes

Idiotypes are the antigenic determinants that distinguish one V region from another V region.[19] These

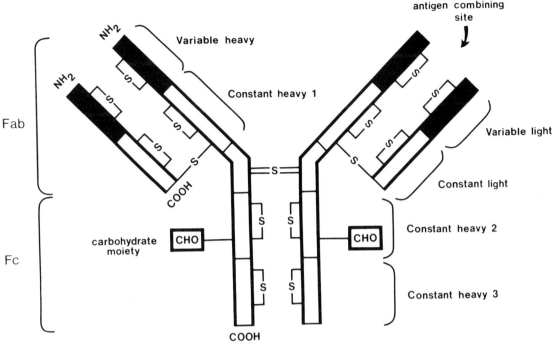

FIGURE 3-7. *Diagram of an immunoglobulin molecule. The 2 large heavy chains and the 2 smaller light chains are linked by disulfide bridges (S). Both heavy and light chains can be divided into 2 segments—a constant region whose amino acid composition varies little among Ig molecules and a variable region with considerable amino acid diversity.*

determinants are commonly located at or near the antigen-binding site because that is the region of the immunoglobulin molecule where the hypervariable segments of the light and heavy chains fold together.

Antigen–Antibody Interactions

Antibody binds antigen with a certain strength that may change during an immune response. This binding strength is known as the affinity of the antibody for the antigen and may be measured by an association constant (K). The affinity of the antibody increases during an immune response; for example, the affinity of rabbit anti-dinitrophenol (DNP) 2 weeks after immunization is 1×10^{-6}, and at 8 weeks post-immunization, it is 250×10^{-6}. The antigen combining site is 500 to 700 A^2 in area, and binding depends upon a close fit between two complimentary areas on the molecule. Binding is noncovalent and reversible and consists of ionic forces, hydrogen bonds, and Van der Waals forces, with energy levels one tenth to one fifth that of covalent bonds.

Valency

A single antibody molecule has the capability of binding two antigen molecules. Pentameric IgM can bind 10 antigen molecules. Antigens may also bind more than one antibody molecule. Such binding properties result in the formation of an antigen–antibody lattice at equivalent concentrations of antibody and antigen. These complexes may become large and visible and form the basis for tests of antibody specificity such as the Ouchterlony test. In this assay, antigen and antibody are placed in small wells punched in agarose a few millimeters apart. As the antibody and antigen migrate through the gel, a precipitin band forms at the line of equivalence.

Complement

If purified antibody against sheep red blood cells is mixed with sheep red blood cells at the optimal concentration, the cells will agglutinate. If fresh normal serum is added to the antibody-coated cells, they will lyse. The activity in the fresh normal serum that causes lysis is known as complement. Complement is composed of approximately 15 separate serum components, some of which are very unstable. The components were labeled in the order of their discovery, not in the order of their activation. The pathway of activation is a cascade, the activation of one component leading to the activation of the next component. Activation by way of the classical pathway requires antigen–antibody complexes, either dimers of complement-fixing IgG or a single molecule of pentameric IgM. Activation can also occur by way of the alternative pathway as a consequence of interactions between agents such as lipopolysaccharide (LPS) and the complement components. The details of the activation pathways can be found elsewhere.[10] During complement activation, a number of pharmacologically active molecules are released. C3a and C5a are anaphylotoxins that can directly cause smooth muscle contraction and mast cell degranulation leading to allergic-type reactions. They are also chemotactic for neutrophils, macrophages, and eosinophils. There are receptors for C3b on neutrophils, macrophages, eosinophils, and B-lymphocytes. Thus, C3b can act as an opsonin-enhancing phagocytosis. C5b67 is also chemotactic for granulocytes. The binding of all the components causes lysis of a cell carrying the antigen bound to the antibody.

Although the earliest antibody produced during the immune response is IgM, as the response develops, there may be a switch in antibody class to either IgG, IgA, or IgE. This switch in immunoglobulin class production occurs at the cellular level, that is, a cell commences producing IgM then switches into the production of a different immunoglobulin class. The switching mechanism appears to be regulated by T cells. Antigen can also play a part in determining the class of immunoglobulin produced, for example, lipopolysaccharide will stimulate the production of IgM, whereas parasitic infection often results in large amounts of IgE production. The molecular basis of this phenomenon is not yet understood.

Antigen-Driven B Cell Activation and Differentiation

The process of B cell activation is still rather poorly understood. The classic experiments of Claman and associates[15] and Mitchell and Miller[44] demonstrated the involvement of T cells in the activation process; for this reason, such T cells came to be known as helper T cells.

Antigen entering the body is processed by APCs and presented to T cells. As discussed previously, this process results in T cell priming. Such T cells are specific for the priming ligand c.x (see Fig. 3-1).

$$Sc.x + T(c.x) \xrightarrow[(2)]{(1)} T'(c.x)$$

While both Class I (K) and Class II (Ia) MHC antigens can act as control molecules under appropriate conditions, when exogenous antigen is processed by the APC, it is presented on the cell surface in the form Ia.x.

$$SIa.x + T(Ia.x) \xrightarrow[(2)]{(1)} T'(Ia.x)$$

Antigen is presented in the form K.x when x is a product of viral particles actively growing within the cell (see above).

Antigen can also interact with and be processed by B cells. The immunoglobulin molecule on the surface of the B cell acts as its antigen-specific receptor (Fig. 3-8). Following binding to this receptor, antigen can be taken up by the B cell and processed.[14] Following processing, degradation products of the native antigen are presented on the surface of the B cell in the form Ia.x. Ia.x then forms the ligand displayed on the B cell, which is specific for the primed T cell. Interaction of this ligand with the T'cell receptor triggers lymphokine production by this cell. The binding of the T' cell to this ligand Ia.x on the surface of the B cell may also signal the B cell itself. The exact details of B cell signaling are not fully understood at this stage; however, both B cell growth factor (BCGF) and B cell differentiation factor (BCDF) are among the lymphokines released when the primed T cell is triggered by the ligand Ia.x on the surface of the B cell. These products are involved in regulating the further proliferation and differentiation of B cells into antibody-secreting plasma cells. Some B cells remain morphologically small B cells to become *memory cells,* which have been clonally expanded and are capable of mounting a rapid response to a second encounter with the priming antigen. Most memory B cells carry IgG on their surface and rapidly differentiate into IgG-secreting cells when triggered by secondary antigen contact (Fig 3-8).

MHC Restriction of T/B Interactions

Because T cells primed against processed antigen are of specificity (Ia.x), they can only interact with B cells that express the ligand Ia.x. This requirement for Class II MHC antigen recognition was discovered experimentally and came to be known as another aspect of the phenomenon of MHC restriction. Thus, it was found that T cells could only collaborate with B cells that express the same Class II antigen as the T cell; T cells and B cells could only interact when they were MHC (Class II antigen) compatible. This phenomenon, MHC restriction of the immune response, was first thought to indicate some strange structural affinity of the T cell receptor for MHC antigen. However, it probably merely reflects the specificity of the immune response; that is, T cells primed to the ligand Ia.x are specific for Ia.x and

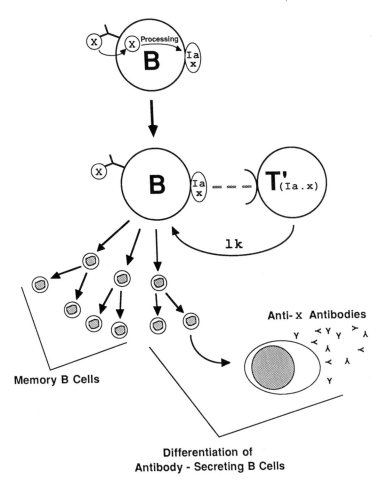

FIGURE 3-8. *Model for antigen processing by B cells with subsequent B cell activation. The immunoglobulin molecule on the surface of the B cell acts as an antigen-specific receptor. Following binding to this receptor, antigen is taken up by the B cell and processed. Following processing, degradation products of the native antigen (X) are presented on the surface of the B cell in the form of Ia.x. Ia.x then forms the ligand which is specific for the primed T cell (helper cell). Interaction of this ligand with the T' cell receptor triggers lymphokine production by this cell. Binding of the T' cell to the ligand Ia.x on the surface of the B cell may also signal the B cell itself. The exact details of B cells signaling are still not fully understood.*

can therefore only collaborate with B cells that also have the capacity to present Ia.x. The unexpected feature of the immune response was that antigen must be processed and presented in the form of Ia.x in order to facilitate the initial step of T cell priming.

Abnormal Induction of B Cells

In certain abnormal situations, allogeneic T cells can interact directly with B cells and induce their differentiation, resulting in antibody secretion. This phenomenon has been observed when animals are undergoing a graft-versus-host (GVH) reaction.[34] In this case, the T' cell interacts with alloantigen, which forms an integral part of the B cell membrane, rather than with processed antigen. The T' cell, which is alloreactive, $^{c1}T'(c)$, has no specificity for processed antigen and thus activates B cells regardless of their receptor specificity. This process results in polyclonal B cell activation and is thought to induce the production of autoantibodies in certain situations.[34]

THE ALLOGRAFT REACTION

Development of Ideas

In the early part of the century, in the West, scientific interest in tissue grafting developed. At this time there was a notion that physiologic incompatibility may be responsible for rejection phenomena. Although never really precisely stated, this idea prompted the suggestion that an organ might be adapted to the new physiologic environment of it's prospective host by maintaining the tissue in the recipient's serum prior to grafting. Medawar[43] led the attack on what he saw as an intellectually soft approach to transplantation biology. His studies had shown graft rejection to have properties of specificity and memory, which were characteristics of the immune response. With the demonstration that specific allograft tolerance could be induced in the newborn, a confirmation of Burnet and Fenner's (1949)[12] theoretical prediction, the notion that graft rejection was an immunologic phenomenon mediated by the recognition and response to genetically encoded transplantation antigens became established.

Any attempt to modify graft immunogenicity prior to transplantation was seen to be theoretically infirm, and such studies were no longer the subject of legitimate experimental investigation.

Yet, as strong as the evidence is on the side of the immunologic concept, there is a nagging problem entwined in this theoretical explanation. This problem is most clearly expressed as the "Transplantation Paradox." Three propositions provide the basis for this paradox:

1. Graft rejection is an immune process initiated by recognition and response to transplantation antigen.
2. The allograft response must be included among the most violent of immune reactions.
3. The transplantation antigens as isolated molecules, regardless of whether they are Class I or Class II MHC antigens, are very weak immunogens.

To solve this paradox, we must answer the following question: How can such weak immunogens initiate such violent immune responses?

The solution to the paradox derives from the new understanding of antigen presentation and the role that the interleukins play in immune induction. This solution, ironically, also leads us back to the notion that graft immunogenicity can be reduced by appropriate treatment of the tissue prior to transplantation.

The Theory of Allogeneic Activity

The theory of allogeneic activity has an important implication—namely, that two quite distinct forms of alloantigen presentation are important for any consideration of allograft immunity: active and passive antigen presentation. Active (direct) antigen presentation occurs when the MHC antigen, on the surface of metabolically active S^+ cells, is recognized by specific T cells (Fig. 3-9). In this situation, activation of alloreactive T cells occurs because the S^+ cell provides both the source of antigen (signal [1]) and CoS activity (signal [2]) required for induction. This reaction has the form

$$^cSc + {}^{c1}T(c) \xrightarrow[(2)]{(1)} {}^{c1}T'(c)$$

where c (MHC) is the control structure on the surface of the APC of c genotype and $^{c1}T(c)$ is a T cell of c1 genotype (allogeneic), which carries a receptor for c. The resultant primed cell, $^{c1}T'(c)$, is unre-

stricted; that is, it is specific for alloantigen alone and has no specificity for c1, the MHC type of the responding T cell. We will refer to this reaction (g) as the direct reaction, because it involves direct presentation of alloantigen to the responsive T cell. When the same antigen (c) is presented on the surface of a cell that cannot provide a source of CoS activity (S^- phenotype), it is presented in a passive form and is therefore nonimmunogenic (Fig. 3-10). This reaction has the form

$$^cP(c) + {}^{c1}T(c) \xrightarrow{(1)} \text{no response}$$

where ^cpc is a passive APC of c genotype, which presents allogeneic MHC antigen c to the potentially responsive T cell $^{c1}T(c)$.

Experimental support for the two-signal model for T cell activation comes from the study of the immunogenicity of tumor cell lines.[37] Tumors of lymphoreticular origin, such as P815 and EL4, express the S^+ phenotype and can actively present alloantigen. Epithelial tumors, on the other hand, express the S^- phenotype[37]; thus, they are unable to produce CoS activity. Both CD4 (Class II MHC antigen-reactive) and CD8 (Class I MHC antigen-reactive) T cells can be activated to alloantigen by the direct pathway.[37]

In the allograft situation, there is no reason why graft antigen cannot be processed by APCs of the host animal and presented in this way to host T cells. In this situation, graft antigen is treated in the same way as exogenous antigen, X (see Fig. 3-9). We call this process *indirect* presentation of graft antigens. Graft antigens, as well as other exogenous antigens, presented in this way require processing by the host APCs and are seen by the T cell in association with the Ia (Class II MHC) antigens of the host. These reactions can be written as follows:

$$X + {}^{c1}SIa1 \longrightarrow {}^{c1}SIa1.x$$

$$^{c1}SIa1.x + {}^{c1}T(Ia1.x) \xrightarrow[(2)]{(1)} {}^{c1}T'(Ia1.x)$$

where Ia1 is the Class II antigen of the host and Ia is the Class II antigen of the graft. Thus, the T cell that is activated will be of specificity (Ia1.x). Such cells are not graft specific; the graft expresses the X set of antigens but cannot express Ia1.x provided that the donor is MHC incompatible with the recipient. However, T cells activated by this indirect reaction could interact with host B cells, which can present processed graft antigens, x, in association with host Class II antigen (Ia1.x). The result of this interaction would be *graft-specific* antibody formation; that is, antigen presentation by way of the

Direct Presentation

ACTIVE

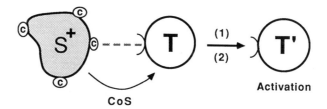

PASSIVE

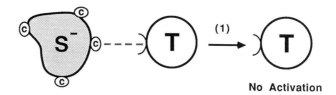

Indirect Presentation

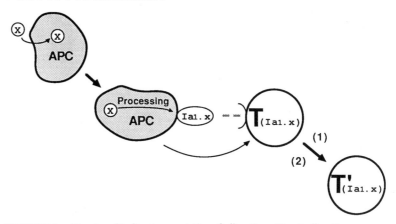

FIGURE 3-9.   Direct *and* indirect *presentation of alloantigen.* Direct *alloantigen presentation occurs in either an* active *or a* passive *form. In the* active *form, antigen is introduced to the T cell on the surface of metabolically active graft* S^+ *cells. Engagement of the control molecule (c) by the T cell receptor provides signal (1) to the T cell, which in turn signals the* S^+ *cell to provide costimulator (CoS) activity that acts as signal (2). These 2 signals are responsible for the shift of the resting T cell into the T' condition (activation).*

Alloantigen is presented in a passive *form when introduced directly to the host's T cell on the surface of graft* S^- *cells. Engagement of the control molecule (c) provides signal (1) for the T cell, however, the* S^- *cell is unable to provide signal (2), and so no activation of the T cell occurs.*

Indirect *presentation of alloantigen occurs following the shedding of any graft antigen, X. Note that the grafted cell's control structure c, once shed, loses its control function and so merely represents a subset of X. The host APC internalizes and processes X and presents the processed product, x, on its surface in association with the host's control structure, Ia1 (distinct from the graft's control structure, Ia). T cells with receptor specificity of (Ia1.x) interact with the Ia1.x complex on the APC, providing signal (1) for the T cell. Costimulator activity, signal (2), is provided by the APC and these 2 signals together result in the production of the primed T cell, T'(Ia1.x).*

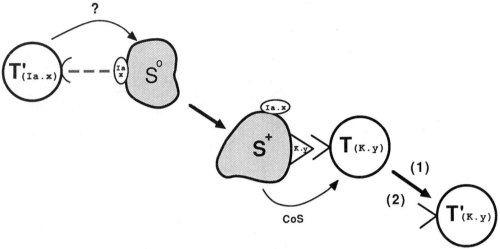

FIGURE 3-10.   *T/T collaboration mediated by indirect induction of the active APC. Primed T cells of specificity (Ia.x) interact with resting APCs and induce CoS production—mechanism unknown. The activated APC can then actively present minor cell surface antigens, y, in association with class I MHC surface antigens (K). The complex K.y cannot of itself act as a control structure because y is a minor antigen and by definition not part of c.*

indirect pathway does not lead to graft-specific T cell activation and may result in the production of antibodies that enhance graft survival.

Immunogenicity of Class II Antigen

There is an erroneous notion associated with current thinking about alloreactivity and the function of the APC—namely, that Class II MHC antigen of itself is highly immunogenic. This idea derives from an alternate two-signal model for T cell activation proposed by Bach and colleagues.[3] These authors suggested that recognition of the Ia epitope on the grafted allogeneic cell activated the host helper T cells, which then provided the second signal for host CTL activation. According to this model, passive presentation of Class II MHC antigen was sufficient for helper T cell activation. We now know that this is not the case.[36] There is also evidence that recognition of Class II antigen is not required for cytotoxic T cell activation in vitro.[2, 54]

This does not mean that Ia-positive cells are unimportant in the process of allogeneic T cell activation. Many cells that express the S[+] phenotype are Ia positive. Inactivation of these cells with anti-I region antibody and complement may remove the stimulating capacity of the cell population.[18] However, not all Ia-positive cells stimulate, and some Ia-negative cells such as P815 and EL4 do stimulate.[37, 54] Although there is a strong correlation between Ia positivity and the expression of the S[+] phenotype, exceptions to the correlation show that

recognition of Ia antigen itself cannot provide the source of the second signal required for cytotoxic T cell activation. Nevertheless, a donor Ia-positive cell is probably the cell responsible for stimulation of both Class I and Class II MHC-reactive T cells of the host. The most likely candidate for the physiologically relevant stimulator is the Ia-rich dendritic cell.

Mechanism of Graft Rejection

There is now evidence that graft rejection is triggered following the interaction of sensitized T-lymphocytes and graft antigen. The transfer of sensitized cells to sublethally irradiated recipient rats carrying heart allografts demonstrated that long-lived, recirculating, immunoglobulin-negative cells were responsible for initiating rejection. Similar experiments showed that memory cells were long-lived, nonrecirculating, immunoglobulin-negative cells. It has also been shown that T cells from sensitized donors can trigger the rejection of skin allografts carried by adult thymectomized, irradiated, bone marrow-reconstituted (ATXBM) mice.[41] T cells are also required for the rejection of metastable islet and thyroid allografts, that is, allografts that have been cultured to reduce their immunogenicity and that survive indefinitely following transplantation into nonimmunosuppressed recipients.[47]

The phenotype of T cells that triggers graft rejection has been a matter of some controversy. The most commonly used model (the first model) involves the transfer of cells, which have been treated to remove one or other cell population, into ATXBM recipients carrying either skin or heart allografts. The second most common model used involves the transfer of sensitized cells into normal animals carrying a metastable islet or thyroid allograft.[37] Pancreatic islets and thyroid tissue can be transplanted to normal allogeneic mice if the tissue is first cultured in an oxygen-rich atmosphere. Such grafts are in a metastable condition. They carry potentially recognizable antigen and are rejected when the host is either actively or passively immunized.[37]

Investigations using the first model found that the transferred CD4 T cells were required for graft rejection.[41] A major problem with this model is the difficulty of ensuring that the ATXBM animals are completely T cell deficient. Recently, it has been shown that ATXBM mice reconstituted with cells that have been treated with anti-Lyt 2 (anti-CD8) antiserum and complement had CD8 T cells of both donor and host origin following graft rejection.[40] It has also been shown that heart grafts in ATXBM animals reconstituted with CD4 T cells contain CD8 cells at the time of rejection.[22] The second model provides more direct evidence that CD8 cells are involved in the rejection process. In this system, the transfer of sensitized CD8 T cells is necessary and is sufficient to initiate the rejection of the metastable graft.[37]

We should emphasize that the phenotype of the cell responsible for graft rejection may be a function of the type of tissue transplant; that is, it may be determined by the type of alloantigen expressed on the graft. Metastable islet and thyroid allografts express only Class I MHC antigens, whereas cells present in skin graft express both Class I and Class II MHC antigens. T cells activated against either class of MHC alloantigen are able to produce lymphokine when appropriately triggered. These cells can also express cytotoxic activity. Therefore, cells of either subclass could mediate graft rejection by one of these processes.

The relative contribution of these two activities (cytotoxicity or lymphokine production) to the rejection process can be determined by using cyclosporine, an agent that inhibits lymphokine release from the primed T cell but has no effect on the expression of cytotoxic activity by these cells. CD8 T cell-dependent rejection of cultured islet allografts is inhibited by cyclosporine, demonstrating a dependence upon lymphokine release. It could be argued that when effector cells are introduced into the systemic circulation, they cannot recirculate and do not reach the graft site. However, under conditions in which lymphocyte recirculation is not required, cyclosporine still inhibits the rejection process.[26] Since lymphokine release is cyclosporine sensitive and cytotoxicity is not, these data suggest that graft rejection mediated by CD8 T cells is a lymphokine-dependent process.

These observations show that the direct cytotoxic activity of the primed CD8 cell is not of itself sufficient for the initiation of graft damage. Graft rejection mediated by primed T cells appears to be a lymphokine-dependent process. It is possible that lymphokine is required for the expression of cytotoxic activity in vivo. IL-2 may be required to maintain a cytotoxic cell in an active proliferating state for a sufficient period of time to cause tissue damage; the proliferation of T cells at the graft site is a feature of rejecting allografts. Gamma-interferon production may be required to raise the antigen density on the target cells to the level required for efficient killing. Another possibility is that the cytotoxic activity of the cell population has little to do with the rejection process. According to this hypothesis, lymphokines released by T cells could activate inflammatory cells and processes that could then mediate tissue damage. This important question awaits further experimental examination.

Role of Antibody in Graft Rejection

Antibody was initially thought to play little part in the rejection process. However, it is now clear that the failure of initial attempts to transfer murine skin graft rejection passively by antibody can be attributed to deficiencies in the complement system of rodents. Antibody-mediated, hyperacute rejection of skin allografts and xenografts has now been demonstrated in rodents, but only when an exogenous source of complement is transferred along with the specific antibody.[37] Different tissues also vary in their susceptibility to antibody-mediated rejection; allografts prepared by primary vascular anastomosis are highly sensitive to antibody and complement and retain the sensitivity for a prolonged period of time. In contrast, with time, skin grafts can show marked variations in their susceptibility to attack by antibody and complement. This effect is related to the replacement of donor endothelium in the skin by host cells. Soon after grafting mice with rat skin, rat cell surface antigens were detected on the graft vasculature. As the graft became less sensitive to anti-rat antibody-mediated damage, mouse cell surface antigens were detected on the endothelium. Eventually, all the graft vasculature was of recipient origin, and the graft was resistant to passively transferred anti-rat antibody.[31]

The administration of immune serum causes rapid rejection of islet allografts in tolerant rats. However, when endothelium is destroyed by a period of organ culture prior to transplantation, grafts are resistant to the action of antibody and complement.[31] These findings suggest that antibody-mediated damage is a vascular phenomenon, a notion supported by the observation that endothelial cells are readily lysed by antibody and complement in vitro. In humans, both Class I and Class II MHC antigens are expressed on endothelial cells and could provide a target for antibody-mediated damage.

A possible mechanism for antibody-mediated graft rejection has been described by Bogman and associates.[6] Small amounts of antibody binding to blood vessel walls fix complement resulting in endothelial cell damage and the release of chemotactic factors. This process results in the attraction and binding, through complement receptors, of PMN, which causes further endothelial damage. Following the exposure of subendothelial tissue, thrombosis occurs. In the situation where animals are naturally deficient in complement, antibody-mediated hyperacute rejection does not normally occur.

ANALYSIS OF THE IMMUNE RESPONSE TO AN ALLOGRAFT

For the detailed analysis of the in vivo response to an allograft, we can use the theory of allogeneic reactivity. This analysis follows three steps:

1. Definition of the cellular composition of the graft.
2. Consideration of how components of the graft interact with the immune system of the host.
3. Consideration of reactivity of T cells activated in the host.

MHC Incompatibility

Let us first consider the host response to an MHC-incompatible graft. Metabolically active S^+ cells of the graft interact with host T cells to generate a graft-specific T cell response, $^cT'(c)$ by way of active presentation and the direct reaction (see Fig. 3-9). Passive APCs (^cPc) do not cause direct T cell activation because they lack a source of signal [2]. However, any graft antigen that we can represent collectively as X can be shed and processed by host APCs, and so activate host T cells by way of the indirect reaction (see Fig. 3-9). The result is the production of T' cells specific for the host Ia associated with processed graft antigens.

We can see that it is only the direct reaction that produces a T cell response specific for the MHC antigens of the graft. The indirect reaction activates T cell specific for the ligand, Ia1.x., where Ia1 is

host Class II antigen. These cells cannot interact directly with the graft but can act as helper cells by virtue of their capacity for lymphokine production (see Fig. 3-9). In this analysis, we make the assumption that T cells must recognize and interact with the cells that they help. Under these conditions, helper cells of specificity (Ia1.x) can interact with host B cells, which present x in association with host Ia, that is, as the ligand Ia1.x. The result of this interaction would be graft-specific antibody formation. Because resting T cells lack Ia antigen and are unable to process antigen, T/T interactions requiring recognition of the ligand Ia1.x cannot occur. On the basis of this analysis, we can see that MHC incompatible APCs carried in the graft provide the major source of tissue immunogenicity. This is the theoretical basis of the concept that passenger leukocytes are a major source of tissue immunogenicity.[37]

This analysis provides a solution to the "Transplantation Paradox." The MHC antigens on the surface of S^+ cells are highly immunogenic because they function as a control molecule. The S^+ cell is the only cell within the graft that can participate in the direct reaction and so generate a strong graft-specific response. Under conditions of indirect antigen presentation, the same antigens are at best only weakly immunogenic. They do not activate a graft-specific T cell response, but may lead to graft-specific antibody formation. Clearly, MHC antigens of the graft are only highly immunogenic when presented to the host on the surface of viable cells expressing the S^+ phenotype, and removal of these cells from the graft prior to transplantation would markedly reduce tissue immunogenicity.

Minor Histocompatibility Differences

Minor histocompatibility antigens are defined as all cell surface antigens other than the MHC antigens. It is implicit in this definition that minor antigens that are constitutive to a particular S^+ cell cannot interact functionally with the MHC antigens of that cell to form part of the control structure. If this were to occur, the "minor" antigens would constitute part of the control structure and thus would no longer be minor antigens.

We can apply the aforementioned analysis to the consideration of allograft reactions across minor histocompatibility differences. In this case, the direct reaction is not activated. The T cell is unable to interact with the control structure alone on the surface of the S^+ cell because it is MHC-identical with the recipient, and, by definition, minor antigens cannot functionally interact with the control system of the APC. Responses to minor antigens must proceed by the indirect pathway to activate T cells of specificity (Ia.x). In this case, the Ia is common to both the donor tissue and the recipient since they are MHC identical. Thus, T cells activated against antigens shed from minor histoincompatible grafts will be *graft specific,* provided that the graft expresses Class II antigen. This analysis predicts that the allograft response to minor antigens will be very much dependent upon the type of tissue transplanted. Tissue rich in Class II MHC antigen (e.g., skin) will present the ligand Ia.x and so provide a target for cells activated by the indirect pathway. These tissues will tend to be rejected acutely when transplanted across minor histocompatibility differences. Tissues that are low in Class II MHC antigen expression will be less sensitive to rejection when transplanted across such minor histocompatibility differences.

Experimental Reduction of Tissue Immunogenicity

In the early 1970s, several groups investigated the effect of organ culture on the immunogenicity of endocrine organs and certain tumor tissues. The idea that organ culture might reduce immunogenicity was not new. In the 1930s, there were reports suggesting clinical benefit when parathyroid tissue was held in organ culture for a period of time prior to transplantation to patients with hypoparathyroidism. These studies were not genetically controlled and were based on the concept that it might be possible to adapt a graft to the recipient by growing it in the recipient serum prior to transplantation. Without the support of an adequate theoretical base, enthusiasm for such experiments rapidly waned. Our interest in organ culture was stimulated by a report from Summerlin and co-workers—subsequently not confirmed—that organ culture prior to transplantation could facilitate the grafting of skin to normal allogeneic recipients. Jacobs and Huseby[28] suggested that antigen expression was modified during the period that it was in organ culture. Such an explanation did not seem very likely, but, against the aforementioned theoretical background, the effect of organ culture could readily be explained if APCs in the tissue died or were inactivated during the culture period.

The organ culture technique has proved spectacularly successful in the case of endocrine organ transplantation. Mouse thyroid can be transplanted under the renal capsule of isogeneic thyroidectomized recipients, where its ability to concentrate radioactive iodine can be used as a measure of graft function.[37] Organ culture of thyroid tissue in an atmosphere of 95% oxygen and 5% carbon dioxide for 3 to 4 weeks enabled successful transplantation to normal allogeneic recipients wherein it func-

tioned indefinitely.[37] This phenomenon has now been demonstrated with parathyroid, pituitary, and islets of the pancreas, in addition to thyroid tissue.

What is the explanation of this phenomenon? Does antigen modulation occur in organ culture as suggested by Jacobs and Huseby,[28] or does the effect result from the postulated loss of passenger leukocytes? During organ culture, there is a rapid degeneration of the vascular bed and blood elements within the cultured tissue. The tissue retains antigen recognizable by immunoferritin labeling and can be rejected when as few as 10^3 viable peritoneal cells of donor origin are injected into the recipient animal at the time that the cultured tissue is transplanted. Clearly, the cultured allograft carries functionally recognizable antigen. Established thyroid allografts are also rejected when a second uncultured thyroid of donor origin is transplanted to the recipient. This effect is antigen specific, since an uncultured third-party graft can be rejected, but its rejection does not affect the integrity of the established cultured allograft.

Hirshberg and Thorsby[25] suggested that vascular endothelium may provide a major stimulus for allograft immunity. Vascular endothelium degenerates during organ culture, and its destruction could account for the reduction in tissue immunogenicity achieved by this procedure. Endothelial cells express MHC antigens (both Class I and Class II) but appear to present these antigens in a passive form. They therefore may provide a primary target for the attack of activated graft-specific T cells or graft-specific antibody. However, the question to be addressed here is whether or not endothelium provides a major source of stimulating activity for the recipient T cells; that is, does Ia-positive endothelium express the S^+ phenotype? The following studies from our laboratory addressed this question.

Cyclophosphamide treatment of animals for 4 days prior to the harvest of tissues caused a profound drop in the capacity of spleen cells to stimulate allogeneic T cells in culture. This treatment of the donor with cyclophosphamide has no obvious effect on thyroid endothelium. However, after this treatment alone, approximately 30% of thyroid allografts functioned normally over a prolonged observation period. Thus, Class II- bearing endothelium cannot be a major source of tissue immunogenicity. Batchelor and colleagues[4] studies of kidney allograft survival after passage through an intermediate host led to a similar conclusion.

Pancreatic Islet Transplantation

Initial attempts to apply the organ culture procedure to pancreatic islet transplantation were frustrated by technical difficulties. The loss of tissue immunogenicity during organ culture is an oxygen-dependent phenomenon, thought to result from the sensitivity of leukocytes to oxygen toxicity. Pancreatic islet tissue cannot be treated in this way. Single islets, isolated from the adult pancreas, are extremely sensitive to oxygen toxicity and rapidly degenerate when cultured in 95% oxygen. This toxicity problem can be overcome by allowing groups of approximately 50 islets to aggregate and fuse together. The islet clusters are more resistant to oxygen toxicity and can be successfully allotransplanted in mice after 1 week of culture under these conditions. Following organ culture in 95% oxygen, islet allografts of from seven to nine clusters have been shown to reverse streptozocin-induced diabetes in mice. Blood sugar levels of transplanted animals rapidly return to normal. The animals become aglycosuric and respond normally to a glucose challenge. Uncultured islets, on the other hand, only temporarily reverse diabetes, and recipient animals usually return to the diabetic state within 4 weeks of transplantation. Lacy's group[35] achieved similar results in the rat. However, in their initial studies, islets were not cultured in 95% oxygen, and allograft acceptance was only achieved when recipient animals were treated with a single dose of anti-lymphocyte serum (ALS) at the time of transplantation. Similar results have been reported in the case of rat islet xenotransplantation to mice. Faustman and colleagues[18] demonstrated a dependence of islet immunogenicity on the presence of Ia-positive cells in the transplanted tissue by achieving allograft survival following anti-Ia serum and complement treatment of donor tissue prior to grafting. Other investigators[20] have been unable to reproduce these findings. However, Ia antigen recognition is not required; Morrow and associates[45] have shown that islet allograft rejection occurs when there is I region compatibility between the donor and recipient. The fact that rejection is dependent upon the presence of an Ia$^+$ cell in the tissues is consistent with the notion that the S$^+$ stimulator cell carries Ia antigen on surface.

Organ Transplantation

Initial attempts to remove passenger leukocytes from organs prior to transplantation were not successful. These attempts involved the induction of leukopenia in the donor tissue by procedures such as whole-body irradiation, cyclophosphamide pretreatment, or treatment with anti-lymphocyte serum. At best, only marginal effects were observed with kidney transplants across MHC barriers and heart allografts transplanted across multiple minor differences. Stuart and co-workers[56] attempted to remove passenger leukocytes by first allografting rat kidneys to passively enhanced intermediate hosts. At 60 to 300 days post-transplantation, the kidney grafts were retransplanted to naive recipient rats isologous to the intermediate host. Only a delay in the onset of rejection was achieved in these studies. These marginal or weak effects led to some confusion over the extent to which passenger leukocytes contribute to tissue immunogenicity.

Studies from Batchelor's laboratory[4] have clarified the role that passenger leukocytes play in renal allografting. This group demonstrated that long-surviving immunologically enhanced (MHC-incompatible) rat kidney grafts, when transplanted from a primary to a secondary recipient of the same genotype, did not elicit T cell alloimmunity in the secondary host. In contrast, normal primary kidney allografts in the relevant donor–recipient combination were regularly rejected in 12 days. The failure of long-surviving kidney grafts to activate a T cell response could not be attributed to a lack of either Class I or Class II MHC antigens, and Batchelor's group suggested that the effect resulted from a loss of passenger leukocytes. They then went on to show quite convincingly that donor-strain dendritic cells, in very low numbers, would trigger rejection of kidneys taken from an intermediate enhanced recipient.[39] The earlier failure to see such a dramatic effect probably resulted from the strain combinations used in those studies.

Response to Minor Histocompatibility Differences

When we studied the effect of organ culture on the immunogenicity of MHC-incompatible allografts, we noticed that some tissues, such as mouse fetal pancreas, were more difficult to prepare for allotransplantation than other tissues, such as islets isolated from adult pancreas. Such tissue-specific differences in immunogenicity can be explained by the extent to which the particular donor tissue is contaminated with lymphoreticular cells. Whereas fetal pancreas is heavily contaminated with lymphoid tissue, isolated islets show no gross contamination. Our theoretical treatment suggests that strong tissue-specific effects will also be seen when tissues are transplanted across minor histocompatibility barriers. Rejection in this situation is seen to result from T cells of specificity (Ia.x) activated by way of the indirect pathway, interacting with Class II MHC antigen-bearing cells in the graft. Thus, tissues rich in Class II MHC antigen would reject more acutely than tissues with relatively low lymphoreticular cell content. Table 3-2 illustrates this effect. When skin, fetal pancreas, fetal proislets, adult islets, and thy-

TABLE 3-2   *Survival of Untreated Balb/c (H-2^d) Tissue Allografts Transplanted Across a Minor Histocompatibility Difference to DBA/2 (H-2^d)-Recipient Mice*

TISSUE GRAFTED	NO. OF GRAFTS	GRAFTS SURVIVING 4–6 WEEKS	% SURVIVAL
Skin	9	0	0
Fetal pancreas	6	0	0
Fetal proislets	11	10	91
Adult islets	5	4	80
Thyroid	27	25	93

(From Simeonovic CJ, Hodgkin PD, Donohue JA et al: An analysis of tissue-specific transplantation phenomena in a minor histoincompatibility system. Transplantation 39:661, 1985.)

roid are transplanted across the minor histocompatibility difference between BALB/c (H-2^d) and DBA/2 (H-2^d)-recipient mice, skin and fetal pancreas are rejected much more acutely than the latter tissues, which may survive indefinitely. These tissue-specific differences in immunogenicity are not due to the expression of tissue-specific antigens by the highly immunogenic tissues (skin and fetal pancreas) or the lack of recognizable antigens on the weakly immunogenic tissues, recipient mice sensitized by allogeneic skin or fetal pancreas reject cultured islet and thyroid allografts taken from the same donor strain. Clearly, the more immunogenic tissues have the capacity to immunize against antigens expressed by the less immunogenic grafts.

A distinctive feature of the highly immunogenic tissues is the presence of associated or fixed lymphoreticular components. Conversely, weakly immunogenic tissues such as thyroid islets and fetal proislets lack gross contamination with lymphoreticular cells. These tissue-specific effects, plus the finding that it is possible to improve the survival of tissues transplanted across minor histocompatibility differences by organ culture prior to grafting, suggest that passenger leukocytes also make a major contribution to tissue immunogenicity when grafting across minor histocompatibility barriers.

The aforementioned findings argue against the notion proposed by Silvers and associates[50] that minor antigens of a graft are efficiently processed and presented in association with Class I MHC antigens of host APCs, which thus activate Class I T cells, which, in turn, mediate rejection. Such a mechanism would not account for the strong tissue-specific effects seen when grafting across minor histocompatibility barriers, and, as pointed out by Silvers and colleagues, removal of stimulator cells from graft by organ culture in oxygen prior to grafting, or by some other procedure, should not alter tissue immunogenicity. However, this is not generally true,

because in most cases organ culture prior to grafting across a minor histocompatibility barrier enhances allograft survival.

We have shown that cultured BALB/c (H-2^d) thyroid survives indefinitely when transplanted to normal DBA/2 (H-2^d)-recipient animals. However, if a skin graft is exchanged between these animals at the time of thyroid transplantation, both grafts reject. The important question is: Why does the skin graft induce a response to antigens on the cultured thyroid that the thyroid tissue is unable to induce of itself? There would appear to be some connection between the high immunogenicity of skin and the presence of Class II antigen-bearing cells in this tissue. Figure 3-10 shows a hypothetical explanation for this phenomenon. According to this model, T' cells of specificity K.y (y is the symbol used to represent minor histocompatibility antigens) are required to initiate cultured thyroid graft rejection because this tissue lacks Class II MHC antigen-bearing cells. T' cells of this specificity (K.y) cannot be activated by direct presentation of minor antigens on the surface of S$^+$ antigen-presenting cells in the skin graft; by definition, minor antigen cannot function as part of the control system. However, T cells of specificity Ia.y, activated by the indirect pathway, could interact with Class II antigen-bearing cells in the graft and activate these cells to CoS production. These activated S$^+$ cells could then present the ligand (K.y) in an immunogenic form without a requirement for the minor antigens to function as part of the control system. This effect has the appearance of a collaborative effect resulting from a T/T interaction. However, as we see it, this should be considered a pseudo-T/T interaction. This model requires only the T' (Ia.y) cell to activate the CoS-producing S$^+$ cell before this cell interacts with T(K.y) (see Fig. 3-10). Here we see expression of the rule: *the T cell must recognize and interact with the cell it regulates* (in this case, the APC). The effect of this interaction is "indirect" induction of the APC, which can now activate the T cell of specificity (K.y).

There are two pieces of experimental evidence that taken together support the notion that activation of the response to minor antigens on a graft represents a pseudo-T/T interaction. The first comes from the study of Keene and Foreman[32] showing that activation of a T cell response to the male-specific antigen (H-y) requires "help" from another T cell specific for the Class I MHC antigen Qa, and that such "help" is only effective when the Qa antigen is expressed on the same cell as that which carries the H-y antigen. The second piece of evidence comes from the Canberra laboratory (Simeonovic, personal communication) and shows that cultured thyroid grafts transplanted across minor histocompatibility difference (BALB/c to DBA/2) are rejected when the recipient is challenged with BALB/c spleen cells. This effect requires the active participation of the APC, because challenge of animals with UV-irradiated spleen cells fails to induce rejection of the cultured thyroid graft. The "indirect" induction model requires active participation of the viable S$^+$ cell (see Fig. 3-9).

IMMUNOLOGIC TOLERANCE

Tolerance is any specifically altered state of reactivity that results in the failure of the animal to express an immune response to the tolerizing antigen, while leaving responses to unrelated antigens intact. Burnet's[11] clonal selection theory postulated that tolerance to "self" developed during the ontogeny of the immune system and resulted from a deletion of self-reactive clones. This suggestion led to the now classical demonstration of neonatally induced transplantation tolerance. Tolerance was induced in strain A mice by the injection of (A × B) F1 bone marrow.[5] Animals treated in this way would then accept skin grafts from strain B animals in adult life but reject skin grafts from third-party animals in a normal manner. Lymphoid cells from such tolerant animals do not respond in the mixed leukocyte reaction (MLR) when stimulated by strain B cells, but they do respond normally to third-party cells. Tolerance of this type cannot be transferred easily from one animal to another and may be due to clonal deletion. Transplantation tolerance of this type may also be induced in adult animals by lethal irradiation followed by the transfer of F1 bone marrow. Such animals behave essentially the same way as neonates injected with bone marrow. Tolerance also develops in animals that have received total lymphoid irradiation (TLI). This treatment, originally developed for the treatment of Hodgkin's disease, involves the administration of fractionated doses of irradiation to animals while shielding the marrow in long bones. This treatment results initially in nonspecific suppression of the immune system followed by the development of tolerance to antigens that are present in the animal during the recovery of the immune system. This type of treatment is being used clinically for immunosuppression of kidney graft recipients and in the treatment of some autoimmune disorders.[55]

A second form of tolerance may be induced by exposure of the immune system to soluble antigen either during neonatal life or, in some cases, following appropriate antigen administration to the adult animal. Neonates injected with antigen at birth are unresponsive to that antigen if antigen administration is maintained. Adult animals injected either with very low doses or very high doses of soluble antigen may become unresponsive to subsequent challenge with this antigen. Tolerance induced in such a manner can often be transferred to a naive animal by T-lymphocytes from the tolerant donor.[42]

It is clear that there can be different forms of immune tolerance. There is strong evidence from the laboratory of Kappler and Marrack (personal communication) that tolerance to "self" components results from the deletion of clones that can be shown to be present during the early phase of thymic T cell maturation. Neonatally induced transplantation tolerance also appears to result from such a deletion mechanism. However, it is equally clear that other forms of tolerance can result from the suppression of immune function. Studies in a number of laboratories have led to the development of complex networks for the positive and negative cellular regulation of immune reactivity.[17,54] It should be noted, however, that there are many ways of suppressing the immune response. For example, the presence of antibody will inhibit the expression of a DTH reaction in a sensitized animal. The rapid removal of antigen will also diminish the response to this antigen, and animals with a highly active reticuloendothelial system tend to mount somewhat lower responses to antigen because of the rapid degradation and removal of antigen from the immune system.

Induction of Allograft Tolerance in Adult Animals

Soon after transplantation, the graft depleted of S$^+$ cells is in a metastable condition; this graft is promptly rejected when the recipient is actively immunized with S$^+$ cells of donor type. However, with the passage of time, the graft enters into a stable interaction with the host and can no longer be rejected by active immunization of the recipient. This stable graft–host interaction results from a specific tolerance induction in the adult animal.[37] In the following discussion, we define this allograft tolerance as *a state of specific altered immune reactivity that allows acceptance of a graft that would otherwise be rejected*. This pragmatic definition makes no assumptions concerning the mechanism of tolerance induction or the procedure used to maintain the tolerant state. The maintenance of tolerance may involve either a passive (clonal deletion) or active (suppression) mechanism or combination of both. The kinetics of spontaneous graft stabilization are characteristic of the particular tissue under study; thyroid allografts stabilize considerably more slowly than islet allografts (350 days and 120 days, respectively).

Graft stabilization could conceivably result from one of two processes. Either the graft has adapted to the host, as, for example, through a loss of antigenicity, or the reactivity of the host has been altered. Results from the study of cultured thyroid allografts suggest that the latter mechanism is responsible for tolerance induction. When cultured thyroid allografts from spontaneously stable animals are retransplanted into a naive recipient animal, the grafts are readily rejected upon host immunization. This demonstrates that the long-established cultured allograft retains antigenicity. Therefore, graft stabilization must involve an adaptive process in the host, that is, the development of specific tolerance. Such a state of specific tolerance has been demonstrated in animals carrying both stable islet and thyroid allografts.[37] These animals accept a second uncultured graft of donor type but reject a third-party graft transplanted at the same time. The acceptance of a graft that would otherwise be rejected, combined with the specificity of this graft acceptance, indicates that a specific state of tolerance has been induced in the recipient of the cultured graft. Although tolerant animals are hyporesponsive in vivo, these animals retain normal mixed leukocyte reactivity in vitro. This latter finding leads to the conclusion that a deletion-type mechanism is not responsible for tolerance induction under these conditions. Some active mechanism must be inhibiting graft rejection in vivo.

THYMIC BIAS OF T CELL SPECIFICITY

It would be unreasonable to leave any general discussion of the immune system without mention of the problem that is currently the focus of intense immunologic debate. This is the thymic bias of immune reactivity. Stated simply, this concept is that the peripheral specificity of T cells is biased by the thymic environment in which these cells differentiate. Thus, when $(A \times B)$ F1 stem cells develop in an A thymus, the reactivity of peripheral T cells is biased toward the MHC of the A thymus; that is, peripheral T cell specificity is of the type $^{F1}T(A.x) > {}^{F1}T(B.x)$. When F1 stem cells develop in a B thymus, $^{F1}T(B.x) > {}^{F1}T(A.x)$. The thymic environment biases the MHC restriction phenotype expressed in the periphery.

When first discovered, this phenomenon was rather simply explained by a dual recognition (receptor) model for T cell reactivity.[6] T cells of specificity (A.x) were thought to express two receptors, one for A and one for x, neither of which could bind either A or x with sufficient affinity to deliver signal [1] to the T cell. However, the binding of A and x together raises the affinity of the interaction above the level required for signal transmission. Using this model and a notion of random generation of T cell receptor diversity, the A thymus will inactivate any developing T cells that bound self-antigen (A) with high enough affinity to signal, and to positively select, in a somewhat mysterious way, those cells that had a low affinity for A. The result being a bias toward A (self-MHC) in the periphery. The problem is to devise a mechanism that will eliminate high affinity A and select for low affinity A at the same time.

Sprent and colleagues[54] came part way to explaining this problem when they showed that different cell populations in the thymus were responsible for clonal elimination (S^+ cells express this function) or thymic bias (S^- thymic epithelial cells express this function). They suggested that the problem could be solved by educating cells first to self by running them through the gauntlet of the thymic epithelium, and subsequently remove any cells with high affinity for self using the S^+ cells of the thymus. Any model requiring both positive and negative selection, at the same time, for self components in the thymus requires considerable special pleading to explain the phenomenon. This is particularly true if we give up the notion of dual receptors on the T cell.

Of course, when we look at the specificity of peripheral T cells, we see that they are of specificity (c.x), which according to the two-signal model is not self because c.x ≠ c; that is, in the thymus, the positive selection is really for "not-self," and any self-reactive clones are eliminated. The problem is to see how the system could select positively for (c.x). One way would be for x to be present in the thymus during T cell development. Singer (personal communication) has suggested such a positive selection model in which x is provided by its corresponding self homologue. The idea of positive selection is attractive, but having a "self" homologue for all potential values of x is a difficult concept to accept.

Another way to expand the T(c.x) repertoire would be to positively select for c1 (allo-MHC) by expressing altered c on the surface of the S⁻ dendritic cells. We know that the alloreactive set subsumes most, but not all, the (c.x) specificities. The expression of alloantigen on the surface of thymic dendritic cells would not be a problem because this tissue is S⁻ and is therefore quite stable in an allogeneic environment. This model states that the thymic epithelium will determine the nature of the expanded peripheral T cell repertoire. Any "holes" in this repertoire, that is, particular missing specificities, will show up as Ir gene effects, and the animal will be a weak responder to those particular (c.x) interactions.

The thymus remains a mystery. Unraveling the secrets of this organ will take us far in the understanding of immunobiology.

GLOSSARY

APC   antigen-presenting cell, which internalizes antigen (X), processes it, and presents processed antigen on its surface in the form (c.x).

c   control structure on the surface of the S^+ cell, which regulates the release of CoS activity.

c.x   complex of c and x on APC surface. It is this complex that is recognized by the T cell receptor.

Class I antigens   Class I MHC antigens are located on all cell types; also written symbolically as K.

Class II antigens   Class II MHC antigens are located predominantly on lymphoreticular cells and may also be expressed on vascular endothelium; also written symbolically as Ia.

CoS   costimulator activity; an inductive molecule necessary for the initial antigen-mediated step in lymphocyte activation. CoS is released by an S^+ cell.

Epitope   an antigenic determinant. The region of a molecule that fits into the combining site of either an antibody or T cell and B cell receptors.

Ia   symbol for Class II antigens.

IL-1   interleukin 1; a soluble factor released from APC providing the second signal for T cell activation.

IL-2   interleukin 2; a lymphokine inducing proliferation of activated T cells.

K   symbol for Class I antigens

lk   lymphokine; soluble factors released by lymphocytes mediating the functions of other cells. A growing group of substances, including IL-2, IL-3, γ-INF, B cell growth factor (BCGF), and B cell differentiation factor (BCDF).

Ligand   a small molecule that can bind to a larger one.

MHC   major histocompatibility complex. Molecules of the MHC are expressed on the cell's surface.

Mitogen   substances that stimulate cell division (mitosis).

S^+ stimulator cell; any cell that has the capacity to release costimulator activity.

T(x)   resting T cell with receptor for x.

T'(x)   activated T cell with receptor for x.

$^c T(x)$ resting T cell of genotype c with receptor for x.

$^c T'(x)$ activated T cell of genotype c with receptor for x.

x   antigen processed and presented on the surface of the APC in association with c.

X   exogenous antigen.

REFERENCES

1. Andrus L, Lafferty KJ: Inhibition of T-cell activity by Cyclosporin A. Scand J Immunol 15:449, 1982
2. Andrus L, Prowse SJ, Lafferty KJ: Interleukin 2 production by both Lyt 2+ and Lyt 2-T cell subsets. Scand J Immunol 13:297, 1981
3. Bach FH, Bach ML, Sondel PM: Differential function

of major histocompatibility complex antigens in T lymphocyte activation. Nature 259:373, 1976

4. Batchelor JR, Welsh KL, Maynard A, Burgess H: Failure of long surviving, passively enhanced allografts to provoke T-dependent alloimmunity. I. Retransplantation of (ASxAUG) F1 kidneys into secondary AS recipients. J Exp Med 150:455, 1979

5. Billingham RE, Brent L, Medawar PB: Actively acquired tolerance of foreign cells. Nature 172:603, 1953

6. Bogman MJ, Berden JH, Hagermann JF et al: Patterns of vascular damage in the antibody mediated rejection of skin xenografts in the mouse. Am J Pathol 100:727, 1980

7. Borel JF (ed): Cyclosporin, Progress in Allergy, Vol 38. K Basel, Switzerland, S. Karger, 1986

8. Bradley B, Prowse SJ, Bauling P, Lafferty KJ: Desferrioxamine treatment prevents chronic islet allograft damage. Diabetes 35:550, 1986

9. Bretcher P, Cohn M: A theory of self-nonself discrimination. Science 169:1042, 1970

10. Brown EJ, Joiner KJ, Frank MM: Complement. In Paul WE (ed): Fundamental Immunology, p 645. New York, Raven Press, 1984

11. Burnet FM: A modification of Jerne's theory of antibody production using the concept of clonal selection. Aust J Sci 20:67, 1957

12. Burnet FM, Fenner F: The Production of Antibodies. London, Macmillan, 1949

13. Butcher EC, Weissman IL: Lymphoid tissues and organs. In Paul WE (ed): Fundamental Immunology, p 109. New York, Raven Press, 1984

14. Chesnut RW, Grey HM: Antigen presentation by B cells and its significance in T-B interactions. Adv Immunol 39:51, 1986

15. Claman HN, Chaperon EA, Triplett RF: Thymus–marrow cell combinations. Synergism in antibody production. Proc Soc Exp Biol Med 122:1167, 1966

16. Coombe DR, Ey PL, Jenkin CR: Haemaglutinin levels in haemolymph from the colonial ascidian *Botrylloides leachii* following the injection of chicken or sheep red blood cells. Aust J Exp Biol Med Sci 60:359, 1982

17. Dorf ME, Benacerraf B: Suppressor cells and immunoregulation. Ann Rev Immunol 2:103, 1984

18. Faustman D, Hauptfeld V, Lacy P, Davie J: Prolongation of murine islet allograft survival by pretreatment of islets with antibody directed to Ia determinants. Proc Natl Acad Sci USA 78:5156, 1981

19. Fleishman JB, Davie JM: Immunoglobulins: Allotypes and idiotypes. In Paul WE (ed): Fundamental Immunology, p 205. New York, Raven Press, 1984

20. Gores PF, Sutherland DER, Platt JL, Bach FH: Depletion of donor Ia⁺ cells before transplantation does not prolong islet allograft survival. J Immunol 137:1482, 1986

21. Granelli–Piperno A, Inaba K, Steinman R: Stimulation of lymphokine release from T lymphoblasts. Requirement for mRNA synthesis and inhibition by cyclosporin A. J Exp Med 160:1792, 1984

22. Hall BM, De Saxe I, Dorsche SE: The cellular basis of allograft rejection in rats III. Restoration of first set rejection of heart allografts in irradiated rats by T helper cells. Transplantation 36:700, 1983

23. Hanafusa T, Pijol–Borrell R, Chiovato L et al: Aberrant expression of HLA-DR antigen on thyrocytes in Grave's disease: Relevance for autoimmunity. Lancet 2:1363, 1981

24. Hildeman WH, Linthicum DS, Vann DC: Transplantation and immunoincompatibility reactions amongst reef building corals. Immunogenetics 2:269, 1975

25. Hirshberg H, Thorsby E: Immunogenicity of foreign tissues. Transplantation 31:96, 1981

26. Hodgkin PD, Agostino M, Sellins K et al: T lymphocyte function in vivo. Ambivalence of the antigen reactive subset. Transplantation 40:288, 1985

27. Hood L, Steinmetz M, Malissen B: Genes of the major histocompatibility complex of the mouse. Ann Rev Immunol 1:529, 1983

28. Jacobs BB, Huseby RA: Growth of tumors in allogeneic hosts following organ culture explantation. Transplantation 5:410, 1967

29. Jerne NK: The natural selection theory of antibody formation. Proc Natl Acad Sci USA 41:849, 1955

30. Jeske DJ, Capra JD: Immunoglobulins: Structure and function. In Paul WE (ed): Fundamental Immunology, p 131. New York, Raven Press, 1984

31. Jooste SV, Colvin RB, Winn HJ: The vascular bed as the primary target in the destruction of skin grafts by antiserum II. Loss of sensitivity to antiserum in long-term xenografts of skin. J Exp Med 154:1332, 1981

32. Keene J, Forman J: Helper activity is required for the in vivo generation of cytotoxic T lymphocytes. J Exp Med 155:768, 1982

33. Kimura H, Wilson DB: Anti-idiotypic cytotoxic T cells in rats with graft-versus-host disease. Nature 308:463, 1984

34. Kotzin BL, Benike CJ, Engleman, EG: Induction of immunoglobulin-secreting cells in the allogeneic mixed leukocyte reaction: Regulation by helper and suppressor lymphocyte subsets in man. J Immunol 127:931, 1981

35. Lacy PE, Davie JM, Finke EH: Prolongation of islet allograft survival following in vitro culture (24°C) and a single injection of ALS. Science 204:312, 1979

36. Lafferty KJ, Andrus L, Prowse SJ: Role of lymphokine and antigen in the control of specific T cell responses. Immunol Rev 51:279, 1980

37. Lafferty KJ, Prowse SJ, Simeonovic CJ: Immunobiology of tissue transplantation: A return to the passenger leukocyte concept. Ann Rev Immunol 1:143, 1983

38. Lafferty KJ, Woolnough JA: The origin and mechanism of the allograft reaction. Immunol Rev 35:231, 1977

39. Lechler RI, Batchelor JR: Restoration of immunogenicity to passenger cell-depleted kidney allografts by the addition of donor strain dendritic cells. J Exp Med 155:31, 1982

40. LeFrancois L, Bevan M: A re-examination of the role of Lyt 2 positive cells in murine skin graft rejection. J Exp Med 159:57, 1984

41. Lovland BE, Hogarth PM, Ceredig RN, McKenzie IFC: Cells mediating graft rejection in the mouse. Lyt 1 cells mediate skin graft rejection. J Exp Med 153:1044, 1981

42. McCullagh P: The transfer of immunological tolerance with tolerant lymphocytes. Aust J Exp Biol Med Sci 51:445, 1973

43. Medawar PB: Introduction: Definition of the immunologically competent cell. In Wolstenholme GEW, Knight J (eds): The Immunologically Competent Cell: Its Nature and Origin, pp 1–3. Ciba Foundation Study Group No. 16. London, Churchill, 1963

44. Mitchell GF, Miller JFAP: Immunological activity of thymus and thoracic duct lymphocytes Proc Natl Acad Sci USA 59:296, 1968

45. Morrow CE, Sutherland DER, Steffes MW et al: Differences in susceptibility to rejection of mouse pancreatic islet allografts disparate for Class I and Class II major histocompatibility antigens. J Surg Res 34:358, 1983

46. Ortaldo JR, Herbeman RB: Heterogeneity of natural killer cells. Ann Rev Immunol 2:359, 1984

47. Prowse SJ, Warren HS, Agostino M, Lafferty KJ: Transfer of sensitized Lyt 2^+ cells triggers acute rejection of pancreatic islet allografts. Aust J Exp Biol Med Sci 61:181, 1983

48. Rao A, Weng–Ping Ko W et al: Binding of antigen in the absence of histocompatibility proteins by arsonate-reactive T-cell clones. Cell 36:879, 1984

49. Schiltnecht E, Ada GL: In vivo effects of cyclosporine on influenza A virus infected mice. Cell Immunol 91:277, 1985

50. Silvers WK, Bartlett ST, Chen H-D et al: Major histocompatibility complex restriction and transplantation immunity. Transplantation 37:28, 1984

51. Simeonovic CJ, Hodgkin PD, Donohue JA et al: An analysis of tissue-specific transplantation phenomena in a minor histoincompatibility system. Transplantation 39:661, 1985

52. Snell GD, Dausset J, Nathenson S: Histocompatibility. New York, Academic Press, 1976

53. Solomon JB, Horton JD: Developmental Immunobiology. New York, Elsevier North-Holland, 1977

54. Sprent J, Schafer M: Capacity of purified Lyt 2^+ T cells to mount primary proliferative and cytotoxic responses to Ia^- tumour cells. Nature 332:541, 1986

55. Strober S: Natural suppressor cells, neonatal tolerance and total lymphoid irradiation: Exploring obscure relationships. Ann Rev Immunol 2:219, 1984

56. Stuart FP, Bastien E, Holter A et al: Role of passenger leukocytes in the rejection of renal allografts. Transplant Proc 3:461, 1971

57. Tada T: Help, suppression, and specific factors. In Paul WE (ed): Fundamental Immunology, p 481. New York, Raven Press, 1984

58. Talmage DW: Immunological specificity. Science 129:1543, 1959

59. Wong GHW, Bartlett PF, Clark–Lewis I et al: Inducible expression of H-2 and Ia molecules. Nature 310:688, 1984

60. Yammura Y, Tada T (eds): Fifth International Congress of Immunology. Tokyo, Academic Press, 1984

CHAPTER 4

Immunobiology of Transplant Rejection

Nancy L. Ascher   Richard L. Simmons

The goal in clinical transplantation is to effect specific graft tolerance, that is, the individual cannot reject his graft but can respond to other foreign antigens. The basis for graft rejection is histoincompatibility between donor and recipient. Transplantation antigens that exist on cell surfaces dictate ease of transplantation. The major histocompatibility complex represents the strongest immunologic barrier to transplantation. Two classes of antigens exist: Class I antigens are expressions of the HLA-A and -B regions and primarily stimulate OKT8[+] cells. Class II antigens are expressions of the HLA-D region and primarily stimulate OKT4[+] cells. The distribution of tissue expression of Class I and Class II antigens varies. The major T-lymphocyte subsets can be identified by their own characteristic antigenic expression.

A variety of rejection mechanisms have been identified that constitute a repertoire of preferred, alternative, or reserve mechanisms, depending upon the nature of the antigen, the route of antigen stimulation, and the immune state of the host.

Coculture of lymphocyte mixtures has delineated the interactive roles of lymphocyte and accessory cells and defined the genetic restrictions that dictate response. Histologic examination of cells infiltrating the graft defines the cell types that actually accumulate at the graft site; functional analysis of these cells indicates how they might affect graft loss. Recipient treatment with agents of known function allows inference of the potential importance of a specific mechanism or cell type.

Reconstitution of animals with cells of known function has greatly expanded the knowledge of allograft rejection. This method has established a role for delayed-type hypersensitivity. The helper/inducer T cell plays a central role in this mechanism as well as in the development of classic T cell cytotoxicity.

THE IMMUNE RESPONSE*

Small lymphocytes constitute the heart of the immune system.[43] Cells of monocyte/macrophage lineage are necessary to modify or present foreign antigens to the lymphocyte, but the immunologic specificity in the reaction resides with the recognition by the lymphocyte of the antigen and the subsequent lymphocyte response.[26] Early in the immune development of an individual, clones or groups of lymphocytes are formed that have discrete target specificities. A single lymphocyte, therefore,

---

* In order to understand the immunobiology of rejection, a summary of normal immune response is necessary. The reader is referred to Chapter 3, Normal Immune Response, for amplification of this process.

can probably recognize only one or a limited number of closely related antigens. The range of possible antigen configurations is, thus, matched by a parallel variety of lymphocyte clones that are reactive against them. It is not known how immune specificity is acquired during development, but small lymphocytes are fully competent cells that are resting and waiting to respond to antigen.

Stimulation of the resting small lymphocyte by antigen transforms it into a large active cell that secretes substances that, in turn, activate or inhibit the functions of other nearby cells.[72] Before the antigen is eliminated or destroyed, many cellular and subcellular events take place. This complex of events offers opportunities for suppression or amplification of the response. For example, it is possible to modify the proliferation and expansion of antigen-sensitive clones of lymphocytes. This has been the key step at which clinical immunosuppression is aimed. Modification of graft antigen, of antigen presentation, or of the effector limb of the response has generally been an ineffective clinical strategy.

Immunosuppression is less effective after the lymphocyte has completed its response to the alloantigen. The immune response is more difficult to control after it has been activated because preformed antibodies, activated cytolytic lymphocytes, and antibody-armed macrophages are difficult to suppress.[38,39] More importantly, multiple mechanisms are involved in the immune response, and suppression of one or two may be ineffective by itself.

Clinical progress will depend on more selective immunosuppression. The goal in transplantation is tolerance of the graft in a fully immunocompetent host. As the complexities of the immune response are better understood, it will become possible to more closely achieve this goal. At present, clinical immunosuppression relies on three general approaches. The first approach involves reducing the number of peripheral lymphocytes by destroying them, the second approach uses a variety of metabolic inhibitors to interrupt the antigen-induced lymphocyte proliferation and differentiation, and the third approach inhibits signal molecules, which activate other cells of the immune cascade.

CONCEPT OF REJECTION

Organ grafts between individuals of the same species (allografts) reject with a vigor proportional to the degree of histocompatibility between individuals. Grafts between different species (xenografts) are rejected even more rapidly. Grafts from identical twins (isografts) or from an individual to himself (autografts) survive indefinitely if the vascular supply has been reestablished. Allografts survive the immediate transplant operation postoperative period as well as do isografts if the individual has not previously been sensitized by antigens within the donor graft. The allograft is, therefore, not morphologically or physiologically distinguishable from the isograft in the early transplant period. The rejection process normally takes several days if the recipient has no prior exposure to donor histocompatibility antigens.

Homan noted that human allogeneic skin grafts did not survive indefinitely in burn patients and attributed this to an immunologic phenomenon.[37] Medawar noted that skin grafts between unrelated rabbits were normal appearing until the fourth or fifth day, at which time inflammation appeared within the graft in the form of a dense leukocyte infiltrate.[62] This led to necrosis of the entire graft by the tenth day. He further demonstrated that rejection was the result of an immunologic mechanism. The first set rejection took place in 10 or 11 days, and, in contrast, a second set rejection from the same donor rabbit resulted in an accelerated response.[61] The reaction was noted to be immunologically specific for the antigens involved in that a third-party graft placed on a sensitized recipient was rejected at the same rate as the first set graft.

Rejection of an allograft is elicited by the foreign histocompatibility antigens on the grafted tissue. Many antigens may act as histocompatibility antigens. For example, ABO blood type antigens may elicit rapid graft rejection in hosts who have natural isoantibody.[51] Similarly, xenografts are rejected rapidly because tissue incompatibilities are so profound between species that preformed antibodies may exist in the recipient. Alloantigenic incompatibilities between members of a species vary, however, and strong antigens can lead to graft rejection within a short period of time, whereas weaker differences may permit long-term graft survival.

IMMUNOGENETICS OF HISTOCOMPATIBILITY

Transplantation (histocompatibility) antigens exist as cell surface structures and constitute the major immunologic barrier to successful transplantation. The strongest of the transplantation antigens is the expression of a single chromosomal region called the major histocompatibility complex (MHC). In humans, MHC is located on the sixth chromosome. All vertebrates have similar MHC, but the nomenclature varies among species. In humans, transplantation antigens were first investigated on leukocytes and therefore were named *human leukocyte antigens (HLA)*. In mice, the strongest antigens are called *H-2 antigens;* in rats, they are called *AGB antigens;* and in dogs, they are known as the *DLA system.* The use of inbred strains of mice has resulted in an enormous amount of knowledge regarding the role of the major histocompatibility antigens in allograft rejection.

The HLA locus has been dissected through immunogenetic analysis. The presence of HLA antigens on a cell surface can be detected in either of two ways. The serologic method uses antigen-specific antisera, which leads to either agglutination or complement-dependent lysis of cells carrying the antigen.[90] Antigens that poorly trigger allogeneic lymphocyte proliferation and were therefore first defined by serologic techniques are called *Class I antigens*. A second method measures the reactivity of host lymphocytes to lymphocytes from potential donors.[7] The responding lymphocytes react to other cellular transplantation antigens. Antigens that can trigger the proliferation of allogeneic lymphocytes are called *Class II antigens*. Both Class I and Class II antigens can now be detected by specific antisera.

Class I antigens are expressions of those portions of the MHC genome known as the HLA-A and HLA-B regions. Class II antigens are expressions of the HLA-D region, which has since been analyzed in the D_Q, D_R, and D_S subregions. HLA-A and HLA-B antigens formed the basis of transplantation tissue typing from many years. Each of them has more than 20 different alleles or antigens. Alleles are the alternate forms of a given gene locus, and the allelic antigens may differ by only one or two amino acids. There are approximately 10 known alleles for each HLA-D_R subregion. Each individual inherits one chromosome and has one set of HLA antigens from each parent. All HLA antigens are expressed (codominant) on the cell surface; therefore, 2-A, 2-B, and 2-D antigens are present for each cell. The known loci in the HLA complex have been mapped on chromosome 6.

The extreme polymorphism of the major histocompatibility locus and the fact that homologous systems exist in all mammalian species suggests that MHC has an important biologic role that is unrelated to transplantation immunology. It is believed that one major role for the MHC is its influence on resistance to infectious diseases. There are a series of levels on which the MHC interacts with the immune system. On the chromosomal level, there must be a sequence of nucleotides in the HLA region that code for immune response genes. These genes code for determinants that appear on a cell surface. Determinants that coat the cell surface interact with pathogens that may invade the body or present themselves as foreign to another host. As a consequence, there is an activation of the immune system that will affect how an organism responds to foreign pathogens.

SEROLOGICALLY DEFINED ANTIGENS

Class I Antigens

The HLA-A, -B, and -C antigens are glycoproteins consisting of a heavy chain of 44,000 dalton that carries the antigenic specificity and a light chain of an 11,600 dalton alpha$_2$ microglobulin subunit. Each Class I heavy chain had multiple "public" antigenic sites (sites that are shared among individuals) and only one "private" HLA-A, -B or -C antigen. These antigens are identified by numbers with the letter of the locus as a prefix (i.e., A-2). Antigens for which good reagents are not yet available have the extra prefix W (from workshop). Class I antigens are present to varying degrees on most tissue parenchymal cells, B- and T-lymphocytes, and platelets but not on mature red blood cells. Studies with radiolabeled alloimmune antibody induced by pregnancy have indicated that each locus determines for about 6,000 antigenic sites on the lymphocyte cell membrane.[25] Thus, each lymphocyte carries 36,000 HLA-A, -B, and -C sites. Capping studies have shown that each antigenic site is carried by a different molecule.[11] Localization of HLA molecules in the membrane architecture can be visualized by electron microscopy using radiolabeled alloimmune antibodies. The amount of HLS antigens in the surface of cells of various organs varies. The presence of either Class I or Class II antigens on the surface of various tissues will affect the immunogenicity of that tissue.[79,89] For example, some immunofluorescent studies have failed to detect HLA-A and -B antigens in sections of kidney tissues, including both epithelial and endothelial cells,[30] but relative paucity does not rule out the presence of these antigens. Since certain cells can be induced to express cryptic antigens under various conditions, one cannot assume that any tissue or cell is totally without alloimmunogenicity.

Class II Antigens

The HLA-D locus was discovered when it was noted that the mixed lymphocyte culture proliferation response was triggered by a locus separate from the HLA-A, -B and -C loci. HLA-D$_r$ determinants are expressed on B cells, monocytes, endothelial cells, epidermal cells, and sperm. Structurally speaking, HLA-D$_r$ determinants have a two-chain structure, both chains of which are glycosylated with molecular weights of 29,000 and 34,000 and each of which is encoded by pairs of genes within the HLA-D$_r$ region. It has not been determined which of the two molecules carries the allospecificity. The total number of Class II alpha- and beta-chain genes is still unknown, although there may be as many as five to seven nonallelic alpha-chain genes and a minimum of nine beta-chain genes.

Chromosomes are paired and each individual receives one set of HLA antigens from each parent. Each set of HLA antigens is referred to as a haplotype. Both sets of antigens are expressed codominantly. Within a given family, 25% of the offspring will share both haplotypes (HLA identical), 50%

will share one haplotype (one haplotype matched), and 25% will share no antigens (haplotype mismatched). Two individuals may be HLA identical and yet ABO compatible, as MHC and ABO antigens are encoded by genes on different chromosomes.

Detection of the HLA-A, -B, and -D alleles for tissue typing requires banks of monospecific antisera. Graft survival when kidneys are transplanted between family members correlates with the closeness of the HLA-A and -B antigen match, particularly if recipient and donor are identical at the A, B locus. The role of the HLA-D sub-locus in transplantation is becoming clearer. Lymphocytes in mixed lymphocyte culture respond to cells with different D antigens by proliferation. Even when the HLA-A and -B antigens are identical, disparity in the HLA-D region results in proliferation in mixed lymphocyte culture. Proliferation induced by HLA-D antigens is essential for the full development of cellular immunity against HLA-A and -B antigens as well. Current studies of large pooled groups of patients have demonstrated an importance of both HLA-D and HLA-A and -B matching in organ transplantation between unrelated (cadaveric) and in living-related donor–recipient pairs,[63,67,74] although it has been difficult to document the beneficial effects of HLA-D and HLA-A and -B matching in small groups of individuals undergoing transplantation at a single center.[21,81]

It is also important to recognize that there are multiple other genes on the sixth chromosome or on other chromosomes that code for histocompatibility antigens (such as vascular endothelial specific antigens) and that may be important in transplant rejection. That such antigen systems are important is obvious from the observation that rejection of organs transplanted between siblings identical at the HLA locus does occur.

HISTOCOMPATIBILITY MATCHING

It is obvious that the less antigenic the graft, the less the host will react against it. In human transplantation when the donor and recipient are identical twins and there is no antigenic difference, the tissue is accepted without immunosuppressive agents. When the donor and recipient are siblings or when a parent donor is used for an offspring, there is greater statistical likelihood for antigens sharing between the donor and the recipient than when a cadaveric or unrelated donor is used.[63,67] Concomitantly, the results are better when either a sibling graft or a parent–child graft is used as compared to a cadaveric transplant.[63,67]

Several methods have been developed for the purpose of demonstrating the antigenic similarities between donor and recipient prior to transplantation so that donor and recipient pairs that are relatively histocompatible may be selected (see Chapter 9, entitled Histocompatibility). This should lessen the need for a large dose of immunosuppressive agents and increase the likelihood for a successful outcome.

THE IMMUNE RESPONSE TO TRANSPLANTATION (HISTOCOMPATIBILITY) ANTIGENS

The Immune Apparatus

The immune response to histocompatibility antigens on cells of transplanted organs triggers the rejection response. The immune system consists of lymphocytes, cells of the monocyte/macrophage lineage, and specialized epithelial cells such as those found in the thymus. These cells are organized into the spleen, lymph nodes, Peyer's patches of the intestine, tonsils, thymus, and bone marrow. Lymphocytes and macrophages contribute to the recirculating pool of cells found in the blood and lymph.

At birth, humans are immunologically competent and have undergone a complex developmental process during embryogenesis. The primordial bone marrow stem cells undergo some early differentiation steps. The daughter stem cells migrate through various centers for further differentiation. Within these centers, progenitor cells for erythrocytes, eosinophils, basophils, neutrophils, and lymphoid cells mature depending on the local microenvironment. It is also likely that proliferation of these progenitor stem cells depends on the actions of stimulating substances that tend to expand the population of sensitive cells in the way that erythropoietin acts on the erythrocyte line.

The lymphoid cell lines first appear within two primary types of lymphoid tissue. The thymus is essential for the development of cellular immunity. In birds, the bursa of Fabricius governs the development of humoral immunity. The equivalent structure in humans has not been identified; however, it may be within fetal liver or bone marrow. In humans, the characteristics of sex-linked agammaglobulinemia of the Bruton type bear low levels of immunoglobulin with normal cellular immunity mediated by thymus-derived lymphocytes, suggesting that the bursa equivalent has failed to develop.

Influence of the thymus and the bursa (or its equivalent) result in the further development of peripheral lymphoid tissue. Certain areas of the lymph node are dependent upon the thymus and others on the bursal equivalent. The paracortical regions of lymph nodes are dependent upon the thymus, whereas the germinal centers are under developmental control of the bursal equivalent. Thymectomy early in the neonatal period or congenital thymic deficiency results in failure of the development of the paracortical region of the lymph node. In chickens, bursectomy leads to failure of the development of the germinal centers and medullary core lymphoid tissues. All cells that were once dependent upon the thymus for their development are called *T cells*. T cells represent the immunocompetent cell population responsible for the development of cellular immunity rather than humoral immunity. These reactions include delayed-type hypersensitivity reactions, direct cytolysis of target cells as well as many of the early reactions responsible for allograft rejection. Other cells (B cells) descend from stem cells in the bone marrow and become responsible for manufacturing circulating immune globulins, that is, humoral immunity. B cells appear to be relatively sessile, but their end products, immunoglobulins and antibodies, can interact with foreign antigens at distant sites. T cells responsible for cell-mediated immunity are of necessity more migratory; they must move to the periphery in order to interact with foreign antigens. Once the lymphocytes have migrated to the peripheral lymphoid tissue, they are fully immunocompetent. The small mature lymphocyte is the control cell in directing the immune response. It appears that a state of preparedness for certain antigens or closely grouped antigens exists within the lymphoid cell so that it is capable of responding only to a narrow range of genetically determined immunospecificities. For this reason, only a small percentage of resting lymphocytes in the body can respond to a specific antigen. It is also likely that the character of the global immune response to an antigen (predominantly cellular or predominantly humoral) may depend upon the number of responder T or B cells encoded to respond to that antigen.

T cells are quite heterogenous. There are not only many clones of cells each differing from one another in the structure of its antigen receptor but also a series of subtypes that differ in the range of their response. Several subtypes mediate important regulatory functions, such as the ability to "help" or "suppress" the development of immune responses, including antibody production. Other T-lymphocytes serve effector functions, such as the production of soluble products that initiate a variety of inflammatory responses (lymphokines). Other T cells act as direct destructive agents to cells bearing antigens ("killer" function). Thus, there is an army of helper T cells, suppressor T cells, killer T cells, and T cells involved in delayed hypersensitivity and related immune phenomena.

In addition, there are lymphocytes that mediate certain "nonspecific" cytotoxic responses. These include the natural killer (NK) cells, which kill certain forms of tumor cells, using recognition systems that may be quite different from those used by T- or B-lymphocytes. Another type of nonspecific killing of target cells is antibody-dependent cellular cytotoxicity (ADCC), which is a function of a lymphocyte (or, in certain circumstances, a variety of other cell types) capable of killing antibody-coated target cells as a consequence of the recognition of a constant portion of the antibody bound to that target cell. Whether ADCC is a function of the cells that mediate NK activity is still uncertain.

A new type of nonspecific cytotoxic T cell has recently been added. These cells are called *lymphokine activated killer cells*, which differ from NK cells in that they can kill fresh (but not cultured) tumor cells, virally infected cells, and lymphoblasts.

The important role of helper and specific cytotoxic T cells in allograft rejection is well founded. The role of the other T cell subtypes is less clear. The major T-lymphocyte populations can be identified because they express characteristic antigens on their membranes. Thus, helper T cells in the mouse express large amounts of the L_3T_4 antigen, whereas suppressor cells and their precursors express the Lyt 2 antigens; cytotoxic T cells and their precursors are also Lyt 2^+. Among human T cells, helper cells express the OKT4 determinant, and suppressor/cytotoxic cells express OKT8.

THE REJECTION RESPONSE

The exact mechanism of allograft rejection has been the subject of much debate. It is clear from a myriad of studies that a variety of mechanisms have been identified and together constitute a vast repertoire of preferred, alternative, or reserve mechanisms depending upon the nature of the antigen (Class I vs. Class II vs. minor) and the route of antigen stimulation (vascularized, intravenous, nonvascularized).[14,29,34,55,59,82–85]

INDUCTION OF IMMUNITY

The Role of the Small Lymphocyte

Mature lymphocytes are small and immunologically prepared. The small lymphocyte can recognize whether or not a molecule is foreign and can react to it. Its reaction consists of proliferation, differentiation, maturation, and production of molecules that can recruit other components of the immune response. In addition, small lymphocytes can carry immunologic memory. Some of these cells have a life span of many years. Most of these functions have now been attributed to the helper T cells, but other subtypes may participate in some of these functions.

The Afferent Arc

Helper T-lymphocytes that recognize immunogenetic determinants translate that recognition into an immunologic response manifested by proliferation, differentiation, division, and release of lymphokines. The first phase of the immunologic response has been called the *afferent arc*. The initial step involves an encounter between the graft histocompatibility antigens in the blood or in the lymphatics or within the tissue itself with an antigen-presenting cell (APC)—itself a product of the monocyte/macrophage differentiation scheme. The antigens are processed in some way by the APC and are presented to the appropriate helper T-lymphocyte that has been genetically programmed to respond to it.[64,76,86,87] Certain differentiated cells of donor type are highly efficient at presenting their alloantigens to host lymphoid cells (Fig. 4-1).

These APC cells tend to be derived from the monocyte/macrophage lineage of the clones (Dendritic cells, Langerhans' cells). They are, in fact, donor APCs and as such can self-process their alloantigens and bypass the need for a host APC.[77] Alloantigens on parenchymal cells of transplanted tissues and organs require host APC for antigen processing and presentation to the host lymphoid cell.

Graft antigens may get to the host by several mechanisms that may differ between grafts. The blood supply and lymphatic drainage of a graft dictate the rapidity with which host cells are exposed to the graft antigens and the host cells that are initially exposed. For vascularized grafts, host cells within the blood compartment will be the first to encounter graft antigens. In contrast, in skin grafts, cells within local lymphatics are first exposed to graft antigens. Thus, much initial sensitization to allografts probably takes place within the peripheral lymphoid tissue of the host by antigens shed from the graft or on donor lymphocytes transplanted with the organ. Importantly, there is good evidence that sensitization can occur within the graft itself by virtue of circulating host lymphocytes that migrate to the graft.[65]

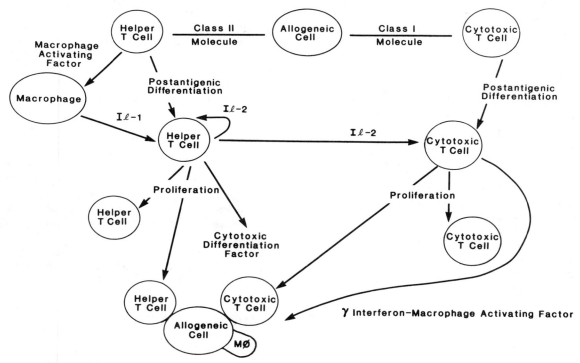

FIGURE 4-1. *Steps involved in the development of mature effector T-lymphocytes. Note the interdependence of different subsets whose mode of communication is via short-acting lymphokines and monokines.*

There is convincing evidence that dendritic cells within whole organs and skin allografts are a major source of antigenic stimuli.[33,50] In studying the allograft effector mechanisms, the immune status of the host must be considered. In the unmodified host, the histologic features of rejection are relatively constant and well described. Animals and humans subjected to immunosuppressive agents and procedure may show a broad spectrum of response depending not only upon the specific agent used but also upon the interaction between that agent and the host. These issues have been well discussed by Hayry and associates.[34] The host species is another important variable in the magnitude and specific type of immune response. The ease with which permanent acceptance of rat cardiac allografts can be achieved with short courses of cyclosporine or with blocking antibodies in the rat is vastly different from the responses seen in other hosts.[24,33] Immunogenetic differences between species in the expression of MHC antigen has been the suggested explanation for these differences, but it remains unclear why these species differences exist.

The mechanism by which an APC presents the antigen to a responsive lymphocyte in an immunogenic form is not clear. Most evidence suggests that it modifies the antigen on its surface to the responder cell. Since the responding host lymphocyte and the host antigen presenting cell must share identical HLA-D/D_r and since the responding T-lymphocytes can recognize HLA-D_r, most investigators agree that the antigen is presented to the lymphocyte "in the context of HLA-D." A double recognition step seems to be involved in which both the processed antigen and HLA-D_r is simultaneously recognized by the responding T cell. Neither recognition step just mentioned is sufficient to trigger a T cell to respond by itself; both are necessary. These statements are true for most T cell–dependent antigens except for the case in which a donor APC can present its own alloantigens directly to a responsive T cell.[77] In a series of experiments, this group has demonstrated two pathways that can initiate the response of the cytolytic T cell—one is dependent upon self-accessory cell via Ia recognition, and the other operates independent of self-Ia. In this way, foreign accessory cells may interact indirectly with a host helper cell to initiate the immune response.

The most striking aspect of the immune response is its specificity. For each unique stimulus, a distinctive population of antibodies or immune cells is elicited. Specificity of the immune response implies that there must be specific antigen receptors on the surface of antigen recognition cells. The receptor site must be at least as discriminatory as the antigen combining sites or the cellular recognition sites on hypersensitive cells. The receptors on B cells are identical to the specific regions of circulating antibodies. Mature B cells, in fact, bear membrane immunoglobulins of the IgM and IgD types. There is no question that T cells also possess specific antigen receptors that show some structural similarity to immunoglobulin. How the recognition molecules on either T or B cells succeed in becoming specific during lymphocyte development is unknown. The clonal selection theory proposes that clones of lymphocytes specifically active to an antigen probably arise by somatic mutation prior to an actual experience with the antigen itself. Thus, lymphocytes are precommitted and equipped with recognition molecules to the antigen before the initial encounter with it. The later encounter does not educate the antigen reactive site of a clone, but it does stimulate the clone to proliferate and mature.

Lymphocyte Transformation

The encounter between host lymphocytes and foreign alloantigen induces a response in those clones in cells precoded to these antigens. The response is manifested by proliferation and differentiation into specifically sensitized cells that actively manufacture and secrete antibody (B cells) or cells with the capability of inflicting damage to the foreign graft by virtue of their presence at close range (T cells). The activation of resting small lymphocytes of both types can be found in regional lymph nodes and the spleen following the placement of allografts. Lymphoid cells enlarge, transform, and divide in response to allogenic stimulation.[71,75] A myriad of subcellular and molecular events accompanies this transformation, which results in changing from resting cells to large active cells. All the subsequent events in the development of a full-fledged rejection response is dependent upon this transformation.

Cell–Cell Interactions

Although lymphocyte activity is central to allograft rejection, extensive cell–cell interaction is needed for the development of maximal lymphocyte activity.[36,71,75,77] Cooperation occurs between T- and B-lymphocytes and between the major T_h-, T_k-, or T_s-defined subpopulations of T cells, which results in an allograft response. This system of cooperation is demonstrated by showing that neither cell population could mount an immune response to certain antigens, whereas mixtures of the two-cell type results in production of high levels of antibody.[44,45] T cells in this system serve as "helper cells," which assist B cells in differentiation and into production of antibody. T cell recognition of antigen is necessary for the production of the specific antibody and response by the B cell. In fact, not all T cells can function in this role. A subgroup of helper T cells carry out this function. The ability to clone T helper cells into populations that carry a specific antigen receptor and that can perform a restricted repertoire of functions has further delineated this distinction. Certain helper T cells can be cloned and induced to release lymphokines, which elicit the differentiation of B cells into antibody producers.[95] Just as T helper cells are necessary for B cell antibody response, other T helper cells are necessary for the development of lymphocyte-mediated cytotoxicity by other clones of effector lymphocytes.[9]

T helper function has been well worked out for B cells but less well worked out for T effectors. T cell help for B cells can be delivered in at least two ways. One way involves the direct interaction of the helper T cell and the responding B cell. The T cell appears to recognize determinants on antigenic molecules already bound to the B cell by its immunoglobulin receptors. These T cells concurrently recognize Class II MHC antigens on the B cell surface. Activation of the helper T cell usually depends upon its co-recognition of antigen and a Class II molecule on the surface of an APC. The APC, in addition to processing the antigen, secretes a monokine Interleukin-I (IL-1), which is essential for T cell proliferation.

The second way in which T cells can help B cell activation is through the production of soluble, nonspecific helper factors (lymphokines). Among these are both growth factors, principally BCGF, which regulates B cell proliferation in response to antigenic stimulation, and differentiation factors (sometimes designated T cell–replacing factors, or TRF), which cause proliferating B cells to develop into antibody-secreting cells. T helper cells play a critical role in the T cell response to an antigen. T_h cells that respond to appropriate antigens presented in APC respond to IL-1 by secreting Interleukin-II (IL-2) and by increasing the number and avidity of IL-2 receptors on the T_h cell surface. IL-2 thus acts as an autocrine stimulating the proliferation of the T_h cells in the vicinity. IL-2 also permits appropriate antigen-specific clones of T effector cells (which cannot themselves secret IL-2, but require it for proliferation) to divide and mature into antigen-specific cytotoxic cells. However, IL-2, in addition, permits the proliferation of all T cells so that nonspecific as well as antigen-specific proliferation of T cells occurs. The T suppressor cell subset can inhibit either the development of antibody-producing B cells or the generation of cytotoxic T cells. Since suppressor cells have not been reproducibly cloned, there is some doubt as to whether this function is carried out by a single cell type.

Cloning of T cytotoxic cells as well as T helper cells has greatly enhanced the knowledge of the function of these cells. Once a lymphocyte subpopulation has been identified, the nature of its interactions can be elucidated. Most interactions seem to involve the manufacturing and release of soluble substances (lymphokines) by stimulated cells that trigger responder cells bearing receptors for these lymphokines.

Lymphocyte Differentiation and Proliferation

A basic question in cell biology is whether a cell must proliferate in order to differentiate. Investigations into transplantation biology have not yet provided an answer to this question. Most evidence, however, supports the idea that B-lymphoid differentiation to antibody-producing cells is accompanied by cellular proliferation. When the B cell proliferates, morphologic differentiation accompanies the functional differentiation and the result is a plasma cell engaged in the production of specific antibody. Conversion from a transformed cell to a plasma cell is seen within a few days after grafting in both organ allografts and lymphoid tissues stimulated by the transplants. It is also apparent that T helper as well as T cytotoxic cells proliferate to varying degrees in order to differentiate. The allogenic stimulation that occurs between two lymphocyte populations in a mixed lymphocyte culture has become the standard model of the alloimmune response in vitro. The amount of immunologic stimulation can be measured by the uptake of tritiated thymidine into DNA or by the mitosis that soon follows. The ability of histocompatibility antigens on the surface of antigen-presenting cells to stimulate lymphocyte proliferation is compelling evidence that similar activation occurs in vivo when an organ is allografted. Further investigations have elucidated that the T helper cell proliferates the most upon recognition of the foreign alloantigen. The T cytotoxic cell proliferates less but differentiates into a cell with the capability to inflict direct cytotoxic damage.

Not only do the two cells respond differently, but their response is elicited by different alloantigens. Class II antigens stimulate helper cells by and large, but, in contrast, Class I antigens are recognized by cytotoxic T cells. Therefore, the precursors of helper cells and cytotoxic cells respond to different alloantigens within the HLA complex, and different T cells appear to accomplish differentiation and proliferation to different degrees. The restriction of effector function to specific surface antigens is not absolute; cytotoxic cells can be generated to Class II antigens.[47] The antigenic markers on these effector cells are of traditional "helper" type (OKT4, Lyt L_3T_4). IL-2 released from helper T cells during their response to Class II antigens enables cytotoxic cells to differentiate in response to Class I antigens.

THE EFFERENT ARC OF ALLOGRAFT IMMUNITY

Expression of Immunity Graft Destruction

The recognition of antigens by sensitized cells or antibodies marks the beginning of the active effort of disposal of the foreign graft. Recognition triggers the activation of several cascading enzyme systems, including the complement clotting and renin pathways. In addition, there are cellular mediators (macrophages, platelets, and polymorphonuclear leukocytes are recruited), both as a consequence of the specific immune reaction itself and as a result of nonspecific subsequent enzymatic events. Consequently, a variety of molecules and cells are active in the destruction of the allograft. The efferent limb of the allograft reaction has both an immunologically specific phase and an immunologically nonspecific effector or amplification phase.

The Role of Specifically Immunized Lymphocytes in Allograft Rejection

Specifically alloimmune T cells probably act as important effectors of allograft rejection. One of the important means through which they do so is by lysing cells bearing alloantigens for which they are specific. Human cytotoxic T cells generally express OKT8 on their membrane. They recognize antigen in a manner akin to that of helper T cells except that they recognize Class I MHC molecules rather than Class II MHC molecules. Recent experiment with human cloned T cells and murine models reveal that the distinction between the function of a cell, its antigenic marker, and its target does not always correlate. Cloned cytotoxic cells can be generated and directed against Class II antigens; they have OKT4 (in the human) or L_3T_4 antigens on their surfaces.[47]

Cytotoxic T cells are derived from T cell precursors, and their replication and differentiation is aided by a type of helper or amplifier T cell that secretes IL-2. Although cytotoxic T cells cannot make IL-2, they need it for proliferation.

Cytotoxic T cells lyse their allogeneic target cells by a complex process. An initial binding stage, presumably representing T cell recognition of Class I molecules on the target cell occurs. This is followed by a second step, referred to as programming for lysis, in which the T cell causes a lesion to develop in the target cell; finally, overt lysis occurs. An individual cytotoxic T cell can engage in several rounds of lysis. It is not itself destroyed in the course of killing its target cells. All T effector cells are not cytotoxic. T cells can play critical roles in a series of very important immune responses, including delayed type (or tuberculin) hypersensitivity (DTH) and contact sensitivity. An important analog of delayed hypersensitivity is the activation of macrophages, which occurs under the influence of T cell products. A consequence of this macrophage activation is the induction of the capacity of the macrophages to induce inflammatory changes, including edema, vascular thrombosis, and so on. The exact mechanism by which DTH destroys a graft is unknown.

MECHANISMS OF GRAFT REJECTION

The specific mechanism(s) of acute graft rejection has been the object of thousands of experiments and remains an issue of active debate. It may be useful to review the basic models used. Variability specific to a particular model may strongly influence the results that are found and the conclusions that are made.

Several basic approaches to the study of graft rejection have been undertaken; the potential advantages and disadvantages of each are worth notation. The simplest model of allograft rejection involves the coculture of two distinct types of lymphocytes to determine the proliferative and cytolytic potential of responder lymphocytes elicited by the stimulator strain. These culture systems have greatly enhanced our knowledge of potential interaction between lymphocytes and accessory cells. The use of congeneic mouse strains helped delineate the genetic restrictions in the generation of response. Optimal cytotoxicity was seen when responder and stimulator lymphocytes differed at both Class I and Class II regions of the MHC; less cytotoxicity was generated in the presence of Class I disparity; and the least cytotoxicity was generated in the presence of a Class II disparity.[6] The coculture model also provided information regarding the important role of the accessory cell in presenting stimulator alloantigen. Differentiation of subpopulations according to antigenic determinants has delineated the cell–cell cooperation that can occur between lymphocytes.[16,93] The problem with the coculture model in predicting in vivo events in graft rejection is that it presumes contact between recipient and donor lymphocytes; recipient lymphoid depots are frequently far removed from donor alloantigen. In some systems, donor alloantigen does not gain access to host cells and rejection can be avoided.

A second approach to the study of rejection is the histologic examination of cells that infiltrate the graft. This approach was used by early investigators[8,42] and more recently by groups who identified subsets of lymphocytes by their surface antigens. Recent investigators have used needle aspiration or core needle biopsy to determine the histology of the rejecting human renal allograft. Ratios of helper T cells to cytotoxic/suppressor T cells have been used to predict recovery after acute allograft rejection. Some investigators have identified increased OKT8[+] cytotoxic/suppressor cells during acute rejection. However, von Willebrand and others have noted increased numbers of OKT4 to helper cells.[15,28,88] This approach infers from the presence and number of a particular cell type its importance in graft rejection. The function of a specific cell is assumed by its known function in vitro; its function within the graft milieu (i.e., the presence of other cells) is unknown. Additionally, histologic examination of the graft provides only a static picture of intragraft events, although some investigators have studied serial biopsies to determine the nature of the changing infiltrate with time and treatment.[58,65] Even with this type of approach, however, cellular interactions are inferred rather than proved by the appearance and disappearance of specific cell types.

A third general approach to the study of the mechanisms of graft rejection is to study the function of cells that accumulate at the site of the allograft. The in vitro–defined function of these cells is presumed to be the function that the cells carry out in vivo. Skin graft models do not apply themselves to this technique because of the difficulty of removing cells for in vitro functional analysis. Whole organ grafts require enzymatic digestion[82,83] or mechanical disruption to retrieve cells; these maneuvers have the potential for adverse effects on the function of cells. Alternatively, the maneuvers may select out subpopulations of infiltrating cells whose function(s) in vivo are normally less prominent. von Willebrand and colleagues have shown that the surface antigens of enzymatically extracted cells is no different from that seen in tissue section.[92] Several groups have attempted to circumvent the problem of enzymatic or mechanical disruption in retrieving cells at the allograft site. The allogeneic tumor model of Berke and Amos[10] involves the peritoneal placement of a spheroid of allogeneic tumor cells. Host cells infiltrating the tumor can be easily achieved by

destruction of donor tumor cells. The sponge allograft model introduced by Roberts and Hayry[73] provided an attractive alternative to the ready retrieval of cells infiltrating an allogeneic graft. Although host cells are easily accessible with squeezing of the sponge, limitations of the technique include (1) slower tempo of the response, which relates to the requirement for revascularization of the sponge graft; (2) the potential for adherent effector cells to stick to the sponge; and (3) most importantly, the lack of an endpoint such as skin graft loss or cessation of a heart beat.

A fourth general approach to the study of allograft rejection involves the treatment of the host with agents. Knowledge of the specific function of an agent enables one to infer the importance of certain mechanisms or cell types. The use of immunosuppressive agents with broad effects limits the utility of this approach; increasing specificity of the treatment used allows for finer delineation of the specific mechanisms involved. Cyclosporine has been used for immunosuppression in a variety of models. The discovery that it inhibits Il-2 production supports the central role of Il-2 in effecting graft rejection. The administration of monoclonal antibody to Il-2 has been shown to prolong rat and mouse cardiac allograft survival.[46,48] Since both helper and cytolytic T cells depend upon Il-2 for growth in vitro, it is not possible to determine from these studies the specific mechanisms by which grafts are rejected. Administering monoclonal antibodies to specific T cell subsets holds great promise in determining which cells result in graft loss and how these subsets interact.[18,19] Specific studies will be discussed in greater detail.

The final general approach to the study of allograft rejection involves reconstitution of animals with cells of known function. Animals are rendered incapable of mounting their own immune response. This is most commonly accomplished by sublethal irradiation or by thymectomy followed by bone marrow reconstitution (depleted of T cell precursors; "B rats," or "B mice"). Cells used to reconstitute these animals are chosen by their in vitro function and enriched by antibody or cloned in vitro. Loveland and associates initiated these types of experiments and reexamined the crucial question of the importance of DTH in allograft rejection.[54,55] There are, however, a number of potential problems with this approach: (1) Injected cells have to traffick to the allograft site or to the central lymphoid depots to be effective—a specific cell may have the potential for effect but may not be able to traffick in the new environment. A number of investigators have shown that trafficking depends upon the state of activation of the transferred cell (O/U) and the immune status of the host.[48] (2) Injected cells may require growth factors to remain viable so that cells with the capability of manufacturing their own growth factors have an advantage over cells that cannot. This concept is supported by the finding that Il-2 administration has a synergistic effect with sensitized cells in restoring the ability to reject an allograft.[17] (3) It is extremely difficult to completely deplete host animals of T cells and T cell precursors. LeFrancois and Bevan[52] showed that B mice reconstituted with L_3T_4 positive cells from congenic donor mice caused skin graft loss, but the cytolytic cells directed against donor alloantigen in the spleens of these mice were of host origin. (4) It is also difficult to completely deplete the reconstituting cell population so that transfer cells may contain small numbers of contaminating cells that can expand the second host and cause graft loss. These issues will be discussed in more detail in the following paragraphs.

In spite of the limitations of the various models just discussed, it appears that allograft can result from a variety of effector mechanisms. The specific mechanism may depend upon the specific experimental or general conditions under which it is studied.

The question of which of the possible T cell–mediated response is actually responsible for graft rejection is still undergoing investigation. Analysis of the cellular components present at the site of allograft rejection reveals that there is a wide variety of inflammatory cells present, including macrophages, lymphocytes, and polymorphonuclear leukocytes. It is believed that all these cells are part of the rejection process. However, in addition to these nonspecific inflammatory cells, there are also sensitized T cells with specificity for the allograft. The specifically sensitized T cells make up only a small portion of the total number of cells that accumulate at the allograft site. Some of the large lymphoid cells exposed to graft alloantigen either within lymphoid deposits or within the graft itself can give rise to clones of immunologically committed cells that can migrate to the graft and respond to it. A small percentage of the cells at the allograft site actively take up tritiated thymidine. These are actively dividing cells, and it is assumed that these actively dividing, sensitized lymphocytes initiate the immune response to the graft.[70]

Histologic Patterns of Graft Rejection

Early investigators who studied the mechanism of graft rejection examined histologic sections. The presence of a specific type of cell was taken as evidence of the role of that cell in allograft rejection.[8,42,69] Since tissue examination is static and does not provide information about cell–cell interactions, interpretations of the histologic patterns must be qualified. The recent development of fine-needle aspiration and serial percutaneous biopsies and the use of monoclonal antibodies to stain subsets of T cells have elucidated events in allograft rejection. Increased OKT8$^+$ cytotoxic suppressor cells compared with OKT4$^+$ helper cells were noted in core-needle biopsies and in fine-needle aspirations of renal allografts undergoing rejection.[31,88,91] On the other hand, in stable renal allografts in humans, OKT4$^+$ helper rather than OKT8$^+$ cytotoxic/suppressor cells are predominant in some studies. Other investigations have resulted in different findings; the majority of cells infiltrating rejection allografts were of helper rather than of cytotoxic/suppressor phenotype.[15,28]

The classic form of acute rejection recognized in the kidney histologically is called *cellular rejection;* it involves cellular infiltration of the renal parenchyma. Small lymphocytes can be identified within hours after transplantation in contact with the peritubular capillary and venular endothelial cells. Two to 3 days later, large lymphocytes with abundant cytoplasm appear adjacent to the endothelial cells lining the small intertubular capillaries and venules. There is also evidence of endothelial cell injury. The initial focal interstitial infiltrate eventually becomes a diffuse interstitial process. The progressive disruption of peritubular capillaries and venules, together with large quantities of fluid accumulation in the interstitium, leads to a fall in renal blood flow and further cellular damage on an ischemic basis.

Hyperacute rejection can be seen in individuals who are presensitized to the allograft antigens as demonstrated by the presence of antidonor antibody in the recipient. Biopsies of hyperacutely rejected kidneys show deposits of IgG and C_3 on the glomerular and peritubular capillary walls. Platelet aggregates are present in the capillary lumen. Polymorphonuclear leukocytes line the capillary walls, with occlusion of intrarenal capillaries and arterioles. This type of antibody-mediated rejection is unusual, however, and first-set grafts to naive recipients are primarily rejected by T cells.

Gradual deterioration of renal function months or years after transplantation usually results from chronic rejection. This histologic pattern involves vascular changes, narrowing of arteries of varying sizes, and thickening of the capillary basement membranes. Although the endothelium is intact, thickened intima and internal elastic lumina are present, particularly in the interlobular and arcuate vessels. Mural deposits containing antibody and complement lead to the gradual thickening of blood vessel walls.

Since direct cytolysis can be documented by in vivo– or in vitro–generated cells, it has been assumed that this is a major mechanism by which allografts can be injured.[10,73] Cytolytic cells with antidonor specificity have been retrieved from rejecting human renal, hepatic, and cardiac allografts as well as from a number of animal transplant and tumor models.[22,41,82,83,85] Our own early work centered on the characterization of cells that infiltrated the murine sponge matrix allograft model of Roberts and Hayry.[3–5] Increasing enrichment of cytolytic T cells with specificity for donor alloantigen was noted.[3] In addition to the specific antidonor cytolytic T cell, other T cells of helper phenotype were present and, in the absence of adherent cells, could proliferate in second-set fashion to donor alloantigen. When the sponge matrix allograft was isolated from the rest of the animal by sublethal irradiation of the animal (with lead shielding of the sponge), we found that by Day 5, precytolytic cells appear in the graft, which, without any further contribution from the host, can develop into mature cytolytic cells with specificity for donor alloantigen. We also observed that when sponge donor and recipient differed at the I region, no cytolytic cells were identified, even though skin grafts exchanged between these mice are readily rejected. We have recently been studying delayed-type hypersensitivity as an alternative pathway operative in this system. We have found that cells infiltrating a sponge allograft can display both cytolytic and DTH function.

As noted previously, another method of determining mechanisms of allograft rejection involves modification of the host by immunosuppressive agents. Knowledge of how the immunosuppressive agents work can elucidate mechanisms of graft loss. For example, although cyclosporine and prednisone or administration of antibody can markedly inhibit rat renal allograft rejection, neither treatment abrogates accumulation of large numbers of mononuclear cells within the graft shortly after engraftment.[23,39,60] Moreover, the mononuclear cells that accumulate in passively enhanced or in cyclosporine-treated hosts have minimal ability to lyse Con A blasts expressing donor alloantigen, whereas mononuclear cells in untreated hosts display strong specific antidonor cytotoxicity.[13] These findings support a central role for cytotoxic T cells in graft rejection but also attest to a potential important interaction between T helper and T cytotoxic cells by means of the lymphokine IL-2, whose function and/ or release can be inhibited by cyclosporine.

In an elegant set of experiments, Kirkman and associates demonstrated that Il-2 receptor–bearing cells were important in graft rejection.[46] They ad-ministered an anti-Il-2 monoclonal antibody to the mouse IL-2 receptors and significantly prolonged vascularized heart allograft survival in two separate H-2 incompatible strains. Kupiec-Weglinski and colleagues performed similar experiments using anti-Il-2 monoclonal antibody in the rat and had comparable results.[48] The Il-2 receptor is expressed on all activated T cells; thus, these experimentals do not delineate a specific mechanism for graft rejection, but they do point to the reliance of a specific immunologic event as the trigger mechanism. It is likely that several mechanisms exist, with the helper T cell as a central initiator of either cytolysis by specifically sensitized cytotoxic T cells or a delayed-type hypersensitivity reaction. Recently, investigators have used monoclonal antibody directed against specific T cell subsets in the mouse to determine the contributions of these subsets to graft rejection. Cobbold and Waldwann found that either monoclonal anti-lyt-2$^+$ antibody or monoclonal anti-L$_3$T$_4$$^+$ antibody had more effect when given early after graft than when administered later.[19] Anti-lyt-2$^+$ antibody had no effect when administered early after skin graft but had a profound effect when administered later. These experiments strongly support the role of the L$_3$T$_4$$^+$ cell in the initiation of the allograft response but also attest to the importance of the cytolytic/suppressor cell in the effector phase of this reaction. These experiments are also of great importance in laying the groundwork for the use of monoclonal antibodies with subset specificity in humans who have received whole organ allografts.

The Role of Delayed-Type Hypersensitivity (DTH) in Allograft Rejection

Recently, several studies have renewed interest in the role of DTH in allograft rejection. This mechanism relies on the recognition of allograft antigen by specifically sensitized helper T cells. These cells proliferate in response to the recognized alloantigen and release lymphokines, which lead to the nonspecific accumulation of nonspecific inflammatory cells. Recent studies have shown that T cell–deprived rats can reject skin, heart, or renal allografts when reconstituted solely with helper T cells.[17,33–35] Loveland and colleagues who led the renewed interest in this field have even identified a unique noncytotoxic T effector cell.[54] These experiments do not exclude the role of cytotoxicity, because T cell–deficient rats contain precursors that develop into cells with cytotoxic potential when provided with helper activity. Additionally, congenitally athymic mice have been shown to contain cytotoxic T cell precursors.[40] Bevan also showed that adult thymectomized, lethally irradiated bone marrow–reconstituted mice bearing skin allografts developed cytotoxic T cells of host origin after injection of helper T cells.[52] This finding attests to the difficulty in totally removing a particular subset using antibody treatment. On the other hand, Lowry and associates showed that rejection of organ allografts in sublethally irradiated rats was mediated with adoptive transfer of specifically primed W 3/25+ splenocytes without any demonstrable cytotoxicity within the grafts.[56,57] Lowry found that depletion of the reconstituting media of either antibody-producing cells or cytotoxic cells failed to alter the tempo of rejection.[57] Further, these investigators identified rat lymphotoxin within rejecting rat renal allografts that could be elicited in a single molecular form. They hypothesized that lymphotoxin may provide the actual tissue injury in delayed-type hypersensitivity reactions. The lymphotoxin they identified is of similar molecular weight to that identified in humans. It has been suggested by other investigators that the cytotoxic effect of human lymphotoxin is augmented in the presence of the lymphokine gamma interferon secreted by helper T cells when they are stimulated by specific antigen.[1] Since gamma interferon is attributed with the increased expression of Class II antigen on parenchymal cells,[78] lymphotoxin and gamma interferon may have synergistic deleterious effects on transplanted tissues. Most experiments that indicate a central role for helper T cell in initiating graft rejection have used a naive or B cell host and the transfer of unsensitized effector cells. This means that the afferent as well as the efferent areas of the immune response are being examined. Hall's group has recently addressed this issue.[27] They found that unsensitized cells of cytolytic phenotypes could not restore cardiac allograft rejection in B rats but that sensitized cells of cytolytic phenotype were more effective than comparable numbers of sensitized or unsensitized cells of helper phenotype. Lafferty's group has shown similar results in mice undergoing thyroid or islet allografts; sensitized cytolytic cells restored allograft immunity.[94] Further evidence for cytolytic cells as effectors comes from Biel and associates,[12] using helper independent cytolytic cell clones, and Tyler and colleagues,[85] using cloned cytolytic cells to cause skin necrosis after intradermal injection.

Other Mechanisms of Allograft Injury

ADCC is another mechanism that can induce cytotoxicity, which is mediated by various cell types, all of which must have surface receptors for the Fc portion of IgG.[68] These cells have no ability to injure targets directly but are stimulated to release lysosomal enzymes or other toxins in the presence of an Fc receptor on an activated T cell. The target, which may be nonspecific, must bear IgG or its surface.

The role of NK cells in allograft rejection is unclear, although they can be found at the allograft site in large numbers.[53] They do not have specificity for donor alloantigen but are reactive to neoplastic and immature cells.

Antibody injury to graft has been identified in a number of models.[2,20,80] In vascularized grafts, the antibody can affect the endothelium directly. Vascular lesions can be identified when a kidney is transplanted into a presensitized host. It is likely that the antibodies exert their effect through a number of nonspecific pathways, which include complement, ADCC, clotting, and kinan-generating systems. Various molecules are released, including kineses, complement fragments that are chemotactic, histamine, and anaphylatoxins. These molecules can change vascular permeability, affect arteriolar spasm, and cause damage to the endothelium. The resultant microthrombi, largely composed of platelet aggregates, contribute to the tissue loss.

In a number of systems, including rejecting human renal allografts, a number of different mechanisms have been identified. These effector mechanisms may be operative simultaneously, causing graft loss. The predominance of one mechanism or another may relate to the specific experimental condition to which the animal is subjected. It is most likely that multiple mechanisms are poised to result in graft loss and that the particular mechanism that is operative depends upon a number of factors, including host, organ allografts, immune state, experimental conditions, and mode of assay.

REFERENCES

1. Aggarwal BR, Moffat B, Harkins RN: Human lymphotoxin. J Biol Chem 259:686, 1984
2. Altman B: Tissue transplantation: Circulating antibody in the homotransplantation of kidney and skin. Ann R Coll Surg Engl 33:79, 1963
3. Ascher NL, Ferguson RM, Hoffman RA et al: Partial characterization of cytotoxic cells infiltrating sponge matrix allografts. Transplantation 27:254, 1979
4. Ascher NL, Chen S, Hoffman RA et al: Maturation of cytotoxic T cells within sponge matrix allografts. J Immunol 131:617, 1983
5. Ascher NL, Hoffman RA, Chen S et al: Specific and

nonspecific infiltration of sponge matrix allografts by specifically sensitized cytotoxic lymphocytes. Cell Immunol 52:38, 1980

6. Bach FH, Bach ML, Sondel PM: Differential function of major histocompatibility complex antigens in T-lymphocyte activation. Nature 259:273, 1976

7. Bach FH, Hirschhorn K: Lymphocyte interaction: A potential histocompatibility test in vitro. Science 143:813–814, 1964

8. Balch CM, Wilson CB, Lee S et al: Thymus-dependent lymphocytes in tissue sections of rejecting rat renal allografts. J Exp Med 138:1584, 1973

9. Baum L, Pilarski L: In vitro generation of antigen-specific helper T cells that collaborate with cytotoxic T cells precursors. J Exp Med 148:1579–1591, 1978

10. Berke G, Amos DB: Mechanism of lymphocyte-mediated cytolysis. The LMC cycle and its role in transplantation immunity. Transplant Rev 17:71, 1973

11. Bernoco D, Cullen S, Scudeller G et al: HL-A molecules at the cell surface. In Dausset J, Comobani J (eds): Histocompatibility Testing, pp 527–537. Copenhagen, Munksgaard, 1972

12. Biel LW, Roopenian DL, Widmer MB et al: Induction of immune skin lesions by T lymphocyte clones of particular subclasses. Transplant Proc 17:610, 1985

13. Bradley JA, Mason DW, Morris PJ: Evidence that rat renal allografts are rejected by cytotoxic T cells and not by nonspecific effectors. Transplantation 39:169, 1985

14. Brent L, Brown JB, Medawar B: Quantitation studies on tissue transplantation immunity. VI. Hypersensitivity reactions associated with rejection of homografts. Proc R Soc Lond (Biol). 156:187, 1962

15. Burdach J, Beschorner W, Smith W et al: Lymphocytes in early renal allograft biopsies. Transplant Proc 17:560–563, 1985

16. Cantor H, Boyse EA: Functional subclasses of T lymphocytes bearing different Li antigens. II. Cooperation between subclasses of Li+ cells in the generations of killer activity. J Exp Med 141:1390, 1975

17. Clason AE, Duarte AJ, Kupiec–Weglinski JW et al: Restoration of allograft responsiveness in B rats by interleukin 2 and/or adherent cells. J Immunol 129:252, 1982

18. Cobbold S, Jayasuriyn A, Wash A et al: Therapy with monoclonal antibodies by elimination of T cell subsets in vivo. Nature 372:548, 1984

19. Cobbold S, Waldmann H: Skin allograft rejection by $L_3/T_4{}^+$ and Lyt 2^+ T cell subsets. Transplantation 41:634, 1986

20. Dubernard JM, Carpenter CB, Busch GJ et al: Rejection of canine renal allograft by passive transfer of sensitized serum. Surgery 64:752, 1968

21. Dyer PA, Tolinson RWG, Mallich NP et al: A single center prospective study showing no benefit of HLA-DR matching between cadaver kidney donors and recipients. Trans Proc 15:137, 1983

22. Engers HA, Glasbrook AL, Sorenson GD: Allogeneic tumor rejection induced by the intravenous injection of Lyt-2 + cytolytic T-lymphocyte clones. J Exp Med 156:1280, 1982

23. Fabre JW, Morris PJ: Studies in the specific suppression of renal allograft rejection in pre-sensitized rats. Transplantation 19:121, 1975

24. Forbes R, Guttmann R: Pathogenetic studies of cardiac allograft rejection using inbred rat models. Immunol Rev 77:5–30, 1984

25. Giphart MJ, Doyer E, Wesse E et al: Quantitative aspects of HL-A2 antigenic surface determinants studied with radiolabelled antibodies. In Kissmeyer-Nielsen F et al (eds): Histocompatibility Testing, pp 739–746. Copenhagen, Munksgaard, 1975

26. Green DR, Flood PM, Gershon RR: Immunoregulatory T-cell pathways. Am Rev Immunol 1:439, 1983

27. Gurley KE, Hall BM, Dorsch SE: The factor of immunization in allograft rejection: Carried by cytotoxic T cells, non–helper-induced T cells. Transplant Proc 18:307, 1986

28. Hall B, Bishop G, Farnsworth A et al: Identification of the cellular subpopulations infiltrating rejecting cadaver renal allografts: Preponderance of the T_4 subset of T cells. Transplantation 37:564–570, 1984

29. Hall BM, de Saxe I, Dorsch SE: The cellular basis of allograft rejection in vivo. III. Restoration of first-set rejection and heart grafts by T helper cells in irradiated rats. Transplantation 36:700, 1983

30. Hall BM, Duggfin GG, Philips J et al: Increased expressed of HLA DR antigens on renal tubular cells in renal transplants: Relevance to the rejection response. Lancet 2:247, 1984

31. Hammer C, Land W, Stadler J et al: Lymphocyte subclasses in rejecting kidney grafts detected by monoclonal antibodies. Transplant Proc 15:356–360, 1983

32. Hart DN: The effects of antibodies on organ allograft survival. Heart Transplant 2:143–150, 1983

33. Hart D, Fabre J: Demonstration and characterization of Ia positive dendritic cells in the interstitial connective tissues of rat heart and other tissues except brain. J Exp Med 154:347–361, 1981

34. Häyry P, von Willebrand E, Parthensas E et al: The inflammatory mechanisms of allograft rejection. Immunol Rev 77:85–142, 1984

35. Heidecke CD, Kupiec–Weglinski JW, Lear PA et al: Interactions between T lymphocyte subsets supported by interleukin 2–rich lymphokines produce acute rejection of vascularized cardiac allografts in T cell deprived rats. J. Immunol 133:582, 1984

36. Hercend T. Ritz J, Schlossman SF et al: Antibody-dependent cytotoxicity and natural killer–like activity mediated by subsets of activated T cells. Clin Immunol Immunopathol 21:134, 1981

37. Homan E: Protein sensitization in Iso-skin grafting. Is the latter of practical value? Surg Gynecol Obstet 38:100, 1924

38. Homan WP, Fabre JW, Millard PR et al: Effect of cyclosporin A upon second-set rejection of rat renal allograft. Transplantation 29:361, 1980

39. Homan WP, Fabre JW, Williams KA et al: Studies on

the immunosuppressive properties of cyclosporin A in rats receiving renal allografts. Transplantation 29:361, 1980

40. Hunig T, Bevan MJ: Specificity of cytotoxic T cells from athymic mice. J Exp Med 152:688, 1980
41. Hurme M, Heterhington CM, Chandler PR et al: Cytotoxic T cell responses to H-Y: Correlation with the rejection of syngeneic male skin grafts. J Exp Med 147:768, 1978
42. Jakobisiaki M: Quantitative data concerning the development of the cellular infiltration of skin allograft in mice. Transplantation 12:364, 1971
43. Katz DH: Lymphocyte differentiation, recognition and regulation. New York, Academic Press, 1977
44. Katz DH, Benacerraf B: The regulatory influence of activated T cells on B cell responses to antigen. Adv Immunol 15:1–94, 1972
45. Katz DH, Dorf ME, Benacerraf B: Control of T-lymphocyte and B-lymphocyte activation by two complementing If-GLo immune response genes. J Exp Med 143:906–918, 1976
46. Kirkman RL, Barrett LV, Gaulton GN et al: Administration of an anti-interleukin 2 receptor monoclonal antibody prolongs cardiac allograft survival in mice. J Exp Med 162:358, 1985
47. Krensky A, Reiss C, Mier J et al: Long-term human cytolytic T cell lines allospecific for HLA DR 6 antigens are OKT4+. Proc Natl Acad Sci USA 79:2365–2369, 1982
48. Kupiec–Weglinski JW, Diananstein T, Tilney N et al: Therapy with monoclonal antibody to interleukin 2 receptors. Proc Natl Acad Sci USA 83:2624–2627, 1986
49. Kupiec–Weglinski JW, Lear PA, Heidecke CD et al: Modification of function and migration pattern of thymocyte populations by cyclosporine after organ transplantation in rats. Transplantation 37:631, 1984
50. Lafferty K, Prowse S, Simeonovic C et al: Immunobiology of tissue transplantation. In Paul WE, Fathman CA, Metzgar H (eds): Annual Review of Immunology, pp 143–173. Palo Alto, California, Annual Reviews, Inc, 1983
51. Landsteiner R, Levine P: On the inheritance of agglutinogens of human blood demonstrable by immune agglutinens. J Exp Med 48:731, 1928
52. LeFrancois L, Bevan MJ: A reexamination of the role of Lyt-2-positive T cells in murine skin graft rejection. J Exp Med 159:57, 1984
53. Lotze MT, Marquis DM, Carey AS et al: Two new assays for the assay detection of transplant rejection: Il-2 response and PHA-augmented NK activity. Transplant Proc 15:1796, 1983
54. Loveland BE, Hogarth PM, Ceredig R et al: Cells mediating graft rejection in the mouse. I. Lyt-1 cells mediate skin graft rejection. J Exp Med 153:1044, 1981
55. Loveland BE, McKenzie IFC: Which T cells cause graft rejection? Transplantation 33:217, 1983
56. Lowry RP, Gurley KE, Forbes RDC: Immune mechanisms in organ allograft. I. Delayed-type hypersensi-

tivity and lymphocytotoxicity in heart graft rejection. Transplantation 36:391, 1983
57. Lowry RP, Marghesco DM, Blackburn JH: Immune mechanisms in organ allograft rejection. Transplantation 40:183, 1985
58. Marboe CC, Knowles DM 2nd, Chess L et al: The immunologic and ultrastructural characterization of the cellular infiltrate in acute cardiac allograft rejection: Prevalence of cells with the natural killer (NK) phenotype. Clin Immunol Immunopathol 27:141, 1983
59. Mason DW: The mechanism of allograft rejection— progress and problems. Trans Proc 15:264, 1983
60. Mason DW, Morris PJ: Inhibition of the accumulation in rat kidney allografts, of specific—but not nonspecific—cytotoxic cells by cyclosporine. Transplantation 37:46, 1984
61. Medawar PB: A second study of the behavior and fate of skin homografts in rabbits. (A report to the War Wounds Committee of the Medical Research Council). J Anat 79:157, 1945
62. Medawar PB: The behavior and fate of skin autografts and skin homografts in rabbits. (A report to the War Wounds Committee of the Medical Research Council). J Anat 78:176, 1984
63. Moen T, Lamm L, Berger L et al: The effect of matching for HLA on cadaveric renal graft survival in Scandiatransplant. Trans Proc 18:13, 1986
64. Moller G (ed): Role of macrophages on the immune response. Immunol Rev 40:1–255, 1978
65. Nemlander A, Soots A, von Willebrand E et al: Redistribution of renal-allograft responding leukocytes during rejection. J Exp Med 156:1087, 1982
66. Oluwole S, Satake K, Kuromoto N et al: Recirculation of indium–111–labeled lymphocytes in normal and allografted rats. Transplantation 36:558, 1983
67. Opelz A, Terasaki PE: Studies on the strength of HLA antigen in related donor kidney transplants. Transplantation 24:106, 1977
68. Perlmann P: Cellular immunity: Antibody-dependent cytotoxicity (K-cell activity). Clin Immunol 3:107, 1976
69. Porter KA: Morphologic aspects of renal homograft rejection. Br Med Bull 21:171, 1965
70. Porter KA, Joseph WH, Rendall JM et al: The role of lymphocytes in the rejection of canine renal hemotransplants. Lab Invest 13:1080, 1964
71. Reinherz EL, Schlossman SF: The differentiation and function of human T-lymphocytes. Cell 19:821, 1980
72. Reinherz EL, Schlossman SF: The characterization and function of human T-lymphocyte subsets. Immunology Today 2:69, 1981
73. Roberts PJ, Hayry P: Sponge matrix allografts. A model for analysis of killer cells infiltrating mouse allografts. Transplantation 21:437, 1976
74. Sanfilippo F, Vaughn WK, Spees EK et al: Benefits of HLA-A and HLA-B matching on graft and patient outcome after cadaveric donor renal transplantation. N Engl J Med 311:358, 1984

75. Schlossman SF, Mauer S, Acuto O et al: Human T-lymphocyte differentiation and function. In Tada T (ed): Progress in Immunology. New York, Academic Press, 1984

76. Schevach EM, Rosenthal AS: Function of macrophages in antigen recognition by guinea pig lymphocytes. II. Role of the macrophages in the regulation of genetic control of the immune response. J Exp Med 138:1213–1229, 1973

77. Singer A, Kruisbeck A, Andrysiak PM: T cell accessory interaction that initiates allospecific cytotoxic T-lymphocyte responses. Existence of both Ia-restricted and Ia-unrestricted cellular interaction pathways. J Immunol 1332:2199, 1984

78. Skoskiewicz MJ, Colvin RB, Schneeberger EE et al: Widespread and selective induction of major histocompatibility complex–determined antigens in vivo by Y-interferon. J Exp Med 162:1645, 1985

79. Steiniger B, Klempnauer J, Wonigiet K: Phenotype and histological distribution of interstitial dendritic cells in the rat pancreas, liver, heart, and kidney. Transplantation 38:169, 1984

80. Stetson CA: The role of humoral antibody in the homograft reaction. Adv Immunol 3:97, 1963

81. Taylor RJ, Andrews W, Rosenthal JT et al: DR matching in cadaveric renal transplantation with cyclosporine. Trans Proc 8:1194, 1976

82. Tilney NL, Garavoy MR, Busch GJ et al: Rejected human renal allografts recovery and characteristics of infiltrating cells and antibody. Transplantation 28:421, 1979

83. Tilney NL, Strom TB, Macpherson SG et al: Surface properties and functional characteristics of infiltrating cells harvested from acutely rejecting cardiac allografts in inbred rats. Transplantation 20:323, 1975

84. Turk JL: Delayed Type Hypersensitivity, p 70. Amsterdam, Elsevier/North Holland Biomedical Press, 1980

85. Tyler JD, Gallis J, Nider ME et al: Cloned Lyt-2 + cytolytic T-lymphocytes destroy allogeneic tissue in vivo. J Exp Med 159:234, 1984

86. Unanue ER, Askonas BA: Persistence of immunogenicity of antigen after uptake of macrophages. J Exp Med 127:915–926, 1968

87. Unanue RE, Cerotinni JC: The immunogenicity of antigen bound to the plasma membranes of macrophages. J Exp Med 131:711–725, 1970

88. Vanes A, Meyer C, Oljans PJ et al: Monoclonal cells in renal allografts. Transplantation 37:134–139, 1984

89. van Rood JJ, de Vries RRP, Bradley BA: Genetics and biology of the HLA system. In Dorf ME (ed): The Role of the Major Histocompatibility Complex in Immunobiology, pp 59–109. Garland St PM Press, 1981

90. van Rood JJ, van Leevwen A, Kevning J et al: The serological recognition of the human MLC determinants using a modified cytotoxicity technique. Tissue Antigens 5:73–79, 1975

91. von Willebrand E: OKT4/T8 ratio in the blood and in the graft during episodes of human renal allograft rejection. Cell Immunol 77:196–201, 1983

92. von Willebrand E, Soots A, Häyry P: In situ effector mechanisms in rat kidney allograft rejection. I. Characterization of the host cellular infiltrate in rejecting allograft parenchyma. Cell Immunol 46:309, 1979

93. Wagner H, Röllinghoff M: T–T–cell interactions during the vitro cytotoxic allograft responses. I. Soluble products from activated Lyl + T cells trigger autonomously antigen–primed Ly23 + T cells to cell proliferation and cytolytic activity. J Exp Med 148:1523, 1978

94. Warren HS, Simeonovig CJ, Dixon JE et al: Sensitized Lyt 2+ T cells trigger rejection. Transplant Proc 18:310, 1986

95. Widmer MB, Roopenian DC, Biel LW et al: Characterization of alloreactive T cell clones in vitro. In von Boehmer H, Haas W (eds) T Cell Clones. New York, Elsevier, 1985

Biological Immunosuppression: Polyclonal Antilymphocyte Sera, Monoclonal Antibody, and Donor-Specific Antigen

Anthony P. Monaco

Polyclonal heterologous antilymphocyte or antithymocyte antibodies (ALS, ALG, or ATG) are extremely effective in prolonging allograft survival. In vivo, ALG causes acute and profound lymphopenia and lymphocyte depletion and a concomitant depression of the allograft reaction. Although ALG is a heterologous protein, it is extremely well tolerated clinically with minimal, attendant allergic reactions. Its major use, is in the treatment of renal allograft rejection, where it has been shown effective when used in conjunction with high-dose steroid therapy or after steroid administration for steroid-resistant rejection, and as a sole rejection treatment. ALG, ATG is used prior to the institution of cyclosporine therapy to prevent cyclosporine nephrotoxicity immediately post-transplantation and to treat steroid-resistant rejection. There has been no significant increase in bacterial sepsis or spontaneous malignancy with ALG therapy, but there is an increased incidence of CMV and other viral infections.

Orthoclone OKT*3 is a monoclonal antibody against the T3 antigen, which is common to all mature human T cells. When administered in vivo, it causes a rapid and concomitant decrease in the number of circulating T3 (CD3) positive as well as T4 and T8 positive T cells. In addition, modulation of the surface T3 antigen is another mechanism by which OKT*3 exerts its in vivo effect. The majority of patients given OKT*3 make some type of antibody response to mouse globulins. OKT*3 is effective in reversing acute renal, cardiac, and hepatic allograft rejection. OKT*3 is also effective in treatment of renal allograft rejection unresponsive to conventional immunosuppressive therapy. The first and/or second dose of OKT*3 is usually accompanied by flu-like symptoms attributable to the release of mediators from the opsonization of T3 positive cells by OKT*3 and their subsequent removal by the RE system.

Modulation of allograft rejection with donor-specific antigen refers to the specific prolongation of allograft survival induced by administration of donor-specific antigen at some time before, during, or after an allograft has been transplanted in association with a transient nonspecific immunosuppression. Although many antigens have been used to induce prolonged survival or specific unresponsiveness, donor bone marrow seems to be a uniquely effective antigen when administered after transient immunosuppression with antilymphocyte globulin. Timing of administration is critical. The unresponsiveness induced in the ALS–bone marrow model is specific and can be modified by administration of various bacterial adjuvants or cyclophosphamide, suggesting that it is a positive immunological response. The cell in the bone marrow associated with the capacity to induce unresponsiveness in ALS-treated mice has the phenotypic characteristics of being Ia negative, Thy-1 negative, complement receptor negative, and Ig negative but is positive for Fc receptors. Specific unresponsiveness similar to that induced by marrow also can be induced by other blood elements (platelets and isolated fractions of peripheral blood lymphocytes). The ALS–bone marrow model has been applied to whole organ allografts in dogs and primates. Whole unstored marrow from donor animals specifically prolongs renal allografts in ALS-treated recipients when administered post-transplantation in a protocol similar to that used in mice. In vitro and in vivo analyses of immune responses showed that unresponsive monkeys were specifically unresponsive to the donor, whereas they retained their reactivity to third-party donor monkeys. The ALS–bone marrow model has been applied in man using one-haplotype disparate, mixed-lymphocyte culture positive living-related donor recipient kidney allograft combinations; some have enjoyed prolonged survival. In these few instances where tried, specific unresponsiveness (as measured by mixed-lymphocyte culture studies) has been achieved in man with the ALS–marrow protocol.

Any type of immunosuppression to modify or attenuate the normal allograft response is in fact biological immunosuppression. The term *biological immunosuppression* is usually used to describe those methods used to suppress allograft immunity that do not utilize chemotherapeutic or hormonal (steroid) agents. Although there are many examples of biological immunosuppression, blood transfusions (both nonspecific and specific) are probably the most widely used. In this chapter, three other well-studied biological suppressive modalities are discussed: (1) polyclonal antilymphocyte sera, (2) monoclonal antibodies to effector lymphocytes, and (3) donor-specific transplantation antigens, administered in a form other than the graft antigens themselves.

POLYCLONAL ANTILYMPHOCYTE, ANTITHYMOCYTE SERA* (ALS, ATS, ALG, ATG)

Antibodies prepared in heterologous species to lymphocytes (antilymphocyte serum, ALS, ALG) and to thymocytes (antithymocyte serum, ATS, ATG) are probably the most effective biological reagents used to prolong allograft and xenograft survival in most experimental animal species studied. Although ALS or ATS or their purified derivatives are invariably superior in experimental studies in prolonging allograft survival compared with such clinically used drugs as azathioprine, prednisone, and, more recently, cyclosporine, the effectiveness of ALG and ATG for clinical immunosuppression was extremely difficult to establish. These efforts spanned a period of more than 10 years. In retrospect, the reasons for this difficulty are numerous. Pharmacologically, there was frequent variability in potency of batches

of ATG or ALG studied, and it is doubtful that adequate dosage schedules were followed. Invariably, most transplant centers that tested ALG or ATG had insufficient patients available to evaluate for study under protocols requiring rigid, randomized appropriate controls. This latter problem led to the use of multicenter clinical trials of ATG with all their attendant problems. Indeed, many of these centers, particularly in the early multicenter trials, were just beginning their transplant programs and were clearly inexperienced. During the recent years of ALG, ATG testing, numerous risk factors (e.g., age, type of donor, blood transfusions, HLA typing) have been identified that influence the outcome of transplantation. Many ATG trials were not appropriately controlled to stratify for these factors in test and control groups. In addition, the ALG products were not standardized, often being produced, purified, and administered by a variety of methods. Furthermore, ATG was invariably tested, until recently, as an adjunctive immunosuppressive agent with Imuran and prednisone, two agents that in combination are reasonably effective in clinical kidney transplantation, especially when patients with certain negative risk factors are excluded. Thus, if ATG improved 1-year functional graft survival 10% to 18%, as it probably does, a large number of appropriate patients for study would be required to demonstrate this difference significantly. Another consideration is that the addition of a highly effective immunosuppressive agent such as ATG to an already effective protocol of Imuran and prednisone could easily partially obscure the beneficial effects of ATG by induction of toxicity through excessive immunosuppression. Thus, it is not surprising that conclusive evidence for the effectiveness of ATG and ALG as immunosuppressive agents in clinical kidney transplantation took several years to achieve.

Production of Antilymphocyte Serum

When one uses the term *antilymphocyte serum* in experimental and clinical immunosuppression, it implies that the antilymphocyte serum is *heterolo-*

---

* In referring to antilymphocyte or antithymocyte antibodies used in various studies and multicenter trials or combined series in which various antilymphocyte or antithymocyte preparations in various states of purification were given, the terms *antilymphocyte serum* or *ALS* or *ALG* will be used. When antithymocyte preparations were used exclusively, the term *ATS* or *ATG* will be used.

gous antilymphocyte serum, that is, antibodies prepared against a given species of lymphocytes or thymocytes prepared in a heterologous species. Allogeneic antilymphocyte sera, as typified by anti-theta sera in mice, are not as immunosuppressive as a heterologous rabbit or goat anti-mouse sera. There are probably many reasons for this. Most important is the fact that many high-affinity antibodies to many subsets of lymphocytes are produced when heterologous species are used for production.

For human use, lymphocytes or thymocytes are used to immunize a heterologous species, such as horse, rabbit, or goat. The sera is appropriately tested for antilymphocyte activity by a number of in vitro immunologic assays,[32–34] and, if acceptable, a production bleeding of the immunized recipient is done. The heterologous sera is then subjected to a number of purification procedures, including isolation of the immunoglobulin (IgG) fraction, followed by various absorption procedures to remove anti-platelet and antierythrocyte antibodies.[52] As currently produced, ALG, ATG are polyclonal antibody preparations. It is estimated that less than 2% of the globulin in antithymocyte globulin preparations currently given for clinical organ transplants are active antilymphocyte globulins—the remaining IgG molecules being directed to nonlymphocyte tissue targets.

There is only one currently available FDA-licensed antithymocyte preparation (ATGAM, Upjohn Co.) for clinical organ transplantation. This is an equine antithymocyte IgG preparation made by immunizing a horse with human thymocytes.[101] A number of centers manufacture their own ALS and ATS preparations, which have been highly effective. Minnesota antilymphoblast globulin is one such preparation, made from immunization of horses with a cultured line of human lymphoblasts.[70] Another preparation commonly used is rabbit antithymocyte globulin. The best and most effective example of this is that produced by Thomas and colleagues.[94] This latter material is produced by immunizing rabbits with human thymocytes.

Mechanism of Action

The exact mechanism of action of ALS or ATS preparations is not known. When ALS or ATS preparations are administered to experimental animals or to humans, there is invariably a rapid and profound decrease in circulating lymphocytes, which recovers when ALS, ATS administration is stopped or if immune elimination develops. In experimental animals, the induced lymphopenia is associated with a profound depletion of the lymphocytes in the paracortical areas of lymph nodes, the areas associated with the peripheral circulation of lymphocytes. As with peripheral lymphopenia, tissue lymphocyte depletion after ALS recovers with cessation of ALS therapy. In rodents, adult thymectomy prior to ALS therapy markedly potentiates and prolongs the lymphopenia, lymphocyte depletion, and concomitant immunosuppression induced by a fixed dose of ALS.[68]

The most likely explanation for the major effect of ALS is that it combines with peripheral circulating lymphocytes, which are rapidly removed from the circulation by the reticuloendothelial system. Another important point to emphasize with regard to the mechanism of action of ALS, ATS is that it is a polyclonal serum containing antibodies to all types of lymphocytes (e.g., T cells, B cells) as well as macrophages, since the immunizing innoculum no doubt contains all of these and many other cells. The fact that ALS, ATS preparations contain antibodies to many of the cellular elements involved in the immune response to allografts accounts for a great deal of their efficacy in modifying allograft rejection.

Clinical Administration

Since ALG, ATG preparations used in humans are heterologous sera, most investigators do not administer these reagents without appropriate skin or conjunctival testing. However, the allergic reactions to these preparations are so relatively infrequent (perhaps because allograft recipients are already immunosuppressed by uremia and/or other immunosuppressive drugs) that some clinical centers no longer perform allergic testing. Equine preparations are given in large dose and volume (10 mg/kg–25 mg/kg) for several days to 3 weeks. Because they are frequently painful if given intramuscularly, they are invariably given intravenously, usually in a high-flow subclavian line, because the material tends to sclerose peripheral veins. Rabbit antithymocyte preparations are usually given in a low dose (100 mg/day) for several injections over a 1- to 2-week period and can be administered intramuscularly. The monitoring of effective ALG, ATG dose by peripheral lymphocyte or T cell analysis varies among centers that use these preparations.

Use of Antilymphocyte Serum as an Adjunctive Immunosuppressive Agent in Organ Transplantation

Numerous review articles by this author and others[59] have discussed the immunosuppressive properties of ATG and ALG used alone or in conjunction with the other immunosuppressive agents. ALG or ATG used alone in human volunteers eliminates delayed hypersensitivity recall reactions to test bacterial antigens and prolongs randomly selected skin allografts.[66] ATG significantly prolongs the survival of skin allografts used to cover excised third-degree burns, resulting in improved patient survival from large (75%) third-degree burns.[15] In spite of this clearcut demonstration of the immunosuppressive potency of ALG and ATG in human skin grafting, the initial results, with the addition of ATG to clinical kidney transplant immunosuppressive protocols utilizing Imuran and prednisone, failed to demonstrate conclusive improvement in patient survival and functional graft survival.[83,93,98,101] Nevertheless, these inconclusive trials invariably demonstrated a reduced incidence and severity of early rejection reactions with greater ease of reversibility by additional conventional therapy. Long-term functional graft survival generally favored the ATG-treated groups; however, statistically significant long-term functional graft survival in patients randomly assigned to ATG groups over control groups was less frequently reported.

The most significant early series was reported by Cosimi and associates[15,61] who studied 104 cadaveric kidney transplant recipients given ATG in conjunction with Imuran and prednisone (60 patients) or Imuran and prednisone alone (44 patients). Significantly fewer early rejection episodes occurred in the ATG-treated group without any increased incidence of infection. A definite decrease in overall steroid requirement, as well as a concomitant reduction in the incidence of avascular necrosis, was identified in the ATG-treated group. Functional graft survival was 10% to 13% higher in the ATG-treated group at all time intervals tested, although the numbers involved had not yet reached clinical significance. Patient survival was the same in ATG-treated and in control groups.

The need for evaluating with statistical significance these kinds of modest differences in allograft survival in large numbers of patients was illustrated by the report of the Kidney Transplant Histocompatibility Study.[2] More than 1500 cadaver kidney transplant recipients enrolled in this collaborative study. Again, at all intervals studied from 3 months to 36 months post-transplantation, allograft survival in patients given antilymphocyte serum treatment was 10% to 11% better than in those who had not received ALS. This study concluded, in view of the large number of patients studied, that the data strongly indicated that antilymphocyte serum is of significant benefit in cadaveric allograft survival.

In another large study from the Southeast Or-

gan Procurement Foundation (SEOPF) group conducted by Spees and associates[87] of more than 1900 cadaveric kidney recipients, the effects of ALS in the overall data (ALS vs. no ALS) showed significant improvement of functional graft survival at 6 months (11% $p = 0.006$) and 12 months (10%, $p = 0.006$) but not at 18 months (7%, $p = $ NS*) or at 24 months (5%, $p = $ NS). Of importance was the finding that when the data were stratified, the effects of ALS were noted to be greater in recipients with good HLA matches in both transfused and nontransfused recipients. The effects in these categories were maintained, that is, the improved survival associated with ALS superimposed on a good HLA match with or without transfusion was maintained for at least 24 months. Interestingly, the overall patient survival rate (ALS or no ALS) was 6% lower in the ALS-treated group at 12 months ($p = 0.007$) but not at 6, 18, or 24 months. This latter adverse effect is the only one that has been found in any large series concerning patient survival in ALS-treated patients. Indeed, in essentially all studies shown, there was no other adverse effect on survival. Nevertheless, this negative effect could have been generated by the possible increased virulence of cytomegalovirus (CMV) infections in ALS-treated patients, which, if not appropriately acknowledged by adjustment of standard immunosuppression of prednisone and Imuran, could lead to increased morbidity and mortality (see the section entitled Clinical Toxicity of ALS).

In a smaller, single center study, Novick and colleagues[74] presented the results of a controlled prospective randomized, double-blind evaluation of Minnesota antilymphoblast globulin as an immunosuppressive adjunct to azathioprine and prednisone in cadaver renal transplantation. There were 31 patients in the ALG group and 36 patients in the control group (Imuran and prednisone only). ALG-treated patients experienced (1) no major side effects, (2) a delayed onset of rejection following transplantation ($p < 0.005$), (3) a reduced total number of rejection episodes ($p < 0.05$), (4) fewer days in hospital ($p < 0.05$), (5) a reduced cost of transplantation ($p < 0.02$), (6) improved graft survival ($p < 0.05$), and (7) equivalent patient survival when compared within the group. They concluded that antilymphoblast ALG is safe, cost-effective, and of definite immunologic benefit in cadaver renal transplantation.

In summary, numerous studies using ALS as an adjunctive immunosuppressive agent in primary cadaveric kidney transplantation show that treatment

* NS = not significant

with ALS results in a 10% to 15% improvement in functional graft survival for 1 to 2 years, with probably no alteration in patient survival. Furthermore, the incidence, severity, and ease of reversibility of early rejection reactions is clearly and significantly improved with adjunctive ALS treatment. This is accomplished with a reduced steroid requirement, which is reflected in a decreased incidence of avascular necrosis.

Use of Antilymphocyte Serum in the Treatment of Rejection

Whereas the use of ALS in the prophylactic treatment of primary cadaveric allograft recipients may be considered by many investigators to be unnecessary, the use of ALS for the actual treatment of rejection is now generally considered highly effective and is becoming accepted and almost routine therapy for rejection. The idea of using ALS for the treatment of rejection rather than as an adjunctive agent makes good sense. It is estimated that 25% of all living-related, non-HLA identical recipients and 20% of cadaveric recipients never show any rejection reaction on conventional immunosuppressive therapy of prednisone and Imuran.[26] Furthermore, it is extremely difficult, if not impossible, to differentiate these potential, nonresponders from those patients destined for rejection by various pretransplant immune indices, for example, mitogen and antigen lymphocyte stimulation, antigen recall, DNCB testing, and so on.[10] The use of additional prophylactic immunotherapy places a significant population (20% to 25%) of nonresponder patients at increased risk owing to excessive immunosuppression. Any gains in allograft survival achieved in the responder population by additional prophylactic therapy may be nullified by the increased morbidity and mortality of overimmunosuppressed nonresponders. The inconsistent conclusions of some studies relative to the effectiveness of the prophylactic use of ALG may be due to this offsetting phenomenon. It therefore seems logical to reserve the use of ALG for those situations in which it is obviously needed, for example, to reverse acute rejection in responder recipients.

Birkeland[5] first observed that ALG therapy (10 mg/kg–20 mg/kg for 21 days) was more effective than steroids in reversing acute rejection episodes, although no long-term advantage to treated patients was achieved with ALG use. Somewhat later, Shields and associates[84] performed a prospective randomized trial comparing ATG (15 mg/kg × 14 days, no increased steroids) with high-dose steroid treatment in a group of recipients of related kidneys

who were experiencing their first rejection crisis. These authors noted more rapid rejection reversal, fewer second rejection episodes, better long-term graft function, and markedly lower steroid dose requirements in the ALS group. Thus, in this study, ATG was shown to be at least as good or better than high-dose steroids, even when the rejection process was previously initiated. Subsequent to these studies, several groups have investigated the use of ALS in the treatment of allograft rejection in cadaveric recipients.

Use of ALG Combined with High-Dose Steroids for Rejection

Hardy's group[35] compared the effectiveness of steroid boosters and ATG (15 mg/kg, ATGAM for 10–21 days) with standard rejection treatment alone (steroids) in cadaveric renal allograft transplantation. First rejection episodes were reversed readily in ALS-treated patients (27/32) and to a lesser extent in patients treated only with steroids (15/20). However, functional graft survival at 6 months and 1 year was 72% and 73%, respectively, for ALS-treated patients but only 45% to 46.6% for steroid-treated patients. Only one patient died (of myocardial infarction) in the ALS group (mortality 3%), but 4 of 20 patients in the steroid-only group died (mortality 20%), mainly from sepsis.

Of 10 patients given 10 doses of ATG, 6 had second rejections, 4 of which were reversed with further use of ALS. No patient in this group lost a graft with the first rejection, and only 2 patients lost a graft with subsequent rejection. Of 22 patients who received ALS for longer periods of time (15–21 doses), 5 lost their grafts with first rejections. Of the remaining 17 patients only 5 had subsequent rejections, 3 of which were successfully reversed with further use of ATG. Of the control (steroid-only) patients, 5 of 20 lost grafts to the first rejection; 12 of the remaining 15 had second rejections, 8 of which were reversed. Second rejections, when they occurred, came much later in the ALS group (average 57.2 days, range 30–141 days) versus 28.3 days average in the control group (range 19–51 days).

Biopsy studies, although incomplete, suggested that the aforementioned patients in whom ALS treatment failed exhibited a significant degree of humoral rejection. These authors concluded that in a randomized controlled study in cadaveric renal allograft recipients, ATG treatment of first and subsequent rejections combined with a standard rejection protocol of high-dose steroids helps to rapidly reverse cellular rejection, decreases the incidence of second rejections when used for 21 days, and increases renal allograft functional survival at 6 months and 1 year by approximately 20% compared with control groups given only standard high-dose steroid rejection therapy.

Filo and colleagues[26] studied the addition of ATG with high-dose steroids for primary allograft rejection (cadaveric and living-related kidney recipients vs. standard antirejection therapy of high-dose steroids). Thus, patients on maintenance Imuran and prednisone who sustained rejection reactions were given ATG (10 mg/kg–15 mg/kg for 15 days) and intravenous (IV) methyl prednisone (30 mg/kg IV every other day for up to 5 days) or increased steroids alone. In cadaveric recipients, 91% of ALS-treated patients had reversal of rejection, whereas only 62% of steroid-treated patients reversed. Likewise, 92% of living-related first rejections reversed with ATG, but only 78% reversed with steroids. The combined results for first rejections was 91% for ATG-treated patients and 67% for steroid-treated patients. When recovery of first rejections occurred, there was no difference in the level of renal function attained by either treatment group. There were, however, no statistically significant differences found for any of these parameters between the two treatment groups for second and third rejections.

Long-term analysis of results showed that ATG-treated patients had superior functional graft survival compared with that of steroid-only–treated patients at 1, 12, 24, and 36 months post-transplantation ($p = < 0.005$), with living-related functional graft survival at 12 months being 74% for ATG treatment versus 63% for steroid-only treatment. Likewise, 67% of ATG-treated cadaveric grafts survived versus 49% of steroid-only–treated grafts. The combined results of living-related and cadaveric transplant recipients showed that an increment of 18.6% functional graft survival was conferred by ATG therapy and that this difference was highly significant at all intervals tested. This was accomplished with only a minimal mortality rate (3%).

The authors concluded that ATG used as an additional agent for rejection along with steroids, compared with steroids alone, produced faster reversal of rejection reactions and was associated with a higher functional graft survival of those kidneys that sustained a rejection reaction (91% vs. 67%). Although ATG did not result in fewer subsequent rejection episodes than standard steroids in this study, long-term survival rates remained significantly higher for the ATG group over the entire 3-year period of the study. The authors also made the interesting observation that even when graft rejection was severe enough to require dialysis—a bad prognostic sign when only high-dose steroids were used—ATG treatment resulted in reversal of rejec-

tion in 70% of such patients. Their finding that ATG failed to influence the incidence of subsequent rejection reactions was at variance with the findings of Nowygrod and associates.[75] This might have been due to the shorter course of ATG therapy used by Filo and colleagues.[26] Nevertheless, long-term survival remained superior for the ATG-treated group. Filo and colleagues' study also emphasized that failure of control of the first rejection episode was the most important factor in long-term allograft survival, because there was a much smaller attrition rate of allografts with subsequent rejections, even when only standard steroid therapy was used successfully.

Howard and associates[38] successfully used a horse antilymphoblast IgG along with high-dose steroids for the treatment of acute rejection. Thirty-three recipients of living-related or cadaveric grafts who experienced their first primary allograft rejection were randomized to a test group given high-dose oral prednisone plus ALG in contrast to a control group given prednisone and a placebo of normal horse IgG. Twenty-four of 33 ALS patients returned to base line creatinine levels within 30 days as opposed to 13 of 31 control patients; significantly, all ALG patients had an initial response to ALG. The number of patients returning to pre-rejection creatinine levels and the number of patients reversing the rejection episode were significantly higher in the ALG groups than in the IgG group ($p < 0.05$). Fewer of the patients in the ALG group (12 of 33 patients) had second rejections than did those in the IgG group (18 of 31 patients; $p < 0.05$). Graft survival was significantly better for the ALG group (82%) than for the IgG group (61%) at 12 months. Fifteen of 20 (75%) cadaver recipients and 12 of 13 (92%) recipients of related grafts in the ALG group had grafts still present at the end of the study. In contrast, only 12 of 18 cadaver recipients (60%) and 7 of 13 (54%) recipients of related grafts in the IgG group retained their kidneys. Patient survival in the ALG group (88%) and in the IgG group (87%) did not differ.

Use of ALG in Steroid-Resistant Rejection

Light and associates[54] extended the use of ALG for rejection to those cases that had resisted initial treatment with steroids. They studied 17 patients who had first rejections. Nine patients reversed rejection reactions following steroid pulses; however, 8 of 9 of these patients had a second rejection, with a mean time of 31 days. None of these 8 patients responded to steroid therapy and irradiation, and 5 patients received ALS at intervals between 20 and 50 days post-transplantation. Four of these 5 patients reversed rejection and went on to long-term functional graft survival; the fifth patient lost the transplant to chronic rejection. The primary rejection episode of the other 8 patients failed to respond to steroid therapy; 6 of these 8 patients received ALS, and 5 responded well with long-term survival. These authors noted that monitoring of rosette-forming cells for ATG dosage did not correlate well with effectiveness; indeed, they believed that reduction of ATG dose because of a low number of rosettes contributed to the failure of ATG in those few cases in which it failed. They noted that the rejection episodes for which ALG was given and was successful were more severe by various criteria than those that responded to steroids alone. In summary, their study showed that only 1 of 17 patients who received steroids alone for rejection reversal had successful long-term graft function; in contrast, 9 of 11 patients who received ALG therapy for graft rejection reversal had successful long-term function. The authors also concluded that ALG therapy was associated with more rapid rejection reversal, an earlier return of serum creatinine to base line, and fewer second rejection reactions when compared with the group of patients with rejection reactions who responded to steroids alone. They believed that ALG was effective in reversing rejection in all patients in whom an adequate dose could be given (minimum amount was probably seven or more daily doses). They emphasized that ALG was particularly effective for severe rejection reactions and should be used for all patients in whom the serum creatinine during the rejection was 3.5 mg or more. Hardy and associates[35] and Streem and colleagues[91] also reported effectiveness of ALG in treating steroid-resistant renal allograft rejection.

Use of ALG as the Sole Treatment for Renal Allograft Rejection

Hoitsma and colleagues[37] studied the effect of rabbit ATG in the treatment of acute rejection of cadaveric kidney transplants. Twenty-eight of 68 cadaveric recipients never rejected and served as a nonrejecting control. The remaining 40 patients were subjected to a prospective, randomized, single-blind trial in which the effect of rabbit ATG, given for 21 days IV in doses to maintain rosette-forming cells between 50 and 150 rosettes/mm^3 without elevation of maintenance steroids, was compared to treatment with high-dose oral prednisone alone. In the ATG group, 15 of 20 patients responded to treatment, and one patient of these lost the kidney to technical failure. In five patients, the rejection was irreversible, despite a subsequent course of high-dose oral prednisone. In the group treated only with prednisone, 13 of 20 patients responded, but 3 of these patients responded only after ATG was also insti-

tuted. The remaining 7 patients underwent transplant nephrectomy before a course of ATG could be given.

Renal function was similar at 6 months in both groups, but fewer infections occurred in the ATG group. The authors concluded that treatment of acute rejections in cadaveric transplant recipients with rabbit ATG was highly efficacious and safe and definitely steroid sparing.

Similarly, Toledo–Pereyra and associates[97] and Streem and colleagues[90] confirmed that ALG or ATG can be used as the sole adjunctive measure to treat acute renal allograft rejection with both immunologic efficacy and steroid-sparing benefits.

Subsequently, Novick and associates[73] reported on their extended experience using ATG only for primary rejection treatment. They used ALG alone (n = 27) versus IV methyl prednisolone (n = 41) as initial antirejection therapy in 68 cadaver transplants. All patients received a maintenance program of prednisone and azathioprine along with an initial prophylactic 2-week course of ALG. Reversal of rejection occurred in 27 (100%) of the ALG-treated patients and in 36 (88%) of IV steroid-treated patients. Subsequent rejections occurred in 11 (41%) of ALG-treated patients and 19 (53%) of steroid-treated patients. One-year graft survival with ALG was 85%; with steroids it was 66%.

In summary, the aforementioned studies show that ATG treatment is extremely effective for the treatment of acute allograft rejection for both living-related and cadaveric kidneys. ATG therapy for rejection is associated with better long-term functional graft survival than standard rejection therapy. Most important, it is effective as either adjunctive therapy or as separate therapy or as sequential therapy (e.g., for steroid-resistant rejections). Reversal of rejection occurs more frequently, more rapidly, and more completely with ALG therapy. More severe rejection episodes, as defined by whatever criteria, respond better if ATG is added to the rejection treatment regimen. Second rejection episodes are usually less frequent after ATG therapy. Most significant is the repeated observation that ATG can be given safely and often effectively for two or three courses. Patient survival is probably the same whether ATG therapy is added or not added to standardized rejection therapies.

Use of ALG, ATG with Cyclosporine

Use of ALG Prior to Institution of CyA Therapy

Cyclosporine is an excellent maintenance immunosuppressive drug. There is experimental evidence that cyclosporine should be started at the time that antigen is introduced, that is, at transplantation.[40] However, the primary nephrotoxic effect of cyclosporine is well known. The damaging effects of cyclosporine were noted early after its introduction by Calne and associates,[8] who found post-transplantation oliguria in 11 of 32 patients given CyA. They attributed this to its inherent nephrotoxicity and advised not starting CyA until an initial diuresis was underway. Likewise, the Canada Multicenter trial[89] showed that primary cadaver renal allograft survival was impaired if CyA was given to recipients of kidneys preserved for more than 24 hours or with a revascularization time of more than 45 minutes. The control group given azathioprine did not show this effect. Another study[76] identified significantly better allograft survival with CyA treatment versus conventional immunosuppression when renal preservation time was less than 36 hours. In contrast, when preservation time was greater than 36 hours, graft survival with CyA treatment was markedly reduced and was no better than that achieved with conventional therapy.

These observations emphasize that the newly transplanted kidney subjected to ischemic insult from the trauma of prolonged harvest or excessive preservation is unusually susceptible to the nephrotoxic effects of CyA. Indeed, although this kind of temporary ischemic insult can frequently be well tolerated with complete recovery, addition of CyA can lead to serious and permanent damage, which may result in diminished overall survival frequently following a high incidence of primary nonfunction.[72] Experimental studies in the rat have shown that the combination of cyclosporine plus ischemia is much more damaging to renal function than is ischemia alone.[42]

Attempts to minimize CyA nephrotoxicity have involved use of CyA at lower doses at the time of transplantation or withholding CyA until adequate renal function has occurred. In both instances, it is now common to use multiple drug therapy combinations, including ALG prior to the introduction of CyA. Ferguson[25] reported a series of 170 cadaveric grafts treated initially with prednisone, azathioprine, and ALG. When adequate renal function was apparent, cyclosporine was substituted for prednisone and azathioprine. Despite the fact that CyA was not given initially during the antigen presentation and recognition phases of the allograft response, only 28% of recipients sustained acute rejection episodes. The incidence of CMV infections was only 4%. Patient and graft actuarial 1-year survival rates were 97% and 82%, respectively.

Many other transplant surgeons (including the author) prefer to treat initially with prednisone, azathioprine, and ALG. Then, when adequate renal function appears, CyA is started, usually at somewhat lower doses. ALG is usually continued for a specified overlap period after starting CyA (usually 3 days). Thereafter, the patient may be continued on maintenance prednisone, azathioprine, and CyA. The Minnesota group has recently reported that they restrict the use of ALG in this protocol to a maximum of 10 days because of a higher incidence of CMV and herpes infections after institution of CyA therapy.[85]

Use of ALG to Treat Steroid-Resistant Rejection in CyA-Treated Patients

Most transplant surgeons treat acute rejection in CyA patients with steroid pulses with excellent results. ALG can be used effectively to treat steroid-resistant rejections in patients receiving CyA. Matas' group[58] used ALG to treat 17 episodes of early steroid-resistant rejection in the setting of discontinuation of CyA therapy during administration of the ALG. Rejection was reversed in 11 of 17 episodes (64%).

Use of ALG in Multidrug Therapy of Nonrenal Organ Allografts

ALG has also been used extensively as part of multidrug therapy in nonrenal allografts, most all of which are treated with CyA and prednisone and/or azathioprine. With liver allografts, it is frequently used as a prophylactic adjunctive drug during periods of renal dysfunction associated with hepatic allografting. In cardiac transplantation, it is frequently added at some time shortly after transplantation when cardiac transplant biopsies suggest rejection activity or when steroid sparing is desired.

Clinical Toxicity of ALG

One of the most surprising observations of the aforementioned studies is the remarkable lack of toxicity associated with ATG therapy. The severe side effects of allergic reactions, anaphylaxis, superinfection, and tissue destruction predicted to be present after this therapy have not materialized. Cosimi[15] provided a summary of the toxic effects, which also reflects the experience of other investigators. He described a situation in which 135 patients were given more than 2500 doses of ATG, 20 patients had two or three courses of ATG. Patients were first skin tested with appropriate dilutions of ATG prior to infusion. Interestingly, they did not report any incidence of sensitization that would have prevented ATG administration.

This author has never had to exclude a patient from ATG treatment because of skin or conjunctival sensitization in dealing with more than 300 patients treated with this agent. On the other hand, Filo and associates[26,27] reported five exclusions after skin testing in 41 patients selected for ATG therapy. Cosimi[15] noted that the most common immediate side effect associated with ALG infusion has been the development of chills and fever, occurring after 15% to 20% of all infusions. Chills and fever can occur repeatedly after each infusion in an individual patient or it may occur only the first few times or even late in the course of therapy, after many previous benign infusions. Fever may be either low-grade or quite high. Invariably, these side effects are controlled by antipyretics and antihistamines. Slowing the rate of ALG infusion in a patient with these symptoms can also render subsequent infusions tolerable and without incident. Intermittent skin rashes with or without pruritus is the second most common toxic effect, occurring in 15% to 18% of patients. Rarely, serum sickness symptoms of joint pain, with or without swelling, have occurred. These symptoms subside with termination of ALG. True anaphylaxis has been rare but has occurred. Leukopenia (< 5000 WBC/mn) and thrombocytopenia (< 100,000 platelets/mn) occur in approximately 10% of treated patients. These side effects respond to delay in treatment or reduction in ALG dose. Neither bleeding secondary to ALG-induced thrombocytopenia nor ALG-induced hemolysis has been reported.

As previously mentioned, there has been no significant increase in bacterial sepsis associated with ALG therapy. However, Cheeseman and associates[13] showed that ATG therapy had an adverse effect on the clinical course of cytomegalovirus (CMV) infection in renal transplant patients, increasing the incidence of viremia and clinical illness attributable to CMV and attenuating the beneficial effects of a prophylactic course of human leukocyte interferon. This was observed when ATG therapy was combined with a standard course of Imuran and prednisone. In an attempt to alleviate this problem, Rubin and associates[82] studied the effect on the incidence of CMV viremia and clinical syndromes in transplant recipients given a standard course of immunosuppressive therapy versus the incidence in patients given 50% of the standard Imuran and prednisone dose plus a course of the ATG. In contrast to previous studies, they found that the incidence of CMV infections was the same in both groups. Thus, even though the study groups were biased against the ATG groups by containing a greater number of cadaveric kidney recipients, a

population at greater risk for serious CMV disease than recipients of kidney from living-related donors, there was no increase in the incidence of CMV viremia or CMV–related clinical disease. Furthermore, these results were achieved without any sacrifice in graft survival, as the 1-year graft survival after cadaveric donor transplantation continued to be 70%, compatible with that achieved with previous ATG protocols with full regimens of Imuran and prednisone.

Similarly, Pass and colleagues[77,78] reported a higher incidence of symptomatic CMV reactivation and viremia in patients receiving high-dose as opposed to low-dose ATG in addition to conventional immunosuppression. Although unsubstantiated as yet in the literature, it is the general belief that ATG-treated patients also have a higher incidence of herpes zoster infection than do patients given conventional immunosuppression alone.

The high incidence of spontaneous neoplasms, especially malignancies of the skin, cervix, and lymphatic organs, in immunosuppressed post-transplantation patients is well established.[79] There have been isolated reports of spontaneous lymphomas at the site of ALG intramuscular injection. Nevertheless, critical analysis of the incidence of all spontaneous malignancies in post-transplantation patients has shown no increased incidence of spontaneous malignancy in ALG-treated patients over that seen in transplantation patients given conventional immunosuppression.

Thus, fairly large experience has shown that significant clinical toxicity from ALG therapy has very rarely occurred. Chills, fever, rash, and/or pruritis occur in approximately 15% of patients, but they are relatively easy to manage and do not preclude therapy. Leukopenia and thrombocytopenia occur in 10% of patients but only rarely interrupt therapy for prolonged periods. Serum sickness is uncommon and anaphylaxis is rare.

Mortality is not increased with ALG, nor is bacterial sepsis or tumor incidence. Although there is an increased incidence and severity of CMV infection in ALG-treated patients, this can be alleviated by reduction in the other immunosuppressive agents.

MONOCLONAL ANTIBODIES

Definition

When a foreign substance enters the body of a vertebrate animal or is injected into it, a complex immune response is initiated. One aspect of most immune responses is the secretion of antibodies by plasma cells. These immunoglobulin molecules have combining sites that recognize the shape and configuration of various determinants on the surface of the foreign substance or antigen in question. The combination of antibodies with these antigenic determinants frequently results in inactivation, destruction, and/or elimination of the foreign substance from the animal's body.

Characteristically, the antibody response to most antigens is extremely heterogeneous. There are perhaps millions of different B-lymphocytes, the precursors of plasma cells (mature antibody-forming cells) in the spleens (and other lymphoid tissues) of mice and humans. Although all different B-lymphocytes are derived from a common stem cell, each line develops an independent capacity to make an antibody that recognizes a different antigenic determinant.

When an immunizing antigen is introduced into an animal, the animal responds by making diverse antibodies detected against different antigenic molecules in the foreign substance, different determinants on a single antigen, and even different antibodies that fit more or less well with a single determinant. Thus, the total response to a foreign substance contains many antibodies. Thus, the total response to a foreign substance contains many antibodies. It is almost impossible to separate the different types of antibody from a serum prepared in response to a complex foreign antigen. Thus, conventional antisera are therefore polyclonal in nature. Additional variability also occurs, since responses vary at different times in the same animal and from animal to animal.

Since each specific antibody is made by a different line of lymphocytes and newly derived plasma cells, one way to achieve a pure antibody preparation is to isolate the lymphocyte secreting the single specific antibody and grow it in long-term tissue culture. The single cell's progeny or clone, therefore, would continually secrete large amounts of identical antibody against a single specific antigenic determinant. Therefore, it would be a monoclonal antibody. Unfortunately, antibody-producing cells cannot be maintained in long-term tissue culture medium. There are, however, certain malignant tumors of the immune system (i.e., myelomas) that produce large amounts of abnormal immunoglobulins (myeloma proteins). Such myeloma tumors are essentially an immortal clone of cells descendent from a single progenitor cell; thus, they can be cultured indefinitely, and all the immunoglobulins that they secrete are identical in chemical structure. They are, in fact, monoclonal antibodies, although one cannot define what antigen they are directed against, and they cannot be induced to make a specific antibody.

In 1975, however, Kohler and Milstein[45] developed a method to fuse mouse myeloma cells with lymphocytes from mice immunized to a particular antigen. The resulting hybrid myeloma, or hybridoma, cells express both the lymphocyte's property of specific-antibody production and the immortal characteristics of the myeloma cells. They can be maintained and manipulated in tissue culture. Individual hybridomas can be cloned, and each derived clone member produces large amounts of identical antibody to a single antigenic determinant. The individual clones can be maintained indefinitely, and, at any time, samples can be grown in culture or injected into animals for large-scale monoclonal antibody production.

Preparation of Monoclonal Antibodies

The basic step in monoclonal antibody production is begun when a recipient animal (usually mice) is immunized with an immunizing antigen (Fig. 5-1). Antibody-producing B cells from the spleen or other lymphatic organs are harvested. These cells are mixed with mouse myeloma cells in a medium (polyethylene glycol) that promotes fusion. The fused cells are then transferred to another medium containing hypoxanthine, aminopterin, and thymidine (HAT) in which only the spleen–myeloma hybrids survive. This is due to the fact that only spleen–myeloma hybridomas can grow in the HAT–containing medium. The individual spleen–myeloma hybridomas are then assayed individually for the specific antibody that one is trying to produce.

Hybridomas producing extraneous antibody are discarded, and specific antibody–producing hybridomas are selected and cloned. Cloned hybridomas can be reassayed for specificity and recloned; they can be frozen for future use. Alternatively, they can be cultured in tissue culture for further antibody production or injected into peritoneal cavities of mice as in vivo ascites forming cultures in which antibody production is amplified and from which ascites fluid containing specific antibody can be obtained and isolated.

Kohler and Milstein[45] have provided a method to achieve an almost immortal cellular factory to produce enormous quantities of specific antibodies manufactured by one cell and its cloned descendents on demand and indefinitely. Since the antibody comes from one cell, it is homogeneous and always the same, with constant defined specificity, isotype, and function. Monoclonal antibodies so produced

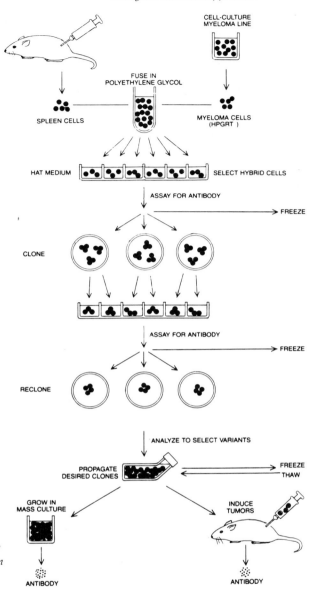

FIGURE 5-1.   Standard procedure for deriving monoclonal antibodies (see text). (From Kohler G, Milstein C: Derivation of specific antibody-producing tissue culture and tumor lines by cell fusion. Eur J Immunol 6:511–519, 1976.)

have the molecular purity and constancy comparable to that of cloned gene products or synthesized manufactured drugs.

Orthoclone OKT3 Monoclonal Antibody

Although several experimental preparations of monoclonal antibodies have been studied and tested for use in organ transplantation,[16,44,92] at the present time, there is only one monoclonal antibody licensed for use in clinical organ transplantation. This is the murine monoclonal antibody, Orthoclone

OKT3 (muromonab-CD3), developed by Gideon Goldstein and associates of the Ortho Pharmaceutical Corporation.[48]

Description

Orthoclone OKT3 (muromonab-CD3) is a murine monoclonal antibody produced according to the technique just described. Human T cells were used to immunize mice, and a hybridoma-producing specific antibody to the T3 (CD3) antigen, which is present on all mature human T-lymphocytes, was isolated and cloned. The antibody is a biochemically purified IgG^{2a} immunoglobulin with a heavy chain of approximately 50,000 daltons and a light chain of approximately 25,000 daltons. It is specifically directed to a glycoprotein with a molecular weight of 20,000 in the human T cell surface, which is essential for T cell functions and is closely associated with the antigenic recognition structure of human T cells.

The proper name for Orthoclone OKT3, muromonab-CD3, is derived from the descriptive term *murine monoclonal antibody*. The CD3 designation identifies the specificity of the antibody as the cell differentiation (CD) cluster 3 defined by the First International Workshop on Human Leukocyte Differentiation Antigens.[71] Since Orthoclone OKT3 is a monoclonal antibody, it is a homogeneous, reproducible antibody product with consistent measurable reactivity to human T cells. The details of the OKT3–producing hybridoma, the characterization of the OKT3 IgG^{2a} antibody, and its preparation as a sterile pyrogen-free solution for parental dosage by weight of immunoglobulin have been described elsewhere.[30,48]

Mechanism of Action In Vitro

The involvement of human T cells in human allograft rejection is well established. T cells recognize the foreignness of allografts by antigen recognition structures on their cell surface.[3,55] This antigen recognition structure is a disulfide-linked heterodimer consisting of two glycosulated polypeptide chains. OKT3 specifically recognizes one of the three associated polypeptide chains in the T3 (CD3) complex (Fig. 5-2).[11,55,99] After the T cell has recognized antigen, the T3 complex transmits an intracellular signal.[39]

In vitro OKT3 reacts with the 20,000 dalton

(CD3) molecule in the human T cell membrane and blocks antigen recognition and signal transduction. In in vitro cytolytic studies, OKT3 blocks both generation and function of effector cells.[56–58] In vitro studies reveal that concentrations of 1000 ng/ml are sufficient to block killing of specific targets by cytotoxic T3$^+$ cells. OKT3 is also a potent mitogen in calf serum, but mitogenicity is markedly reduced in human serum.

In Vivo Action and Clinical Pharmacology

Serum levels of OKT3 are measured by using an enzyme-linked immunosorbent assay (ELISA). After a single intravenous bolus of OKT3 (5 mg), there is a rapid achievement of mean plasma levels of 1002 ng/ml at 1 hour, which decline to 104 ng/ml at 24 hours. During treatment with the usual daily dose of 5 mg/ml, mean serum trough levels of the drug rise over the first 3 days and then average 0.9 mg/ml on Days 3 to 14. These levels obtained on daily IV therapy are those shown to block T cell effector functions in vitro.

In vivo, OKT3 reacts with most peripheral blood T cells, but it has not been found to react with other hemotopoietic elements or other tissues of the body. Following a single IV 5-mg dose of OKT3 in humans, there is a rapid and concomitant decrease in the number of circulating T3 (CD3) positive, T4 (CD4) positive, and T8 (CD8) positive T cells. With continued daily IV dosage of OKT3, CD3 positive cells usually remain undetectable, although between Days 2 and 7, increasing numbers of CD4 and CD8 positive cells have been observed despite continued OKT3 administration. Appearance of CD4 and CD8 positive cells has not been associated with diminished clinical effectiveness.

The binding of OKT3 with CD3 positive cells

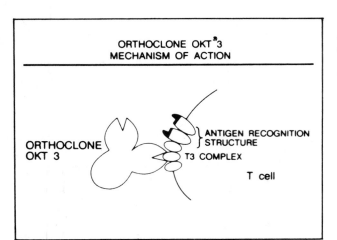

FIGURE 5-2.   *OKT3 reacts with the T3 (CD3) antigen on human T-lymphocytes, effectively blocking the function of the T3 molecule in the membrane of human T cells. (Courtesy of G. Goldstein; reprinted with permission from Dialysis and Transplantation, Volume 15, Number 12, December 1986.)*

in the circulation and their subsequent opsonization and elimination by way of the reticuloendothelial system is probably the primary mechanism of removal of CD3 positive cells from the circulation. As previously stated, this mechanism becomes saturated during repeated injection of OKT3, so that near steady state 24-hour serum trough levels (902 ng/ml) after the third daily dose approximate the levels required to block T cell function in vitro. In addition, CD3 positive cells reappear rapidly and reach pretreatment levels within a week following termination of OKT3 therapy. This finding and the appearance of CD4 and CD8 positive cells in the absence of detectable CD3 positive cells during OKT3 therapy suggest that modulation of the surface T3 (CD3) antigen is another mechanism by which OKT3 exerts its in vivo effect.[12,29] A third mechanism of action may involve the blocking of T cell function by OKT3 antibody without the modulation or opsonization mechanisms being involved.

Antibody Response to OKT3

When OKT3 is administered in conjunction with low-dose prednisone and Imuran during treatment of acute renal allograft rejection, the majority of treated patients make some type of antibody to mouse globulins, usually beginning after 10 days of therapy, when the OKT3 therapy is being discontinued. Indeed, increasing numbers of CD3 positive cells have been observed in some patients during the second week of daily OKT3 therapy, possibly as a result of the development of neutralizing antibodies to OKT3. IgM antibodies occurred with an incidence of 21%, IgG antibodies with an incidence of 80%, and IgE antibodies with an incidence of 29%. The mean time of appearance of IgG antibodies was approximately 3 weeks (20 ± 2 days). Early IgG antibodies occurred at the end of the second week of therapy in 3% of patients.

Studies have been carried out to identify allotypic, isotypic, and anti-idiotypic antibodies, that is, antibodies that were made specifically against the OKT3 variable region. Most patients had anti-idiotypic antibody in the presence of other types of antibody. It should be noted that when OKT3 was given as a sole immunosuppressive agent with no prednisone and Imuran by Kreis and colleagues,[46] rejection reactions occurred, and continued administration was limited by development of host antibodies in most patients. With the addition of prednisone and Imuran, antibody formation was reduced, and administration could be continued for 30 days.

In most studies using OKT3 to treat rejection, the appearance of antibody prevents further useful therapy because there is immune elimination of the OKT3; thus, therapeutic serum levels have not been able to be maintained. Interestingly, when OKT3 is administered in the presence of anti-OKT3 antibody, significant allergic or anaphylactic reactions do not occur, but therapeutic effect, especially in experimental animals, has been lost. For this reason, treatment schedules have usually been limited to one treatment program. Addition of Cytoxan as OKT3 was being discontinued reduced the number of patients making an antibody response from 75% to 80% down to 35% to 40%. Several centers have reported a few instances of retreatment with OKT3, either after the antibody levels formed in response to the first course have become undetectable or when they are still present. Reversal of rejection in these circumstances has been alleged to have occurred in isolated cases. Most important, there have been no instances of allergic or anaphylactic responses in these limited number of cases. The usefulness of retreatment with OKT3 for recurrent rejection remains undefined, although immune elimination of the OKT3 will probably render this form of treatment relatively ineffective. However, monitoring the appearance and presence of CD3 positive cells and the amount and type of anti-OKT3 antibody formed should permit determination of the pharmacologic effectiveness of continued administration or readministration of OKT3.

Clinical Administration

At the present time, OKT3 monoclonal antibody has been documented to be effective in reversing acute renal allograft rejection. It has also been effective in reversing hepatic and cardiac allograft rejection.

Dosage and Administration. Orthoclone OKT3 is supplied as a sterile solution in 5-ml ampules containing 1 mg/ml anti-T3 (CD3) monoclonal antibody. It is given by IV administration only. The material is stable between 2°C and 8°C for over 1 year. The usual treatment course is 5 mg OKT3 administered as a daily IV bolus injection for 10 to 14 days. Treatment should begin as soon as allograft rejection is diagnosed, although appropriate preparation of the patient (fluid overload) must be considered. As previously mentioned, treatment schedules are suggested as a one-time treatment course only, but good results with retreatment and with extended treatment schedules with appropriate monitoring of CD3 circulating cells have been reported. Patients should be monitored carefully, particularly during the first 48 hours of treatment for adverse reaction.

Intravenous methyl prednisolone (1.0 mg/kg)

given prior to Orthoclone OKT3 administration and IV hydrocortisone (100 mg) given 30 minutes post OKT3 administration are strongly recommended to decrease the incidence of reactions to the first dose. Acetaminophen and antihistamines can be given concomitantly with OKT3 to reduce early reactions (Table 5-1).

In general, it has been the practice to lower conventional immunosuppressive therapy (prednisone and Imuran) during OKT3 administration. Maintenance immunosuppression is usually resumed to previous pre-rejection levels approximately 3 days prior to cessation of OKT3 therapy. Although this was the general protocol of administration in the initial trials of OKT3, there is not total consensus that this is the optimal method of treatment. Many investigators now believe that maintenance immunosuppression should not be reduced during OKT3 therapy for bouts of rejection. Indeed some believe that the incidence of recurrent rejection (see below) is reduced if maintenance immunosuppression is not lowered during OKT3 therapy. In patients undergoing OKT3 treatment for rejection while on cyclosporine, the cyclosporine dose may be maintained, lowered transiently, or discontinued temporarily. To date, no drug interactions have been observed with all the other drugs commonly taken by transplant patients that would alter the efficacy or safety of OKT3. An important attraction of OKT3 is daily simplicity of administration. With polyclonal ALG or ATG preparations, administration usually requires an indwelling IV catheter in a high-flow venous tributary, frequently in a hospitalized setting. In contrast, OKT3 is administered by rapid IV push, usually into an antecubital vein. The first few doses are usually given in the hospital, but, thereafter, once initial adverse reactions have

occurred (first few days), it can easily be administered on a daily outpatient basis.

Clinical Safety and Adverse Reactions.   After the first and/or second dose of OKT3, there are usually a number of acceptable adverse reactions that are predictable and manageable. These first-dose adverse reactions are attributable to release of mediators from the opsonization of T3 positive cells by OKT3 and their subsequent removal by the reticuloendothelial system. Adverse reactions do not prevent subsequent OKT3 administration. The most common early adverse reaction is a self-limited acute febrile syndrome consisting of pyrexia, chills, and tremor, occurring in varying degree in more than 90% of the patient (see Table 5-1). Respiratory symptoms such as dyspnea, chest pain, and wheezing occur in less than 25% of patients, whereas gastrointestinal symptoms (e.g., diarrhea, nausea, rarely vomiting) occur in less than one third of patients.

A small number of patients evince some insignificant cardiovascular symptoms of fluid retention, hypotension, hypertension, and/or tachycardia. Likewise, less than 20% of patients show some evidence of transient leukopenia, headache, dizziness, and agitation. The very important complication of pulmonary edema was noted in 5 of the first 107 patients treated (4.7%). It was found that fluid overload seemed to predispose these patients to the development of pulmonary edema, with the respiratory responses associated with the first or second dose of OKT3. It was reasoned that pulmonary hemodynamic changes induced by released mediators resulted in development of acute pulmonary edema in patients with fluid overload. The protocol of administration was subsequently modified to include

TABLE 5-1   *Suggested Prevention and Treatment of Orthoclone OKT3 First Dose Effects*

ADVERSE REACTION	EFFECTIVE PREVENTION OR PALLIATION	SUPPORTIVE TREATMENT
1. Severe pulmonary edema	Clear chest x-ray within 24 hr preinjection	Prompt intubation and oxygenation
	Weight restriction to < 3% gain over 7 days preinjection	24 hr close observation
2. Fever, chills	1.0 mg/kg methylprednisolone sodium succinate preinjection	Cooling blanket
	Fever, reduction below 37.8°C (100°F) preinjection	Acetaminophen prn
3. Respiratory effects	100 mg hydrocortisone sodium succinate 30 min postinjection	Additional 10 mg hydrocortisone sodium succinate prn

a clear chest x-ray, no clinical signs of fluid overload, and a restriction of body weight gain to 3% of body weight from that of the week prior to OKT3 administration. With the introduction of these measures, there have been no instances of pulmonary edema post OKT3 administration.

OKT3 administration does not appear to increase the risk of infection over other antirejection protocols. In randomized multicenter trials, the evidence of infection was comparable in patients treated with OKT3 and in those treated with high-dose steroids. Likewise, there is no evidence that OKT3 therapy used as just described is associated with an increase in malignant complications post-transplantation.

Clinical Effectiveness of Orthoclone OKT3

OKT3 monoclonal antibody has been shown to be effective in modifying allograft rejection in a number of clinical organ graft situations.

Treatment of Acute Primary Cadaveric Renal Allograft Rejection. Goldstein and associates[30] reported use of Orthoclone OKT3 in 123 patients undergoing acute rejection in primary cadaveric renal allografts. Patients were treated with OKT3, 5 mg IV, daily for a mean period of 14 days, with simultaneous lowering of azathioprine and prednisone (63 patients) or with conventional high-dose steroid therapy (60 patients) (Fig. 5-3). Similar programs

FIGURE 5-3. *Plan of daily immunosuppressive drug regimens for patients randomly assigned to OKT3 or steroid treatment for acute renal-allograft rejection. During OKT3 treatment, dosages of steroids and azathioprine were reduced, with resumption of the prerejection dosage of steroids and azathioprine when OKT3 was discontinued. By contrast, steroid treatment alone involved a high steroid dosage, with maintenance of the azathioprine dosage (I.V. = intravenous). (From Goldstein G, Schindler J, Tsai H et al: A randomized clinical trial of OKT3 monoclonal antibody for acute rejection of cadaveric renal transplants. N Engl J Med 313:337–342, 1985; reprinted by permission of the New England Journal of Medicine.)*

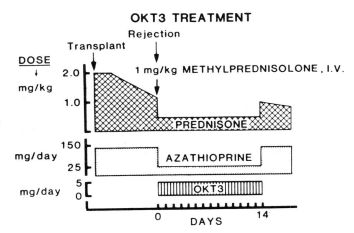

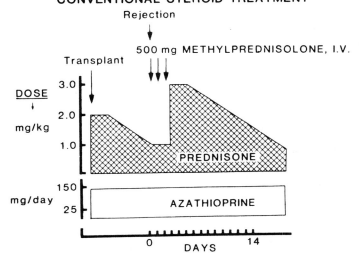

of maintenance immunosuppression of prednisone and azathioprine were given to both groups, and later recurrent rejection episodes were similarly treated with high-dose steroids or polyclonal anti-lymphocyte globulin. Reversal of rejection was significantly better in the OKT3-treated group (94%) versus that observed in the high-dose steroid-treated group (75%). Recurrent rejections were common in both groups—66% in patients initially given OKT3, and 73% in patients with initial high-dose steroid treatment. Percentage of subsequent loss of renal allografts to repeated rejection episodes was the same in both groups—33% in OKT3-treated patients, and 38% in high-dose steroid-treated patients. However, because of the initial higher rejection reversal rate, the OKT3-treated group had a higher 1-year survival rate than the primary steroid-treated group. It must be remembered that these are 1-year survival rates of patients who had undergone an initial rejection reaction. Furthermore, this was

accomplished with an overall reduced amount of conventional immunosuppression in the OKT3-treated group (Tables 5-2 and 5-3).

Treatment of Renal Allograft Rejection Unresponsive to Conventional Immunosuppressive Therapy. There has been extensive experience in the use of OKT3 in renal allografts in which rejection has been unresponsive to conventional immunosuppression or in which conventional therapy with high-dose steroid or polyclonal antisera was contraindicated or unavailable.[63] In short, these patients were treated with OKT3 for rejections for which no other effective therapy was available and in situations in which no further attempts to alter the course of rejection reaction could be made. Treatment was the same as treatment for primary graft rejection— 5 mg OKT3 daily IV push for 10 to 14 days.

This study was a noncontrolled, multicenter experience involving 173 patients who rejected ca-

TABLE 5-2   *Mean Cumulative Dosage of Immunosuppressive Medications Over the First 28 Days of Treatment for Patients Randomly Assigned to OKT3 or Steroids for Acute Renal Allograft Rejection*

MEDICATION	OKT3 (63 PATIENTS) Mean Cumulative Dosage	STEROIDS (60 PATIENTS) Mean Cumulative Dosage
	mg	mg
Prednisone	1218	2042
Methylprednisolone sodium succinate	965	2019
Azathioprine	1765	2711

(Revised from Goldstein G, Schindler J, Tsai H et al: A randomized clinical trial of OKT3 monoclonal antibody for acute rejection of cadaveric renal transplants. N Engl J Med 313:337–342, 1985; used by permission of the New England Journal of Medicine)

TABLE 5-3   *Efficacy of Treatment with OKT3 or Steroids for Acute Renal Allograft Rejection*

	OKT3	STEROIDS INCIDENCE (%)	p VALUE
Reversal of rejection			
Serum creatinine level alone	55/62 (89)	37/60 (62)	< 0.001
One-year follow-up			
Patient survival			
Actual	53/62 (85)	52/58*(90)	0.47(NS†)
Kidney survival			
Actual	36/53 (68)	25/52 (48)	0.029

* Two patients were lost to follow-up

† NS = not significant

(Revised from Goldstein G, Schindler J, Tsai H et al: A randomized clinical trial of OKT3 monoclonal antibody for acute rejection of cadaveric renal transplants. N Engl J Med 313:337–342, 1985; used by permission of the New England Journal of Medicine)

daver or living-related grafts (140 patients rejecting first grafts, 28 rejecting second grafts, 4 rejecting third grafts, and 1 rejecting fourth graft). Reversal was achieved in 49/66 (74%) of patients in whom increased steroids and polyclonal serum had failed, in 67/100 (67%) in whom increased steroids alone had failed, and 5/7 (71%) in whom polyclonal serum only had failed. Thus, reversal was achieved in 70% of patients, with no real difference regardless of what conventional immunosuppressive therapy had previously failed. Actuarial 6-month graft survival was 62% for all grafts treated. Considering that all the grafts in this study would probably have been rejected, that is, no further treatment would have been attempted if OKT3 were not available, this is an impressive result.

Gaber and colleagues[28] reported a smaller, single-center study that demonstrated more dramatically the effectiveness of OKT3 treatment for steroid-resistant renal allograft rejection. They used OKT3 to treat steroid-resistant rejection in patients who received ALG as part of their baseline treatment and were then maintained on various combinations of CyA, prednisone, and azathioprine. They treated 37 (65%) of 67 rejection episodes successfully with outpatient steroid boluses (5 mg/kg–10 mg/kg IV methyl prednisolone for 3 days). The remaining 20 steroid-resistant episodes were admitted and treated with OKT3 (5 mg IV for 10 days). Nineteen of 20 (95%) rejections were reversed by this program. The mean interval to reversal of steroid-resistant rejection was 6.7 days, which was longer than that seen when OKT3 was used for primary rejection treatment (3.2 days). Only 3 (16%) recurrent rejection episodes were encountered in the follow-up period (2–9 months).

This study admittedly limited, suggests that rapid introduction of OKT3 therapy after short-term steroid bolus treatment may be the most effective treatment for steroid-resistant rejection.

Use of OKT3 Monoclonal Antibody for Primary Hepatic Allograft Rejection.

OKT3 has been used successfully in a multi-institutional, randomized, prospective protocol, comparing it with conventional steroid treatment for primary hepatic allograft rejection.[17] All recipients initially received CsA and steroids post-transplantation. At the time of acute rejection, high-dose steroids were added. If after two steroid boluses (250 mg–1000 mg) biopsy-confirmed rejection was not reversed, the patients were randomly assigned to OKT3 or continued high-dose steroids. "Rescue" therapy with OKT3 (for the second group) or further conventional therapy (for the OKT3 group) was prescribed if the patient failed to respond. Twenty patients were randomized. Two of 10 patients in the steroid group responded and had continued good function. The remaining 8 patients required OKT3 rescue therapy. One patient failed to respond to OKT3 and died of hepatic failure; rejection was reversed in the remaining 7 patients.

In the OKT3 group, improved allograft function occurred in 9 of 10 patients in 72 hours. In 8 of 10 patients assigned to the OKT3 group, the original allograft was functional at 1 to 14 months following transplantation. The authors noted that although liver function and histologic appearance improved rapidly, serum bilirubin levels did not always return to normal following OKT3 therapy. They documented failure to clear OKT3-coated lymphocytes from the circulation in these patients, suggesting that this mechanism of OKT3 suppression might be impaired in these patients.

Treatment of Rejection of Extrarenal Organ Allografts not Responsive to Conventional Immunosuppressive Therapy.

OKT3 has been useful in rescuing patients undergoing rejection of liver and heart allografts unresponsive to various conventional immunosuppressive treatments and in patients in whom reversal of such rejection constituted a lifesaving measure. Starzl's group[88] has accumulated data in patients requiring OKT3 rescue therapy at various times after liver transplantation. Group I patients were treated 2 to 9 days post-transplantation; Group II, 10 to 90 days after transplantation; and Group III over 90 days post-transplantation, with a median in the latter group of 230 days. These patients were evaluated for the cause of hepatic dysfunction post-transplantation including biopsy when possible. If technical causes could be ruled out, they were treated with a recycle of steroids. If they failed to respond to steroids, OKT3 was started as described above in rescue therapy for rejecting renal allografts.

Overall, with a 1-year follow-up, 22% of patients had no response, approximately 1 of 4 had a partial response, and over half had a complete response. The best responses were seen in patients in Group II with a high incidence of biopsy-proven cell-mediated rejection; here fewer than 1 in 10 did not respond. Results were good but less dramatic in Group III, probably because of a high incidence of chronic rejection. Group I had a response rate in approximately two thirds of patients; these patients tended to be much sicker and have more aggressive cellular rejection. Use of OKT3 in this group significantly reduced early post-transplantation mortality and facilitated enhanced long-term survival. The number of recurrent rejection reactions in OKT3 liver transplant recipients followed for more than 1 year post therapy have been lower than with OKT3-treated kidney transplant recipients, that is, about 20%. Starzl and colleagues[88] concluded that OKT3 has made a significant contribution to increasing survival post liver transplantation and reducing the necessity for liver allograft retransplantation. A limited experience has also been achieved with acute cardiac allograft rejection. Early trials have shown that in the limited instances in which OKT3 has been used for rescue, a significant number of cardiac allografts have been rescued.

Use of OKT3 Monoclonal Antibody Prophylactically in Renal Allograft Rejection.

At the present time, studies are underway to determine the efficacy of prophylactic use of OKT3 monoclonal antibody in both renal and hepatic transplantation. The most common period for serious acute rejection of both organs is in the first 30 days. It will be of interest if prophylactic OKT3 in association with other conventional immunosuppressive agents can significantly prevent early rejection and lead to improved patient and graft survival. An alternative goal is achieving the equally good patient and graft survival with reduced steroids and/or eliminating the need for cyclosporine.

Kreis and colleagues[46,47] demonstrated that OKT3 alone cannot be used as a prophylactic immunosuppressive agent. They randomized 13 patients to azathioprine and high-dose steroids (7 patients) versus OKT3 alone (6 patients). All OKT3-treated patients had rejection episodes necessitating introduction of steroids within 2 weeks of transplantation (12.8 ± 2.9 days). Rejection was related to appearance of anti-OKT3 antibodies leading to disappearance of detectable OKT3 in the serum. Thus, in the patient not receiving any other concomitant immunosuppression, OKT3 is highly immunogenic, thus restricting the effectiveness of this type of protocol.

Future Considerations Relative to the Use of Monoclonal Antibodies for Immunosuppression

The T3 (CD3) antigen is common to all mature T cells, that is, helper/inducer, suppressor/cytotoxic subclasses. Ideally one would like to inactivate and/or eliminate helper/inducer cells, sparing suppressor cells and eliminating cytotoxic T cells. It is hoped that future monoclonal antibodies will be directed to the specific subclass of lymphocytes involved in the destructive arm of the allograft rejection reaction while sparing the suppressor cells that may facilitate tolerance of the organ allograft.

MODULATION OF ALLOGRAFT REJECTION WITH DONOR-SPECIFIC ANTIGEN

Medawar and colleagues[4] were the first to demonstrate that donor-specific antigen itself could be used to attenuate or eliminate the allograft rejection reaction. In their classic studies, they injected living-replicating lymphoid cells into in utero or neonatal recipients—a time when the recipients were naturally immunosuppressed by virtue of their underdeveloped immune system. They demonstrated that such recipients were rendered specifically unresponsive to grafts from the lymphocyte donors as adults. This phenomenon was called *acquired immunologic tolerance.* These tolerant adults were lymphoid cell chimeras—they rejected third party grafts and could reject donor specific grafts if their immune system was reconstituted with adult syngeneic lymphoid cells that had not been exposed in utero to the donor antigens. The exact immunologic basis for the observation has not been completely defined. However, this experiment has served as an impetus that has persisted for decades to induce specific nonreactivity to tissue allografts without the use of chronically administered nonspecific immunosuppression.

It should be noted that Medawar and colleagues used F1 hybrid cells as the donor-specific inoculum to avoid graft-versus-host reactions that would have occurred when these immunologically competent cells were injected as homozygous allogeneic cells.

All attempts to translate Medawar's experiment to adult animals have been more or less based on the assumption that it must be done in immunologically mature adult animals if it is to be clinically useful. Therefore, almost all attempts to use donor-specific antigen to modulate the allograft response have used an initial period of transient nonspecific immunosuppression (to mimic the neonatal state) during which exposure to donor specific antigen was superimposed. Early studies utilized total body irradiation or chemotherapeutic drugs followed by various forms of donor antigen prior to or after a donor-specific test allograft, usually a skin graft. These early studies provided only minimal, augmented specific prolongation, most likely owing to the fact that the degree of transient immunosuppression was not very profound.

Definition of Specific Unresponsiveness

With the advent of antilymphocyte serum or globulin (ALS, ALG) as an experimental immunosuppressive agent, the ease with which specific unresponsiveness could be induced experimentally was greatly increased. The use of ALG to induce unresponsiveness in a number of experimental systems has been reviewed elsewhere.[60] In the following studies, the principles underlying the development of a clinically applicable model to induce specific allograft unresponsiveness will be reviewed. It is now generally recognized that the term *specific unresponsiveness to allografts* be used in experiments on immunologically competent adult animals rather than *actively acquired immunologic tolerance to allografts*, because the latter refers to a phenomenon obtained by a defined experimental protocol in neonatal animals.

Specific unresponsiveness to tissue allografts or specific suppression of an allograft response may be defined as suppression of the immune response to donor-specific alloantigens without suppression of the immune responses to other antigens (e.g., bacterial, viral, other alloantigens of a different donor graft), leading to prolonged survival of the given specific allograft while retaining the ability to reject a different (third-party) allograft and to make normal immune responses to other antigens. Conversely, nonspecific suppression of the immune response, as it relates to allograft rejection, involves generalized suppression of the immune response, usually with methods selected for effectiveness against the allograft rejection mechanism but invariable suppressing other immune responses. Nonspecific suppression implies that responses to other allografts (third-party) are also depressed, as are bacterial and viral responses to varying degrees.

Examples of Unresponsiveness Produced by Graft and Antigen Modifications

The extraordinary experiments of other investigators showing that modified antigen and grafts can be presented to the intact immune system in such a way that unresponsiveness is induced will not be described here in detail. Included in these studies are those in which thyroid[49] or islet cell grafts[6,86] are cultured in vitro under various conditions and transplanted across strong histocompatibility barriers with indefinite survival. Although the mechanism by which culturing leads to unresponsiveness (i.e., apparent permanent graft acceptance) is not known, one explanation is that culturing leads to elimination of dendritic and other antigen-presenting components rich in Class II antigens. This idea is consistent with the finding that treatment of islets with anti-Ia antibodies and complement prior to transplanation produces extended allograft survival.[24]

Another example of the importance of antigen presentation is found in the allograft response to vascularized grafts in miniature swine.[80] In this model, both the class of antigen disparity and the form in which antigen is presented are important. Skin grafts across either a Class I or Class II difference cause sensitization and rejection. In contrast, vascularized kidney grafts across Class I differences enjoy long-term acceptances and induce a systemic state of unresponsiveness that extends to subsequently placed skin grafts across Class I differences that also enjoy prolonged survival.

Other examples of unresponsiveness associated with differences in antigen presentation include the tolerance (rather than sensitization) induced by vascularized liver allografts in the rat, even when complete MHC differences are involved. Liver allografts in rats across MHC barriers survive and also lead to long-term survival of heart allografts.[41] Likewise, the acceptance of liver allografts in swine without immunosuppression described by Calne's group represents a similar example.[7]

Induction of Unresponsiveness Using Donor Antigen (Bone Marrow) and Transient Immunosuppression with ALG

The ideal system for inducing unresponsiveness for clinical cadaveric organ transplantation would involve use of donor antigen *after* organ grafting, since it would be unlikely that adequate amounts of donor antigen would be available for significant periods prior to organ availability *unless* better methods of organ preservation become available.

Early Studies in Mice

This discussion will focus on the use of intact (unmodified) specific donor antigen in the transiently immunosuppressed but otherwise immunologically competent adult animal to induce specific allograft unresponsive. It will describe in detail the use of one form of transient immunosuppression, ALS or ALG, and predominantly one form of donor antigen, bone marrow harvested from adult animals. In the broadest sense, specific unresponsiveness in these studies refers to the specific prolonged allograft survival achieved in animals given transient, nonspecific immunosuppression and donor antigen over allograft survival seen in animals given only transient immunosuppression. Obviously, other types of transient immunosuppression and other kinds of donor antigen can and have been used. The principles elaborated and defined in the following studies apply in general to the use of other types of immunosuppression and donor antigen. In the studies that follow, donor antigen has been used in un-modified form.

Early studies clearly suggested that ALG would be unusually effective in inducing specific unre-sponsiveness. ALG is an extraordinarily potent im-munosuppressive agent for prolongation of allo-grafts.[68] Furthermore, when adult animals are thymectomized and given ALG, the induced im-munosuppression is markedly prolonged and poten-tiated.[65]

Monaco and associates[67] showed very early in their series that if adult-thymectomized ALS-treated mice are infused with F1 hybrid lymphoid cells, specific immunologic unresponsiveness to the donor strain could be produced that was similar in every way to the actively acquired tolerance produced by Medawar and colleagues.[4] This observation served as the basis for extensive study of ALG to prepare adult animals for induction of unresponsiveness. Since F1 hybrid lymphoid cells would never be available for cadaveric organ transplant studies, the first attempts involved infusion of homozygous donor-specific lymphoid cells in adult-thymecto-mized, ALG-treated recipients. As might be ex-pected, severe graft-versus-host reactions were in-duced, and no clinically effective unresponsiveness was obtained.

Attempts to use nonreplicating immunologi-cally incompetent cells (e.g., epidermal kidney and hepatic cells) failed to induce any unresponsive-ness.[62] Use of cell-free antigen preparations gave some specific prolongation but was not long-last-ing.[1] Subsequently, Lance and Medawar[50] showed that specific unresponsiveness in adult mice treated with ALG but not thymectomized could be pro-duced with injections of low doses of F1 hybrid cells. Our group subsequently systematically studied the use of low doses of non-F1 hybrid, homozygous allogeneic lymphoid cells for efficacy in inducing specific unresponsiveness.

The Bone Marrow–ALG Model in Mice

This model system was designed to be immediately applicable to experimental rodent systems. Implicit in this design was that it could be extended to large organ grafts in large animals and was then appli-cable to human cadaver transplants.

The Standard Protocol. In the standard experi-ment, recipient mice receive ALS (ALG) on Day −1 and +2 relative to skin allografting on Day 0, fol-lowed by infusion of donor-specific antigen on Day +8, that is, after transplantation. Lymphoid cells (25×10^6 cells per mouse) from lymph nodes, spleen, thymus, and bone marrow were compared

as the tolerance-conferring inoculum in this stan-dard protocol (Fig. 5-4). At this dose, lymph node–derived lymphocytes, splenocytes, or thymus in-duced very little augmented graft survival over ALS alone. In contrast, bone marrow cells induced sig-nificant augmented survival, some ALG–BM-treated mice bearing grafts for more than 100 days.[105]

Effect of Dose. When 50×10^6 lymphoid cells were used in the standard protocol, there was little effect using lymph node cells or thymus cells, whereas bone marrow cells were more effective than at 25×10^6 cell dose. Splenocytes were as effective as bone marrow at the 50×10^6 cell dose. At 100×10^6 cell dose, lymph node–derived lymphocytes cur-tailed graft survival (i.e., in sensitized animals), thy-mocytes *prolonged* grafts slightly, but marrow was still the superior tolerogen, although splenocytes were almost as effective. In all studies, there was no suggestion of clinical graft-versus-host reactions. In addition, the prolongation of graft survival was spe-cific, that is, third-party bone marrow cells did not prolong test allografts, and animals bearing long-surviving grafts after ALG and BM cells rejected third-party grafts.

As previously noted, increases in lymph node–derived lymphocytes as the tolerance conferring in-oculum produced a shortened graft survival at the higher doses. Also, BM doses of 10, 25, 50 × 10⁶ and 100 × 10⁶ were clearly tolerogenic, with 50 × 10⁶ being most tolerogenic.[103] Most importantly, there was a clear decrease in tolerogenic effect at 1×10^8 dose, but no obvious sensitization (Fig. 5-5). If larger doses were tested, the survival curve (relative to ALS alone) may have been shortened, that is, sensitization induced. The important consid-eration for future clinical application is that the to-lerogenic effect does not increase progressively with increased dose. Above a maximal effective level, decreased effectiveness and possible sensitization may follow BM infusion in ALG-treated animals.

The Effect of Timing of Bone Marrow Cell Infusion on Subsequent Induction of Unresponsiveness. When a standard dose of donor-specific bone mar-row cells (25×10^6) was injected IV into ALS-treated recipients (also given on Days −1 and +2 relative to test skin allografting on Day 0) on Days +1, +2, +3, +4, +8 (the standard protocol), or +16, *or* +23, profoundly different results were obtained. Figure 5-6 shows that infusion on Day +8 as well as +4 were highly tolerogenic, whereas BM given on Day +3 (24 hours post ALS injection) was sig-nificantly tolerogenic, but less so than that given on Day +4 or +8. Cells given on Day +2 failed to induce any specific unresponsiveness and, in fact,

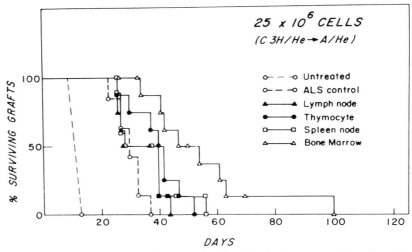

FIGURE 5-4. *Effect of 25 × 10⁶ C3H/He lymph node cells, thymocytes, spleen cells, and bone marrow cells on C3H/He graft survival in ALS-treated A/He mice. A/He mice received 0.5 ml ALS i.p. on days −1 and +2 relative to C3H/He grafting on Day 0 and cell infusion on Day +8.*

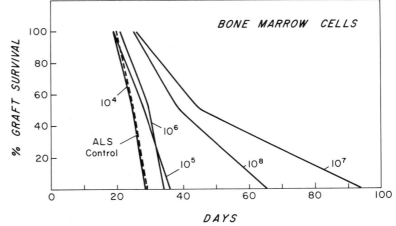

FIGURE 5-5. *Effect of various doses (1 × 10⁴ − 1 × 10⁸) of C3H bone marrow cells on C3H/He graft survival in ALS-treated A/He mice. A/He mice received 0.5 ml ALS i.p. on Day −1 and +2 relative to skin grafting on Day 0 and cell infusion on Day +8.*

may have sensitized some recipients. One of the most striking effects was that marrow given on Day +1 had a sensitizing effect. This is probably due to an effect of subsequent ALS on Day +2 on the marrow cells. Infusion on Day +16 or +23 failed to induce any significant unresponsiveness. Thus, for eventual clinical application, not only would the dose of bone marrow be important—the timing of marrow infusion relative to ALG administration would also be significant.

Modification of Allograft Survival in ALS-Treated, Marrow-Infused Mice with Bacterial Adjuvants and Cyclosphosphamide. The unresponsiveness

induced with ALS and marrow in adult immunologically competent mice differs in a number of respects from the classical actively acquired immunologic tolerance described by Medawar and colleagues. First, it is of interest that the IV route is not obligatory. In certain instances, donor marrow given IP or even intraorgan injection (e.g., intrasplenic, intrahepatic) induced long-lived specific unresponsiveness.[64] Also, in vitro treatment of recipients with various bacterial adjuvants dramatically alters the unresponsiveness induced.[14] The adjuvants *Bordetella pertussis*, Bacillus Calmette-Guerin (BCG), and *Corynebacterium parvum* abrogated the prolongation when given 5 days after grafting, but

B. pertussis produced a striking increase in prolongation when given 7 days before skin grafting wih ALS and subsequent marrow injection. This effect was not found with BCG or *C. parvum. B. pertussis* may exert this unique effect by the extraordinary changes it produces in regional nodes (see mechanism of action below). Another interesting observation is the differential effect that the immunosuppresive drug cyclophosphamide has in the ALS– bone marrow model. If cyclophosphamide is given before marrow in the standard protocol, that is, on Day +4 or +6, the specific graft-prolonging effect of marrow was clearly abrogated. On the other hand, if cyclophosphamide was given after marrow, the graft-prolonging effect of marrow was definitely potentiated if the drug was given within 1 week of marrow injection. Although bacterial adjuvants and drugs such as cyclophosphamide have many possible effects on the immune response, subsequent experiments (see mechanism of action below) suggest the explanation for their effect is mediated through modification in the generation of suppressor cells.

Induction of Specific Unresponsiveness by Donor Marrow in ALS-Treated Mice Involves Generation of Suppressor Cells.

Early studies have clearly shown that unresponsive ALS-treated mice are not lymphoid cell chimeras after marrow infusion as determined by the Mitchison Chimera assay. However, Liegeois and colleagues[53] subsequently showed by elegant chromosomal analysis studies using the T6T6 system that ALS-treated, marrow-injected mice retained donor lymphoid cells in their spleen in very low numbers (< 1.5%) at least to 146 days. The term *microchimerism* was used to describe this phenomenon. It should be noted that unresponsiveness could never be transferred with serum from unresponsive mice. Subsequently, Wood and Monaco[102] studied the capacity of spleen cells from unresponsive ALS-treated, marrow-infused mice to transfer specific unresponsiveness (i.e., for the presence of suppressor cells) to syngeneic recipients. ALS-treated, B6AF$_1$ recipient mice were grafted with C3H/He skin (Day 0) and infused with C3H/He marrow on Day +8. Spleen cells were obtained from unresponsive mice at various times and assayed for suppressor cells.

In any in vivo suppressor cell assay, it is necessary for recipients to be initially immunosuppressed in order to demonstrate a suppressor cell effect. Graft survival in test animals was compared with graft survival seen in ALS-treated B6AF$_1$ controls injected with normal B6AF$_1$ spleen cells.

C3H/He skin graft survival was prolonged in secondary B6AF$_1$ recipients receiving syngeneic spleen cells removed on Day 13 from ALS-treated donors who had received either a C3H/He skin graft and marrow combined or a C3H/He skin graft alone when compared with controls receiving normal syngeneic spleen cells. This result showed that administration of ALS and a skin graft with or without donor-specific bone marrow resulted in the production of suppressor-type cells by Day 13 post-grafting. Although the MST of the grafts in the group injected with cells from donors treated with marrow alone was not significantly different from controls, 25% of these recipients had grafts that showed marked prolongation (50–150 days). No graft prolongation was observed in the group injected with syngeneic spleen cells compared to the donor group treated with ALS alone.

When cells were transferred from unresponsive mice on Day +42, significant suppression of the allograft response, as indicated by prolonged graft survival, was achieved only in the group that received syngeneic spleen cells from the ALS-treated donor group that had received both a graft and marrow, that is, the donor group bearing enhanced grafts. Spleen cells from donors who had received a graft alone transferred immunity, whereas graft survival in the recipients injected with cells from donors treated with marrow alone or ALS alone was similar to that in controls.

It is known that suppressor cells are a T cell population sensitive to anti-theta serum and complement. Spleen cells from donors bearing enhanced grafts were treated with anti-theta serum and complement *before* transfer in the aforementioned suppressor cell assay. In these studies, the ability of anti-theta-treated spleen cells to transfer unresponsiveness was totally abrogated, confirming that the cellular mechanism of unresponsiveness was most likely a T suppressor cell. Furthermore, specificity of the suppression transferred with syngeneic spleen cells from ALS-treated, marrow-infused mice was demonstrated in that spleen cells from B6AF$_1$ ALS-treated C3H/He marrow-infused mice transferred unresponsiveness only to C3H/He skin grafts in the suppressor assay but not to third-party DBA/2 skin grafts.

Considerable evidence suggests that a population of T cells exists as part of the normal regulatory mechanism of the immune response that suppresses both humoral and cellular immunity. Suppressor T cells have been implicated in graft-versus-host responses, mixed lymphocyte reactions, and delayed hypersensitivity, as well as in unresponsiveness to protein antigens. Specific suppressor cells have also been identified in rats made unresponsive to skin allografts by neonatal injection of donor bone marrow cells and in adult mice made unresponsive to skin allografts by ALS treatment and injection of donor antigen. In the studies just described, cells capable of transferring suppression of the allograft response appeared on Day 13 in mice that had received either a graft alone or both a graft and donor marrow and, to a lesser degree, in mice given marrow alone. After mice recovered from the immunosuppressive effects of ALS, suppressor cells persisted only in the spleens of mice bearing enhanced grafts after marrow injection, suggesting an active response to marrow on the part of the host to induce suppression.

Suppressor cells can be both antigen-specific and nonspecific, but in specific suppression, the induction of suppressor activity appears to be a direct result of antigenic stimulation. In nonimmunosuppressed animals, there are at least two target cells in the T cell population available for antigenic stimulation: (1) the mature immunocompetent cell, which proliferates into either an effector or helper cell, and (2) the precursor of the suppressor cell, which is thought to be more immature and short-lived than the effector cell. Antigenic stimulation results in proliferation of both effector and suppressor cells, but under normal conditions, the immune (effector) response usually predominates. Suppressor cells do not prevent the immune response but limit its intensity.

The ability of an ALS-treated animal to make a cell-mediated response is impaired as the pool of long-lived immunocompetent T cells is significantly depleted. In contrast, the pool of short-lived suppressor cells is not affected by ALS. Therefore, in an ALS-treated animal, the balance would be in favor of suppression after antigenic stimulation. As previously described, the finding of suppressor cells in the spleens of ALS-treated mice 13 days after grafting suggests that a graft alone generates an excess of suppressor cells in an ALS-treated animal.

The nature of the response that marrow elicits in an ALS-treated animal to enhance graft survival beyond the time of ALS immunosuppression is not clear. Spleen cells from ALS-treated mice injected with marrow alone do not show strong suppressive activity after transfer. It is possible that marrow injected into skin-grafted mice initiates a "second set" suppressive response. There is a proliferation of donor strain cells after the injection of marrow into ALS-treated mice bearing skin grafts.[53] This proliferation does not occur after marrow injection in ALS-treated mice that have not been grafted. This proliferation of donor cells could be an added antigenic stimulus for activation of suppressor cells.

The injection of marrow could also elicit an antibody response, which might in turn stimulate generation of suppressor cells.

Evidence that suppressor cells are generated in response to injection of marrow also comes from experiments with cyclophosphamide-treated mice. Precursors of suppressor cells are sensitive to cyclophosphamide, and immune responses are increased in cyclosphosamide-treated animals. Prolongation of graft survival is decreased in ALS-treated mice given cyclophosphamide before injection of marrow, whereas cyclophosphamide has no effect on graft survival in ALS-treated mice not given marrow. It is possible that cyclophosphamide removes a population of (? suppressor) cells whose response to marrow results in enhancement of the graft. Enhanced proliferation of suppressor cells after marrow injection could protect the graft by delaying sensitization of the host. Suppressor cells are most efficient in suppressing the early stages of differentiation of cytotoxic cells into mature cells, whereas cytotoxic cells that have differentiated beyond a certain stage can no longer be suppressed.

Kinetic Studies of Suppressor Cells in the ALS–Marrow Model.

The presence of suppressor cells in other lymphoid tissues of unresponsive mice in the ALS–marrow model has been confirmed.[103] Suppressor cell assays performed on cells taken from the spleen, bone marrow, lymph nodes, and thymus of unresponsive mice at various times showed that suppressor cells can be found only in the spleen of ALS-treated, marrow-injected mice on Day +13 but not in other lymphatic tissues (Fig. 5-6). By Day +42, suppressor cells were still present in the spleen, and also appeared in the lymph nodes, emphasizing that the suppressor cells in this model were not restricted to the spleen only.

The role of the spleen in the induction and maintenance of unresponsiveness to skin allografts and in the generation of suppressor cells has been studied in ALS-treated B6AF$_1$ mice grafted with C3H/He skin and injected with C3H/He marrow.[104] B6AF$_1$ mice were splenectomized either before the induction of unresponsiveness or after unresponsiveness was induced. Graft survival was prolonged equally in all splenectomized groups and in the nonsplenectomized controls. To study the effect of the spleen on the generation of suppressor cells, lymph node cells were removed at Day +42 from splenectomized ALS-treated, marrow-injected B6AF$_1$ mice bearing C3H/He skin grafts and were transferred to ALS-treated B6AF$_1$ recipients grafted with C3H/He skin. Suppressor cell activity could be detected in the nodes of splenectomized mice, but a higher dose

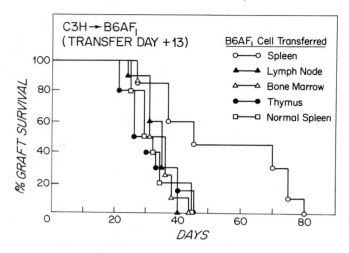

FIGURE 5-6.   *Graft survival curves (suppressor cell assay) of C3H/He skin on ALS-treated B6AF$_1$ mice injected with syngeneic spleen, lymph node, bone marrow, or thymus cells removed Day +13 from ALS-treated B6AF$_1$ donors that had received both C3H/He skin and bone marrow (20 mice/recipient group).*

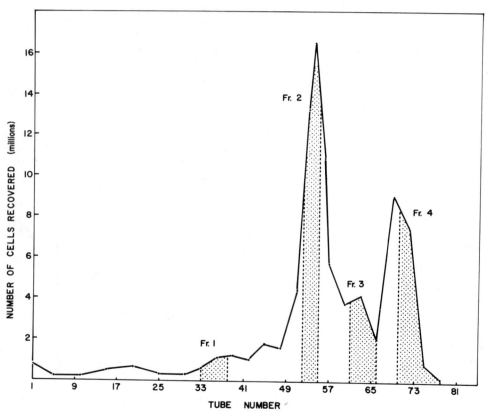

FIGURE 5-7.   *Elution profile of 2.5 × 10^6 C3H/He bone marrow cells fractionated on a 1 g 2.0% to 4.0% BSA gradient. Each tube contains 200 drops of the BSA cell mixture and is plotted against the total number of cells in each tube.*

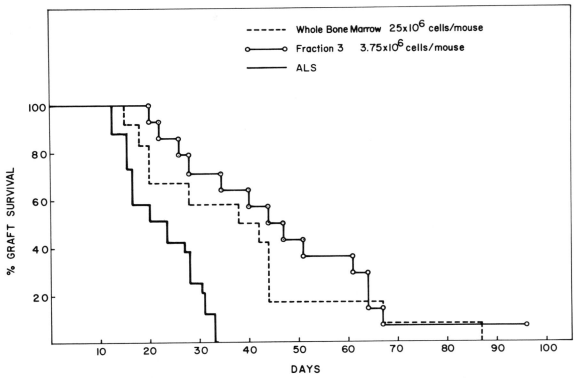

FIGURE 5-8.   *ALS and allografted B6AF₁ mice were infused with either 25 × 10⁶ unfractionated whole marrow cells or 3.75 × 10⁶ cells from fraction 3. The control group was treated with only ALS.*

of lymph node cells was required to transfer unresponsiveness from splenectomized donors compared to that required of nonsplenectomized donors. These results indicate that the spleen is not necessary for the induction or maintenance of unresponsiveness to skin allografts in ALS-treated, marrow-injected mice. In addition, suppressor cells can be generated in the lymph nodes of unresponsive mice in the absence of the spleen, although the production of suppressor cells appears to be less effective in splenectomized mice than in mice with intact spleens.

The Nature of the Cell in Bone Marrow Associated with Induction of Unresponsiveness in ALS-Treated Mice.   If bone marrow could be fractionated and the active unresponsiveness-producing fraction could be isolated, the ability to infuse small numbers of active fractionated donor marrow cells would be advantageous, because infusion of whole unfractionated marrow can be associated with a number of complications. Gozzo and associates[31] showed that whole murine marrow could be fractionated into four distinct fractions in a 1 × g velocity sedi-

mentation chamber using a linear bovine serum albumin density gradient. Figure 5-7 shows a typical fractionation profile of such a separation. Groups of B6AF₁ mice treated with ALS and grafted with C3H/He skin (Day 0) were infused with 25 × 10⁶ whole marrow cells or the cells of each fraction isolated from 25 × 10⁶ whole marrow. Fraction 3 was as effective as whole marrow in inducing specific unresponsiveness (Fig. 5-8). When the dose of fraction 3 was increased, significant graft prolongation was achieved compared to that achieved in mice given 25 × 10⁶ whole marrow cells. Fraction 3 contains 93% small lymphocytes when examined by Wright's stained smears.

Phenotypic Characteristics of Active Bone Marrow Cells for Unresponsiveness Induction.   The phenotypic characteristics of active bone marrow cells necessary for induction of unresponsiveness have been studied by exposing whole marrow cells to various specific antisera prior to infusion in the standard protocol.[18]

Cells that adhere to anti-Ia-coated plates extend graft survival only slightly better than ALS alone, whereas nonadherent (Ia-depleted) cells, as well as cells treated with anti-Ia and complement, retain good prolonging activity. Likewise, panning on anti-immunoglobulin (Ig)-coated plates produces an active, Ig$^+$-depleted population and an inactive adherent population, and killing Thy-1$^+$ cells with antibody and complement does not compromise the ability of marrow to prolong graft survival. Complement receptor–positive (EAC$^+$) and Fc receptor-positive cells (EA$^+$) were separated by panning on plates coated with sheep erythrocyte/antibody/complement and erythrocyte/7S antibody, respectively. Adherent, EAC$^+$-enriched cells were only slightly active, whereas the nonadherent, EAC-depleted population was fully active in graft prolongation. However, both the Fc R$^+$ (EA$^+$)-enriched and depleted populations were active—the enriched fraction producing significantly better prolongation than the depleted population. Thus, active marrow cells that prolong skin graft survival in ALS-treated mice appear to be Ia$^-$, Thy.1$^-$, largely complement receptor-negative and Ig$^-$, but are largely positive for Fc receptors. Active cells in marrow co-fractionated during sedimentation in Ficoll at unit gravity with populations that were reduced in Ia$^+$, Ig$^+$, and Thy.1$^+$ cells but that had modest percentages of FcR$^+$ cells. The active bone marrow cells may be natural suppressor or natural regulatory cells.

The fractionation of active marrow extended using velocity sedimentation in Ficoll.[19] This method permitted resolution of previously active fraction 3 into fractions c and d. When fraction c or d were injected into ALS-treated mice, only fraction c induced considerable specific graft survival. Fraction c contained small percentages of Ia$^+$ cells (10%) and moderate percentages of EA$^+$ and EAC$^+$ cells (15%).

Density Gradient Fractionation of Active Bone Marrow Cells.

Although velocity sedimentation at unit gravity can be used for active marrow fractions, it is not useful where large volumes of cells are required. A rapid high-capacity method is required. Therefore, density gradient fractionation can be applied to the fractionation of large volumes of marrow cells.[22] The top interface is designated fraction 4, followed by fractions 3, 2, 1 and the discarded cell pellet, which contains erythrocytes and a few nucleated cells. Fraction 3 is the most enriched fraction for cells active in graft prolongation and contains small- to medium-sized lymphocytes. Two of the four fractions (fractions 2 and 3) have good prolonging ability.

It is possible to estimate the density of a major portion of the cells active in graft prolongation as being in the range of 1.061 g/liter to 1.066 g/liter

and to produce one fraction with superior graft-prolonging activity (fraction 3). This fraction, which constitutes only 10% of the recovered cells, is enriched for small- to medium-sized lymphocytes, Ia$^+$, Thy-1$^+$ and IgM$^+$ cells, and contains cells bearing a marker known to be present on active cells (Fc R).

Effect of Age, Storage, and Freezing on Ability of Marrow to Induce Unresponsiveness.

It is obvious that for application of the ALS–marrow model to clinical cadaver transplantation, the marrow will have to be harvested with the cadaver organ and stored for approximately 2 to 3 weeks before infusion, since infusion at the time of grafting is ineffective. Storage for this length of time will undoubtedly require freezing. In addition, donors of all ages are used for cadaver organ sources; the effectiveness of bone marrow from very young or older donors must be confirmed.

Suspensions of marrow from juvenile (6 weeks) to adult-aged (25–35 weeks) donors were compared for their ability to prolong graft survival (induce unresponsiveness) in ALS-treated mice. 5×10^6 nucleated marrow cells prolonged graft survival significantly over ALS alone regardless of the age of the donor. Thus, donor marrow from adult as well as juvenile animals is equally effective in inducing unresponsiveness in ALS-treated recipients.[20]

Survival of active graft-prolonging bone marrow cells under several storage conditions was investigated. Bone marrow cells retained their graft-prolonging effect if stored at 4°C in 10% fetal calf serum for 18 hours prior to infusion, but did not retain this effect if maintained for 18 hours at 37°C under standard lymphocyte culture conditions. Bone marrow cells retained their unresponsiveness-inducing capability after freezing and thawing or overnight refrigeration.[21] Thus, the model could be applied clinically to cadaver grafts using frozen, stored marrow.

Use of Other Blood Elements to Induce Unresponsiveness in ALS-Treated Mice.

As noted previously, bone marrow cells are the most effective and efficient donor antigen versus other lymphoid cells to induce unresponsiveness in ALS-treated mice. However, as the dose of cells is increased, splenocytes are also effective in ALS-treated mice. This suggests that spleen cells could be used as a source for the active cells in clinical application. The use of spleen or other tissue as a source for the active tolerance–inducing cell would be attractive, since harvesting of marrow from cadavers or living-related donors is a time-consuming procedure. Kapnick and Monaco[43] were able to induce modest degrees of unresponsiveness to skin allografts in ALS-treated mice using blood platelets, although they had to be injected later (usually 2 weeks post-grafting) and in association with adjuvants.

De Fazio and associates (unpublished observations) also showed that peripheral blood lymphocytes were effective using the standard protocol. The peripheral blood lymphocytes (PBLs) active in graft prolongation are Thy-1 negative and display a density in Percoll gradients similar to that of previously demonstrated active marrow cells. When PBLs were injected in combination with bone marrow cells, the length of graft survival was shortened compared with that produced by marrow alone. The cells associated with abrogation appear to be mature T cells. This abrogation cannot be produced by PBLs treated with anti-thy-1 plus complement or by thymocytes, but it is a property of lymph node cells enriched for T cells by nylon wool fractionation. Thus, it would appear that peripheral blood lymphocytes, although they specifically prolong graft survival in ALS-treated mice, contain mature T cells that can also abrogate this effect. These studies show that if whole marrow is used clinically, the degree of contamination with blood should be minimized.

In Vitro Analysis of the Mechanism of Unresponsiveness in ALS-Treated, Marrow-Infused Mice.
The previously discussed in vivo studies in mice show that the specific unresponsiveness induced in mice is associated with the generation of suppressor cells. The in vitro analysis of the immune responses in this model emphasizes that the generation of suppressor cells is achieved in several steps.[56]

Responses to mitogens in standard protocol animals and in controls was studied first. To evaluate the functional properties of T cells and B cells, spleen cells (SPC) obtained at various times from three groups of B6AF$_1$ mice, that is, (1) ALS, (2) ALS-Graft, and (3) ALS-Graft-BM groups, were stimulated by optimal concentrations of PHA, concanavalin A (Con A), or LPS. The proliferative response to T cell mitogens was markedly suppressed in all groups given ALS treatment. Although an initial suppression (approximately 10% of normal B6AF$_1$ SPC) of Con A response was seen immediately followed by gradual recovery in the ALS and ALS-Graft groups, more prolonged suppression of Con A responsiveness was observed in the ALS-Graft-BM group. By Day 56, reactivity to PHA and Con A returned to normal levels in all groups. On the other hand, reactivity to the B cell mitogen, LPS, was minimally suppressed in all groups throughout the time course studied.

Direct lymphocyte-mediated cytotoxicity (LMC) was also determined. To evaluate the presence of cytotoxic lymphocytes generated in B6AF$_1$ recipients against C3H alloantigens, SPC obtained from the ALS-Graft and the ALS-Graft-BM groups were tested directly against Cr-labeled L929 and EL-4 lymphoma targets.[51] Lymphocytes obtained from the ALS-Graft group exhibited high LMC against L929 target cells at Day 21, before any grafts showed macroscopic signs of rejection. On the other hand, the LMC in the ALS-Graft-BM group remained low until the time of allograft rejection.

A similar analysis of proliferative responses and generation of cell-mediated lympholysis (CML) in the mixed-lymphocyte culture (MLC) was performed. To evaluate the ability of cells to respond to the alloantigens of the skin donors, SPC obtained from the Graft-only, ALS-Graft, and ALS-Graft-BM groups were sensitized to C3H stimulator cells in a MLC. Figure 5-9 demonstrates the prolonged inability of SPC taken from the ALS-Graft-BM group to respond proliferatively to C3H alloantigens. SPC obtained from the ALS-Graft group exhibited suppressed proliferative response (MLR) for 3 weeks, followed by a high "secondary-type" response on Day 28 when the skin grafts were rejected. In contrast, the SPC of the ALS-Graft-BM group exhibited a markedly prolonged suppression of the MLR. Even at the time of rejection, the stimulation index rose only moderately.

Although ALS treatment induces nonspecific impairment of T cell reactivity, as evidenced by a low proliferative response to PHA and Con A and by the initial low MLR and CML to C3H and DBA/2 alloantigens, ALS treatment alone failed to inhibit the eventual generation of cytotoxic reactivity against donor alloantigen, that is, SPC obtained at Day 21 from the ALS-Graft group already exhibited high LMC and CML despite continued low MLR against C3H stimulators. In contrast, donor marrow injection in the ALS-Graft-BM group led to the further inhibition of generation of effector activity as illustrated by prolonged low LMC in this group.

These results indicate that the specific unresponsiveness induced in ALS-treated, marrow-injected mice is not due to the classical actively acquired tolerance by clonal deletion. In addition, these results seem to be in agreement with the previous reports by Wagner and Rollinghoff[100] and Engers and colleagues[23] that alloantigen-primed memory T cells differentiate into cytotoxic T cells in the absence of cell proliferation in the secondary MLC.

Initially, the administration of ALS alone probably results in the production of ALS-induced antigen nonspecific suppressor cells. Maki and associates[57] showed that mere administration of rabbit anti-mouse lymphocyte serum results in the development of suppressor cells that can be detected

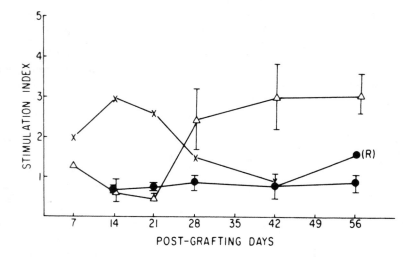

FIGURE 5-9. *Sequential changes of proliferative responses to C3H alloantigens. Results of three separate series of experiments ± SD. 7.5 × 10⁶ spleen cells of mice from Graft-only, ALS-Graft, or ALS-Graft-BM group were co-cultured with 2.5 × 10⁶ mitomycin-C–treated C3H spleen cells for 4 days. (R indicates the proliferative response exhibited by spleen cells of mice in the ALS-Graft-BM group that had already rejected C3H skin allografts.)*

by co-culture mixed lymphocyte culture experiments. The putative suppressor cells inhibit nonspecifically the proliferative response as well as the generation of cytotoxicity of normal responder cells. Suppressor activity is dose dependent and is not attributable to cell crowding, shifting of peak activity, or release of cell-bound ALS. Subsequently, additional antigenic stimulation by skin allografting in ALS-treated mice shifts the specificity of suppressor cells from nonspecific to specific for the skin donor alloantigen (Tables 5-4). ALS-induced suppressor cells are Lyt-1^+2^- T cells, whereas suppressor cells present in ALS-treated, skin allograft–bearing mice are Lyt-1^-2^+ T cells.

The exact mechanism of induction of suppressor cells by ALS is not known. ALS may stimulate a subset of T cells to differentiate into suppressor cells, as has been shown in the case of Con A–induced suppressor cells. ALS may contain various anti-T cell receptor antibodies, which may trigger induction of polyclonal suppressor cells. Finally, ALS, which is cytotoxic to some subpopulations of T cells, may spare suppressor cells or suppressor cell precursors. In similar experiments, Maki and associates[56] compared the suppressor cell activity in vitro of SPC removed from B6AF$_1$ mice given ALS and a C3H skin graft versus those from B6AF$_1$ mice given ALS and C3H marrow and skin grafts. They showed that SPC from the ALS-Graft group were capable of inhibiting the anti-C3H MLR of normal B6AF$_1$ responders early after grafting (Day 14), but they lost suppressive activity when grafts showed signs of rejection (Day 35). On the other hand, SPC obtained either at Day 14 or Day 42 from mice of the ALS-Graft-BM group bearing intact skin graft exhibited marked suppression of anti-C3H MLR. By complex genetic analysis, they were able to show

that specific suppressor cells were derived at least in part from the donor marrow.

In view of the present findings, the following hypothesis concerning the induction and maintenance of the unresponsiveness in the ALS-treated, C3H marrow-injected B6AF$_1$ mice is suggested. ALS-treatment depresses the activity of immunocompetent T cells. Antigenic stimulation by C3H skin allografting may lead to the generation of suppressor cells of host B6AF$_1$ origin. These suppressor cells are most efficient in suppressing the early recognition phase of reaction, thus limiting the expansion of cytotoxic T-lymphocytes. In addition, the presence of donor antigen specific and/or nonspecific suppressor cells at the time of C3H marrow injection would prevent the rejection of donor marrow and allow its proliferation in the recipient's thymic and/or splenic environment. By yet unknown mechanisms, the generation of marrow-derived GVH responsive cells is hampered, and the marrow cells give rise to suppressor T cells. The C3H marrow-derived suppressor cells are specific for self (C3H)-antigens, thus further limiting the host (B6AF$_1$) response to the skin grafts as well as to the surviving marrow cells that bear C3H alloantigens. Skin grafts are rejected after the balance between the suppressor cell activity and cytotoxic activity shifts toward the latter.

The Bone Marrow–ALS Model in Dogs

Effect of Whole, Unstored Marrow in Prolonging Renal Allografts. The studies that have been completed in dogs have shown that the marrow–ALS model is totally applicable to whole organ grafts in large species. The canine experiments were designed as follows: Immunosuppressive regimens and timing of bone marrow infusion were chosen in order

TABLE 5-4   *Effect of Skin Allografting on Antigen Specificity of Suppressor Cells*

RESPONDER CELLS*	^{3}H-THYMIDINE UPTAKE (CPM $\times$ 10^{-3})			
	Day +5		Day +16	
	Anti-BALB/c	Anti-B6	Anti-BALB/c	Anti-B6
SPC$_N$ (0.5)	18.5 ± 0.6	13.2 ± 1.3	52.9 ± 7.9	18.1 ± 1.6
SPC$_N$ (1.0)	24.4 ± 4.6	19.2 ± 4.2	135.3 ± 16.2	45.2 ± 7.3
SPC$_{ALS}$ (0.5)	NT†	NT	9.4 ± 1.1	9.2 ± 2.2
SPC$_N$ (0.5) + SPC$_{ALS}$ (0.5)	4.1 ± 0.6	3.2 ± 0.5	21.1 ± 1.1	13.2 ± 0.3
SPC$_{A-G}$ (0.5)	NT	NT	8.0 ± 0.3	7.3 ± 0.2
SPC$_N$ (0.5) + SPC$_{A-G}$ (0.5)	5.1 ± 0.4	4.1 + 0.2	25.3 ± 1.2	18.0 ± 0.3

* Spleen cells of C3H mice given ALS alone (SPC$_{ALS}$ or ALS and BALB/c skin grafts (SPC$_{A-G}$) were obtained on Day +5 or +16 and sensitized against 0.5 $\times$ 10^6 BALB/c or B6 stimulators with or without normal C3H spleen cells (SPC$_N$).

† NT = not tested.

(From Maki T, Gottschalk R, Wood ML et al: Specific unresponsiveness to skin allografts in anti-lymphocyte serum-treated marrow-injected mice: Participation of donor marrow–derived suppressor cells. J Immunol 127:1433–1438, 1981; © American Association of Immunologists)

to reproduce in dogs the critical timing that had been demonstrated in mice, that is, injection of bone marrow 2 to 5 days following completion of ALS treatment.[9]

The study was carried out in eight groups of dogs (Table 5-5). In the control (no treatment) group, rejection occurred within 10 to 14 days. Dogs (Group A) given only low doses of ALS had modest renal allograft prolongation, in that they succumbed in 14 to 24 days. When bone marrow obtained from the kidney donor was infused on Day +10 after low-dose ALS treatment (Group B, 1 ml/kg and 2–4 $\times$ 10^6 cells/kg), a slight prolongation of kidney allograft survival over that seen in Group A was achieved, with the dogs succumbing in 14 to 33 days. All animals died of rejection.

It was therefore concluded that a more profound immune suppression was required prior to bone marrow infusion in order to achieve a tolerogenic effect. In an attempt to produce such a state, the RADLS dose was increased to 2 ml/kg (Group C). Under this increased RADLS regimen, all dogs had a normal BUN level on Day +10, the time of bone marrow infusion in the protocol. It was thought, therefore, that such dogs were sufficiently immunosuppressed to be satisfactory recipients of potentially tolerogenic bone marrow. In Group D, in which six dogs were given 2 ml/kg of RADLS followed by 2 to 4 $\times$ 10^8 cells/kg on Day +10, survival ranged from 20 to 78 days. Of these six animals, three died of rejection on Days +28, +41, and +56. The other three died of infection with no evidence of rejection (BUN < 20 mg/ml).

Experimental work with cell-free antigens and with cellular antigens has produced evidence that specific immunosuppression may be reinforced by postinfusion of antigen. It was thought, therefore, that further pulsation with bone marrow cells on Day +20 might yield still better results. This procedure was carried out in the five dogs of Group E that received 2 ml/kg of RADLS followed by 2 to 4 $\times$ 10^8 cells/kg on Days +10 and +20. In this group, survival ranged from 114 to 204 days. Bone marrow cells (2–4 $\times$ 10^8 kg) given on Day +2 (Group F) or Day +5 (Group H) to dogs not treated with ALS were not effective, in that the survival of these two groups was similar to that of the untreated controls.

Of interest is the report by Rowinski and colleagues,[81] who induced additional prolonged canine renal allograft survival with donor-specific platelets in ALS-treated dogs. They clearly showed that the augmented survival was specific, since a third-party renal allograft transplanted to the neck was rejected while the test allograft from the platelet donor remained well tolerated.

Use of Fractionated and Frozen-Stored Bone Marrow Cells.
It is obvious that for the marrow model to be applied clinically to cadaver transplantation, marrow would have to be harvested and stored for various periods of time to be infused post-grafting. Thus, it was important to establish the efficacy of stored marrow in a large animal, whole-organ allograft model. Gozzo and colleagues[36] demonstrated the effectiveness of fractionated and frozen-stored canine bone marrow cells in prolonging renal allograft survival in ALS-treated dogs.

Renal allografts were performed in histoincompatible outbred dogs treated daily with anti-dog ALS

TABLE 5-5 *Survival of Canine Renal Allografts After ALS and Bone Marrow Treatment*

GROUP	NUMBER OF DOGS	ALS	BONE MARROW	SURVIVAL
Control	6	—	—	10, 10, 11, 12, 14, 14
A	7	1 ml/kg	—	14, 15, 16, 16, 16, 17, 24
B	6	1 ml/kg	2–4 × 10⁸/kg (day +10)	14, 17, 19, 28, 31, 33
C	7	2 ml/kg	—	14*, 17*, 23, 23, 24, 25, 31
D	6	2 ml/kg	2–4 × 10⁸/kg (day +10)	20*, 28, 38*, 41, 56, 78*
E	5	2 ml/kg	2–4 × 10⁸/kg (days +10 and +20)	114, 142, 163, 172, 204
F	6	—	2–4 × 10⁸/kg (day +2)	9, 9, 11, 12, 12, 13
G	3	—	2–4 × 10⁸/kg (day +5)	12, 13, 13

* No clinical or histologic evidence of rejection at time of death.

(From Caridis T, Liegeois A, Barrett I et al: Enhanced survival of canine renal allografts of ALS-treated dogs given bone marrow. Transplant Proc 5:671–674, 1973)

from Day −6 to Day +7, relative to kidney allografting on Day 0. Fresh, whole, unfractionated donor-specific bone marrow or a bone marrow fraction (BMFr3) was infused IV into recipients on Day +13 or Day +14. Alternatively, frozen/thawed (F/Th) bone marrow or BMFr3 was infused after storage at −80°C for 2 weeks. BMFr3 and unfractionated bone marrow significantly ($p < 0.005$) prolonged the median allograft function time (MST) beyond the controls treated only with ALS (46 and 35 days vs. 18 days). F/Th marrow was as effective as fresh bone marrow in prolonging graft survival. Reduced MLR responses to the specific donor as well as third-party cells and markedly reduced responsiveness to Con A, PHA, and pokeweed mitogens suggested that animals were nonspecifically immunosuppressed at this time. However, by 60 days post-transplantation, two dogs treated with BMFr3 showed normal MLR responses to third-party cells but not to specific donor cells. The responses to mitogens had also returned to pre-ALS treatment values. Thus, in vitro studies in two animals suggested that long-term specific immunosuppression was induced by fractionated bone marrow. Furthermore, in vivo confirmation of this specific unresponsiveness suggested by in vitro studies was achieved when third-party renal allografts placed in the neck of dogs with well-tolerated renal allografts after ALS and marrow treatment were rejected, while the original marrow donor graft remained unrejected. This suggests that application of this model to human transplantation may be effective using fresh or F/Th bone marrow fractions obtained from living-related or cadaver donors.

The ALS–Marrow Model in Primates

The use of the ALS–bone marrow model has been applied with great success to renal allografts in primates by the Thomases.[95,96] J.M. Thomas and colleagues[94] enhanced skin allograft survival in Rhesus monkeys with ATG and donor lymphoid cells over that achieved with ATG alone. Encouraged by these results, they extended their studies to renal allografts in highly incompatible outbred Rhesus monkeys (Macacca mulatta). Four groups of recipients received either (1) no treatment, (2) ATG only, (3) ATG plus donor marrow on Day 12, or (4) ATG plus donor marrow on Days +12 and +20. *Monkeys received no other immunosuppression.* Untreated monkeys rejected kidneys in 6 to 14 days, and ATG only monkeys rejected kidneys in 28 to 42 days. Recipients receiving ATG plus one infusion of marrow did not reject grafts from 140 to 400 days, at the time of reporting, with normal serum creatinines.

Monkeys given ATG and two marrow injections showed a bimodal survival curve; one half had survival equivalent to ATG alone, while one half had extended survival from 73 to 127 days. Monkeys given ATG and a single marrow infusion were initially nonspecifically unresponsive to polyclonal mitogens and allogeneic cell stimulation. Eventually, the MLR-to-allogeneic cell stimulation reversed to normal, but the MLR-to-the-*specific donor* stimulation was consistently negative, as the kidneys remained unrejected. Co-culture experiments of lymphocytes from nonspecific donors with normal allogeneic cells and donor-stimulating cells resulted in reduced MLR reactions. If stimulating cells came from indifferent donors, MLR suppression was not found. These extraordinary observations strongly suggested that a state of donor-specific unresponsiveness in the MLR was related to the presence of antigen-specific suppressor cells.

The ALS–Marrow Model in Humans

Preliminary Studies. Prior to the recent demonstration that stored, frozen marrow is effective in prolonging renal allograft survival in ALS-treated dogs, use of bone marrow as donor-specific antigen could not be applied in clinical cadaver organ grafting post-transplantation where use of stored marrow is mandatory. For this reason, the model has been applied in a preliminary series of living-related kidney transplants of one-haplotype-mismatched, high mixed-lymphocyte culture-positive patients. It is likely that this subgroup of living-related transplants has a poor outcome unless donor-specific blood transfusions, cyclosporine, or some other additional immunosuppressive regimen beyond the standard conventional immunosuppressive regimens is used.

In this preliminary study,[69] living-related donor–recipient pairs that were one-haplotype-mismatched, high mixed-lymphocyte culture (MLC)-positive were entered into the protocol after informed consent from recipient and donor. In brief,

the recipient received the living-related transplant with standard Imuran, prednisone, and ATG treatment. One week after the ATG treatment was finished, donor marrow was given to the recipient.

Immunosuppression involved prednisone (60 mg/day from the day of transplant, tapered 5 mg/week to 10 to 15 mg/day maintenance), Imuran (2 mg/kg daily as tolerated), and ATG (10 mg/kg/day to 15 mg/kg/day from Days 0 to 14 and then discontinued). Kidney transplantation was performed by standard techniques—Day 0 taken as the day of transplantation. Donor bone marrow was harvested from the previous kidney donor on postoperative Day 21 by multiple iliac crest aspiration and the marrow was infused with careful physiologic monitoring during and immediately postinfusion.

In the six patients who completed the protocol and received marrow infusion, three are 20 to 40 months postoperative, with good renal function. A fourth patient sustained total rejection shortly after 1 year and returned to dialysis. The fifth patient rejected in the second postoperative month, probably secondary to noncompliance in taking his maintenance prednisone and Imuran, after an excellent early course. The sixth patient died of a CVA 1 week post-marrow infusion. This was deemed unrelated to the marrow infusion. Two long-term survivors after marrow infusion have never had an acute rejection episode, and one survivor has had only one. MLC analysis (Table 5-6) has shown that specific anti-donor reactivity has remained depressed, whereas anti-third-party reactivity, initially nonspecifically depressed after ATG treatment, recovered

TABLE 5-6   Post-operative MLC-reactivity

TIME POST-TRANSPLANTATION	SERUM CREATININE	RDx	RCx
Pre-op	—	8.7	42.0
3 wk (post marrow)	0.9	1.0	11.3
1 mo	0.8	1.0	24.1
2 mo	0.9	2.2	25.4
3 mo	1.2	1.0	2.8
5 mo	1.3	1.0	1.4
7 mo	1.3	2.2	7.4
9 mo	1.7	0.4	2.8
10 mo	1.6	1.7	14.3
11 mo	1.5	0.9	6.0
13 mo	1.7	0.7	25.8
18 mo	1.7	1.1	59.9
20 mo	2.1	1.0	31.6
28 mo	2.6	—	—
35 mo	2.3	2.3	22.7

At various times postoperatively, the patient's peripheral blood lymphocytes (PBL) were sensitized against frozen or fresh kidney and marrow donor (PBL) (RDx) and frozen or fresh third-party PBL (RCx). Results are expressed as stimulation index (SI). MLC-stimulating ability of frozen donor cells was always confirmed by their ability to stimulate normal third-party cells (data not shown).

to pretransplantation levels. Analysis of lymphocyte subpopulations showed that successful bone marrow–infused patients had reduced T4 to T8 ratios through the first postoperative year, a finding observed in the monkey model of this protocol.[96]

Future Considerations. The previously discussed preliminary studies in humans with the ALS–marrow model are encouraging in two aspects. First, specific MLR nonreactivity to the specific donor has been demonstrated for a long period of time posttransplantation, whereas third-party MLR reactivity after an initial period of nonspecific suppression (related to ATG administration) returned to normal. Second, it is highly significant that in the three successful patients, only one bout of acute rejection has been encountered in 100 patient-months posttransplantation. On the other hand, these patients have been maintained on low-dose prednisone and Imuran (for ethical considerations), so it has not been proved that the degree of specific unrespon-

siveness indicated by donor-specific nonreactivity in MLR is sufficient to maintain the graft without continued maintenance immunosuppression. Indeed, specific immune suppression might not be an all-or-none phenomenon. In future studies or trials, the effectiveness of donor-specific antigen may be evaluated not only by improved patient and graft survival but also by other salutary effects such as steroid sparing, reduced rejections, and minimization of maintenance immunosuppression requirements.

The use of bone marrow as the specific donor antigen is cumbersome because of the difficulty in harvesting from both living-related donors and cadavers. In this regard, the studies in mice that suggest that the putative effective cell associated with unresponsiveness induction in the marrow can be isolated from the spleen and peripheral blood are most encouraging studies. Indeed, if this cell can be isolated in sufficient numbers from blood and/or spleen, the application of this model to human clinical organ transplantation will be greatly facilitated.

REFERENCES

1. Abbott WM, Monaco AP, Russell PS: Antilymphocyte serum and cell-free antigen loading. Transplantation 7:291, 1969
2. Barnes BA, Olivier D: Analysis of NIAID kidney transplant histocompatibility study (KTHS): Factors associated with transplant outcomes I. Transplant Proc 13:65–72, 1981
3. Biddison WE, Rao PE, Talle MA et al: Possible involvement of the OKT3 molecule in T cell recognition of class II HLA antigens: Evidence from studies of cytotoxic T-lymphocytes specific for SB antigens. J Exp Med 156:1065–1076, 1982
4. Billingham RE, Brent L, Medawar PB: Acquired immunological tolerance. Nature (London) 172:603, 1953
5. Birkeland SA: The use of antilymphocyte globulin in renal allograft rejection: A controlled study. Postgrad Med J 52 (Suppl 5):82, 1976
6. Bowen KM, Andrus L, Lafferty KJ: Survival of pancreatic islet allografts. (Letter) Lancet 2:585, 1979
7. Calne RY: In Calne R (ed): Immunologic Aspects of Transplantation Surgery, p 296. New York, John Wiley & Sons, Inc, 1973
8. Calne RY, Rolles Y, White DJG et al: Cyclosporine A initially as the immunosuppressant in 34 recipients of cadaver organs. Lancet 2:1033, 1979
9. Caridis T, Liegeois A, Barrett I et al: Enhanced survival of canine renal allografts of ALS-treated dogs given bone marrow. Transplant Proc 5:671–674, 1973
10. Carpenter CB, Morris PJ: Immunological monitoring of transplant patients. Transplant Proc 11:1153–1159, 1980
11. Chang TW, Kung PC, Gingras SP et al: Does OKT3 monoclonal antibody react with an antigen-recognition structure on human T cells? Proc Natl Acad Sci 78:1805–1808, 1981
12. Chatenoud L, Baudrihaye MF, Kreis H et al: Human in vivo antigenic modulation induced by the anti-T cell OKT3 monoclonal antibody. Eur J Immunol 12:979–982, 1982
13. Cheeseman SH, Rubin RH, Stewart JA et al: Controlled clinical trial of prophylactic human leukocyte interferon in renal transplantation. N Engl J Med 300:1345–1349, 1979
14. Clark AW, Monaco AP: The effect of bacterial adjuvants on allograft survival after antilymphocyte serum (ALS) and donor bone marrow. Immunology (British) 27:887–893, 1974
15. Cosimi AB: The clinical value of antilymphocyte antibodies. Transplant Proc 13:462–468, 1981
16. Cosimi AB, Burton RC, Colvin RB et al: Treatment of acute renal allograft rejection with OKT3 monoclonal antibody. Transplantation 32, 535–539, 1981
17. Cosimi AB, Cho SI, Delmonico FL et al: A randomized clinical trial comparing OKT3 and steroids for treatment of hepatic allograft rejection. Transplantation 43:91, 1987
18. De Fazio SR, Hartner WC, Monaco AP et al: Mouse skin graft prolongation with donor strain bone marrow of the active bone marrow cells. J Immunol 135:3034, 1985
19. De Fazio SR, Hartner WC, Monaco AP et al: Prolongation of graft survival in ALS-treated mice by donor-specific bone marrow: density gradient fractionation of the active bone marrow cells. Transplantation vol 43, 1987
20. De Fazio SR, Hartner WC, Monaco AP et al: Mouse

skin prolongation with donor strain bone marrow and antilymphocyte serum. Effect of donor age. Transplantation 40:563, 1985

21. De Fazio SR, Hartner WC, Monaco AP et al: Mouse skin graft prolongation with donor strain bone marrow and antilymphocyte serum: Effect of bone marrow cell storage. Transplantation 41:26, 1986

22. De Fazio SR, Kowlenko M, Gozzo JJ: Isolation by continuous density gradient centrifugation and characterization of bone marrow cells active in prolonging allograft survival in antilymphocyte serum–treated mice. Transplant Proc 19:547, 1987

23. Engers HD, Thomas K, Cerottini JC et al: Generation of cytotoxic T-lymphocytes in vitro. V. Response of normal and immune spleen cells to subcellular alloantigens. J Immunol 115:356, 1975

24. Faustman D, Hauptfeld V, Lacy P et al: Prolongation of murine islet allograft survival by pretreatment of islets with antibody directed to Ia determinants. Natl Sci USA 78:5156, 1981

25. Ferguson RM: Strategy IV—Quadriple drug therapy. Transplantation and Immunology Letter 2(2):3, 1985

26. Filo RS, Smith EJ, Leapman SB: Therapy for acute cadaveric renal allograft rejection with adjunctive antithymocyte globulin. Transplantation 30(6):445, 1980

27. Filo RS, Smith EJ, Leapman SB: Reversal of acute renal allograft rejection with adjunctive ATG therapy. Transplant Proc 13:482–490, 1981

27a. Fung J, Iwatsuki S, Gordon R et al: Other organ transplant experiences with Orthoclone OKT3. Nephron (in press)

28. Thistethwaite JR Jr, Gaber AO, Haag BW et al: OKT3 as either primary or secondary treatment for renal allograft rejection. Transplantation 43:176, 1987

29. Giorgi JV, Cosimi AB, Colvin RB et al: Monitoring immunosuppression following renal transplantation. 1:174–178, 1983

30. Goldstein G, Schindler J, Tsai H et al: A randomized clinical trial of OKT3 monoclonal antibody for acute rejection of cadaveric renal transplants. N Engl J Med 313:337–342, 1985

31. Gozzo JJ, Litvin DA, Monaco AP et al: Fractionated bone marrow: Use of lymphocyte containing fraction for skin prolongation in antilymphocyte serum (ALS) treated mice. Transplant Proc 13:592, 1981

32. Gozzo JJ, Wood ML, Monaco AP: In vitro antilymphocyte serum cell-binding affinity as an indicator of in vivo immunosuppressive ability. Surg Forum 23:298–300, 1972

33. Gozzo JJ, Wood ML, Monaco AP: Studies on heterologous antilymphocyte serum in mice. IX. In vitro assay by indirect leukoagglutination. Transplantation 14:358–362, 1972

34. Gozzo JJ, Wood ML, Monaco AP: Indirect leukoagglutination: An in vitro assay for antilymphocyte serum. Surg Forum 22:277–280, 1971

35. Hardy MA, Nowygrod R, Elberg A et al: Use of ATG in treatment of steroid-resistant rejection. Transplantation 39:162, 1980

36. Hartner WC, De Fazio SR, Maki T et al: Prolongation of renal allograft survival in antilymphocyte serum-treated dogs by post-operative injection of density gradient-fractionated donor bone marrow. Transplantation 42:593, 1986

37. Hoitsma AJ, Reekers P, Kreeftenberg JG et al: Treatment of acute rejection of cadaveric renal allografts with rabbit antithymocyte globulin. Transplantation 33:12, 1982

38. Howard RJ, Condie RM, Sutherland DER et al: The use of antilymphoblast globulin in the treatment of renal allograft rejection. Transplantation 24(6):419, 1977

39. Imboden JB, Stobo JD: Transmembrane signaling by the T cell antigen receptor. J Exp Med 161:446–456, 1985

40. Kahan BD: Individualization of cyclosporine therapy using pharmacokinetic and pharmacodynamic parameters. Transplantation 40:457–475, 1985

41. Kamada N, Wight DG: Antigen-specific immunosuppression induced by liver transplantation in the rat. Transplantation 38:217, 1984

42. Kanazi G, Stowe N, Steinmuller D et al: Effect of cyclosporine upon the function of ischemically damaged kidneys in the rat. Transplantation 41:782, 1986

43. Kapnick SJ, Monaco AP: Induction of unresponsiveness to skin allografts with donor strain platelets in antilymphocyte serum–treated mice. Transplant Proc 11:982–985, 1979

44. Kirkman RL, Aranjo JL, Busch GJ et al: Treatment of acute renal allograft rejection with monoclonal anti-T12 antibody. Transplantation 36:620–626, 1983

45. Kohler G, Milstein C: Derivation of specific antibody-producing tissue culture and tumor lines by cell fusion. Eur J Immunol 6:511–519, 1976

46. Kris H, Chkoff H, Vigeral PH et al: Prophylactic treatment of allograft recipients with a monoclonal anti-T3+ cell antibody. Transplant Proc 17:1315–1319, 1985

47. Kreis H: See Vigeral P et al.

48. Kung PC, Goldstein G, Reinberg EL et al: Monoclonal antibodies defining distinctive human T cell surface antigens. Science 206:347, 1979

49. Lafferty KJ, Booes A, Dart G et al: Effect of organ culture on the survival of thyroid allografts in mice. Transplantation 22:138, 1976

50. Lance EM, Medawar PB: Quantitative studies in tissue transplantation immunity. IX. Induction of tolerance with antilymphocyte serum. Proc Roy Soc B 173:447, 1969

51. Landegren V, Ramstedt V, Axberg I et al: Selective inhibition or initiation of lysis by mono 'onal OKT3 and Leu-2a antibodies. J Exp Med 155:1579–1584, 1982

52. Latham WC, Cooney RM, Brown KJ et al: Preparation of purified antilymphocyte serum on an immuno-absorbent column. In Proceedings of a Symposium on Standardization of Antilymphocyte Serum, Vol 16, pp 171–178, 1970

53. Liegeois A, Escourrow J, Ouvre E et al: Microchimerism: A state of low ratio proliferation of allogeneic bone marrow. Transplant Proc 9:272, 1977

54. Light JA, Alijan MR, Biggers JA et al: Antilymphocyte globulin (ALG) reverses "irreversible" allograft rejection. Transplant Proc 13:475, 1981

55. Mak TW, Yanagi Y: Genes encoding the T cell antigen receptor. Immunol Rev 81:221–233, 1984

56. Maki T, Gottschalk R, Wood ML et al: Specific unresponsiveness to skin allografts in antilymphocyte serum-treated, marrow-injected mice: Participation of donor marrow–derived suppressor cells. J Immunol 127:1433–1438, 1981

57. Maki T, Simpson M, Monaco AP: Development of suppressor T cells by antilymphocyte serum treatment in mice. Transplantation 34:376–381, 1982

58. Matas JG: Personal communication

59. Monaco AP: Antilymphocyte globulin: A clinical transplantation research opportunity. Am J Kidney Dis 2:67, 1982

60. Monaco AP: Antilymphocyte serum and other methods of lymphocyte depletion. In Najarian JS, Simmons RL (eds): Transplantation, Chap 6, Section IV, pp 222–251. Philadelphia, Lea & Febiger, 1972

61. Monaco AP, Codish S: Collective review: Antilymphocyte serum. Surg Gynecol Obstet 142:419–423, 1976

62. Monaco AP, Wood ML: Studies on heterologous antilymphocyte serum in mice. VII. Optimal cellular antigen for induction of immunologic tolerance with antilymphocyte serum. Transplant Proc 2:489–496, 1970

63. Monaco AP, Goldstein G, Barnes L: Treatment of acute renal allograft rejection unresponsive to conventional immunosuppressive therapy with OKT3 monoclonal antibody. Transplant Proc (in press)

64. Monaco AP, Gozzo JJ, Wood ML et al: Use of low doses of homozygous allogeneic bone marrow cells to induce tolerance with antilymphocyte serum (ALS): Tolerance by intraorgan injection. Transplant Proc 3:680–683, 1971

65. Monaco AP, Wood ML, Russell PS: Adult thymectomy: Effect on recovery from immune depression in mice. Science 149:432, 1965

66. Monaco AP, Wood ML, Russell PS: Some effects of purified heterologous anti-human lymphocyte serum in man. Transplantation 5:1106, 1967

67. Monaco AP, Wood ML, Russell PS: Studies on heterologous antilymphocyte serum in mice. III. Immunologic and chimerism produced across the H-2 locus with adult thymectomy and antilymphocyte serum. Ann NY Acad Sci 129:190, 1966

68. Monaco AP, Wood ML, Gray JG et al: Studies on heterologous antilymphocyte serum in mice. II. Effect on the immune response. J Immunol 96:229, 1966

69. Monaco AP, Wood ML, Maki T et al: Attempt to induce unresponsiveness to human renal allografts with antilymphocyte globulin and donor-specific bone marrow. Transplant Proc 17:1312–1314, 1985

70. Najarian JS, Simmons RL, Condie R et al: Seven year's experience with antilymphoblast globulin for renal transplantation. Ann Surg 184:352, 1976

71. Nomenclature Subcommittee Differentiation human leukocyte antigens: A proposed nomenclature. Immunology Today 5(6) 158–159, 1984

72. Novick AC, Ho-Hsieh H, Steinmuller D et al: Detrimental effect of cyclosporine on initial function of cadaver renal allografts following extended preservation: Results of a randomized prospective study. Transplantation 42:154, 1986

73. Novick AC, Khauli RB et al: Improved results of cadaver renal transplantation with azathioprine, prednisone, and antilymphoblast globulin. J Urol 131:636, 1984

74. Novick AC, Steinmuller D et al: A controlled prospective randomized double blind study of antilymphoblast globulin in cadaver renal transplantation. Transplantation 35:175, 1983

75. Nowygrod G, Appel P, Hardy MA: Use of ATG for reversal of acute allograft rejection. Transplant Proc 13:469–472, 1981

76. Opelz G: The influence of ischemia times and HLA-Dr matching in cyclosporine-treated cadaver kidney grafts. Transplant Proc 17:1478, 1985

77. Pass RF, Long WK, Whitley RJ et al: Productive infection with cytomegalovirus and herpes simplex virus in renal transplant recipients: Role of source of kidney. J Infect Dis 137:556–563, 1978

78. Pass RF, Whitley RJ, Diethelm AG et al: Cytomegalovirus infection in patients with renal transplant: Potentiation by antithymocyte globulin and an incompatible graft. J Infect Dis 142:9–17, 1980

79. Penn I: Malignant lymphomas in organ transplant recipients. Transplant Proc 13:736–738, 1981

80. Pescovitz MD, Thistlethwaite JR Jr, Auchincloss H Jr et al: Effect of Class II antigen matching on renal allograft survival in miniature swine. J Exp Med 160:1495, 1984

81. Rowinski W, Ryffa T, Ruke M et al: Platelet-induced donor-specific unresponsiveness to kidney allografts in mongrel dogs treated with ALG. Transplant Proc 13:536–588, 1981

82. Rubin RH, Cosimi AB, Hirsch MS et al: Effects of antilymphocyte globulin on cytomegalovirus infection in renal transplant recipients. Transplantation 31:143–145, 1981

83. Sheil AGR, Mears D, Johnson JE et al: Antilymphocyte globulin in patients with renal allografts from cadaveric donors: Late results of a controlled trial. Lancet 2:227, 1973

84. Shields CF, Cosimi AB, Tolkoff–Rubin N et al: Use of antilymphocyte globulin for reversal of acute allograft rejection. Transplantation 28(6):461, 1979

85. Simmons RL: Personal communication

86. Sollinger HW, Burkholder PM, Rasmus WR et al: Prolonged survival of xenografts after organ culture. Surgery 81:74, 1977

87. Spees EK, Vaughn WK, Niblack G et al: The effects of blood transfusion on cadaver renal transplanta-

tion: A prospective study of the Southeastern Organ Procurement Foundation. Transplant Proc 13:155–160, 1981

88. Starzl T: See Fung J et al.

89. Stiller RY, Rolles K, White DJG et al: The Canadian trial of cyclosporine: Cyclosporine therapy compared to standard immunosuppression in renal transplants, an exploration of nephrotoxicity. Transplant Proc 15:2479, 1983

90. Streem AB, Novick AC et al: Low-dose maintenance of acute rejection: A steroid-sparing approach to immunosuppressive therapy. Transplantation 35:420, 1983

91. Streem SB, Novick AC, Braun WE et al: Antilymphoblast globulin for treatment of acute renal allograft rejection. Transplant Proc 15:590, 1983

92. Takahashi H, Okasaki H, Terasaki PI et al: Reversal of transplant rejection by monoclonal antiblast antibody. Lancet 2:1155–1158, 1983

93. Taylor HE, Ackman CFD, Horowitz I: Canadian clinical trial of antilymphocyte globulin in human cadaver renal transplantation. Can Med Assoc J 115:1205, 1976

94. Thomas JM, Carver FM, Burnett CM et al: Enhanced allograft survival in Rhesus monkeys treated with antihuman thymocyte globulin and donor lymphoid cells. Transplant Proc 13:599–602, 1981

95. Thomas F, Carver FM, Foil MB et al: Long-term incompatible kidney survival in outbred higher primates without chronic immunosuppression. Ann Surg 198:370, 1983

96. Thomas JM, Carver FM, Foil MB et al: Renal allograft tolerance induced with ATG and donor bone marrow in outbred Rhesus monkeys. Transplantation 36:104, 1983

97. Toledo–Pereyra LH, Mittal VK, Baskin S et al: Nonsteroid treatment of rejection in kidney transplantation: A new approach including long-term treatment of rejection with antilymphoblast globulin in a high-risk population. Transplantation 33:325, 1982

98. Turcotte JG, Feduska NJ, Haines RF et al: Antilymphocyte globulin in renal transplant recipients: A clinical trial. Arch Surg 106:484, 1973

99. Van den Elsen P, Shepley BA, Borst J et al: Isolation of cDNA clones encoding the 20K T3 glycoprotein of human T cell receptor complex. Nature 312:413–418, 1984

99a. Vigeral P, Chkoff N, Chatenoud L et al: Prophylactic use of OKT3 monoclonal antibody in cadaver kidney recipients. Transplantation 41:730, 1986

100. Wagner H, Rollinghoff M: Secondary cytotoxic allograft response in vitro. II. Differentiation of memory T cells into cytotoxic lymphocytes in the absence of cell proliferation. Eur J Immunol 6:15, 1976

101. Wechter WJ, Morell RM, Bergan et al: Extended treatment with antilymphocyte globulin (ATGAM) in renal allograft recipients. Transplantation 28:354, 1979

102. Wood ML, Monaco AP: Adoptive transfer of specific unresponsiveness to skin allografts by spleen cells from ALS-treated, marrow-injected mice. Transplant Proc 11:1023–1027, 1979

103. Wood ML, Monaco AP: Suppressor cells in specific unresponsiveness to skin allografts in ALS-treated, marrow-injected mice. Transplantation 29:196, 1980

104. Wood ML, Gottschalk R, Monaco AP: Effect of splenectomy on specific unresponsiveness to skin allografts induced in ALS-treated, marrow-injected mice. Transplantation 29:320, 1980

105. Wood ML, Monaco AP, Gozzo JJ et al: Use of homozygous allogeneic bone marrow for induction of tolerance with antilymphocyte serum: Dose and Timing. Transplant Proc 3:676–679, 1971

CHAPTER 6

Chemical Manipulation of the Immune Responses

Nicholas L. Tilney   T.B. Strom

If there are histocompatibility differences between donor and host, the immune responses must be altered for graft acceptance; thus, knowledge of the steps in the cascade has helped in determining specific mechanisms of action of various immunosuppressive agents. Class I molecules are found on virtually all cell surfaces; Class II HLA molecules are present on the surface of T- and B-lymphocytes, some monocytes, and antigen-processing cells.

The distinct role of each of the cell subpopulations in unmodified rejection is still undefined, although it is clear that macrophages and cytotoxic and helper cells play a role.

Several antiproliferative drugs have been used with varying degrees of success as immunosuppressive agents in clinical transplantation. Azathioprine, an imidazole derivative of 6-mercaptopurine, has been the linchpin of immunosuppressive treatment. It inhibits the primary immune responses but has little effect upon the secondary responses. Complications include jaundice, anemia, alopecia, and, most importantly, leukopenia.

Cyclosphosphamide is of a class of drugs derived from nitrogen mustard. It depresses the cellular immune responses and prolongs survival of skin allografts in several animal species. In contrast, it has been reported to abolish the effects of immunologic enhancement in prolonging allograft survival in several experimental models, possibly by its selective destruction of suppressor lymphocytes. In clinical transplantation, it is probably less effective than azathioprine and may be exceedingly toxic, particularly regarding leukopenia and thrombocytopenia.

An imidazole derivative, niridazole, is an antihelmintic that has been shown to decrease cell-mediated immunity in laboratory animals. It has little effect on the antibody-mediated responses. This agent increases graft survival in mice and rats, although its immunosuppressive effectiveness in clinical trials has been marginal.

Corticosteroids inhibit both cellular and humoral immunity as well as having profound anti-inflammatory activity. They reduce migration of neutrophils into infected tissues and reduce inflammation by inhibiting lysosomal enzyme release by these cells. Their activity in the immunologic cascade has also been defined. They directly inhibit antibody-driven T cell population by mechanisms different from those of azathioprine.

Most transplant groups treat episodes of acute rejection with short bursts of methylprednisolone. However, some rejection episodes are not sensitive to steroids, particularly repeat rejections or episodes occurring during infection with opportunistic organisms. Such treatment is ineffectual in antibody-mediated rejections, including hyperacute rejections and chronic rejections. It is clear that because of their profound side effects, steroids should be used judiciously.

Cyclosporine either facilitates activation of or spares selectively allospecific suppressor T cells while blunting overall effector T cell proliferation; the resultant cellular imbalance may render an allograft recipient functionally unresponsive to the allograft. Multiple clinical studies have consistently improved graft survival rates in cyclosporine-treated patients compared with patients given conventional immunosuppression with azathioprine and prednisone. Regimens using low doses of cyclosporine in combination with doses of prednisone, combination therapy with azathioprine, or conversion to azathioprine after an induction period of several months, emerge as reasonable alternative approaches in providing effective immunosuppression and diminishing nephrotoxicity. Graft dysfunction remains a critical problem, particularly in differentiating between acute rejection, drug nephrotoxicity, and acute tubular necrosis.

The production of indefinite and specific host tolerance toward a foreign graft has been the primary goal of those involved in organ transplantation for many years. This concept has a compelling basis in biology. Different ABO blood types can reside together in bone marrow and peripheral blood of twins,[98] and skin grafts are not rejected in freemartin cattle, animals with placental cross circulation.[125] Similarly, a fetus exposed to allogeneic tissue will develop lifelong tolerance to the specific antigen.[13] A markedly prolonged survival of a parental skin graft was obtained in a child who had been injected with his father's leukocytes at birth.[190]

Despite this success in humans, these findings remained biological peculiarities for many years, irrelevant to clinical use. It was not until the later 1950s, when the salvage of terminally ill patients with renal failure by kidney isografts was clearly demonstrated, that the need for modifying the host immune responses for successful transplantation with allografts become obvious.[109] At first, the only available means of immunosuppression was total body x-radiation, used with some success in animal allograft recipients, with less success clinically.[68,97] Then, in 1959, in a landmark article that showed that the immune responses could indeed be altered chemically, Schwartz and Dameshek[155] described depression of the antibody response to antigens in rabbits using a new antimetabolite drug, 6-mercaptopurine. An imidazole derivative of this compound, azathioprine, was then quickly noted to be a more powerful immunosuppressant in dogs and then in patients by Calne, Murray, and Zukoski.[24,27,194] When corticosteroids, whose immunosuppressive anti-inflammatory effects on the allograft response had first been described by Billingham,[15] were used in conjunction with azathioprine in 1962, effective suppression of recipient immunity became reality.

Many immunosuppressive modalities other than azathioprine and steroids have been attempted, the majority of which have proved unsuccessful. However, in recent years, accelerating advances in therapy have included the advent of cyclosporine, the use of antilymphocyte serum to combat rejection, and the increasing potential for monoclonal anti-T cell antibodies. In this chapter, we review the types of chemical immunosuppression that are or have been used in clinical transplantation. Their mechanisms of action, both in vitro and in vivo, and their effectiveness in allograft recipients are assessed.

HOST IMMUNORESPONSIVENESS

Because of remarkable recent advancements in basic immunobiology, it seems reasonable to preface a discussion of chemical immunosuppression by briefly summarizing existing concepts of the host responses against allografted tissues. With this as background, it will be easier to detail the particular steps of immunologic cascade affected by the various pharmacologic agents. A detailed analysis of the normal immune response is presented elsewhere in this book.

Histocompatibility Antigens and Receptors

Clearly, the immune responses must be altered for graft acceptance if histocompatibility differences exist between donor and host. All mammals have a single chromosomal region encoded for major transplantation antigens, highly polymorphic cell surface structures whose recognition allows the host to distinguish between self and non-self.[3] Genes for the major histocompatibility complexes are aligned closely on the 6th chromosome in humans and are named the human leukocyte antigen (HLA) system. HLA antigens are glycoproteins expressed in varying quantities on most cell surfaces, except for mature erythrocytes. Class I HLA molecules are expressed on virtually all cell surfaces; Class II HLA molecules are present on the surface of only a few cell types, including B-lymphocytes, some monocytes and other antigen-presenting cells (dendritic cells, Langerhans' cells in skin), as well as T-lymphocytes that have become "Class II positive" when activated.[3,174]

Clinical histocompatibility testing has shown that recipients with preformed antibodies against Class I but not Class II donor antigens are at high risk of hyperacute rejection. In addition, host responses against HLA molecules, particularly Class II, are a formidable barrier to successful organ transplantation, because the cellular responses against such antigens are T cell dependent. However, many recent studies on the cellular constituents and molecular basis of the allograft response have allowed progressive dissection into T cell functions, with increased understanding as to why Class II HLA matching is of such great potential importance in clinical transplantation.

All mature T-lymphocytes bear the T3 protein as a distinctive surface marker; the two complementary and essentially nonoverlapping T helper and cytotoxic cell subsets bear either the T4 or T8 surface protein.[135] Perhaps the most important functional differences in these subpopulations lie in their differential reactivity toward various classes of HLA molecules. Thus, T4 + helper T-lymphocytes respond to Class II molecules such as DR, DP, and DQ, whereas T8+ cytotoxic T-lymphocytes preferentially recognize Class I HLA A, -B and -C locus molecules.[12,110] Indeed, the T8 protein and the T4 protein bind to nonpolymorphic regions of HLA Class I and Class II proteins, respectively. Anti-T3 monoclonal antibodies such as OK T3 essentially define the entire immunocompetent human T cell population.[92,134,184] Interaction of low concentrations of these antibodies with circulating leukocytes results in T cell mitogenesis and suggests a central role for the T3 protein in the event of cell activation.

The T cell antigen receptor protein is a 92,000 dalton heterodimer that is not associated with T4 or T8 but is noncovalently linked to the T3 membrane protein.[47,89] Hence, T cells recognize antigen by both stereospecific receptors and adjunctive binding proteins. The elements that the T cell uses to bind antigen are increasingly well understood; a dual receptor model for T cell recognition of antigen appears valid. The T cell receptor binds the antigenic portion of HLA antigens, although its attachment to antigen is often insufficiently avid to support T cell activation. Accordingly, adjunctive binding proteins are required; T4 and T8 proteins expressed upon cytotoxic T-lymphocytes fulfill the role of adjunctive target cell binding proteins.

The Sequence of T Cell Activation

Activation of T helper cells by Class II major histocompatibility complex antigens such as HLA-Dr probably effect the release of a macrophage stimulant (perhaps the same molecule as colony stimulating factor[113]) as well as the formation of receptors for transferrin,[180] insulin,[71–73] interleukin 1 (IL-1),[62] and interleukin 2 (IL-2).[36,138] Cytotoxic T-lymphocytes stimulated by Class I HLA antigens develop IL-2 receptors.[138] At the same time, macrophages and other accessory cells, activated by T cell products,[113] release IL-1, which, in turn, stimulates the release of IL-2 by activated helper cells (Fig. 6-1).[160] This lymphokine interacts with specific IL-2 receptors expressed on activated helper and cytotoxic T cells.[29,30,160] causing the initiation of DNA synthesis and driving clonal proliferation of the IL-2 receptor bearing cell populations. The proliferative rate of antigen-activated T cells is governed both by the ambient concentration of IL-2 and the density of IL-

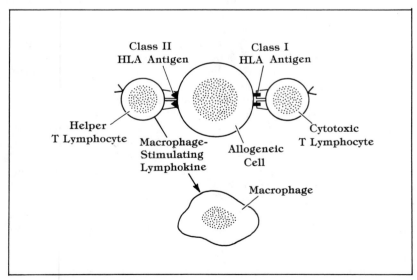

FIGURE 6-1.   *The T cell activation sequence and the impact of immunosuppressive therapy; activation of T cell subsets by HLA Class I and II molecules.*

2 receptor proteins upon the activated cells.[29,159,160] Moreover, the continued viability of activated T cell clones is IL-2 dependent. IL-2 also causes release of gamma interferon by activated T cells, which stimulates macrophages for allograft destruction.[51,127] This may initiate a vicious cycle as these products induce both expression of Class I molecules upon endothelial cells and certain Class II negative macrophages.[83,132] IL-2 also causes release of B cell growth factors, which stimulate proliferation of antigen- activated B cells.[77,79] The release of cytotoxic differentiation factor, another product of antigen-activated T cells, is also probably stimulated by IL-2. Whereas IL-2 activates clonal growth of cytotoxic T cells, cytotoxic differentiation factor evokes the cytotoxic potential of noncytotoxic T8+ T cells.

Thus, activation of helper cells by alloantigen and IL-1 stimulates their release of several lymphokines, which, in turn, activate macrophages, cytotoxic T cells, antibody-releasing B cells, as well as increasing the immunogenicity of the graft by inducing further expression of Class I molecules. These factors also support clonal expansion and viability of antigen-activated T and B cells. Unmodified rejection has been thought to result primarily from the cytodestructive effects produced by cytoxic T-lymphocytes, activated macrophages, and antibody. Although cytotoxic cells are prominent among cells that infiltrate the allograft during graft rejection both in experimental animals and in man, the transcendent importance of helper cells in the event of rejection may derive from the "endocrine" role of these cells in providing various soluble growth and activation signals required during the allograft response.[70,170,171,177] That both subsets together are critical in acute rejection of vascularized organ grafts has been proved by re-establishing allograft immunity following selective cell transfer into T cell–deficient experimental animals.[177]

IMMUNOSUPPRESSIVE DRUGS

The immunosuppressive activities of each of the chemical agents used in clinical transplantation directly interfere with one or another of the several steps in the "allograft response." Unfortunately, the majority of such therapy is nonspecific and decreases all immune responses in general, including those against bacteria, fungi, viruses, or even malignant tumors; hence, the continuing search for more selective and specific agents. The various types of drugs used in clinical transplantation and their general classes are listed in Table 6-1 and will be discussed individually. Other chemical agents used in

TABLE 6-1   Chemical Immunosuppressive Agents Used in Transplantation

I. Antiproliferative agents—act on cells synthesizing DNA
   A. Antimetabolites
      6-Mercaptopurine
      Azathioprine
   B. Alkalating agents
      Cyclophosphamide
   C. Imidazoles
      Niridazole
II. Glucocorticosteroids—anti-inflamatory effects
III. Anti-lymphocytic agents
   Cyclosporine

the earlier stages of clinical transplantation will not be mentioned here because of their lack of effectiveness.

Azathioprine

This S-imidazole derivative of 6-mercaptopurine has been the lynchpin of immunosuppressive treatment for renal transplantation since its first clinical use in 1961. An antimetabolite, its importance in depressing immune reactivity can be traced to the seminal investigations on 6-mercaptopurine (6-MP).[38] Although the original work on 6-MP demonstrated important suppression of antibody formation in rabbits,[157] the immunosuppressive potential of this drug and of other purine analogs were also noted in several species, including chickens, rats, rabbits, dogs, monkeys, and humans.[153,156] In addition to its effects on antibody production, the drug was found to suppress specific delayed hypersensitivity responses as well as influencing skin graft survival.

Azathioprine was synthesized by Hitchings and Elion[76] specifically to provide an analog of 6-MP suitable for parenteral administration. It was then found to be a more potent immunosuppressive agent than 6-MP in several transplant models.[26] It possesses several critical activities. Its metabolites, including 6-MP, are incorporated into cellular DNA, which inhibits the synthesis and metabolism of purine nucleotides and influences synthesis and function of RNA. Its general antiproliferative activity allows it to effect rapidly dividing activated B and T cells during the proliferative cycle of effector lymphocytes. As antigen stimulation causes cell division and proliferation, the predominant immunosuppressive effect of azathioprine is to interdict mitosis of immunologically competent lymphoid cells by interfering with nucleotide synthesis. (Fig. 6-2).

Although the drug inhibits the primary immune responses, it has little effect upon the secondary responses; thus, it is useful in preventing acute

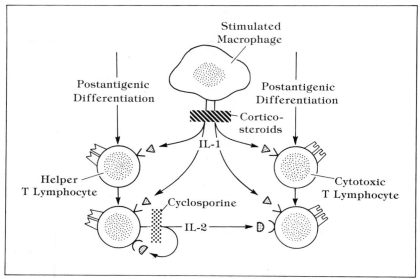

FIGURE 6-2.   *The T cell activation sequence and the impact of immunosuppressive therapy; IL-1 release is blocked by corticosteroids, and IL-2 release is inhibited by cyclosporine.*

rejection but not in reversing ongoing rejection. Indeed, pretreatment with the agent for 48 hours before grafting produces optimal suppression in various experimental models. As a result, many groups have generally begun treatment 2 to 3 days before transplantation in recipients of kidney allografts from living-related donors, although, by necessity, it is initiated immediately preoperatively when cadaver kidneys are used. With this type of regimen, the results of graft survival in patients receiving a standard combination of azathioprine and steroids have been about 50% by the end of the first year for cadaver grafts and about 75% for grafts from non-HLA identical living-related donors.[173]

Azathioprine is administered initially in our unit at a loading dose of 4 mg/kg/day for 4 days. If renal function is satisfactory, it is then reduced to 3 mg/kg/day; if the patient is oliguric, 2 mg/kg/day is used. The drug is then continued indefinitely at maintenance doses of 2 mg/kg/day to 3 mg/kg/day, depending upon allograft function, because even transient discontinuation early in the post-transplantation period has produced a high rate of graft failure.[67] Because the agent is metabolized rapidly by the liver, its dose has little direct relevance on renal function per se, although some persons, especially if their graft function is compromised, are particularly sensitive to its myelosuppressive effects. In such patients, the dose should be decreased or stopped until the leukopenia resolves—the peripheral leukocyte count being the most consistent measure of azathioprine toxicity. Unfortunately, interruption of treatment with this drug because of leukopenia may at the same time allow the occurrence of rejection episodes. As cyclosporine is not myelosuppressive, persons faced with this complication may be converted from azathioprine to cyclosporine with relative safety.

Other complications of azathioprine treatment include jaundice, anemia, and alopecia. The increased potential for malignancy in transplant recipients, especially the lymphoproliferative disorders, may also relate to drug toxicity.[130] Although cyclophosphamide has been substituted for azathioprine in persons with evidence of hepatocellular damage, it seems clear that those with active hepatitis do not require cytotoxic drug therapy for allograft maintenance; the grafts may continue to function for indefinite periods of time without immunosuppression.[86,188] In addition, a high rate of opportunistic infections occurs in patients with liver disease on normal maintenance doses of azathioprine. Finally, those receiving this agent should never be treated coincidentally with allopurinol for gout. As allopurinol blocks the catabolism of azathioprine and other purines, the combination of the two drugs is devastating and several deaths from bone marrow aplasia have occurred.[86]

Cyclophosphamide

Cyclophosphamide is one of the alkalating agents—a class of drug derived from nitrogen mustard. The two armed dichlorethyl moieties of the molecule attach to nucleic acid chains or enzyme macromolecules and interfere with their function. The agent affects dividing cells; its lack of activity on resting cells may explain its relative lack of hepatotoxicity despite being concentrated highly in liver cells.[55]

The anticancer and potent immunosuppressive activity of cyclophosphamide has been well documented.[153] It is most effective when administered up to 48 hours following the antigenic stimulus, during stages of cell proliferation and/or differentiation.[8,59,152] It strongly affects humoral immunoresponsiveness. Stender and associates[165] first reported that it suppressed antibody formation in rats following the appearance of detectable antibody in the serum. Results were confirmed in several other animal species as well as in humans.[8,101,133] The drug also depresses the cellular immune responses, particularly delayed hypersensitivity reactions in tumor systems,[121,193] and decreases the induction of tuberculin and contact sensitivity in guinea pigs.[100,181] It also inhibits the development of large pyroninophilic cells in lymph nodes draining such site, cells that are a prominent feature in delayed hypersensitivity.[182] This is in contrast, for instance, to the effect of methotrexate, a folic acid antagonist that does not inhibit the appearance of such cells but prevents their maturation into small lymphocytes. The survival of skin allografts in several species, including mice, rabbits, rats, and guinea pigs,[7,20,56,151,172] can be prolonged, particularly when the first dose of the drug is administered within several days of grafting.

In contrast to these immunosuppressive qualities, cyclophosphamide has been reported to abolish the effects of immunologic enhancement in prolonging the survival of liver allografts in baboons[117] and of cardiac allografts in rats.[105] These enigmatic observations have also been noted in cyclosporine-treated rat recipients bearing indefinitely surviving heart grafts.[95] Acute rejection could be initiated in well-established, long-term, functioning heart grafts in cyclosporine-modified recipients only when cyclophosphamide was added to an infusion of sensitized spleen cells. Cyclophosphamide was then necessary to override the immunologic process that was responsible for the long-term graft acceptance.

The activity of suppressor cells may be a specific immunologic effect that is, in large part, responsible for indefinite prolongation of organ allografts in the aforementioned models. This has particularly been shown in graft recipients treated with cyclosporine.[93] Cyclophosphamide is reputed to destroy suppressor T cells[96,126,141]; once this protective host mechanism has been abrogated, the grafts undergo acute rejection. The suggestion that IL-2 inhibitor activity is controlled by cyclophosphamide sensitive T suppressor cells has also been examined.[93] The sera of cyclosporine-treated grafted hosts was found to contain high levels of IL-2 inhibitor; administration of cyclophosphamide resulted in dramatic reduction of this mediator.[95] Thus, the concept that increased cell-mediated responsiveness may result from selective elimination of cyclophosphamide-sensitive suppressor T cells or their precursors may have important theoretical implications in immunosuppression. Thus, if long-term graft maintenance or a quasi "tolerant" state is mediated through activity of suppressor cells, cyclophosphamide may be exactly the wrong immunosuppressive agent to use, either early during the development of such cells or late during their maintenance phase.

There is rather scanty information on the use of cyclophosphamide in clinical transplantation. In 1971, Starzl suggested that the drug might be more effective than azathioprine in renal and liver transplantation; however, follow-up was brief, and no control group was apparent.[162] Few other clinical reports have accrued subsequently, probably because the agent may be exceptionally toxic. Indeed, leukopenia and thrombocytopenia can be profound as well as causing nausea, vomiting, alopecia, and other unpleasant side effects. In animal models, a combination of azathioprine, prednisolone, and cyclophosphamide has been found effective,[58] although when tried clinically, such combination therapy was remarkably toxic.[10] The use of cyclophosphamide in treating rejection episodes was described by Uldall[183] in 1971, although more recent controlled trials have shown such treatment to be of little help.[147] However, it is still used relatively routinely to prepare recipients for bone marrow transplantation.[168]

Niridazole

The imidazoles, particularly the benimidazoles subclass, have been shown to modulate the immune responses. First described in the late 1960s as possessing immunosuppressive properties,[50] benimidazole derivatives were noted to suppress both humoral and cellular immune responses in mice[167] when administered in considerably smaller doses than azathioprine. One such derivative, niridazole, profoundly suppressed granuloma formation in a *Schistosoma mansoni* egg granuloma model,[103] as well as inhibiting foot pad swelling in mice that had been sensitized with parasitic eggs. This agent was later found to depress cell-mediated immunity in a skin allograft model in mice,[104] then in rats. It also diminished cell-mediated immunity in murine tumor systems.[142] It has little effect on antibody-mediated responses,[129] either primary or secondary, or ongoing production of antibody.[111] In initial studies in mouse recipients of skin grafts, a dose of 100 mg/kg of body weight of niridazole increased allograft survival from 10 to 18 days; more importantly, a synergistic effect was noted when this drug was administered together with anti-thymocyte globulin.[39,102,145] Using a heterotopic heart graft rat model, Salaman[142] noted that niridazole, given orally at a dose of 50 mg/kg, tripled the median graft survival time; this effect was not increased by administering concurrent prednisolone or azathioprine. However, when all three drugs were combined, six of eight grafts survived indefinitely. Unfortunately, when the immunosuppressive qualities of niridazole were later tested in a controlled clinical trial, they showed no benefits for its use in combination with azathioprine and steroids in recipients of cadaver transplants. When niridazole was given in conjunction with concurrent high doses of steroids alone, the results were slightly superior to those of control patients.[145] Thus, based on both clinical and experimental data, high-dose steroids plus niridazole seem to be marginally effective immunosuppressive therapy.

The immunosuppressive activity of the agent has been reasonably defined. Immunosuppression in vitro had been thought to result from an active metabolite of this antihelmintic drug; thus, antigen-induced inhibition of migration of sensitized peritoneal exudate cells can be decreased markedly by serum from treated guinea pigs.[39] However, this effect cannot be produced by the drug itself. Niridazole is metabolized primarily in the liver; the active metabolite has now been identified and synthesized. Indeed, other synthetic imidazoles have shown similar immunosuppressive properties as well as being useful antihelmintic agents.[111] However, based on existing knowledge, although immunosuppressive activity can certainly be demonstrated in animal models, there is little explanation for increased graft survival in terms of solubility, drug structure, metabolism, absorption, or excretion. As noted, however, although clinically of little immunosuppressive potency when used alone, the imidazoles may be marginally useful in transplant recipients when combined with other agents, particularly high-dose steroids.

CORTICOSTEROIDS

In the quarter century during which chemical agents have been used for immunosuppression of patients with tissue allografts, it has become clear that ad-

ministration of adjunctive maintenance corticosteroids, at least in the early period after transplantation, is almost mandatory for continued graft success. Indeed, although early in the clinical transplant experience it was recognized that azathioprine alone was relatively successful in preventing rejection, a combination of azathioprine plus steroids was considerably more effective.[65] Despite compelling experimental evidence to suggest that the corticosteroids might have important immunosuppressive potential,[15] cortisone alone was ineffectual in prolonging kidney graft survival in dogs.[40] The drug was noted to effect both cellular and humoral immunity as well as other aspects of the host responses. Some initial studies showed that the responsiveness of mice to sheep erythrocytes could be inhibited when the animals were pretreated with prednisone,[9,19] while others suggested that these agents might block the antigen-processing steps.[42] Although chronic steroid administration decreases synthesis of IgG, primary or secondary antibody responses to antigens are unaffected by late short pulses of the material.[23]

In general, the effects of steroids on cellular immunity are more powerful than on humoral immunity. They depress powerfully delayed hypersensitivity responses in animals and in humans, although much of this action may be due to their local anti-inflammatory effects.[45,60,124] However, both systemic and local steroid administration prolong survival of skin allografts in rats, mice, guinea pigs, and rabbits, although not in other species, including man.[14,90,91,161,189,191] In vitro, they dampen the generation of cytotoxic T cells following transplantation of tissue allografts and inhibit effector cells in the antibody-dependent cytotoxicity assay.[4] They impair the production of gamma interferon, an activity consistent with their primary effect, which is directed at IL-1-producing monocytes.[69] The diminished production of IL-2 and gamma interferon may also be due to decreased IL-1 production secondary to administration of these drugs (Fig. 6-3).

The anti-inflammatory activities of these agents are well known. Glaser and colleagues,[63] the first to appreciate the anti-inflammatory properties of adrenocortical extracts, noted that they reduced migration of neutrophils into infected tissues, although the chemotactic response of neutrophils and monocytes with bacteriocidal and fungicidal activity seemed to be somewhat improved.[37,136] Steroids also reduce inflammation by inhibiting lysosomal enzyme release by neutrophils.[64]

The effects of these agents on the immunologic cascade have been well worked out. They directly inhibit antigen-driven T cell proliferation, although

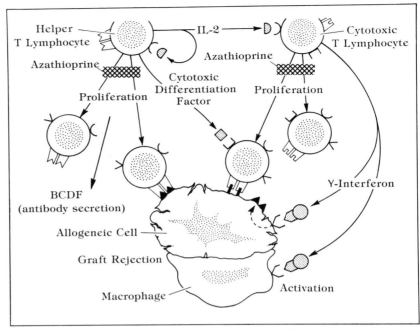

FIGURE 6-3. *The T cell activation sequence and the impact of immunosuppressive therapy; IL–2-dependent proliferation is blocked by azathioprine.*

by mechanisms quite different from those of aza-thioprine. A brief and brisk lymphocytopenia occurs in humans following steroid administration, although human lymphocytes are more refractory to steroid-induced lympholysis than are those of mouse, rat, or rabbit.[32] T and B peripheral blood lymphocyte counts decrease maximally 4 to 6 hours following oral prednisone (60 mg) or intravenous methylprednisolone (1 g), with T lymphocytopenia being more profound primarily through sequestration of recirculating lymphocytes into lymphoid tissues rather than lysis.[33,52,53,187,192] High concentrations of corticosteroids lyse mouse T cells more profoundly than human T cells; nonetheless, T cell proliferation is inhibited in human tissue culture.[44] Steroids have been shown in vitro to prevent the production of IL-2, thus denying essential trophic factors for activated T cells[61]; this may explain their ability to reverse rejection episodes in vivo. Although they do not act directly on the IL-2-producing T cell, they inhibit production of this lymphokine by preventing monocytes from releasing IL-1,[160] thereby blocking IL-1-dependent release of IL-2 from antigen-activated T cells (Fig. 6-3).

In most series, corticosteroids have been found necessary as immunosuppressive adjuncts to maintenance azathioprine or cyclosporine, as well as being the most effective agent for reversal of rejection when given in high doses for short periods of time. Until relatively recently, in our unit, 1.0 mg/kg/day to 1.5 mg/kg/day of prednisone was administered immediately before or at the time of transplantation, with reduction in dosage to maintenance levels of 10 mg/day to 20 mg/day occurring over a period of 2 to 3 months. However, the important adverse effects of these drugs, particularly predisposition to infection, impairment of wound healing, and probable increase in gastrointestinal complications, made it desirable to give as small a dose as possible, both initially and as maintenance therapy. Thus, based on the results of several trials, we now start prednisone at a dose of 50 mg/day in patients receiving azathioprine or 30 mg/day in those treated with cyclosporine. No patient takes more than 25 mg/day of prednisone 3 months after transplantation, with the dose reduced further to as low levels as possible (approximately 10 mg/day or less) commensurate with continued satisfactory graft function.

In 1977, McGeown and associates[107] first suggested that low-dose maintenance steroids used in combination with azathioprine could be as effective as the more generally accepted higher doses. Although such a change was not based on compelling clinical or experimental evidence, the results were encouraging.[148] Indeed, this concept held true in subsequent experimental studies using rat and baboon recipients,[35,146] and in several controlled clinical trials that compared tapered low and high dosages of steroids administered to persons receiving cadaver renal transplant.[21,128,144] In all trials, graft survival was identical in both high- and low-dose groups; however, all trials reported increased numbers of complications associated with the higher doses. In contrast, the results of a Finnish study disagreed, showing that there was marginal improvement in the high-dose group.[46] In our own experience with low-dose (20 mg/day) maintenance steroids administered to patients receiving azathioprine, the results were also disappointing, with a large incidence of graft loss compared with our standard (50 mg/day initial treatment) protocol. In contrast, since cyclosporine therapy has become routine in our institution, we are able to keep the maintenance dose of prednisone at 30 mg/day for the first 2 months with satisfactory results.[178] However, various centers in Europe and in the United Kingdom use no adjunctive steroids in allograft recipients treated with cyclosporine and report results comparable to those obtained in the United States.

The timing of the dosage and the concept of alternate-day therapy has also been debated. Because of diurnal variations in the endogenous production of corticosteroids,[88] the time of taking the daily dose may be important. This may be difficult to ascertain, however, particularly as there is wide variation in drug administration between transplantation units.[106] Few data have been generated on this point, either experimentally or clinically. Several short-term studies have suggested that alternate-day steroid therapy may reduce steroid toxicity as well as providing adequate immunosuppression in some transplant patients.[5,41,150] A lower incidence of osteonecrosis of the hip has been described in a recent controlled trial in patients randomized to alternate-day steroid therapy.[43] However, because most of the persons in these studies were treated with initial high-dose steroids, a decreased starting dose may have been equally effective.[148] In addition, particularly in recipients of cardiac transplants, large doses of corticosteroids are administered at the time of the transplant operation. Although there is some evidence in rats that allograft survival can be prolonged by such a maneuver,[6,143] clinical trials have not borne this out.[82] Few data are available on initial high-dose steroids combined with subsequent low maintenance doses.

Treatment of Rejection

In many centers, episodes of acute rejection are treated with methylprednisolone, 250 mg to 1 g, intravenously for 3 days immediately upon diag-

nosis. At the present time, increasing options for treatment of rejection include the use of polyclonal anti-lymphocyte serum and various monoclonal antibodies, including OKT3[123] and anti-T12.[85] When the rejection episode is sensitive to steroids, results are usually apparent within 48 to 96 hours. Some groups have used oral steroids (approximately 3 mg/kg/day) in lieu of intravenous steroids in the treatment of rejection with good success.[66,122] In rats, the two approaches give comparable results, and the effects of oral steroids and intravenous steroids on the mixed lymphocyte reaction are similar.[57]

Much of the morbidity surrounding organ transplantation has been directly attributable to immunosuppressive protocols using high-dose steroids; therefore, it has become increasingly clear that these drugs must be administered prudently so as to minimize their potentially lethal side effects.[179] Indeed, not all rejection episodes are sensitive to steroids (Table 6-2), particularly repeated rejections or episodes occurring in the presence of opportunistic infections or significant leukopenia. However, improved patient survival can be achieved through judicious use of immunosuppressive steroid therapy without sacrificing graft success.[149,179]; thus, we never treat patients for more than three rejection episodes occurring within the first year after transplantation, fearing the risks of oversuppression. However, steroids can be successful in reversing early acute rejection episodes, typically those occurring within the first month following transplantation. Such early crises are often characterized by mononuclear leukocyte infiltration of the graft with minimal glomerular and arteriolar immunoglobulin deposits. In contrast, hyperacute rejection, which may occur shortly after engraftment in patients preimmunized against the transplant and who exhibit circulating cytotoxic anti-HLA antibodies, is completely refractory to steroids. This type of rejection is characterized by rapid development of an intense antibody-mediated vasculitis with microvascular thrombosis. Chronic humoral rejection, presumably also an antibody-mediated process, which

TABLE 6-2   Contraindications of Steroid Use As Antirejection Treatment

Steroid-resistant rejections (2 previous failures)
Important leukopenia
Opportunistic infection
Antibody-mediated rejection with vasculitis (biopsy proven)
Chronic rejection with fibrosis (biopsy proven)

occurs over months or years, is also resistant to steroid therapy.

CYCLOSPORINE

Cyclosporine was discovered in 1972 by workers at Sandoz Ltd (Basel, Switzerland) while screening for agents with anti-microbial properties. This drug was subsequently shown to possess remarkable immunosuppressive capabilities in a variety of animal models as well as in humans. Its effectiveness has been shown so clearly in clinical transplantation that, at present, it has virtually replaced azathioprine as primary immunosuppression. Since many of its attributes and clinical effects have been well reviewed,[16,34,114,166] the present discussion will concentrate primarily on its immunologic effects and current clinical results.

Immunosuppressive Activity

Cyclosporine blocks humoral and cellular effector mechanisms participating in rejection by interfering with lymphocyte activation. Although the agent inhibits activation of both B and T cells as well as various macrophage functions, its predominant effect appears to be interference with the function of helper T-lymphocytes. While B-lymphocytes *participate* in the acute rejection process, the role of T-lymphocytes is *critical;* indeed, for most antibody-mediated responses, activation of antibody-producing B cells requires signals from T helper cells. The sites of its influence upon the effector cascade are shown in Figure 6-3. It shares with corticosteroids the capacity to block the entry of activated T-lymphocyte into the S phase of the cell cycle.[18] In contrast to corticosteroids, however, cyclosporine does not inhibit the capacity of all accessory cells to release IL-1 but blocks IL-2 release from activated helper T-lymphocytes.[22,75] The release by activated T cells of other lymphokines such as gamma-interferon, B cell differentiation, and cytotoxic differentiation factor is also inhibited by the drug,[81] whereas the expression of IL-2 receptors[81] and the responsiveness of activated T-lymphocytes to lymphokines are not blocked in vitro or in vivo.[112] Thus, under the influence of the drug, T helper–dependent T cytotoxic cells, B cells, and macrophages are not fully activated owing to a lack of necessary helper cell stimulants (Fig. 6-3).

Ample experimental evidence has also demonstrated that cyclosporine does not interfere, at least grossly, with activation and proliferation of suppressor T-lymphocytes; indeed, the agent spares this lymphocyte subpopulation in vivo, while the presence of a suppressor factor in the supernatants of cyclosporine-treated mixed lymphocyte cultures, which promotes suppressive cell activation in vitro, has been described.[185,186] In vivo, the drug has been shown to inhibit both release of IL-1 and Il-2 in heart allografted rats and to allow the release of a soluble mediator, which may also be linked to the activation of suppressor T cells.[1,2] Thus, while cyclosporine blocks the expansion of helper and cytotoxic T cells by interference with IL-2 release, liberation of suppressor cell inducing factors are not affected.[74] The preferential activation or selection sparing of suppressor cells under the umbrella of cyclosporine therapy may be the key to induction of a state of tolerance in experimental animals, as well as explaining, at least partially, the efficacy of this agent in clinical renal transplantation.[78,94]

Serum Levels

Cyclosporine is a metabolite of the fungal species *Tolypocladium inflatum* (previously termed *Trichoderma polysporum*).[17,18] The drug is a neutral hydrophobic cyclic peptide consisting of 11 amino acids, including a previously unknown amino acid in position 9. The immunosuppressive activity depends upon the presence of the carbon chains of the amino acids in positions 1 and 11. For oral use, the drug is dissolved in olive oil, whereas for intravenous administration, a gelenic formulation is used.

Native cyclosporine is immunosuppressive; some of its defined metabolites may also have some suppressive properties. Plasma or whole blood levels of the drug can be measured either by radioimmunoassay (RIA), which detects the parent drug and its metabolites, or high pressure liquid chromatography (HPLC), which selectively measures the parent compound.[84,120] The correlation between the two techniques is excellent, although values obtained by RIA are approximately 1.3 times higher than those obtained by HPLC. The rate and degree of absorption after oral administration are extremely variable. Forty percent to 60% of the drug concentration in whole blood is bound to red cells, lymphocytes, and granulocytes; each bind approximately 5%, while the remaining drug is associated with lipoproteins.[120] Because drug binding to red cells is temperature dependent, plasma must be separated from the erythrocytes at 37°C to obtain reproducible plasma levels. Thus, for convenience, the drug concentration of lysed whole blood is often determined, because this technique avoids the temperature-dependent erythrocyte-binding phenomenon. In addition, since the agent is metabolized primarily by the liver and excreted by way of bile and feces, liver dysfunction causes it to accumulate and serum levels to rise. Approximately 10% of the metabolites of the parent compound are excreted in the urine; however, only 0.1% of the native drug is detected in the urine. These characteristics explain why impaired renal function does not grossly affect plasma or whole blood levels. Liver dysfunction does, however, cause accumulation of cyclosporine.

Considerable controversy exists as to whether serial determinations of drug concentration aid in the management of renal transplant recipients. In our view, pro forma measurements of drug levels add little to patient management and cannot be used reliably to measure nephrotoxic or immunosuppressive effects.

Several kidney transplant groups initially adopted a policy of keeping plasma cyclosporine levels between 100 ng/ml and 400 ng/ml. Although these levels have been shown to be sufficient to prevent donor-specific immunoreactivity in in vitro assays, which quantify recipient anti-donor lymphocyte proliferative and cytotoxic functions, it soon became apparent that almost all patients experienced drug-induced nephrotoxicity.[84] Some clinical groups that still screen circulating drug levels recommend therapy aimed at producing even lower levels and do not exceed plasma trough levels of 150 ng/ml to 200 ng/ml; they believe that such levels are rarely associated with nephrotoxicity. Utilization of "low"-dose cyclosporine treatment does not seem to hamper the success rate of either living-related or cadaver donor kidney grafts, although, in our unit, many rejection episodes occur in patients treated in this manner.[178] In a very successful program,[175] cyclosporine levels were monitored so low as to have been considered, at least in first generation cyclosporine studies, to be beneath the therapeutic range; comparable levels are ineffective in vitro. Other units have adopted a policy of administering low-dose cyclosporine, but they use both azathioprine and corticosteroids as an adjunct. Clearly, there is no general consensus as to the single optimal regimen.

Catabolism of the drug is accelerated by coincident administration of rifampicin and phenytoin, which lower plasma levels by inducing degradative hepatic enzymes. Cyclosporine, in turn, affects the metabolism of prednisolone by reducing hepatic clearance through reduction of functional liver mass or by competitive inhibition of the hepatic cytochrome B 450. Concurrent therapy with aminoglycosides, trimethoprim/sulfa, ketoconazole, and amphotericin B also elevate plasma drug levels and result in increased nephrotoxicity.

Clinical Efficacy

The application of cyclosporine may be one of the most important developments in clinical transplantation since the first use of azathioprine as chemical immunosuppression at the Peter Bent Brigham Hospital in 1962. Calne's group[25] was the first to test the drug in recipients of mismatched cadaver kidney grafts; the 1-year graft survival rate of patients receiving cyclosporine alone reached 86%, a number clearly superior to historical controls receiving azathioprine and steroids. Similar results were obtained by Starzl and co-workers,[163] who recommended combining cyclosporine and prednisone. However, in both groups, a substantial number of patients demonstrated acutely impaired graft function, particularly protracted initial oliguria.

The drug was subsequently tested in a number of randomized controlled multicenter[28,48,49] and single-center[54,108,119,176,178] studies in which it was compared with different established standard treatment protocols. The actuarial rate of patient survival at 1 year exceeded 90%, although graft survival differed considerably among the centers. However, 70% to 90% of grafts placed into cyclosporine-treated hosts functioned after 1 year, whereas the standard treatment protocols yielded survival rates ranging from 50% to 85%.

In general, conventional therapy with azathioprine and corticosteroids has invariably produced results inferior to those achieved with cyclosporine ± corticosteroids. A recent analysis of HCFA data (the International Collaborative Transplant Study, Krakower H, unpublished data) revealed a 9% advantage in the rate of engraftment at 1 year for patients receiving cyclosporine (74%) as compared with patients receiving conventional therapy (65%). However, these results were obtained during the prolonged learning period during which most clinicians were unfamiliar with this very difficult drug; indeed, results have improved as familiarity with the agent has increased. Because cyclosporine has only recently been approved by the FDA in the United States, the results obtained in the five U.S. centers gaining experience with the drug during its trial phase of treatment were 18% better than those for the conventional treatment groups. Following this initial learning period, the excellent results (82% first year engraftment) obtained in experienced centers have become more general throughout the transplant community. Thus, later analysis of HCFA data of the outcome of more than 9000 primary cadaver renal transplants has demonstrated a 12% advantage in the rate of engraftment at 1 year for patients treated with cyclosporine ± corticosteroids compared with persons treated with standard azathioprine and steroids.

Combination treatment has also been tested. In general, the effect of prophylactic antilymphocyte globulin as an adjunct to conventional therapy reveals the following hierarchy of results: cyclosporine; conventional treatment + antilymphocyte globulin; conventional treatment alone. It should be noted that several centers have used azathioprine, corticosteroids, and certain heterologous antilymphocyte globulin preparations and have produced results comparable to cyclosporine ± corticosteroids.[119,158] Even in these studies, however, several categories of high-risk patients, including recipients of haploidentical living-related donor kidneys with high anti-donor antibody titers,[80] patients with prior immunologic loss of a renal allograft, and aged persons[137] experience a pronounced improvement in graft survival with cyclosporine therapy with an increase of the 1-year graft survival from 40% to more than 70%.

The combination of cyclosporine and corticosteroids ± antilymphocyte globulin appears to be particularly effective, possibly because of the ability of both the former two agents to abrogate IL-2 release through different sites of action, as well as the general inactivation of T cells by antilymphocyte globulin. Whereas cyclosporine acts predominantly on the release of IL-2 by activated helper cells, corticosteroids prevent IL-1 release from antigen-stimulated accessory cells (see Fig. 6-3). It is also of interest that although a combination of antilymphocyte globulin, azathioprine, and steroids provide superior results to azathioprine and steroids alone at 1 year of follow-up, the advantage of the antilymphocyte globulin–containing protocol is lost by 2 years (Sanfillippo, personal communication). It is obvious that additional long-term follow-up studies are needed before firm conclusions can be made regarding combination therapy. Nonetheless, in our series, the benefits of cyclosporine and steroid therapy appear to be maintained through 2 years of follow-up.[178]

Conversion Treatment

Conversion from maintenance cyclosporine to azathioprine has been undertaken by several investigators for two reasons: (1) the financial considerations of this expensive treatment, and (2) the unknown long-term nephrotoxic effects of the drug. At what financial cost has the improved graft function been obtained? As first noted in the Minnesota trial,[119] the HCFA analysis showed that the increased costs for cyclosporine are offset by the reduced costs

of hospitalization. Total costs for the first year for patients treated with cyclosporine are equal to costs among azathioprine-treated patients, particularly when a 10% to 20% improvement in the rate of engraftment is achieved. However, there is no doubt that after the first year, continued cyclosporine therapy increases total costs for successfully transplanted patients. No systematic study has been performed to evaluate whether the drug needs to be administered in perpetuity following transplantation or whether patients may be safely switched from cyclosporine to azathioprine at some interval post-transplantation.

In consideration of the potential nephrotoxic effects of the drug, the Oxford group[31,116] and, more recently, we at the Brigham and Women's and Beth Israel Hospitals[139] have switched from maintenance cyclosporine to azathioprine in many patients. The results are very promising. The Oxford study described a significant fall in serum creatinine by 45%, indicating the presence of a nephrotoxic component in almost all patients converted to azathioprine 3 to 4 months after transplant; however, this change in immunosuppression was followed in about one third of patients by an acute rejection episode that led to graft loss only in persons with a concurrent compromising situation, such as primary graft nonfunction. A more benign course was seen in our center following conversion to azathioprine in 57 patients following treatment with cyclosporine and steroids for 3 to 6 months. Improved renal function occurred in 65%, 21% had stable function, and 14% showed declined function. The occurrence of uncontrollable rejection was minor, although 18 patients (32%) developed 20 episodes of rejection, which resulted in one case in the loss of the graft. The relative safety of delayed cessation of cyclosporine treatment has also been confirmed in persons treated at other centers.

Allograft Dysfunction

Despite the improved rate of engraftment among cyclosporine-treated patients compared with those receiving azathioprine and prednisone alone, graft dysfunction remains an important problem. It is still somewhat controversial as to whether most poorly functioning grafts experience smoldering rejection or actual drug-induced nephrotoxicity. Biopsies of poorly functioning renal allografts often show lymphocytic infiltrates throughout the parenchyma, which, when associated with local tissue necrosis, occur secondary to rejection and not to nephrotoxicity. Prominent cellular infiltration has not been noted in the native kidneys of heart graft recipients given high doses of cyclosporine, although a severe and irreversible form of nephrotoxicity marked by an intense interstitial fibrosis has been described.[118]

Nephrotoxic effects of cyclosporine are readily observed in humans but not in most animal models. Nephrotoxicity may become manifest in the early postoperative course as acute renal failure or later as an insidious decrease in glomerular filtration rate. In the original Cambridge experience, several patients with a brisk initial diuresis become oligoanuric after institution of cyclosporine.[25] It was thus suggested that administration of the drug be delayed for 6 hours postoperatively to keep these recipients of cadaver allografts with primary oliguria from experiencing potentially nephrotoxic cyclosporine treatment. This policy was then adopted in the European multicenter trial.[48,49] In contrast, after a prolonged clinical experience, most researchers now believe that the agent can be used safely in all kidney recipients regardless of initial graft function, although early oligoanuria can be protracted in patients taking cyclosporine.[178]

In the Canadian multicenter trial,[48] machine perfusion time longer than 24 hours and prolonged rewarming times longer than 45 minutes were noted as special risk factors for cyclosporine-treated patients with initial oliguria. These factors also included an increased incidence of primary nonfunction as well as a higher number of acute rejection episodes resulting in more frequent prednisone pulses for antirejection treatment. A subsequent study has revealed that primary nonfunction was actually associated with prolonged warm but not cold ischemic time (Stiller, personal communication). Hence, the risk of nonfunction for cyclosporine-treated patients is primarily associated with prolonged surgical anastomotic time.

Each transplant group using cyclosporine has had to struggle to learn how drug-related nephrotoxicity can be distinguished from acute rejection, because both conditions usually become manifest only by impairment of graft function. Cyclosporine-treated recipients undergoing rejection episodes often lack the classical signs of fever, graft tenderness, and hypertension. Indeed, the presence of other side effects may cause suspicion that worsening graft function is due to cyclosporine toxicity; for instance, hyperbilirubinemia is invariably correlated with high cyclosporine blood levels and can be an indicator of nephrotoxicity. Nonetheless, drug-induced toxicity, including nephrotoxicity, does not rule out concomitant rejection, as both conditions may commonly coexist. Direct correlation of plasma or whole blood cyclosporine trough levels with toxicity is poor, however, because there is no drug concentra-

tion that excludes with certainty the diagnosis of nephrotoxicity. On the other hand, acute rejection may occur despite high blood levels.

The only useful clinical sign is the absence of hypertension in progressive azotemia; hypertension is extremely common during acute rejection, whereas many but certainly not all nephrotoxic patients are normotensive in the euvolemic state. Some groups report that much lower doses of cyclosporine than originally recommended in conjunction with prednisone yield a high graft survival rate with a low incidence of nephrotoxic episodes.[166] Thiel and co-workers[175] found in a group of 23 recipients of cadaver kidneys that serum creatinine concentrations did not differ from those of an historical control group receiving azathioprine and prednisone. Similar results have been obtained using low-dose cyclosporine plus azathioprine and corticosteroids.

Other Drug Toxicities

Cyclosporine affects the liver by an unknown mechanism, with serum bilirubin levels increasing in proportion to the sustained cyclosporine plasma trough concentrations.[87,99] Trough levels above 500 ng/ml are accompanied by elevated serum bilirubin, a phenomenon observed in about 20% of kidney graft recipients. Serum transaminase levels occasionally rise in a dose-dependent fashion. An intriguing finding is the persistent elevation of alkaline phosphatase in about one third of the patients,[99,140] which occurs within the first 3 weeks of treatment and remains increased despite reductions in drug dosage; the bone-specific isoenzyme fraction is elevated, not the liver-specific fraction. Although other indices of chronic cholestasis remain normal in renal graft recipients, cholestasis cannot be absolutely excluded, because heart transplant recipients exhibit dramatically increased serum concentrations of bile acid (cholyglycine and sulfolithocholylglycine).[154] Further studies, including bone and liver biopsies, must assess the impact of cyclosporine on these two organs.

It is well known that the risk among immunosuppressed transplant recipients for the development of malignancies is increased, especially those of lymphoreticular origin.[131] If cyclosporine is used alone or in combination with low doses of prednisone, the incidence of lymphoproliferative disease is 0.4% compared with 0.8% when other immunosuppressive adjuncts are added to these agents. As a result, the manufacturer now recommends keeping plasma trough levels in a range of 50 ng/ml to 200 ng/ml.[11] Starzl and co-workers[164] recently analyzed the outcome in 17 cyclosporine-treated organ recipients who developed a lymphoproliferative disorder 2 to 68 months after transplantation. The disease became manifest within 8 months in 16 of the 17 recipients. In 10 patients, the disease was localized to the gastrointestinal tract; 11 of the 17 are alive and symptom-free after surgical treatment and reduction of cyclosporine dosages. Epstein–Barr virus (EBV) infection may be important in the genesis of these lymphoproliferative disorders; several tumors have been found to express EBV proteins. Indeed, excessive inhibition of T cell surveillance has been shown to favor uncontrolled proliferation of EBV–infected B cells.

Hirsutism occurs in approximately 30% to 40% of patients and sometimes poses a cosmetic problem, especially in women. It is, however, a completely dose-dependent phenomenon, which disappears after conversion to azathioprine. So far, no hormonal abnormalities have been implicated. Tremor is fairly frequent as long as higher doses of cyclosporine are used. Paresthesias and burning sensations primarily in the fingers are other neurologic side effects that respond to lower drug doses.

Overall, the incidence of infectious complications is comparable in standard and cyclosporine-treated groups. However, in our experience, *Pneumocystis carinii* pneumonia is more common in cyclosporine-treated kidney recipients. Consequently, our patients now receive long-term, low-dose trimethoprim/sulfa prophylaxis when the serum creatinine falls below 3 mg/dl.

REFERENCES

1. Abbud–Filho M, Kupiec–Weglinski JW, Araujo JL et al: Cyclosporine therapy of rat heart allograft recipients and release of interleukins (IL-1, IL-2, IL-3): A role for IL-3 in graft tolerance? J Immunol 133:2582, 1984

2. Abbud–Filho M, Kupiec–Weglinski JW, Araujo JL et al: Interleukins and suppressor cells during Cyclosporin A-induced route of tolerance. Transplant Proc 17:1384, 1985

3. Bach FH, van Rood JJ: The major histocompatibility complex—genetics and biology. N Engl J Med 295:806, 1976

4. Balow JE, Hunninglake GW, Fauci AS: Corticosteroids in human lymphocyte mediated cytotoxic reactions. Transplantation 23:322, 1977

5. Bell MJ, Martin LW, Gonzalez LL et al: Alternate day single dose prednisone therapy: A method of reducing steroid toxicity. J Pediatr Surg 7:223, 1972

6. Bell PRF, Briggs JD, Calman KC et al: The immunosuppressive effect of large doses of intravenous prednisolone in experimental heterotopic rat heart and human renal transplantation. Surgery 73:147, 1973

7. Berenbaum MC: Effect of cyclophosphamide on the homograft response in the guinea pig. Transplantation 3:671, 1965

8. Berenbaum MC: The effect of cytotoxic agents on the production of antibodies to TAB vaccine in the mouse. Biochem Pharmacol 11:29, 1962

9. Berglund K: Inhibition of antibody function by prednisone: Location of a short sensitive period. Acta Path Microbiol (Scand) 55:187, 1962

10. Berlyne GM: Danovitch GM: Cyclophosphamide for immunosuppression in renal transplantation. Lancet 2:924, 1971

11. Beveridge T, Krupp P, McKibbin C: Lymphomas and lymphoproliferative lesions developing under cyclosporine therapy. Lancet 1:788, 1984

12. Biddison WE, Rao PE, Talle MA et al: Possible involvement of the T4 molecule in T cell recognition of class II HLA antigens: Evidence from studies of proliferative responses to SB antigen. J Immunol 131:152, 1983

13. Billingham RE, Brent L, Medawar PB: Actively acquired tolerance of foreign cells. Nature 172:603, 1953

14. Billingham RE, Krohn PL, Medawar PB: Effect of cortisone on survival of skin homografts in rabbits. Br Med J 1:1157, 1951

15. Billingham RE, Krohn PL, Medawar PB: Effect of locally applied cortisone acetate on survival of skin homografts in rabbits. Br Med J 2:1049, 1951

16. Bordes–Aznar J, Tilney NL: Cyclosporin A: A nonspecific immunosuppressive agent? J Clin Surg 1:53, 1982

17. Borel JD: Comparative study of in vitro and in vivo drug effects on cell-mediated cytotoxicity. Immunology 31:631, 1976

18. Borel JF, Feurer C, Gubler HV et al: Biological effects of Cyclosporin A: A new antilymphocyte agent. Agents Action 6:468, 1976

19. Borum K, Berglund K (cited by Berglund K): Studies on the induction phase of antibody function: Effects of corticosteroids and lymphoid cells. In Starzl J, coworkers (eds): Molecular and Cellular Basis of Antibody Formation, p 405. New York, Academic Press, 1965

20. Brody GL, Jones JW, Haines RF: Influence of cyclophosphamide on homograft rejection. JAMA 191:297, 1965

21. Buckels JAC, Mackintosh P, Barnes AD: Controlled trial of low versus high dose oral steroid therapy in 100 cadaveric renal transplants. Proc Eur Dial Transplant Assoc 18:394, 1981

22. Bunjes D, Hardt C, Rollinghoff M, Wagner H: Cyclosporin A mediates immunosuppression of primary

cytotoxic T cell responses by impairing the release of interleukin-1 and interleukin-2. Eur J Immunol 11:657, 1981

23. Butler WT, Rosser RD: Effect of corticosteroids on immunity in man. I. Decreased serum IgG concentration caused by 3 or 5 days of high doses of methylprednisolone. J Clin Invest 52:2629, 1973

24. Calne RY, Alexandre GPJ, Murray JE: A study of the effects of drugs in prolonging survival of homologous renal transplants in dogs. Ann NY Acad Sci 99:743, 1962

25. Calne RY, White DJG, Thorin S et al: Cyclosporin A in patients receiving renal allografts from cadaver donors. Lancet 2:1323, 1978

26. Calne RY: Inhibition of the rejection of renal homografts in dogs by purine analogues. Transplant Bull 26:65, 1961

27. Calne RY: The rejection of renal homografts. Inhibition in dogs by 6-mercaptopurine. Lancet 1:417, 1960

28. Canadian Multicentre Transplant Study Group: A randomized clinical trial of cyclosporine in cadaveric renal transplantation. N Engl J Med 309:809, 1983

29. Cantrell DA, Smith KA: Transient expression of interleukin-2 receptors. Consequences for T cell growth. J Exp Med 158:1895, 1983

30. Cantrell DA, Smith KA: The interleukin-2 T cell system: A new cell growth mode. Science 224:1312, 1984

31. Chapman JR, Griffiths D, Harding NG, Morris PJ: Reversibility of cyclosporine nephrotoxicity after three months' treatment. Lancet 1:128, 1985

32. Claman HN: Corticosteroids and lymphoid cells. N Engl J Med 287:388, 1972

33. Cohen JJ: Thymus-derived lymphocytes sequestered in the bone marrow of hydrocortisone-treated mice. J Immunol 108:841, 1972

34. Cohn DJ, Loertscher R, Rubin MF et al: Cyclosporine: A new immunosuppressive agent for organ transplantation. Ann Intern Med 101:667, 1984

35. Cooper DKC, Rose AG: Low-dose versus high-dose steroid therapy in the prevention of acute rejection in baboon heterotopic cardiac allografts. Transplantation 34:107, 1982

36. Cotner T, Williams JM, Christenson L et al: Simultaneous flow cytometric analysis of human T cell activation, antigen expression, and DNA content. J Exp Med 157:461, 1983

37. Dale DC, Fauci AS, Wolff SM: Alternate-day prednisone, leukocyte kinetics and susceptibility to infections. N Engl J Med 291:1154, 1974

38. d'Apice AJF: Non-specific immunosuppression: Azathioprine and steroids. In Morris PJ (ed): Kidney Transplantation, 2nd ed, p 239. London, Grune & Stratton.

39. Daniels JC, Warren KS, David JR: Studies in the mechanism of delayed hypersensitivity by the antischistosomal compound niridazole. J Immunol 115:1414, 1975

40. Dempster WJ: The effects of cortisone on the homotransplanted kidney. Arch Int Pharmacodyn Ther 95:253, 1953

41. Diethelm AG, Sterling WA, Hartley MW, Morgan JM: Alternate-day prednisone therapy in recipients of renal allografts. Arch Surg 111:867, 1976

42. Dukor P, Dietrich FM: Characteristic features of immunosuppression by steroids and cytotoxic drugs. Int Arch Allergy 34:32, 1968

43. Dumler F, Leven NW, Szego G et al: Long-term alternate day steroid therapy in renal transplantation. A controlled study. Transplantation 34:78, 1982

44. Dupont E, Berkenboom G, Leempoel M, Potliege P: Failure of dexamethasone to induce in vitro lysis of human mononuclear cells. Transplantation 30:387, 1980

45. Ebert RH: In vivo observations on the effect of cortisone on experimental tuberculosis using the rabbit ear chamber technique. Am Rev Tuberc 65:64, 1952

46. Eklund B, Ahonen J, Hayry P et al: Comparison of two different immunosuppressive dosages of methylprednisone in renal transplantation. Scan J Urol Nephrol 64:179, 1981

47. Engleman EG, Benoke CJ, Grumet FC, Evans RL: Activation of human T lymphocyte subsets: Helper and suppressor T cells recognize and respond to distinct histocompatibility antigens. J Immunol 127:2124, 1981

48. European Multicentre Trial Group: Cyclosporin A as sole immunosuppressive agent in recipients of renal allografts from cadaver donors. Preliminary results of a European Multicenter Trial. Lancet 2:57, 1982

49. European Multicentre Trial Group: Cyclosporine in cadaveric renal transplantation: One year follow-up of a multicentre trial. Lancet 2:896, 1982

50. Faigle JW, Keberle H: Metabolism of niridazole in various species including man. Ann NY Acad Sci 160:544, 1969

51. Farrar WL, Johnson HM, Farrar JJ: Regulation of the production of immune interferon and cytotoxic T lymphocytes by interleukin-2. J Immunol 126:1129, 1981

52. Fauci AS, Dale DC: The effect of in vivo hydrocortisone on subpopulations of human lymphocytes. J Clin Invest 53:240, 1974

53. Fauci AS: Mechanism of corticosteroid action on lymphocyte subpopulations. I. Redistribution of circulating T and B lymphocytes to the bone marrow. Immunology 28:669, 1975

54. Ferguson RM, Ryansiewicz JJ, Sutherland DER et al: Cyclosporin A in renal transplantation: A prospective randomized trial. Surgery 92:175, 1983

55. Floersheim GL: Pharmacological immunosuppressive agents. Transplant Proc 12:315, 1980

56. Fox M: Studies of homotransplantation of mouse skin and human kidney. In Fairley GH, Simister JM (eds): Cyclophosphamide, p 136. Baltimore, Williams & Wilkins, 1965

57. Frey BM, Frey FJ, Holford NHG et al: Prednisolone pharmacodynamics assessed by inhibition of the

mixed lymphocyte reaction. Transplantation 33:578, 1982

58. Friedman EA, Ueno A, Beyer MM, Micastri AD: Combination drug treatment in immunosuppression. Transplantation 15:619, 1973

59. Frisch AW, Davies GH: Inhibition of hemagglutinin synthesis by cytoxan. Cancer Res 25:745, 1965

60. Gell PGH, Hinde IT: The histology of the tuberculin reaction and its modification by cortisone. Br J Exp Pathol 32:516, 1951

61. Gillis S, Crabtree GR, Smith KA: Glucocorticoid-induced inhibition of T cell growth factor production. II. The effect on the in vitro generation of cytolytic T cells. J Immunol 123:1632, 1979

62. Gillis S, Mizel SBN: T cell lymphoma model for the analysis of interleukin-1 mediated T cell activation. Proc Natl Acad Sci USA 78:1133, 1981

63. Glaser RJ, Berry JW, Loeb LH, Woods WB: The effect of cortisone in streptococcal lymphadenitis and pneumonia. J Lab Clin Med 38:363, 1951

64. Goldstein IM: Effect of steroids on lysosomes. Transplant Proc 7:21, 1975

65. Goodwin WE, Kouffman JJ, Mims MM et al: Human renal transplantation. I. Clinical experiences with six cases of renal homotransplantation. J Urol 89:13, 1963

66. Gray D, Shepherd H, Daar A et al: Oral versus intravenous high-dose steroid treatment of renal allograft rejection. The big shot or not? Lancet i:117, 1978

67. Haessleim AC, Pierce VC, Lee HM, Hume DM: Leukopenia and azathioprine management in renal homotransplantation. Surgery 71:598, 1972

68. Hamburger J, Crosnier J, Tubiana M et al: Transplantation d'un rein entre jumeaux non monozygotes. La Presse Medicale 67:1773, 1959

69. Hardt C, Rollinhoff M, Pfizenmaier K et al: Lyt-23 + cyclophosphamide-sensitive T cells regulate the activity of an interleukin-2 inhibitor in vivo. J Exp Med 154:262, 1981

70. Hayry P, von Willebrand E, Parthenis E et al: The inflammatory mechanisms of allograft rejection. Immunol Rev 77:85, 1984

71. Helderman JH, Strom TB: Specific insulin binding site on T and B lymphocytes as a marker of cell activation. Nature 174:62, 1978

72. Helderman JH, Strom TB: Role of protein and RNA synthesis in the development of insulin binding sites on activated thymus-derived lymphocytes. J Biol Chem 254:7203207, 1979

73. Helderman JH, Strom TB, Garovoy MR: Rapid mixed lymphocyte culture testing by analysis of the insulin receptor on alloactivated T lymphocytes: Implications for human tissue typing. J Clin Invest 67:509, 1981

74. Hess AD, Tutschka PJ, Santos GW: Effect of Cyclosporin A on human lymphocyte responses in vitro. II. Induction of specific alloantigen unresponsiveness mediated by a nylon wool adherent suppressor cell. J Immunol 126:961, 1981

75. Hess AD, Tutschka PJ, Santos GW: Effect of Cyclo-

sporin A on human lymphocyte responses in vitro. III. CsA inhibits the production of T lymphocyte growth factors in secondary mixed lymphocyte responses but does not inhibit the response of primed lymphocytes to TCGF. J Immunol 128:355, 1982

76. Hitchings GH, Elion GB: The role of antimetabolites in immunosuppression and transplantation. Accounts Chem Res 2:202, 1969

77. Howard M, Matis L, Malek TR et al: Interleukin-2 induces antigen-reactive T cell lines to secrete BCGF-1. J Exp Med 158:2024, 1983

78. Hutchinson IF, Shadur CA, Duarte AJS et al: Cyclosporin A spares selectively lymphocytes with donor specific suppressor characteristics. Transplantation 32:210, 1981

79. Inaba K, Granelli–Piperno G, Steinman RM: Dendritic cells induce T lymphocytes to release B cell-stimulating factors by an interleukin-2-dependent mechanism. J Exp Med 158:2040, 1983

80. Kahan BD, Van Buren CT, Flechner SM et al: Cyclosporine immunosuppression mitigates immunologic risk factors in renal allotransplantation. Transplant Proc 15:2469, 1983

81. Kalman VK, Klimpel GR: Cyclosporin A inhibits the production of gamma interferon but does not inhibit production of virus-induced alpha–beta interferon. Cell Immunol 78:122, 1983

82. Kauffman HM, Sampson D, Fox PS, Stawicki AT: High dose (bolus) intravenous methylprednisolone at the time of kidney transplantation. Ann Surg 186:631, 1977

83. Kelley VE, Fiers W, Strom TB: Cloned human interferon-gamma, but not interferon-beta or -alpha, induces expression of HLA-DR determinants by fetal monocytes and myeloid leukemia cell lines. J Immunol 132:240, 1984

84. Keown PA, Stiller CR, Ulan RA et al: Immunological and pharmacological monitoring in the clinical use of Cyclosporin A. Lancet 1:686, 1981

85. Kirkman RL, Araujo JL, Busch GJ et al: Treatment of acute renal allograft rejection with monoclonal anti-T12 antibody. Transplantation 36:620, 1983

86. Kirkman RL, Strom TB, Weir MR, Tilney NL: Late mortality and morbidity in recipients of long-term renal allografts. Transplantation 34:347, 1982

87. Klintmalm GBG, Iwatzuki S, Starzl TE: Cyclosporin A hepatotoxicity in 66 renal allograft recipients. Transplantation 32:488, 1981

88. Knapp MS, Byrom NP, Pownall R, Mayor P: Time of day of taking immunosuppressive agents after renal transplantation: A possible influence on graft survival. Br Med J 281:1382, 1980

89. Krensky AM, Reiss CS, Mier JW et al: Long-term cytolytic T cell lines allospecific for HLA-DR6 antigen are OKT4 + . Proc Natl Acad Sci USA 79:2365, 1982

90. Krohn PL: The effect of ACTH on the reaction to skin homografts in rabbits. J Endocrinol 11:71, 1954

91. Krohn PL: The effect of ACTH and cortisone on the survival of skin homografts and on the adrenal glands in monkeys. J Endocrinol 12:220, 1955

92. Kung PC, Goldstein G, Reinherz EL, Schlossman SF: Monoclonal antibodies defining distinctive human T cell surface antigens. Science 206:347, 1979

93. Kupiec–Weglinski JW, Filho MA, Strom TB, Tilney NL: Sparing of suppressor cells: A critical action of cyclosporine. Transplantation 38:97, 1984

94. Kupiec–Weglinski JW, Heidecke CD, Araujo JL et al: Behavior of helper T lymphocytes in cyclosporine-mediated long-term graft acceptance in the rat. Cell Immunol 93:168, 1985

95. Kupiec–Weglinski JW, Lear PA, Strom TB, Tilney NL: Population of cyclophosphamide-sensitive T suppressor cells maintain cyclosporine-induced allograft survival. Transplant Proc 15:2357, 1983

96. Kupper TS, Green DR, Chanchy IH et al: A cyclophosphamide-sensitive suppressor T cell circuit induced by thermal injury. Surgery 95:699, 1984

97. Kuss R, Legrain M, Mathe G et al: Premices d'une homo-transplantation renale de soeur a frere non jumeaux. Press Med 68:755, 1960

98. Lillie FR: The theory of the freemartin. Science 43:611, 1916

99. Loertscher R, Thiel G, Harder F, Brunner FP: Persistent elevation of alkaline phosphatase in Cyclosporin A treated renal transplant recipients. Transplantation 36:115, 1983

100. Maguire HC Jr, Maibach HI: Effect of cyclophosphamide, 6-mercaptopurine, actinomycin D and vincaleukoblastine on the acquisition of delayed hypersensitivity (DNCB) contact dermatitis in guinea pigs. J Invest Dermatol 37:427, 1961

101. Maguire HC Jr, Maibach HI: Specific immune tolerance to anaphylactic sensitization (egg albumin) induced in the guinea pig by cyclophosphamide (Cytoxan). J Allergy 32:406, 1961

102. Mahmoud AAF, Mandel MA, Warren KS, Webster LT Jr: Niridazole II. A potent long-acting suppressant of cellular hypersensitivity. J Immunol 114:279, 1975

103. Mahmoud AAP, Warren KS: Anti-inflammatory effects of tartar emetic and niridazole: Suppression of schistosome egg granuloma. J Immunol 112:222, 1974

104. Mandel MA, Mahmoud AAF, Warren KS: Marked prolongation of skin homograft survival with niridazole. Plast Reconstr Surg 55:75, 1975

105. Marquet R, Heysteek G: The induction and abolition of specific immunosuppression of heart allografts in rats by use of donor blood and cyclophosphamide. J Immunol 115:405, 1975

106. McGeown MG: Immunosuppression for kidney transplantation. Lancet ii:310, 1973

107. McGeown MS, Kennedy JA, Loughridge WGG et al: One hundred kidney transplants in the Belfast City Hospital. Lancet ii:648, 1977

108. McMaster P, Haynes IG, Michael J et al: Cyclosporine in cadaveric renal transplantation: A prospective trial. Transplant Proc 15:2543, 1983

109. Merrill JP, Murray JE, Harrison H et al: Successful homotransplantation of the kidney between non-identical twins. N Engl J Med 262:1251, 1960

110. Meuer SC, Schlossman SF, Reinherz EL: Clonal analysis of human cytotoxic T-lymphocytes: T4+ and T8+ effector T cells recognize products of different major histocompatibility complex regions. Proc Natl Acad Sci USA 79:43959, 1982

111. Miller JJ: The imidazoles as immunosuppressive agents. Transplant Proc 12:300, 1980

112. Miyawaki T, Yachie A, Ohzeki S et al: Cyclosporin A does not prevent expression of Tac antigen, a probably TCGF receptor molecule on mitogen-stimulated human T cells. J Immunol 130:2737, 1983

113. Moore RN, Oppenheim JJ, Farrar JJ et al: Production of LAF (IL-1) by macrophages activated with colony stimulating factors. J Immunol 125:1302, 1980

114. Morris PJ: Cyclosporin A. Transplantation 32:349, 1981

115. Morris PJ, Chan L, French ME, Ting A: Low dose oral prednisolone in renal transplantation. Lancet ii:525, 1982

116. Morris PJ, French ME, Dunnill MS et al: A controlled trial of cyclosporine in renal transplantation with conversion to azathioprine and prednisone after three months. Transplantation 36:273, 1983

117. Myburgh JA, Smit JA: Passive and active enhancement in baboon liver allografting. Transplantation 14:227, 1972

118. Myers BD, Ross J, Newton L et al: Cyclosporin-A associated chronic nephropathy. A potentially reversible renal injury. N Engl J Med 311:699, 1984

119. Najarian JS, Strand M, Fryd DS et al: Comparison of cyclosporine versus azathioprine—antilymphocyte globulin in renal transplantation. Transplant Proc 15:2463, 1983

120. Niederberger W, LeMaire G, Maurer K et al: Distribution and binding of cyclosporine in blood and tissues. Transplant Proc 15:2419, 1983

121. North RJ: Cyclophosphamide-facilitated adoptive immunotherapy of an established tumor depends on elimination of tumor induced suppressor T cells. J Exp Med 155:1063, 1982

122. Orta–Sibu N, Chantler C, Bewick M, Haycock G: Comparison of high-dose intravenous methyprednisolone with low-dose oral prednisolone in acute renal allograft rejection in children. Br Med J 285:258, 1982

123. Ortho Multicenter Transplant Study Group. A randomized clinical trial of OKT3 monoclonal antibody for acute rejection of cadaveric renal allograft. N Engl J Med 313:337, 1985

124. Osgood CK, Favour CB: The effect of adrenocorticotrophic hormone on inflammation due to tuberculin hypersensitivity and turpentine and on circulating antibody levels. J Exp Med 94:415, 1951

125. Owen RD: Immunogenetic consequence of vascular anastomoses between bovine twins. Science 102:400, 1945

126. Ozer H, Cowens JW, Colvin M et al: In vitro effects of 4-hydroperoxycyclophosphamide on human immunoregulatory T subset function. J Exp Med 155:276, 1982

127. Pace JL, Russell SW, Schreiber RD et al: Macrophage activation: Priming activity from a T-cell hybridoma is attributable to gamma-interferon. Proc Natl Acad Sci USA 80:3782, 1983

128. Papadakis J, Brown CB, Cameron JS et al: High versus "low" dose corticosteroids in recipients of cadaveric kidneys: Prospective controlled trial. Br Med J 286:1097, 1983

129. Pelley RP, Pelley RJ, Stavitsky AB et al: Niradazole, a potent long acting suppressant of cellular hypersensitivity III. Minimal suppression of antibody responses. J Immunol 115:1477, 1975

130. Penn I: Cancer as a complication of clinical transplantation. Transplant Proc 9:1121, 1977

131. Penn I: Lymphomas complicating organ transplantation. Transplant Proc 15:2790, 1983

132. Pober JS, Gimbrone MA, Cotran RS et al: Ia expression by vascular endothelium is inducible by activated T cells and by human gamma interferon. J Exp Med 157:1339, 1983

133. Potel J: Influence of cyclophosphamide on the formation of antibodies. In Fairley GH, Simister JM (eds): Cyclophosphamide, p 147. Baltimore, Williams & Wilkins 1965

134. Reinherz EL, Meuer SC, Schlossman SF: The human T cell receptor: Analysis with cytotoxic T cell clones. Immunol Rev 74:81, 1983

135. Reinherz EL, Schlossman SF: Regulation of the immune response—inducer and suppressor T lymphocyte subsets in human beings. N Engl J Med 303:370, 1980

136. Rinehart JJ, Sagone AL, Balcerzak SP et al: Effects of corticosteroid therapy on human monocyte function. N Engl J Med 292:236, 1975

137. Ringden O, Ost L, Klintmalm GBG et al: Improved outcome in renal transplant recipients above 55 years of age treated with cyclosporine and low doses of steroids. Transplant Proc 15:2507, 1983

138. Robb RJ, Munch A, Smith KA: T cell growth factor receptors—quantitation, specificity and biological relevance. J Exp Med 154:1455, 1981

139. Rochet LL, Milford EL, Kirkman RL et al: Conversion from cyclosporine to azathioprine in renal allograft recipients. Transplantation 38:669, 1984

140. Rodger RSC, Turney JH, Haines I et al: Cyclosporine and liver function in renal allograft recipients. Transplant Proc 15:2754, 1983

141. Rollinhoff M, Starzinski-Powitz A, Pfizenmaier K, Wagner H: Cyclophosphamide-sensitive T lymphocytes suppress the in vivo generation of antigen specific cytotoxic T lymphocytes. J Exp Med 145:455, 1977

142. Salaman JR, Bird M, Godfrey AM et al: Prolonged allograft survival with nirizadole, azathioprine, and prednisolone. Transplantation 23:29, 1977

143. Salaman JR, Couhig E: Timing of antirejection therapy. Transplantation 29:468, 1980

144. Salaman JR, Griffin PJA, Price K: A controlled clinical trial of low-dose prednisolone in renal transplantation. Transplant Proc 14:103, 1982

145. Salaman JR, Griffin PJA, Johnson RWJ: A controlled clinical trial of miridazole in cadaver renal transplantation. Transplant Proc 12:297, 1980

146. Salaman JR: Influence of steroid dosage on the survival of cardiac allografts in the rat. Transplantation (in press).

147. Salaman JR: Non-specific immunosuppression. In Morris PJ (ed): Tissue Transplantation, p 60. Edinburgh, Churchill Livingston, 1982

148. Salaman JR: Steroids and modern immunosuppression. Br Med J 286:1373, 1983

149. Salvatierra O, Feduska NJ, Cochrum KC et al: The impact of 100 renal transplants at one center. Ann Surg 186:424, 1977

150. Sampson D, Albert DJ: Alternate day therapy with methylprednisolone after renal transplantation. J Urol 109:345, 1973

151. Santos GW, Owens AH Jr: A comparison of the effects of selected cytotoxic agents on allogeneic skin graft survival in rats. Bull Johns Hopkins Hosp 116:327, 1965

152. Santos GW, Owens AH Jr: A comparison of selected cytotoxic agents on the primary agglutinin response in rats injected with sheep erythrocytes. Bull Johns Hopkins Hosp 114:384, 1964

153. Santos GW: Chemical immunosuppression. In Najarian JS, Simmons RL (eds): Transplantation, pp 212–213. Philadelphia, Lea & Febiger, 1972

154. Schade RR, Guglielmi A, Van Thiel DH et al: Cholestatis in heart transplant recipients treated with cyclosporine. Transplant Proc 15:2757, 1983

155. Schwartz R, Dameshek W: Drug-induced immunological tolerance. Nature 183:1682,1959

156. Schwartz RS, Eisner A, Dameshek W. The effect of 6-MP on primary and secondary immune responses. J Clin Invest 38:1394, 1959

157. Schwartz RS, Stack J, Dameshek W: Effect of 6-MP on antibody production. Proc Soc Exp Biol Med 99:164, 1958

158. Sheil AGR, Hall BM, Tiller DJ et al: Australian trial of cyclosporine in cadaveric donor renal transplantation. Transplant Proc 15:2485, 1983

159. Smith KA, Lachman LB, Oppenheim JJ, Favata MF: The functional relationship of the interleukins. J Exp Med 151:1551, 1980

160. Snyder DS, Unanue ER: Corticosteroids inhibit murine macrophage Ia expression and interleukin-1 production. J Immunol 129:1803, 1982

161. Sparrow EM: The behavior of skin autografts and skin homografts in the guinea pig, with special references to the effect of cortisone acetate and ascorbic acid on the homografts reaction. J Endocrinol 9:101, 1953

162. Starzl TE, Halgrimson GC, Penn I et al: Cyclophosphamide and human organ transplantation. Lancet 2:70, 1971

163. Starzl TE, Nalesnik MA, Porter KA et al: Reversibility of lymphomas and lymphoproliferative lesions developing under cyclosporine therapy. Lancet 1:583, 1984

164. Starzl TE, Weil R III, Iwatzuki S et al: The use of Cyclosporin A and steroid therapy in 66 cadaver

kidney transplants. Surg Gynecol Obstet 151:17, 1980

165. Stender HS, Ringlieb D, Strauch D, Winter H: Die beeinflussung der antikorpebildung durch zytostatika und rontgenbestrahlung. Strahlentherapie 43:392, 1959

166. Stiller CR, Keown PA: Cyclosporine therapy in perspective. In Morris PJ, Tilney NL (eds): Progress in Transplantation, Vol 1, p 61. Edinburgh, Churchill Livingstone, 1984

167. Stone RL, Wolfe RN, Culbertson CG, Paget J: Studies on frenazole—a novel immunosuppressive agent. Fed Proc 333:1976

168. Storb R, Thomas ED: Allogeneic bone marrow transplantation. Immunol Rev 71:77, 1983

169. Strom TB, Tilney NL: Immunobiology and immunopharmacology of graft rejection. In Schrier RW, Gottschalk CW: The Kidney, 4th ed. Little, Brown & Co, (in press)

170. Strom TB, Tilney NL, Carpenter C, Busch GJ: Identity and cytotoxic capacity of cells infiltrating renal allografts. N Engl J Med 292:1257, 1975

171. Strom TB, Tilney NL, Paradysz JM et al: Cellular components of allograft rejection: Identity, specificity, and cytotoxic function of cells infiltrating acutely rejecting allografts. J Immunol 118:2020, 1977

172. Sutton WT, VanHagen F, Griffith BH, Preston FW: Drug effects on survival of homografts of skin. Arch Surg 87:840, 1963

173. Terasaki PI: Presidential Address: Transplantation Society 1982. Transplant Proc 15:14, 1983

174. Termijtelen A, van Leeuwen A, van Rood JJ: HLA-linked lymphocytes activating determinants. Immunol Rev 66:79, 1982

175. Thiel G, Harder F, Loertscher R: Cyclosporin A used alone or in combination with low dose steroids on cadaveric renal transplantation. Klin Urschr 61:991, 1983

176. Tilney NL, Kirkman RL, Araujo JL et al: Use of cyclosporine and monoclonal antibodies in clinical renal transplantation. Transplant Proc 15:2889, 1983

177. Tilney NL, Kupiec—Weglinski JW, Heidecke CD, Strom TB: Mechanisms of rejection and prolongation of vascularized organ allografts. Immunol Rev 77:185, 1984

178. Tilney NL, Milford EL, Aranjo J-L et al: Experience with cyclosporine and steroids in clinical renal transplantation. Ann Surg 200:604, 1984

179. Tilney NL, Strom TB, Vineyard GC, Merrill JP: Factors contributing to the declining mortality rate in renal transplantation. N Engl J Med 299:1321, 1978

180. Trowbridge IS, Omary MB: Human cell surface glycoprotein related to cell proliferation is the receptor for transferrin. Proc Natl Acad Sci USA 78:3039, 1981

181. Turk JL: Studies on the mechanism of action of methotrexate and cyclophosphamide on contact sensitivity in the guinea pig. Int Arch Allergy 24:191, 1964

182. Turk JL, Stone SH: Implications of the cellular changes in lymph nodes during the development and inhibition of delayed type hypersensitivity. In Amos B, Koprowski H (eds): Cell Bound Antibodies, p 51. Philadelphia, Wistar Institute Press, 1963

183. Uldall R, Taylor R, Swinney J: Cyclophosphamide in human organ transplantation. Lancet 2:258, 1971

184. van Wauwe JP, DeMey JR, Goosens JG: OKT3: A monoclonal anti-human T lymphocyte antibody with potent properties. J Immunol 124:2708, 1980

185. Wang HB, Heacock EH, Zheng CX et al: Evidence for the presence of suppressor T lymphocytes in animals treated with Cyclosporin A. J Immunol 128:1382, 1982

186. Wang BS, Zheng CX, Heacock EH et al: Inhibition of the production of a soluble helper mediated by Cyclosporin A results in the failure to generate alloreactive cytolytic cells in mixed lymphocyte culture. Clin Immunol Immunopathol 27:160, 1983

187. Webel ML, Ritts RE Jr, Taswell HF: Cellular immunity after intravenous administration of methylprednisolone. J Lab Clin Med 83:383, 1974

188. Weir MR, Kirkman RL, Strom TB, Tilney NL: Chronic liver disease in recipients of long-term renal allografts; analysis of morbidity and mortality. Kidney Int (Suppl) 28:839, 1985

189. Weisman PA, Quinby WC, Wright A, Cannon B: The adrenal hormones and homografting: Exploration of a concept. Ann Surg 134:506, 1951

190. Woodruff MFA: Can tolerance to homologous skin be induced in the human infant at birth? Transplant Bull 4:26, 1957

191. Woodruff MFA, Llaurado JG: The effect of systemic administration of fluoro- and chloro-cortisone, and the local application of fluoro-cortisol on skin homografts in rabbits. Plast Reconstr Surg 18:251, 1956

192. Yu DTY, Clements PJ, Paulus HE et al: Human lymphocyte subpopulations: Effect of Corticosteroids. J Clin Invest 53:565, 1972

193. Yu S, Lannin DR, Tsui—Collins AL, McKhann CF: Effect of cyclophosphamide on mice bearing methylcolanthrene-induced fibrosarcomas. Cancer Res 40:2756, 1980

194. Zukoski CF, Lee HM, Hume DM: The prolongation of functional survival of canine renal homografts by 6-mercaptopurine. Surg Forum 11:470, 1960

CHAPTER 7

Manipulation of the Immune Response: Other Methods

James A. Schulak   Robert J. Corry

Manipulation of the immune response in clinical transplantation can be achieved by many different methods.

Numerous early uncontrolled studies on the clinical value of splenectomy revealed conflicting results. Whether or not any benefit is long-lived remains unclear. In one study, graft survival in splenectomized patients, although better in the first 3 years after transplantation, was not different from that in nonsplenectomized patients at 5 to 6 years. Splenectomy places the patient at an increased risk for developing life-threatening sepsis. Considering the continued controversy regarding its clinical effect, the well-recognized risk of post-splenectomy sepsis, and the lack of strong experimental data to support its use, splenectomy is not generally recommended for routine use in clinical transplantation.

Radiation can be used to modify the donor, the graft, or the recipient. Moreover, it can be used therapeutically to treat rejection crises. Donor and graft irradiation prior to transplantation are primarily experimental tools used to deplete the graft of passenger leukocytes or prevent subsequent graft-versus-host disease. Recipient whole-body irradiation is not currently used because of its attendant lethal bone marrow toxicity. Total lymphoid irradiation (TLI), on the other hand, has been demonstrated to be a very effective immunosuppressive therapy. Its use, however, requires urgent transplantation within several weeks of administration and therefore is somewhat impractical. Therapeutic graft irradiation for the treatment of acute rejection has been reported to be successful in one prospective study and possibly deleterious in two others and is therefore not widely used in clinical transplantation.

Thoracic Duct Drainage (TDD) is a technique by which the recipient is rendered lymphopenic by removal of circulating lymphocytes from thoracic duct lymph. Short-term studies of cadaver graft recipients prepared by pretransplant TTD have routinely revealed a graft survival advantage. However, the long-term benefit of this cumbersome procedure has not been clearly established.

Plasmapheresis is used to remove antibodies from the blood of transplant patients who are experiencing acute allograft rejection. Although theoretically attractive, plasmapheresis has not been demonstrated to be more successful in reversing steroid-resistant rejection crisis than supplemental immunosuppression alone in any controlled trials to date. Other applications of plasmapheresis have included pretransplant removal of anti-ABO antibodies, thereby permitting successful transplantation across these barriers, and attempted reduction of panel-reactive antibodies in highly presensitized patients.

Donor pretreatment with pharmacologic immunosuppression in the form of cyclophosphamide and methylprednisolone may reduce immunogenicity of the graft. Most trials of this regimen have not demonstrated a graft survival advantage for the pretreated whole-organ grafts. Removal of Class II antigen–bearing passenger leukocytes can be achieved by short-term tissue culture and treatment with ALG in the case of tissue grafts yielding long-term experimental graft survival. It is doubtful, however, whether these techniques can be applied to primarily vascularized organs because Class II antigen is present on vascular endothelium.

Manipulation of the immune response to favor the transplanted graft has been the elusive goal of transplant immunologists ever since allograft rejection was first recognized. The most widely used methods of immune manipulation are reviewed in other sections of this book. Rather, in this chapter, the more controversial and somewhat less efficacious techniques of immunologic manipulation will be reviewed. In the recipient, these include (1) splenectomy, (2) depletion of circulating lymphocytes by thoracic duct drainage, (3) removal of circulating anti-donor antibodies by plasmapheresis, and (4) host irradiation. Techniques of donor and graft immune manipulation prior to transplantation include graft or donor irradiation and donor treatment with immunosuppressive drugs.

SPLENECTOMY

The spleen constitutes approximately 25% of the total body lymphoid mass and is therefore the largest solid immune organ in the body. Consequently, it has long been hypothesized that splenectomy may alter the immune response to favor allograft survival. Although its use in clinical transplantation was first reported by Starzl in 1963[91] and laboratory evaluation was reported even earlier, the usefulness of splenectomy as a method of host immune manipulation remains somewhat controversial to this day. Most clinical reports have described noncontrolled and nonrandomized series and often used nonconcurrent patient groups for comparison. Moreover, laboratory investigations have utilized various species and types of grafts, differing times of splenectomy in relation to grafting, and multiple adjuvant immunosuppressive regimens, thereby further confusing the issue. Nevertheless, a consensus is beginning to evolve that recognizes splenectomy as a method of achieving at least partial immunologic ablation that may come, however, with the expense of increased patient morbidity and mortality and whose salutory effect may be short-lived.

Effect of Splenectomy on the Immune System

The spleen has several important functions, not all of which involve the immune system. Injured and old red blood cells are cleared by the spleen, as are thrombocytes and leukocytes. Consequently, asplenic persons often exhibit morphologically aberrant cells as well as both leukocytosis and thrombocytosis. This latter consequence of splenectomy provided the rationale for its use in many patients by countering immunosuppression-related bone marrow depression. In addition to scavaging the abnormal formed elements of blood, the spleen is an important site for the clearance of blood-borne foreign antigens such as bacteria in the case of infection and passenger leukocytes in the case of organ allotransplantation. The spleen therefore serves a dual role as both a cellular trap in the reticuloendothelial system and as a site for early recognition of foreign antigens, recruitment of appropriate immunologic effector cells, and elaboration of the humoral immune response. Most important in this latter regard may be the production of opsonizing and cytophilic antibodies, which are critically important in the host defense against sepsis owing to the encapsulated variety of bacteria.

The fact that splenectomy causes immunologic impairment in both laboratory animals and humans has been well established. Rowley[78] reported as early as 1950 that splenectomized persons exhibited decreased levels of circulatory antibody in response to intravenous challenge with allogeneic erythrocytes. Claret and associates[15] documented serial quantitative changes in immunoglobulin concentration following splenectomy in children and observed that IgM levels were significantly decreased, IgA levels were significantly increased, and IgG levels were only minimally greater than in spleen intact controls. Opsonin activity is decreased following splenectomy, as are levels of tuftsin, a peptide with phagocytosis-stimulating activity.[53] These deficits are currently believed to be responsible for the well-recognized problem of overwhelming post-splenectomy sepsis. The effect of splenectomy on the cellular arm of host immunity is less well understood and has been evaluated primarily in experimental allograft models. The spleen, however, is believed to be a primary site for suppressor cell generation and amplification, raising the question of whether splenectomy would be harmful in situations in which this type of response is the desired result of immunologic manipulation.

Splenectomy in Experimental Transplantation

Early attempts to achieve prolongation of allograft survival in experimental animals yielded varied results. Improved skin graft survival was reported in nonimmunosuppressed splenectomized mice but not in rabbits. In canine models where recipients also received pharmacologic immunosuppression, splenectomy did not significantly prolong either skin[101] or renal[46] allograft survival when compared to that achieved in drug-treated animals alone. In the rat, splenectomy in conjunction with thymectomy, antilymphocyte globulin, cyclosporine, or total lymphoid irradiation prolongs survival of heart grafts when compared with nonsplenectomized but otherwise similarly treated recipients.[19,20,74] Splenectomy has also been reported to be beneficial in rat renal allotransplantation, although this may be somewhat dependent upon the degree of histocompatibility between donor and recipient.[21] It has also been suggested that, in the rat, splenectomy may be more effective if delayed until after transplantation.[88] Splenectomy, however, does not significantly prolong survival or rat pancreas allografts whether delayed or used adjuvantly with cyclosporine.[82]

Further confusing the issue is the hypothesis that the presence of the spleen may be advantageous rather than deleterious in transplanted patients. Several investigators have reported that the salutory effect of donor-specific blood transfusion (DST) in murine allotransplantation models is dependent upon the spleen being present at the time of blood administration.[55,84] Also, splenectomy prior to immune manipulation has been demonstrated to prevent both active and passive enhancement but does not abrogate such responses if delayed until the time of transplantation.[9,22] Although these experiments suggest that splenectomy may be disadvantageous in transplantation, clinical data are not available to adequately analyze this possibility.

Splenectomy in Clinical Transplantation

Starzl's[91] inaugural report in 1963 described a successful outcome for four of five recipients of living-related donor (LRD) renal transplants who also underwent thymectomy, total body irradiation, and pharmacologic immunosuppression, thereby making it difficult to attribute the outcome solely to removal of the spleen. Nevertheless, this experience served as an impetus for others to evaluate splenectomy. Unfortunately, early reports were contradictory in that some described a salutory effect whereas others did not,[31,101] depending upon whether the grafts were of LRD or cadaver (CAD) origin. Pierce and Hume,[71] failing to observe a salutory effect of splenectomy in either LRD or CAD primary renal transplant recipients, were the first to report that splenectomized recipients of second renal transplants enjoyed better graft survival than their nonsplenectomized counterparts.

Subsequent single- and multicenter studies involving larger numbers of patients failed to settle the controversy. Opelz and Terasaki[68] reported a series of 1618 patients from 51 centers in which 487 recipients were splenectomized prior to transplantation and 1131 were not. One- and 2-year graft survivals for CAD recipients were marginally better for those in the splenectomized group, but this difference was not statistically significant. Moreover, they also failed to observe a beneficial effect of splenectomy in second transplants. Consequently, this report is often cited as proof that splenectomy is not beneficial. Caution must be exercised in the interpretation of these data, however, because comparisons were made between centers that exclusively performed splenectomy and those that did not, thereby introducing the variable of "center effect." Subsequently, another multicenter study has suggested a salutory effect of splenectomy in CAD transplantation.[2] One variable in most of these studies that has not been controlled is the timing of splenectomy in regard to transplantation. This may be important. Kauffman and colleagues[43] reported that CAD recipients splenectomized prior to transplantation experienced significantly better 1- and 2-year graft survival than did those patients who were splenectomized either simultaneously with transplantation or at a later date.

Since 1980, four single-center studies of splenectomy in renal transplantation have demonstrated a favorable effect. Stuart and co-workers[95] reported a prospective but only partially randomized series of first CAD transplants in which splenectomy significantly improved patient and graft survival. Although this study combined patients who were randomized with those in whom splenectomy was performed because of pretransplant leukopenia, the data clearly demonstrated splenectomy to be beneficial. Splenectomized patients enjoyed a 52% 4-year graft survival compared with 23% for those with intact spleens. Graft survival advantage for the splenectomized patients in this series has persisted for 5 years.[77] Studying a similar patient population, Mozes and colleagues[61] reported that splenic ablation, achieved by either conventional splenectomy or by transcatheter partial splenic embolization, also significantly improved graft survival. Although in this study splenectomized patients had a better outcome when prophylactic antilymphocyte globulin (ALG) was used, the trend for longer graft survival in splenectomized patients was present even in the absence of this drug. The impact of splenectomy on high-risk patients who were either older than 50 years or diabetic was reviewed by Okiye and associates[66] at the Mayo Clinic in a single-center study of 165 patients. Splenectomy was associated with better 5-year CAD graft survival in both subsets of patients and for the combined high-risk group as a whole when compared with their nonsplenectomized cohorts. Conversely, splenectomy again was not found to be beneficial in HLA-identical LRD renal transplantation.

Fryd and co-workers[30] reported the University

of Minnesota's experience with the only truly prospective and randomized study of splenectomy versus no splenectomy in renal transplantation. Splenectomy performed prior to transplantation in 56 patients and concomitantly in 91 patients significantly improved 1- and 2-year graft survival for recipients of either HLA-nonidentical LRD or CAD grafts, whereas recipients of HLA-identical LRD kidneys faired equally well irrespective of their splenectomy status. Long-term follow-up of the Minnesota series, however, has revealed that the benefit of splenectomy was present only for the first 3 years after transplantation; graft survival rates for their splenectomized patients were not significantly better after that time.[96]

Finally, a relatively novel application of splenectomy in human transplantation has been proposed by Alexandre and colleagues,[4] who have reported that splenectomy along with plasmapheresis and donor-specific platelet transfusion has permitted successful LRD renal transplantation to be performed across ABO red blood cell incompatibility barriers. Although confirmation of these results by other centers is necessary before use of the technique can be endorsed, it provides a possible alternative to categorically refusing all ABO incompatible LRD donors.

The risk of post-splenectomy sepsis remains the major drawback to use of this adjuvant method of immunosuppression. Typically, these patients have a fulminant course with systemic toxicity, fever, chills, vascular collapse, and a rapid demise. Although many studies with short-term follow-up have failed to observe this syndrome in transplantation patients, longer periods of evaluation have made this increased risk apparent in both children[13,56] and adults.[3,70] Of interest is Alexander's[3] observation that a graft survival advantage without increased patient mortality in splenectomized patients is present up to 2 years after transplantation, but that afterward, graft survival curves converge, whereas the patient survival curves diverged in favor of the spleen-intact patients. In view of the increased mortality apparently associated with splenectomized transplant patients, a good argument can be made for long-term use of prophylactic antibiotics in splenectomized patients and for immediate administration of broad-spectrum coverage as soon as the syndrome is suspected.

In summary, splenectomy cannot be generally advised as a method for manipulating the immune response in transplant patients. Nevertheless, selected use of splenectomy may be prudent in patients with hypersplenism and persistent azathioprine-associated leukopenia and in candidates for retransplantation when use of cyclosporine and/or ALG is precluded.

GRAFT IRRADIATION

Radiation of the allograft for the purpose of modifying the immune response has been under investigation since the earliest days of clinical transplantation. More specifically, radiotherapy has been used in three different ways. First, grafts have been radiated for a brief course immediately after transplantation with the hope of achieving prophylactic immunosuppression. More commonly, graft irradiation has been used as an adjuvant component of antirejection therapy. A third variant of graft radiotherapy is pretransplantation, ex vivo graft irradiation, performed in order to alter the immunogenicity of the organ. The first two methods have been evaluated in both the clinics and the laboratory, whereas the latter method is primarily a research endeavor.

Prophylactic Irradiation

Empiric administration of low-dose radiation to the transplanted allograft was described by Hume and colleagues in 1963; however, its usefulness was not evident in that small series. Kauffman and associates[42] and Wolf and colleagues,[104] working in Hume's laboratory, subsequently evaluated prophylactic graft irradiation in canine renal transplant models. Both investigative teams demonstrated moderate improvement in graft survival and a decreased lymphocytic infiltrate in the irradiated organs. The effect of prophylactic graft irradiation on the immune response is a relatively weak effect, however, in that neither indefinite nor long-term survival was achieved in these experiments. In 1971, Birch and co-workers[10] observed better 3- and 12-month graft survival for a small group of patients in whom 600 rads in fractionated doses were administered to the graft after transplantation when compared with patients who did not receive local radiation. Carefully controlled studies of prophylactic graft irradiation, however, have not been performed.

Therapeutic Irradiation

Local graft irradiation for the treatment of acute allograft rejection has also been used since the early days of renal transplantation, although only several controlled studies are available for review. Godfrey and Salaman[32] observed a trend toward increased reversibility of acute rejection for grafts treated with both steroid pulses and graft irradiation when compared with those treated with steroids alone, although the difference was not statistically significant. Surprisingly, however, 1-year graft survival for the irradiated grafts (26%) was significantly worse than that for those not irradiated (50%). Similar data have also been reported by Pilepich and colleagues.[72] In their randomized, prospective, double-blind study, reversibility of rejection episodes was not significantly improved by the addition of radiotherapy, and long-term graft survival was also adversely affected. In contrast, Johnson and colleagues[41] reported that low-dose local radiotherapy used in conjunction with antithymocyte serum to treat acute renal allograft rejection does markedly, but not significantly, improve long-term graft survival (61% vs. 34%). A clear explanation for the discrepancy in outcome between these three studies has not been made. However, decreased long-term graft survival in the first two studies may have been due to nonimmunologic dysfunction, as low-dose irradiation has been reported to be deleterious to the transplanted kidney.[59]

In view of these conflicting data, the use of local graft irradiation for the treatment of acute rejection episodes cannot be given an unqualified endorsement. Rather, unless it is further evaluated by protocol, its use may be most appropriate for patients who either have life-threatening infection that precludes use of systemic immunosuppression or have already received their limit of the more proven methods of antirejection therapy. Typically, such therapy consists of 3 to 4 doses of 150 rads to 175 rads administered directly to the graft on alternating days.

Donor and Graft Irradiation

Irradiation of the donor prior to organ harvest or of the graft before implantation for the purpose of altering its immunogenicity has not been routinely performed in clinical transplantation; however, investigative interest in this technique has continued. Donor irradiation has been successfully used to deplete the graft of passenger leukocytes prior to transplantation, thereby decreasing its ability to stimulate the host immune response.[94] Donor irradiation also decreases or prevents development of lethal graft-versus-host disease (GVHD) in recipients of experimental allogeneic small intestine[60] or combined pancreas–spleen grafts.[83] In addition, ex vivo graft irradiation prior to transplantation prevents subsequent GVHD in small bowel and spleen recipients, although larger doses of radiation are necessary.[52,83]

Similarly, irradiation of rat islets with ultraviolet (UV) light prior to allotransplantation is an effective method of altering this graft's subsequent immunogenicity, presumably by inactivating the Class II antigen–bearing dendritic cells. For example, in experiments reported by Lau and co-workers,[51] highly histoincompatible Lewis islets irradiated ex vivo with a dose of 900 J/m^2 subsequently maintained normoglycemia for 75 days in diabetic ACI rats without use of other immunosuppressive therapy.

Irradiation of Donor and Recipient Blood

Lau, Reemstma, and Hardy[50] have also demonstrated that UV irradiation may be used to alter the immunogenicity of donor-specific blood when the latter is used as part of pretransplant preparation for allotransplantation. In their experiments, rats transplanted with highly histoincompatible islets enjoyed indefinite graft survival when they had previously received three irradiated donor-specific transfusions, whereas graft survival in all control groups was approximately 8 days. Again, it appears that UV irradiation may inactivate the contaminating Class II antigens in such a way that presensitization does not occur, whereas induction of a suppressor cell response does. Clearly, clinical evaluation of this phenomenon is indicated in view of the fact that the greatest disadvantage to DST protocols currently in use is their propensity to sensitize 10% to 30% of the patients, thereby precluding subsequent transplantation with that donor.

Direct irradiation of host blood for the purpose of manipulating the immune response has also been evaluated. Hume and co-workers[38,39] described a technique for extracorporeal irradiation of blood (ECIB) using an external arteriovenous shunt in which the tubing was passed through a self-contained strontium 90 source. They reported that this therapy may have been responsible for reversal of renal allograft rejection in several patients. ECIB was studied in greater detail by Weeke and Sorensen,[103] who reported that it resulted in lymphopenia and decreased immunologic function of circulating lymphocytes as measured by their in vitro response to tuberculin and allogeneic cells but not to the mitogen phytohemaglutinin. In addition, they also suggested that ECIB resulted in fewer rejection episodes in the treated patients. Further confirmation of the immunosuppressive effect of ECIB was reported by Chana and associates,[14] who, using a ^{137}Cr source of radiation, were able to double renal allograft survival in goats not receiving other forms of immunosuppression. Despite these preliminary data that demonstrate an immunodulatory effect for ECIB, the technique has never gained widespread clinical use and currently is not being further evaluated.

RECIPIENT LYMPHOID IRRADIATION

Recipient whole-body irradiation for the purpose of achieving immunosuppression was the first method of immune manipulation attempted in clinical renal transplantation. Although somewhat successful, the dosage requirements necessary to achieve immunosuppression also resulted in prohibitive patient morbidity and mortality owing to bone marrow and gastrointestinal toxicity.[35,39] Consequently, clinical use of whole-body irradiation was quickly abandoned in favor of a more selective approach to radiotherapy (description follows). Nevertheless, Rapaport and colleagues[75] extensively evaluated whole-body irradiation and recipient hemopoietic reconstitution with autologous bone marrow in dogs. These investigators demonstrated that when renal transplantation was delayed only 12 to 30 hours after irradiation and marrow replacement in dog leukocyte antigen (DLA)-identical dogs, permanent acceptance of the kidney occurred in approximately 60% of the recipients without use of other forms of immunosuppression. Unfortunately, when attempted with DLA-nonidentical donor–recipient pairs, all grafts ultimately rejected, thereby dampening enthusiasm for attempting clinical trials in human transplantation.

Total Lymphoid Irradiation

Kaplan and colleagues at Stanford University first demonstrated that selective irradiation of the lymphoid mass alone was possible with relatively little significant morbidity. Using a technique called *total lymphoid irradiation (TLI)* for the treatment of Hodgkin's disease, they demonstrated that up to 4000 rads could be administered safely in fractions to the cervical, axillary, mediastinal, para-aortic, iliac, and inguinal nodes as well as to the thymus and spleen. Other radiosensitive tissues such as the lungs, kidneys, bone marrow, and central nervous system are protected during TLI by lead shields. As a result, the morbidity associated with TLI is negligible when compared with that of whole-body radiotherapy. Although, constitutional symptoms such as nausea, anorexia, diarrhea, fatigue, and malaise are transiently experienced by some patients, life-threatening infection has generally not been a problem.

The immunosuppressive effect of TLI has been well documented in both experimental and clinical transplantation. TLI induces a marked decrease in the peripheral lymphocyte count, which persists for 1 to 2 years following therapy. There appears, however, to be a longer lasting reduction of T cells, which may account for the depressed immune function attributed to this lymphocyte subset, such as nonreactivity in mixed lymphocyte culture, reduced ability to mount a delayed hypersensitivity reaction, and reduced ability to proliferate when stimulated by various mitogens. In addition, use of monoclonal antibodies to T cell subset surface antigens has demonstrated a reversal of the normal T helper to T suppressor cell ratios following allogeneic transplantation in recipients pretreated with TLI. Overall, observations such as these have suggested that TLI may be useful in clinical transplantation.

Experimental TLI

The use of TLI in experimental models of murine transplantation was first described by Strober, Slavin, and colleagues[93] and has been extensively reviewed elsewhere. These investigators were able to induce donor-specific tolerance for allogeneic bone marrow grafts in mice by pretreating the recipients with TLI. Stable chimerism was demonstrated in these animals who later were able to reject third-party skin grafts but not those of the donor strain. Subsequently, the same effect was reproduced in rat experiments when the secondary graft was a donor strain heart.[87] Attempts, however, to achieve similar results in a canine model were unsuccessful when the TLI and donor bone marrow model of chimerism was studied. On the other hand, the Stanford group has achieved long-term canine heart allograft survival with a regimen of pretransplantation TLI and post-transplantation immunosuppression with ATG and azathioprine.[45]

Myburgh and colleagues[62] in Johannesburg have extensively studied the use of TLI in experimental primate transplantation models. Their experiments in outbred baboons were designed to evaluate various fractionation regimens for radiation administration, fields of irradiation, necessity for donor bone marrow transplantation, concomitant use of pharmacologic immunosuppression, as well as the efficacy of TLI in presensitized hosts. With TLI alone, donor-specific tolerance was achieved for renal allografts in a small number of animals using weekly fractions of 200 rads to a cumulative dose of 600 rads to 3000 rads. Acute rejection episodes could be prevented in kidney and liver recipients with total doses of 2000 rads and 1000 rads, respectively, although radiation-related mortality was encountered frequently when the cumulative dose was greater than 2000 rads. Subsequently it was discovered that cumulative doses of as little as 600 rads also resulted in significant improvement in long-term graft survival, especially when transplantation was delayed until 2 to 3 weeks after irradiation. Administration of donor bone marrow did not appear to be necessary in order to achieve the salutory effect of TLI in these experiments. Of clinical importance, however, was their observation that concomitant use of ATG was synergistic with TLI, whereas post-transplantation administration of cyclosporine was not and may actually have been deleterious. The Stanford group also evaluated combined use of TLI and cyclosporine in a heart transplant model in outbred cynomolgus monkeys and similarly failed to observe a synergistic effect between TLI and cyclosporine.[69] Conversely, TLI and low-dose rather than conventional-dose cyclosporine has been reported to be synergistic in rat heart allotransplantation.[79] Lymphoma did occur in several animals receiving both TLI and cyclosporine in the Stanford experience but was not encountered in any of Myburgh's experiments. Nevertheless, the potential for overimmunosuppression when TLI is used adjunctively with other methods of immune modulation must be recognized.

An innovative approach to achieving selective lymphoid irradiation of the transplant recipient has been studied extensively by Hardy and colleagues at Columbia University.[36] They demonstrated that a beta-emitting radioisotope of palladium (^{109}Pd), when chelated with hematoporphyrin, forms a complex (Pd-H) that localizes preferentially in the reticuloendothelial tissues and lymphoid organs while sparing the thymus, bone marrow, and intestine. Short-term perioperative treatment with Pd-H has induced transplantation tolerance between weakly histoincompatible rat strains. However, unless coupled with donor bone marrow administration, adjunctive immunosuppression with ALG, or cyclosporine, subsequent allograft survival was not significantly prolonged in the context of strong histoincompatibility.[47,67] These latter studies did demonstrate that Pd-H therapy may decrease initial dosage requirements for cyclosporine, as suboptimal doses of CsA, when combined with this type of selective lymphoid irradiation, were more effective than either modality alone. It has also been suggested that use of Pd-H and concomitant immunosuppressive agents may be useful in the presence of donor-specific presensitization.[37] Clinical studies with Pd-H, especially in this latter context, may be warranted in view of its apparent safety and ease of administration.

Clinical TLI

Despite growing experience with TLI in experimental transplantation, clinical trials have not been widely attempted. The largest series was reported by Najarian and colleagues,[64] who reserved its use for retransplantation patients who suffered early immunologic loss of their previous renal allograft. TLI, administered in daily fractions of 100 rads to 125 rads with a total dose range of 1050 rads to 4050 rads, was complicated by leukopenia, nausea, vomiting, and infection that required temporary cessation of therapy in many patients. Transplantation followed as soon as an organ was available, which in most cases was less than 40 days. All patients in this series were splenectomized and received azathioprine and prednisone. Two-year graft survival for this high immunologic risk group was 74%, which compared very favorably with the 35% survival rate for their historical control group. Unfortunately, 2 of the 22 patients studied developed disseminated lymphoma; however, overall patient survival was not different from the non-TLI cohort. Immunologic analysis of the TLI patients revealed a marked decrease in circulating T-lymphocytes, reduced responsiveness to both mitogen and allogenic cell stimulation, and reversed OKT4 to OKT8 cell ratios. Of interest was the observation that if TLI-treated patients maintained in vitro immunodeficiency, they did not experience chronic rejection, whereas those in whom immune reactivity returned did experience chronic rejection.

Cortesini and associates[18] at the University of Rome similarly evaluated the efficacy of TLI used with either conventional immunosuppression or cyclosporine in high-risk renal transplant patients, the latter being defined as strong immunoresponders, diabetics, and those undergoing retransplantation. Both high-dose (2500 rads–3500 rads) and low-dose (1500 rads–2000 rads) TLI protocols were studied. Prophylactic ALG, prednisone, and azathioprine were used with the former; cyclosporine alone was used with the latter. Both regimens proved to be successful—only 3 of 14 grafts were lost to rejection in the first year in the TLI-conventional immunosuppression group, and none of 14 grafts were irreversibly rejected in the TLI-cyclosporine group. TLI-associated morbidity was frequently encountered with the high-dose regimen but did not occur with low-dose TLI and cyclosporine. Furthermore, no cases of lymphoproliferative neoplasia were observed. A smaller series of 10 diabetic patients prepared for renal transplantation with TLI was reported by Vanrenterghem and colleagues[99] in Leuven, Belgium. A salutory effect of TLI in this

series was evidenced by reduced doses of both steroids and azathioprine, with use of the latter being
totally eliminated in some patients.

A preliminary experience with the use of TLI
in non–high-risk renal transplant recipients was reported by Sampson and colleagues.[80] Fractionated
TLI was combined with a short course of postoperative antithymocyte globulin and low-dose prednisone. Of 19 grafts at risk for immunologic loss, 17
have survived for longer than 1 year, 12 never having sustained a rejection episode. Early in this series,
an attempt was made to completely eliminate prednisone therapy, but because this was followed by
several late rejections, the remaining patients have
been maintained on low-dose steroids. TLI-induced
leukopenia and thrombocytopenia were common
and necessitated a temporary interruption of therapy in many patients; however, other types of morbidity were minimal, and no cases of lymphoma
have occurred. This study again demonstrates the
immunosuppressive potential for TLI in clinical
transplantation by achieving excellent cadaver allograft survival without use of azathioprine and cyclosporine and without the need for pretransplantation
blood transfusions.

In summary, both laboratory and clinical evidence demonstrate that TLI is a potent method of
immune manipulation. With TLI, concomitant
pharmacologic immunosuppression may be either
reduced or curtailed, even in patients who traditionally are poor risks. A major disadvantage to TLI,
however, is the necessity for acquiring a crossmatch
negative organ within a relatively short period of
time following completion of the radiotherapy. Consequently, TLI may ultimately be better suited for
use in LRD than in CAD transplantation. However,
additional clinical studies are necessary in order to
better define both the optimal irradiation–immunosuppression regimen and the long-term morbidity
before TLI can be endorsed for widespread use.

THORACIC DUCT DRAINAGE

Thoracic duct drainage (TDD) requires creation of
an external lymphatic fistula through which 2 to 5
liters of lymph can be removed daily for a period of
3 to 5 weeks or more. During this time, billions of
lymphocytes may be extracted through the fistula,
which is created by surgical exposure of the thoracic
duct in the neck and cannulation of the duct with
a silastic multilumen catheter. Following removal,
the lymph is separated into its cellular and liquid
components, with the latter being reinfused in a
cell-free state during the next day. Originally, lym-
pocytes were eliminated through lysis by hypotonic

exposure; currently, however, this is accomplished
by centrifugation. Complications with TDD include
catheter-related infection, sepsis from reinfusion of
contaminated lymph, fluid electrolyte and protein
deficiencies, and premature closure of the fistula.
TDD has been thoroughly evaluated in experimental
as well as clinical transplantation. These studies all
demonstrate an immunomodulatory effect of TDD,
the extent of which is dependent upon many factors,
such as the duration of lymphatic drainage, degree
of histoincompatibility between donor and recipient, and concomitant use of pharmacologic immunosuppression.

The immunologic consequences of TDD have
been well characterized.[54] Initially, TDD produces a
rapid fall in circulating small lymphocytes, the majority of which are T cells. Although depletion lasts
as long as the fistula is maintained, lymphocyte
counts eventually return to normal after discontinuation. TDD-induced lymphopenia is evidenced by
lymphocyte depletion in the cortex of lymph nodes.
In addition, using monoclonal antibodies to T cell
surface antigens, reduced OKT3 cells, increased
OKT10 cells (immature lymphocytes), and a decrease in the OKT4 to OKT8 ratio have been demonstrated.[8] Functionally, decreased responsiveness
to both T cell mitogens and allogeneic lymphocytes
have been reported along with impaired cell-mediated lympholysis.[76]

B-lymphocytes, on the other hand, are removed at a slower rate; therefore, a relative increase
in their number may occur. The effect of TDD on
circulating antibody levels is less well documented.
Immunoglobulin levels have been reported to be
unchanged by TDD[76] or to undergo selective decrease in IgA and IgG.[54] Fish and colleagues[24] suggested that IgM is short-lived and not primarily
found in lymph and, therefore, not subject to the
dilutional decreases that occur with prolonged TDD,
whereas IgG levels are decreased not only because
of dilution, as in serum albumin and total protein,
but also because of decreased synthesis. TDD may
interfere with the primary humoral response but
does not effectively prevent anamnestic antibody
production. Because experimental models of TDD
have been difficult to maintain and because clinical
TDD is always accompanied by adjuvant use of immunosuppression, a clearer picture of the effect of
this technique of immune modulation is difficult to
obtain.

Experimental TDD

Removal of the majority of circulating small lymphocytes from the rat by means of a thoracic duct
fistula was first demonstrated by Gowans in 1959.[33]

Shortly thereafter, Gowans and colleagues reported on the immunosuppressive potential of lymphocyte depletion by TDD. The primary antibody response to either tetanus toxoid or sheep erythrocytes was blunted by short-term (5 days) TDD, but a secondary response was not.[57] With minor histocompatibility differences between donor and recipient, McGregor and Gowans[58] observed prolonged skin graft survival when grafting closely followed 8 days of TDD, whereas graft rejection ensued promptly if transplantation was delayed for 18 days or more. Conversely, TDD produced only minimal graft prolongation if major antigenic differences were present between donor and recipient. Similar data have been reported by others.[105] In canine models, both skin and renal allograft survival can be prolonged by simultaneous creation of a lymphatic fistula and transplantation; however, graft rejection does occur as the circulating pool of lymphocytes is repleted.[81,86] Because of the difficulties in creating and maintaining thoracic duct fistulae in experimental animals and because of the advent of other similar techniques for reduction of the lymphocyte pool, such as with use of antilymphocyte serum, continued laboratory investigation of TDD has not occurred.

Clinical TDD

Use of TDD in clinical transplantation was introduced by Franksson in 1964, when he reported a salutary effect for combined therapy with azathioprine, prednisone, and post-transplantation TDD. Tilney and Murray[98] followed by describing use of pretransplantation TDD for 2 to 7 days as a method of preparing their patients for renal transplantation. Fewer rejection episodes and later occurrence was observed in the patients who had a well-draining fistula when compared with those in whom fistula function was poor. Fish, Sarles, and colleagues[25,26] also reported favorable experiences with TDD in renal transplantation, especially when it was performed prior to transplantation rather than after grafting.

During the next decade, several centers reported larger series of renal transplant patients treated with TDD. Walker and colleagues[102] at Vanderbilt University achieved 76% 1-year graft survival for poorly matched cadaver renal allografts and only 48% for their non-TDD controls. Fish and co-workers,[27] in an update of their experience, reported a 1-year graft survival rate of approximately 80% for TDD patients also treated with azathioprine and steroids, an outcome that was twice as good as that achieved without TDD. Combination of ATG with TDD, however, proved to be too immunosup-

pressive, resulting in a marked increase in patient mortality. Franksson and associates,[29] on the other hand, reported a salutory effect of post-transplant TDD when used adjunctively with ALG and thymectomy but not in patients treated by TDD alone. They too, however, have reported a high rate of infection with this combination.

Starzl and colleagues[90] enthusiastically endorsed use of TDD in human transplantation while reporting significantly improved short-term graft survival rates for both liver and renal allografts. Subsequent reports further characterized their early experience with TDD and established that the optimal regimen of lymphatic drainage was pretransplant therapy for more than 20 days.[92] Long-term follow-up of Starzl's patients, however, revealed a somewhat less beneficial effect.[89] Although the percentage of grafts lost to rejection and the number of rejection episodes were markedly less in the optimally prepared recipients compared with those in the non-TDD control group, these authors reported a continued fall in graft survival during the ensuing months, suggesting that the salutory effect of TDD may be short-lived.

TDD has also been evaluated as a method of achieving successful transplantation in the presence of presensitization, although with inconsistent results. The Vanderbilt group reported that TDD can prevent hyperacute rejection when transplantation is performed in patients who have a positive T cell crossmatch with their donor.[65] Transplantation in this situation was also attempted by Starzl and co-workers[89] who conversely did observe hyperacute rejections in 3 of 6 patients. In a larger series that included only patients who were T cell crossmatch negative with their donor, Fish and associates[24] observed hyperacute or early antibody-mediated irreversible rejection in 14 of 107 grafts in patients pretreated with TDD. It appears, then, that the usefulness of TDD as a method of blunting the humoral immune response in clinical renal transplantation has not proved to be as effective as was once hoped.

In summary, TDD is an effective method for achieving at least short-term manipulation of the immune response by significantly depleting the host of circulating T-lymphocytes and by decreasing immunoglobulin levels, albeit if only through dilution. As a consequence, early renal allograft survival has been improved in most clinical trials of TDD. Whether or not TDD provides a long-lasting benefit with regard to graft survival, however, is not clear. TDD is relatively difficult to perform, is cumbersome to both the patient and nursing staff, and greatly prolongs patient hospitalization if used prior to transplantation. Considering all these factors, it is easy to understand why TDD neither has been widely practiced nor is currently being endorsed for widespread future use.

PLASMAPHERESIS

Both plasmapheresis and plasmaleukapheresis have been used in an attempt to alter the host immune response to allograft transplantation. "Apheresis" is performed by removing relatively large amounts (3–5 liters) of blood from the patient, separating it into its various components, eliminating unwanted elements and reinfusing that which remains. Most commonly, this procedure is used for removal of plasma, thereby eliminating plasma-borne substances such as antibodies, immune complexes, and toxic materials. This is accomplished by use of extracorporeal perfusion with either continuous centrifugation or by passage of the blood through various filtration devices. The cellular constituents are then reconstituted with various solutions and reinfused. Although plasmapheresis is facilitated by the presence of a hemodialysis type of vascular access, it can be performed effectively through any central venous catheter.

The usual duration of therapy for short-term plasmapheresis is in the range of 5 to 10 treatments given in 7 to 14 days. It has been calculated that approximately 90% of a pathogenic substance may be removed in this short period of time.[85] Because overall success is dependent upon many factors, such as rate of resynthesis or reaccumulation and equilibriation between the extravascular and vascular space, therapeutic regimens often need to be individualized. Although serious complications related to plasmapheresis have been reported, most authors report that it is a safe procedure.

Plasmapheresis has been demonstrated to be effective in ameliorating antibody-mediated hematologic disorders, hyperviscosity syndrome, myesthenia gravis, Goodpasture's syndrome, and certain autoimmunity-type syndromes. Its use, however, in the treatment of allograft rejection has not been widely studied, either in the laboratory or in the clinic. Moreover, the clinical data are conflicting in their results and, for the most part, anecdotal in nature.

The rationale for use of plasmapheresis or plasma exchange (PE) as therapy for allograft rejection is based upon the assumption that unrelenting rejection is often due to the presence of anti-donor antibody, which cannot be removed by immunosuppression alone. Consequently, the majority of trials of plasmapheresis in clinical transplantation have been limited to patients who were "steroid resistant," as defined by failure to achieve improved or stabilized renal function after a short course of supplemental steroid administration. The first use of plasmapheresis in this setting was reported by Cardella and associates[11] in 1977 when they described rejection reversal in four of seven patients. Subsequently, several additional noncontrolled reports, either supporting[23,63] or refuting[73] the beneficial effect of plasmapheresis in refractory rejection, have appeared. For the most part, these have been small series except for a report by Adams and colleagues,[1] who observed a salutory effect of PE in 33 of 51 (65%) patients for whom serum creatinine values continued to rise despite 3 consecutive days of supplemental methylprednisolone administration.

A major deficit of all of the aforementioned studies is that they were not controlled. This is an important criticism not only because most of the reports included small numbers of patients but also because PE was often initiated on the heels of steroid pulse therapy, rendering it difficult to discern between a salutory effect of plasmapheresis and a "delayed" response to steroid supplementation. Several controlled trials of plasmapheresis in renal allograft rejection are available for scrutiny. Kirubakaran and associates[44] reported a small study comprised of 12 control and 11 test patients, the latter receiving eight PE treatments. There was no improvement in either short- or long-term outcome in the treated group. Similar data were reported by Allen and colleagues,[6] who, in addition to the usual criteria for diagnosing rejection, required histologic verification of the humoral nature of the episode. Fourteen patients received their standard therapy; 13 were additionally treated with plasmapheresis. PE resulted in decreased levels of IgG, IgA, and IgM, with a cumulative fall during the time of therapy to approximately 10% of pretreatment levels. These immunoglobulin concentrations returned to normal in 4 weeks. Despite this significant decrease in circulating antibodies, long-term graft survival was not prolonged in the PE group.

In contrast to these two relatively small controlled studies of PE, Cardella and colleagues[12] have reported a much larger trial of this therapy for kidney rejection. All rejections were included in this later study without determining whether they were steroid-resistant. Forty-two patients receiving PE had significantly better 1- and 3-year graft survival than the 43 patients not undergoing plasma exchange (74% and 68% vs. 56% and 47%, respectively, $p = 0.05$). Although many of the patients in both groups did not have a predominantly humoral rejection, the data suggest a beneficial effect for the therapy in renal allograft rejection.

One additional use for plasmapheresis in clinical transplantation is to prepare the difficult-to-graft person for subsequent transplantation. Pretransplant PE has been used to remove specific anti-HLA antibodies in highly presensitized potential cadaver kidney recipients, thereby decreasing their panel-reactive antibody (PRA) levels and consequently facilitating their subsequent transplantability.[97] Similarly, PE has been used with splenectomy prior to transplantation in order to permit LRD grafting between ABO incompatible donors and recipients.[4] Although both of these applications of PE are appealing, neither have been confirmed by trials in other centers. Plasmaleukapheresis, a variant of apheresis that includes removal of lymphocytes as well as plasma, has also been reported to be effective in reversing renal allograft rejection, but not in controlled trials.[5]

In summary, plasmapheresis, although theoretically an attractive method of manipulating the immune system, has not gained widespread popularity in clinical circles. This is not only because of the lack of controlled data to support its use but also because of the added inconvenience and cost to the patient attendant with its use. Nevertheless, in view of the conflicting evidence available, additional controlled evaluations of PE in the setting of humorally mediated allograft rejection may be warranted. Also, plasmaleukapheresis may be a useful alternative to the post-transplantation use of either TDD or ALG as a method of achieving lymphocyte depletion. Routine use of plasmapheresis in clinical transplantation, however, cannot be advised.

DONOR PRETREATMENT

The concept that both Class I and Class II antigens are necessary in order to stimulate the host immune response to alloantigens is well accepted.[100] Because in many grafts, Class II antigens are not present on the parenchymal cells themselves, rather, they are manifested by leukocytes trapped within the interstitial spaces, many investigators have attempted to rid the graft of these immunostimulating cells prior to transplantation. Techniques used to eliminate these so-called passenger leukocytes include graft irradiation, tissue culture, and pharmacologic pretreatment of the donor.

The role of graft and donor irradiation has been discussed previously. Tissue culture of allogenic islets and thyroid has been demonstrated by several investigators to effectively eliminate passenger leukocytes from the graft such that subsequent allotransplantation in murine models routinely results in extended survival.[48,49] It has also been demonstrated, albeit not as conclusively, that elimination of passenger cells will prolong experimental kidney allograft survival.[94] Experiments such as these have led to trials of donor pretreatment in human renal transplantation, with the goal of rendering the allograft less immunogenic.

Clinical trials evaluated the use of high-dose methylprednisolone and cyclophosphamide, usually administered 5 to 20 hours prior to organ harvest.[34,106] Zincke and Woods[107] reported that donor pretreatment resulted in a nearly 40% improvement in 3-year actuarial cadaver graft survival when compared with grafts that were not treated. This study, however, was not randomized in that the nontreated kidneys were not obtained locally, whereas the pretreated grafts were. Corry and colleagues[16,17] evaluated a similar pretreatment regimen in a prospective manner and likewise demonstrated a graft survival advantage for the treatment group that was, however, not statistically significant. Of interest in this latter study was the observation that transfused recipients of pretreated kidneys enjoyed an exceptionally good result, with 88% 1-year graft survival compared with 50% or less for the remaining three possible group combinations. Conversely, other investigators have failed to demonstrate any salutory effect for donor pretreatment in clinical renal transplantation.[7,40]

Because vascularized grafts may also harbor Class II antigens on the vascular endothelium, it is unlikely that donor pretreatment with pharmacologic agents will be able to permanently alter graft immunogenicity to the extent that would warrant the added cost and inconvenience incurred by the requisite delay in actual organ harvest. Tissue grafts that are not primarily revascularized, however, such as islets of Langerhans, parathyroid and thyroid glands, skin, and bone marrow, may indeed be altered successfully prior to allotransplantation, and it is in this context that further research and clinical trials with donor or graft pretreatment may prove to be most fruitful.

REFERENCES

1. Adams MB, Kauffman HM, Hussey CV et al: Plasmapheresis in the treatment of refractory renal allograft rejection. Transplant Proc 13:491, 1981
2. Advisory Committee to the Renal Transplant Registry. The Thirteenth Report of the Human Renal Transplant Registry. Transplant Proc 9:9, 1977
3. Alexander JW, First MR, Majewski JA et al: The late adverse effect of splenectomy on patient survival fol-

lowing cadaver renal transplantation. Transplantation 37:467, 1984

4. Alexandre GPJ, Squifflet JP, DeBruyere M et al: Splenectomy as a prerequisite for successful human ABO-incompatible renal transplantation. Transplant Proc 17:138, 1985

5. Alijani MR, Pechan BW, Darr F et al: Treatment of steroid-resistant renal allograft rejection with plasmaleukapheresis. Transplant Proc 15:1063, 1983

6. Allen NH, Dyer P, Geoghegan T et al: Plasma exchange in acute renal allograft rejection. A controlled trial. Transplantation 35:425, 1983

7. Barry JM, Bennett WM: Primary cadaver kidney transplant survival after donor pretreatment with cyclophosphamide and methylprednisone. Transplantation 26:202, 1978

8. Bell JD, Marshall GD, Shaw BA et al: Alterations in human thoracic duct lymphocytes during thoracic duct drainage. Transplant Proc 15:677, 1983

9. Birinyi LK Jr, Hendry WS, Baldwin WM III, Tilney NL: The effects of splenectomy and thymectomy on enhanced cardiac allograft survival. Fed Proc 38:1102, 1979

10. Birtch AG, Carpenter CB, Tilney NL et al: Controlled clinical trial of antilymphocyte globulin in human renal allografts. Transplant Proc 3:762, 1971

11. Cardella CJ, Sutton D, Uldall PR, DeVeber GA: Intensive plasma exchange and renal-transplant rejection. Lancet 1:264, 1977

12. Cardella C, Sutton D, Uldall P et al: Factors influencing the effect of intensive plasma exchange on acute transplant rejection. Transplant Proc 17:2777, 1985

13. Cerilli J, Jones L: A reappraisal of the role of splenectomy in children receiving renal allografts. Surgery 82:510, 1977

14. Chana AD, Cronkite EP, Joel DD, Stevens JB: Prolonged renal allograft survival: Extra corporeal irradiation of blood. Transplant Proc 3:838, 1971

15. Claret I, Morales L, Montaner A: Immunological studies in the postsplenectomy syndrome. J Pediatr Surg 10:59, 1975

16. Corry RJ, Patel NP, West JC, Schanbacher BA: Pretreatment of cadaver donors with cyclophosphamide and methylprednisolone: Effect on renal transplant outcome. Transplant Proc 12:348, 1980

17. Corry, RJ, West JC: Combined effect of recipient blood transfusion and donor pretreatment with cyclophosphamide and methylprednisolone. Transplant Proc 13:161, 1981

18. Cortesini R, Renna Molanjoni E, Monari C et al: Total lymphoid irradiation in clinical transplantation. Experience in 30 high risk patients. Transplant Proc 17:1291, 1985

19. Downing TP, Reitz BA, Aziz S et al: Increased efficacy of Cyclosporin A with splenectomy prolonging the survival of rat heart allografts. Transplantation 32:76, 1981

20. Downing TP, Sadeghi AM, Reitz BA, Shumway NE: Cardiac allotransplantation in rats supported with preoperative total irradiation, low-dose cyclosporine and splenectomy. Transplantation 37:636, 1984

21. Enomoto K, Lucas ZL: Immunological enhancement of renal allografts in the rat. Transplantation 15:8, 1973

22. Fabre JW, Batchelor JR: The role of the spleen in the rejection and enhancement of renal allografts in the rat. Transplantation 20:219, 1975

23. Fassbinder W, Ernst W, Stutte HJ et al: Reversal of acute vascular rejection by plasma exchange. Int J Artif Organs 6:57, 1983

24. Fish JC, Flye W, Williams A et al: Inability of thoracic duct drainage to prevent hyperactive rejection. Transplantation 36:134, 1983

25. Fish JC, Sarles HE, Remmers AR Jr et al: Circulating lymphocyte depletion in preparation for renal allotransplantation. Surg Gynecol Obstet 128:777, 1969

26. Fish JC, Sarles HE, Remmers AR Jr: Thoracic duct fistulas in man. Surg Gynecol Obstet 131:869, 1970

27. Fish JC, Sarles HE, Remmers AR Jr et al: Renal transplantation after thoracic duct drainage. Ann Surg 193:752, 1980

28. Franksson C: Surivival of homografts of skin in rats depleted of lymphocytes by chronic drainage from the thoracic duct. Lancet 1:1331, 1964

29. Franksson C, Lundgren G, Magnusson G, Ringden O: Drainage of thoracic duct lymph in renal transplant patients. Transplantation 21:133, 1976

30. Fryd DS, Sutherland DER, Simmons RL et al: Results of a prospective randomized study on the effect of splenectomy versus no splenectomy in renal transplant patients. Transplant Proc 13:48, 1981

31. Gleason RE, Murray JE: Report from the kidney transplant registry; analysis of variables in the function of human kidney transplants. I. Transplantation 5:343, 1967

32. Godfrey AM, Salaman JR: Radiotherapy in treatment of acute rejection in human renal allografts. Lancet 1:938, 1976

33. Gowans JL: The recirculation of lymphocytes from blood to lymph in the rat. J Physiol 146:54, 1959

34. Guttmann, RD, Beaudoin JG, Morehouse DD et al: Donor pretreatment as an adjunct to cadaver renal allotransplantation. Transplant Proc 7:117, 1975

35. Hamburger J, Vaysse J, Crosnier J et al: Renal homotransplantation in man after radiation of the recipient. Am J Med 32:854, 1962

36. Hardy MA, Fawwaz R, Oluwole S et al: Selective lymphoid irradiation. I. An approach to transplantation. Surgery 86:194, 1979

37. Hardy MA, Oluwole S, Fawwaz R et al: Selective lymphoid irradiation. III. Prolongation of cardiac xenografts and allografts in presensitized rats. Transplantation 33:237, 1982

38. Hume DM, Lee HM, Williams GM: Comparative results of cadaver and related donor renal homografts in man, and immunologic implications of the outcome of second and paired transplants. Ann Surg 164:352: 1966

39. Hume DM, Wolf JS: Modification of renal homograft

rejection by irradiation. Transplantation 5:1174, 1967

40. Jeffrey JR, Downs A, Graham JW et al: A randomized prospective study of cadaver donor pretreatment in renal transplantation. Transplantation 25:287, 1978

41. Johnson HK, Malcolm A, Al-Abdulla S et al: The effect of local graft irradiation upon the reversal of cadaveric renal allograft rejection. Transplant Proc 17:29, 1985

42. Kauffman HM, Cleveland RJ, Dwyer JJ et al: Prolongation of renal homograft function by local graft radiation. Surg Gynecol Obstet 120:49, 1965

43. Kauffman HM, Swanson MK, McGregor WR, Rodgers RE: Splenectomy in renal transplantation. Surg Gynecol Obstet 139:33, 1974

44. Kirubakaran MG, Disney APS, Norman J et al: A controlled trial of plasmapheresis in the treatment of renal allograft rejection. Transplantation 32:164, 1981

45. Koretz SH,, Gottlieb MS, Strober S et al: Organ transplantation in mongrel dogs using total lymphoid irradiation (TLI). Transplant Proc 13:443, 1981

46. Kountz SL, Cohn R: Prolonged survival of a renal homograft by simultaneous splenectomy and homotransplantation. Surg Forum 13:59, 1962

47. Kuromoto N, Hardy MA, Fawwaz R et al: Selective lymphoid irradiation and Cyclosporin A in rat heart allografts. J Surg Res 36:428, 1984

48. Lacy PE, David JM, Finke EH: Prolongation of islet allograft survival following in vitro culture (24°C\ and a single injection of ALS. Science 204:312, 1979

49. Lafferty KJ,, Cooley MA, Woolnough K, Walker Z: Thyroid allograft immunogenicity is reduced after a period in organ culture. Scince 188:259, 1975

50. Lau H, Reemtsma K, Hardy MA: Pancreatic islet allograft prolongation by donor-specific blood transfusions treated with ultraviolet irradiation. Science 221:754, 1983

51. Lau H, Reemtsma K, Hardy MA: Prolongation of rat islet allograft survival by direct ultraviolet irradiation of the graft. Science 223:607, 1984

52. Lee KKW, Schraut WH: In vitro allograft irradiation prevents graft-versus-host disease in small-bowel transplantation. J Surg Res 38:364, 1985

53. Likhite VV: Immunological impairment and susceptibility to infection after splenectomy. JAMA 236:1376, 1976

54. Machler HI, Paulus H: Clinical and immunological alterations observed in patients undergoing long-term thoracic duct drainage. Surgery 84:157, 1978

55. Martin DC, Hewitt CW, Dowdy S et al: Transfer of the beneficial blood transfusion effect on rat renal allograft survival by spleen isografts. Transplantation 37:319, 1984

56. McEnery PT, Flanagan J: Fulminant sepsis in splenectomized children with renal allografts. Transplantation 24:154, 1977

57. McGregor DD, Gowans JL: The antibody response

58. McGregor DD, Gowans JL: Survival of homografts of skin in rats depleted of lymphocytes by chronic drainage from the thoracic duct. Lancet 1:629, 1964

59. Meakins JL, Smith EJ, Aron BS, Alexander JW: Delayed recovery from acute tubular necrosis following radiation. Transplant Proc 3:494, 1971

60. Monchik GJ, Russell PS: Transplantation of small bowel in the rat: Technical and immunological considerations. Surgery 70:693, 1971

61. Mozes MF, Spigos DG, Thomas PA Jr et al: Antilymphocyte globulin (ALG) and splenectomy or partial splenic embolization (PSE): Evidence for a synergistic beneficial effect on cadaver renal allograft survival. Transplant Proc 15:613, 1983

62. Myburgh JA, Smit JA, Browde S, Stark JH: Current status of total lymphoid irradiation. Transplant Proc 15:659, 1983

63. Naik RB, Ashlin R, Wilson C et al: The role of plasmapheresis in renal transplantation. Clin Nephrol 11:245, 1979

64. Najarian JS, Ferguson RM, Sutherland DER et al: Fractionated total lymphoid irradiation as preparative immunosuppression in high risk renal transplantation. Ann Surg 196:442, 1982

65. Niblack GD, Johnson HK, Richie RE et al: Preformed cytotoxic antibody in patients subjected to thoracic duct drainage. Proc Dial Transplant Forum 5:146, 1975

66. Okiye SE, Zincke H, Engen DE et al: Splenectomy in high-risk primary renal transplant recipients. Am J Surg 146:594, 1983

67. Oluwole S, Fawwaz R, Satake K et al: Effect of bone marrow cells on induction of tolerance with selective lymphoid irradiation and ALG in rats. Surg Forum 31:382, 1980

68. Opelz G, Terasaki PI: Effect of splenectomy on human renal transplants. Transplantation 15:605, 1973

69. Pennock JL, Reitz BA, Bieber CP et al: Survival of primates following orthotopic cardiac transplantation treated with total lymphoid irradiation and chemical immune suppression. Transplantation 32:467, 1981

70. Peters TG, Williams JW, Harmon HC, Britt LG: Splenectomy and death in renal transplant patients. Arch Surg 118:795, 1983

71. Pierce JC, Hume DM: The effect of splenectomy on the survival of first and second renal homotransplants in man. Surg Gynecol Obstet 127:1300, 1968

72. Pilepich MV, Sicard GA, Breaux SR et al: Renal graft irradiation in acute rejection. Transplantation 35:208, 1983

73. Power D, Nichols A, Muirhead N et al: Plasma exchange in acute renal allograft rejection: Is a controlled trial really necessary. Transplantation 32:162, 1981

74. Racelis D, Martinelli GP, Schanzer H: Prolongation of cardiac allograft survival in rats by combined pretransplant thymectomy, splenectomy, and antithy-

of rats depleted of lymphocytes by chronic drainage from the thoracic duct. J Exp Med 117:303, 1963

mocyte globulin treatment. Transplantation 33:96, 1981

75. Rapaport FT, Bachvaroff RJ, Dicke K, Santos G: Total body irradiation and host reconstitution with stored autologous marrow: An experimental model for the induction of allogeneic unresponsiveness in large mammals. Transplant Proc 11:1028, 1979

76. Richie, RE, Niblack G, Johnson HK, Tallent MB: Thoracic duct drainage in transplantation. Transplant Proc 12:483, 1980

77. Rohrer R, Meller J, Reckard CR et al: Splenectomy revisited: More restricted indications for pretransplant splenectomy. Transplant Proc 17:132, 1985

78. Rowley DA: The formation of circulating antibody in the splenectomized human being following intravenous injection of heterologous erythrocytes. J Immunol 65:515, 1950

79. Rynasiewicz JJ, Sutherland DER, Kawahara R, Najarian JS: Total lymphoid irradiation: Critical timing and combination with Cyclosporin A for immunosuppression in a rat heart allograft model. J Surg Res 30:365, 1981

80. Sampson D, Levin BS, Hoppe RT et al: Preliminary observations on the use of total lymphoid irradiation, rabbit antithymocyte globulin, and low-dose prednisone in human cadaver renal transplantation. Transplant Proc 17:1299, 1985

81. Samuelson JS, Fisher B, Fisher ER: Prolonged survival of skin homografts in dogs with thoracic duct fistula. Surg Forum 14:192, 1963

82. Schulak JA, Engelstad KM: Splenectomy in experimental pancreas transplantation. Transplantation 40:564, 1985

83. Schulak JA, Sharp WJ: Graft irradiation abrogates GVHD in combined pancreas–spleen transplantation. J Surg Res 40:326, 1986

84. Shelby J, Wakely E, Corry RJ: Splenectomy abrogates the improved graft survival achieved by donor-specific transfusion. Transplant Proc 17:1083, 1985

85. Shumak KH, Rock GA: Therapeutic plasma exchange. N Engl J Med 310:762, 1984

86. Singh LM, Vega RE, Makin GS, Howard JM: External thoracic duct fistula and canine renal homograft. JAMA 191:1009, 1965

87. Slavin S, Reitz BA, Bieber CP et al: Transplantation tolerance in adult rats using total lymphoid irradiation: Permanent survival of skin, heart, and marrow allografts. J Exp Med 147:700, 1978

88. Souther SG, Morris RE, Vistnes LM: Prolongation of rat cardiac allograft survival by splenectomy following transplantation. Transplantation 17:317, 1974

89. Starzl TE, Klintmalm G, Iwatsuki S, Weil R: Late follow-up after thoracic duct drainage in cadaveric renal transplantation. Surg Gynecol Obstet 153:377, 1981

90. Starzl TE, Koep LJ, Weil R et al: Thoracic duct drainage in organ transplantation: Will it permit better immunosuppression? Transplant Proc 11:276, 1979

91. Starzl TE, Marchioro TL, Talmage DW, Waddell WR: Splenectomy and thymectomy in human renal homotransplantation. Proc Soc Exp Biol Med 113:929, 1963

92. Starzl TE, Weil R, Koep LJ et al: Thoracic duct drainage before and after cadaver kidney transplantation. Surg Gynecol Obstet 149:815, 1979

93. Strober S, Slavin S, Gottlieb I et al: Allograft tolerance after total lymphoid irradiation (TLI). Immunol Rev 46:87, 1979

94. Stuart FP, Bastien E, Holter A et al: Role of passenger leukocytes in the rejection of renal allografts. Transplant Proc 3:461, 1971

95. Stuart FP, Reckard CR, Ketel BL, Schulak JA: Effect of splenectomy on first cadaver kidney transplants. Ann Surg 192:553, 1980

96. Sutherland DER, Fryd DS, So SKS et al: Long-term effect of splenectomy versus no splenectomy in renal transplant patients. Reanalysis of a randomized prospective study. Transplantation 38:619, 1984

97. Taube DH, Cameron JS, Ogg CS et al: Renal transplantation after removal and prevention of resynthesis of HLA antibodies. Lancet 1:824, 1984

98. Tilney, NL, Murray JE: The thoracic duct fistula as an adjunct to immunosuppression in human renal transplantation. Transplantation 5:1204, 1967

99. Vanrenterghem Y, Waer M, Ang K et al: Cadaveric kidney transplantation in diabetics after total lymphoid irradiation (TLI). Transplant Proc 16:636, 1984

100. van Schilfgaarde R, Brom HLF, van Breda Vriesman PJC: Passenger cells in organ transplantation: A review of current concepts. Heart Transplant 2:58, 1982

101. Veith FJ, Luck RJ, Murray JE: The effect of splenectomy on immunosuppressive regimens in dog and man. Surg Gynecol Obstet 121:299, 1965

102. Walker WE, Niblack GD, Richie RE et al: Use of thoracic duct drainage in human renal transplantation. Surg Forum 28:316, 1977

103. Weeke E, Sorensen SF: Extra corporeal irradiation of the blood: Lymphocyte transformation tests and clinical results after renal transplantation. Transplant Proc 3:387, 9171

104. Wolf JS, McGavic JD, Hume DM: Inhibition of the effector mechanism of transplant immunity by local graft irradiation. Surg Gynecol Obstet 128:584, 1969

105. Woodruff, MFA, Anderson NA: Effect of lymphocyte depletion by thoracic duct fistula and administration of antilymphocyte serum on the survival of skin homografts in rats. Nature 200:702, 1963

106. Zincke, H, Woods JE: Attempted immunological alteration of canine renal allograft donors. Transplantation 18:480, 1974

107. Zincke H, Woods JE: Immunological donor pretreatment in combination with pulsatile preservation in cadaveric renal transplantation. Transplantation 26:207, 1978

CHAPTER 8

The Role of Blood Transfusions in Transplantation

Oscar Salvatierra, Jr.

Under conventional immunosuppression, third-party blood transfusions are one of the simplest methods of improving the graft survival in recipients of cadaver kidneys. In the post-cyclosporine immunosuppression era, there has been some controversy regarding the beneficial effect of pretransplant transfusions prior to cadaver transplantation. Despite the improved graft survival rates achieved with cyclosporine therapy, a large collected series and the evaluation of graft survival at our own center have shown a beneficial effect of pretransplant transfusions with post-transplant cyclosporine therapy.

With living-related transplantation, third-party blood transfusions before transplantation appear to confer a beneficial effect in HLA-identical siblings and one haplotype-matched donor recipient pairs with conventional immunosuppression. There are currently few data in regard to a possible transfusion effect in living-related transplantation treated with cyclosporine immunosuppression.

The most impressive results of a definite transfusion effect continue to be seen with the donor-specific blood transfusion (DST) protocol under conventional immunosuppressive therapy. At present, DST appears to be efficacious not only in all 1-haplotype-matched donor–recipient pairs but also in 0-haplotype-matched donor–recipient pairs where DST graft survival is now essentially the same as that achieved with HLA-identical transplants.

The principal problem with the DST protocol has related to donor-specific sensitization. Imuran coverage during DST administration has its maximal effect with a first transplant and with a pre-DST PRA $< 10\%$ (sensitization $\approx 12\%$). DST is most effective before third-party transfusions are administered and the PRA is increased. The highest sensitization rate occurred in patients undergoing a secondary transplant; in this group, Imuran had no influence.

Only 4% of patients who receive DST alone develop more than a 10% increase in T-warm panel cytotoxins from baseline compared with 23% of patients who receive both DST and third-party transfusions ($p = 0.01$).

Probably the most negative aspect of blood transfusions relates to third-party transfusions where the past medical history of the blood donor may not have been ascertained accurately. A significant small percentage of transfused patients are expected to develop hepatitis (mostly non-A, non-B), and some of these patients may eventually develop severe chronic liver disease. The risk of acquired immune deficiency syndrome (AIDS) is another consideration with random third-party blood transfusions, even though current screening tests may rule out infectious units in almost all, but yet not all, instances.

The ultimate objective of organ transplantation is to obtain maximal graft and patient survival. Of all the therapeutic innovations introduced in transplantation, blood transfusions have proved to be one of the simplest and safest methods of improving the outcome of transplant recipients. Most of the experimental work in clinical experience assessing the role of pretransplant blood transfusions in organ transplantation has pertained to the kidney. The role of pretransplant blood transfusions and their influence on the outcome of cardiac and hepatic transplantation have been less clear. The most attractive aspect of transfusion therapy has been that it has improved graft survival without simultaneously suppressing the recipient's immune response to infectious organisms. In this chapter, we review the role of pretransplant blood transfusions in both cadaver and living-related renal transplant patients. The enhancement effect on graft survival in cadaver kidney transplantation will be assessed in regard to the pre-cyclosporine and post-cyclosporine eras of immunosuppression.

At this time, literature on the possible influence of pretransplant blood transfusions on cardiac and liver transplantation is limited. It would be difficult to extrapolate the results achieved with blood transfusions in kidney transplantation to cardiac or liver transplantation because of two primary considerations.[34] First, potential kidney recipients receive their transfusions while they are uremic, which, in itself, confers a degree of depressed immune responsiveness that may affect the ultimate outcome of the transfusion. Second, uremia reduces the undesirable humoral sensitization to histocompatibility antigens. Ferrera and associates[7] demonstrated sizeable humoral responses in 50 of 62 nonuremic volunteers who were challenged with third-party transfusions. This occurrence of detectable cytotoxic antibodies in nonuremic persons is much greater than that seen in uremic dialysis patients.

In 1973, Opelz and co-workers[24] reported that blood transfusions were associated with improved graft survival in cadaver transplantation. Since then, studies from many centers have confirmed the beneficial effects of blood transfusions in cadaver renal transplantation under conventional immunosuppression (pre-cyclosporine use). Currently, in the post-cyclosporine era, controversy appears to focus on whether pretransplant blood transfusions have any influence on ultimate graft survival in cadaver transplantation. Third-party blood transfusions have been used in living-related transplantation, but the most significant influence appears to have resulted in 1978 from the introduction of the donor-specific blood transfusion (DST)protocol, in which blood from the prospective kidney donor is deliberately administered at specified times to the intended recipient prior to transplantation, resulting in a significant increase in graft survival.[30,32]

INFLUENCE OF PRETRANSPLANT BLOOD TRANSFUSIONS ON CADAVER GRAFT SUCCESS

In the late 1960s, renal transplant candidates were freely transfused. However, when it appeared that transfusion-induced sensitization against a random leukocyte panel might lead to a high rate of graft failure, the universal policy of withholding blood from dialysis patients was adopted in the early 1970s. A subsequent comparison of transfused and nontransfused recipients showed, surprisingly, that the best graft survival occurred in patients with previous blood transfusions.[24]

Pre-Cyclosporine Era

Clearly in the pre-cyclosporine era of conventional immunosuppression, various multifactorial analyses, both single-center and with collective data, have shown pretransplant blood transfusions to emerge as the most important factor affecting ultimate cadaver graft survival.

In our own analyses of the graft survival of more than 1000 primary cadaver transplants performed at the University of California, San Francisco (UCSF) center during the pre-cyclosporine period of conventional immunosuppression (1970–1982), pretransplant third-party transfusions did have a significant beneficial effect on graft survival ($p < 0.0001$). However in our study, this effect appeared to be achieved equally well with smaller numbers of transfusions; larger numbers of transfusions appeared to afford no additional benefits (Fig. 8-1).[24] Several other prospective studies confirm these results.[9,44] In contrast, Opelz and Terasaki[23,25,43] reported that in their collected series, patients with more than 20 third-party transfusions had the highest 1-year graft survival rate. However, recipients with only one packed-cell transfusion had a 59% 1-year graft survival rate compared with 41% in the nontransfused group ($p < 0.001$). Although the transfusion effect was dose-related in their series, more than half the maximal observed beneficial effect with more than 20 units (compared with the nontransfused group) was achieved with a single unit of blood.

Post-Cyclosporine Era

In the post-cyclosporine immunosuppression era, there has been some controversy regarding the beneficial effect of pretransplant transfusions prior to cadaver transplantation. Despite the improved graft survival rates achieved with cyclosporine therapy, Opelz,[22] in his analysis of the transfusion effect with cyclosporine treatment in almost 4000 patients, showed an incremental beneficial effect that correlated with the numbers of transfusions received. Again, one unit of blood appeared to achieve half the beneficial effects achieved with a larger number

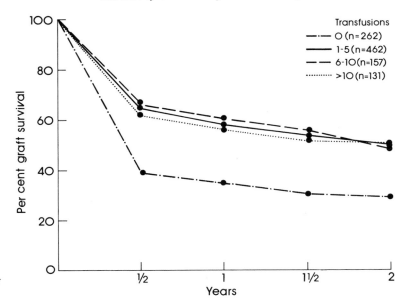

FIGURE 8.1. Influence of pretransplant third-party transfusions on the survival of primary cadaver grafts performed from 1970 through 1982 under conventional immunosuppression.

of units of blood. There was no difference between those patients receiving 2 to 10 units of blood and those receiving more than 10 units of blood. The experience at our center (UCSF) corroborates the findings from Opelz's series. Graft survival in 183 consecutive recipients of primary cadaver kidneys treated with cyclosporine was evaluated with respect to the effect of pretransplant blood transfusions (Table 8-1). Further analysis based on the number of pretransplant blood transfusions demonstrates an incremental favorable trend in various outcome parameters (Table 8-2).

The results of these two series appear somewhat different than those presented at a Cyclosporine Conference in late 1984, when the use of this drug was first assessed after various clinical trials by five centers and a report of the initial national experience following FDA release of the drug. Three of the five reporting institutions with the pre-FDA-released clinical trials had shown no transfusion effect in their series, and no longer routinely pretransfuse their recipients of cadaveric renal grafts.[6,12,14] The other two centers did not study the effects of transfusions but have continued to routinely multiply transfuse their recipients as was the protocol under conventional immunosuppressive therapy.[20,40] Results of the national data in a large collective series show a trend toward a transfusion effect but did not reach statistical significance.[13] Obviously additional studies must be pursued in regard to the transfusion effect in recipients of cadaver grafts.

Complications of Pretransplant Blood Transfusions

Sensitization

The rate of sensitization with pretransplant blood transfusions appears to increase in proportion to the transfusion exposure even though Opelz and Terasaki[25] indicated that the most favorable graft survival in a pre-cyclosporine conventional immunosuppression group was obtained in the group that received more than 20 pretransplant blood transfusions. Most investigators agree that it is the multiply transfused patient who has experienced the greatest sensitization rate. Terasaki[42] found that among cadaver graft recipients who were given more than 20 pretransplant blood transfusions, 54% demonstrated lymphocytotoxic antibodies, and about 26% had an antibody level (PRA) of more than 80%. This study did not include those patients with more than 20 blood transfusions who may not have been transplanted. Other studies have also shown that antibody levels increase progressively with additional transfusions.[5,44]

Hepatitis

Post-transfusion hepatitis remains the most serious complication of blood transfusions. Although fewer than 5% of transfused patients are expected to contract this disease, some of these patients may eventually develop severe chronic liver disease. This is particularly evident at a later date, when the major cause of morbidity and mortality following trans-

TABLE 8-1   The Effect of Transfusions in Patients Treated with Cyclosporine

GRAFT SURVIVAL (%)	1 year	2 year
Cyclosporine without pretransplant blood transfusions (n = 44)	64 + 7	56 + 8
	(p = 0.03)	(p = 0.008)
Cyclosporine with pretransplant blood transfusions (n = 139)	84 + 3	82 + 3

TABLE 8-2   Influence of Number of Pretransplant Blood Transfusions

		0	1–5	6–10	>10
Number of patients		44	102	25	12
% Patients with severe first rejection episode (creatinine greater than 2 mg/dl)		31	27	22	0
% Patients with creatinine normalized post-rejection		85	88	100	100
% Graft survival	1 yr	64 ± 7.9	80 ± 4.2	96 ± 3.9	91 ± 8.3
	2 yr	56 ± 8.8	77 ± 4.7	96 ± 3.9	91 ± 8.3
% Patient survival	1 yr	88 ± 5.1	91 ± 3.0	96 ± 3.9	100 ± 0
	2 yr	84 ± 6.1	89 ± 3.8	96 ± 3.9	100 ± 0
Creatinine, mean	1 yr	3.14 ± 0.95	1.69 ± 0.12	1.61 ± 0.11	1.47 ± 0.03

plantation is hepatic dysfunction. Pirson and associates[27] have understood the long-term consequences of chronic HBs antigenemia in renal transplant recipients. In their series, HBs antigenemia was associated with a high incidence of severe liver disease and impaired patient and graft survival primarily after the third year post-transplantation. However, the major cause of liver disease in patients with renal transplantation may be non-A, non-B hepatitis. It has been suggested that chronic liver disease, presumably caused by non-A or non-B hepatitis virus, is associated with modest morbidity and mortality.[15] These findings emphasize that screening of blood donors for hepatitis B antigen alone does not preclude the subsequent development of hepatic dysfunction and that some caution must be exercised in advocating a large number of pretransplant third-party blood transfusions prior to cadaver transplantation.

Acquired Immune Deficiency Syndrome (AIDS)

The risk of AIDS is another consideration with random third-party blood transfusions. Of 15,948 cases of AIDS reported in the United States as of December 31, 1985, 286 (1.8%) were related to transfusions. Theoretically, recipients of kidney transplants may be at increased risk for AIDS because of frequent blood transfusions and immunosuppression,

and, in addition, kidney transplants can undoubtedly serve as a vehicle of transmission. Because the incidence of AIDS per capita in the region of our center (UCSF) appears to be the highest in the world (147 cases per 100,000 population—47 times that for the rest of the United States, or 1744 total cases, as of December 31, 1985), the risk of AIDS to our recipient population has been critically analyzed. In our series of 2600 transplants, 1500 of which were performed since 1978, there has been only a single case of AIDS that has occurred in our recipient population, despite the fact that most of our recipients have been transfused prior to transplantation. The single case of AIDS occurred in a homosexual male recipient of a cadaver kidney transplant who had received only one blood transfusion 3 years earlier. Neither the donor of this blood transfusion nor the donor of this kidney transplant was believed to have been the source of AIDS. The recipient died of AIDS at approximately 10 months following transplantation, with both Kaposi's sarcoma and *Pneumocystis carinii* pneumonia. The recipient of the other kidney transplant from the same cadaver donor continues to enjoy excellent health and normal renal function at 2 years.

The risk of AIDS and other possibly related conditions in recipients of kidney transplants is probably very small in spite of direct and indirect exposure to numerous blood transfusions, immunosuppression, and the possibility that some transplant donors may have the AIDS virus (although present methods of screening should rule out this occurrence). However in view of the apparently long incubation period for AIDS, it will undoubtedly be years before the validity of this statement can be proved. However, when AIDS does occur in the kidney transplant recipient, the patient's course is likely to be adversely affected by immunosuppression.

LIVING DONOR TRANSPLANTATION

Influence of Third-Party Blood Transfusions

Random third-party transfusions before transplantation also appear to have a beneficial effect prior to transplantation of organs from living-related donors. An analysis of 314 HLA-identical siblings and 585 1-haplotype-matched transplant recipients showed that pretransplant third-party blood transfusions had a significant 10% improvement in 1-year graft survival in each of these living-related categories when compared with nontransfused recipients.[21] Also, graft survival in 1-haplotype living-related pairs is significantly improved after random pretransplant third-party blood transfusions.[2] A more current and similar study evaluating single haplotype living-related recipients also showed enhanced graft survival in this group.[26] All of these studies were conducted with patients under conventional immunosuppressive therapy, and none of these studies enumerated segregated 1-haplotype recipients by mixed lymphocyte culture (MLC).

Most 1-haplotype-related donor–recipient pairs exhibit a high reactive MLC. In our experience, transplantation in this group resulted in a 56% 1-year graft survival rate, but when this group was analyzed according to pretransplant third-party transfusions, there was a 73% 1-year graft survival rate in the group that had received transfusions compared with the lower (56%) graft survival rate in the nontransfused group ($p < 0.002$).[35]

All of the aforementioned studies relate to a transfusion effect with third-party blood transfusions in living-related transplantation prior to the cyclosporine era of immunosuppression. Currently, there are essentially no data in regard to a possible transfusion effect in living-related transplantation treated with cyclosporine immunosuppression.

Donor-Specific Blood Transfusions (DST)

In order to select MLC-incompatible 1-haplotype-related donor–recipient pairs that might achieve

better graft survival, and in an effort to alter the recipient immune response, the DST protocol was introduced at our center in 1978.[28,32] Because donor blood transfusions given to recipients before renal allografting might result in sensitization to the donor and subsequent hyperacute rejection, clinicians had previously been hesitant to use this technique in renal transplantation. With the early good results, the indications for the DST protocol have been expanded, and, in addition, considerations for its use and for its maximal efficacy have been better defined. In 1982, it was decided to pretreat all non-HLA-identical donor–recipient pairs with DST, regardless of the MLC, since the results in the DST-treated MLC-incompatible group were better than those in the non-DST-treated low-reactive MLC group.[33]

In addition, DST pretreatment has included a recent group of 0-haplotype-matched donor–recipient pairs, and the influence of low Imuran coverage during DST administration has been evaluated, as well as the effect of flow cytometry (fluorescence-activated cell sorter [FACS]), in discriminating harmless from harmful positive B-warm crossmatches.[30]

The current DST procedure is essentially the same as that first introduced and involves administration to the recipient of 200 ml of fresh whole donor-specific blood or packed-cell equivalent on three separate occasions at 2-week intervals.[32] Small children receive blood volumes in proportion to their weight. Immunosuppression had not been given during the transfusion process except when a recent group received DSTs under Imuran coverage, in which a maximum of 1 mg/kg Imuran was administered beginning 1 week prior to transfusion. The Imuran dosage is titrated by the white cell count and is scaled down with evidence of leukopenia. Until the time that transplantation is performed, potential recipient sensitization against blood donor lymphocytes is closely monitored by weekly crossmatch testing of recipient sera obtained before, during, and after the blood transfusion period. The time of transplantation has generally been about 4 weeks after the last transfusion, and the criteria for proceeding with transplantation are a negative T-warm and a B-warm donor-specific crossmatch, although it has recently been possible to select out cases with a positive B-warm donor-specific crossmatch where transplantation was possible using flow cytometry.

Patient and graft survival are calculated as consecutive transplants without any exclusions. Immunosuppression has primarily consisted of Imuran, prednisone, and ATGAM or ALG for steroid-resistant rejection. The primary consideration in the use of immunosuppression at this center is in placing a ceiling on the amount of medication administered and a limitation on the number of rejection episodes treated.[31]

Graft and Patient Survival

Graft and patient survival in recipients pretreated with DST prior to transplantation has been essentially the same as that achieved in the concurrent HLA-identical group since the introduction of the DST protocol in 1978. Graft and patient survival rates in patients transplanted from 1978 through 1984 and with a minimum of 5 months follow-up are shown in Table 8-3.[30]

It was initially feared that the DST effect might dissipate with time, but an analysis of graft survival in 174 consecutive nondiabetic DST recipients with a minimum of 5 months follow-up shows that the transfusion effect persists for at least 4 years (Table 8-4).[30] The corresponding graft function in this same group, as determined by mean serum creatinine of functioning grafts through 4 years, is excellent and remains stable.[30]

These results have now been confirmed by a number of reports from other centers.[1,11,16,17,19,38,41,45]

DST With Living 0-Haplotype-Matched Pairs

Since only about one-third of the 200 or more transplants performed yearly at our center have living-related donors with either an HLA-identical match or with DST pretreatment and, with a shortage of donor organs that cannot meet an increasing cadaver waiting list of more than 500 patients, an effort has been undertaken to use the DST protocol in well-informed 0-haplotype-matched donor–recipient pairs. Graft survival in 24 such patients pretreated with DST has been 100% at 18 months. The Wisconsin group[38] also shows similar graft survival in the 0-haplotype-matched group.

Cyclosporine Versus DST

The cyclosporine experience with living-related transplantation at our center is limited. In the 1-haplotype-matched group, the percentage of graft survival in the cyclosporine group (n = 31) was 87 ± 6%, 82 ± 7%, and 76 ± 8% at 6 months, 1 year, and 2 years, respectively.

The question of whether DST or cyclosporine is the best therapy for incompatible donor–recipient pairs is probably settled with regard to 0-haplotype-matched donor–recipient pairs but remains to be established in 1-haplotype-matched living-related donor–recipient pairs. What appears promising is the use of DST in 0-haplotype-matched donor–recipient pairs, which would include not only siblings but also distant relatives and spousal transplants. Our results of DST in this group and the Wisconsin series[38] show graft survival similar to the DST-treated 1-haplotype-matched living-related donor–recipient pairs and HLA-identical siblings. The only

TABLE 8-3   Living-Related Graft and Patient Survival (1978–1984)

GRAFT SURVIVAL (%)	6 months	1 year	2 years	3 years	4 years
DST 0- and 1-Haplotype (n = 221)	97 ± 1	94 ± 2	90 ± 2	85 ± 3	82 ± 4
HLA-identical (n = 186)	92 ± 2	90 ± 2	87 ± 3	85 ± 3	84 ± 3
PATIENT SURVIVAL (%)					
DST 1- and 0-Haplotype (n = 221)	98 ± 1	97 ± 1	95 ± 2	95 ± 2	95 ± 1
HLA-identical (n = 186)	99 ± 1	97 ± 1	95 ± 2	94 ± 2	93 ± 2

TABLE 8-4   Nondiabetic-Related Graft Survival (%) (1978–1984)

	6 months	1 year	2 years	3 years	4 years
DST 1- and 0-Haplotype (n = 174)	98 ± 1	96 ± 1	91 ± 1	88 ± 3	88 ± 3
HLA-identical (n = 143)	91 ± 2	89 ± 3	87 ± 3	85 ± 1	83 ± 4

experience with cyclosporine in a somewhat similarly matched group relates only to cadaver transplants, in which graft survival is lower. If long-term follow-up establishes that there is no significant attrition in graft survival rate in DST-pretreated 0-haplotype-matched pairs, this may clearly be the treatment of choice in this group.

With regard to the 1-haplotype-matched living-related donor–recipient pairs, only a prospective study of DST- and cyclosporine-treated patients with long-term follow-up will establish the optimal regimen. There is, to date, only one significant series with separately defined 1-haplotype-matched living-related donor–recipient pairs treated with cyclosporine as the principal therapy.[8] It is hoped that further extension of our concurrent 1-haplotype cyclosporine-treated group will provide information regarding the most appropriate therapy. Of concern is the possible deleterious effect of cyclosporine on long-term kidney function because of its potential nephrotoxicity. However, it should be noted that cyclosporine immunosuppression following DST pretreatment may possibly eliminate the beneficial effects of DST.[39]

Sensitization After DST

The incidence of donor-specific sensitization and changes in panel cytotoxins following DST were previously evaluated in the initial 172 patients who received blood from their potential kidney donors.[29,33] Seventy percent of the patients who received DST prior to primary transplantation were accepted as potential recipients of a kidney from their blood donor on the basis of an appropriate negative T-warm and B-warm donor-specific crossmatch. The sensitization rate was greater in patients who had already rejected a previous transplant. In essence, if sensitization occurred, the planned transplant was aborted, and a cadaver transplant was later performed in most cases.

Three patterns of donor-specific sensitization have emerged: (1) Approximately one half of the patients who became sensitized to their blood donor had a positive T-warm crossmatch pattern; (2) one fourth of the patients had an initially positive B-warm crossmatch, which later converted to a positive T-warm crossmatch; and (3) another one fourth of the patients had a persistently positive B-warm crossmatch. There was approximately equal distribution in the percentage of patients who developed a positive crossmatch after the first, second, and third DSTs.

It is important to define and differentiate the favorable effects of DST from the capacity to immunize potential kidney recipients. The same weekly sera that were evaluated for specific humoral response to the blood donor by crossmatch testing were also prospectively screened against a panel of 30 potential unrelated donors in the first 131 patients undergoing DST prior to primary transplantation.[29,33] Only 4% of the patients who received DST alone developed more than a 10% increase in T-warm panel cytotoxins from baseline compared with 23% of those patients who received both DST and third-party transfusions ($p = 0.01$). The effect of third-party transfusions was unpredictable. In those who received them, neither the number nor the timing of the transfusions appeared to influence the rate of increased panel sensitization. Only the absence of third-party transfusion was significant. This suggests that when sensitization to DST alone occurs, it is usually specific and narrow, as might be expected from exposure to a limited number of transplantation antigens. However, exposure to a larger variety of foreign histocompatibility antigens, in the form of additional random third-party transfusions, has resulted in a greater degree of panel sensitization in some patients. In the final analysis, however, the DST process itself does not appear to produce an unfavorable degree of panel sensitization that would preclude transplantation from another donor source if necessary.

The observation that some persons exposed to other transfusions in addition to DST are at higher risk of developing increased levels in T-warm panel cytotoxins is further corroborated by the study of Scornik and co-workers,[36] who demonstrated amplification of previous antigenic exposure by the development of broadly reactive cytotoxic antibodies following blood transfusions. It should also be noted that the DST protocol is not the only mechanism for the development of a positive crossmatch between a potential kidney recipient and a potential donor. A group of 16 potential recipients did develop a positive crossmatch to their potential donor immediately prior to the start of the DST protocol at our center (UCSF). All patients had previously demonstrated a negative crossmatch at the time of their initial evaluation, but administration of third-party transfusions in the interval between the negative and the positive crossmatches most likely produced the sensitization.

Influence of Imuran Coverage on DST Sensitization

Even though the donor-specific sensitization rate with DST should not, by itself, make patients non-transplantable, efforts are underway to reduce this sensitization possibility. Anderson and associates[1] and Glass and colleagues[11] have lowered their donor-specific sensitization rate to approximately 10% by using Imuran during DST administration. In our center, Imuran coverage has not produced the overall 10% sensitization rate; however, this is probably the result of the lower Imuran dose, initially 1 mg/kg, with an immediate decrease on manifestation of even mild leukopenia. Our dosage is approximately half the initial dose used by the other two groups, but it has not been accompanied by any infections during the dialysis period when renal failure patients are at high risk.

The influence of Imuran in decreasing donor-specific sensitization in two concurrent groups receiving or not receiving Imuran was evaluated.[30] Table 8-5 shows results from an evaluation of patients for a primary transplant and indicates a trend toward a beneficial effect against sensitization in persons with a PRA less than 10% prior to DST under Imuran coverage.[30] Imuran conferred no protective effect against sensitization in the smaller group of patients in whom the PRA was greater than 10%.

Following a high sensitization rate in a previous report of 15 patients receiving DST prior to second or third grafts,[33] a subsequent experience with 18 patients for second or third transplants resulted in 50% becoming sensitized to the blood donor. Imuran did not reduce the sensitization rate. In the patients being considered for second or third transplants, PRA levels had no influence on the subsequent development of a positive crossmatch. What appeared to be most important was the fact that the patient had a failed first transplant.

Thus, it appears that Imuran has its maximal effect on patients undergoing their first transplant with a pre-DST PRA less than 10%. Fortunately, this is by far the largest group of patients to undergo DST. These results encourage early DST and transplantation in this particular group of patients before

TABLE 8-5 *Primary Living Transplant—DST Pretreatment*

PRA*	Positive	Crossmatch (%)
PRA < 10% (n = 144)		
Imuran	9/74	12
No Imuran	15/70	21
PRA > 10% (n = 22)		
Imuran	7/9	78
No Imuran	4/13	31

* PRA = percentage of reactive antibody against a panel of 40 selected cells.

third-party transfusions are administered and the PRA is increased. The Imuran protocol appears to have an attractive theoretical basis because it interferes with DNA synthesis and may therefore inhibit the development of primary antibody responses in persons without previous allogeneic exposure by preventing the proliferation of antigen-activated lymphocyte clones during the transient, repetitive exposure of blood from the potential kidney donor. Imuran coverage, however, does not appear to confer any beneficial effect on primary transplants with higher pretransplant PRAs and in persons undergoing a second or third transplant. In these cases, blood transfusions (DST or third-party transfusions) seem only to amplify previous response to exposed foreign histocompatibility antigens.

Positive B-warm Crossmatches

The clinical significance of B-warm antibodies in the recipient pretransplant has been uncertain. Pretransplant B-warm antibodies have, in the past, been considered by many not to be harmful, but early and severe rejection in such patients was reported. One fourth of patients with a positive crossmatch following DST pretreatment had B-warm antibodies alone.[29,33] In an attempt to decrease the number of patients that might be excluded from subsequent transplantation because of a positive B-warm crossmatch alone, flow cytometry was used to accurately exclude anti-donor Class I antigen activity in the recipient.[10]

This procedure has provided a means of detecting previously unrecognized anti-T-lymphocyte (Class I antigen) activity in patients with a positive B-warm crossmatch without requiring prior platelet absorption of sera or physical separation of T- and B-lymphocytes.[10] The latter feature was made possible because of the presence of two peaks on FACS histograms. The first was a large low-intensity peak consisting of T-lymphocytes; the second was a smaller high-intensity peak of immunoglobulin-positive B cells. Binding of expressed B-warm antibody to T-lymphocytes was considered indicative of anti-HLA-A, -B, or -C antibodies and was demonstrated by a rightward shift of the T cell peak proportional to the increased number of bound antibody molecules. In those patients with a positive B-warm crossmatch alone, 73% had a subsequent negative FACS crossmatch.[30] Of the FACS-negative crossmatch patients, all but one had a B-warm antibody titer of 1:4 or less; one had a titer of 1:8. In those patients with a B-warm titer of 1:4 or less and a negative FACS crossmatch, only one graft has been lost; the single patient with a 1:8 titer also lost his graft.

DST Summary

For the potential kidney donors in the DST protocol, the process of preliminary blood donation has been harmless and has spared many donors the possibility of donating a kidney that probably would have been rejected at a later time. The blood donor who has been excluded from renal donation because of a positive donor-specific crossmatch has experienced increased self-esteem in attempting to identify a compatible kidney for his family member. For the blood transfusion donor who eventually undergoes an operation, the process of renal donation is being accomplished with excellent prospects of success, and the donor is able to approach the surgical procedure with more confidence and less anxiety. An additional advantage of the donor-specific blood transfusions is that the family history of the blood donor is known, with essentially no risk of hepatitis, AIDS, and so on to the recipient.

In conclusion, (1) DST provides excellent long-term graft survival in 1-haplotype-mismatched pairs; (2) excellent short-term graft survival has also been obtained in a limited 0-haplotype-match experience; (3) Imuran coverage appears to decrease DST sensitization to the blood donor in nonsensitized patients undergoing a first transplant, encouraging early DST and transplantation in this group; (4) flow cytometry has been extremely helpful in excluding subliminal anti-Class I antigen activity in patients with positive B-warm crossmatches; (5) DST, in itself, does not appear to preclude subsequent cadaveric transplantation in patients sensitized to their blood donor; and (6) further assessment of cyclosporine in 1-haplotype-related transplantation is still needed. In these cases, consideration of nephrotoxicity and cost may be major factors in determining the therapy of choice.

As a strategy for preparing a patient with end-stage renal disease for living-related transplantation, choosing an HLA-identical sibling match is ideal. DST pretreatment in this group may provide some benefit that will be determined by a larger experience with greater follow-up, but transfusions of some sort, DST or third-party, appear to enhance graft survival in this group. In the 1-haplotype group, DST with Imuran coverage is probably preferable in nonsensitized or low-sensitized patients being considered for a first transplant. In highly sensitized patients, DST may be used, but probably without Imuran, or cyclosporine may be considered. In patients being evaluated for a second or third transplant, cyclosporine and not DST may possibly be the therapy of choice. If living-related or unrelated transplantation is to be considered with a 0-haplotype match, DST with Imuran coverage appears, at present, to be the only logical consideration.

MECHANISM OF THE TRANSFUSION EFFECT

The beneficial effect of blood transfusions prior to both cadaver and living-related transplantation has been confirmed by many studies, yet the mechanisms of action are not well understood. The immune response in itself is extremely complex with many interrelated interactions; thus, it is not unreasonable to expect that there are probably a number of mechanisms for graft enhancement that need to be better elucidated. Approximately 20% of the patients who receive multiple transfusions before cadaver transplantation are strong responders and become hyperimmunized; thus, they are eliminated by crossmatch testing. In this group of patients, selection is a consideration. There is, however, strong immunologic evidence suggesting that blood transfusions primarily act by inducing enhancement or active immunologic unresponsiveness to donor alloantigens. This appears to be a more attractive mechanism to explain a prominent effect achieved with just one unit of blood where a negligible sensitization rate excludes selection as the predominant mechanism. For example, immunologic unresponsiveness could be induced by and include suppressor T cells or antibodies directed against the T cell antigen-specific receptor, the anti-idiotypic antibodies.[4,37] Further evidence that blood transfusions induce some degree of immunologic unresponsiveness has been provided by improved graft survival rates in the transfused HLA-identical siblings, in whom, by definition, selection cannot be a consideration.

In regard to the DST protocol, initially it was thought that by careful monitoring of the specific humoral response to the blood donor, there appeared to be a segregation of responders from nonresponders, that is, the high responders became sensitized and were not transplanted with that donor. However, recent experience with administering DST under Imuran coverage has resulted in a very low donor-specific sensitization rate without a decrease in graft survival, which seems to exclude selection as a primary mechanism. The excellent graft survival and generally benign post-transplant course achieved by many patients who eventually receive a kidney from their crossmatch negative blood donor requires other explanations. Because immunogenic exposure has involved the repetitive transfusion of donor-specific antigens in a modest dose, it can be theorized that there has been an induction of some degree of specific unresponsiveness to these same antigens on a subsequently transplanted kidney. The DST effect probably involves a complex of various immunologic mechanisms, where, for example, suppressor cells may play an important role,[18] as could anti-idiotypic antibodies.[38]

The data from Burlingham and associates[3] and Terasaki[42] favor an idiotypic network model and clonal deletion as the primary mechanisms responsible for the DST effect and where T cell priming by DST exposure is a central feature of both mechanisms. The correlation of plasma-enhancing factors as shown by Burlingham and associates[3] with early DST-type rejection episodes could be consistent with an idiotypic network model for the control of initiation of a rejection response. The reversal of these early rejections by immunosuppressive therapy may, in turn, also result in deletion of responding alloreactive clones. Thus, a combination of the clonal deletion and idiotypic network mechanisms, as well as the induction of suppressor cells, may be involved in the DST effect.

Of great interest are the mice skin allograft experiments of Okazaki and colleagues.[21] If these animal experimental results transcend species differences, they may theoretically indicate that the DST effect may be of greatest benefit in donor–recipient pairs with the greatest disparity. Their experiments showed that graft prolongation was superior with nonspecific blood in donor–recipient pairs with weak histocompatibility differences, but that in strong histocompatible combinations, graft prolongation was associated only with transfusion of donor–specific blood. The latter results may explain the excellent clinical results obtained in a growing 0-haplotype- match experience.

CONCLUSION

Pretransplant blood transfusions appear to have a definite role in improving the graft survival of both cadaver and living-related organs in kidney transplantation. In cadaver transplantation, there appears to be evidence of a salutory effect, even in the current cyclosporine immunosuppression era. The DST protocol has allowed the use of living donors with excellent results—results similar to those achieved with HLA-identical sibling transplantation. Although the role of blood transfusions prior to other organ transplantation is not clear at this time, certain major differences between the kidney and other organ allograft recipients would caution against the expectation of a precisely similar result in extrarenal transplantation. Only after further studies have increased our understanding of the mechanism of action of blood transfusions can we develop an even better and optimal transfusion protocol for both cadaver and living-related renal transplant patients. This might possibly also include the consideration of the use of transfusions in some way in extrarenal organ transplantation.

REFERENCES

1. Anderson CB, Tyler JD, Sicard GA et al: Pretreatment of renal allograft recipients with immunosuppression and donor-specific blood. Transplantation 38:664, 1884
2. Brynger H, Frisk B, Ahlmen J et al: Graft survival and blood transfusions. In Robinson BHB (ed): Proceedings of the XIVth Congress of the European Dialysis and Transplant Association. Kent, England, Pitman Medical Publishing Co., Ltd., 14:290–295, 1977
3. Burlingham WJ, Grailer A, Sparks–Mackety EMF et al: Improved renal allograft survival following donor-specific transfusions; in vitro correlates of early (DST-type) rejection episodes. Transplantation 43:41–46, 1987
4. Fagnilli L, Singal DP: Blood transfusions may induce anti-T cell receptor antibodies in renal patients. Transplant Proc 14:319–321, 1982
5. Fehrman I Groth c-G, Lundgren G et al: Improved renal graft survival in transfused uremics. Transplantation 30:324–327, 1980
6. Ferguson RM, Sommer BG: Cyclosporine in renal transplantation: A single institution experience. Am J Kidney Dis 5:296–306, 1985
7. Ferrera GB et al: HLA unresponsiveness induced by weekly transfusions of small aliquots of whole blood. Transplantation 17:194–200, 1974
8. Flechner SM, Kerman RH, Van Buren CT et al: The use of cyclosporine in living-related renal transplantation. Transplantation 38:685, 1984
9. Frisk B, Brynger H, Sandberg L: Two random transfusions before primary renal transplantation—four years' experience from a single center. Transplant Proc 14:386–388, 1982
10. Garovoy M, Colombe BW, Melzer J et al: Flow cytometry crossmatching for donor-specific transfusion recipients and cadaveric transplantation. Transplant Proc 17:693, 1985
11. Glass NR, Miller DT, Sollinger HW Belzer FO: Comparative analysis of the DST and Imuran-plus-DST protocol for live donor renal transplantation. Transplantation 36:636, 1983
12. Gordon RD, Iwatsukii S, Shaw BW et al: Cyclospor-

ine–steroid combination therapy in 84 cadaveric renal transplants. Am J Kidney Dis 5:307–312, 1985

13. Hunsicker LG: Impact of cyclosporine on cadaveric renal transplantation: A summary statement. Am J Kidney Dis 5:335–341, 1985

14. Kahan BD, Kerman RH, Wideman CA et al: Impact of cyclosporine on renal transplant practice at the University of Texas Medical School at Houston. Am J Kidney Dis 5:288–295, 1985

15. LaQuaglia MP et al: Impact of hepatitis on renal transplantation. Transplantation 32:504–507, 1981

16. Leivestad T, Flatmark A, Hirschberg H, Thorsby E: Effect of pretransplant donor-specific transfusions in renal transplantation. Transplant Proc 14:370, 1982

17. Light JA, Metz SJ, Oddenino K: Donor-specific transfusion with minimal sensitization. Transplant Proc 15:917, 1983

18. Maki T, Okazaki H, Wood MA et al: Induction of suppressor cells by donor-specific blood transfusions in mice with skin allografts. Surg Forum 32:396, 1981

19. Mendez R, Iwaki Y, Mendez RG et al: Antibody response and allograft outcome with deliberate donor-specific blood transfusions. Transplant Proc 14:378, 1982

20. Milford EL, Kirkman RL, Tilney NL et al: The clinical experience with cyclosporine and azathioprine at Brigham and Women's Hospital. Am J Kidney Dis 5:313–317, 1985

21. Okazaki H, Maki T, Wood ML: Effect of blood transfusions on skin allograft survival in immunosuppressed mice. Transplant Proc 13:515–517, 1981

22. Opelz G: Effect of HLA matching, blood transfusions, and presensitization in cyclosporine-treated kidney transplant recipients. Transplant Proc 17(6):2179–2183, 1985

23. Opelz G, Mickey MR, Terasaki PI: Blood transfusions and kidney transplants: Remaining controversies. Transplant Proc 13:136–141, 1981

24. Opelz G, Sengar DPS, Mickey MR et al: Effect of blood transfusions on subsequent kidney transplants. Transplant Proc 5:253–259, 1973

25. Opelz G, Terasaki PI: Dominant effect of transfusions on kidney graft survival. Transplantation 29:153–158, 1980

26. Pfaff WW, Fennell RS, Howard RJ et al: Planned random donor blood transfusion in preparation for transplantation. Transplantation 38:701–703, 1984

27. Pirson Y, Alexandre GP, van Ypersele de Strihou C: Long-term effect of HBs antigenemia on patient survival after renal transplantation. N Engl J Med 296:194–196, 1977

28. Salvatierra O, Amend WJC, Vincenti F et al: Pretreatment with donor-specific blood transfusions in related recipients with high MLC. Transplant Proc 13:142, 1981

29. Salvatierra O, Iwaki Y, Vincenti F et al: Incidence, characteristics, and outcome of recipients sensitized after donor-specific blood transfusions. Transplantation 32:528, 1981

30. Salvatierra O, Melzer J, Potter D et al: A seven-year experience with donor-specific blood transfusions: Results and considerations for maximum efficacy. Transplantation 40:654–659, 1985

31. Salvatierra O, Potter D, Cochrum KC et al: Improved patient survival in renal transplantation. Surgery 79:166, 1985

32. Salvatierra O, Vincenti F, Amend WJC et al: Deliberate donor-specific blood transfusions prior to living related transplantation—a new approach. Ann Surg 192:543, 1980

33. Salvatierra O, Vincenti F, Amend WJC et al: Four-year experience with donor-specific blood transfusions. Transplant Proc 15:924, 1983

34. Salvatierra O, Vincenti F, Amend WJC et al: The enhancement of graft survival with pretransplant blood transfusions. Heart Transplant 2:181–187, 1983

35. Salvatierra O, Vincenti F, Amend WJC et al: What about blood transfusions in living related transplantation? Abstracts of the American Society of Nephrology Twelfth Annual Meeting, pg 178A. Boston, 1979

36. Scornik JC, Ireland JE, Howard RJ, Pfaff WW: Assessment of the risk for broad sensitization by blood transfusions. Transplantation 37:249–253, 1984

37. Singal DP, Joseph S, Szewczuk MR: Possible mechanism of the beneficial effect of pretransplant blood transfusions on renal allograft survival in man. Transplant Proc 14:316–318, 1982

38. Sollinger HW, Burlingham WJ, Sparks EMF et al: Donor-specific transfusions in unrelated and related HLA-mismatched donor-recipient combinations. Transplantation 38:612, 1984

39. Sommer BG, Ferguson RM: Mismatched living-related donor renal transplantation: A prospective, randomized study. Surgery 98(2):267–274, 1985

40. Sutherland DER, Fryd DS, Strand MH et al: Results of the Minnesota randomized prospective trial of cyclosporine versus azathioprine–antilymphocyte globulin for immunosuppression in renal transplant recipients. Am J Kidney Dis 5:318–327, 1985

41. Takahashi I, Otsubo O, Nishimura M et al: Prolonged graft survival by donor-specific blood transfusion (DSBT). Transplant Proc 14:367, 1982

42. Terasaki PI: The beneficial transfusion effect on kidney graft survival attributed to clonal deletion. Transplantation 37:119, 1984

43. Terasaki PI, Perdue S, Ayoub G et al: Reduction of accelerated failures by transfusion. Transplant Proc 14:251–259, 1982

44. Werner–Favre C, Jeannet M, Harder F et al: Blood transfusions, cytotoxic antibodies, and kidney graft survival. Transplantation 28:343–346, 1979

45. Whelchel JD, Curtis JJ, Barger BO et al: The effect of pretransplant stored donor-specific blood transfusion on renal allograft survival in one-haplotype living-related transplant recipients. Transplantation 38:654, 1984

CHAPTER 9

Molecular, Genetic, and Clinical Aspects of the HLA System

William E. Braun

The human lymphocyte antigen (HLA) system consists of the glycoprotein gene products of loci in the major histocompatibility complex (MHC) located on the short arm of the 6th chromosome. Along with the ABO red blood cell system, it constitutes the major transplantation antigen system in humans.

There are several ways of designating the HLA antigens, including Class I versus Class II, serologic versus cellular, public versus private specificities, definition of allogenotypes through the digestion of DNA by restriction endonucleases, and identification of a new population of interlocus epitopes by means of monoclonal antibodies. The most commonly used classification of HLA antigens, Class I and Class II, is based on a number of distinctive features.

Whereas Class I antigens are found on essentially all nucleated cells as well as in soluble form in the serum, saliva, seminal fluid, urine, and breast milk, Class II antigens have a relatively restricted expression on B-lymphocytes, monocytes, some macrophages, epidermal Langerhans' cells, dendritic cells, activated T-lymphocytes in both normal and disease states, epithelium of a variety of organs, including the gastrointestinal tract and urinary bladder, bone marrow precursor cells, certain neoplasms, as well as capillary and glomerular vascular endothelium. However, Class II antigens are absent from platelets, unstimulated T cells, and other somatic cells.

HLA antigen expression is decreased by a number of substances, including chloramphenicol, glucocorticoids, cyclosporine, prostaglandin E, ultraviolet light and immune complexes. Other stimuli have been shown to induce or increase the expression of HLA antigens on the cell surface. These include nitrogens, activated T cells, allograft rejection, microbial antigens, autoimmune states, and interferons. Class II antigens vary in their expression on developing cell lines and therefore can be considered as differentiation antigens. Class II antigens in the kidney do not normally appear on either the proximal or distal tubular epithelial cells except when an immunologic stimulus such as rejection or local graft-versus-host reaction has taken place.

There are approximately 20 to 30 Class I genes in humans, including many pseudogenes. The loci for these genes are only partly in the established HLA-A, -B, and -C subregions; the majority exist in sites telomeric to the HLA-A locus.

Class II antigens are products of loci in the D region and its three subregions, DR, DQ, and DP. Within the subregions, there are genes for at least seven β and six α chains.

The HLA antigen system in humans has not been easily stratified into a hierarchy of strong and weak histocompatibility antigens. Evidence from two widely divergent sources, oligonucleotide mapping and cadaver renal transplant success, raise the possibility that the two broad serologic entities DRw52 (MT2) and DRw53 (MT3) may have a very significant influence on allograft survival.

The mixed lymphocyte culture (MLC) has been used in renal transplantation to (1) confirm serologically HLA-identical pairs, (2) detect possible recombinants in the D region, (3) discriminate further degrees of incompatibility prior to transplant between living-related and cadaver donor–recipient pairs (e.g., low responders and high responders), (4) prognosticate concerning steroid withdrawal, (5) assess the level of immune responsiveness following transplantation and determine whether it is donor- specific or nonspecific and whether it is modified by suppressor cells or by anti-idiotypic antibody.

Haplotype matching for living-related transplants has shown that the best near-term and long-term survivals can be achieved when both haplotypes are matched, an event expected in 25% of siblings but occasionally found between parent and child. Still, some of these HLA-identical transplants have been lost because of delayed hyperacute rejections that may be based upon the presence of vascular endothelial cell antibodies. But they have also failed because of technical problems, infection, recurrent disease, and incompatibility of certain minor antigen systems such as H-Y.

Patient survival 5 years following a first cadaver renal transplant has shown improvement based upon better HLA matches in at least two major studies.

The effect of HLA matching on short-term (1–2 yr) cadaver allograft survival has received strong support from several multicenter studies, two of which reported a significant matching effect even with cyclosporine. However, in two other multicenter studies no matching effect was found when cyclosporine was used. Some single-center studies have shown a beneficial effect on cadaver allograft survival initially with HLA-A and -B matching, and later for DR.

Since 1980, at least eight large studies have shown that the major effect of HLA matching is on long-term cadaver allograft outcome.

For patients who are to receive a repeat transplant, particularly a cadaver transplant, and whose first allograft was lost in less than 6 months, the degree of HLA matching was of major importance for the success of the second graft.

Re-exposure to the same mismatched antigen has been reported to have both no effect and an adverse effect on the outcome of the second graft. These apparently conflicting findings may be explained by differences in the causes of failure and the duration of the first graft, as well as by the presence or absence of a positive B lymphocyte crossmatch, and the interval to the second graft.

The proposition that DRw6 in a transplant recipient identified that person as a "high responder," one more likely to make antiendothelial antibodies and to have a worse cadaver allograft outcome, remains controversial.

The multifactorial "center" effect has had a significant influence on cadaver renal allograft success.

The human lymphocyte antigen (HLA) system consists of the glycoprotein gene products (antigens) of loci in the major histocompatibility complex (MHC) located on the short arm of the 6th chromosome. Its evolution over the past 33 years was triggered by the crucial description of leukocyte antibodies by Jean Dausset in 1952.[45] His work in humans and that of George Snell and Baruj Benacerraf[17] in the murine histocompatibility systems merited them the Nobel Prize in medicine in 1980. Since that time, which seemed as though it could be the ultimate point in histocompatibility, a new wave of molecular biology has sent HLA soaring. Consequently, the dramatic progress in understanding the human MHC that has already been documented in a series of nine international workshops will expand further in the molecular biology and structure of HLA in the next international workshop in 1987.

The introduction of HLA in the field of clinical transplantation began in the 1960s when the era of identical twin transplants that had begun in 1954 began to experience a natural decline. Methods other than extensive red blood cell testing, intradermal lymphocyte transfer tests, and reciprocal or third-party skin grafts were needed in order to identify compatible non-twin living-related as well as unrelated cadaver donors. Complement-dependent cytotoxicity (CDC) techniques using well-defined parous female sera as typing reagents rapidly became the standard approach for serologic testing throughout the world.[112] Similarly, mixed lymphocyte cultures (MLC), both bidirectional and unidirectional, became the standard method for determining cellularly defined compatibility in living-related transplants.[36,76] Subsequently, a wide variety of other methodologies and scientific advances enhanced the assessment of histocompatibility, including cellular typing using homozygous typing cells (HTC)[48]; cell-mediated lympholysis (CML)[63]; primed lymphocyte testing (PLT)[168]; tissue-specific antigen systems such as those on epidermal, endothelial, dendritic, renal tubular, and glomerular cells; serum antibody analyses by computer; hybridoma production of monoclonal antibodies[23]; T cell cloning[55a]; flow cytometry analysis for antibody detection[59]; immunochemical isolation, purification, and analysis of HLA antigens[93,104]; DNA clones[135]; radiation-induced HLA mutant cell lines[88]; restriction fragment length polymorphisms (RFLP) and specific α and β chain probes[37]; and studies with labeled oligonucleotides.[106]

Notwithstanding the technologic advances, the crux of clinical matching for renal allografting remains serologic typing for Class I HLA-A and -B and Class II HLA-DR antigens. Data from large continuing collaborative studies are providing new insight into the interaction of histocompatibility matching with other transplant factors, particularly blood transfusions and cyclosporine.[51,54,122,148,179,182]

HLA NOMENCLATURE

Following the 1984 International HLA Workshop, the new nomenclature for the HLA system was published (Table 9-1). The HLA system consists of seven series of antigens (HLA-A, -B, -Cw, -DR, -DQ, -DP, and -Dw).[118] Except for the Dw series, which is more diffusely represented by a "region," each antigen series has a mapped or proposed "subregion" on the short arm of the 6th chromosome with loci for its component chains (Fig. 9-1). These loci as well as those for the complement components (C2, C4, and Bf) reside in an area on the 6th chromosome known as the MHC. At least three subregions (DR, DQ, and DP) contribute to the definition of Dw by mixed lymphocyte culture using HTCs.[109,158] The DR subregion, which includes two former broad MT specificities, DRw52 and -53, was named that because it was "D-related," whereas DQ was previously called "DS," "DC," and "MB," and DP was known as "SB" for "secondary B" locus.

Each antigen is designated by the prefix HLA followed by the locus, and then by an Arabic number for the antigen specificity, for example, HLA-A28, HLA-B7, and HLA-DR3. If an antigen has not been officially accepted by the World Health Organization Nomenclature Committee or must be distinguished from other nomenclature systems, as in the case of the Cw specificities to avoid confusion with complement components,[118] a "w" for "workshop" is inserted between the letter of the locus and the antigen number, for example, HLA-Cw1 and HLA-DRw8. As the genes for the Class II antigens are defined, their nomenclature will eventually in-

clude a designation of the α and β genes involved. Unfortunately, ambiguities may arise because a term such as "HLA-A" can be used in referring to a subregion, locus, and antigen. Several other useful ways of designating HLA antigens are described in the following sections.

Class I Versus Class II

This classification of the HLA antigens is based on their biochemical and functional differences. The Class I antigens include HLA-A, -B, and -Cw, whereas Class II antigens include HLA-DR, -DQ, -DP, and -Dw. Although more detailed descriptions are given elsewhere in this chapter regarding the features of Class I and Class II antigens, in brief, the Class I antigens:

1. Consist of a heavy chain of 44,000 daltons noncovalently bound to β_2-microglobulin of 11,700 daltons.
2. Have a broad distribution on virtually all the nucleated cells of the body.
3. Activate and act as targets of cytotoxic T-lymphocytes.
4. Provide restriction elements for (i.e., their proximity is necessary for the recognition of) minor histocompatibility antigens such as H-Y, most viral antigens, and haptens.
5. Can function by themselves as alloantigens or in a restricted fashion with Class II antigens.
6. Effectively stimulate an antibody response.
7. Function reliably in cell-mediated lympholysis.
8. Contribute little to mixed lymphocyte culture or graft-versus-host reactions.
9. Have certain strong disease associations, such as A3 and hemochromatosis or B27 and ankylosing spondylitis.
10. Are analogous to the H2D and H2K gene products of the mouse.

In contrast, Class II antigens:

1. Consist of a 34,000 dalton α chain noncovalently bound to a 29,000 dalton β chain.
2. Are distributed on a restricted number of cell types in the body such as B-lymphocytes and antigen presenting cells.
3. Activate T helper lymphocytes.
4. Provide restriction elements for alloantigens and certain viruses such as measles and herpes simplex I.
5. Can function by themselves as alloantigens.
6. Can evoke an antibody response.
7. Are the primary stimulators in the mixed lymphocyte culture and graft-versus-host reaction.

TABLE 9-1   Complete Listing of Recognized HLA Specificities

A	B	C	D	DR	DQ	DP
A1	B5	Cw1	Dw1	DR1	DQw1	DPw1
A2	B7	Cw2	Dw2	DR2	DQw2	DPw2
A3	B8	Cw3	Dw3	DR3	DQw3	DPw3
A9	B12	Cw4	Dw4	DR4		DPw4
A10	B13	Cw5	Dw5	DR5		DPw5
A11	B14	Cw6	Dw6	DRw6		DPw6
Aw19	B15	Cw7	Dw7	DR7		
A23(9)	B16	Cw8	Dw8	DRw8		
A24(9)	B17		Dw9	DRw9		
A25(10)	B18		Dw10	DRw10		
A26(10)	B21		Dw11(w7)	DRw11(5)		
A28	Bw22		Dw12	DRw12(5)		
A29(w19)	B27		Dw13	DRw13(w6)		
A30(w19)	B35		Dw14	DRw14(w6)		
A31(w19)	B37		Dw15			
A32(w19)	B38(16)		Dw16	DRw52		
Aw33(w19)	B39(16)		Dw17(w7)	DRw53		
Aw34(10)	B40		Dw18(w6)			
Aw36	Bw41		Dw19(w6)			
Aw43	Bw42					
Aw66(10)	B44(12)					
Aw68(28)	B45(12)					
Aw69(28)	Bw46					
	Bw47					
	Bw48					
	Bw49(21)					
	Bw50(21)					
	B51(5)					
	Bw52(5)					
	Bw53					
	Bw54(w22)					
	Bw55(w22)					
	Bw56(w22)					
	Bw57(17)					
	Bw58(17)					
	Bw59					
	Bw60(40)					
	Bw61(40)					
	Bw62(15)					
	Bw63(15)					
	Bw64(14)					
	Bw65(14)					
	Bw67					
	Bw70					
	Bw71(w70)					
	Bw72(w70)					
	Bw73					
	Bw4					
	Bw6					

PUBLIC SPECIFICITIES

Bw4: B5, B13, B17, B27, B37, B38(16). B44(12), Bw47, B49(21), B51(5), Bw52(5), Bw53, Bw57(17), Bw58(17), Bw59, Bw63(15).

Bw6: B7, B8, B14, B18, Bw22, B35, B39(16), B40, Bw41, Bw42, B45(12), Bw46, Bw48, Bw50(21), Bw54(w22), Bw55(w22), Bw56(w22), Bw60(40), Bw61(40), Bw62(15), Bw64(14), Bw65(14), Bw67, Bw70, Bw71(w70), Bw72(w70), Bw73.

DRw52: DR3, DR5, DRw6, DRw8, DRw11(5), DRw12(5), DRw13(w6), DRw14(w6)

DRw53: DR4, DR7, DRw9.

8. Contribute little to cell-mediated lympholysis.
9. Have certain disease associations, such as DR4 and rheumatoid arthritis or DR3 and DR4 with insulin-dependent diabetes mellitus.
10. Are analogous to the immune response gene products of the I region in the mouse, particularly DQ with I–A and DR with I–E.

Serologically vs. Cellularly Defined Antigens

The HLA-A, -B, -Cw, -DR, -DQ, and some -DP antigens are serologically defined by sera derived from parous females, allograft recipients, and transfused persons, as well as by some monoclonal antibodies. In the A series of antigens, a new specific-

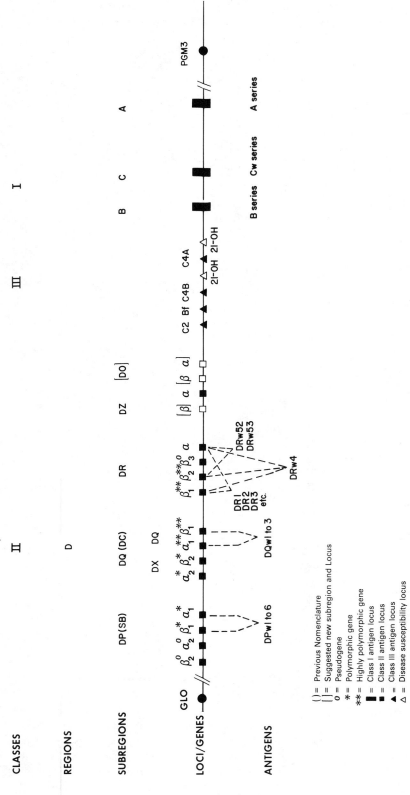

FIGURE 9-1. *Molecular, genetic, and clinical aspects of the HLA system.*

ity, Aw69, a split of A28, is the first example of an officially recognized specificity identified primarily by a monoclonal antibody. The DP specificities, now numbering six, were initially identified by secondary MLCs using PLTs, but now a monoclonal antibody has been produced that corresponds to some PLT-determined specificities[166] (see section entitled Primed Lymphocyte Testing).

The Dw antigens are cellularly defined by HTCs. Since the 1980 International HLA Workshop, the number of HLA-Dw determinants has risen officially from 12 to 19, with 3 more proposed. However, the gene frequency of the Dw blank still remains in the range of 33%. The gene frequencies of the individual HLA-Dw determinants vary among different ethnic groups, paralleling what occurs with serologically defined HLA antigens.[66] The HLA-Dw specificities are not exclusively associated with any one of the three D subregions (DR, DQ, DP), although they most closely resemble HLA-DR.[55a,158] In some cases, Dw antigens correspond very closely to the DR specificities determined by alloantibody (e.g., Dw1 with DR1), and in other cases (e.g., Dw18 and Dw19 with DRw13), they do not. The Dw-DR-DQ equivalencies become more complex because different Dw specificities, such as Dw2 and Dw12, can express the same DR and DQ antigens, DR2 and DQw1, respectively. Finally, some Dw specificities, such as Dw4 and Dw6, have their subspecificities ("splits") defined by monoclonal antibodies that have no apparent relationship to DR, DQ, or DP.

In any event, because DR, DQ, and DP molecules are all stimulatory to varying degrees in the primary MLC, in order for two persons to be Dw compatible they will probably have to be identical with one another not only for HLA-DR but also for -DQ, -DP and possibly other molecules as well.[55a,109,158]

Public vs. Private Specificities

Private specificities are all of the individual antigens shown in Table 9-1 except Bw4 and Bw6, and DRw52 and DRw53. Public antigens were constructed initially on the basis of cross-reacting groups (CREGS) exemplified by such cross-reacting antibodies as those to HLA-1, -3, and -11.[38] Sequential immunoprecipitation studies later showed that a public antigen called "X" was common to the heavy chain of the B7-CREG comprised of HLA-B7, -22, -27, -40, and -42.[162] Similarly, the B5-CREG consisting of HLA-B5, -15, -18 and -35 was found to have a common determinant called "Y."[161] The public determinants can function as target antigens in cell-mediated cytotoxicity. The clinical relevance

of such CREGS or public specificities has been shown in recent studies of renal allografts in which matching for the better defined HLA-A and HLA-B CREGS continued to yield a significant correlation with allograft success and simplify prospective donor–recipient matching.[54,149] (See Clinical Studies of HLA Matching in Renal Allografting.)

Another type of public specificity consists of Bw4 and Bw6, which relate exclusively to groups of B series antigens (see Table 9-1). In fact, the B series antigens and, most importantly, difficult subspecificities ("splits") of these antigens can be partitioned by the Bw4/Bw6 distinction.[118] For example, the B38 split of B16 is associated with Bw4, whereas the B39 split of B16 is associated with Bw6. An additional practical use of the Bw specificities can be appreciated when just a single B locus antigen has been identified and the presence of Bw4 or Bw6 indicates that still another B locus antigen is present, although yet undetected.

Similarly, DRw52 and DRw53, formerly called MT2 and MT3, respectively, are associated with certain groups of DR antigens: DR3, DR5, DRw6, and DRw8 with DRw52, and DR4, DR7, and DRw9 with DRw53 (see Table 9-1).[118] These specificities are believed to be a distinct subset of DR-like antigens comprised of polypeptides coded by the DR_α and $DR2_\beta$ genes of the DR subregion (see Fig. 9-1).[39] Matching for DRw52 and -53 has recently been reported to have a significant benefit on the outcome of cadaver allografts.[54]

Allogenotopes

Cleavage of a person's DNA by a variety of endonucleases results in different patterns of DNA fragments, called restriction fragment length polymorphisms (RFLPs), detected with the Southern blotting technique.[173] A fragment produced in such a system, described by its size in kilobases, by the enzyme used to produce it, and by the probe used to identify it is called an *allogenotope*.[37] Further details of this methodology are presented in the section entitled Molecular Genetics.

Interlocus

Antibody molecules have been thought to be exclusively reactive with just one series of antigens or another. The basis for this was the mistaken belief that there were no epitopes (specific amino acid sequences) common to antigens of different HLA loci. However, monoclonal antibodies have shown definitively that shared or interlocus epitopes are present on antigens of two different loci, such as

HLA-A and -B.[140] The initial reports involved antibodies reacting with HLA-A and Bw4 or Bw6 specificities, but in 1982, an antigenic determinant was found that was shared by HLA-A2 and B17.[35] Since monoclonal antibodies are epitope specific, the dual reactions of such monoclonal antibodies have solidly established the commonality of epitopes between A2 and B17; A32 and B27; Aw19, B40, and Bw41; Aw33 and B8; A9 and Bw4; and A2 and B16.[140]

DISTRIBUTION AND EXPRESSION OF HLA ANTIGENS

Class I and Class II antigens have different tissue distribution and expression. Class I antigens are found on essentially all nucleated cells, on reticulocytes, in very low density on mature erythrocytes, and probably on trophoblasts and sperm.[24,47,52,75,103,165] At a time when the HLA antigens were not specified as to class, early studies demonstrated that they occurred with decreasing density on spleen, lung, liver, intestine, kidney, heart, aorta, fat, and brain.[19] Class I antigens could also be detected in soluble form in serum, saliva, seminal fluid, urine, and breast milk.[4,85,191]

In contrast, the Class II antigens have a relatively restricted expression on B-lymphocytes, monocytes, some macrophages,[71,194] epidermal Langerhans' cells,[177] dendritic cells,[175] activated T-lymphocytes in both normal and disease states,[195] epithelium of the gastrointestinal tract and urinary bladder, bronchial glands, thymic reticuloendothelial cells, epithelium of the mammary gland, parotid acinar cells, astrocytes, alveolar macrophages, Kupffer's cells, endometrium,[116] bone marrow precursor cells,[102,138] certain neoplasms (some melanomas, lymphoid malignancy, and colonic carcinomas),[40,80,137,156] and capillary and glomerular vascular endothelium,[58,163] but they are absent from platelets, unstimulated T cells and other somatic cells.[4,71,102,194]

Various substances can alter HLA antigens or their H-2 murine counterparts, one group decreasing their expression or depressing their induction or metabolically active state,* and the other inducing or increasing their expression† (Table 9-2). Chloramphenicol decreases the expression at least of Class I antigens on cell surface membranes.[16] Glucocorticoids do not influence the expression of Class I antigens (HLA-A, -B, Cw) or β_2-microglobulin, but do decrease the expression of Class II antigens.[108] Of further interest is the fact that in vitro treatment of peripheral blood lymphocytes with dexamethasone does not alter the expression of DR, so that the decrease in DR expression is apparently an indirect effect occurring exclusively in vivo.[108] Cyclosporine inhibits the induction of both Class I and Class II antigens.[6,98] Prostaglandins of the E series in physiologic doses inhibit the expression of Class II antigens on mature macrophages in mice, an effect probably mediated by cyclic AMP (analogs of which also inhibit Class II antigen expression) and one antagonized by thromboxane B_2 and indomethacin.[170] There appears to be, at least in certain tumors, a reciprocal expression between Class I or Class II histocompatibility antigens and presumed tumor antigens. A reciprocal relationship was described between the H2 and TL antigen in the mouse,[120] as well as between Class I antigens and sarcoma cells[164] and the presence of a lymphoma.[21] In rat baby kidney cells, the oncogenicity of cells transformed by adenovirus 12 is specifically correlated with the absence of the heavy chain of the rat Class I antigens. The oncogenicity develops because

---

* References 6,16,21,97,98,108,120,157,164,170,192
† References 10,13,18,33,69,70,72,77,91,133,134,143,150, 155,189

TABLE 9-2　*Factors Modifying the Expression of Histocompatibility Antigens*

Decreased By	Increased By
Chloramphenicol (16)	Interferons (13,80,134)
Glucocorticoids (108)	Activated T-lymphocytes (134)
Cyclosporine (6,98)	Mitogens (33,133)
Prostaglandin E (170)	Prolactin (97)
Ultraviolet light (97)	Allograft rejection (18,69,70,77)
Immune complexes (192)	Graft-vs.-host reaction (10,70)
Certain neoplasms (21,80,120,157,164)	Microbial antigens (155)
	Autoimmune states (72)
	Genetic control (143)
	G2 phase of cell cycle (150)

intact Class I antigens are not present to focus Class I-restricted cytotoxic lymphocytes (CTLs) on the adjacent viral antigen and thereby lead to rejection of the tumor in vivo.[157]

The factors that increase the expression of HLA antigens can have a differential effect on Class I versus Class II antigens, and, even among the Class II antigens, a discordancy may occur among DR, DQ, and DP. For example, all three classes of interferon enhance expression of Class I antigens on lymphocytes, but only gamma interferon increases the synthesis and expression of DR antigens and β_2-microglobulin.[13] Although γ-interferon usually induces DR, DP, and DQ, some Class II gene products, such as DX_α and DZ_α, are not induced.[93] Discordancy has also been described in neoplasms in which Class II antigen expression has been neatly classified as constitutive (as in certain melanomas), γ-interferon inducible (as in carcinoma of the breast, colon, pancreas, bladder, kidney, ovary and brain, other melanoma lines, as well as fibroblasts, kidney epithelia, and epidermal keratinocytes), and γ-interferon noninducible (as in teratocarcinoma, choriocarcinoma, neuroblastoma, and a few other melanoma cell lines).[80] Although γ-interferon fails to induce Class II antigens on the latter three neoplasms, Class I antigens are induced.[80] When T-lymphocytes are activated in MLC, by phytohemagglutinin or concanavalin A, the majority of cells express DR but not DQ and DP.[33,133,134] Vascular endothelial cells, when tested in MLC, do not express Class II antigens at the outset but show it by 30 minutes and express it on about one-third of the cells at 24 hours.[133] Under hormonal influence, epithelium of the lactating, but not the resting, mammary gland in guinea pigs expresses Class II antigen.[91]

At a more basic level, the normal regulation of Class II antigen expression appears to be controlled by two genes located outside the MHC.[143] There is also a cell cycle–dependent expression of HLA-DR antigens in that their expression is lowest in the quiescent state and highest in the G2 phase.[150] HLA-A and -B antigens, on the other hand, maintain a relatively constant surface density throughout the entire cell cycle.

Of particular importance is the distribution and changeable expression of histocompatibility antigens within the kidney itself. Based on several studies, it would appear that Class I antigens are present on cells in the glomerulus, endothelium of large vessels and capillaries, interstitial dendritic cells, and proximal and distal tubules[58,69,70,77,163] (Table 9-3). Class II antigens are most abundantly expressed on dendritic cells in the interstitium and appear on glomerular endothelial and some mesangial cells, but they are absent from the epithelial cells in Bowman's capsule and are either undetectable or barely detectable on the endothelium of large vessels. Perhaps their most useful characteristic is the fact that they do not appear normally on either the proximal or distal tubular epithelial cells, but when an immunologic stimulus occurs, such as rejection or a local graft-versus-host reaction, these cells exhibit Class II antigens that are demonstrable in renal biopsies and that may appear on lymphocytes in the urinary sediment.[10,18,69,70,77] This alteration appears to be mediated by γ-interferon.[70] It is likely that the appearance of Class II DR antigens on renal tubular cells in response to immunologic stimuli may provoke allograft rejection. Moreover, the expression of HLA-DR has been noted on peripheral T-lymphocytes assayed by flow cytometry in allograft recipients who suffered rejection episodes or had cytomegalovirus infection.[189]

In autoimmune disorders, Class II antigens are also known to be expressed on cells that usually do not express them.[72] When Class II antigens are elicited, possibly in response to γ-interferon, they initiate immunologic responses, such as autoantibody

TABLE 9-3   HLA Antigens in the Kidney

	VASCULATURE		GLOMERULUS				TUBULE		INTERSTITIUM
	Large	Cap	Endo	Mesang	Epi	Bowman's Cap	Prox	Distal	Dendritic
Class I (HLA-A, -B, -C)	+ +	+ +	+ +	0/+	0/+	+	+	+	+ +
Class II (HLA-DR)	0/+	+ +	+ +	+	0	0	(Intracellular) 0/+*	0*	+ + +

* Inducible (see text)

(Large = large vessels; Cap = capillaries; Endo = endothelial; Mesang = mesangial; Epi = epithelial; Bowman's Cap = Bowman's capsule; Prox = proximal)

production, where presumably none had existed earlier.

In addition to their altered expression on differentiated cells in response to the factors just described, Class II HLA antigens (DP, DQ, and DR) vary on developing cells and can therefore be considered as differentiation antigens. Although not entirely clear, the pattern of expression of Class II antigens on normal and malignant cells suggests that during differentiation, the first to be expressed may be DP, then DR, and finally DQ.[67] HLA-DR and -DP can be detected on stem cells (CFU$_{GEMM}$, CFU$_{G/M}$, CFU$_c$, BFU$_e$, and CFU$_{meg}$) that eventually mature into B- and T-lymphocytes, monocytes, granulocytes, erythrocytes, and megakaryocytes, many of which do not remain DR positive.[102,138] For example, when B-lymphocytes become antibody-secreting plasma cells, they too lose DR expression. HLA-DP expression is similar to that of HLA-DR not only on stem cells but also on peripheral B-lymphocytes and monocytes. The most striking differences are between the expression of HLA-DQ when compared with HLA-DR and -DP. HLA-DQ is expressed only on DR-positive B-lymphocytes, macrophages, and DR-positive monocytes but is absent on peripheral T-lymphocytes. In other tissues, DR and DQ also differ in their distribution. Although both DR and DQ antigens are present on thymic epithelium, parotid acinar cells, and renal glomerular cells, only DR antigens are found on the epithelium of the stomach, small intestine, and colon. On malignant cells, DR and DP expression usually coincide, whereas DR and DQ are divergent.[138]

CLINICAL GENETICS OF HLA

The HLA antigens are products of linked loci, A, B, Cw, DR, DP, and DQ, and are inherited codominantly as a genetic unit called a *haplotype*. Each parent contributes to an offspring a single haplotype consisting of one antigen from each of the six loci. Consequently, a fully typed person would have two haplotypes with a total of 12 antigens, two from each series. For clinical purposes, however, the HLA-A, -B, and -DR antigens are most frequently used. The seventh series of antigens, Dw, represents a combined contribution of several loci, at least DR, DP, and DQ, and is measured as a composite result expressed by the level of stimulation in the MLC.

The inheritance patterns of these antigens in a family is shown in Tables 9-4 and 9-5. In the first example, the parents share no haplotype, or even antigen (Table 9-4). Under this circumstance, there

TABLE 9-4   *Inheritance Pattern of HLA Antigens*: No Shared Haplotype*

		DP	DQ	DR	B	Cw	A		
FATHER	a	1	2	2	7	5	3	Child 1	ac
	b	3	1	14	44	6	2	Child 2	ad
								Child 3	bc
MOTHER	c	2	3	3	8	7	1	Child 4	bd
	d	5	3	7	35	3	32	Child 5	ac

* The letters a, b, c, and d denote an entire haplotype. For a given child (e.g., child 1), there is a 25% chance that a sibling will share either two haplotypes (child 5) or no haplotype (child 4), and a 50% chance that a sibling will share one haplotype (children 2 and 3).

TABLE 9-5   *Inheritance Pattern of HLA Antigens*: Shared Parental Haplotype*

		DP	DQ	DR	B	Cw	A		
FATHER	a(= c)	2	3	3	8	7	1	Child 1	ac
	b	3	1	14	44	6	2	Child 2	ad
								Child 3	bc
MOTHER	c(= a)	2	3	3	8	7	1	Child 4	bd
	d	5	3	7	35	3	32	Child 5	ac

* The letters a, b, c, and d denote an entire haplotype. A mating in which the parents share a haplotype (a = c) creates new compatibility possibilities: The father and child 3 are HLA identical, as are the mother and child 2; children 2 and 3 now have a 75% chance of a one haplotype match and a 25% chance of a two haplotype match; children 1, 4, and 5 have the same chances of compatibility as shown in Table 9-4. Additionally, children 1 and 5 could be used as donors for homozygous typing cells (HTC's).

is a 25% possibility of an HLA-identical sibling pair among their offspring, a 25% possibility of a totally incompatible sibling pair, and a 50% chance of a one-haplotype-matched sibling pair. In a second situation, in which the parents share a haplotype, there is not only the possibility of HLA-identical siblings but also of HLA-identical parent–child matches (Table 9-5). A rarer phenomenon in which there has been a recombination between the B and DR loci is shown in Table 9-6. These genetic variations in typing as well as the need to verify homozygosities make it essential to perform a thorough family study in living-related transplants and a complete typing of cadaver allograft recipients with family members if necessary.

The principle of linkage exhibited by the HLA-loci is straightforward. The occurrence of a different phenomenon, linkage disequilibrium, can be seen in both the paternal and maternal haplotypes used in Table 9-4. Linkage disequilibrium can be defined as the occurrence of two or more antigens together more frequently than would be expected on the basis of their individual gene frequencies. For example, the paternal "a" haplotype has antigens A3, B7, and DR2 that show linkage disequilibrium, just as A1, B8, and DR3 do in maternal haplotype "c" (Table 9-4). The degree of linkage disequilibrium can be quantitated and is expressed as a delta value. For the A3, B7 combination, the actual delta value for North American Caucasians is 228 ($p < 0.01$); for A1, B8 484 ($p < 0.001$); for B7, DR2 392 ($p < 0.001$), and for B8, DR3 628 ($p < 0.001$). Linkage disequilibrium may be either positive, as just shown, or negative for antigens found together *less* frequently than expected, (e.g., A1, Bw44, $p < 0.001$). Furthermore, antigens exhibiting linkage disequilibrium can vary from race to race (e.g., A29, B7 in American blacks, $p < 0.001$ vs. no significant disequilibrium in Caucasians). Knowledge about linkage dis-

equilibrium can be helpful clinically, because in cadaver donors, where haplotype information from family studies is not available, the occurrence of two antigens in strong positive linkage disequilibrium suggests that they may actually be on the same chromosome, thereby permitting not just antigen matching but possibly haplotype matching approximating what is routinely available in living-related transplants.

MOLECULAR GENETICS OF CLASS I HLA ANTIGENS (GENES, LOCI, SUBREGIONS, AND ANTIGENIC POLYMORPHISM)

There have been tremendous advances enabling better understanding of the molecular basis for the composition and complexity of HLA antigens. It will ultimately be through such exquisitely detailed analyses of these antigens that we will be able first to understand and then to manipulate them so that those antigenic sites that (1) differentially provoke cytotoxic vs anti-idiotype antibody formation on one hand and cytotoxic vs suppressor T-lymphocytes on the other, (2) represent shared sequences with one another as well as other cell surface molecules or microbial agents, or (3) are susceptible to perturbation by physical, chemical, or radiologic immunosuppression can be used to decrease the antigenicity of beneficial grafts and augment the antigenicity of undesired neoplasms.

Although some of the Class I loci are the well-known loci in the HLA-A, -B, and -C subregions, the majority are in other sites telomeric (i.e., located away from the centromere) to the HLA-A locus where they appear to be analogs of the murine T1 and Qa genes.[43,79,84] Class I as well as Class II gene products show a striking similarity to those of the

TABLE 9-6   *Inheritance Pattern of HLA Antigens: Recombinant Maternal Haplotype**

		DP	DQ	DR	B	Cw	A		
FATHER	a	1	2	2	7	5	3	Child 1	ac
	b	3	1	14	44	6	2	Child 2	ad
								Child 3	bc
MOTHER	c	2	3	3	8	7	1	Child 4	bd
	d	5	3	7	35	3	32	Child 5	ac:d

* The letters a, b, c, and d denote an entire haplotype. A recombination between the B and DR loci has occurred in child 5. Consequently, child 5 has not only the intact paternal "a" haplotype but also a recombinant maternal haplotype "c:d" with the c haplotype antigens for HLA-B, Cw, and A (8, 7, and 1, respectively) but the d haplotype antigens for HLA-DP, -DQ, and -DR (5, 3, 7, respectively). Because of this, children 1 and 5 would mistakenly appear to be HLA-identical if typed only for HLA-A, -B, and -Cw antigens. But their MLC should be stimulatory, and a full family typing with further testing for HLA-DP, -DQ, and -DR would reveal the recombinant haplotype.

immunoglobulin gene(s). This is borne out in amino acid sequencing of these molecules, described later, and suggests a common ancestral gene modified by gene duplication or deletions.

In humans, the genes for Class I antigens number approximately 20 to 30 and include many pseudogenes (i.e., genes without a known protein product). The typical gene for the Class I heavy chain has eight exons: The first exon encodes a 5' untranslated sequence of 18 nucleotides; both the second and third exons contain about 270 nucleotides, are the most polymorphic of the large exons, and encode the α_1 (1–90 amino acid sequence) and α_2 domains (91–182 amino acid sequence), respectively; the fourth exon, with 270 nucleotides, is the most conserved, resembles a domain of the immunoglobulin constant region, and encodes the α_3 domain (amino acid sequence 183–274); the fifth exon, with its 122 nucleotides, encodes a transmembrane segment consisting of hydrophobic amino acids and flanking residues that interact with the phosphates of the membrane phospholipids; the sixth and seventh exons are small coding regions, and the eighth exon is the largest, with its 400 residues.[84,174] Although the extracellular domains play a direct role in immune reactions, the cytoplasmic domains coded by exons 6, 7, and 8 may also have an important role yet to be explored. They have been thought to be the carrier or transmitter of the cytoplasmic signals of immune response and/or anchoring devices for proper orientation in the cytoskeletal matrix.

The ultimate method of histocompatibility testing would be through analysis of the DNA of the histocompatibility genes. For example, Class I genes have been studied by means of their DNA cleavage products that are created by treatment with different endonucleases. In this procedure, DNA prepared from a person's blood cells is digested by a restriction endonuclease having a specific recognition site. This generates DNA fragments of various lengths that are separated by gel electrophoresis and then transferred onto a nitrocellulose membrane. A radiolabeled DNA sequence used as a probe will hybridize with DNA fragments showing sequence complementarity with it. The radiolabeled DNA fragment is then developed by autoradiography. When applied to DNA studies, this technique is called *Southern blotting*.[173] Molecular cloning of genes from the HLA region has made various probes available for such studies.

Changes in the patterns of these fragments reflect differences in the location of restriction sites that were recognized by the specific endonuclease used. The end result is called a restriction fragment length polymorphism (RFLP), which is simply a polymorphism in the distribution of restriction sites revealed by such fragment patterns. An RFLP of such a system, one not found invariably in all persons tested, is called an *allogenotope*.[37] Through studies of RFLPs between 15 and 25 bands have been detected for Class I antigens, depending upon the enzyme used to produce the RFLPs. This number of bands is compatible with the estimate of 20 to 30 Class I genes. However, there can be discrepancies by this technique, since several bands may correspond to a single gene (intragenic site), or several genes may correspond to a single band (several fragments of the same size).[37]

The majority of allogenotopes, whether single or clusters, correlate with HLA-A, -B, or -Cw specificities. HLA-A specificities usually have about 12 allogenotopes, with a range of 4 for A9 haplotypes, to 18 for Aw19 haplotypes.[37] The majority of Class I allogenotopes are correlated with HLA-A alleles (63%), and only a few correlate with -B or -Cw alleles (13% and 5%, respectively). This is just the opposite of serologic analyses, which show a greater degree of polymorphism for the B series. Further differences exist between serologic specificities and allogenotopes. Although allogenotopes do correlate with the cross-reacting antigens A1-A11, no allogenotopes are found to correlate with the strongly cross-reacting antigens A2-A28, and still another allogenotope correlates with A3 and A9 that are not known to be cross-reactive serologically.[37] It therefore seems that analysis of HLA genes will need to go beyond determination of their DNA by RFLPs alone and will ultimately involve the use of oligonucleotide probes and even DNA nucleotide sequencing.

The biochemistry of the Class I antigens has been studied extensively. Class I antigens are highly polymorphic cell surface glycoproteins consisting of a polymorphic heavy chain of about 44,000 daltons that is noncovalently bound to β_2-microglobulin, a nonpolymorphic 11,700 dalton polypeptide (Fig. 9-2).[104] The heavy chain is coded for by genes in the MHC of the 6th chromosome, whereas β_2-microglobulin is coded for by a gene on the 15th chromosome.[65] The heavy chain is composed of an aminoterminal extracellular portion, a transmembrane segment, and a carboxyterminal intracellular portion. The extracellular portion has been divided into three domains (α_1, α_2, and α_3), each containing approximately 90 amino acid residues. There is conservation of the protein sequence in the α_3 domain that is the main interaction site for β_2-microglobu-

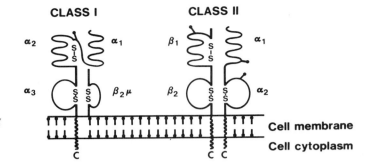

FIGURE 9-2. *Schematic model for class I and II HLA antigens. (S-S = disulfide bond; C = carboxy terminus, = carbohydrate side chain). (Adapted from Kaufman JF: Cell 36:1, 1984)*

lin, and more variability in the α_1 and α_2 domains that carry the polymorphic determinants for antibodies and cytolytic T-lymphocytes. The majority of the variable residues are clustered in seven segments, three of them located in α_1 (residues 9–12, 40–45, and 62–83), and four in α_2 and the α_2/α_3 interdomain (residues 94–97, 105–116, 137–163, and 173–194). Even the most polymorphic positions have only a low number of different residues, frequently only two.

Comparison of the amino acid sequences have helped to establish the molecular basis for the serologic specificity as well as cross-reactivity seen not only with alloantibodies used for clinical tissue typing but also with monoclonal antibodies.[104] For example, the amino acid sequence of HLA-A2 differs from that of the cross-reactive HLA-A28 by approximately 11 amino acids. Because five of them are in the hypervariable region 62 to 74, and two are at positions 107 and 114, these may be the alterations responsible for the allospecificity of each. The B locus sequences that have been analyzed from the cross-reacting antigens HLA-B7, -B27, and -40 are more complex because they differ from one another in at least 19 positions.[104] Nevertheless, segment 62 to 83 is the most variable and has been thought to be the major contributor to the allospecificities of these three antigens. An antiserum developed against a synthetic peptide with the sequence of residues 62 to 83 of HLA-B7 specifically reacts with this antigen and thereby provides direct evidence that this is the critical region for the B7 allospecificity.[104]

On the other hand, cross-reactivity is promoted by the restricted variability in the polymorphic regions, because many epitopes are common to different Class I molecules. Antigenic polymorphism may also be generated by the combination of several regions with low variability. As a result, antibodies

produced to Class I HLA antigens are often directed against structures that are not unique to a single gene product, that is, cross-reactive determinants.

The allodeterminants defined by serologic reagents appear to be different from those for HLA-restricted CTLs recognizing Class I antigen plus a virus.[104] In fact, at least six HLA-A and -B specificities have been split into subtypes by CTLs. Variants detected by CTLs all seem to express differences in the segment 145 to 157 with only a rare exception.[94] This area, surprisingly, is one of low polymorphism as a whole, but one in which a conformational change occurs, namely an α-helix, that brings residues 152 and 156 into proximity with one another.[104] Remarkably, it is residues 152 and 156 that represent the points of all known substitutions. Another special feature of CTL variants is that they all have at least one amino acid substitution involving a difference in charge.

MOLECULAR GENETICS OF CLASS II HLA ANTIGENS (GENES, LOCI, SUBREGIONS, AND ANTIGENIC POLYMORPHISMS)

The D region for Class II antigens has at least three subregions, DR, DQ, and DP (Fig. 9-1).[39,43,186] Within the subregions are at least seven β and six α genes that code for the α and β chains of the Class II molecules, sequences of which resemble one another more so within each locus than they do analogous chains of other Class II loci.[186] Some general statements can be made about the characteristics of Class II genes: they are numerous, include several pseudogenes, and may differ in number in various haplotypes.[106] The DP subregion has two α and two β genes, the DQ subregion has two α and two β genes, and the DR subregion has one α and at least three β genes. An additional locus called DZ_α, possibly nonfunctional, has also been described but is not formally mapped.[186] The α_1 and β_1 DP genes encode the DP antigens, whereas the α_2 and β_2 genes are unexpressed and appear as pseudogenes.[186] Similarly, in the DQ subregion, one pair of α and β genes encodes the DQ antigens, whereas the second α gene (DX_α) and the second β gene (DX_β) have not yet been demonstrated to be expressed and may be pseudogenes.[186] In the DR subregion, the α gene is expressed and nonpolymorphic, but the β genes include an unexpressed pseudogene (β_3) and at least two other expressed β genes that may occur singly or together (e.g., DR4 cell lines have two β chains that form heterodimers with DR_α).[93] Polymorphism is imparted primarily by the expressed β genes, and DQ_α, but DX_α, and $DP_\alpha 1$ are polymorphic as well.[186]

The six exons coding for the Class II glycoprotein chains are those for the signal sequence(s), the first domain (1), the second domain (2), the membrane spanning portion (M), the cytoplasmic segment (C), and the 3' untranslated region (3').

Both murine and human Class II gene products have the same basic biochemical structure. Each Class II antigen has two chains, an α (heavy) chain of approximately 34,000 daltons, and a β (light) chain of 29,000 daltons, and each chain has two extracellular domains (the first or distal domain, α_1 and β_1, respectively; and the second or proximal domain, α_2 and β_2, respectively) as well as transmembrane and cytoplasmic portions (See Fig. 9-2).[15] The first β chain domain has 90 amino acids and two cysteines that form a disulfide loop, but the first α chain domain is shorter and has no disulfide loop. Both the α and β chain second domains have disulfide loops, are highly conserved, and exhibit homologies with the immunoglobulin constant region (CH3).[15] The α chain, at least of DR, is responsible for the autologous MLC response.[128] The hydrophobic transmembrane portions are joined to the proximal domains by a hydrophilic 12 amino acid sequence. The cytoplasmic portion varies in length, and for DQ_β, it is shorter by eight amino acids. The α and β chains are noncovalently bound to each other and reside on the surface of a restricted number of cells, described earlier (Distribution and Expression of HLA Antigens).

The antigens encoded by genes in the Class II region of the major histocompatibility complex (MHC) have been shown to be highly polymorphic by techniques that began with the mixed lymphocyte culture (MLC) and alloantisera,[76,118] and have progressed in sophistication and depth to include homozygous typing cells (HTC),[48,66] primed lymphocyte typing (PLT),[168,193] monoclonal antibodies,[23] protein sequencing,[39,186] cDNA clones,[93,135,186] mutant cell lines,[88] restriction fragment length RFLP,[37,43] and labeled oligonucleotides.[106]

The important question of how polymorphisms arise in Class II molecules and at how exquisitely basic a level they may exist is unfolding with studies of the molecular genetics of the DR genes. At the functional level, serologic reagents and HTCs have detected differences in reactivity patterns that have been used to identify polymorphisms within the DR subregion. But, often, what appeared to be a single antigen in these assays was found to be more complex. More discriminating distinctions between such functionally single antigenic determinants were provided by studies of RFLPs. Because the enzymes used to produce the RFLPs usually cut the DNA in noncoding areas, or introns, it was suspected that subtle differences in the exons could still be overlooked. That suspicion has recently been confirmed. Studies using labeled oligonucleotides revealed that what appeared to be a single specificity even by RFLP analysis could actually be two different specificities distinguished only by a single nucleotide difference.[106] As a result of this type of molecular probing, it seems that the polymorphisms that are so abundant even at the functional level of serologic and cell typing will be shown to be even more prolific because of exquisitely minute alterations consisting of single nucleotide differences. Protein sequencing of the molecule, a much more laborious task, can confirm the amino acid differences resulting from the nucleotide variations.

However, the antigenicity of Class II molecules is engendered not only by certain highly variable portions of the amino acid sequences but also by the proximity of amino acids in a tertiary structure as they approximate one another in the outer domains. One could visualize, then, that by itself, a conformational alteration of the chain without any structural change would be sufficient to destroy the antigenicity of a particular set of determinants.

VARYING STRENGTHS OF HLA ANTIGENS

Although H-2 histocompatibility antigens in the mouse have been characterized as strong and non-H-2 histocompatibility antigens as weak, the distinction for human histocompatibility antigens has been much less clear. Data from skin and renal allograft survivals,[46,145,180] antibody production,[119] MLC,[83] and CML studies[50] suggest that HLA-A2 is a strong histocompatibility antigen and that HLA-1,

-3, and -11 are weak histocompatibility antigens. HLA-A2 incompatibility was also focused upon by the Stanford cardiac transplant team as being associated with recurrent atherosclerosis, which may also be another manifestation of chronic rejection.[22]

The HLA-Cw antigens are believed to be the weakest set of antigens and to have barely any relevance in clinical human allografting.[3] Even intentional immunizations specifically for HLA-Cw antigens have generally been unsuccessful.[53]

The HLA-B locus antigens as a group were thought to represent stronger Class I incompatibilities in some studies of human renal allografting primarily because of the proximity of the B locus to the D region, which was originally marked only by MLC reactivity.[14,41,121,122,153] After the D region began to be redefined serologically initially by HLA-DR antigens, the DR antigens emerged as perhaps the strongest set of HLA antigens marking for compatibility in the human MHC.[*] It was the DR antigen, DRw6, that was later thought to be an especially strong transplantation antigen since it might characterize a hyperresponder type of recipient.[78,87,100] (See Clinical Studies of HLA Matching in Renal Allografting; 8. DRw6 and Renal Allograft Rejection.)

The most remarkable insight into the hierarchy of HLA antigenic strengths has recently been provided through the use of labeled oligonucleotides to do "DNA typing."[106] By this technique, DR3 appears to have arisen by gene conversion from the same primordial genes found in DRw6 and to have only very minor differences in its β chains, whereas DR4 seems to have had different primordial genes and substantial differences in its β chains. In fact, two major clusters have evolved by this technique: DR3, 5, w6, and DR4, 7.[106] It is remarkable that these two clusters derived by oligonucleotide typing are already represented to a substantial degree by the serologic entities DRw52 (MT2) and DRw53 (MT3).[118] Consequently, from this molecular information, one can speculate that donor DR antigen mismatches could be evaluated according to the recipient's antigens in general terms as minor (e.g., a DR3-DRw6 disparity), or major (e.g., a DR3-DR4 difference).[106]

Also important in the concept of antigenic strength is the finding that more global regulatory genes exist that control the expression of Class II antigens, a process often mediated by γ-interferon.[13,106] The regulatory gene(s) responsible for the expression of Class II molecules appears to be located outside the MHC, possibly even on another chromosome.[143]

MIXED LYMPHOCYTE CULTURE (MLC)

From MLC studies in animals, it was shown that the Class II antigens (also known as Ia antigens in the mouse) are responsible for stimulating the proliferation of unprimed clones of T cells.[117] Further, it was shown that antibodies to the Ia antigens can effectively block the response that would normally be provoked by the Ia antigens of the stimulatory cells.[110]

Clinically, the MLC has been used to (1) confirm serologically HLA identical pairs,[4,99] (2) detect possible recombinants for the D region,[4] (3) project allograft success in serologically mismatched recipients (i.e., low responders vs. high responders) for both living-related and cadaver allografts,[9,20,36,82,90,96,136,146,151,185] (4) evaluate steroid withdrawal,[55,57,176,187,197] and (5) assess the posttransplant mechanisms of recipient immune responsiveness that may be either donor-specific or donor nonspecific[57] and mediated by suppressor cells[101] or by putative anti-idiotype antibody.[169] The level of stimulation in both two-way and one-way MLCs has been described by the stimulation index (S.I.), the percent relative response (R.R.), and absolute counts per minute). The exact cutoff for nonstimulation, low stimulation, and high stimulation may vary somewhat in different laboratories using these three parameters.

Serologically HLA-identical sibling pairs will have nonstimulatory MLCs that confirm the identity of the Class II loci involved in generating the MLC response, namely, DR, DQ, and DP, and possibly others not yet identified.[109,158] In the event of a recombination between the loci responsible for the MLC and the serologically defined ones, an event that happens in fewer than 1 of every 100 gametes, stimulation in the MLC can be seen in siblings identical for HLA-A, -B, and -Cw; or, conversely, MLC compatibility could occur despite HLA-A, -B, -Cw differences (see Table 9-6). In the former recombination, there is not full 2 haplotype matching, and, in the latter, there is more than 1 haplotype matching (see Table 9-6). With just 1 or 0 haplotype matched, the MLCs would typically be stimulatory. Occasionally, persons who would be expected to have only a single haplotype shared, such as parent and child combinations, may actually share both haplotypes because one haplotype is common to both parents (see Table 9-5).[99] It has recently been shown that even in unrelated persons, matching for

---

[*] References 30,64,81,105,107,111,113,122,123,184

common "extended" haplotypes containing identical B and DR specificities as well as the same complotypes (genes for the complement components) for Bf, C2, C4A, and C4B specificities creates a very high probability of finding nonstimulatory MLCs.[9] Since about 30% of normal Caucasians will have 1 such common extended haplotype and 9% will have 2, this information may be extremely important in selecting the best donor from an unrelated living or cadaver population. A suggestion of this was brought out by earlier work showing that partially related or even unrelated persons matched for HLA-A and -B or for HLA-B and -DR had lower mixed lymphocyte reactivity when the HLA combinations were ones known to be in positive linkage disequilibrium.[136] (See Clinical Genetics of HLA.)

Projections of allograft success in serologically mismatched recipients have been based on the degree of stimulation in MLC. The classic study relating allograft survival to MLC responsiveness used human skin grafts in living-related pairs matched for 1 HLA haplotype. In six cases in which the MLC was nonstimulatory, the survival time was significantly prolonged. But stimulation in the MLC lacked total predictive value, because 8 of 35 persons showing MLC stimulation had skin graft survival times that were also remarkably prolonged.[151] In renal transplantation, the degree of stimulation in MLC has been used in nonidentical living-related donor–recipient pairs in order to distinguish high from low responders.[20,36,90,146,185] Those with low stimulation (S.I. <6.5–10) had allograft survival rates of approximately 80% compared with about 40% to 60% for those with stimulation indices above that range.[36,90,146,185] The poor allograft survival in the high stimulation group led to the use of donor-specific transfusions (DST), a strategy that then raised their level of success to approximately 90%.[146] Numerous other studies have also confirmed the fact that patients with low MLC reactivity have better survival of living-related allografts, although some have failed to find such a correlation.[185] In addition to a low S.I. or an R.R. of 20% or less,[20] a low responder population has also been identified before transplantation based on less than 28,000 cpm in MLC in conjunction with less than 36.5% active T rosette-forming cells, anergy to microbial skin test antigens, and in vitro spontaneous blastogenesis less than 14,600 counts per minute.[90] In cadaver graft recipients in which the results are necessarily retrospective, there is more uncertainty about the association between a low MLC response and better graft survival.[82,96]

The prospect for successful steroid withdrawal has also been measured by MLC responsiveness. In 19 HLA-identical sibling renal allograft recipients, prednisone was gradually discontinued an average of 13.2 months after transplantation, and 18 of the recipients, with follow-up for 14 to 82 months, have had normal renal function irrespective of whether or not they had had acute rejection episodes early after transplantation.[55] Among another five recipients of successful living-related transplants who stopped azathioprine and prednisone against medical advice, two who were nonidentical by serologic typing and MLC developed renal failure in 2 to 6 months, whereas none of the three recipients of HLA-identical kidneys who were MLC nonstimulatory developed changes in renal function despite being off medication from 7 to 30 months.[187] Although similar results could be obtained without using MLC information in both living-related and cadaver graft recipients,[176] a retrospective study in the United States failed to identify a single patient with a cadaver kidney who was able to maintain stable renal function for longer than 2 years without immunosuppression.[197] In cyclosporine-treated living-related renal recipients, the MLC has also been used to evaluate steroid withdrawal.[57] Of seven HLA-identical recipients on cyclosporine who had steroids withdrawn 6 to 9 months after transplantation, six have had stable renal function for 9 to 12 months, whereas one patient who also stopped cyclosporine experienced a severe rejection with only partial reversal.[57] Of nine haploidentical (one haplotype-matched) recipients with low MLC stimulation (<6.5 S.I.) who had steroid withdrawal attempted, five on cyclosporine alone had stable renal function without a rejection episode for 13 to 18 months, two others on low-dose alternate-day prednisone had stable renal function, and two others had serious rejections.[57]

The MLC has also been used to examine possible mechanisms of immunosuppression, such as the appearance of suppressor lymphocytes after donor-specific transfusions,[101] as well as serum suppressor substances following random blood transfusions,[169] and during cyclosporine therapy posttransplantation.[57] The reduction of donor-specific one-way MLC response by the addition of putative suppressor cells or serum factors has been the cornerstone of such assay systems.[57,101,169]

PRIMED LYMPHOCYTE TESTING (PLT)

Despite its rapidity and conceptual advantage that was based on having an established library of lymphocytes specifically primed to respond maximally only to rechallenge with the same set of Class II determinants, the PLT was only rarely used in clinical renal typing.[168,172] It had even been demonstrated in a random panel of 53 unrelated persons that PLT typing could predict MLC reactivity.[188] Pairs of the panel members who shared PLT specificities had threefold lower MLC responses, whereas an increasing number of disparate PLT specificities on the stimulator cell coincided with significant increases in MLC reactivity.

The antigenic determinants responsible for PLT reactivity are now known to be primarily, if not exclusively, the DP molecules (formerly SB).[167,193] Slowly but surely, monoclonal antibodies are being developed that can detect some of these DP antigens.[166] Unless the PLT cellular determinants and the DP serologic determinants significantly diverge in their specificity, as did the HTC-determined Dw specificities from the DR serologic specificities, it is likely that serologic reagents will eventually be the method of choice for identifying the DP/PLT determinants.

CELL-MEDIATED LYMPHOLYSIS (CML)

Information provided by the CML is an extension of that derived from the MLC. Whereas the MLC measures the recognition or proliferative phase of the immune response, the CML test measures the effector phase that is manifested by antibody-*inde*pendent destruction of the stimulating or target cells. The effector cells require sensitization by a D region antigen but exert their effect against the stimulating cells based on differences in Class I antigens (HLA-A, -B, and -Cw).[50]

Cell-mediated lympholysis has been used as a cellular typing method to identify surface molecules recognized by cytotoxic T-lymphocytes (CTLs).[63,154] (See also *Molecular Genetics of Class I HLA Antigens.*) CTLs can identify target molecules that represent both Class I and Class II antigens as well as determinants that do not correspond to known serologic specificities. For example, some CTL-defined specificities represent Class I molecular variants corresponding to HLA-A2, -B27, and -B44.[154] Still other CTLs have lysed allogeneic target cells that have no known Class I specificities shared with the sensitizing cells.

In the most recent International HLA Workshop experience, the CTL responses were found to be more complex than or different from those predicted on the basis of defined HLA antigens.[154] In most situations, predicted reactions were not missed by CTLs, rather, CTLs had extra reactions. Several splits of otherwise well-defined antigens have also been detected using CTL techniques.[154] It is hoped that the use of cloned CTLs and transfected target cells expressing cloned HLA genes will yield better information on the genetic basis for CTL recognition.

CLINICAL STUDIES OF HLA MATCHING IN RENAL ALLOGRAFTING

Although a vast number of studies have been done in this area dating back to 1965, the most relevant studies are those published in the 1980s because of the introduction of clinical DR typing, the almost universal use of pretransplant blood transfusions, a decrease in technical failures and complications owing to excessive immunosuppression, and the availability of cyclosporine. Based primarily on studies during this period, histocompatibility matching in human renal allografting will be examined in terms of its effect upon (1) allografts from living-related donors, (2) allografts from unrelated living donors, (3) patient survival in those receiving cadaver allografts, (4) short-term (1–2 yr) cadaver allograft survival with or without cyclosporine or transfusions, (5) long-term (4–10 yr) cadaver allograft survival, (6) waiting time for and success of repeat cadaver transplants, (7) modification of steroid or azathioprine dosage in cadaver and living-related allograft recipients, (8) allograft survival in recipients with DRw6, (9) the ''center'' effect in allograft survival, and (10) developing strategies for cadaver donor matching.

Histocompatibility between recipient and donor can be evaluated according to either the number of HLA antigens matched or mismatched. Different results can occur from these two approaches in circumstances in which not all of the *donor* antigens can be identified (i.e., ''blanks'' exist).[64] For example, mismatching presumes that a blank represents either an homozygous antigen or an identical antigen between donor and recipient, whereas matching presumes that a blank is an unidentified and universally incompatible antigen.[64] As a result of these differences, the dominant effect of calculating by mismatching is to raise the survival rate of the poorest matches. For example, even cadaver donors with no detectable DR antigens or one undetectable and one antigen identical with the recipient's would be considered 0 mismatches, just as those with two identical antigens. Conversely, the dominant effect of calculating by matching is to lower the survival of the better matches. For example, cadaver donors with one identified DR antigen that is a true homozygosity identical with a recipient's DR antigen would be considered a 1 DR match rather than the actual 2 DR. When only fully phenotyped or genotyped donors are used for analysis, this problem should disappear.

Living-Related Transplants

Histocompatibility of living-related transplant pairs is graded by the number of haplotypes matched (0, 1, or 2) and the degree of stimulation in MLC. Two-haplotype identities can be expected in 25% of siblings, but they may occasionally be found between a parent and child (see Tables 9-4 and 9-5).[99] Unless a recombinant event has occurred between the D region loci responsible for MLC reactivity, such as DR, DQ, or DP, and those loci whose genes code for the Class I antigens (HLA-A, -B, -C) (see Table 9-6), two-haplotype-matched living-related pairs will show essentially no stimulation in MLC. The likelihood of a recombination occurring is less than 1 per 100 gametes.

Two-haplotype-matched living-related pairs have the best early graft survivals and the best long-term prognosis.[126] In 1977, HLA identical grafts had a two-year success rate of 93% as well as a further excellent prognosis indicating that 50% of the grafts would still be functioning at 34 years.[126] HLA-identical sibling transplants continue to show excellent two-year patient and allograft survival in the range of 95% to 98% and 87% to 90%, respectively.[144,181] Despite the overall excellent prognosis for HLA-identical sibling transplants, some have still failed because of recurrent disease, technical problems, and "delayed hyperacute rejections."[25,115] The majority of "delayed hyperacute rejections" have been said to be caused by monocyte antibodies that also have reactivity against vascular endothelial cells.[32] Because of the cross-reactivity of staphylococcal and HLA antigens, it is perhaps relevant to note that staphylococcal infections were present in at least two of the HLA-identical siblings who lost their allografts because of delayed hyperacute rejections.[115,139] Accelerated rejection has also been reported in a female recipient of an HLA-identical male kidney with its H-Y antigen.[132] In this case, 2 weeks following transplantation, the female recipient developed HLA-A2-restricted cellular cytotoxicity against her male donor's and other male A2-positive lymphocytes. Allograft failure may also happen because certain immunologically mediated renal diseases are more likely to recur in HLA-identical recipients and could easily be confused with rejection.[28] In fact, recurrent glomerulonephritis was a major finding in untreated human isografts.[60]

One- or zero-haplotype-matched living-related recipients initially had decidedly worse allograft survival. Such recipients were categorized as high or low responders, depending upon the MLC S.I.; those with a low S.I. (<6.5–10) had nearly a doubling of allograft survivals to approximately 80% (see Mixed Lymphocyte Culture).[36,90,146,185] As the success of donor-specific transfusions (DST) became apparent, virtually all mismatched living-related recipients, whether high or low responders in MLC, began to receive DSTs, third-party transfusions, or cyclosporine. The survival curves of mismatched living-related recipients who have received DSTs,[5,144] third-party transfusions,[131] or cyclosporine[56] have approached or duplicated at least the early survival rates of HLA-identical siblings. However, diminished long-term success and a lower chance for total discontinuation of immunosuppression at a later date may yet be found to occur more frequently in mismatched living-related allograft recipients, just as it has in poorly matched recipients of cadaver allografts. Although antigen systems are not usually evaluated individually in living-related transplants, the DQ system has been studied. Its importance may lie in the fact that it is one of the contributors to MLC reactivity. Unconfirmed work on the influence of this Class II antigen system, previously called MB, showed that among 21 patients who had received a 1-haplotype intrafamilial transplant, all 8 of the rejected kidneys were from MB-incompatible donors, whereas 12 of 13 successful transplants were from MB-compatible donors.[49]

Living Unrelated Transplants

The initial experience with living unrelated donors was uniformly poor.[1,68] It has perhaps been forgotten that in the 1960s, 166 living unrelated renal transplants were performed with approximately a 25% survival rate at 1 year post-transplantation, a figure slightly worse than the 36% success rates seen in 1074 cadaver grafts performed during the same period.[1] No matching information was available in that era. In another early study of 18 unrelated volunteer donors, only 2 of the 18 grafts survived to 1 year.[68]

The success of cyclosporine and various transfusion protocols has recently stimulated new trials.[12,142,171] Eighty-seven cases of living unrelated donors, 20 of whom received DSTs, exhibited a 40.3% graft loss that was approximately the same whether or not the patient received DSTs.[142] Histocompatibility information was meager and included only the fact that all cases except one had different HLA phenotypes, and most had two or more HLA incompatibilities for HLA-A, -B, and

-Cw. In a small series that included seven unrelated donor–recipient pairs (six spouses and one friend), apparently 2-haplotype mismatched, all were treated with DSTs and all had functioning grafts with follow-ups ranging from 2 to 30 months.[171] After the DSTs but before transplantation, the plasma of the three patients who were tested showed a donor-specific MLC inhibitor as well as a nonspecific inhibitor 6 to 8 weeks following transplant.[171] Another two patients, the first matched for HLA-A2 and B40 and the second for HLA-A2, were also treated with DSTs and both still had functioning allografts 13 and 17 months after transplantation.[12] No MLCs were reported.

Patient Survival

Two major studies have shown improved patient survival associated with better HLA-A and -B matching.[130,184] At 5 years post-transplantation, among 2522 recipients of a first cadaver allograft, the 471 patients without any HLA-A or -B mismatches had a survival rate of 72%, compared with 55% in recipients with 3 or 4 mismatched antigens ($p = 0.001$).[130] Similarly, among 305 first cadaver recipients, those patients who received an HLA-A and -B compatible kidney had a 97% 5-year survival rate compared with 80% for those receiving 3 to 4 A and B mismatched grafts.[184] However, in a third study, there was no significant improvement in patient survival when one progressed from the worst to the best match, a result that may have been affected by a sudden decrease in the success rate of just the best matched patients despite a consistent correlation of success with matching before that point.[148]

Short-Term (1–2 Year) Cadaver Allograft Survival (Table 9-7)

Reports concerning the effect of HLA matching on short-term (1–2 yr) cadaver allograft survival can be divided into two groups: (1) multicenter or collaborative studies, and (2) single or dual institution studies with much smaller numbers, particularly in the subsets of patients. Most of these studies, particularly the larger collaborative ones, show an advantage to HLA matching in cadaver transplantation.

Multicenter and Collaborative Studies

Of the seven multicenter studies from 1983 to 1986 (Table 9-7), all six having patients not treated with cyclosporine reported an advantage to HLA matching, five for HLA-A, -B matching,[30,51,54,122,148] and three for HLA-B, -DR matching.[41,54,123] Of the four studies having patients on cyclosporine, the two largest studies with the greatest number of well-matched patients both reported significant correlations between allograft success and better matching.[30,123] Highlights of these studies are summarized in Table 9-7, and further descriptions are offered here.

In the International Collaborative Transplant Study, first cadaver allograft recipients with or without cyclosporine had 1-year graft survival rates improve nearly 20% with no mismatches for HLA-B and -DR antigens compared with those grafts having 4 mismatched antigens.[123] Specifically, 161 transplant recipients with cyclosporine treatment and no mismatches for HLA-B or -DR antigens had a 1-year graft survival rate of 86% ± 3%, whereas 181 recipients of grafts with 4 HLA-B and -DR antigen mismatches had a graft survival rate of 67% ± 4% ($p < 0.001$).[123] Without cyclosporine, the corresponding 1-year graft survival rates were 75% ± 2% and 57% ± 3% for transplants with 0 or 4 mismatched HLA-B or -DR antigens, respectively ($p < 0.0001$). This study clearly showed the significant advantage of HLA matching with or without cyclosporine and emphasized the fact that these two elements are additive in improving cadaver allograft success rates. In the longest American multicenter study, among cyclosporine-treated patients, those with 0 to 1 HLA-A, -B mismatches had an 80% 1-year graft survival rate compared with 70% in those with 3 or 4 incompatibilities ($p < 0.02$).[30] With conventional therapy, the corresponding values were lower overall and showed 69% survival with 0 to 1 HLA-A, -B mismatch and 60% survival with 3 to 4 mismatches ($p < 0.005$).[30] Matching for DR antigens in patients receiving cyclosporine achieved an 85% cadaver graft survival at 1 year compared with 74% with zero DR antigens matched ($p < 0.004$).[30] This study supports the findings of the International Collaborative Transplant Study, both in terms of an independent HLA matching effect and an additive effect with cyclosporine.

A third large collaborative study by the Southeastern Organ Procurement Foundation (SEOPF), although not yet having results on the effect of DR matching or cyclosporine, has provided extensive data on the effects of HLA-A and -B matching. One year following cadaver transplantation, success rates for those with only 0 to 1 HLA-A or -B matched antigen were 47% and 51%, respectively, compared with 58% and 59%, respectively, for those with 3 or 4 HLA-A and -B antigens matched ($p = 0.052$ by the Breslow method and $p = 0.0007$ by the Mantel-Cox test).[148] When only those allografts lost to re-

TABLE 9-7   Cadaver Renal Allograft Short-Term (1-Year) Survival
(Recent Multicenter and Collaborative Studies)

STUDY (ref)	BEST MATCH SURVIVAL (%)	BEST MATCH (n)	TYPE OF BEST HLA MATCH	CYCLO-SPORINE	DIFFERENCE IN SURVIVAL BETWEEN BEST AND WORST MATCH*(%)	P
Festenstein et al, 1986[54]	86	144	A,B 3–4 matches	no	+26	0.0001
	84	128	B,DR 0–1 mismatch	no	+29	0.03
	82	194	B,MT 0–1 mismatch	no	+58	0.03
Opelz, 1985[123]	86 ± 3	161	B,DR 0 mismatch	yes	+19	0.001
	75 ± 2	381	B,DR 0 mismatch	no	+18	0.0001
Cats, 1985[30]	80	145	A,B 0–1 mismatch	yes	+10	0.02
	69	590	A,B 0–1 mismatch	no	+9	0.005
	85	85	DR 2 matches	yes	+11	0.004
Sanfilippo et al, 1984[148]	59 ± 4	141	A,B 4 matches	no	+8	0.05
D'Apice et al, 1984[41]	83 ± 15	6	B,DR 4 matches	no	+43	0.002
Klintmalm et al, 1985[92]†	61	6	A,B 0 mismatch	yes	−13	NS
	78	71	DR 0 mismatch	yes	−5	NS
European Multi-centre, 1983[51]	89	9	A,B 0 mismatch	no	+43	‡
	27	11	A,B 0 mismatch	yes	−48	0.001

* When histocompatibility is reported according to the number of HLA antigens *matched,* the worst match will be 0 antigens matched; when reported according to the number of antigens *mismatched,* the worst match will be all or all but one (in the case of 4 antigens) antigen mismatched.

† 6-month survival.

‡ Data not reported.

jection were compared, the results were even more significant, with 1-year success rates of 71% and 70% for those with 3 or 4 HLA-A or -B antigens matched, respectively, compared with 59% and 65% for those with 0 to 1 HLA-A or -B antigen matched ($p = 0.0077$) by the Breslow test and $p = 0.0001$ by the Mantel-Cox test).[148] Of additional practical value is the fact that when public antigens or cross-reacting groups (CREGS) for the HLA-A and -B series were considered rather than all the individual specificities, a significant correlation of matching remained and was particularly apparent in those grafts lost because of rejection.[149] In the Australian and New Zealand combined dialysis and transplant registry, 187 primary cadaver allograft recipients with no incompatible HLA-A or -B antigens had a 1-year success rate of 63% ± 4% compared with 50% ± 3% in the 133 recipients having 3 or 4 incompatibilities.[14] The effect appeared to be mostly the result of B locus antigens, because at 1 year, primary grafts with no B locus mismatches had success rates of 61% ± 2%, those mismatched for 1 B antigen had success rates of 54% ± 1%, and those mismatched for 2 B antigens had success rates of 48% ± 2%.[14] Subsequently, 22 transplant units in Sydney and Melbourne, Australia reported on a prospective and randomized trial of matching in 352 recipients of a cadaver renal transplant without the use of cyclosporine.[41] Matching for HLA-B and -DR were

shown to have approximately equal, significant, independent, and additive effects on graft survival. One-year graft survival rates for 0, 1, 2, 3, and 4 HLA-B and -DR matched grafts were 40% ± 12.6%, 46.8% ± 4.9%, 54.0% ± 4.2%, 61.3% ± 5.9%, and 83.3% ± 15.2%, respectively ($p = 0.002$).[41]

The London Transplant Group recently reported that in 1341 recipients of a cadaver allograft not treated with cyclosporine, the beneficial effect of HLA-A and -B matching was seen long-term, whereas the combined HLA-B plus -DR or -MT effect occurred by 1 year post-transplantation.[54] For the 309 transplants since 1978, the success rate was 84% when no DR or B antigen was mismatched, 82% when no MT or B antigen was mismatched, and 80%, 76%, and 74% when no DR, MT, or B antigen alone was mismatched, respectively.[54] For a single antigen system, the worst results (59% survival) occurred when the two MT antigens (MT2 and MT3), now named DRw52 and DRw53, were mismatched.[54] With only two such broad antigens to consider, the clinical feasibility of MT matching becomes great. Furthermore, this clinical approach now has a newly appreciated molecular basis.[106]

Although two multicenter studies have found a matching effect when cyclosporine was used,[30,123] two others did not.[51,92] In the Scandinavian Multicentre Trial, in which individual centers had cadaver graft survivals ranging from 69% ± 5% to 86% ±

6%, there was no significant difference in cadaver graft survival according to the degree of matching for HLA-A, -B, or -DR, but some of the subgroups were very small and the follow-up was only 6 months.[92] For 0, 1, and 2 DR mismatches, the 6-month graft survival was approximately 78% for 71 patients, 70% for 46 patients, and 83% for 22 patients, respectively. For 0, 1, 2, 3, and 4 A and B mismatches, the 6-month graft survival rates were 61% for 6 patients, 70% for 23 patients, 79% for 57 patients, 79% for 42 patients, and 74% for 12 patients, respectively.[92] Because these patients were all treated with cyclosporine, it was concluded that HLA matching for A, B, or DR had no effect in the presence of cyclosporine. This study also found no adverse effect on renal transplant outcome at 6 months from lack of transfusions, high MLC reactivity, or longer ischemia times.[92] The European Multicentre study was compromised by having small numbers of patients in the best matched cohorts.[51] It did show an advantage to A and B matching in conventionally treated patients who had an 89% 1-year graft survival rate in 9 cases with no A,B mismatches, 50% survival in 78 cases with 1 to 2 mismatches, and 46% survival in 28 patients with 3 to 4 mismatches.[51] However, in the cyclosporine-treated group, there was a reverse matching effect, with only a 27% graft survival rate in the 11 patients with no mismatches, 77% in the 70 patients with 1 to 2 mismatches, and 75% success in the 36 patients with 3 to 4 mismatches ($p<0.001$).[51] This study's data on DR mismatching also showed a reverse effect, even in the conventionally treated group in which there was a 43% survival rate in the 14 patients with 0 mismatches, 53% in the 38 with 1 mismatch, and 83% in the 6 patients with 2 mismatches.[51] In the cyclosporine-treated group, there was again a reverse effect of DR mismatching in that success rates were 57% in the 21 patients with 0 mismatches, 71% in the 14 patients with 1 mismatch, and 67% in the 6 patients with 2 mismatches.[51]

Single- or Dual-Center Studies

A large number of single- or dual-center studies have also examined the effect of HLA matching on cadaver graft survival, highlights of which are presented in Table 9-8. Eleven of these studies reported an advantage to HLA matching,[*] and three did not.[73,86,178] The University of Minnesota reported that HLA matching for 2 or more antigens resulted in significantly superior 2- to 4-year patient and cadaver graft survival compared with that of recip-

ients matched for only 0 or 1 HLA antigen.[8] In 149 nondiabetic recipients of a first cadaver allograft performed before September, 1975, there was at 2 years 95% patient and 87% graft survival rate in those matched for 2 or more HLA-A and -B antigens compared with 72% and 65%, respectively, in those matched for only 0 to 1 antigen ($p<0.05$).[8] In Leiden, among 208 transfused cadaveric allograft recipients, there were 6-month graft survival rates of 87% in 23 patients with 4 antigens identical with their cadaver donor, 79% in 33 patients with no mismatched antigens, 68% in 95 patients with 1 mismatch, and 49% in 57 patients with 2 or more mismatched A or B antigens ($p<0.001$).[190] In recipients of first cadaver grafts at the National Hospital in Oslo, an improvement was seen in graft survival based on matching for HLA-A and -B.[2] Although the graft survivals rates were relatively low in these 373 cadaver recipients, the graft survival at 1 year was 58% in those with 0 mismatches, 47% in those with 1 to 2 mismatches, and 35% in those with 3 to 4 mismatched HLA-A and -B antigens ($p<0.05$).[2] At Vanderbilt, where transplants were not done with less than a 2 antigen match, there was also a beneficial effect of HLA matching on cadaver allograft survival, so that at 1 year, there was a 69% ± 8% survival rate in those recipients with 4 antigen matches, 61% ± 4% in those with 3 antigen matches, and 46% ± 7% in those with just 2 HLA-A and -B matches.[141]

Since 1980, numerous single-center studies have focused on the effect of HLA-DR matching in the context of conventional immunosuppression (azathioprine, prednisone, and antilymphocyte globulin), cyclosporine, and blood transfusions (see Table 9-8). The earliest large study came from Oslo and reported that in 170 prospectively typed cadaveric recipients, there was a beneficial effect derived from avoiding DR antigen mismatches primarily, and A and B incompatibilities secondarily, among those who had DR incompatibilities as well.[113] The effect of mismatching was stronger than that of matching for the DR antigens.[113] In the University of Iowa's report of first cadaver renal allografts, those receiving 2 DR matched grafts had a 1-year actuarial graft survival rate of 92%, whereas those matched for 1 DR had a 65% survival rate, and those with 0 DR matched had only a 41% survival rate.[64] The feasibility of using DR matching was also highlighted by this same group, which specifically analyzed the question of how long a patient would wait in order to get a DR matched kidney.[62] For a recipient with 2 DR antigens identified, it was estimated that there would be an additional wait of approximately 78 days for a 0 DR mismatched graft,

---

* References 2,8,64,81,105,107,111,113,141,160,190

TABLE 9-8   Cadaver Renal Allograft Short-Term (1–2-Year) Survival
(Recent Single or Dual Center Studies)

STUDY (ref)	BEST MATCH SURVIVAL (%)	BEST MATCH (n)	TYPE OF BEST HLA MATCH	CYCLO-SPORINE	DIFFERENCE IN SURVIVAL BETWEEN BEST AND WORST MATCH* (%)	P
Ascher et al[8]	87	41	A,B ≥2 matches	no	+22	<0.05
van Hooff et al[190]†	79	33	A,B 0 mismatch	no	+30	<0.001
Albrechtsen et al[2]	58	68	A,B 0 mismatch	no	+23	<0.05
Richie et al[141]	69	36	A,B 4 matches	no	+23	‡
Moen et al[113]	80	45	DR 0 mismatch	no	+39	<0.05
Goeken et al[64]	92	12	DR 2 matches	no	+51	<0.005
Ting & Morris[184]	80	92	DR 0 mismatch	no§	+18	<0.006
Madsen et al[107]	72	57	DR 2 matches	no‖	+35	<0.001
Jakobsen et al[81]	72	97	DR 0 mismatch	no	+31	‡
Middleton et al[111]	94	17	A,B,DR 4–6 matches	no	+22	<0.05
Lucas et al[105]	84	43	DR 0 mismatch	no	+20–51	<0.05
Kahan et al[86]	59	79	DR 0–1 mismatch	no	+28	0.05
	78	69	DR 0–1 mismatch	yes	−2	NS
Taylor et al[178]	67	12	DR 2 matches	yes	−9	NS
Harris et al[73]	75	24	DR 0 mismatch	no	+38	0.01
	83	21	A,B,DR 0–1 mismatch	no	+47	—
	64	58	DR 0 mismatch	yes	−36	<0.001
	53	20	A,B,DR 0–1 mismatch	yes	−47	—

* When histocompatibilty is reported according to the number of HLA antigens *matched*, the worst match will be 0 antigens matched; when reported according to the number of antigens *mismatched*, the worst match will be all or all but one (in the case of 4 antigens) antigen matched.
† 6-month survival.
‡ Data not given.
§ 52 of 305 patients received cyclosporine.
‖ 6 of 201 patients received cyclosporine.

whereas with 1 recipient DR antigen identified, there would be an additional 180-day wait.[62] Even though the number of DR antigens has increased from the initial group of 8 specificities to the 14 shown in Table 9-1, the feasibility of matching is hampered primarily by the failure to share a well-matched kidney, a process that forces local patients to draw their kidneys only from a local pool, which necessarily will have a much smaller probability of providing a well-matched graft. The Iowa team had also made the remarkable observation earlier that if one were able to genotype the cadaver donor, having already genotyped the recipient, the results of such haplotype matching rather than individual antigen matching yielded results comparable to what was seen with living-related, haplotype-matched donor–recipient pairs.[183] In 31 cadaver donors genotyped by typical family studies, the survival rate at 1 year was 77% compared with 33% in those receiving completely mismatched kidneys.[183]

Certain single-center studies emphasized the effect of matching and transfusion. The Oxford, England group reported that in 305 recipients of first cadaver allografts, 52 of whom received cyclosporine, the beneficial effect of HLA-DR matching was seen at 3 months and that of A and B matching 3 years after transplantation.[184] Similar to what had been reported earlier from Oslo,[113] they found that HLA-A and -B matching did not influence the survival of grafts already well matched for HLA-DR, but did have a significant effect on graft survival when 1 or 2 DR antigens were mismatched (*p*<0.02).[184] DR matching exerted a significant effect in both transfused and untransfused patients (*p*<0.02, and <0.04, respectively), but there was an augmented matching effect with transfusion, the highest graft survival rate of 87% occurring in transfused recipients of a DR compatible graft and the lowest graft survival rates of 47% in untransfused recipients of a DR incompatible kidney.[184] Allograft survival rates were similar in untransfused recipients who received a DR compatible graft and in those who were transfused but received a DR incompatible graft (70% and 73% at 1 year, respectively).[184]

The combined HLA compatibility and transfusion effect has also been found in numerous other studies.[3,31,81,107,114,122,160] An analysis of 201 consecutive cadaveric renal transplants from Aarhus, Denmark has shown that at 6 months, 57 recipients of 2 DR matched grafts had a 72% survival rate compared with 52% in 98 recipients with 1 DR antigen matched and 37% in 46 recipients with 0 DR antigen matched ($p = 0.001$).[107] The effect of DR matching was apparent even in transfused patients among whom there was 71% graft survival at 6 months in those with 2 DR antigens matched compared with 55% and 33% in those with only 1 or 0 DR antigens shared ($p = 0.0005$).[107] From two transplant centers in Copenhagen that were not using cyclosporine for their patients, the 1-year cadaver graft survival rate was 72% for 97 HLA-DR compatible recipients compared with 41% for 49 incompatible recipients ($p = 0.0007$).[81] This effect persisted even when the data were stratified for transfusion status.[81]

Exceptionally high allograft success rates of 89% and 84% have been reported in renal allograft recipients with more than four transfusions who had complete matching for HLA-A, -B, and -DR or HLA-B and -DR, respectively.[31] Similarly, in the recent Iowa experience, survivals of 91% and 89% could be achieved in 1 or 0 DR mismatched recipients if they had 2 or more A and B antigens matched and had received transfusions pretransplantation.[160] The poor survivals, ranging from 0% to 67%, occurred in those DR mismatched recipients who had only one or neither of these factors present.[160] A similar potentiating effect of matching and blood transfusions had also been reported earlier from the Medical College of Virginia.[114]

Other reports of extraordinary cadaver graft success rates in well-matched, transfused recipients have come from Belfast, Ireland and the University of Kentucky.[105,111] The transplant unit in Belfast, Ireland, which was also the first to show the safety and efficacy of low-dose steroid therapy in cadaver recipients, in a study of 72 primary cadaver allograft recipients who did not receive cyclosporine, achieved a 90% graft survival rate in 10 recipients with 0 DR mismatches, 89% success in 36 recipients with 1 DR mismatch, and 65% success in 26 recipients with 2 DR mismatches.[111] Using combined A, B, and DR matching, there was 94% graft survival in 17 recipients with 4 to 6 shared antigens, 83% success in 23 recipients with 3 shared antigens, and 72% success in 32 recipients with only 0 to 2 shared antigens.[111] The University of Kentucky at Lexington reported that in first cadaver recipients not receiving cyclosporine, there was an 84% graft survival rate in 43 recipients with no DR mismatch,

64% success in 11 recipients with 1 DR mismatch, and 33% success in 3 patients with 2 DR mismatches.[105]

Three other single-center studies in which cadaver allograft recipients were treated with cyclosporine, however, failed to find any advantage to DR matching, although the matching effect usually persisted in conventionally treated patients.[73,86,178] The group from Houston has reported that in conventionally treated patients, HLA-A and -B matching slightly improved 1-year graft function with a 44% success rate in the 55 recipients of grafts having more than 2 incompatibilities compared with a 59% success rate in 56 recipients with fewer incompatibilities ($p = 0.05$).[86] HLA-DR compatibility was more effective with only a 31% graft survival rate in 32 recipients with 2 DR mismatches compared with 59% success in 79 recipients with 0 to 1 antigen mismatches ($p = 0.05$).[86] In the group with fewer than 2 HLA-A or -B mismatches and only 0 to 1 DR incompatibilities, there was 70% graft survival in 40 recipients compared with 31% to 46% success in those with greater incompatibility ($p = 0.01$).[86] However, with cyclosporine, 63 recipients of allografts with fewer than 2 A,B mismatches had 82% 1-year graft survival compared with 79% in 37 recipients of grafts with more than 2 A,B mismatches.[86] Similarly, there was virtually no difference based on DR mismatching, since 69 recipients with 0 to 1 DR mismatch had 78% graft survival compared with 80% in 31 recipients with 2 DR mismatches.[86] Even the best combined matching of fewer than 2 A,B and 0 to 1 DR mismatches in 39 recipients that produced an 80% graft survival rate was slightly less than the 82% survival rate seen in 54 recipients with either 2 DR mismatches or more than 2 A,B mismatches.[86]

In the Pittsburgh study, the 12-month cumulative actuarial graft survival for 2 DR matches was 67%, for 1 DR match it was 78%, and for 0 DR match it was 76%.[178] When the data were examined according to DR mismatching, there was 74% graft survival in 11 recipients with no mismatches, 77% in 34 recipients with 1 mismatch, and 76% in 35 recipients with no DR matching.[178] There was also no significant difference in the number of rejections per patient based on the degree of DR mismatching.[178] Some of the most surprising results appeared in the report of 275 renal allografts performed in Portsmouth, England.[73] In the 128 recipients treated with conventional therapy, there was a correlation between better matches and higher graft survival, whereas in the 147 recipients treated with cyclosporine, the reverse effect was found.[73] With azathioprine, there was 75% 1-year actuarial graft survival in 24 recipients with no DR mismatch, 45% success in 67 recipients with 1 DR mismatch, and 37% success in 37 recipients with 2 DR mismatches.[73] Combining A, B, and DR mismatching, there was 83% success in 21 patients with only 0 or 1 mismatch, 47% success in 98 patients with 2, 3, or 4 mismatches, and 36% success in 9 patients with 5 or 6 mismatches.[73] But the opposite effect was seen in those recipients treated with cyclosporine; there was 64% success in 58 patients with no DR mismatches, 66% success in 68 patients with 1 DR mismatch, and 100% success in 21 patients with 2 DR mismatches.[73] The combined effect of A, B, and DR mismatching was similar in cyclosporine-treated recipients in that 20 patients had 53% success with 0 or 1 mismatch, 105 patients had 64% success with 2, 3, or 4 mismatches, and 22 patients had 100% success with 5 or 6 mismatches.[73] This group noted that pretransplant blood transfusions also had a deleterious effect on graft survival in those patients who were receiving cyclosporine.[73]

In conclusion, although there are conflicting short-term results in some single-center studies that use cyclosporine, the impressive findings of the International Transplantation Study, the UCLA collaborative study, and others substantiate a significant matching effect even in the presence of cyclosporine. Moreover, studies such as those from the University of Kentucky and Belfast have shown that cadaver allograft success rates from 84% to 94% can be achieved with HLA matching and excellent clinical care in the absence of cyclosporine.[105,111] There is little doubt that in conventionally treated cadaver allograft recipients, there is a significant matching effect that may be augmented by transfusions.

Long-Term (4–10 Year) Cadaver Allograft Survival (Table 9-9)

The eight major studies that have addressed the effect of HLA matching on long-term cadaver allograft outcome have all shown a significant advantage for its use.[8,14,42,54,130,141,148,184] In the 1980 annual report of France Transplant, the 8-year graft survival in 2069 recipients of a first cadaver allograft was approximately double in those recipients who were matched for 3 or 4 A and B series antigens (38%) and those matched for 2 A and B antigens (34%) compared with those matched for just 0 or 1 A or B antigen (20%) ($p<0.001$).[42] Similar results in the United States have been obtained by SEOPF in a study that showed that at 4 years there was 44% allograft survival for those with 4 antigens of the A and B series antigens matched compared with only 18% for those with 0 matched A or B anti-

gens.[148] In the Oxford experience, at 5 years, HLA-A and -B antigens had their effect when DR mismatching had occurred.[184] Among 195 patients who received 1 or 2 DR antigen mismatched kidneys, there was, at 5 years, 63% survival in those with no A, B mismatches, 52% in those with 1 or 2 A, B mismatches, and 33% in those with 3 or 4 A and B mismatches ($p<0.02$).[184] However, in 92 recipients with no DR mismatches, the survival rates only slightly decreased from 75% with no A, B mismatches to 73% with 1 or 2 mismatches, and 66% with 3 or 4 A, B mismatches.[184] After recalculation for the DR effect only, it appears that 0 DR mismatches would yield approximately 70% 5-year graft survival and 1 or 2 DR mismatches only 45% survival.[184] The initial benefit of HLA-A, -B matching seen at 2 years in the Minnesota experience was also apparent at 4 years when there was 82% success in those with 2 or more antigens matched compared with approximately 57% for those with fewer than 2 antigens matched.[8] Follow-up data of the European Dialysis and Transplant Association and of the Eurotransplant Foundation showed that in 2522 recipients of a first cadaver graft, the 5-year survival rate in recipients of a kidney with 0 A or B antigens mismatched was 51% compared with 32% when all 4 antigens were mismatched.[130] In 2648 cadaver kidney transplants from Australia, there was also a significant matching effect for HLA-A and -B at 5 years, with a 54% graft survival rate in the 187 recipients with no antigen mismatched compared with a 32% to 40% survival rate in those with 2 to 4 mismatched antigens.[14] In a single-center study in which all the kidneys were matched for at least 2 HLA-A and -B antigens, the effect of matching at 5 years was apparent even at the higher degrees of matching: 64% ± 9% in 36 patients with 4 antigens matched, 52% ± 4% in 181 patients with 3 antigens matched, and 32% ± 6% in 54 patients with 2 antigens matched.[141] With follow-up to 12 years, the London Transplant Group has reported significant advantages for HLA-A and -B matching at 5 and 10 years ($p=0.0001$) and for DR matching at 5 years ($p=0.02$).[54]

Because the fall-off in allograft survival with time in cyclosporine-treated patients has thus far not differed significantly from that seen in conventionally treated patients, it is likely that there will also be a long-term matching effect here.[27]

Repeat Cadaver Transplants (Table 9-10)

Approximately 15% of all transplants performed each year in the United States are retransplants. A number of factors, particularly the duration of func-

TABLE 9-9   *Cadaver Renal Allograft Long-Term (4–10-Year) Survival*

STUDY (ref)	YEARS AFTER TRANSPLANT	TYPE OF BEST HLA MATCH	BEST MATCH SURVIVAL (%)	(n)	WORST MATCH SURVIVAL (%)	(n)	P
Festenstein et al, 1986[54]	10	A,B 3–4 matches	47	144	19	51	0.001
	5	A,B 3–4 matches	54	144	32	51	0.001
Dausset, 1980[42]	8	A,B, 3–4 matches	38	679	20	361	0.00001
Ting & Morris, 1984[184]	5	A,B 0 mismatch (with 1–2 DR mismatches)	63	19	33	77	0.02
	5	DR 0 mismatch	70*	92*	45	195	†
Persijn et al, 1982[130]	5	A,B 0 mismatch	51	471	32	92	0.0005
Bashir et al, 1982[14]	5	A,B 0 mismatch	54	187	40	133	0.005
Richie et al, 1979[141]	5	A,B 4 matches	64 ± 9	36	32 ± 6	54	†
Sanfilippo et al, 1984[148]	4	A,B 4 matches	44 ± 7	141	18 ± 4	542	0.05
Ascher et al, 1979[8]	4	A,B ≥2 matches	82	41	57	108	0.05

* Calculated from reported data.

† Data not reported.

TABLE 9-10   *Effect of HLA Matching on the Outcome of Repeat Cadaver Renal Transplants*

STUDY (ref)	BEST MATCH SURVIVAL (%)	BEST MATCH (n)	TYPE OF BEST HLA MATCH	CYCLO-SPORINE	DIFFERENCE IN SURVIVAL BETWEEN BEST AND WORST MATCH (%)	TIME AFTER TRANS-PLANTA-TION (yr)	P
Sanfilippo et al[184]	48 ± 17	*	A,B 4 matches	no	+36	4	*
Bashir et al[14]	47	100	B 2 matches	no	+14	5	<0.005
Lucas et al[105]	80	10	DR 0 mismatch	no	+51	1	*
Perdue[129]	*	*	A,B 3–4 matches	no	*	1	<0.005
Opelz[123]	80	49	A,B,DR 0 mismatch	no	+25	2/3	*
	68	97	B,DR 0 mismatch	no	+18	1	*
	66	124	A,B 0 mismatch	no	+16	1	*

* Data not reported.

tion and cause of the first graft failure, have been examined for their influence on the outcome of the second renal graft at varying post-transplant periods. For those grafts lost in less than 6 months, the degree of HLA matching (3 to 4 A and B matches vs. 0 to 1) was of major importance ($p<0.005$) in the success of the second graft from the first month to the end of the period of analysis at 12 months.[129] However, a more dominant matching effect occurred in later post-transplant periods, especially in those recipients whose first graft had a long duration. In the SEOPF study, the benefit of matching was even more impressive in patients receiving repeat allografts, notably at 4 years, when the differ-

ence in survivals widened to 48% ± 17% for those with 4 antigens matched compared with only 12% ± 7% for those with 0 matched HLA-A and -B antigens.[148] In the Australian experience, the poor survival of secondary grafts was related to mismatching for HLA-B antigens.[14] Significant improvement in graft survival that began by 1 year and persisted to 5 years after transplantation was seen in 100 recipients with no mismatched HLA-B antigen who maintained approximately a 10% to 19% advantage over those with 1 or 2 mismatched HLA-B antigens.[14] Specifically, at 1 year, the survivals were 62% versus 43% and 52%, respectively, and at 5 years, 47% versus 28% and 33%, respectively (*p*<0.05 and <0.005, respectively).[14] In a small number of retransplanted patients, none of whom received cyclosporine, a beneficial effect of DR matching was suggested with an 80% 1-year graft survival rate in the 10 patients with no DR mismatches, 50% in the 6 patients with 1 DR mismatch, and only 29% in the 7 patients with 2 DR mismatches.[105]

In the International Collaborative Transplant Study, second cadaver allografts at 8 months had an 80% survival rate in 49 recipients with no A, B, or DR antigen mismatches compared with a 55% survival rate in 95 recipients with 5 or 6 mismatches.[124] In this same study, 97 retransplanted patients with 0 mismatches for B and DR antigens had 1-year graft survival rates of 68% compared with 50% in 60 recipients with all 4 of these antigens mismatched. Even A and B matching was important because 66% of 124 second cadaver allografts with no A or B mismatches survived to 1 year compared with 50% of 95 grafts with all 4 A and B antigens mismatched.[124]

Special considerations in retransplantation are re-exposure to the same mismatched antigen and the existence of recipient antibody to a mismatched antigen of the repeat transplant, either of which would be expected to have an adverse effect on allograft survival. But the mixed results indicate that the initial sensitization may fade with time or evoke suppressor as well as cytotoxic mechanisms. Thirteen patients who had at least one mismatched antigen that was the same in the first and second donor had the same allograft survivals (54%) as those without repeated mismatched antigens.[7] A similar result was seen in Terasaki's collaborative study in which the repetition of the same HLA antigen mismatch in 180 second graft recipients did not appear to lessen the survival rate when compared with 925 grafts with no such repeated incompatibility.[127] However, in a recent collaborative study, 9 of 15 patients re-exposed to the same mismatched donor antigen have lost their allografts.[61] Moreover, additional data from both the International Collaborative Study[125] and from the survey by the American Society for Histocompatibility and Immunogenetics[61] indicate that persons receiving a second transplant have a sharply lower success rate (52% and 48%, respectively) than those receiving a first graft (67% and 65%, respectively) when they have a remote positive but current negative T cell crossmatch or a positive current B-lymphocyte crossmatch (*p*<0.01).[61] Similarly, among recipients sensitized to greater than 25% of a lymphocyte panel, despite a negative donor crossmatch, second allografts had significantly worse survival (*p* = 0.02).[41]

An extremely important but previously ignored aspect of HLA matching for cadaver organ recipients is the detrimental effect that poor matching of a first graft has on recipient sensitization levels and retransplantation rates. In a combined study of 397 first cadaver renal allograft recipients transplanted at four centers from 1978 to 1982 in which the same percentage of patients with poorly matched (0 to 1 antigen match) and well matched (3 to 4 antigens matched) first grafts were placed on the waiting list (46% and 47%, respectively), those who had had a well-matched first cadaver graft subsequently had lower panel reactive antibody (PRA) levels (37% ± 4% vs. 51% ± 6%, respectively; *p*<0.05) and were more likely to be retransplanted (67% vs. 47%, respectively; *p*<0.004).[147] Thus, the consequences of poor matching include not only lower success rates for the first cadaver graft but also more difficulty in retransplantation.

Modification of Steroid or Azathioprine Dosage

The recent SEOPF study provided data showing that both in first transplants and repeat transplants, there was a significantly lower amount of prednisone and methylprednisolone used in better-matched recipients than in the poorer-matched recipients.[148] For example, the first-year cumulative prednisone dose decreased from 11,206 mg in the poorly matched first cadaver recipients to 10,572 mg in the better-matched recipients (*p* = 0.04), and methylprednisolone dosage decreased from an average of 5,548 mg to 3,634 mg (*p* = 0.0001), respectively.[148] Similar significant differences were apparent in repeat transplants. In another approach to the steroid question, gradual attempts to stop prednisone in patients who left the hospital with a functioning cadaver allograft were successful in 12 patients who had an average of only 0.58 incompatible antigens, temporarily successful in another 24 patients with mean mismatch antigen levels of 0.83, and impossible in 66 patients with the highest average level of incompatible antigens at 1.29.[95]

In patients requiring the discontinuation of azathioprine because of severe liver disease or cancer, 10 of the 30 cadaver kidney recipients showed subsequent deterioration in graft function, an outcome significantly more frequent in recipients of an allograft mismatched for 2 to 4 HLA-A or -B antigens (*p* = 0.02).[29] In another series of 305 recipients of first cadaver allografts, 54% of those with no DR mismatches were able to receive low-dose steroids, compared with 31% and 33% of those with 1 and 2 DR mismatches, respectively, yet the 0 DR mismatched recipients had better graft survival (79%) than those with 1 or 2 DR mismatches (62%).[184]

The role of MLC reactivity in determining steroid reduction or withdrawal was discussed earlier (see Mixed Lymphocyte Culture).

DRw6 and Renal Allograft Rejection

The initial report of this effect described a 1-year allograft survival rate of 75% in 130 DRw6-negative recipients compared with just 59% success in 44 DRw6-positive patients whose graft failure typically occurred in the first 3 months ($p = 0.01$).[78] This finding suggested that DRw6-positive recipients were "high responders." The more remarkable finding was that DR matching significantly improved allograft survival only in DRw6-positive patients who had a 95% graft survival rate with no mismatched DR antigens and only a 38% survival rate with 2 DR antigens mismatched ($p = 0.009$).[78] In contrast, in DRw6-negative patients, there was only a slight effect of DR matching with an 83% 1-year allograft survival rate in those with no DR mismatching compared with 72% in those with 2 DR mismatches.[78]

The concept of DRw6 positivity characterizing a "hyperresponder" received additional support from the finding that the formation of endothelial/monocyte antibodies in recipients who rejected their first allograft was almost entirely restricted to those who had DRw6.[78] Other support of the high responder capability of persons with DRw6 was suggested by the fact that DRw6-positive lymphocytes bound streptococcal antigen and optimally elicited helper factor in the dose range of 1 or 10 ng compared with a much higher dose of 1,000 ng for cells bearing DR1, 2, 3, 4, or 5.[100]

However, since those initial reports, many studies have failed to support the DRw6 hyperresponder concept.[54,74,87,89] In a series of 271 recipients of a cadaver graft, the presence of DRw6 either in the recipient or the donor had no significant effect on overall graft survival irrespective of whether cyclosporine or azathioprine was used.[74] In 339 allograft cases in which 18% of the recipients and 17% of the cadaver donors were positive for DRw6, the 1-year actuarial graft survival rate was 70% overall, 67% in the 60 DRw6-positive recipients, and 71% in the 279 DRw6-negative recipients.[89] Whether their donors were DRw6-positive or -negative made no difference. An evaluation of the DRw6-positive patients for their immune responsiveness showed that only 25% had a strong responder status compared with 85% of the DRw6-negative recipients.[89] The UCLA Collaborative Study also could not confirm the association between DRw6 and high immune responsiveness.[87] Rather than detecting a DRw6-positive high-responder group, this study found that patients with DR1 produced the lowest levels of cytotoxic antibody and that patients who were either homozygous for DR1 or were DR1 and DR5 had the best 1-year graft survival rates of 74% and 80%, respectively.[87] In the International Collaborative Transplant Study, when DRw6-positive recipients had DRw6-positive donors, their 6-month graft survival rate was 80%, whereas with DRw6-negative donors, the survival rate dropped to 58%.[122] Surprisingly, DRw6-negative recipients of DRw6-positive kidneys had intermediate and relatively good survival rates of 68%, the same result seen in both DRw6-positive and DRw6-negative recipients alone.[122] In the Australian study in which 67 of 276 cadaver recipients had DRw6, there also was no significant difference in the 1-year graft survival between the groups, DRw6-positive being 54.3% ± 6.2%, and DRw6-negative being 53.7% ± 3%.[41]

The explanation for these conflicting results involves both clinical and serologic areas. First, part of the difficulty in assigning a high-responder status to recipients with DRw6 may be that in some laboratories, the DRw6 antigen may be inadequately defined. Furthermore, DRw6 has several subdivisions, only two of which, namely, DRw13 and DRw14, are identifiable with available serologic reagents.[118,159] It is possible that one of these subdivisions of DRw6 is the critical antigen. Second, allograft survival is a relatively crude measure of a single antigen effect. However, the data do indicate that the DRw6 antigen by itself in the recipient does not necessarily identify a hyperresponder, because DRw6-positive recipients showed both the best and the worst graft survivals, depending upon whether their donor was matched or mismatched, respectively, for DRw6.[122] Alternatively, the presence of DRw6 in a donor may impart only weak immunogenicity.

Center Effect

One of the strongest influences on the outcome of cadaver allograft success and the one with the least explanation is the "center" effect. Perhaps the first description of this in the renal transplant literature was the Kidney Transplant and Histocompatibility Study conducted from 1974 to 1976.[11] In this study, the observed-to-expected risk of patient and allograft loss among the 20 largest contributing centers showed a threefold difference between the extremes of those centers, a finding not explained by chance and not unexpected in view of the experience in other scientific collaborative studies.[11] At least two other major collaborative renal transplant studies have also documented the significant influence of a center effect in cadaver transplantation.[34,122] In the International Collaborative Transplant Study, major contributing centers were able to be grouped into "good centers," with average 1-year allograft cadaver survivals of nearly 80%; "medium" centers, with allograft survival approximating 70%; and "poor" centers, with allograft survival averaging 60%.[122] Within each of these transplant center rankings, there was a stratification based on DR matching, so that in the good centers, 0 and 1 DR mismatched grafts had identical survivals of 80% and the 2 DR mismatched grafts 73%; in the medium centers, the 0 DR mismatched grafts had 71% survival, those with 1 mismatch 66% survival, and those with 2 mismatches 57% survival; in the poor centers, the 0 DR mismatched grafts had 61% 1-year survival, those with 1 mismatch 52% survival, and those with 2 mismatches 50% survival. It can be seen that the best survival of 71% in the medium group was nearly that of the worst survival in the good centers, namely 73%, and that the best survival of 61% in the poor centers was close to the worst results in the medium group, namely, 57%.[122]

A more extensive analysis of the "center" effect has recently been reported.[34] Transplant centers that had performed at least 100 first cadaver transplants were classified as "excellent, good, or fair" based on their overall cadaver graft survival rates at 1 year of 62%, 51%, and 39%, respectively, from 1965 through 1984. There was a constant 10% difference in graft survival between the centers during any time period. In the first 3 months after transplantation, the "fair" centers lost 60% to 80% more kidney grafts and from 6 to 48 months 80% to 100% more grafts than did the excellent centers, even though the loss diminished to just 1.1% per month in the "fair" centers compared with 0.6% per month in the "excellent" centers.[34] This same center effect also held for the different success achieved in second cadaver grafts and living-related transplants. In both univariate and multivariate analyses, the center effect was more important than the transfusion effect, HLA matching, or the other traditional factors thought to contribute to allograft success.

Certain practices were noted in the different types of centers. For example, "excellent" centers transfused more of their patients with a higher number of units, matched their patients for HLA-A, -B, and -DR, and achieved a greater degree of success with cyclosporine therapy.[34] Even though "fair" centers had an improvement in graft survival with more than four transfusions, the transfused recipients at "fair" centers had poorer graft survivals than did nontransfused patients at "excellent" centers (53% and 56%, respectively).[34] With respect to matching, almost twice the percentage of patients were matched for 1 or 2 DR antigens at the "excellent" and "good" centers compared with the "fair" centers (31%, 31%, and 17%, respectively).[34] Furthermore, a remarkable 92% graft survival rate was achieved in "excellent" centers when there was no mismatching for A, B, or DR antigens, 81% when there was no mismatching for the A or DR antigens, and 84% when there was no mismatching for B or DR antigens.[34] Two major clinical factors implicated in graft survival were the immunosuppression used and the management of graft rejection episodes. The "excellent" and "good" centers had 11% and 8% increases, respectively, in their graft survival when cyclosporine was used, while the "fair" centers actually had a 3% decrease.[34]

The center effect for patient mortality was detected only during the first year after transplant and not beyond.[34] Although there was a 20% difference in 1-year graft survival from the "fair" to the "excellent" centers between 1978 and 1984, there was only a 3% difference in patient mortality.[34] Consequently, the center effect on patient survival has virtually disappeared.

Other factors such as race, recipient age, original disease, warm ischemia time, cold ischemia time, and the level of cytotoxic antibody did not contribute significantly to the center effect.[34]

Strategies for Cadaver Donor Matching

There is no doubt that matching for both HLA haplotypes, a task that requires genotyping the donor and recipient, is accompanied by exceptionally good short-term and long-term allograft survival with less immunosuppression as documented in living-related transplants. In cadaver transplantation without cyclosporine, the best matching, namely, that approaching two haplotypes, can itself achieve graft survivals in the range of 84% to 94%.[31,54,105,111,123,160,184] Assuming that recipient genotyping can be done, the problem is how to approximate two haplotype matches when cadaver donors are only phenotyped. The first strategy, then, is directed at estimating or establishing the cadaver haplotypes. There seems little likelihood that the genotyping of cadaver donors once accomplished by the University of Iowa team will be duplicated.[183] Currently, partial haplotype matching by means of HLA-B and -DR antigens provides the greatest contribution of any two HLA antigen series with or without cyclosporine.[54,123] As more of the D region antigens other than HLA-DR that contribute to MLC reactivity become routinely typed, such as DQ and DP, the matching effect should become even stronger. Extended haplotype matching that includes the complement components already can predict MLC compatibility for some donor–recipient pairs.[9]

The second strategy is aimed at taking advantage of information about the way that a patient responds to blood transfusions in order to select the best of mismatched donors. If the recipient makes no antibody to blood transfusions, a better subsequent kidney donor would theoretically be one matched for Class II antigens as a priority over A and B identities.[44] The basis for this is that such persons have already demonstrated that by not making antibody to the HLA-bearing cells in blood transfusions, they have the capability to make a T suppressor factor that will mitigate the effects of additional incompatible A and B antigens.[152] On the other hand, if the recipient has made antibody to transfusion challenges, priority should be given to A and B identity because this person has had a predominant response by T helper lymphocytes primed to respond to Class I antigens in general.[44]

For retransplants, a third strategy for those losing a graft to early rejection involves matching with more emphasis on HLA-A and -B compatibility, being more suspect of the usually safe remote positive-current negative T cell crossmatch circumstance, and avoiding positive B cell crossmatches.[14,61,105,124,148]

A fourth strategy applies to an extremely critical area, the successful transplantation of highly sensitized recipients. This can be done by defining the specificity of the recipient antibodies (and thereby the corresponding unacceptable potential donor antigens in the population) so that a "safe" donor antigen profile can be established for each patient. Furthermore, by knowing the population frequencies of the "safe" donor HLA antigens and acceptable red cell antigens, one can calculate the cumulative probability of transplantability (P_c) that predicts the needed size of a donor pool for rapid transplantation.[196] Ultimately this solution will depend upon a sharing mechanism linking the full resources of the national organ pool to the clearly defined requirements of sensitized recipients that include not just the avoidance of a positive crossmatch but also the achievement of better matching.[26,105,124,147,148,196]

A fifth strategy centers on expanding the molecular[106] and early clinical[54] evidence that the MT antigens (DRw52 and DRw53) are distinct and important broad transplantation antigens. There would be an immense practical advantage achieved in matching if only two such broad antigens were responsible for the majority of the histocompatibility or matching effect. Further molecular studies may provide not only new and firmer foundations for understanding histocompatibility in human transplantation but also simpler and more practical approaches for its use.

REFERENCES

1. Advisory Committee of the Human Kidney Transplant Registry. 7th Report of the Human Kidney Transplant Registry. Transplantation 8:721, 1969
2. Albrechtsen D, Bratlie A, Kiss E et al: Significance of HLA matching in renal transplantation. Transplantation 28:280, 1979
3. Albrechtsen D, Moen T, Flatmark A et al: Influence of HLA-A, B, C, D, and DR matching in renal transplantation. Transplant Proc 13:924, 1981
4. Amos DB, Ward FE: Immunogenetics of the HLA system. Physiol Rev 55:206, 1975
5. Anderson CB, Sicard GA, Etheredge EE: Pretreatment of renal allograft recipients with azathioprine and donor-specific blood products. Surgery 92:315, 1982
6. Antenried P, Halloran PF: Cyclosporine blocks the induction of Class I and Class II MHC products in mouse kidney by graft-vs-host disease. J Immunol 135:3922, 1985
7. Ascher NL, Ahrenholz DH, Simmons RL et al: 100 second renal allografts from a single transplantation institution. Transplantation 27:30, 1979
8. Ascher NL, Simmons RL, Fryd D et al: Effects of HLA-A and B matching on success of cadaver grafts at a single center. Transplantation 28:172, 1979
9. Awdeh ZL, Alper CA, Eynon E et al: Unrelated individuals' matched MHC extended haplotypes and HLA-identical siblings show comparable responses in mixed lymphocyte culture. Lancet 2:853, 1985
10. Barclay AN, Mason DW: Induction of Ia antigen in rat epidermal cells and gut epithelium by immunological stimuli. J Exp Med 156:1665, 1982
11. Barnes BA, Olivier D: For the principal investigators of the KTHS. Analysis of NIAID kidney transplant histocompatibility study (KTHS): Factors associated with transplant outcomes. I. Transplant Proc 13:65, 1981
12. Barry JM, Hefty T, Fischer SM et al: Donor-specific blood transfusions and successful spousal kidney transplantation. J Urol 133:1024, 1985
13. Basham TY, Merigan TC: Recombinant interferon-γ increases HLA-DR synthesis and expression. J Immunol 130:1492, 1983
14. Bashir HV, d'Apice A, on behalf of a committee:

Cadaver renal transplantation and HLA matching in Australia from 1971–1980: A report of the Australian and New Zealand combined dialysis and transplant registry. Transplantation 34:183, 1982

15. Bell JI, Denny DW Jr, McDevitt HO: Structure and polymorphism of murine and human Class II major histocompatibility antigens. Immunol Rev 84:51, 1985

16. Ben-David A, Orgad S, Danon Y et al: HL-A antigen changes in patients treated with chloramphenicol. Tissue Antigens 3:378, 1973

17. Benacerraf B: Role of MHC gene products in immune regulation. Science 212:1229, 1981

18. Benson EM, Colvin RB, Russell PS: Induction of Ia antigens in murine renal transplants. J Immunol 134:7, 1985

19. Berah M, Hors J, Dausset J: A study of HL-A antigens in human organs. Transplantation 9:185, 1970

20. Berg B, Groth CG, Lundgeen C et al: The influence of HLA-D matching on the outcome of interfamilial kidney transplantation with special emphasis on the predictive value of the relative response in MLC. Scand J Urol Nephrol (Suppl) 64:46, 1981

21. Bertrams J, Kuwert E, Gallmeier WM et al: Transient lymphocyte HL-A antigen "loss" in the case of irradiated M. Hodgkin. Tissue Antigens 1:105, 1971

22. Bieber CP, Hunt SA, Schwinn DA et al: Complications in long-term survivors of cardiac transplantation. Transplant Proc 13:207, 1981

23. Bodmer JG, Kennedy LJ, Aizawa M et al: HLA-D region monoclonal antibodies. In Albert ED, Baur, MP, Mayr WR (eds): Histocompatibility Testing 1984. Berlin, Springer-Verlag, 1984

24. Boettcher B: Haploid expression of HLA genes on spermatozoa. Lancet 1:363, 1977

25. Braun WE: Histocompatibility testing in clinical renal transplantation. Urol Clin 10:231, 1983

26. Braun WE: Management of the sensitized patient awaiting a cadaver allograft. Artif Organs (in press)

27. Calne RY, Wood AJ: Cyclosporin in cadaveric renal transplantation: 3-year follow-up of a European Multicentre Trial. Lancet 2:549, 1985

28. Cameron JS: Glomerulonephritis in renal transplants. Transplantation 34:237, 1982

29. Campos H, Kreis HA, Rioux P et al: Azathioprine withdrawal in renal transplant recipients: A long-term follow-up. Transplantation 38:29, 1984

30. Cats S: Effect of Cyclosporin A in kidney transplantation. In Terasaki PI (ed): Clinical Kidney Transplants 1985, pp 217–226. Los Angeles, UCLA Tissue Typing Laboratory, 1985

31. Cecka M, Cicciarelli J: The transfusion effect. In Terasaki PI (ed): Clinical Kidney Transplants 1985, pp 73–92. Los Angeles, UCLA Tissue Typing Laboratory, 1985

32. Cerilli J, Brasile L, Clarke J et al: The vascular endothelial cell-specific antigen system three years' experience in monocyte crossmatching. Transplant Proc 17:567, 1985

33. Chen YX, Evans RL, Pollack MS et al: Characteri-

zation and expression of the HLA-DC antigens defined by anti-Leu 10. Human Immunol 10:221, 1984

34. Cicciarelli J: Transplant center and kidney graft survival. In Terasaki PI (ed): Clinical Kidney Transplants 1985, pp 93–110. Los Angeles, UCLA Tissue Typing Laboratory, 1985.

35. Claas F, Castelli-Visser R, Schreuder I et al: Alloantibodies to an antigenic determinant shared by HLA-A2 and B17. Tissue Antigens 19:388, 1982

36. Cochrum KC, Salvatierra O, Perkins HA et al: MLC testing in renal transplantation. Transplant Proc 7(Suppl 1):659, 1975

37. Cohen D, Paul P, LeGall I et al: DNA polymorphism of HLA Class I and Class II regions. Immunol Rev 85:87, 1985

38. Colombani J, Colombani M, Degos L et al: Effect of cross reactions on HL-A antigen immunogenicity. Tissue Antigens 4:136, 1974

39. Crumpton MJ, Bodmer JG, Bodmer WF et al: Biochemistry of Class II antigens: Workshop report. In Albert ED, Baur MP, Mayr WR (eds): Histocompatibility Testing 1984, pp 29–37. Berlin, Springer-Verlag, 1984

40. Daar AS, Fuggle SV, Ting A et al: Anomalous expression of HLA-DR antigens on human colo-rectal cancer cells. J Immunol 129:447, 1982

41. D'Apice AJF, Sheil AGR, Tait BD et al: A prospective randomized trial of matching for HLA-A and B versus HLA-DR in renal transplantation. Transplantation 38:37, 1984

42. Dausset J: France-Transplant Annual Report, 1980

43. Dausset J, Cohen D: HLA at the gene level. In Albert ED, Baur MP, Mayr WR (eds): Histocompatibility Testing 1984, pp 22–28. Berlin, Springer-Verlag, 1984

44. Dausset J, Contu L: MHC in general biological recognition: Its theoretical implications in transplantation. Transplant Proc 13:895, 1981

45. Dausset J, Nenna A: Presence d'une leuco agglutine dans le serum d'un cas d'agranulocytose chronique. C R Biol (Paris) 146:1539, 1952

46. Dausset J, Rapaport FT, Legrand L et al: Skin allograft survival in 238 human subjects. Role of specific relationships at the four gene sites of the First and Second HL-A loci. In Terasaki PI (ed): Histocompatibility Testing 1970, pp 381–397. Copenhagen, Munksgaard, 1970

47. Doughty RW, Goodier SR, Gelsthorpe K: Further evidence for HL-A antigens present on adult peripheral red blood cells. Tissue Antigens 3:189, 1973

48. Dupont B, Jersild C, Hansen GS et al: Typing for MLC determinants by means of LD-homozygous and LD-heterozygous test cells. Transplant Proc 5:1543, 1973

49. Duquesnoy RJ, Annen KB, Marrari MM et al: Association of MB compatibility with succesful intrafamilial kidney transplantation. N Engl J Med 302:821, 1980

50. Eijsvogel, VP: The cellular recognition in vitro of

antigens related to human histocompatibility. Semin Hematol 11:305, 1974

51. European Multicentre Trial Group. Cyclosporin in cadaveric renal transplantation: One-year follow-up of a multicentre trial. Lancet 2:986, 1983

52. Fellous M, Dausset J: Probable haploid expression of HL-A antigens on human spermatozoon. Nature 225:191, 1970

53. Ferrarra GB, Tosi RM, Longo A et al: Low immunogenicity of the third HLA series. Transplantation 20:340, 1975

54. Festenstein H, Doyle P, Holmes J: Long-term follow-up in London Transplant Group recipients of cadaver renal allografts. N Engl J Med 314:7, 1986

55. First MR, Munda R, Kant KS et al: Steroid withdrawal following HLA-identical related donor transplantation. Transplant Proc 13:319, 1981

55a. Fitch FW: T-lymphocyte clones having defined immunological functions. Transplantation 32:171, 1981

56. Flechner S, Kerman RH, van Buren CT et al: The use of Cyclosporin A for high MLC haploidentical living-related transplants. Transplant Proc 15:442, 1983

57. Flechner SM, Kerman RH, van Buren C et al: Mixed lymphocyte culture hyporesponsiveness as a marker for steroid withdrawal in cyclosporine-treated living-related renal transplants. Transplant Proc 17:1260, 1985

58. Fuggle SV, Errasti P, Daar AS et al: Localization of major histocompatibility complex (HLA-ABC and DR) antigens in 46 kidneys: Differences in HLA-DR staining of tubules among kidneys. Transplantation 35:385, 1983

59. Garovoy MR, Reinschmidt MA, Bigos M et al: Flow cytometry analysis (FCA): A high technology cross-match technique facilitating transplantation. Transplant Proc 15:1939, 1983

60. Glassock RJ, Feldman D, Reynolds ES et al: Human renal isografts: A clinical and pathologic analysis. Medicine 47:411, 1968

61. Goeken NE: Outcome of renal transplantation following a positive crossmatch with historical sera: The second analysis of the ASHI survey. Transplant Proc 17:2443, 1985

62. Goeken NE, Schulak JA, Nghiem DD et al: Feasibility of optimal HLA-DR matching: A retrospective view. Transplantation 34:297, 1982

63. Goeken NE, Thompson JS: Functional cell mediated lympholysis: II. Genetics Tissue Antigens 17:411, 1981

64. Goeken NE, Thompson JS, Corry RJ: A 2-year trial of prospective HLA-DR matching. Effects on renal allograft survival and rate of transplantation. Transplantation 32:522, 1981

65. Goodfellow PN, Jones EA, van Heynigen V et al: The β_2-microglobulin gene is on chromosome 15 and not in the HLA region. Nature 254:267, 1975

66. Gross-Wilde H, Doxiadis I, Brandt H: Definition of HLA-D with HTC. In Albert ED, Baur MP, Mayr WR (eds): Histocompatibility Testing 1984, pp 249–264. Berlin, Springer-Verlag, 1984

67. Guy K, van Heyningen V: An ordered sequence of expression of human MHC Class-II antigens during B-cell maturation? Immunol Today 4:186, 1983

68. Halgrimson CG, Penn I, Booth C et al: Eight-to-ten year follow-up in early cases of renal homotransplantation. Transplant Proc 5:787, 1973

69. Hall BM, Bishop GA, Duggin GG et al: Increased expression of HLA-DR antigens on renal tubular cells in renal transplants: Relevance to the rejection response. Lancet 2:247, 1984

70. Halloran PF, Jephthah-Ochola J, Urmson J et al: Systemic immunologic stimuli increase Class I and Class II antigen expression in mouse kidney. J Immunol 135:1053, 1985

71. Hammerling GJ: Tissue distribution of Ia antigens and their expression on lymphocyte subpopulations. Transplant Rev 30:64, 1976

72. Hanafusa T, Pujol-Borrel R, Chiovato L et al: Aberrant expression of HLA-DR antigen on thyrocytes in Graves' disease: Relevance for autoimmunity. Lancet 2:1111, 1983

73. Harris KR, Digard N, Gosling DC et al: Azathioprine and cyclosporine: Different tissue matching criteria needed? Lancet 2:802, 1985

74. Harris KR, Digard NJ, Gosling DC: HLA-DR matching in renal transplant patients on cyclosporine. Transplant Proc 17:42, 1985

75. Harris R, Zervas JD: Reticulocyte HL-A antigens. Nature 221:1062, 1969

76. Hartzman RJ, Segall M, Bach ML et al: Histocompatibility matching. VI. Miniaturization of the mixed leukocyte culture test: A preliminary report. Transplantation 11:268, 1971

77. Hayry P, von Willebrand F, Ahoren J et al: Do well-to-do and repeatedly rejecting renal allografts express the transplantation antigens similarly on their surface? Scand J Urol Nephrol (Suppl)64:52, 1981

78. Hendriks GFJ, Schreuder GMTh, Claas FHJ et al: HLA-DRw6 and renal allograft rejection. Br Med J 286:85, 1983

79. Hood L, Steinmetz M, Malissen B: Genes of the major histocompatibility complex in the mouse. Ann Rev Immunol 1:529, 1983

80. Houghton AN, Thomson TM, Gross D et al: Surface antigens of melanoma and melanocytes. Specificity of induction of Ia antigens by human γ-interferon. J Exp Med 160:255, 1984

81. Jakobsen BK, Langhoff E, Platz P et al: The impact of HLA-DR compatibility on cadaver kidney graft survival in a prospective study with special emphasis on the quality of typing. Tissue Antigens 23:94, 1984

82. Jeffery JR, Cheung K, Masniuk J et al: Mixed lymphocyte culture response: Lack of correlation with cadaveric renal allograft survival and blood transfusions. Transplantation 38:42, 1984

83. Johnson AH, Amos DB, Noreen H: Strong mixed lymphocyte reaction associated with the LA or first locus HLA. Transplantation 20:291, 1975

84. Jordan BR, Caillol D, Damotte M et al: HLA Class I genes: From structure to expression, serology, and function. Immunol Rev 84:73, 1985

85. Kachru RB, Mittal KK: Serological detection of HL-A antigens in human mammary secretion. In Kissmeyer-Nielsen F (ed): Histocompatibility Testing 1975, pp 404–413. Copenhagen, Munksgaard, 1975

86. Kahan BD, van Buren CT, Flechner SM: Cyclosporine immunosuppression mitigates immunologic risk factors in renal allotransplantation. Transplant Proc 15:2469, 1983

87. Katz DV, Mickey MR, Cecka M et al: The immune response and HLA. In Terasaki PI (ed): Clinical Kidney Transplants 1985, pp 205–215. Los Angeles, UCLA Tissue Typing Laboratory, 1985

88. Kavathas P, Bach FH, DeMars R: Gamma-ray-induced loss of expression of HLA and glyoxalase I alleles in lymphoblastoid cells. Proc Natl Acad Sci USA 77:4251, 1980

89. Kerman RH, Flechner SM, van Buren CT: DRw6 phenotype, immune responder status, and renal allograft outcome. Transplant Proc 17:44, 1985

90. Kerman RH, Floyd M, van Buren CT et al: Improved allograft survival of strong immune responder–high-risk recipients with adjuvant antithymocyte globulin therapy. Transplantation 30:450, 1980

91. Klareskog L, Forsum U, Peterson PA: Humoral regulation of the expression of Ia antigens on mammary gland epithelium. Eur J Immunol 10:958, 1980

92. Klintmalm G, Brynger H, Flatmark A et al: The blood transfusion, DR matching, and mixed lymphocyte culture effects are not seen in cyclosporine-treated renal transplant recipients. Transplant Proc 17:1026, 1985

93. Korman AJ, Boss JM, Spies T et al: Genetic complexity and expression of human Class II histocompatibility antigens. Immunol Rev 85:45, 1985

94. Krangel MS, Biddison WE, Strominger JL: Comparative structural analysis of HLA-A2 antigens distinguishable by cytotoxic T lymphocytes. II. Variant DK1: Evidence for a discrete CTL recognition region. J Immunol 130:1856, 1983

95. Lange H, Michalik R, Himmelmann GW: Withdrawal of steroids after kidney transplantation: A prospective study. 9th International Congress of Nephrology, June 16, 1984, Los Angeles, CA

96. Langhoff E, Jakobsen BK, Platz P et al: The impact of low donor-specific MLR vs HLA-DR compatibility on kidney graft survival. Transplantation 39:18, 1985

97. Lau H, Reemtsma K, Hardy MA: Pancreatic islet allograft prolongation by donor-specific blood transfusions treated with ultraviolet irradiation. Science 221:754, 1983

98. Leapman SB, Strong DM, Filo RS et al: Cyclosporin-A prevents the appearance of cell surface "activation" antigens. Transplantation 34:94, 1982

99. Lebrun A, Sasportes M, Dausset J: Role of MLC locus and related genes of the chromosomal HL-A region. Transplant Proc 5:363, 1973

100. Lehner T: Antigen-binding human T suppressor cells

and their association with the HLA-DR locus. Eur J Immunol 13:370, 1983

101. Leivestad T, Thorsby E: Effects of HLA-haploidentical blood transfusions on donor-specific immune responsiveness. Transplantation 37:175, 1984

102. Linch DC, Nadler LM, Luther EA et al: Discordant expression of human Ia-like antigens on hematopoietic progenitor cells. J Immunol 132:2324, 1984

103. Loke YW, Joysey VC, Borland R: HL-A antigens on human trophoblast cells. Nature 232:403, 1971

104. Lopez de Castro JA, Barbosa JA, Krangel MS et al: Structural analysis of the functional sites of Class I HLA antigens. Immunol Rev 85:149, 1985

105. Lucas BA, Jennings CD, Thompson JS et al: Prospective DR matching for first cadaver donor renal allografts and retransplantation. Transplantation 39:39, 1985

106. Mach B: Molecular expression for the polymorphism and regulation of HLA Class II genes. American Society for Histocompatibility and Immunogenetics Annual Meeting, October 14, 1985

107. Madsen M, Graugaard B, Fjeldborg O et al: HLA-DR antigen matching in cadaveric renal transplantation: An analysis of 201 consecutive transplants performed in Aarhus from 1978 to 1983. Transplant Proc 17:47, 1985

108. Madsen M, Kissmeyer-Nielsen F, Rasmussen P et al: Decreased expression of HLA-DR antigens on peripheral blood B lymphocytes during glucocorticoid treatment. Tissue Antigens 17:195, 1981

109. Matsui Y, Alosco SM, Awdeh Z et al: Linkage disequilibrium of HLA-SB1 with the HLA-A1, B8, DR3, SCO1 and of HLA-SB4 with the HLA-A26, Bw38, Dw10, DR4, SC21 extended haplotypes. Immunogenetics 20:623, 1984

110. Meo T, David CS, Rijnbeck AM et al: Inhibition of mouse MLR by anti-Ia sera. Transplant Rev 7:127, (Suppl 1) 1975

111. Middleton D, Gillespie EL, Doherty CC et al: The influence of HLA-A, B, and DR matching on graft survival in primary cadaveric renal transplantation in Belfast. Transplantation 39:608, 1985

112. Mittal KK, Mickey MR, Singal DP et al: Serotyping for homotransplantation. XVIII. Refinement of microdroplet lymphocyte cytotoxicity test. Transplantation 6:913, 1968

113. Moen T, Albrechtsen D, Flatmark A et al: Importance of HLA-DR matching in cadaveric renal transplantation. N Engl J Med 303:850, 1980

114. Mohanakumar T, Ellis TM, Dayal H et al: Potentiating effect of HLA matching and blood transfusion on renal allograft survival. Transplantation 32:244, 1981

115. Montoliu J, Cheigh JS, Mouradian JA et al: Delayed hyperacute rejection in recipients of kidney transplants from HLA identical sibling donors. Am J Med 67:590, 1979

116. Natali PG, DeMartino C, Quaranta V et al: Expression of Ia-like antigens in normal human nonlymphoid tissues. Transplantation 31:75, 1981

117. Niederhuber JE, Frelinger JA: Expression of Ia an-

tigens on T and B cells and their relationship to immune-response functions. Transplant Rev 30:101, 1975

118. Nomenclature for factors of the HLA system 1984. In Albert ED, Baur MP, Mayr WE (eds): Histocompatibility Testing 1984, pp 4–8. Berlin, Springer-Verlag, 1984

119. Oh JH, Maclean LD: Comparative immunogenicity of HLA antigens: A study in primiparas. Tissue Antigens 5:33, 1975

120. Old LJ, Stockert E, Boyse EA et al: Antigenic modulation. Loss of TL antigen from cells exposed to TL antibody. Study of the phenomenon in vitro. J Exp Med 127:523, 1968

121. Oliver RTD, Sachs JA, Festenstein H: A collaborative scheme for tissue typing and matching in renal transplantation: VI. Clinical relevance of HLA matching in 349 cadaver renal transplants. Transplant Proc 5:245, 1973

122. Opelz G: International Collaborative Transplant Study. Ninth International HLA Workshop, Munich, May 6–11, 1984

123. Opelz G, for the Collaborative Transplant Study: Correlation of HLA matching with kidney graft survival in patients with or without cyclosporine treatment. Transplantation 40:240, 1985

124. Opelz G: International Transplant Study Newsletter, April, 1984

125. Opelz G: International Transplant Study Newsletter, December, 1985

126. Opelz G, Mickey MR, Terasaki PI: Calculations on long-term graft and patient survival on human kidney transplantation. Transplant Proc 9:27, 1977

127. Opelz G, Terasaki PI: Absence of immunization effect in human kidney retransplantation. N Engl J Med 299:369, 1978

128. Palacios R, Claesson L, Moller G et al: The alpha chain, not the β chain of HLA-DR antigens participates in activation of T cells in autologous mixed lymphocyte reaction. Immunogenetics 15:341, 1983

129. Perdue ST: Risk factors for second transplants. In Terasaki PI (ed): Clinical Kidney Transplants 1985, pp 191–203. Los Angeles, UCLA Tissue Typing Laboratory, 1985

130. Persijn GG, Cohen B, Lansbergen Q et al: Effect of HLA-A and HLA-B matching on survival of grafts and recipients after renal transplantation. N Engl J Med 307:905, 1982

131. Pfaff WM, Fermell RS, Howard RJ et al: Planned random donor blood transfusions in preparation for transplantation. Transplantation 38:701, 1984

132. Pfeffer PF, Thorsby E: HLA-restricted cytotoxicity against male-specific (H-Y) antigen after acute rejection of an HLA-identical sibling kidney. Transplantation 33:52, 1982

133. Pober JS, Gimbrone MA Jr: Expression of Ia-like antigens by human vascular endothelial cells is inducible in vitro: Demonstration by monoclonal antibody binding and immunoprecipitation. Proc Natl Acad Sci USA 79:6641, 1982

134. Pober JS, Gimbrone MA, Cotran RS et al: Ia expression by vascular endothelium is inducible by activated T cells and by human γ-interferon. J Exp Med 157:1339, 1983

135. Poegh HL, Orr HT, Strominger JL: Molecular cloning of a human histocompatibility antigen cDNA fragment. Proc Natl Acad Sci USA 77:6081, 1980

136. Pollack MS, Chin-Louie J, Callaway M et al: Unrelated bone marrow transplantation donors for patients with HLA-B/DR haplotypes with significant genetic disequilibrium. Transplant Proc 15:1420, 1983

137. Pollack MS, Chin-Louie J, Moschief R: Functional characteristics and differential expression of Class II DR, DS, and SB antigens on human melanoma cell lines. Hum Immunol 9:75, 1984

138. Radka SF, Charron DJ, Brodsky FM: Review: Class II molecules of the major histocompatibility complex considered as differentiation markers. Hum Immunol 16:390, 1986

139. Rapaport FI, Chase RM Jr: The bacterial induction of homograft sensitivity. II. Effects of sensitization with Staphylococci and other microorganisms. J Exp Med 122:733, 1965

140. Richiardi P, Cambron-Thomsen A, Menicucci A: HLA-A, B interlocus specificities. In Albert ED, Baur MP, Mayr WR (eds): Histocompatibility Testing 1984, pp 237–238. Berlin, Springer-Verlag, 1984

141. Richie RE, Johnson HK, Tallent MB et al: The role of HLA tissue matching in cadaveric kidney transplantation. Ann Surg 189:581, 1979

142. Sabbaga E, Ianhez LE, Chocair PR et al: Kidney transplants from living nonrelated donors: An analysis of 87 cases, including 20 cases with specific blood transfusions from the donor. Transplant Proc 17:1741, 1985

143. Salter RD, Alexander J, Levine F et al: Evidence for two trans-acting genes regulating HLA Class II antigen expression. J Immunol 135:4235, 1985

144. Salvatierra O: Advantages of continued use of kidney transplantation from living donors. Transplant Proc 17:18, 1985

145. Salvatierra O Jr, Perkins HA, Cochrum KC et al: HLA typing and primary cadaver graft survival. Transplant Proc 9:495, 1977

146. Salvatierra O Jr, Vincenti F, Amend W et al: Deliberate donor-specific blood transfusions prior to living-related renal transplantation: A new approach. Ann Surg 192:543, 1980

147. Sanfilippo F, Goeken N, Niblack G et al: The effect of first cadaver renal transplant HLA-A, B match on sensitization levels and retransplant rates following graft failure. Transplantation 43:240, 1987

148. Sanfilippo F, Vaughn WK, Spees EK et al: Benefits of HLA-A and HLA-B matching on graft and patient outcome after cadaveric-donor renal transplantation. N Engl J Med 311:358, 1984

149. Sanfilippo F, Vaughn WK, Spees EK et al: The effect of HLA-A, -B matching on cadaver renal allograft rejection comparing public and private specificities. Transplantation 38:483, 1984

150. Sarkar S, Glassy MC, Ferrone S et al: Cell cycle and the differential expression of HLA-A, B and HLA-DR antigens on human B lymphoid cells. Proc Natl Acad Sci USA 77:7297, 1980

151. Sasportes M, Lebrun A, Rapaport FT et al: Skin allograft survivals in relation to HLA-A incompatibilities and responses in MLC. Transplant Proc 5:353, 1973

152. Sasportes M, Wollman E, Cohen D et al: Suppression of the human allogeneic response in vitro with primed lymphocytes and suppressive supernates. J Exp Med 152:2705, 1980

153. Scandiatransplant Report: HLA matching and kidney graft survival. Lancet 1:240, 1975

154. Schendel DJ, Jennert W, Bickert K et al: CML: A method for cellular typing. In Albert ED, Baur MP, Mayr WR (eds): Histocompatibility Testing 1984, pp 306–312. Berlin, Springer-Verlag, 1984

155. Scher MG, Beller DI, Unanue ER: Demonstration of a soluble mediator that induces exudates rich in Ia-positive macrophages. J Exp Med 152:1684, 1984

156. Schlossman SF, Chess L, Humphreys RE et al: Distribution of Ia-like molecules on the surface of normal and leukemic human cells. Proc Natl Acad Sci USA 73:1288, 1976

157. Schreier PI, Bernards R, Vaessen RTMJ et al: Expression of Class I major histocompatibility antigens switched off by highly oncogenic adenovirus 12 in transformed rat cells. Nature 305:771, 1983

158. Schreuder GMT, Degos L: HLA-DR, DQ, and Dw relationships. In Albert ED, Baur MP, Mayr WR (eds): Histocompatibility Testing 1984, p 243. Berlin, Springer-Verlag, 1984

159. Schreuder GMTh, Parlevliet J, Termijtelen A et al: Reanalysis of the HLA-DRw6 complex. Tissue Antigens 24:62, 1983

160. Schulak JA, Goeken NE, Nghiem DD et al: Successful DR-incompatible cadaver kidney transplantation: Combined effect of HLA-A and B matching and blood transfusion. Transplantation 38:649, 1984

161. Schwartz BD, Luehrman LK, Lee T et al: A public antigenic determinant in the HLA-B5 cross-reacting group: A basis for cross-reactvity and a possible link with Behçet's disease. Hum Immunol 1:37, 1980

162. Schwartz BD, Luehrman LK, Rodey GE: A public antigenic determinant on a family of HLA-B molecules. A basis for cross-reactivity and a possible link with disease predisposition. J Clin Invest 64:938, 1979

163. Scott H, Brandtzaeg P, Hirschberg H et al: Vascular and renal distribution of HLA-DR-like antigens. Tissue Antigens 18:195, 1981

164. Seigler HF, Kremer WB, Metzgar RS et al: HL-A antigenic loss in malignant transformation. J Natl Cancer Inst 46:577, 1971

165. Seigler HF, Metzgar RS: Embryonic development of human transplantation antigens. Transplantation 9:478, 1970

166. Shaw S, DeMars R, Schlossman SF et al: Serologic identification of the human secondary B cell antigens. J Exp Med 156:341s, 1980

167. Shaw S, Johnson AH, Shearer GM: Evidence for a new segregant series of B cell antigens that are encoded in the HLA-D region and that stimulate secondary allogeneic proliferative and cytotoxic responses. J Exp Med 152:565, 1980

168. Sheehy MJ, Sondel PM, Bach ML et al: HLA LD (lymphocyte defined) typing: A rapid assay with primed lymphocytes. Science 188:1308, 1975

169. Singal DP, Joseph S: Role of blood transfusions on the induction of antibodies against recognition sites on T lymphocytes in renal transplant patients. Human Immunol 4:93, 1982

170. Snyder DS, Beller DI, Unanue ER: Prostaglandins modulate macrophage Ia expression. Nature 299:163, 1982

171. Sollinger HW, Burlingham WJ, Sparks EMF et al: Donor-specific transfusion in unrelated and related HLA-mismatched donor–recipient combinations. Transplantation 38:612, 1984

172. Sondel PM, Sparks EM, Glass NR et al: Prospective renal allograft matching by pool primed lymphocyte. Transplantation 33:224, 1982

173. Southern EM: Detection of specific sequences among DNA fragments separated by gel electrophoresis. J Mol Biol 98:503, 1975

174. Srivastava R, Duceman BW, Biro PA et al: Molecular organization of the Class I genes of human major histocompatibility complex. Immunol Rev 84:93, 1985

175. Steinman RM, Kaplan G, Witmer MD et al: Identification of a novel cell type in peripheral lymphoid organs in mice. V. Purification of spleen dendritic cells, new surface markers, and maintenance in vitro. J Exp Med 149:1, 1979

176. Steinman TI, Zimmerman CE, Monaco AP et al: Steroids can be stopped in kidney transplant patients. Transplant Proc 13:323, 1981

177. Stingl GK, Tamaki K, Katz SI: Origin and function of epidermal Langerhans cells. Immunol Rev 53:149, 1980

178. Taylor RJ, Andrews W, Rosenthal JT et al: DR matching and cadaveric renal transplantation with cyclosporine. Transplant Proc 17:1194, 1985

179. Terasaki PI (ed): Clinical Kidney Transplants 1985. Los Angeles, UCLA Tissue Typing Laboratory, 1985

180. Terasaki PI, Mittal KK, Singal DP: Serotyping for homotransplantation: XXI. The role of the Mac(LA2) antigen in kidney transplantation. Symposium on Immunologic and Clinical Questions of Organ Transplantation, Bonn, May 26–28, 1968

181. Terasaki PI, Toyotome A, Mickey MR et al: Patient, graft, and functional survival rates: An overview. In Terasaki PI (ed): Clinical Kidney Transplants 1985, pp 1–27. Los Angeles, UCLA Tissue Typing Laboratory, 1985

182. The Canadian Multicentre Transplant Study Group. A randomized clinical trial of cyclosporine in cadaveric renal transplantation. N Engl J Med 309:809, 1983

183. Thompson JS, Bonney WW, Lawton RL et al: Effect

of HLA-A haplotype matching on renal transplantation. Transplantation 17:438, 1974

184. Ting A, Morris PJ: The influence of HLA-A, -B and -DR matching and pregraft blood transfusions on graft and patient survival after renal transplantation in a single centre. Tissue Antigens 24:256, 1984

185. Tiwari JL, Sasaki N: Mixed lymphocyte culture response and graft survival in living-related kidney transplants. In Terasaki PI (ed): Clinical Kidney Transplants 1985, pp 227–232. Los Angeles, UCLA Tissue Typing Laboratory, 1985

186. Trowsdale J, Young JAT, Kelley AP et al: Structure, sequence, and polymorphism in the HLA-D region. Immunol Rev 85:5, 1985

187. Uehling DDT, Hussey JL, Weinstein AB et al: Cessation of immunosuppression after renal transplantation. Surgery 79:278, 1976

188. Valentine-Thon E, Bach FH: Primed lymphocyte typing predicts MLC reactivity between unrelated individuals. Tissue Antigens 21:336, 1983

189. vanEs A, Baldwin WM, Oljans PJ et al: Expression of HLA-DR on T lymphocytes following renal transplantation, and association with graft-rejection episodes and cytomegalovirus infection. Transplantation 37:65, 1984

190. van Hooff JP, van Hooff-Eijkenboom YEA, Kalff MW et al: Kidney graft survival, clinical course, and HLA-A, B, and D matching in 208 patients transplanted in one center. Transplant Proc 11:1291, 1979

191. Vincent C, Revillard J-P, Betuel H: Purification of HLA antigens from urine. Transplantation 22:500, 1976

192. Virgin HW IV, Wittenberg GF, Unanne ER: Immune complex effects on murine macrophages. I. Immune complexes suppress interferon-γ induction of Ia expression. J Immunol 135:3735, 1985

193. Wank R, Schendel DJ: Genetic analysis of HLA-D region products defined by PLT. In Albert ED, Baur MP, Mayr WR (eds): Histocompatibility Testing 1984, pp 289–299. Berlin, Springer-Verlag, 1984

194. Winchester RJ, Kunkel HG: The human Ia system. Adv Immunol 28:22, 1980

195. Yu DTY, McCune JM, Fu SM et al: Two types of Ia-positive T cells. Synthesis and exchange of Ia antigens. J Exp Med 152:89s, 1980

196. Zachary AA, Braun WE: Calculation of a predictive value for transplantation. Transplantation 39:316, 1985

197. Zoller KM, Cho SI, Cohen JJ et al: Cessation of immunosuppressive therapy after successful transplantation: A national survey. Kidney Int 18:110, 1980

CHAPTER 10

Sensitization and Its Role in Transplantation

Paul I. Terasaki   James Cicciarelli

Sensitization or immunization to transplantation antigens is a fundamental immunologic concept in the field of transplantation. In actual clinical practice, its impact has been considerably blunted by immunosuppression. Thus, the expected effect of sensitization has been limited following pregnancies, transfusions, and graft rejection. Even the use of the same immunizing donor for subsequent transplants, such as grafts from child to mother or from the same donor used for blood transfusion (DST), has not resulted in low survival rates.

Sensitization does, however, result in some instances in humoral antibodies. Although not all antibodies are harmful, some are extremely dangerous and can initiate an immediate rejection of a graft. Evidence is cited that, aside from hyperacute rejection, complete nonfunction of grafts can also be induced by antibodies. To avoid such transplants, effective crossmatching procedures are necessary. Procedures that currently exist and those that need to be developed are:

	CURRENT	FUTURE
Sensitization	Panel testing by lymphocyte cytotoxicity	Panel testing of cellular immunity; Panel testing using other target cells

Crossmatch test	1. Lymphocyte cytotoxicity
	  a. long incubation
	  b. T, B monocyte target
	  c. IgG (by DTT treatment)
	2. Antiglobulin test
	
	3. Flow cytometry
		Cellular crossmatch
		More sensitive tests
		Elimination of autoantibody reactions
		Reaction with other targets such as monocytes
		Tests for anti-idiotype or regulatory immunoglobulins and cells

SENSITIZATION: OVERVIEW

Sensitization, or immunization to allografts, was the key observation that ushered in the modern era of transplantation. It was Medawar's observation that a second graft would be rejected more rapidly than the first graft, which first clearly showed that immunologic rejection was responsible for skin graft and other allograft failures.[36] The "second set" phenomenon could not be explained in any other way. Once it was recognized that tissue transplantation between individuals of the same species was analogous to infections with microorganisms, immunologic approaches came to be used extensively. Thus, sensitization, as it is generally used, means the immunization of patients before their actual transplant. The phenomenon is clinically important because it is often difficult to avoid sensitization, and once the patient has been sensitized, the effect is long-lasting and difficult to neutralize. The adverse effect of sensitization is primarily manifested in the first 2 months after transplantation.[28]

We shall first discuss how sensitization is detected. In experimental animals, the classical method has been to simply retransplant and demonstrate shorter regraft survival time. Obviously, in clinical transplantation, other means of detecting sensitization is required. Although the need is great, it is noteworthy that, at the practical level, there is only a single test that is commonly used to detect sensitization. This test, which was introduced in 1971,[59] is the lymphocyte cytotoxicity test, using a panel of cells from random individuals. It was shown that kidney transplant patients who were sensitized, that is, those who had cytotoxic antibodies to random donor lymphocytes, tended to have lower kidney transplant survival rates than patients who did not have such antibodies. After 15 years of extensive research, this measure remains the most widely used "standard" measure of sensitization. Patients who have lymphocytotoxic antibodies are denoted as sensitized and those who do not are denoted as nonsensitized.

There are reasons why classification on the basis of cytotoxic antibody might be expected to be defective in measuring sensitization. Most importantly, if transplant rejection is a cellular, as well as an antibody, mediated rejection, a test that measures the reactivity of cells should be more appropriate, as well as a test that measures the antibody level. Yet, to date, no cellular test has been widely used to measure sensitization in clinical kidney transplantation. Cell-mediated lympholysis (CML) has been shown to increase in patients who were rejecting kidney allografts.[26] The test would seem useful to measure sensitization, but the requirement of large numbers of cells precludes its use in its present form for large-scale clinical testing. In addition, leukocyte migration-inhibiting lymphokine[15] and direct lymphocyte-mediated cytotoxicity[8] have been used, albeit infrequently, as measures of cell-mediated immunity sensitization. Mixed lymphocyte culture (MLC) does not measure presensitization and therefore cannot be used as a sensitization test.

If we assume that cells that reject grafts are localized within the graft and may not circulate, cell samples from peripheral blood may give an inadequate index of the patient's immune status. Perhaps an even more difficult problem is that memory cells specific for a given antigen immunization may not be circulating at certain times after the initial immunization. For example, a woman immunized by pregnancy 20 years previously may not have circulating memory cells. Yet after transplantation, primed cells could be activated from sequestered sites. The number of memory cells may be below the threshold of measurement, although their effect could be considerable after stimulation and expansion. Although these are some difficulties associated with measuring cellular presensitization, development of such a test should be important.

There are various reasons why the humoral antibody test yields either false-positive or false-negative results. The most common reason for a false-positive conclusion on sensitization is reactions produced by autoantibodies. Although lymphocytotoxic antibodies were initially said to be directed against HLA antigens on lymphocytes, it was first shown in 1970 that some lymphocytotoxic antibodies reacted to determinants other than HLA.[39] These antibodies occurred under various conditions that did not involve alloimmunization, such as in patients with infectious mononucleosis, systemic lupus erythematosus (SLE),[60] many viral diseases, and autoimmune diseases[45] and even in normal subjects.[46] These antibodies often were cytotoxic to autologous lymphocytes with the use of rabbit complement.[46] They were mostly IgM in nature and usually reacted more strongly in the cold or at room temperature than at 37°C.[13,30] These autoantibodies also reacted more frequently with B-lymphocytes than with T-lymphocytes,[46] although autoreactive T cell antibody does occur and does not contraindicate transplantation.[12a] Many reactions of B-lymphocyte targets are autoimmune reactions with no relation to antibodies against HLA.

Various means have been proposed to distinguish between autoantibodies and HLA antibodies. The simplest is the use of different incubation temperatures. Antibodies that react at 5°C but do not react at 22°C or 37°C are called *cold antibodies* and do not indicate sensitization to transplantation antigens.[31] On the other hand, antibodies that react at 37°C are generally antibodies directed to HLA. Reactions at 22°C, which is the most commonly used temperature for testing for lymphocyte cytotoxicity, yield ambiguous results, since some cold antibodies tend to react at that temperature. Because incubation temperature is not very discriminating, use of mercaptoethanol or dithiothreitol (DTT) has been suggested.[3,41] Adding these reagents to the microcytotoxicity test is a simple and convenient way to rule out IgM antibodies. In a recent survey, as many as 20% of patients who were thought to have antibodies against 100% of a random panel actually had no antibodies that were IgG class.[29] This means that some patients, although they had waited for several years for transplants, could have been transplanted with any donor.

Another method of distinguishing autoantibodies has been proposed by Ting and Morris[65] using cells from patients with chronic lymphocytic leukemia (CLL). Since CLL cells did not react with autoantibodies, sera that reacted with B-lymphocytes but that did not react with CLL cells were assumed to contain autoantibodies. The Oxford group has recently proposed a further improvement in using monoclonal antibodies against HLA to distinguish the two types of antibodies. Fab fragments of a goat antimurine antibody used in conjunction with a monoclonal antibody to the common determinant of HLA were used to block the reaction against HLA.[12] This may currently be the most specific way by which the two antibodies can be distinguished. What remains to be shown, however, is whether a simple test using DTT might also accomplish the same purpose.

There are various technical errors that could result in false-positive reactions in the cytotoxicity test. Most important is the low viability of test cells resulting from toxicity of the rabbit complement. The reactions must be reviewed carefully to rule out such false-positive tests. The use of a frozen panel of cells[52] has made it easier to test for panel reactive antibodies, but they should be used cautiously to avoid errors introduced by some cells with poorer viability. It is important to know whether a patient has preformed antibodies. This is particularly true for liver and heart transplant patients in whom it might be decided to proceed without a prospective crossmatch in those who have no preformed antibodies. The classification is also important when shipping kidneys long distances. Shipment to patients with no cytotoxic antibodies can be done more readily than to those with antibodies who may subsequently have a positive crossmatch test. Another source of a false-positive classification of patients results from use of a small cell panel, because a single false-positive result will categorize a patient as sensitized. Generally, a random panel of approximately 50 cells should be used to avoid such technical errors.

The false-negative conclusion of sensitization is often the result of using too few donors of panel cells to detect sensitization. Since the number of HLA specificities is so numerous, it is difficult to assemble cells having all the specificities. With a small panel, if a false-negative reaction occurs with a single cell, sensitization could be overlooked. The conclusion of sensitization or nonsensitization could rest on the reaction of a few cells. Attention to technical details in performing the test, such as ensuring that the reagents are mixed, that complement is strong, and that readings are recorded accurately are important. Another aspect of false-negative sensitization is that a patient may have been previously sensitized but could have lost the antibodies by the

time that the test was done. This problem is discussed in the following section.

LATENT SENSITIZATION

Dossetor and Olsen,[18] in 1972, first called attention to the phenomenon of latent sensitization in which a patient could have been sensitized previously but lost his antibodies at the time of transplantation. The phenomenon is well known in immunology. After sensitization, antibodies are lost, but memory cells remain. Upon restimulation, an anamnestic response occurs, which is generally higher than the primary response. Thus, if a previously sensitized patient appears not to be sensitized at the time of transplantation, he should be considered to be latently sensitized. This concept was widely accepted, resulting in storage of periodically collected samples from the time that recipients are entered onto the various waiting lists. Crossmatching is generally done using the sera samples with the highest activity as well as the serum sample collected just before transplantation.

There is recent evidence, however, suggesting that this policy may require reevaluation, that is, patients who have lost their sensitization appear to accept transplants as though they previously had never been sensitized. Cardella, Falk, and Nicholson[7] reported that patients who had a current negative crossmatch, but a historic positive crossmatch, had graft survival rates that were equivalent to patients who previously never had antibodies. This finding was subsequently modified to apply mainly to first transplant patients but not to second graft recipients.[22] Although this work has drawn considerable attention, several comments might be made. First, in most waiting recipient pools, there are sufficient numbers of patients who are negative by both current and prior antisera to not warrant the transplantation of historically positive crossmatch patients. Second, it is important to exclude patients who may have had autoantibodies that subsequently disappeared, since they may have been transplantable regardless of current or peak levels of antibody. It is possible that in many of those patients who converted from historic positive to current negative had autoantibody and not anti-HLA antibody. Until this has been excluded, it may be inappropriate to transplant any historic positive current negative combination, particularly because the results with second transplants are not as good as in patient–donor combination without any detectable antibody at any time. Therefore, until it is clear that such autoantibodies are not involved, one might question the need to change transplantation policies.

SOURCES OF SENSITIZATION

The most common source of sensitization is pregnancy. In almost all pregnancies, there is an incompatibility between the fetus and the mother. Since HLA is extremely polymorphic, the father almost always has a different HLA haplotype from the mother. In large families, the mother may be immunized repeatedly to the same haplotype from the father. This would then result in repeated immunization to the same antigens. In fact, pregnant women are the primary source of alloantibodies used in HLA typing.[48,49,68] Pregnancies could render a women sensitized. Many years subsequently, when no antibodies exist in her sera, another stimulus, such as a transfusion, may elicit an anamnestic response. Women produce cytotoxic antibodies twice as often as men, almost certainly because of prior sensitization from pregnancy.[42] Abortion after HLA antigens are developed in the fetus could readily result in immunization, just as carrying the fetus to full term. Even an unrecognized early abortion or seminal fluid could possibly immunize women. It is interesting that despite the fact that women are clearly sensitized by pregnancies, evidence for a deleterious effect of pregnancies on transplantation has been difficult to obtain.[4,23] Moreover, a harmful effect of pregnancies on subsequent pregnancies is also not clearly shown. If pregnancies sensitize, some effect on future pregnancies or transplants should be demonstrable.

Transfusions are also a major source of sensitization.[42] Lymphocytes contain the highest quantity of HLA antigens, although platelets also have an abundant quantity of HLA-A, -B, -C antigens. Plasma contains some HLA antigens.[50] There is recent evidence that red cells contain a small quantity of HLA per cell, but since there are a thousand times more red cells than white cells, the total quantity of HLA antigens in red cells may be similar to that contained on lymphocytes.[21] Thus, attempts to use buffy coat–free blood or washed cells may not solve the problem. Fresh whole blood may be even more antigenic than the commonly used products from the blood bank, which are often as much as 3 weeks old.

We have shown that approximately 10% of patients were sensitized by a single transfusion and that this rate increases to 20% and 40% with 10 transfusions for males and females, respectively.[42] After multiple transfusions, there is a steady increase in sensitization, which gradually levels off (Table 10-1). The sensitization rate is lower when tested against T cells than against B-lymphocytes. Aside from sensitivity to HLA-A, -B, -C, it is likely that sensitivity to B cells also takes into account sensitization to the Dr and DP specificities. The complication of also having reactivity to autoantigens has been discussed earlier. Nevertheless, most of the response to transfusions is likely to be against the HLA antigens. Usually, multiple transfusions result in increasing antibody titers, although a few instances have been reported in which multiple transfusions result in decreased levels of antibodies.[30]

Patients with end-stage renal disease often require transfusions as part of their medical care since production of erythropoietin by their diseased kidneys is curtailed. It is only in polycystic kidney disease that blood transfusions are usually not needed. With the risks of hepatitis and AIDS, transfusions

TABLE 10-1   Frequency of Panel-Reactive Antibody Associated with Transfusion and Graft Rejection*

	1st CADAVER GRAFT			2nd CADAVER GRAFT			3rd CADAVER GRAFT		
NO. OF TRANS-FUSIONS	Sensitized Patients (N)	No. With >50% Antibody	%	Sensitized Patients (N)	No. With >50% Antibody	%	Sensitized Patients (N)	No. With >50% Antibody	%
0	127	17	13.4	35	13	37.1	3	1	33.3
1–5	590	144	24.4	174	65	37.4	15	5	33.3
6–10	364	94	25.8	175	71	40.6	29	23	79.3
11–20	277	93	33.6	158	77	48.7	33	19	57.6
>20	230	83	36.4	190	97	51.1	48	32	66.7

* Analysis of UCLA Transplant Registry.

Note: Of patients who have never been transfused, 13.4% have become sensitized presumably through pregnancy, unreported transfusions, or nonspecific etiologies. With a second or third transplant, sensitization rate increases to about 33.3% to 37.1%; the 20% increase from the first transplant representing that caused by retransplantation. Similarly, sensitization rate rises with each grouping of increased number of transfusions, yielding an observed rise of about 20% (13.4%–36%) for first transplants and about 30% (33%–66.7%) for third transplants.

are not given as liberally as in the past. Transfusions are, however, given deliberately to increase kidney transplant survival rates. Since the demonstration in 1973[43] that transfusions can increase graft survival rates, there have been more than 69 studies confirming this effect.[67] Because of this evidence, 90% of patients transplanted in 1985 had been transfused before transplantation.[57,62] Some indication of the proportions of deliberate transfusions can be gained by assuming that usually not more than five deliberate transfusions would be given and that any excess would be for medical reasons. Under this assumption, about one third of the patients are deliberately transfused, and about one half require transfusions. Transfusions will therefore be difficult to eliminate completely as a source of sensitization.

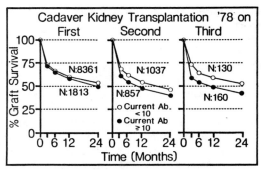

FIGURE 10-2.   *Two-year graft survivals are given for first, second, and third transplants. Note that the difference in graft survival becomes more marked between antibody-positive and antibody-negative patients only as the number of transplants increases. (Analysis of U.C.L.A. Transplant Registry.)*

Sensitization by Prior Transplantation

Perhaps the strongest source of sensitization is rejection of a prior transplant (Fig. 10-1). After rejection of a kidney transplant, approximately one half of the patients develop cytotoxic antibodies to HLA antigens.[38] It appears that these antibodies are more effective in causing nonfunction of subsequent kidney transplants than are antibodies induced by transfusions.[28] The antibodies present in patients who had rejected a prior transplant are more often IgG in nature and generally higher in titer. Because these antibodies are more strongly associated with subsequent kidney destruction, either there are other undetected antibodies that are more damaging or the HLA antibodies are themselves of greater strength than antibodies produced by pregnancies

or transfusions. Transplants into patients who have previously rejected a graft have consistently had a 10% or more lower survival rate than first grafts (Fig. 10-2).[62] Sensitization produced by transplant rejection probably results in the most difficult sensitization to abolish or attenuate. It is surprising, however, that the difference in survival rates between first and second grafts is usually 10% at 1 year, indicating that sensitization by rejection of a graft results in only a 10% lower survival than in patients not previously immunized.

Sensitization by Nonspecific Agents

It has been reported sporadically that lymphocytotoxic antibodies are produced by various infections or agents other than alloimmunizations.[19] Antibodies to HLA cross-react with M proteins of streptococci.[27] These examples are rare, and we are inclined to attribute lymphocyte cytotoxic activity to the presence of autoantibodies, which are known to be produced by nonspecific stimuli.[45,47] If we can be assured that only alloimmunization results in sensitization, it would not be necessary to test dialysis patients for the presence of cytotoxic antibodies unless the patient had become pregnant or had a transfusion. The routine monitoring of dialysis patients for sensitization is probably not required in the absence of allogeneic stimuli. However, since errors could occur in reporting transfusions, some routine method of checking for antibodies would be desirable. For this reason, some set interval for testing of cytotoxic antibodies should be instituted for patients who are reported as not transfused. Antibodies produced by nonspecific stimuli are generally weak and probably can be ignored.

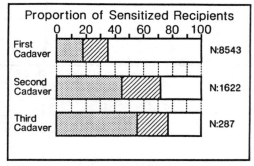

FIGURE 10-1.   *Proportion of sensitized recipients in first, second, and third cadaveric kidney transplants. Stippled area is sensitization rate at the time of transplant. Crosshatched area is the percentage of patients who were sensitized but became negative by the time of transplantation. Note the increased sensitization rate with increased number of prior transplants. (Analysis of U.C.L.A. Transplant Registry.)*

ABSENCE OF SENSITIZATION

We have previously called attention to evidence from clinical kidney transplants that sensitization may actually have a rather minor effect.[44] We have discussed the three major sources of immunization and the interesting finding that these three sources do not result in dire consequences to the patient. First, pregnant women do not necessarily have a higher risk of undergoing transplant rejection than men who have never been exposed to alloantigens. Second, patients who are exposed to transfusions actually have a higher graft survival rate than those who were never preimmunized by transfusions. Third, even patients who previously rejected a transplant have graft survival rates that are almost the same as those of patients with first transplants.[44] Thus, in clinical kidney transplantation, the effect of sensitization is actually not as great as one might expect on purely theoretic grounds. A patient who rejects an HLA-A2 incompatible transplant and is retransplanted with a subsequent HLA-A2 incompatible graft has almost the same survival rate as those patients transplanted with different HLA incompatible antigens.[44] Although it is common practice to try to avoid mismatching of the same antigens, there are relatively few data indicating that such repeated mismatching is associated with poorer graft survival. In fact, a recent study shows that there was some effect of mismatching for the same antigens twice, but generally the effect was not as marked or as strong as one might expect. Among 400 regrafts with the same mismatch, an overall 1-year graft survival rate of 47% was noted, which was not statistically different from regrafts with no HLA-A, -B antigens mismatched twice.[14]

The data do not disprove the concept of sensitization, but they show that with the use of immunosuppression, some of the basic concept of sensitization may not be supported by the clinical data. One explanation of these observations follows from the clonal deletion theory discussed in the following section.

Clonal Deletion Theory

The immunization process consists of stimulation of selected immunocompetent cells and consequent expansion of the clones. The sensitized individual simply has more preprogrammed cells or clones of cells than a nonsensitized person. This conclusion derives from experimental studies of transplant immunity. Thus, in a sensitized person, certain selected clones have been stimulated and memory cells were accumulated against the specific immunizing antigens. Immunosuppression was postulated to act by deletion or reduction of rapidly expanding clones of cells following stimulation.[56] It was postulated that transfusions immunize the patient and that the transplant serves as a secondary stimulus against which an anamnestic response is generated by expansion of clones. Immunosuppression, which is given at its highest dosage at the time of transplantation, serves to inactivate the rapidly dividing cells. If the treatment is sufficient, only small numbers of these cells remain, and they can be kept under control by constant immunosuppression. Thus, according to this hypothesis, presensitization can actually be helpful to the outcome of transplantation since it serves to prestimulate the relevant clones.

According to this theory, sensitized patients benefit more from immunosuppression given at the time of transplant than nonsensitized patients, because their rejection reaction starts earlier than that in nonsensitized recipients. Maximal immunosuppression is conventionally given at the time of transplant in all protocols used today. This theory explains why transplants have been performed successfully with the same mismatches, why sensitization with transfusions could result in a higher graft survival rate, and why secondary transplants have almost the same survival rate as first grafts. In other words, immunosuppression is timed well to overcome sensitization.

IMMUNOLOGIC RESPONSIVENESS

Immunologic responsiveness is a concept that is related to sensitization. It assumes that individuals vary in their ability to respond to allografts. The responsive patient would reject almost any transplant, and a nonresponsive patient would not react against numerous HLA incompatibilities. The strongest evidence for this concept comes from deliberate transfusions of healthy volunteers.[24] These studies, originally performed to produce HLA antibodies, showed that some patients would respond to even a single transfusion, whereas others would not produce antibodies even after multiple transfusions. This phenomenon has also occurred in dialysis patients who are transfused.[42] Today, when 90% of the patients transplanted are transfused, essentially all of them have been challenged, but those who did not make antibodies are denoted as nonsensitized, and those with antibodies are denoted as sensitized. Actually, those without antibodies are patients who are nonresponsive, although they were in fact sensitized. This distinction is an important one, because responsiveness may actually be the critical factor governing the fate of transplantation, rather than whether the patient is "sensitized" or "nonsensitized." A nonsensitized patient would not respond to a transfusion with production of antibody and, according to this idea, would also not respond to a transplant. On the other hand, a responsive patient would vigorously respond to a transfusion and may repeatedly reject multiple transplants.

We have pointed out the interesting fact that although 90% of the patients are transfused, 80% of transplanted patients have no preformed cytotoxic antibodies.[57] This means that although most of the patients who are transplanted have in fact been sensitized in the sense of being pre-exposed to alloantigens, most have not responded to the transfusion challenge. Today, division of waiting patients into responsive and nonresponsive groups is being done unconsciously by transplant centers when they transfuse the patients. They also use the absence of cytotoxic antibodies in selecting recipients. Although many centers admit to the use of preformed cytotoxic antibodies as a selection criterion, they are unconscious of using this criterion as a measure of responsiveness. In most of the waiting pools, approximately half of the patients are presensitized; that is, they have cytotoxic antibodies reactive to the panel. Yet only 20% of the transplant patients come from the sensitized group, and 80% are "nonsensitized." Much of this selection is also based on convenience, especially when kidneys are shipped longer distances. In addition, since the crossmatch test eliminates the sensitized patients, more opportunities are routed toward those who do not have antibodies. These patients are actually nonresponsive patients, since most of them have been prechallenged by transfusions. Thus, as more patients who have not been transfused are transplanted, it will be interesting to see to what extent such a policy will affect the overall kidney transplant survival rates.

It is important to realize that responsiveness is a hidden component of what we normally think of as sensitization. Future tests of responsiveness could be developed completely independent of tests for sensitization. The MLC reaction would seem to be ideally suited as a responsive test. Perhaps if the test could be standardized and modified to be more reproducible, it could reveal basic differences in responsiveness among different persons. Obviously, responsiveness is unlikely to be completely dichotomous. It is likely that grades of responsiveness exist, particularly to certain alloantigens. Thus, the patient can be a responder to certain mismatches and a nonresponder to other incompatibilities.

THE CROSSMATCH TEST

In practical terms, over the past 20 years, the most important contribution of tissue typing to clinical kidney transplantation has been the crossmatch test. Exactly how valuable it has been is difficult to determine in terms of the number of hyperacute failures it has prevented. Hyperacute failure rates in patients who are transplanted without any crossmatching cannot be determined readily, because the procedure has been widely used for more than 15 years. In the very early studies in which crossmatching was done retrospectively, the approximate hyperacute rate was 6% for first grafts and 41% for second grafts.[47,61] From what we know now, the hyperacute failure rate would be expected to increase with increasing sensitization, such as with transfusions and regrafts. Because at present it appears that there is no way of reversing a hyperacute rejection, any method by which this dreaded rejection can be avoided is valuable for transplantation. Among 25,000 transplants in the last 10 years, the hyperacute rejection rate was 0.5% for first grafts and 1% for regrafts.[29] For these transplants, the standard lymphocytotoxicity crossmatch test was used. This indicates that, for most practical purposes, the hyperacute rejection has been reduced to low levels by standard means.

In the first recorded lymphocytotoxicity crossmatch, the patient had been previously pregnant, and the kidney transplant from a brother failed to function.[58] The patient's serum was cytotoxic to the brother's lymphocytes. Kissmeyer-Nielsen[34] subsequently showed leukoagglutinating antibodies in two patients with kidneys that did not function. The lymphocytotoxicity crossmatch was predictive of hyperacute rejection in two subsequent studies.[47,61] Of the positive crossmatch patients, 80% had kidneys that never functioned. Thus, even in the early studies, some false-positive crossmatches were noted. There appears to be agreement that following the initial triggering produced by the preformed antibody in the patient against donor antigens, coagulation processes are initiated, causing early vascular damage to the kidney.[55,70] For practical purposes, determining that the recipient has preformed antibodies against the donor is sufficient to prevent hyperacute rejection.

Starzl and associates[55] recently reported that the liver transplant can absorb the HLA antibodies to such an extent that a positive crossmatch for the kidney transplant became negative in five patients. Following transplantation of the liver in four of the five kidney transplants performed, immediate function was noted. The one failed kidney occurred in a patient whose crossmatch did not become completely negative. It appears, therefore, that the liver is not subject to hyperacute rejection as is the kidney, perhaps because of its mass or ability to neutralize the HLA antibodies. However, the statement that liver transplants can be done across a positive crossmatch may be an oversimplification, inasmuch as certain types of antibody as well as certain strengths of antibodies may not be surmountable by the liver transplant. Primary nonfunction of liver transplants occurs in approximately 6% of grafts. If some of these failures can be avoided by effective crossmatching, the desperate search for a donor liver and the subjection of the recipient to another operation can be avoided.

Although it has been stated that crossmatching may not be necessary for heart transplants in patients without panel-reactive antibodies,[6] there have been some clear examples of primary nonfunction following heart transplantation across a positive crossmatch.[69] Again, because of the seriousness of immediate failure in a heart transplant, any crossmatch test that would avoid these failures would be valuable. In heart transplant recipients, sensitization can be examined against a panel before transplantation, and patients who have antibodies should be crossmatched. The crossmatching procedure should also invoke looking for autoantibodies, because a false-positive crossmatch can also result in a patient unnecessarily being denied a transplant.

CROSSMATCHING AND EARLY NONFUNCTION

Although crossmatching was first shown to affect hyperacute rejections, there is also the possibility that by using more sensitive crossmatch techniques, early acute rejections can be predicted. We recently called attention to the fact that there are many kidneys that never function after transplantation. These kidneys do not manifest the classical signs of hyperacute rejection, although they never function. We have denoted such transplants as suffering unrecognized hyperacute or nonclassical hyperacute rejections.[28] The reason that these failures are similar to hyperacute rejection is that they occur more often in immunized patients; the incidence of primary nonfunction for kidneys is 8% for nonsensitized patients, and 13% for sensitized first transplants. Thus, the mere fact that the patients have

cytotoxic antibodies increases the rate of nonfunction for 1 month. This rate increases to 22% in patients transplanted for the second time. In those recipients receiving third grafts, the 1-month nonfunction rate is as high as 25%. Thus, there is a clear correlation between nonfunction and levels of immunization. Although these kidneys are often thought to fail because of preservation or donor factors, many fail because the recipient had been preimmunized. Thus, it is important to have tests that detect this preimmunization state by more sensitive crossmatch tests.

METHODS OF CROSSMATCHING

The standard method of lymphocytotoxicity crossmatching has been used for 20 years. As noted earlier, the hyperacute failure rate is 0.5% when the test is used throughout this country in an extremely large number of transplants. Thus, for practical purposes, the method can be assumed to be well established. To eliminate the 0.5% failures, there have been many attempts to make the test more sensitive and to detect certain antibodies, such as antibodies against Class II antigens or to vascular endothelial cells (VEC).[10] In addition, there have been attempts to make the crossmatch less sensitive, so that antibodies against autoantigens, for example, would not react. We consider these proposed modifications below.

First, the standard lymphocytotoxicity crossmatch consists of reacting the serum of the potential recipient against the lymphocytes of the donor for 30 minutes at room temperature followed by 1 hour with rabbit complement. These conditions are obviously arbitrary and were originally agreed upon at a meeting at the NIH (hence the name, NIH test).

SENSITIVE CROSSMATCH TEST

Long Incubation

The simplest means by which the test could be made more sensitive is a longer incubation period resulting in considerable gain in sensitivity.[64] Its only drawback may be the requirement for more time, especially in crossmatching for cadaver donor transplants.

Antiglobulin Test

The antiglobulin test detects a wider range of antibodies than the simple complement-fixation test, since noncomplement-fixing antibodies are also detected.[40]

Because different lots of antiglobulin vary considerably in their activity, it is important to use well-tested ones that are noncytotoxic and that produce specific reactions. The most commonly used is polyvalent goat or rabbit antihuman IgG,[33] but other reagents such as anti-kappa chain antiglobulin reagent are used.[32] It is clear that the antiglobulin test detects more antibodies than the cytotoxic test. However, the evidence that the extra reactions represent hyperacute rejections is not very convincing. We are not aware of any wide-scale studies that show that the rate of hyperacute rejections will be reduced by using the antiglobulin test. This is difficult to accomplish because the incidence of hyperacute rejection is very low with the standard test. Moreover, the frequency with which patients are not transplanted because of an antiglobulin-positive crossmatch may be considerable. Thus, patients could be denied transplantation or may lose the opportunity of being transplanted with a given donor based on assumptions from a positive test result. This problem is especially acute in patients who are said to be highly sensitized on the basis of having levels of noncomplement-fixing antibodies and who may, in reality, be transplantable. It is important to generate data showing that noncomplement-fixing antibodies do trigger hyperacute rejections. The necessity of performing antiglobulin crossmatch testing would depend upon these data.

Flow Cytometry Crossmatch

Fluorescence-activated cytometry (FCXM) has introduced a new dimension of sensitivity and specificity to crossmatching. Garovoy and associates[25] first demonstrated that there was a higher incidence of nonfunctioning kidneys in patients with positive FCXM than in those with negative FCXM. It is interesting that this correlation is with early function and not with hyperacute rejection; that is, patients with a positive flow crossmatch do not undergo hyperacute rejection but, nevertheless, have kidneys that either fail to function or function only briefly. As mentioned previously, these are patients who may have unrecognized or nonclassical hyperacute rejections.[28] Thus, FCXM appears to detect low levels of sensitization against the donor, which, often, but not inevitably, leads to nonfunctional grafts. In a large recent study involving more than 200 patients, a similar correlation of a positive FCXM with nonfunction was noted.[16] In this study, among 44 positive FCXM recipients, the 1-month nonfunction rate was 36%, compared with 9% for 187 recipients with negative crossmatches. However, when the pa-

tients were differentiated as to whether or not they previously had a panel-positive reaction, in those with greater than 10% panel-positive reactions, 45% had nonfunction with a positive FCXM, whereas 15% had 1-month nonfunction with a negative FCXM. The FCXM was particularly useful in regrafted patients, because among positive-crossmatched patients, 64% had 1-month failures, compared with 25% for those with negative FCXM. Thistlewaite and colleagues[63] reported similar data for FCXM. Thus, although a positive FCXM does not necessarily result in hyperacute or early nonfunction, FCXM helps to reduce early nonfunctional grafts.

We conclude that the FCXM test is an extremely useful new tool in crossmatching. It is particularly important in patients already judged to have antibodies and in those who have previously rejected transplants. These conclusions are based on early studies of T-cell antibodies. Further refinement in testing for other kinds of antibodies may prove to be useful in the future.

T-Cell Crossmatch

Since T cells have HLA-A, -B, -C antigens but lack the HLA-Dr antigens, they are better targets to detect the HLA-A, -B, -C antigens than are B cells, which have, in addition, HLA-Dr antigens. Standard crossmatching uses nonseparated lymphocytes, although T cells are the predominant cell population and most of the results can be attributed to anti-T-cell activity. However, some weak crossmatch reactions could be produced by antibodies directed against B cells in the lymphocyte preparation. Therefore, it is preferable to use pure T-lymphocytes for crossmatching in order to obtain a more specific result. Most laboratories do not make this separation because whole lymphocytes are predominantly T cells, and preparation of the T cells requires an extra step. Purification of lymphocytes by passage through a nylon wool column is not very difficult. Also, Lymphokwik, which is a reagent composed of monoclonal antibodies to B cells, platelets, and red cells permits the one-step isolation of cells. Separation of T-cell crossmatches is important, since the role of B cells in crossmatching is still not completely understood.

B-Cell Crossmatch

B-lymphocytes, which have HLA-Dr antigens in addition to HLA-A, -B, -C antigens, are routinely used for HLA-Dr typing. Since the Class II Dr antigens are important in transplantation, it is somewhat surprising to find that B cell-positive crossmatches do not generally result in hyperacute rejection,[20,35] albeit a few cases of hyperacute or accelerated rejection have been reported.[1,5] In general, it seems clear that antibodies mainly against the HLA-A, -B, -C antigens produce hyperacute rejections. Why the reaction against Dr antigens may not trigger the same reaction is not immediately clear. One possibility is that the HLA antibodies reacting against platelets, which do not have Dr antigens, constitute the initial trigger reaction. If this were the case, it would seem that complete perfusion of the donor kidney would obviate hyperacute rejections.

Next, we might ask whether preformed antibodies to the HLA-Dr antigens might indicate sensitization and whether patients with B cell–positive crossmatches could be expected to have accelerated rejections. We were again surprised that, in general, the graft survival rate was similar for patients who had no antibodies and for those who had B cell–positive crossmatches.[29] Several studies have arrived at the same conclusion.[35,37,66] There are, however, some investigations indicating the B cell–positive crossmatches are associated with lower graft survival.[2,17,53] We suspect that some of this discrepancy can be explained by further subdivision of the B cell–positive crossmatches, as explained in the following paragraphs.

As noted earlier, B-lymphocytes are very good targets for autoimmune antibodies. Thus, autoantibodies are best detected on B-lymphocytes rather than on T-lymphocytes,[47] and the incidence of autoantibodies to B-lymphocytes in normal persons is as high as 5%. We believe that this is because B-lymphocytes have IgM on their surface and that autoantibodies react to the IgM.[13] Thus, the B cell–positive crossmatch can result from antibodies to HLA-Dr antigens as well as from antibodies to IgM. The particular sensitivity of B-lymphocytes to cytotoxic reactions is also evident by the fact that it is the cell that is most sensitive to the action of complement, and, often, special complement selected as nontoxic to B cells must be used. In addition, antibodies that are cytotoxic to B cells in the cold are the most frequent antibodies found in human sera. If one wished to test a patient under the most sensitive conditions, it would be against B-lymphocytes in the cold. It has now been demonstrated repeatedly that patients who have exclusively B cold antibody do not have a graft survival rate lower than nonsensitized patients.[29,31] Thus, at least this type of autoantibody reactive against B-lymphocytes is

not associated with poor transplant outcome. It is important to distinguish B cell–positive crossmatches produced by autoantibodies from B cell–positive crossmatches produced by HLA-Dr. One method is to test with sera treated with DTT. Such DTT-treated sera would be devoid of IgM antibodies.[3,41]

Once the distinction between the allo- and autoantibody is made, the role of the B cell–positive crossmatch may become more clear.

Vascular Endothelial Crossmatch

It is possible that the crossmatching technique used today still fails to detect other antigens responsible for hyperacute or acute failures. One possible antigen is the VEC antigen, which is present on monocytes and vascular endothelial cells.[9] The wide adoption of this method is limited by the difficulty of producing pure monocytes on a routine basis for cadaver donors and the infrequency with which the VEC crossmatch is positive when all the other test results are negative. The frequency of the VEC antibodies in prospective recipients has been found to be approximately 7% or less.[11] If antibodies to these antigens produced hyperacute rejections, it would be important, obviously, to incorporate this test into the routine. In addition, it will be valuable to define the VEC antigens by exchange of relevant antisera that contain pure antibodies to these antigens.

Conclusions

The lymphocyte cytotoxicity crossmatch test was shown to be associated with hyperacute rejections 20 years ago. Widespread usage of the standard lymphocyte cytotoxicity test results in a rate of approximately one hyperacute rejection per 500 transplants. Crossmatching may, when used at a more sensitive level, serve to detect low levels of sensitization and thereby prevent the occurrence of nonfunctional kidneys. FCXM appears to identify sensitized patients who have a higher rate of nonfunctional kidneys. Although there has been some hope that crossmatching might even be able to detect helpful enhancing antibodies,[29] we are not certain now, after studies of larger numbers of patients, that the B cold antibodies act as enhancement antibodies. Whether helpful anti-idiotypic antibodies can be detected[51] has also not yet been established.

REFERENCES

1. Ahern AT, Artuc SB, Della Pelle P et al: Hyperacute rejection of HLA-AB identical renal allografts associated with B lymphocytes and endothelial reactive antibodies. Transplantation 33:103–106, 1982

2. Ayoub G, Park M, Terasaki P et al: B-cell antibodies and crossmatching. Transplantation 29:227–229, 1980

3. Ayoub G, Terasaki P, Tonai R: Improvement in detection of sensitization. Transplant Proc 15:1202–1207, 1983

4. Beleil OM, Mickey MR, Terasaki PI: Comparison of male and female kidney transplant survival rates. Transplantation 13:493–500, 1972

5. Berg B, Moller E: Immediate rejection of HLA-AB compatible HLA-Dr incompatible kidney with a positive donor recipient B-cell crossmatch. Scand J Urol Nephrol (Suppl), 54:36, 1980

6. Bolman RM, Anderson RN, Elich B et al: Cardiac transplantation without a prospective crossmatch. Transplant Proc 17:209–211, 1985

7. Cardella CJ, Falk JA, Nicholson MJ et al: Successful renal transplantation in patients with T-cell reactivity to donor. Lancet, 2:1240–1248, 1982

8. Carpenter CB, Morris PJ: The detection and measurement of pretransplant sensitization. Transplant Proc 10(2):509–513, June 1978

9. Cerilli J, Brasile L, Clarke J et al: The vascular endothelial cell specific antigen system three years experience in monocyte crossmatching. Transplant Proc 17:567–570, 1985

10. Cerilli J, Brasile L, Galozis T et al: Clinical significance of anti-monocyte antibody in kidney transplant recipients. Transplantation 32:495–497, 1981

11. Cerilli J, Brasile L, Lempert B et al: An overview of vascular endothelial cell antigen system. 17:2314–2317, 1985

12. Chapman JR, Taylor CJ, Ting A et al: The positive crossmatch: Antibody class and specificity correlate with graft outcome. Transplant Proc 19:725–726, 1987

12a. Chapman JR, Taylor CJ, Ting A et al: Immunoglobulin class and specificity of antibody causing positive T cell crossmatches. Transplantation 42(6): 608, December 1986

13. Cicciarelli JC, Chia D, Terasaki PI et al: Human IgM anti-IgM cytotoxin of E lymphocytes. Tissue Antigens 15:275–282, 1980

14. Cicciarelli JC, Cho R. Regraft kidney transplant survival. In Terasaki PI (ed): Clinical Transplants 1986, pp 223–230. Los Angeles, UCLA Tissue Typing Laboratory

15. Cochrum C, Haynes DM, Salvatierra O, et al: Leukocyte migration inhibiting factor (LIF) as an indicator of presensitization and allograft survival. Transplant Proc 10(2):445–458, June 1978

16. Cook D, Terasaki P, Iwaki Y: Flow cytometry crossmatch and kidney graft survival. (submitted)

17. Deierhoi M, Radvany R, Wolf JS: Correlation of B-cell antibodies and clinical course in DrW-typed renal allograft recipients. Transplant Proc 13:942–944, 1981

18. Dossetor JB, Olsen LA: Evidence of latent sensitization to HLA antigens. Transplantation 13:576–579, 1972

19. Ebringer A, Avakian H, Cowling P et al: Ankylosing spondilitis, HLA-B27, and Klebsiella crossreactivity studies with rabbit antilymphocyte sera and human tissue typing sera. Ann Rheum Dis 39:194, 1980

20. Ettinger R, Terasaki PI, Opelz G: Successful renal transplant across a positive crossmatch for donor B-lymphocyte alloantibodies. Lancet 2:56, 1976

21. Everett ET, Kao KJ, Scornik J: Class I HLA molecules on human erythrocytes. Quantitation and transfusion effects. Transplantation (in press)

22. Falk J, Cardella CJ, Halloran P et al: Graft outcome in multiple transplant patients with a positive donor crossmatch on noncurrent serum. Transplant Proc 1987 19:720–721, 1987

23. Fauchet R, Wattelet J, Genetet B et al: Role of blood transfusions and pregnancies in kidney transplantation. Vox Sang 37:222–228, 1979

24. Ferrara GB, Tosi RM, Azzolina G et al: HLA unresponsiveness induced by weekly transfusions of small alloquots of whole blood. Transplantation 17:194–198, 1974

25. Garovoy MR, Colombe BW, Melzer J et al: Flow cytometry crossmatching for donor-specific transfusion recipients and cadaveric transplantation. Transplant Proc 17:693–695, 1983

26. Haisch CE, Deepe RM, Gordon DA et al: Quantitation of immune responsiveness pretransplant by recipient in vitro generation of cytotoxic T effector cells. Transplant Proc 15:1148–1150, 1983

27. Hirata A, Terasaki P: Crossreaction between streptococcal M proteins and human transplantation antigens. Science 168:1095–1096, 1970

28. Iwaki Y, Iguro T, Terasaki PI: Effect of sensitization on kidney allografts. In Terasaki PI (ed): Clinical Kidney Transplants 1985, pp 139–146. Los Angeles, UCLA Tissue Typing Laboratory, 1985

29. Iwaki Y, Terasaki PI: Sensitization effect. In Terasaki PI (ed): Clinical Transplants 1986 pp. 257–265. Los Angeles, UCLA Tissue Typing Laboratory

30. Iwaki Y, Terasaki PI, Heintz R et al: Desensitization following donor-specific transfusions. Heart Transplant 1:203–207, 1982

31. Iwaki Y, Terasaki PI, Park MS et al: Enhancement of human kidney allografts by cold B-lymphocyte cytotoxins. Lancet 1:1228–1229, 1978

32. Johnson AH: Antiglobulin crossmatch for transplantation. In Rose N (ed): Manual of Clinical Immunology, pp 814–820. Washington, DC, American Society for Microbiology, 1976

33. Johnson AH, Rossen RD, Butler WT: Detection of aloantibodies using a sensitive antiglobulin microcytotoxicity test: Identification of low levels of preformed antibodies in accelerated allograft rejection. Tissue Antigens 2:215–226, 1972

34. Kissmeyer-Nielsen F, Olsen S, Peterson P et al: Hyperacute rejection of kidney allografts associated with preexisting humoral antibodies against donor cells. Lancet 2:662–665, 1966

35. Lobo PI, Westervelt F, Rudolf L: Kidney transplantability across a positive crossmatch. Lancet 1:925–

928, 1977

36. Medawar PB: The behavior and fate of skin allografts and skin homografts in rabbits. J Anat 78:176, 1944

37. Morris P, Ting A, Daar AS et al: B-cell alloantibodies and renal allografts. Lancet 2:312–313, 1976

38. Morris PJ, Williams GM, Hume DM et al: Serotyping for homotransplantation XII. Occurrence of cytotoxic antibodies following kidney transplantation in Man. Transplantation 6:392–399, 1968

39. Mottironi VD, Terasaki PI: Detection of non-HLA antibodies In Terasaki PI (ed): Histocompatibility Testing 1970, pp 301–308. Copenhagen, Munksgaard, 1970

40. Nelken D, Cohen I, Furcaig I: A method to increase the sensitivity of the lymphocyte microcytotoxicity test. Transplantation 10:346–347, 1970

41. Okuro T, Kondelis N: Evaluation of dithiothreitol (DTT) for inactivation of IgM antibodies. J Clin Pathol 31:1152–1155, 1978

42. Opelz G, Graver B, Mickey MR et al: Lymphocytotoxic antibody responses to transfusions in potential kidney transplant recipients. Transplantation 32:177–183, 1981

43. Opelz G, Sengar DPS, Mickey MR et al: Effect of blood transfusions on subsequent kidney transplants. Transplant Proc 4:253–259, 1973

44. Opelz G, Terasaki PI: Absence of immunization effect in human kidney transplantation. N Engl J Med 299:369–374, 1978

45. Ozturk G, Terasaki PI: Non-HLA lymphocyte cytotoxins in various diseases. Tissue Antigens 14:58, 1979

46. Park MS, Terasaki PI, Bernoco D: Autoantibody against B lymphocytes. Lancet 2:465–468, 1977

47. Patel R, Terasaki P: Significance of positive crossmatch test in kidney transplants. N Engl J Med 280:735–739, 1969

48. Payne R: Leukocyte agglutinins in human sera: Correlation between blood transfusions and their development. Arch Intern Med 99:587, 1958

49. Payne R: The development and persistence of leukoagglutinins in parous women. Blood 19:411–424, 1962

50. Pellegrino M, Ferrone S, Pellegrino A et al: Evaluation of two sources of soluble HLA antigens: Platelets and serum. Eur J Immunol 4:250, 1974

51. Reed E, Hardy M, Brensilver J et al: Antiidiotypic antibodies prevent early allograft rejection in patients transplanted with an historical positive crossmatch. Transplant Proc 19:762–763, 1987

52. Sollmann P, Nathan P: Improved method of preparing refrozen rethawed human lymphocytes on plates for microcytotoxicity studies. Cryobiology 16:118–124, 1979

53. Soullilou J, deMouzon A, Pegrot M et al: Role of anti-donor B-lymphocyte in definitive graft rejection. Transplant Proc 11:770–775, 1979

54. Starzl TE: Multi-organ transplants in renal failure. In Proceedings 5th International Capri Uremia Conference. J Urol (in press)

55. Starzl TE, Boehmig HK, Amemiya H et al: Clotting changes, including disseminated intravascular coagulation, during rapid renal-homograft rejection. N Engl J Med 283:338–390, 20 August 1970

56. Terasaki PI: The beneficial transfusion effect on kidney graft survival attributed to clonal deletion. Transplantation 37:119–125, 1985

57. Terasaki P, Himaya N, Cecka M et al: Overview. In Terasaki PI (ed): Clinical Transplants 1986, pp 367–392. Los Angeles, UCLA Tissue Typing Laboratory

58. Terasaki PI, Marchioro T, Starzl T: Serotyping of human lymphocytes antigens preliminary trials on long-term kidney homograft survival. Natl Acad Sci Monograph on Histocompatibilty Testing, Washington, DC, 1965, pp 83–96.

59. Terasaki PI, Mickey MR, Kreisler M: Presensitization and kidney transplant failures. Postgrad Med J 47:89–100, 1971

60. Terasaki PI, Mottironi VD, Barnett EV: Cytotoxins in disease. Autocytotoxins in lupus. N Engl J Med 283:724–728, 1970

61. Terasaki P, Thrasher DL, Hawber H: Serotyping for homotransplantation XIII: Immediate kidney transplant rejection and associated preformed antibodies. In Dausset J (ed): Advances In Transplantation, pp 225–229. Baltimore, Williams & Wilkins, 1967

62. Terasaki PI, Toyotome A, Mickey MR et al: Patient, graft, and functional survival rates: An overview. In Terasaki PI (ed): Clinical Kidney Transplants 1985, pp 1–27. Los Angeles, UCLA Tissue Typing Laboratory, 1985

63. Thistlewaite JR, Buckingham M, Stuart JK et al: The T-cell immunofluorescence flow cytometric crossmatch: Correlation of the results with rejection and graft loss in cadaver renal transplant recipients. Transplant Proc 19:722–724, 1987

64. Ting A, Hasegawa T, Ferrone S et al: Presensitization detected by sensitive crossmatch tests. Transplant Proc 5:813–817, 1973

65. Ting A, Morris PJ: Reactivity of autolymphocytotoxic antibodies from dialysis patients with lymphocytes from chronic lymphocytic leukemia (CLL) patients. Transplantation 25:31–33, 1978

66. Ting A, Morris P: Development of donor-specific B-lymphocyte antibodies after renal transplantation. Transplantation 28:13–17, 1979

67. Tiwari J: Review: Kidney transplantation and transfusion. In Terasaki PI (ed): Clinical Kidney Transplantation 1985, pp 257–273. Los Angeles, UCLA Tissue Typing Laboratory, 1985

68. Van Rood JJ, von Leeuwen A, Ernise JG: Leukocyte antibodies in sera of pregnant women. Vox Sang 4:427–444, 1959

69. Weil R, Clarke DR, Iwaki Y et al: Hyperacute rejection of a transplanted human heart. Transplantation 32(1):71–72, 1981

70. Williams GM, Hume DM, Hudson RP Jr et al: Hyperacute renal-homograft rejection in man. N Engl J Med 279:611–618, 1968

Tissue-Specific Antigens— A Role in Organ Transplantation Theory for the Existence of Tissue-Specific Antigens

G. James Cerilli   Lauren Brasile

The potential significance of tissue-specific antigens in organ transplantation is supported by several clinical observations, including (1) a spectrum of allograft survival for various organs, (2) morphologic and immunologic evidence that the microvasculature within a transplanted organ is a primary target of rejection, and (3) HLA identical, living-related combinations result in approximately 10% irreversible rejection. Therefore, the role of tissue-specific antigens in clinical transplantation appears to be important.

The tissue-specific antigens expressed by vascular endothelial cells (VEC) are definitely a major source of transplant immunogen in renal and cardiac transplantation and probably in every vascularized graft. The VEC-restricted antigens are polymorphic and appear to be linked to the major histocompatibility complex. Antibody to the VEC-specific antigens is the most commonly encountered antibody in patients rejecting a renal allograft.

Two antigenic systems restricted to epidermal cells play a significant role in skin graft transplantation. The generation of cytotoxic T cells specific to epidermal cells document the cellular-mediated response to alloantigens restricted to epidermal cells.

Antigens distinct from the systemic HLA antigens are also present in the kidney, on the renal tubular cell, and on both the glomerular and tubular basement membranes. Reports linking these antigens with kidney allograft rejection are few.

The tissue-specific antigens identified in pancreas, heart, and liver have not been studied extensively, so the relevance of these alloantigens in clinical transplantation remains to be elucidated.

The study of tissue-specific antigens in bone marrow is complicated by (1) the observation that antigen expression on precursor cells is different from the antigen expression of fully differentiated bone marrow cells, and (2) the complexity of the different polymorphic antigen systems expressed on the bone marrow–derived cells. The lymphocyte has been used as the standard target cell in evaluating histocompatibility based on the assumption that all the relevant transplant antigens were well expressed on the lymphocyte.

The response to this concept has been to develop more sensitive testing methods to detect subthreshold levels of antibody to lymphocytes. In the past, antibodies to tissue-specific antigens have rarely been considered to be a cause of rejection despite the well-documented existence of tissue-specific antigens. However, this is changing, particularly as the knowledge relative to the immunologic role of VEC antigens expands. Although further study is necessary to clearly delineate the role of these tissue-specific alloantigens, many studies, particularly with VEC, highlight the immunogenicity and transplant relevance of these antigens.

Tissue-specific antigens are defined as an antigen system that is expressed on only one type of organ, tissue, or cell. These tissue-specific antigens are independent from the systemic antigens such as HLA or ABH antigens, which have a wide distribution throughout the body. Tissue-specific antigens have either been characterized or theorized for almost every organ of the body. The identification of tissue-specific antigens had been anticipated since cell differentiation results in the development of molecules that serve specialized biological functions. Therefore, it is logical that such specialized molecules would have polymorphic antigenic structures, because anthropologic diversity is recognized to lead to antigenic polymorphism. What is less clear is the biological role of antigenic polymorphism. Among the theories that account for tissue-specific antigenic polymorphism, the most appealing are those in which, through evolution, tissue-specific antigens have mutated, giving rise to polymorphism. Polymorphism would be necessary in the recognition of self as part of immune surveillance. This latter mechanism may also be important in the monitoring and controlling of the embryologic development and maturation of individual organs and cells.

OBSERVATIONS SUPPORTING THE EXISTENCE OF TISSUE-SPECIFIC ANTIGENS

The potential significance of tissue-specific antigens in organ transplantation is supported by several observations. In 1969, Calne[9] first described the phenomenon of differential allograft survival between organs from the same donor. Whereas skin and kidney allografts were acutely rejected, liver allograft survival seemed to be prolonged in untreated pigs. A spectrum of allograft survival may exist involving skin, kidney, heart, pancreas, and liver allografts. Several cases of multiple organ transplants have been reported in which one organ is rejected while another continues to function. This spectrum of survival varies; generally, skin is considered to be the most aggressively rejected organ, whereas liver may be the least. One possible explanation for this observation is the relative immunologic effect of tissue-specific antigens. If all relevant transplant antigens were ubiquitous, graft survival should be fairly uniform in recipients receiving multiple organs from a single donor. It has been postulated that close compatibility in the HLA system between the recipient and the donor may prevent sensitization to the tissue-specific antigens. However, HLA identity and a negative mixed lymphocyte culture does not prevent an immune response to the increasingly well-studied VEC-specific antigens. In fact, 78% of recipients of HLA identical, living-related renal allografts who irreversibly reject their allografts develop antibody to their donors' VEC-specific antigens. Thus, compatibility for the HLA system does not guarantee compatibility for tissue-specific antigens.

Despite our understanding of the potential significance of tissue-specific antigens, for almost 20 years HLA compatibility has been the standard for evaluating recipient–donor antigenic compatibility in human organ transplantation. Although HLA identity in siblings leads to a high rate of success in renal transplantation (90%), an immunosuppressive regimen is necessary to prevent rejection, which can still occur in spite of the regimen. Likewise, prolonged graft survival can occur in cases of HLA mismatched organs. All these observations support the potential significance of non-HLA, tissue-specific antigens in organ transplantation.

If the role of tissue-specific antigens is potentially so significant in organ transplantation, why have these antigen systems not been as intensively studied as the traditional HLA antigens? The study of tissue-specific antigens is technically difficult. The isolation of pure cell populations from within a whole organ is imprecise. Often, there are no parameters to determine the purity of the cell preparations from the organ to be studied. Even if the methodology could be standardized to isolate the different classes of cells within a complex organ, isolation techniques such as enzymatic digestion of the tissue could affect the cell membranes, thereby making characterization of surface antigens difficult. In addition, the restrictive expression and distribution of tissue-specific antigens is not conducive to the development or identification of antibody to tissue-restrictive antigens. Tissue-specific antigens would not be an immunogen in transfusions, because they are most likely not in the circulation in high concentration. Likewise, antibodies to tissue-specific antigens would not be frequently encountered in multiparous sera, because tissue-specific antigens would not be likely to cross the placental barrier in significant amounts during pregnancy. The main mechanism by which sensitization to the tissue-specific antigens would occur is through an autoimmune mechanism or through transplantation of the organ containing the tissue-specific antigens. Therefore, the potential sources of alloantibodies to be used in the study of tissue-specific antigens are limited.

ALLOANTIGENS SPECIFIC TO VASCULAR ENDOTHELIUM

The vascular endothelial cells (VEC) of the transplanted organ are at the interface between the graft and the recipient blood containing immunocompetent cells. Pathologic appraisal of both early and late graft rejections place the VEC in an important role in the rejection process. VEC not only represent a transplant barrier but also are an endocrine-like organ capable of synthesizing clotting factors and inactivating hormones. VEC can also serve as antigen-presenting cells; they are able to phagocytize and are partly responsible for the normal function of platelets.[50,92] All these functions and observations, coupled with the now established presence of an antigen system unique to VEC, support the conclusion that the VEC is extremely important in the pathogenesis of the rejection process.

The specialized functions of VEC naturally implied the existence of specialized surface receptors. The first evidence suggesting the existence of such specialized receptors that could serve as transplant immunogens was provided by Vetto and Burger in the early 1970s.[91] These early studies in which antibody specific to the VEC was developed highlighted the role of vascular endothelium as the sensitizing milieu in a transplanted organ where the initial recognition occurs. The recognition of grafted endothelium being immunologically potent led to studies evaluating the clinical significance of the VEC-specific antigens.

Moraes and Stastny,[58,59] Paul et al,[63] and Cerilli et al[15,16] provided evidence for VEC and peripheral blood monocytes sharing restricted non-HLA antigens that were clinically significant in renal transplantation. The discovery that the expression of this important transplant immunogen is restricted to VEC and monocytes has sparked speculation about its biological role; monocytes have been shown to be capable of substituting for VEC under certain circumstances. Williams et al[93] demonstrated that bone marrow derived cells, presumably monocytes, can lodge among normal VEC and appear as morphologically identical to VEC. Our studies as well as those of other investigators indicate approximately 90% concordance between VEC and monocyte reactivity, that is, about 90% of sera reacting to a monocyte react to the concordant VEC in the absence of any anti-HLA activity (Table 11-1). The difference, 10%, is due to a monocyte-specific antigen system. Recent unpublished data from our laboratory strongly suggest that there is also a VEC antigen system totally restricted to the VEC and not located on concordant monocytes. It appears from

TABLE 11-1   Monocyte and VEC Correlation Studies

NUMBER OF SERA	CYTOTOXICITY*	
	Monocytes†	VEC†
42	Positive	Positive
12	Negative	Negative
4	Positive	Negative
1	Negative	Positive

* T- and B-lymphocyte negative
† Concordant VEC and monocytes

Note: Studies using concordant cells indicate that the peripheral blood monocyte also expresses the VEC-specific antigens; therefore, the monocyte can be used as an alternative target cell.

our preliminary observations that an immunologic response to this VEC-restricted antigen system may also play an important role in transplant rejection.

Other studies provide further evidence that supports the importance of the VEC antigen system in allograft transplantation.[10,12,17,64] Antibody specific to VEC is the most commonly encountered antibody in patients rejecting a renal allograft (Table 11-2). Ninety-six percent of the patients who experienced accelerated rejection and 94% of the patients who experienced chronic rejection developed anti-VEC antibody. Antibody to VEC is rarely encountered in normal controls and only in low frequency in patients experiencing a benign clinical posttransplantation course. The results of retro- and prospective testing in human renal transplantation have shown that patients who develop donor-specific antibody directed against the VEC antigens have a high incidence of rejection regardless of the degree of HLA matching. Seventy-eight percent of the patients who reject their HLA identical living-related renal allograft exhibit donor-specific anti-VEC antibody.[13] Most of these patients had anti-VEC antibody present in their pretransplantation sera in the absence of any anti-HLA antibody to the donor. This VEC antigen system appears to be an important immunogen in non-HLA-identical combinations as well. Many such patients who experience irreversible rejection exhibit anti-VEC antibody in their posttransplantation nephrectomy sera. (Table 11-3). In fact, anti-VEC antibody is more frequently encountered than anti-HLA antibody in the sera of patients rejecting a cadaver renal transplant. In contrast, antibody to VEC is detected in only approximately 7% of patients with a benign clinical course. In a prospective study of the frequency of anti-VEC antibody in patients awaiting renal transplantation, a minimum of 7% of prospective living-related or cadaveric donor recipients had donor-

TABLE 11-2 *Percent Positive Reactions Against Various Cell Types*

PATIENT GROUP	VEC	RENAL CELL	LYMPHOCYTE
Normal	0	0	0
Sensitized dialysis	49	46	60
Posttransplant, good function	4	0	3
Chronic rejection	94	40	49
Accelerated rejection	91	18	26

Note: VEC-specific antigen(s) are immunogeneic, and antibodies to these antigens are frequently developed in recipients of allografts. Antibody to VEC is the most frequently encountered antibody in patients who reject an allograft.

TABLE 11-3 *Screening Studies Using Posttransplantation Nephrectomy Sera**

NUMBER OF PATIENTS	VEC PANEL REACTIVITY† (%)	LYMPHOCYTE PANEL REACTIVITY (%)
27	8–83 (median panel, 28)	0–100 (median panel, 33)

* A positive reaction is scored with greater than 50% kill of the allogeneic cells.

† After absorption with pooled platelets and B cells to remove all HLA antibody

Note: In non-HLA-identical transplants, the development of anti-VEC antibody occurs as an independent coevent to the development of anti-HLA antibody. The values represent the percent reactivity of sera from patients who have rejected a renal allograft to a panel of vascular endothelial cells after sera absorption and lymphocyte preabsorption.

specific anti-VEC antibody (Table 11-4). It is important to note that the specific anti-VEC antibody found in these patients cannot be absorbed with pooled T- or B-lymphocytes (HLA antigens) and can be removed only with pooled VEC or monocytes. Thus, it is thought that the VEC contains on its cell surface Class I, Class II, ABO, and the VEC/monocyte antigen systems. Because the monocyte also expresses the VEC-specific antigens, prospective screenings can now be performed using the peripheral blood monocyte as an alternative and easily available target cell in crossmatching. Using the monocyte crossmatch would avoid transplanting patients with antibody to donor VEC antigens.

More recently, the VEC-specific antigens have also been shown to play an important role in cardiac transplantation.[7] Patients experiencing acute cardiac dysfunction immediately following transplantation, as well as patients who died during the first 24 hours posttransplantation, have been found to exhibit anti-VEC antibody without HLA antibody to the donor (Table 11-5). In one well-studied patient who experienced hyperacute cardiac rejection, donor-specific anti-VEC antibody was present in the pretransplantation sera in the total absence of donor-specific HLA antibody. In controls, anti-VEC antibody is very rarely detected in the cardiac allograft recipients with benign clinical courses. Thus, in both

renal and cardiac transplantation, antibody to donor VEC correlates with graft rejection and to a greater degree than donor-specific HLA antibody.

UBIQUITY, SPECIFICITY, AND LINKAGE TO THE MAJOR HISTOCOMPATIBILITY COMPLEX

The VEC antigens are expressed in abundance throughout the renal vasculature. There is a particularly high concentration of these antigens along the peritubular capillaries and veins.[3] In the extrarenal vasculature, the VEC antigens are expressed on the endothelial cells of all the major abdominal vessels, both arterial and venous. We have noted the concentration of these VEC antigens to be highest on the venous side of the vasculature, as have other investigators.

The results of sera screening analysis have led to the initial identification of several VEC antigen specificities. Moraes and Stastny[59] defined eight clusters of reactivity and designated these specificities as E-M antigens. Our group has identified six VEC antigens and assigned them the nomenclature VEC 1 through 6.[5,6] The role of these VEC antigens in graft outcome was analyzed in 14 HLA identical living-related donor transplants. In the seven pa-

TABLE 11-4   Sequential Prospective Screening Studies

		POSITIVE CROSSMATCHES	
GROUP	NUMBER OF DONORS	B Cell and Monocyte	Monocyte*
Cadaveric	83	29/83 (35%)	6/83 (7%)
Living-related	70	15/70 (21%)	5/70 (7%)

* All positive monocyte reactions reflected anti-VEC antibody.

Note: The frequency of anti-VEC antibody in patients awaiting a renal allograft is approximately 7%. However, this may actually represent an underestimate, since the patients with positive B cell crossmatches have not been retested after absorption to remove HLA antibody.

TABLE 11-5   Analysis of Anti-VEC Antibody in Cardiac Allograft Recipients*

NUMBER OF PATIENTS	GROUP	MONOCYTES (%)	VEC (%)
4	Hyperacute rejection	20–89	20–89
8/9	Accelerated rejection	20–78	20–78
17	Benign course	0	0

* Range of panel reactivity

Note: VEC-specific antigens are ubiquitous and appear to serve as an important target of rejection in cardiac transplantation. Patients with accelerated or benign courses were studied in a blinded fashion. All patients with hyperacute rejection and most with accelerated rejection had anti-VEC antibody. One patient (hyperacute rejection) had documented anti-VEC antibody to the specific donor without any anti-T or -B cell antibody.

tients with a benign clinical course the VEC antigens were similar in the donor and recipient. All seven patients who did poorly following transplantation were mismatched for at least one VEC antigen. (Fig. 11-1).

Antisera that identify these six VEC antigens have been used in our laboratory to perform pedigree studies. In 24 meioses studied, the VEC antigens were always found to segregate in association with parental HLA haplotypes (Fig. 11-2). These results support the VEC antigen system being a part of, or closely linked to, the major histocompatibility complex (MHC).[6] The results of cytotoxicity inhibition studies performed by Moraes and Stastny[58,59] suggest that the VEC antigens are associated with β_2-microglobulin. The association of the VEC antigens with β_2-microglobulin and the apparent linkage of these antigens with the MHC suggest that these antigens are a new Class I–like alloantigen.

CELLULAR-MEDIATED RESPONSE

A cellular-mediated mechanism for VEC damage in renal transplantation is suggested by the discovery of lymphocytes in direct contact with the endothelium of grafted organs. Acute cellular rejection, as well as chronic rejection, is frequently characterized by cell infiltration without immunoglobulin deposition.[8] Endothelial cells were first shown to be capable of stimulating allogeneic lymphocytes in mixed lymphocyte endothelial cultures by Hirschberg et al[35] in 1974. Resting VEC express Class I antigens but usually express little Class II antigens. T-lymphocytes are capable of modulating surface receptors on VEC, thereby inducing Class II antigen expression.[68] The VEC are then capable of activating T-lymphocytes. Subsequently, Groenewegen et al[28] have been able to generate cytotoxic cells specific for VEC antigens. However, allogeneic cells were used; therefore, antigens other than those specific (restricted) to VEC could have been the stimulating antigen. Further evidence for the VEC-specific antigen stimulating a blastogenic response was provided by a recipient–donor combination in which the only detectable antigen disparity was found in the VEC antigen system. The blastogenic response stimulated by the donor's VEC antigen, although positive, was considerably lower than the response detected by stimulation with Class II disparate cells.[4]

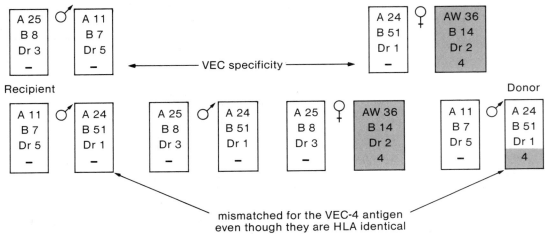

FIGURE 11-1. *When HLA identical, living-related recipient/donor combinations experience irreversible rejection, VEC antigen typing results indicate that they are mismatched for the VEC specific antigen(s).*

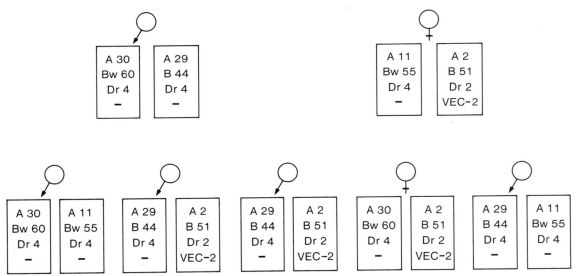

FIGURE 11-2. *Pedigree from segregation studies showing genetic linkage of the VEC antigen system with the Major Histocompatibility Complex. In this example, VEC-2 antigens segregate with the A2, B51, Dr2 haplotype. (A LOD, corrected for e_1, equals 0.04, which would place the genes coding for the VEC antigen system approximately four recombination units from the major histocompatibility complex.)*

These studies indicate that VEC-specific antigens distinct from the MHC antigens might play a role in lymphocyte stimulation, and this may initiate a cellular immune response.

SUMMARY—VEC ANTIGEN SYSTEM

This unique antigen system on the VEC is shared only with the peripheral blood monocyte and is a powerful immunogen that initiates an immune response that may explain the rejection of most HLA-identical renal transplants. There is growing evidence that the immune responses to the VEC antigens are important in cardiac transplantation, cadaveric renal transplantation, and living-related donor transplantation. It is conceivable that the immune response to the VEC antigen system may be more important in the pathogenesis of rejection than the immune response to the HLA system, but it has been overlooked in the past because of the difficulty in studying this system.

There is strong evidence for the presence of a tissue-restricted antigen system on the VEC as evidenced by the following: (1) There is a documentable antibody cytotoxic to VEC in the absence of any cytotoxicity to the same donor lymphocytes. (2) This antibody can be absorbed only with pooled VEC and not with the concordant lymphocytes. (3) VEC specificities have been documented by appropriate sera screening and statistical analysis. (4) Cytotoxic T cells specific to VEC and nonreactive to lymphocytes can be generated. (5) Patients who rejected a renal allograft frequently have anti-VEC antibody in the absence of anti-HLA antibody.

What is the current role, therefore, and possible future significance of the VEC antigen system? First, all patients about to undergo transplantation should have pretransplantation screening performed for the presence of anti-donor VEC antibody, using the monocyte crossmatch technique. If the monocyte crossmatch is positive, appropriate cell panel analysis should be performed to determine whether the antibody is VEC or monocyte specific. Second, it is becoming increasingly clear that some anti-donor antibody detected using the lymphocyte as the target cell may represent sensitization to lymphocyte-restricted antigens and not sensitization to the transplant-relevant antigens, either HLA or VEC antigens. These can be identified by appropriate screening techniques, and such recipient–donor combinations could possibly be transplantable. Third, the better definition of the VEC specificities may improve the selection of the most appropriate donor because the VEC antigens could be the most potent immunogen in the rejection process. Fourth, the VEC-specific antigen system appears to play an important role in the pathogenesis of idiopathic vasculitis and even possibly atherosclerosis.[14] Almost all patients with active vasculitis have an autoantibody to their VEC, and more than one third of patients with peripheral vascular disease have an autoantibody to their VEC antigens.[14] A knowledge of the antigen system and immunologic process involved in the pathogenesis of these two diseases widens the therapeutic options. Most importantly, the now documented role of the VEC antigens in transplantation and other disease states will encourage investigation into the role of other organ-specific antigen systems.

SKIN-SPECIFIC ANTIGENS

Skin is the most abundant and accessible tissue for the study of tissue-specific antigens. It can be differentiated into epithelial and stromal components by trypsin digestion.[54] Skin, therefore, like the VEC, is well suited for the study of tissue-specific antigens.

Excluding VEC and muscle tissue, skin consists of four major cell types: (1) the keratinocyte (the major epithelial cell), (2) the dermal fibroblast (the major cell type of the stromal component), (3) the melanocyte (which provides pigment), and (4) the Langerhans' cell (part of the reticuloendothelial system). Skin is one of the most susceptible tissues to rejection.[61] In the mouse, the Ia antigens of the MHC are believed to play a role in the rejection of skin grafts.[42] Although not all skin cells express the Ia antigens,[78] all types of skin cells can stimulate in a mixed lymphocyte–skin reaction.[36] Studies such as those previously described suggest that antigens specific to skin may be involved in the rejection of skin grafts. Two antigenic systems restricted to epidermal cells have been described: the serologically defined SK antigens, and the cellularly defined Epa antigens. The skin-specific alloantigens of the mouse were first described in 1972 and were found to be encoded by genes outside the H2 complex.[73]

The human equivalent of the Epa antigens is also capable of stimulating lymphocyte proliferation and further supporting the existence of skin-specific antigens. When proliferating lymphocytes in allogeneic mixed lymphocyte reactions were removed by H3 thymidine pulsing, the residual lymphocytes were still capable of responding to the epidermal-specific antigens in the absence of any proliferation to the same donor lymphocytes. Since the lymphocytes responded to epidermal cells in the absence of any proliferation to the lymphocytes from the same donor, the stimulating antigens were specific to epidermal cells. This observation supports the presence of tissue-specific antigens on epidermal cells, which are capable of stimulating-lymphocytes to blastogenesis.[37] When mice are immunized with epidermal cells, cytotoxic T-lymphocytes can be generated that exhibit a marked specificity for donor epidermal cells in comparison with lymphocytes.[77] Steinmuller and Tyler[77] have interpreted this observation as being indicative of the generation of multiple clones, where some clones are directed against the antigens shared by lymphocytes and epidermal cells. In addition, some clones would be specifically directed against epidermal cell antigens. The generation of cytotoxic T-lymphocytes specific for epidermal cells documents the cellularly defined response to alloantigens unique to epidermal cells. Thus, the skin does contain tissue restrictive antigens capable of eliciting an immune response, and this immune response seems capable of a significant role in skin rejection.

KIDNEY-SPECIFIC ANTIGENS

Glomerular

Historically, the study of tissue-specific antigens in the kidney has centered predominantly on the glomerular antigens involved in nephrotoxic serum nephritis and antigens on the renal tubule cells. The original interest in nephrotoxic serum nephritis stemmed from its similarity to the morphology of glomerulonephritis in humans. These early animal models demonstrated that a single injection of specific anti-kidney serum in animals could produce acute nephritis. The acute nephritis caused by an antibody–antigen reaction can also lead to chronic disease. In subsequent studies, the glomerular cortex was demonstrated to be the site of this immune reaction.[33,75] Subsequently, the nephrotoxic antigen capable of producing the nephrotoxic sera was localized to the glomeruli because isolated glomerular fractions preferentially absorbed the nephrotoxic activity of antisera.[76] Further evidence supporting the tissue-specific immunogenicity of glomeruli was later provided by using a nephrotoxic serum produced by immunization in rabbits with isolated dog glomeruli.[26] Other cortical components free of glomeruli were relatively nonimmunogenic. The isolated structures within the glomeruli were studied in order to further define the source of the nephrotoxic antigen.[27] The parietal capsule and parietal epithelial cells were subsequently found to be relatively nonimmunogenic. Although nephrotoxic sera reacted with isolated glomerular cells, reactions were much stronger with the glomerular basement membrane preparations. Later chemical studies indicated that this nephrotoxic antigen is a protein-polysaccharide complex localized on the glomerular basement membrane.[25,49,97] Interestingly, the "expression" of nephrotoxic antigen in various tissues of the dog correlates with the degree of vascularization.[42] Nonvascularized tissues such as cartilage and cornea lack this antigen, and poorly vascularized tissue such as heart valves and tendons expressed very little nephrotoxic antigen.

Tubular Cell Antigens

A difference between antigens localized in the cytoplasm of tubular cells and basement membrane antigens of glomeruli was first noted in 1953.[34] Rabbit anti-rat kidney sera, absorbed with rat lung, stained only the cytoplasm of renal tubule cells by immunofluorescence techniques. Antisera to glomeruli failed to stain tubules and reacted only with the tubule basement membrane. Rabbits immunized with mitochondrial and microsomal fractions of hamster kidney produce antibodies to renal tubular cell cytoplasm after the antisera was absorbed with cytoplasmic particles from liver, lung, and red cells. These observations support the presence of a distinct antigen system in the renal tubular cell.

Relationship of Renal Cell Antigens to Graft Rejection

Antigens distinct from the systemic HLA antigens are present in the human kidney. Glomerular basement membranes, renal tubular epithelial cells, and tubular basement membranes are thought to represent the main potential sources of tissue-specific antigens in a renal allograft. Correspondingly, the search for detrimental antibodies in the sera from renal allograft recipients has centered on these three renal structures. Unfortunately, the study of kidney-specific antigens is technically very difficult because of the lack of methodology to definitively identify renal cells or to purify basement membranes. Despite the technical difficulties, kidney-specific antigens have occasionally been documented to affect the outcome of renal transplantation. The first evidence of anti-donor kidney-specific antibody being associated with a detrimental clinical outcome was reported in 1968.[93] Subsequently, several studies have supported the existence of renal cell antigens and their potential importance on graft outcome. Some caution is necessary in the interpretation of these early studies, because the proper identification and isolation of renal cells was not clearly established. Despite the technical difficulties, the results of several studies suggest that renal cells express antigens not found on concordant lymphocytes and that these restrictive antigens play a role in the rejection process. For instance, eluates from 14 rejected renal allografts were analyzed for the presence of cytotoxic antibodies.[57] The eluates were screened against a panel of T- and B-lymphocytes, as well as primary renal cell cultures. After appropriate absorption, sera that reacted only with renal cells were developed. These results, along with another study,[67] support the existence of unique renal cell antigens that are distinct from the antigens of the MHC and a role in rejection for these antigens.

These renal cell–specific antigens have been linked persuasively to a case report of hyperacute rejection.[94] The recipient exhibited preformed antibody cytotoxic to the donor's kidney cells in the absence of reactivity to the same donor's lymphocytes. Although the techniques necessary to perform screenings for donor-specific anti-renal cell antibody are difficult to perform routinely and are beyond the scope of most laboratories, these studies also support the potential clinical significance of renal cell–specific antigens in graft outcome.

Renal Basement Membrane Antigens and Graft Rejection

Both glomerular and tubular basement membranes contain non-HLA antigens. Occasionally, a renal allograft has been reported to contain basement membrane antigens of a particular specificity that is lacking in the recipient. There is evidence that these basement membrane antigenic differences can serve as a source of immunogen that induces antibasement membrane antibodies after transplantation. This antitubular basement membrane antibody can lead to glomerulonephritis or tubulointerstitial nephritis in the transplanted organ just as autoantibody can lead to these disease states.[22,66,96] It must be noted, however, that these antigenic differences are rare and do not represent a common problem in transplantation. Progress in the study of basement membrane antigens has been limited by technical difficulties in isolating purified basement membranes.

Chronic renal allograft rejection has also been associated with the presence of antitubular basement membrane antibody.[41,53,95] In one study, all the patients experiencing acute rejection episodes were found to develop antitubular basement membrane antibodies.[96] The presence of antitubular basement membrane antibody correlated with the onset and severity of the rejection episodes.

Cellular-Mediated Response to Kidney-Specific Antigens

A cellular response to kidney-specific antigens was demonstrated when only kidney cells could reduce the in vitro cellular-mediated response of T cells sensitized to kidney cell antigens. The results of these target inhibitor studies suggest that kidney cells express restricted antigens that are recognized by a selected population of cytotoxic lymphocytes. Evidence for renal allograft rejection being at times mediated by a cellular response toward kidney restricted antigens is provided by the work of Manca and co-workers.[51] Sensitized cytotoxic lymphocytes that were specific for the donor kidney fibroblasts and did not kill the donor's peripheral blood lymphocytes, were isolated in the human donor's kidney. A salient point is that if one looks for cytotoxic

cell activity in the peripheral blood exclusively, the relevant sensitization directed against tissue-specific antigens that is occurring within the graft could be overlooked. The recipient's peripheral blood lymphocytes do not reflect the sensitized T cell population sequestered in the transplanted organ.

It has been pointed out that the reports linking antitubular basement membrane or tubular cell antibodies with kidney allograft rejection are few. Most studies, as well as morphologic evidence, support the major source of immunogen in the kidney being the VEC. Also in support of this interpretation is the finding that the stimulation in the mixed lymphocyte–kidney cell reaction is probably due to contaminating VEC, because flomerular cell suspensions failed to stimulate lymphocytes to blastogenesis.[90] Freshly isolated or cultured tubular cells also failed to stimulate lymphocytes. In contrast, VEC stimulate allogenic lymphocytes to blastogenesis.[36] Thus, although there are isolated reports that imply that non-HLA or non-VEC antigens are important in renal allograft rejection, these reports are few, and the data are susceptible to other interpretation as a result of methodological difficulty.

PANCREAS-SPECIFIC ANTIGENS

Pancreas-specific antigens were, presumably, first detected serologically in rabbits in 1960.[71] Rabbits immunized with pooled allogeneic pancreatic extracts produced pancreas-specific antibodies that did not react with autologous pancreatic extracts, although they did react with allogeneic pancreatic extracts.[71] Immunofluorescent analysis indicated that these alloantibodies bind to the exocrine, acinar cells. The antibodies do not bind to the endocrine cells.[55] Subsequently, sera from newly diagnosed insulin-dependent diabetic children were found to contain antibodies to human islet cell antigens.[1] These antigens were detected on islets but not on the lymphocytes from all the pancreas donors studied. The high frequency of autoantibody to islets present in newly diagnosed diabetics suggests that these tissue-specific antibodies are involved in the pathogenesis of diabetes mellitus, because they react primarily with the islet cells.[89] Characterizing the targeted cell–restricted antigens has been difficult because of the complexity of the endocrine pancreas. The endocrine pancreas is structurally complex; it includes both the islets of Langerhans and the extra-islet endocrine cells.[47] The endocrine tissue is made up of at least four cell types—B, A, D, and F cells (which produce insulin, glucagon, somatostatin, pancreatic polypeptide), capillary endothelial cells, and connective tissue. It was originally thought that the absence of VEC in an isolated islet allograft would make the islet less antigenic. Unfortunately, isolated islets are not immunologically privileged and are equally susceptible to rejection.[61] Isolated islet cells contain antigens of the MHC as well as islet-specific determinants. Matching for the HLA antigens has not prevented the rejection of islet transplants.[60] If islet-specific antigens and an autoimmune mechanism play a role in the pathogenesis of diabetes mellitus, it is now generally recognized that these antigens can also serve as a source of immunogen in a pancreas transplant.[52]

Human islets are capable of stimulating allogeneic T-lymphocytes to blastogenesis[70] and therefore contain antigens that are recognized by T-lymphocytes. However, these lymphocyte-stimulating antigens are not HLA, because when the responding lymphocytes are first primed with lymphocytes, there is no subsequent response to the islets from the same donor. This observation indicates that the lymphocytes are responding to antigens on the lymphocytes that are not shared by the islet cell. Therefore, the T-lymphocyte stimulation caused by the islet cells is probably due to non-HLA antigens. These results not only provide evidence for the existence of tissue-specific antigens on isolated islet cells, but also indicate a potential role for these antigens as a source of immunogen capable of stimulating lymphocyte blastogenesis.

Clearly, pancreatic islets contain cell-restricted antigens that play a role in diabetes and probably play a role in rejection. The role of acinar cell–restricted antigens in rejection is unclear.

BONE MARROW

Significance of Graft-Versus-Host

Despite HLA identity, rejection of the bone marrow transplanted from a sibling occurs frequently, particularly in patients with aplastic anemia.[29] Rejection of a bone marrow allograft has been reported to range from 25% to 60% in recipients who are sensitized by transfusion.[23,80] Bone marrow transplantation is further complicated by the occurrence of graft-versus-host disease (GVHD). Bone marrow is the only organ transplantation in which the donor's immune response plays a significant role in the graft outcome. GVHD is generally characterized into two categories: acute and chronic. Acute GVHD is most likely mediated by mature T-lymphocytes present in the bone marrow graft.[69,81,88] The im-

munologic process is targeted predominately against antigens present in the skin, liver, and intestine. Acute GVHD usually develops within 100 days after transplantation and is associated with a high mortality rate. Chronic GVHD is most likely to develop in patients experiencing the acute form of this disease.[81] Like the acute disease, chronic GVHD is thought to be cellularly mediated[79] and develops after 100 days post-transplantation. Chronic GVHD can be severely disabling and occurs in about 20% of cases.[83] It resembles the clinical features of autoimmunity, but it is multiorgan.

Cell-Mediated Antigens

The high frequency of rejection and GVHD in bone marrow transplantation between HLA-identical living-related siblings suggests that antigens other than those of the MHC may serve as an important source of immunogen. Incompatibility for these non-HLA antigens could occur frequently in HLA-identical combinations if inheritance of these antigens is independent of the MHC. In the recipient sensitized through transfusions, the non-HLA cell–specific antigens that are the target for the rejection would have to be shared between the mature hematopoietic cells in the blood and their early myeloid component in the bone marrow. This consideration highlights the potential difficulty in studying the role of non-HLA antigens in bone marrow transplantation. Support for the differences between antigen representation on mature cells and the antigens expressed on early myeloid components is provided by the finding that alloimmune neonatal neutropenia is caused by neutrophil-specific antibodies crossing the placenta. However, bone marrow cells are spared because these early myeloid cells lack the neutrophil-specific antigens.[45] Further complicating the study of non-HLA antigens in bone marrow transplantation is the complexity of the different polymorphic antigen systems expressed on the bone marrow–derived cells. Antigens with restricted cell expression have been reported for the granulocyte[46,84] and the monocyte.[2,11,62] In addition to these restricted antigens of the granulocyte and monocyte, antigens have been reported with shared expression on the monocyte and granulocyte,[72,85,86] such as the HGA-1 and HMC-2 antigens. There are also the antigens shared exclusively by the VEC and monocyte described previously. Lastly, antigens have been described with expression restricted to the granulocyte, monocyte, or VEC.[87] Similar to the non-HLA antigens studied in other tissues, very little is known of the genetics of these polymorphic systems. However, antibodies to some of these non-

HLA antigens in bone marrow transplantation seem to have a detrimental influence.

Monocyte-Specific Antigens

Several studies have demonstrated a correlation between anti-monocyte-specific antibody and bone marrow graft rejection. In one study, 51 bone marrow recipients with aplastic anemia were screened for the presence of antibody to monocytes and B-lymphocytes using a panel of allogeneic donors.[24] There was no association between the pretransplantation presence of the anti-monocyte-specific antibody and the patient's subsequent clinical course. However, the development of anti-monocyte antibody post-transplantation was found to correlate with rejection. Anti-monocyte antibodies to allogeneic cells (not donor specific) were also found in patients experiencing good clinical courses. The results of this study indicated that there was no predictive value in any individual case. These observations can possibly be explained by the lack of donor-specific testing. In another study, it was demonstrated that rejection was more likely in the recipients of HLA-identical bone marrow transplants who developed anti-monocyte antibody than in patients who never developed these antibodies.[18] The presence of anti-monocyte antibody could be irrelevant to graft outcome if the antigen specificity to which the antibody is directed is absent in the donor. These studies emphasize the importance of the polymorphism of cell-restricted antigens. If the recipient develops antibody to the monocyte-restricted antigens of the specific donor, rejection would seem more likely. If the recipient develops or has pretransplantation antibody to monocyte-restricted antigen specificities not represented in the donor, outcome seems unaffected. This is not unlike the observations with the HLA antigen system in renal transplantation.

Other Cell-Specific Antigens

Antigens expressed on mature, as well as immature, granulocytes and monocytes may play a significant role in bone marrow transplantation.[38,44,87] Although the nomenclature varies from group to group, HGA-1, HMC-2, HMA-1 and HMA-2, and 9a antigens are probably similar. In fact, HMA-1 and 9a have been shown to have the same specificity and are probably situated on the same molecule.[38, 44] Differences in the reported reactivity to these antigens may be attributable to various testing techniques for their detection. While several groups have reported a significant effect of antibodies to the granulocyte and monocyte antigens in bone marrow transplantation,[18,38,87] others have found matching for monocyte/granulocyte antigens not to be statistically significant.[44]

Antibodies to specific cell components of bone marrow, therefore, do develop posttransplantation. There is some evidence, particularly with antimonocyte antibody, that such antibody correlates with graft rejection. However, the evidence that such humoral responses to specific marrow components impact on graft survival is still very preliminary. Typing for a limited number of cell-specific antigens in the marrow has not proved useful in marrow transplantation.

Cardiac-Specific Antigens

The ability of heart tissue to induce organ-specific alloantibodies was first demonstrated through immunofluorescence studies on fixed and unfixed tissue that detected antibodies specific for heart tissue.[40] Absorption of these antisera with various tissue extracts failed to remove the anti-heart activity. The sites of immunofluorescence detected with the anti-heart sera were localized in sites rich in lipid material. Also supporting the existence of heart-specific alloantigens is the finding that administration of cell-free extracts of donor-specific heart resulted in prolonged graft survival.[82] The heart extracts were thought to contain not only the major histocompatibility antigens but also cardiac specific antigens. This interpretation was developed on the basis that heart extracts produced longer allograft survival than did donor-specific cell-free extracts from the liver and spleen. This apparent tolerance may have been induced by blocking antibodies that were developed in response to the donor-specific antigens in the extracts.[82] The results of these early studies suggested the existence of heart-specific antigens localized to the intermyofibrillar region of cardiac sarcoplasm.

A correlation between the presence of anti-heart-specific antibodies and acute rejection episodes in cardiac transplants was first reported in 1970.[21] The presence of anti-heart-specific antibodies is associated with a slightly higher incidence of acute rejection episodes.[30] After transplantation, 69% of the patients developed antibodies that bound to heart tissue. Anti-heart antibody was found in four of six patients who died from acute cardiac allograft rejection.

However, other studies have found that heart-specific antigens have little impact in transplantation. Heart-specific alloantigens, which are encoded by genes outside the mouse MHC, have been detected in the rat. The alloantigens are present on the myocardial cell membrane and the T tubule system. Indirect evidence suggests that heart-specific antigens do not appear to serve as an important source of transplant immunogen in the rat. By using back-cross donors, it was shown that cardiac allograft rejection time was not influenced by the expression of heart-specific antigens. Therefore, with the exception of VEC-specific antigens, a role for organ-specific antigen has not yet been clearly established in heart transplantation.

Liver-Specific Antigens

Liver-specific antigens were described in the 1960s.[20,48,56] Liver-specific antigens became of interest when it was discovered that autoantibody to these antigens was frequently found in the sera from patients with chronic hepatitis.[74] The autoantibody could not be absorbed with antigens from other organs and thus appeared to be organ specific. More recently, alloantibodies to liver-specific antigens have been identified.[32] Using a rat model, antibodies

can be detected with specificity for liver alloantigens located on the external and intracellular membranes of the hepatocytes. The genes coding for these liver-specific antigens are encoded by a locus outside the MHC. The existence of these alloantigens can be determined by the serologic analysis of liver homogenates as well as from sera from allograft recipients. Although this study documented the existence of liver-specific alloantigens, the possible relevance of these alloantigens in clinical liver transplantation was not determined.

Liver cells can elicit an immune response. For instance, isolated human liver cells stimulate lymphocytes to blastogenesis, although liver cells lack the expression of Ia-like antigens.[19,31] Liver cells are capable of inducing lymphocyte stimulation in some animals that are identical for the MHC antigens and inbred for four generations.[65] These results suggest that liver antigens distinct from the antigens of the MHC are capable of eliciting blastogeneic responses. However, their role is unknown in liver graft rejection.

REFERENCES

1. Baekkeshov S, Nielsen JH, Marner B et al: Autoantibodies in newly diagnosed diabetic children immunoprecipitate human pancreatic islet cell proteins. Nature 298:167, 1982
2. Baldwin WM, Claas FHJ, Paul LC et al: All monocyte antigens are not expressed on renal endothelium. Tissue Antigens 21:254, 1983
3. Baldwin WM, Claas FHJ, van Es LA et al: Distribution of endothelial-monocyte and HLA antigens on renal vascular endothelium. Transplant Proc 13:103, 1981
4. Brasile L, Clarke J, Cerilli J: The ability of the VEC antigen system to elicit a blastogenic response in HLA identical combinations. Transplant Proc 17:2322, 1985
5. Brasile L, Clarke J, Galouzis T et al: The clinical significance of the vascular endothelial cell antigen system: Evidence for genetic linkage between the endothelial cell antigen system and the major histocompatibility complex. Transplant Proc 17:741, 1985
6. Brasile L, Galouzis T, Clarke J et al: Clinical significance of vascular endothelial cell antigen system and the MHC. Transplant Proc 17:2318, 1985
7. Brasile L, Rabin B, Clarke J et al: The identification of antibody to vascular endothelial cells (VEC) in patients undergoing cardiac transplantation. Transplantation 40:672, 1985
8. Busch GJ, Garovoy MR, Tilney NL: Variant forms of arteritis in human renal allografts. Transplantation 11:100, 1979

9. Calne RY, Sells RA, Pena JR et al: Induction of immunological tolerance by porcine liver allografts. Nature 223:472, 1969
10. Cerilli J, Brasile L: Endothelial cell alloantigens. Transplant Proc 12:37, 1980
11. Cerilli J, Brasile L, Clarke J et al: The vascular endothelial cell-specific antigen system: Three years' experience in monocyte crossmatching. Transplant Proc 17:567, 1985
12. Cerilli J, Brasile L, Galouzis T et al: Clinical significance of antimonocyte antibody in kidney transplant recipients. Transplantation 32:495, 1981
13. Cerilli J, Brasile L, Galouzis T et al: The vascular endothelial cell antigen system. Transplantation 39:286, 1985
14. Cerilli J, Brasile L, Karmody A: Role of the vascular endothelial cell antigen system in the etiology of atherosclerosis. Ann Surg 202:329, 1985
15. Cerilli J, Holliday JE, Fesperman DP: The role of antivascular endothelial antibody in predicting renal allograft rejection. Transplant Proc 9:771, 1977
16. Cerilli J, Holliday JE, Koolemans-Beynen A: An analysis of the cell specificity of the antibody response accompanying human renal allograft rejection. Surgery 83:726, 1978
17. Claas FHJ, Paul LC, van Es LAS et al: Antibodies against donor antigens on endothelial cells and monocytes in eluates of rejected kidney allografts. Tissue Antigens 15:19, 1980
18. Claas FHJ, van Rood JJ, Warren RP et al: The detec-

tion of non-HLA antibodies and their possible role in bone marrow graft rejection. Transplant Proc 11:423, 1979

19. Davies H, Taylor JE, White DJG et al: Major transplantation of antigens of the pig kidney and liver. Comparisons between the whole organs and their parenchymal constituents. Transplantation 25:290, 1978

20. Dorner M, Simon EJ, Miescher PA: Studies on a liver-specific antigen. Fed Proc 21:43, 1962

21. Ellis RJ, Lillehei CW, Fischetti VA et al: Heart-reactive antibody: An index of cardiac rejection in human heart transplantation. Circulation 42:91, 1970

22. Ende N, Orsi EV, Britton TL et al: Anti-kidney cytotoxic antibodies in human renal allografts. Am J Clin Pathol 66:395, 1976

23. Gluckman E, Devergia A, Marty M et al: Allogeneic bone marrow transplantation in aplastic anemia—report of 25 cases. Transplant Proc 10:141, 1978

24. Gluckman JC, Gluckman E, Azoquieo et al: Mono-cytotoxic antibodies after bone marrow transplantation in aplastic anemia. Transplantation 33:599, 1982

25. Goodman HC, Baxter JH: Nephrotoxic serum nephritis in rats; preparation and characterization of soluble protective factor produced by trypsin digestion of rat tissue homogenetics. J Exp Med 104:487, 1956

26. Greenspon SA, Krakower CA: Direct evidence for antigenicity of glomeruli in production of nephrotoxic serums. AMA Arch Pathol 49:291, 1950

27. Greenspon SW, Krakower CA: Localization of nephrotoxic antigens within isolated renal glomerulus. AMA Arch Pathol 51:629, 1951

28. Groenewegen G, Buurman WA, Jeunhomme GMAA et al: In vitro stimulation of lymphocytes by vascular endothelial cells. Transplantation 37:206, 1984

29. Hansen JA, Clift RA, Thomas ED et al: Histocompatibility and marrow transplantation. Transplant Proc 11:1924, 1979

30. Harkiss GD, Cave P, Brown DL et al: Anti-heart antibodies in cardiac allograft recipients. Int Arch Allergy Appl Immunol 73:18, 1984

31. Hart DNJ, Fabre JW: Quantitative studies on the tissue distribution of IA and SD antigens in the DA and Lewis rat strains. Transplantation 27:110, 1979

32. Hart DNJ, Fabre JW: Antibody response after alloimmunization with heart tissue in the rat. Transplantation 31:174, 1981

33. Heymann W, Gilkey C, Salehar M: Antigenic property of renal cortex. Proc Soc Exp Biol Med 73:385, 1950

34. Hill AGS, Cruichshank B: Histochemical identification of connective tissue antigens in rats. Br J Exp Pathol 34:27, 1953

35. Hirschberg H, Evensen SA, Henriksen T et al: Stimulation of human lymphocytes by allogeneic endothelial cells in vitro. Tissue Antigens 4:257, 1974

36. Hirschberg H, Evensen SA, Thorsby E et al: Stimulation of human lymphocytes by cultured allogeneic skin and endothelial cells in vitro. Transplantation 19:454, 1975

37. Hirschberg H, Thorsby E: Lymphocyte activating al-

loantigens on human epidermal cells. Tissue Antigens 6:183, 1975

38. Jager MJ, van Leeuwen A, Claas FHJ et al: Histocompatibility Testing, p 148. Springer-Verlag, Berlin, Heidelberg, 1984

39. Jonker M, van Leeuwen A, Koch CT et al: Influence of matching for HLA-DR antigens on skin graft survival. Transplantation 27:91, 1979

40. Kaplan MH: Immunologic studies of heart tissue. J Immunol 80:254, 1958

41. Klassen J, Kano K, Milgrom F et al: Tubular lesions produced by autoantibodies to tubular basement membrane in human renal allografts. Int Arch Allergy Appl Immunol 45:675, 1973

42. Klein J, Hamptfeld M, Haupfeld V: Evidence for a third, IR-associated histocompatibility region in the H-2 complex of the mouse. Immunogenetics 1:45, 1974

43. Krakower CA, Greenspan SW: The localization of the "nephrotoxic" antigen(s) in extraglomerular tissue. AMA Arch Pathol 66:364, 1958

44. Lalezari P: Organ-specific and systemic alloantigens: Interrelationships and biologic implications. Transplant Proc 12:12, 1980

45. Lalezari P: Alloimmune neonatal neutropenia and neutrophil-specific antigens. Vox Sang 46:415, 1984

46. Lalezari P: In Greenwalt TJ, Jamieson GA (eds): Granulocyte Function and Clinical Utilization, p 209. New York, Alan R. Liss, Inc., 1977

47. Larsson LI, Sundler F, Hakanson R: Pancreatic polypeptide—a postulated new hormone: Identification of its cellular storage site by light and electron immunocytochemistry. Diabetologia 12:211, 1976

48. Licht E: Zur frage leberstezisischer antigene beim menschen. Klin Wochenschr 44:833, 1966

49. Liu CT, McCrory WW, Flick JA: Cytotoxic effect of nephrotoxic serum on rat tissue culture. Proc Soc Exp Biol Med 95:331, 1957

50. Majno G, Joris I: Endothelium 1977: A review. Adv Exp Med Biol 104:169, 1978

51. Manca F, Barocci S, Kunkl A et al: Recognition of donor fibroblast antigens by lymphocytes homing in the human grafted kidney. Transplantation 36:670, 1983

52. Mashimo S, Sakai A, Ochiai et al: The mixed kidney cell—lymphocyte reaction in rats. Tissue Antigens 7:291, 1976

53. McCoy RC, Johnson HK, Stone WJ et al: The kidney in progressive systemic sclerosis: Immunohistochemical and antibody elution studies. Lab Invest 34:325, 1976

54. Medawar PB: Sheets of pure epidermal epithelium from human skin. Nature 148:783, 1941

55. Metzgar RS: Immunologic studies of pancreas-specific isoantigens. J Immunol 93:176, 1964

56. Meyer Zum Buschenfelde KH, Schrank CH: Untersuchungen zur frage organspezifischer antigene der leber. Klin Wochenschr 44:654, 1966

57. Mohanakumar T, Phibbs M, Haar J et al: Alloantibodies eluted from rejected human renal allografts: Reac-

tivity to primary kidney cells in culture. Transplant Proc 12:65, 1980

58. Moraes R, Stastny P: A new antigen system expressed in human endothelial cells. Clin Invest 60:449, 1977

59. Moraes R, Stastny P: Human endothelial cell antigens: Molecular independence from HLA and expression in blood monocytes. Transplant Proc 9:1211, 1977

60. Najarian JS, Sutherland DER, Matas AJ et al: Human islet transplantation: A preliminary report. Transplant Proc 9:233, 1977

61. Nash JR, Peters M, Bell PRF: Comparative survival of pancreatic islets, heart, kidney and skin allografts in rats with and without enhancement. Transplantation 24:70, 1977

62. Paul LC, Baldwin WM, Claas FHJ et al: In Vookman A (ed): Mononuclear Phagocyte Biology, p 151. New York, M. Dekker, Inc., 1982

63. Paul LC, Claas FHJ, van Es LAS, et al: Accelerated rejection of a renal allograft associated with pretransplantation antibodies directed against donor antigens on endothelium and monocytes. N Engl J Med 300:1258, 1979

64. Paul LC, van Es LAS, Kaliff MW et al: Intrarenal distribution of endothelial antigens recognized by antibodies from renal allograft recipients. Transplant Proc 11:427, 1979

65. Pawelee G, Davies HffS, Pearson JD et al: Stimulation of lymphocyte proliferation by non-lymphoid porcine tissue cells. Tissue Antigens 14:367, 1979

66. Perkins HA, Gantan Z, Siegel S et al: Reactions of kidney cells with cytotoxic antisera: Possible evidence for kidney-specific antigens. Tissue Antigens 5:88, 1975

67. Pierce JC, Kay S, Lee HM: Donor-specific IgG antibody and the chronic rejection of human renal allografts. Surgery 78:14, 1975

68. Pober JS, Gimbrone MA, Collins T et al: Interactions of T lymphocytes with human vascular endothelial cells: Role of endothelial cells surface antigens. Immunobiology 168:483, 1984

69. Prentice HG, Blacklock HA, Janossy G et al: Use of anti-T-cell monoclonal antibody OKT3 to prevent acute graft vs. host disease in allogeneic bone marrow transplantation for acute leukemia. Lancet 1:700, 1982

70. Rabinovitch A, Fuller L, Mintz D et al: Responses of canine lymphocytes to allogeneic and autologous islets of Langerhans in mixed cell cultures. J Clin Invest 67:1507, 1981

71. Rose NR, Metzgar RS, Witebsky EJ: Studies on organ specificity. Immunology 85:575, 1960

72. Russ GR, Churcher H, Sato M et al: A murine monoclonal antibody recognizing a polymorphic determinant on monocytes and granulocytes. Transplant Proc 16:944, 1984

73. Scheid M, Boyse EA, Carsell EA et al: Serologically demonstrable alloantigens of mouse epidermal cells. J Exp Med 135:938, 1972

74. Schumacher K, Koch W: Nachweis zirkulierender autoantikorper bei chronisch-progressiver hepatitis. Klin Wochenschr 46:925, 1968

75. Smadel JE: Experimental nephritis in rats induced by injection of anti-kidney serum; preparation and immunological studies of nephrotoxin. J Exp Med 64:291, 1936

76. Solomon DH, Gardella JW, Fanger H et al: Nephrotoxic nephritis in rats; evidence for glomerular origin of kidney antigens. J Exp Med 90:267, 1949

77. Steinmuller D, Tyler JD: Evidence of skin-specific alloantigens in cell-mediated cytotoxicity reactions. Transplant Proc 12:107, 1980

78. Stingl G, Katz SI, Abelson LD et al: Immunofluorescent detection of human B cell alloantigens on S-Ig-positive lymphocytes and epidermal Langerhans' cells. J Immunol 120:661, 1978

79. Storb R: Advances in Immunobiology: Blood Cell Antigens and Bone Marrow Transplantation, p 337. New York, Alan R. Liss Inc, 1984

80. Storb R, Thomas ED: Human marrow transplantation. Transplantation 28:1, 1976

81. Storb R, Thomas ED: Allogeneic bone marrow transplantation. Immunol Rev 71:77, 1983

82. Stuart FP, Fitch FW, Rowley DA: Specific suppression of renal allograft rejection by treatment with antigen and antibody. Transplant Proc 2:483, 1970

83. Thomas ED, Storb R, Clift RA et al: Bone marrow transplantation. N Engl J Med 292:832, 895, 1975

84. Thompson JS, Blaschke J, Birney S et al: Detection of allospecific granulocyte antigens by capillary agglutination and microgranulocytotoxicity. Transplant Proc 9:1895, 1977

85. Thompson JS, Herbick JM, Burns CP et al: Granulocyte antigens detected by cytotoxicity (GCY) and capillary agglutination (CAN). Transplant Proc 10:885, 1978

86. Thompson JS, Herbick JM, Burns CP et al: Granulocyte-specific antigen detected by microgranulocytotoxicity. Transplant Proc 11:431, 1979

87. Thompson JS, Overlin V, Severson CD et al: Demonstration of granulocyte, monocyte, and endothelial cell antigens by double fluorochromatic microcytotoxicity testing. Transplant Proc 12:26, 1980

88. Vallera DA, Soderling CB, Carlson GJ et al: Bone marrow transplantation across major histcompatibility barriers in mice. Effect of elimination of T cells from donor grafts by treatment with monoclonal Thy-1.2 plus complement or antibody alone. Transplantation 31:218, 1981

89. Van Dewinkel M, Smets G, Gepts W et al: Islet cell surface antibodies from insulin-dependent diabetics bind specifically to pancreatic B cells. J Clin Invest 70:41, 1982

90. Vegt PA, Buurman WA, van der Linden CJ et al: Cell-mediated cytotoxicity toward canine kidney epithelial cells. Transplantation 33:465, 1982

91. Vetto R, Burger D: The identification and comparison of transplantation antigens on canine vascular endothelium and lymphocytes. Transplantation 11:374, 1971

92. Wagner C, Vetto R, Burger D: The mechanism of an-

tigen presentation by endothelial cells. Immunobiology 168:453, 1984

93. Williams M, Han R, Parks L et al: Rejection and repair of endothelium in major vessel transplants. J Cardiovasc Surg 17:94, 1976

94. Williams GM, Hume DM, Hudson RP et al: "Hyperacute" renal-homograft rejection in man. N Engl J Med 279:611, 1968

95. Wilson CB: Individual and strain differences in renal basement membrane antigens. Transplant Proc 12:69, 1980

96. Wilson CB, Lehman DH, McCoy RC et al: Antitubular basement membrane antibodies after renal transplantation. Transplantation 18:447, 1974

97. Yagi Y, Korngold L, Pressman DJ: Purification of kidney components capable of neutralizing kidney localizing anti-rat kidney antibodies. Immunology 77:287, 1956

CHAPTER 12

Significance of the ABO Antigen System

G.P.J. Alexandre   J.P. Squifflet

Blood group substances A and B behave as transplantation antigens in humans. When considering donor–recipient ABO combinations, two categories must be distinguished: (1) *Safe combinations,* which include group 0 transplants into non-group 0 recipients or group A or B transplants into AB recipients; these combinations involve only minor consequences.

(2) *Unsafe donor–recipient combination,* such as A to non-A, B to non-B, and AB to non-AB often result in postoperative hyperacute irreversible vascular rejection.

A method to perform living donor kidney transplantation across the ABO barrier has been developed, which includes preoperative administration of specific donor platelets and elimination of natural anti-A and anti-B isoagglutinins by plasmapheresis, splenectomy of the recipient, and a quadruple immunosuppressive regimen (antilymphocyte serum, cyclosporine, Imuran, and steroids).

Eighteen ABO-incompatible living donor kidney transplantations are now functioning 3.5 years to 2.5 months post-transplantation. Thus, ABO incompatibility with a living kidney donor is no longer a contraindication for kidney transplantation.

It has been known for many years that the HLA antigen system and for the last few years that the antigen system specific to the vascular endothelial cell (VEC) are important transplant immunogens that affect the immune response to the transplanted kidney. The HLA antigens are widely distributed throughout the body in nucleated cells. For many years, it has also been assumed that the blood group substances, antigens A and B, which are also widely distributed in the human body, have an impact on allograft survival. These blood groups are located in the VEC of all vessels of all sizes, irrespective of the presence or absence of secretor (S,s) genes. The blood group antigens are also located in the collecting tubules of the kidney, but they are found in these instances only in the nonsecretors.[36] There is little doubt that the ABO blood group antigens do function as transplantation antigens in humans and influence the clinical course of vascularized grafts. Rapaport et al[25] showed that one could hyperimmunize normal, healthy human volunteer recipients to blood group A or B antigens. Such hyperimmunized recipients will reject ABO incompatible skin grafts in an accelerated or white graft manner. The

fact that this effect is dependent upon the blood group antigen and not upon other HLA antigens was clear from those experiments as well as those of other investigators. Group A recipients who were pretreated with Group A erythrocytes did not show accelerated rejection of skin allografts. This, therefore, indicates that the allograft hypersensitivity that was developed by the incompatible human erythrocytes was specific for the blood group antigens and not representative of other alloantigens.

BACKGROUND

The exact role and impact of the AB antigens on transplantation, however, was never totally defined, although it was, as previously indicated, strongly suggested that they impacted on graft survival. In the field of kidney transplantation, Jacobson and Najarian[20] clearly showed that when pretreated with group incompatible erythrocytes, you could decrease the survival of dog renal allografts if the donor kidney shared blood groups compatible with the sensitizing erythrocytes. These observations appear to be paralleled in humans when the earliest transplants, which were performed in the mid-1950s by Hume et al,[19] indicated that the blood group antigens did impact on graft survival. They concluded, based on the early loss post-transplantation of a B kidney transplanted into an O recipient, that renal transplantation would be strongly inadvisable in the presence of ABO incompatibility. Nevertheless, the exact role of ABO antigens in transplantation remained uncertain and was reported quite extensively by Starzl in the early 1960s.[30,33,34] Although one of Starzl's reports indicated that it was safe to transplant across the ABO barrier, the overall conclusion was that safe donor–recipient combinations were the same as those to be used for blood transfusions, that is, O could be regarded as a universal donor and AB as a universal recipient. Incompatible or unsafe combinations were A to non-A, B to non-B, or AB to non-AB, because they generally resulted in a form of rejection that was classified as acute vascular rejection with early thrombosis of the vessels of the graft. The issue was not clear because sporadic reports as early as the mid-1960s indicated that for unknown reasons, it was possible to transplant across the ABO barrier as evidenced by a blood group A patient who received a blood group B kidney from a sister in 1963 and who still has a functional graft 24 years later.[31]

Nevertheless, the overall impression beginning around the mid-1970s was that irreversible vascular rejection as reported by Wilbrandt et al[37] occurred in about 75% of ABO incompatible renal allografts within a few months after transplantation and that the rapidity and aggressiveness of the rejection process was related quite significantly to the titer and pretransplantation anti-A or anti-B isoantibodies in the recipient.[39] For these reasons, for many years ABO incompatibility has been thought to be an absolute prerequisite and requirement for human renal and other organ transplantation. The only possible clinical exception to this, as indicated, were the occasional successful outcomes of ABO incompatible cadaver kidneys[21,29] or liver[8] transplants that have been sporadically reported during the last 5 years. It should be indicated that the utilization of A2 donors transplanted into O recipients[11,12] has been associated not infrequently with excellent graft survival without any special immunologic therapeutic manipulation of the recipient prior to transplantation. The reason for this has been thought to be the relative rarity and low density of the A determinant on erythrocytes of the A2 antigen group.[28] Because such reports were sporadic and inconsistent, for the last 20 years, the practice in transplan-

tation has been to avoid transplantation across the ABO barrier. This has limited flexibility of transplantation, particularly with living-related donors. The availability of O blood group kidneys appears to be more limited than that of A or B, and the waiting list for patients of O blood group is substantially longer than that for A or B blood groups. The ability to transplant across the ABO barrier with living-related donors would be a very useful addition to the therapeutic armamentarium of the transplant surgeon.

BEGINNING OF ABO INCOMPATIBLE BLOOD GROUP TRANSPLANTATION

In March of 1981, a patient in our group with a blood group O inadvertently received a kidney from a cadaver with an A blood group. Immunosuppression was standard—Imuran, steroids, and antilymphocyte serum—and the patient did not have a splenectomy. With the exception of a classic rejection crisis, which responded to the usual antirejection therapy of steroids, the patient's postoperative course was remarkably benign. Postoperatively, his IgM anti-A isohemagglutinins increased to 1/2048, but by the 16th day post-transplantation, he had normal renal function, and his renal function has remained normal since then. This observation, coupled with the sporadic reports in the literature of successful transplantation across incompatible ABO mismatches, as well as the frequent successes of ABO incompatible bone marrow transplantation,[13,17] stimulated us to consider a program of evaluating the feasibility of performing living-related ABO incompatible renal transplantation by using a method similar to that which had been reported for ABO incompatible bone marrow transplantation. This protocol, which has proved so successful in bone marrow transplantation, consisted of standard immunosuppression but, most importantly, pretransplantation plasmapheresis to eliminate the circulating recipient isohemagglutinins directed against donor blood group antigens. The protocol consisted of (1) a donor-specific platelet transfusion, (2) plasmapheresis, (3) splenectomy, (4) injection of substance A or B blood group antigen, and (5) standard immunosuppression with cyclosporine, Imuran, steroids, and antilymphocyte serum.

Platelet transfusions were used in attempt to mimic the beneficial immunologic effect of donor-specific blood transfusions, which could not be used because of the obvious ABO incompatibility between the donor and the recipient. Three donor-specific platelet transfusions were given to the recipient at five weekly intervals simultaneously with Imuran in order to parallel the immunologic effect of whole blood transfusions. These platelet transfusions contained approximately 200 lymphocytes per mm^3 in an attempt to augment the beneficial immunologic effect. It has been subsequently shown by other researchers that platelets can be an effective immunogen, inducing beneficial immunomodulation, as does whole blood.

We have published in great detail the preoperative preparation and the perioperative procedures[1,2,3] to which these recipients were subjected. The recipient isohemagglutinins are transiently eliminated by plasmapheresis, which requires a minimum of three or four plasmapheresis treatments per patient. The amount of plasma exchange per plasmapheresis varies from 1 to 4 liters. In an attempt to remove residual isohemagglutinins and possibly to induce a tolerogenic effect, substance A or B or both (BENASIL Corporation, Miami) was injected, depending upon the donor's incompatible ABO blood type. This was given after the last plasmapheresis, and the method of administration has been described.[2] With this approach, it is possible to lower serial isohemagglutinin levels to essentially undetectable levels.

The initial five patients in this series were splenectomized. Because of the results in three unsplenectomized patients who did poorly, splenectomy was made a permanent part of the protocol.[3]

The drug therapy in these patients is similar to that of our standard transplantation population. The patients receive a quadruple immunosuppressive regimen consisting of antilymphocyte serum (ALG, Behringwerke, Germany), cyclosporine, Imuran, and steroids.[2] ALG administration begins 3 days prior to transplantation and is continued for 11 days post-transplantation, at which time the triple drug regimen is continued with cyclosporine, Imuran, and low-dose steroids. Piracetam (Nootropyl, I.C.B., Belgium) is given intravenously to the donor during the nephrectomy procedure and is also given to the recipient for the first 2 postoperative weeks at a dose of 50 mg/kg every 8 hours. This drug is used as a prophylactic agent in sickle cell disease.[23] Its application to the ABO incompatible transplantation is based on its effectiveness as an antiplatelet agent in humans.[6,9,18] In addition, it interacts with red cell membrane, increasing its deformability and decreasing its adherence to endothelial cells.[14,38] For these reasons, the drug may act to minimize the adhesive tendency of the incompatible red cells to the endothelium of the vascularized organ.

RESULTS

Patient Population

By December 31, 1986, 29 patients had entered the series to be considered for ABO incompatible living donor renal transplantation (Table 12-1). Three of these patients, while being prepared with donor-specific platelet transfusions, developed a positive T-cell crossmatch against the donor and were thus eliminated from the protocol. A fourth patient could not be transplanted with the respective donor, because during nephrectomy, significant and unexpected vascular anomalies were encountered that prevented utilization of the organ. Three consecutive patients who were not splenectomized lost their graft from acute vascular irreversible rejection before the end of the first postoperative week.[3] In each of these three cases, the transplant became rapidly necrotic after rejection and needed to be removed after a few days. The consecutive success of the first five patients who were splenectomized and the consecutive failure of the three cases who were not led to the conclusion that splenectomy was an important factor in avoiding irreversible vascular rejection of these ABO incompatible kidneys; therefore, splenectomy became a permanent part of this clinical protocol. One patient received successively two ABO incompatible kidney transplants. The first transplant, donated by his mother, functioned for 22 months and was eventually rejected; the patient was retransplanted with a second ABO incompatible kidney from an uncle. Both transplants shared the same ABO incompatibility with the recipient.

In the entire series, one patient died 2 months after transplantation from cytomegalovirus infection. Among the 23 kidney transplants performed in the series of 22 recipients who were splenectomized, two grafts were lost from acute vascular irreversible rejection on the 7th and 19th postoperative days, respectively. Two other grafts were lost from chronic rejection in the 7th and 22nd postoperative months. Eighteen transplants are thus functioning 5 years to 6 months post-transplantation.

Based on these observations, we have determined that no factor other than splenectomy was able to predict successful long-term function in those patients who are susceptible to acute irreversible vascular rejection in the early postoperative pe-

TABLE 12-1 ABO-Incompatible Splenectomized Living Donor Renal Allografts

	TRANSPLANT DATE	PATIENT AGE	DONOR	DONOR RECIPIENTS — HLA ANTIGENS	ABO	Rh	Se/se	FOLLOW-UP NOVEMBER 1986 CREATININE (mg %)
1	06/30/82	18	Mother	D : A1, A 26, B 38, B 35, —, DR 5 R : A1, A 30, B 18, B 35, DR 3, DR 5	A_1 / O	+ / +	SE / se	1,25
2	11/11/82	13	Mother	D : A 11, A 25, B 7, B 51, DR 1, DR 2 R : A 24, A 25, B 7, B 18, DR 1, DR 2	A_1 / O	+ / +	SE / SE	0,84
3	11/17/82	24	Mother	D : A 11, A 24, B 18, B 377, DR 2, — R : A 2, A 24, B 18, B 37, DR 2, DR 5	A_1 / O	+ / +	se / SE	1
4	12/08/82	17	Mother	D : A 2, A 1, B 8, B 62, DR 4, DR 1 R : A 2, A 23, B 14, B 62, DR 4, DR 9	B / O	+ / −	SE / SE	1,22
5	02/02/83*	23	Husband	D : A 26, A 11, B 14, B 18, DR 5, DR 7 R : A 2, A 30, B 45, —, DR 5, DR 7	A_1 / O	− / −	se / se	1,30
6	09/09/83	38	Wife	D : AW 19, A 30, B 50, B 55, DR 5, DR 7 R : A 2, A 24, B 51, B 8, DR 3, DR 4	A_1 / B	+ / −	se / SE	Chronic rejection RD 3/27/84
7	11/16/83†	31	Mother	D : A 3, —, B 7, —, DR 5, DR 2 R : A 3, A 24, B 7, B 35, DR 5, —	B / O	+ / +	SE / SE	1,46
8	11/30/83	27	Sister	D : A 3, A 32, B 8, B 7, DR 3, — R : A 1, A 32, B 8, B 63, DR 3, DRW 6	B / O	+ / +	SE / SE	1,8
9	05/09/84	20	Mother	D : A 11, A 30, B 35, B 13, DR 7, DRW 6 R : A 11, A 24, B 35, —, DR 5, DRW 6	A_1B / B	+ / +	SE / SE	1,96
10	07/04/84	9	Mother	D : A 2, A 30, B 14, B 35, DR 1, DRW 10 R : A 2, A 24, B 14, B 35, DR 1, DRW 10	A_1 / B	+ / +	SE / SE	1,1
11	07/18/84	33	Mother	D : A 28, A 23, B 49, B 35, DR 2, DRW 6 R : A 28, A 3, B 51, B 35, DR 2, DR 1	A_2 / O	+ / −	se / SE	1,7

No.	Date	Age	Relation	HLA antigens	Blood group		SE/se	Outcome
12	09/26/84	10	Father	D : A 9, A 28, B 21, B 35, DRW 6, DR 2 R : A 3, A 28, B 5, B 35, DR 1, DR 2	A₁ O	+ −	SE se	0,95
13	12/05/84	19	Mother	D : A 1, A 11, —, B 35, DRW 6, DR 5 R : A 1, A 2, B 12, B 35, DRW 6, —	A₁ O	− +	se se	Acute rejection Ty 12/14/1984
14	01/23/85	24	Wife	D : A 32, A 23, B 49, B 27, DR 2, DR 7 R : A 2, A 24, B 35, B 39, —, DRW 6	A₁ O	+ +	se SE	1,09
15	03/20/85	17	Father	D : A 28, A 19, B 27, B 50, DR 3, DRW 6 R : A 2, A 19, B 17, B 50, DR 3, DR 7	A₁ O	+ +	SE SE	1,64
16	06/05/85	36	Wife	D : A 1, A 24, B 35, B 49, DR 5 DRW 6 R : A 11, A 32, B 35, B 52, DR 2, DRW 6	A₁ O	+ +	SE SE	0,8
17	07/03/85	11	Mother	D : A 1, A 28, B 7, B 35, DR 2, DRW 6 R : A 3, A 28, B 44, B 35, DR 5, DRW 6	A₁ O	+ +	SE SE	0,9
18	10/16/85	21	Mother	D : A 1, —, B 51, B 55, DR 2, DR 5 R :: A 1, —, B 8, B 55, DR 2, DR 3	A₁,B A₁	+ +	SE SE	1,80
19	12/4/85	43	Wife	D : A 2, —, B 44, —, DR 7, DR 5 R : A 2, A 1, B 49, —, DR 4, DR 5	A₁ O	+ +	SE SE	Acute rejection Ty 12/23/85
20	04/16/86	51	Wife	D : A 23, —, B 49, B 58, DR 5, DRW6 R : A 28, —, B 35, B 44, DR 1, —	A₂ O	+ +	se SE	Death from CM after 2 months
21	07/16/86	72	Mother	D : A 2, A 3, B 7, B 18, DRW 11, DR 7 R : A 2, —, —, B 18, DRW 11, —	B O	+ +	SE SE	0,8
22	10/15/86*	11	Uncle	D : A 2, A 24, B 58, B 18, DR 2, DRW 11 R : A 2, A 24, B 14, B 35, DR 1, DRW 10	A₁ B	+ +	SE SE	0,7
23	10/22/86	12	Father	D : A 2, A 24, B 7, B 35, DR 2, DR 3 R : A 1, —, B 7, B 8, DR 2, DR 3	B O	+ +	SE SE	0,9

* = secondary graft

† = tertiary graft

D = donor; R = recipient; Ty = transplantectomy; RD = return to dialysis; SE/se = secretor status

Note: Underlined HLA antigens are incompatible antigens

riod. Nevertheless, splenectomy clearly does not afford a complete guarantee against this early aggressive form of rejection, because two splenectomized patients still experienced early aggressive irreversible rejection. However, the rejection in these patients was more delayed than that in the nonsplenectomized patients, again supporting the role of splenectomy in ABO incompatible transplants.

With this protocol, none of the patients developed immediate on-the-table hyperacute vascular rejection as has been reported by Starzl and associates,[34] and all regained a normal function in the first few postoperative days. This is probably the result and consequence of eliminating all the isohemagglutinins by plasmapheresis and by injection with the donor blood group antigens. Clearly, these isohemagglutinins have a capacity for returning in the postoperative period to their preoperative level. The rate at which their preoperative level is achieved seems to correlate with the likelihood of acute rejection. Those who have a rapid return of their isohemagglutinin levels are more likely to experience early acute rejection. At the time of the acute rejection crisis, there is always a clear increase of the isohemagglutinins, and it is a very consistent immunologic parameter accompanying the rejection process in these categories of patients. The magnitude of the titer of the isohemagglutinins achieved does not, however, appear to predict the severity of the rejection episode and the likelihood for long-term successful graft function. The 11th case of this series demonstrates this point, as the isohemagglutinin level increased up to 1/65.536 at the time of the rejection crisis. This graft, which was the sole A2 to O transplant of the series is still functioning well at the present time. Therefore, high isohemagglutinin levels do not indicate a totally dismal prognosis.

Role of HLA Antigens in ABO Incompatible Transplants

An obvious question is whether the degree of HLA incompatibility influences the likelihood of success or failure of ABO incompatible transplants. Unfortunately, the definitive answer to this question cannot be presented.

There is no HLA identical match in the series. Three of the four patients who received a full-house DR identical transplant and all three who received a DR compatible transplant have normal renal function.

The two patients whose grafts were acutely and irreversibly rejected in the early postoperative period were DR incompatible with the donor. Five of the six patients who were transplanted with an ABO graft from a nonrelative (spouse) and who were not well matched did not do as well as the patients transplanted with a related transplant. The less good results obtained in DR incompatible subgroup compared with the well-matched subgroup (DR compatible and DR identical transplants) suggest that DR compatibility impacts on graft survival in ABO incompatible transplants with living-related donors. However, one patient (patient 14) with blood group O who received an A₁ kidney from his wife still has a normally functioning graft, even with total HLA-A, B, and DR incompatibility.

In addition, this particular recipient not only was HLA incompatible but also contained the DRW 6 antigen in the absence of such an antigen in the donor. The aforementioned observations suggest, but certainly do not prove, that HLA matching in ABO incompatible transplants may play a role in the likelihood of graft success. This is not a surprising assumption, because the two systems may elicit quite different immunologic responses from the recipient and therefore may act by totally independent mechanisms on graft function.

Analysis of Data

Based on our observations and that of other investigators, several conclusions can be presented. There are certain safe ABO combinations, for example, group O transplants into non-group O recipients, or group A or B transplants into AB recipients. It is important to indicate that although such transplants reflect a minimal impact of such ABO incompatibility, in some instances there is an immunologic effect of ABO mismatching. This results from the lymphocytes that are transplanted along with the graft producing isohemagglutinins against recipient AB blood groups. This can lead to hemolytic anemia because of these ABO antibodies produced by the lymphocytes of the transplanted organ. This has been observed following kidney,[10,16,35] lung,[7] liver,[24] and spleen[27,32] transplantation. Generally, the production of these antirecipient AB antibodies persists for a few weeks and the hemolytic anemia is transient. However, in the case of spleen transplantation, they produce significant hemolysis, which can be severe enough to necessitate the removal of the transplanted organ.[27,32]

The experimental protocol of transplanting patients across the ABO barrier provides an opportunity for evaluating the possibility that the ABO blood groups impact on immunologic reactivity of the recipient. In other words, are either matched or unmatched kidney transplants dependent upon or influenced by the blood group of the recipient? It appears that if this is the case, the major difference observed favors group O recipients.[15] Patients with blood group O seem to have a somewhat better graft survival, but determining this definitively is extremely difficult because of the other well-known factors that influence graft survival. For instance, blood group O patients will wait a significantly longer period of time before obtaining a cadaver kidney because of the shortage of O blood group kidneys. Dialysis influences the likelihood of graft success in that patients who are on prolonged dialysis seem to do better. In addition, patients on prolonged dialysis tend to receive more blood transfusions, which also favorably influence results. Therefore, it is impossible to dissect out the role of the blood group O antigens as an etiologic factor in improved graft survival. However, it has been suggested that an association does exist between ABO antigens and immune response genes.[22] For instance, type O recipients are less frequently positive for cytomegalovirus (CMV) than are recipients of other ABO blood types, as reported by Andrus et al.[4,5] Minor mismatches in group A recipients seem to impact on survival as reported by Rosenthal and colleagues,[26] who found that graft survival in blood group A2 recipients was significantly poorer than that in all other groups. Nevertheless, these influences of ABO blood groups in ABO compatible mismatched donor–recipient combinations are quite small compared with the impact of the HLA antigens in such transplants.

CONCLUSIONS

The ABO differences can thus be overcome by appropriate immunologic manipulation of the recipient, permitting to a limited extent the transplantation of ABO incompatible kidneys with results that are equivalent to ABO compatible transplants. Such ABO incompatible combinations are not limited to A2 donors; successful transplantation can be accomplished with B blood groups into O donors, A1 blood groups into O donors, and A to B and the reciprocal. It is also clear that successful transplantation across the ABO barrier can occasionally occur in the absence of manipulation of the donor, based on the sporadic reports in the literature, the success of bone marrow transplantation, and the recent observation of Starzl (personal communication) in large numbers of liver transplants across the ABO barrier. In a series of 671 liver transplants, 31 were performed in ABO incompatible combinations with a 35% graft function compared with 55% in ABO compatible combinations. Why liver transplants can be successful to such a high frequency with ABO incompatibility is unknown. Some researchers believe that the liver is less immunogenic than other organs. These two observations suggest that the antigen systems represented on the VEC of the liver, that is, HLA, ABO, and vascular endothelial specific, may be present in much less density or quantity than in other organs. Confirmation of this observation would certainly explain the clinical observations that have been reported.

The technique of using ABO incompatible donors not only increases our flexibility of transplantation of living-related donors but also provides encouragement for the possibility of successfully transplanting xenografts. Xenografts almost uniformly fail very rapidly because of the presence of preformed anti-donor antibody in the recipient in significant concentrations. The experience with the ABO incompatible series suggests that a transient decrease of anti-donor antibody can effectively prevent the early graft rejection. Subsequent reestablishment of anti-donor antibody titers does not uniformly lead to graft loss in ABO incompatible combinations, and it is hoped that it will not result in graft loss either in xenograft transplants or possibly the transplantation of patients who have significant anti-HLA antibody. Thus, this experience, while limited to date, opens the door for exciting new explorations in the field of transplantation.

REFERENCES

1. Alexandre GPJ, De Bruyère M, Squifflet JP et al: Human ABO-incompatible living donor renal homografts. Neth J Med 28:231, 1985
2. Alexandre GPJ, Squifflet JP, De Bruyère M et al: ABO-incompatible related and unrelated living donor renal allografts. Presented at Second International Symposium on Organ Procurement, Detroit, MI, October 3–5, 1985. Transplant Proc (in press)
3. Alexandre GPJ, Squifflet JP, De Bruyère M et al: Splenectomy as a prerequisite for successful human ABO-incompatible renal transplantation. Transplant Proc 17:138, 1985
4. Andrus CH, Betts RF, May AG et al: Better allograft survival in erythrocyte type O recipients correlates with resistance to cytomegalovirus infections. Transplant Proc 13:120, 1981

5. Andrus CH, Betts RF, May AG et al: Cytomegalovirus infection blocks the beneficial effect of pretransplant blood transfusion on renal allograft survival. Transplantation 28:451, 1979

6. Barnhart MI, Penner J, Walz DA et al: Plaquettes hyperréactives et maladie thromboembolique. Essentialia UCB 6:12, 1981

7. Beck H, Haines R, Oberman H: Unexpected serologic findings following lung homotransplantation (abstract). American Association of Blood Banks, 24th Annual Meeting, Chicago, 1971

8. Beelen JM: Responses to donor antigens in liver transplantation. In Progress in Living Transplantation, pp 119–123. Boston, Martinus Nijhoff, 1985

9. Bick RL: In vivo platelet inhibition by piracetam. Lancet II:752, 1979

10. Bird G, Wingham J: Anti-A autoantibodies with unusual properties in a patient on renal dialysis. Immunol Commun 9:155, 1980

11. Brynger H, Blohme I, Lindholm L et al: Transplantation of cadaver kidneys from blood groups A_2 donors. Transplant Proc 14:195, 1982

12. Brynger H, Rydberg L, Samuelsson B et al: Renal transplantation across A blood group barrier—A_2 kidneys to O recipients. Proc Eur Dial Transplant Assoc 19:427, 1982

13. Buckner CD, Clift RA, Sanders JE et al: ABO-incompatible marrow transplants. Transplantation 26:233, 1978

14. Bureck CL, Digho CA, Taylor G et al: Diminished adherence of sickle erythrocytes to rat and human vascular endothelium by piracetam. Hematological and metabolic aspects of piracetam. International Congress Heidelberg, Oct. 22–25, 1981

15. Cecka M: ABO blood group antigens and kidney transplantation. In Terasaki PI (ed): Clinical Kidney Transplants 1985. Los Angeles, UCLA Tissue Typing Laboratory, 1985

16. Contreras M, Hazelhurst G, Armitage S: Development of "auto-anti-A_1 antibodies" following alloimmunization in an A_2 recipient. Br J Haematol 55:657, 1983

17. Gali RP, Feig S, Ho W et al: ABO blood group system and bone marrow transplantation. Blood 50:185, 1977

18. Henry RL, Nalbandian RM, Hermann GE et al: Inhibition of PF-4 and β-TG from platelets by piracetam. Thromb Haemostas 42:477, 1979

19. Hume DM, Merrill JP, Miller BF et al: Experiences with renal homotransplantation in the human: Report of nine cases. J Clin Invest 26:327, 1955

20. Jacobson E Jr, Najarian JS: Role of the red blood cell antigens in homograft rejection. Surg Forum 15:138, 1964

21. Kramer P, Broyer M, Brunner FP et al: Combined report on regular dialysis and transplantation in Europe, XII, 1981. Proc Eur Dial Transplant Assoc 19:4, 1982

22. Kreis H: Selection of a donor. In Hamburger J, Crosnier J, Bach JF et al (eds): Renal Transplantation, p 36. Baltimore, Williams & Wilkins, 1981

23. Nalbandian RM, Henry RL, Murayama M: Sickle-cell disease: Two new therapeutic strategies. Lancet ii:570, 1978

24. Ramsey G, Nusbacher J, Starzl TE et al: Isohemagglutinins of graft origin after ABO-unmatched liver transplantation. N Engl J Med (in press)

25. Rapaport FT, Dausset J, Legrand L et al: Erythrocytes in human transplantation: Effects of pretreatment with ABO group-specific antigens. J Clin Invest 47:2206, 1968

26. Rosenthal RL, Sochnev AM, Bitsans I et al: Dependence of survival rate of kidney allotransplants on the histocompatibility of donor and recipient ABO antigens. Probl Genatol Pereliv Krovi 27:34, 1982

27. Salamon DJ, Ramsey G, Nusbacher J et al: Anti-A production by a group O spleen transplanted to a group A recipient. Vox Sang 48:309, 1985

28. Schachter H, Tilley CA. In Manners DJ (ed): Biochemistry of Carbohydrates II, p 209. Baltimore, University Park Press, 1978

29. Slapak M, Naik RB, Lee HA: Renal transplant in a patient with major donor-recipient blood group incompatibility. Transplantation 31:4, 1981

30. Starzl TE: Patterns of permissible donor-recipient tissue transfer in relation to ABO blood groups. In Starzl TE (ed): Experience in Renal Transplantation, p 37. Philadelphia, WB Saunders, 1964

31. Starzl TE: Personal communication

32. Starzl TE, Iwatsuki S, Shaw BW et al: Pancreaticoduodenal transplantation in humans. Surg Gynecol Obstet 159:265, 1984

33. Starzl TE, Marchioro TL, Hermann GG et al: Renal homografts in patients with major donor-recipient blood group incompatibility. Surg Forum, 14:214, 1963

34. Starzl TE, Marchioro TL, Holmes JH et al: Renal homografts in patients with major donor-recipient blood group incompatibilities. Surgery 55:195, 1964

35. Stevens J, Callender C, Jilly P: Emergence of red blood cell agglutinins following renal transplantation in a patient with systemic lupus erythematosus. Transplantation 32:398, 1981

36. Szulman Aron E: The histological distribution of blood group substances A and B in man. J Exp Med 111:785, 1960

37. Wilbrandt R, Tung KSK, Deodhar SD: ABO-blood group incompatibility in human renal homotransplantation. Am J Clin Pathol 51:15, 1969

38. Williams GA: The effects of piracetam on erythrocyte deformability and adherence in sickle-cell anemia and diabetes. 10th International Symposium on Nootropic Agents, Paris, October 1982

39. Wilson WEC, Kirkpatrick CH: Immunological aspects of renal homotransplantation. In Starzl TE (ed): Experience in Renal Transplantation, p 239. Philadelphia, WB Saunders, 1964

ABO Incompatibility in Transplantation

A. BANNETT

At the *ABO Incompatibility in Transplantation* meeting held in Philadelphia, Pennsylvania, in March 1987, an internationl forum of clinicians and researchers presented current data to refine the clinical and theoretical aspects of ABO incompatible transplantation. A summary of the symposium's findings by its organizer follows. —G.J.C.

Interest in performing ABO incompatible allografts has spanned most areas of transplantation, including bone marrow, liver, kidney, and heart. Deliberate transplantation across the ABO barrier is common in bone marrow transplantation and has proven to be quite successful. The major complication in this type of transplantation is destruction of the donor red cells, resulting in hemolysis and anemia. Bensinger[4] reviewed various techniques available for reduction of ABO isohemagglutinins in bone marrow recipients and the effect of ABO incompatible transplantation in 292 patients. The following were reviewed: (1) no treatment; (2) RBC removal; (3) plasmapheresis; (4) *in vivo* adsorption; or (5) extracorporeal immunoadsorption. All of the procedures were viable forms of therapy allowing for successful bone marrow engraftment. Plasma exchange was more effective for antibody removal than was immunoadsorption, but recent modifications of the synthetic antigen and the physical conformation of the immunoadsorbent material have improved antibody binding. Similar observations were made by Tichelli[26] in 11 patients who received ABO incompatible bone marrow transplants. In order to reduce titers, *in vivo* adsorption with incompatible RBC transfusions were performed. This methodology was as effective in reducing titers as plasma exchange or extracorporeal immunoadsorption.

Liver transplants are probably not affected by the ABO barrier. However, there are occasional problems with hemolysis due to the presence in the graft of B cells, which produce anti-ABO isohemagglutinins. The urgency involved in transplanting this organ sometimes necessitates crossing the ABO barrier. Gordon[9] reviewed 1016 liver transplants and found that, while there was a significant advantage to graft survival in ABO matched transplants, a surprising number of ABO incompatible grafts were successful. Similarly, in a review of 79 orthotopic liver transplants, 25% of which were between ABO unmatched pairs, the graft survival between matched and unmatched pairs was not significantly different although there was a tendency

for unmatched pairs to develop a hemolytic syndrome.[10] Also, Angstadt[2] reported the same major complication of the hemolytic syndrome in 6 ABO unmatched liver grafts not noted in 13 ABO matched transplanted livers.

Renal transplantation across the ABO barrier probably involves the greatest challenge and complexity. In an analysis of 2125 kidney transplants, an ABO effect was found even in mismatched compatible kidney grafts.[25] This effect is small but significant and can be easily overcome with current immunosuppressive therapies. Alexandre (see preceding text) has a current series of 26 ABO incompatible living donor renal allografts.[1] Immunologic preparation of the recipient includes donor-specific platelet transfusions, splenectomy, plasmapheresis, and the administration of ABO soluble substance to effectively eliminate ABO antibodies. This approach indicates that ABO incompatible living donor transplantation is a feasible procedure but that plasmapheresis and splenectomy of the recipient are prerequisites for a successful outcome. Similarly, five ABO incompatible but HLA identical living donor renal allografts were performed by Bannett.[3,3a] All patients were splenectomized, and, unlike Alexandre's series, ABO incompatible isohemagglutinins were removed by immunoadsorption utilizing a column of synthetic antigen (Bio-Synsorb) produced by Chembiomed of Canada.

Four of five transplants were successful and uneventful. The fifth resulted in a hyperacute rejection, probably related to sensitization by the donor ABO antigens causing a precipitous rise in IgG anti-ABO antibodies. There is little question that some form of recipient manipulation is required for successful renal transplantation across the ABO barrier. Cook[8] evaluated 25 inadvertent transplants of cadaver kidneys into unmodified, ABO incompatible recipients. Only one of these survived longer than 12 months, confirming the importance of either avoiding ABO incompatibilities or modifying the ABO titer in the recipients. An exception to this is an A2 to an O allograft. The results of 40 such transplants indicate that transplantation of blood group A2 kidneys into recipients of "incompatible" blood groups is feasible and may lead to long-term function.[5,14]

Not all ABO incompatible grafts are successful; ABO incompatible kidney transplant failures manifested by delayed hyperacute rejection are probably due to hyperimmunization and the formation of high affinity IgG antibodies to the mismatched ABO antigens.[7,13]

There is clear evidence that ABO antigens serve as targets of rejection in human tissues and organs owing to their wide dissemination. For instance, volunteers injected with A or B substance have an accelerated graft rejection of subsequent skin grafts. This hyperacute rejection is mediated by antibody to target antigens located in the vascular bed. The end result is caused by the effector cascade of secondary and nonspecific events, including inflammation and coagulation, resulting in devascularization and destruction of the transplanted organ. Points of emphasis for therapeutic intervention are now apparent.[24] Antibody reduction is important. Probably more important would be the modification of the nonspecific effector cascade. During the effector phase of the immune response, the endothelium constitutes the most accessible and important site for immune injury.[16] These sites are probably of greatest importance during hyperacute or accelerated acute rejection in relation to preexisting antibodies to target antigens. The greatest damage is caused by activation of the cascade events in response to the primary insult. Natural isohemagglutinins to donor ABO antigens would be one of the best sources of such a primary insult due to the expression of ABO antigens in renal vessel endothelium. Kemp and associates[11] have described methods to deal effectively with the cascade reactions that are the primary adverse phenomenon seen in hyperacute rejection, especially in xenograft rejection. Intravascular platelet aggregation is the predominant finding. Vasodilating agents and ACE inhibitors delay hyperacute rejection in a rabbit–cat xenograft model, whereas conventional immunosuppressive therapy has no effect. Most impressive was cobra venom factor (an anti-complement drug), which could delay graft rejection for several days. The role of the cascade reactions in antibody-mediated immunologic insults of the hyperacute or accelerated acute type has been noted by others.[12] Platelet activating factor (PAF) seems important in the cascade effect. A significant abrogation of a very rapid and violent form of hyperacute rejection can be achieved solely by the phrmacologic manipulation of the platelet effector cascade.

In dealing with a patient receiving an ABO

incompatible transplant, much of the success seems to be in the preparation of the patient. In renal and cardiac transplants, the preparation primarily involves the reduction and/or removal of the offending ABO isohemagglutinins. This requires an understanding of the physical and biologic nature of the isohemagglutinins and a clear understanding of the chemical makeup of the target ABO antigens. Studies of ABO titers in 125 blood group O patients awaiting kidney transplant who were highly sensitized to HLA antigens showed that more than two-thirds of the O patients who had been waiting 2 years or longer for a kidney transplant had low titer isohemagglutinins (less than 1:4) and might therefore be *ideal* candidates for ABO incompatible transplant with proper modification of the ABO titers.[6]

Chembiomed, Ltd., manufacturer of Bio-Synsorb, the synthetic ABO antigen used in the immunoadsorbent columns, has now chemically synthesized trisaccharides having A or B specificities. Since these trisaccharides represent only one blood group epitope per molecule, a hapten-like behavior would be expected *in vivo,* resulting in neither immunogenicity nor complement activation upon antibody binding. These synthetic sugars may be of medical utility in situations where antibody neutralization is desirable *in vivo.* Extracorporeal immunoadsorption columns from Chembiomed, Ltd., can be inserted in the lines during dialysis.[17] Adsorption of specific ABO antibodies using whole blood passing through the BioSynsorb matrix was an effective procedure in preparing a kidney recipient for an ABO incompatible transplant. Trisaccharide-A and -B have a greater affinity for the isohemagglutinins anti-A or anti-B than did the RBCs themselves, actually out-competing the RBCs for the antibody.[19] Because of the solubility of the trisaccharide, a greater number of molecular binding sites could be presented than those of the RBCs themselves. These results support the concept that the administration of trisaccharide-A or -B presents a rational treatment modality for the *in vivo* neutralization of anti-A and/or anti-B antibodies. Administration of 100 mg of trisaccharide-A to an ABO group O volunteer reduced the A group titer from 1:512 to 1:64 within 3 hours.[20] No adverse effects were observed, complement was not activated, and there was no sensitization of the immune system to A substance as measured by IgG production. Titers returned to normal 24 hours later. A group A volunteer was administered the same 100 mg with no adverse effects. There was no change in the anti-B titer, and all the trisaccharide was excreted in the urine.

Treatment with larger doses of the trisaccharide

and/or combined with plasma extracorporeal immunoadsorption using group-specific trisaccharides coupled to solid matrix could be very successful for anti-A and anti-B neutralization.

The Old World primate is the most appropriate experimental model for ABO incompatible transplantation, since it is the most similar genetically to man and since the genetic control of these antigens dictates their presence in similar locations, such as the erythrocyte and the vascular endothelium.[15] Although each of the other animal models (pig, dog, rabbit, rats, and mice) affords some interesting characteristics, they fail to provide the appropriate target that would define an acceptable model. Both Old and New World monkeys have developed some form of ABO type blood group specificities with varying degrees of cross-over reactivity with the human system.[23] Of these, the Old World monkeys, especially the chimpanzee, would serve well as an experimental model for xenotransplantation. What seems to be particularly important is that, not unlike the situation in man, the dominant A, B, and H group substances are omnipresent in vascular endothelium. Equally important is that following immunization, the titer of IgG antibodies usually increases similar to that probably resulting from an ABO incompatible graft. Recent studies also show experimental transplantation between some species of Old World monkeys to be similar to xenotransplantation encountered between man and chimpanzee.

The role of the Lewis blood antigens is still controversial. Lewis-negative regrafted kidney transplant recipients may have a survival rate below that expected.[21] However, Smith[22] noted that only Lewis-negative patients with preexisting anti-Lewis antibody should be excluded from regrafting with a Lewis-positive donor. Others have concluded that the Lewis alloantigens are not a significant factor in liver transplantation[18]

Therefore, it seems that the ABO barrier in transplantation, which has been an accepted criteria for over 20 years, may soon be a barrier no longer, thereby opening up a greater number of clinical options for the transplant community.

REFERENCES

1. Alexandre GPJ, Squifflet JP, De Bruzere M et al: Present experiences of a series of 26 ABO incompatible living donor renal allografts. Transplant Proc 1987

2. Angstadt J, Jarrell B, Maddrey W et al: Hemolysis in ABO incompatible liver transplantation. Transplant Proc 1987

3. Bannett A: Experiences with known ABO mismatched renal transplants in humans. Transplant Proc 1987

3a. Bannett AD, Bensinger WI, Raja R et al: Immunoadsorption and renal transplant in two patients with a major ABO incompatibility. Transplantation 1987 (in press)

4. Bensinger WI, Buckner CD, Clift RA et al: Comparison of techniques for dealing with major ABO-incompatible marrow transplants. Transplant Proc 1987

5. Brynger H: Specific ABO-incompatible transplantation in the unmodified recipient: A2-O blood types. Transplant Proc 1987

6. Cecka JM, Breidenthal SE, Terasaki PI: Low anti-A and anti-B titers in some type O patients may permit renal transplantation across the ABO barrier. Transplant Proc 1987

7. Chopek MW, Simmons RL, Platt JL: ABO incompatible kidney transplantation: Initial immunopathologic evaluation. Transplant Proc 1987

8. Cook DJ, Graver B, Terasaki PI: ABO incompatibility in cadaver donor kidney allografts. Transplant Proc 1987

9. Gorden RD, Iwatsuki S, Esquivel CO et al: The effect of ABO blood group matching on graft outcome in liver transplantation. Transplant Proc 1987

10. Jenkins RL, Georgi BA, Gallik-Karson CA et al: ABO mismatch and liver transplantation. Transplant Proc 1987

11. Kemp E, Steinbriichel D, Starklint H et al: Renal xenograft rejection. Prolonging effect of captopril, ACE-inhibitors, prostacyclin and cobra venom factor. Transplant Proc 1987

12. Makowka L, Miller C, Chapchap P et al: Management of hyperacute rejection by modification of the platelet response. Transplant Proc 1987

13. McAlack RF, Bannett AD, Romano E et al: Delayed hyperacute rejection in an ABO incompatible renal transplant. Transplant Proc 1987

14. Nelson PW, Helling TS, Pierce GE: Successful transplantation of blood group A2 kidneys into non-A recipients. ASTS 1987

15. Oriol R: Tissular expression of ABH and Lewis antigens in man and animals. Expected value of different animal models in the study of ABO incompatible organ transplants. Transplant Proc 1987

16. Paul LC, Baldwin WM III: Humoral rejection mechanisms and ABO incompatibility in renal transplantation. Transplant Proc 1987

17. Raja R, McAlack RF, Mendez M et al: Technical aspects of antibody immunoadsorption (IA) prior to ABO incompatible transplant. Transplant Proc 1987

18. Ramsey G, Wolford J, Boczkowski DJ et al: The Lewis blood group system in liver transplantation. Transplant Proc 1987

19. Romano EL, Soyano A, Linares J et al: Neutralization of ABO blood group antibodies by specific oligosacchandes. Transplant Proc 1987

20. Romano EL, Soyano A, Linares J: Preliminary human study of synthetic trisaccharide representing blood substance-A. Transplant Proc 1987

21. Roy R, Terasaki PE, Chia D et al: Low kidney graft survival in Lewis negative patients after regrafting and newer matching schemes for Lewis. Transplant Proc 1987

22. Smith WJ, Hopkins KA, Schaefer KL et al: Failure of Lewis blood group matching to influence renal allograft outcome. Transplant Proc 1987

23. Socka WW, Marboe CC, Michler RF et al: Primate animal model for the study of A-B-O incompatibility in organ transplantation. Transplant Proc 1987

24. Starzl TE, Tzakis A, Makowka L et al: the definition of ABO factors in transplantation: Relation to other humoral antibody states. Transplant Proc 1987

25. Stock PG, Sutherland DER, Fryd DS et al: ABO compatible mismatching decreases 5 year actuarial graft survival after renal transplantation. Transplant Proc 1987

26. Tichelli A, Grativohl A, Wenger R et al: ABO-incompatible bone marrow transplantation: In vivo adsorption, and old forgotten method. Transplant Proc 1987

PART THREE

Renal Transplantation

CHAPTER 13

The Role of Dialysis in the Management of End-Stage Renal Disease

Christopher R. Blagg

Dialysis remains the usual form of treatment for most patients with end-stage renal disease (ESRD) in the United States. The patient population treated by dialysis and transplantation has changed; it is now older and includes more patients with multiple medical problems than previously. Long-term dialysis has proved very successful.

The most common complications of dialysis include hypotension, cramps, nausea, and malaise during the dialysis; these are usually due to short dialysis with removal of a large volume of fluid by ultrafiltration or use of acetate-containing dialysate. Episodes of hypotension are also sometimes related to hemorrhage. Other complications include the disequilibrium syndrome, hemorrhage, air embolism, fever, infections, problems associated with improperly prepared dialystate, and aluminum intoxication.

Peritoneal dialysis became practical as a long-term treatment with development of continuous ambulatory peritoneal dialysis (CAPD) and continuous cycling peritoneal dialysis (CCPD).

Complications associated with peritoneal dialysis include mechanical problems such as pain, bleeding, leakage, and bowel perforation; metabolic effects such as protein loss, hyperglycemia, and hyperlipidemia; and pulmonary complications, including atelectasis and pleural effusion. Infection remains the major problem with all forms of peritoneal dialysis, and recurrent episodes of peritonitis are frequently the factor limiting the long-term use of this treatment.

The optimal timing to start dialysis or to consider an elective renal transplant remains uncertain. There has been recent renewal of interest in better dietary management of the patient with chronic renal failure, including dietary supplementation with essential amino acids and ketoacids, and the importance of control of hypertension before the onset of ESRD has also been emphasized.

A major advance in the comparison of different modalities of treatment is use of the Cox proportional hazards model. Data based on more than 1000 patients aged 15 to 55 years confirm that in both nondiabetic and diabetic patients, patient survival is best with related donor transplantation, but there is no significant difference in survival with cadaver transplantation and hemodialysis when allowance is made for age, cause of renal disease, number of associated diseases, and year of treatment. Patient survival with CAPD is comparable to that with hemodialysis, but, with intermittent peritoneal dialysis, long-term survival may be less.

Because there appears to be no difference in patient survival between dialysis and cadaver transplantation, patients and physicians must consider the complications associated with both in making a decision on treatment. The lack of vitality in dialysis patients is one marked difference between patients with a successful transplant and most patients treated by dialysis. Renal osteodystrophy is more readily controlled, but osteomalacia related to aluminum bone disease has become more significant. The effects of steroids and malignancies are a problem in transplanted patients.

The quality of life and the opportunity for rehabilitation are best in patients with a successful transplant; home hemodialysis patients do significantly better than patients treated by in-center hemodialysis.

Both dialysis and kidney transplantation are expensive treatments. Initial transplantation charges are higher, in part because of costs associated with graft injection and death of some patients; thus, a successful transplant does not result in overall cost-saving until about 3 years after transplantation. Improved rehabilitation in transplant patients decreases transplant costs.

Recent availability of the immunosuppressive agent cyclosporine has resulted in a significant increase in the transplantation of hearts, livers, heart-lungs, pancreases, and other organs and has stimulated both scientific and public interest in transplantation. This, in turn, has resulted in an increase in the number of all organs available for transplantation. In particular, the number of kidney transplants in the United States has increased by more than 10% in each of the last 2 years, so that in 1986 approximately 8800 kidney transplants were performed. Apart from the various surgical and technical differences, perhaps the greatest contrast between kidney transplantation and the transplantation of other solid organs is that, with the possible exception of the use of an artificial heart (which is clearly still experimental), end-stage renal disease (ESRD) is the only major organ failure for which an alternative long-term maintenance therapy is available in addition to transplantation. In fact, it was the development of maintenance dialysis in the early 1960s, occurring at the same time as the initial developments in immunosuppressive therapy, which made possible the rapid evolution of kidney transplantation as a definitive form of treatment for chronic kidney failure during the course of the 1960s and early 1970s.

When one looks back at the approximately 10,000 patients who were treated by dialysis in the United States in 1973, most had been selected to a greater or lesser degree as suitable candidates for a long-term dialysis program. As a result of this selection, most of these patients would certainly have been candidates for both living-related donor and cadaveric donor transplantation if organs had been available. However, following institution of coverage for the treatment of ESRD under the Medicare program in July 1973, the patient population treated by dialysis changed to a great degree,[25] and these changes have continued. Thus, the patient population now is significantly older, sicker, and more disadvantaged than 12 years ago; and, in the United States at least, almost all patients with ESRD are now offered either dialysis and/or transplantation. Total enrollment of new patients in the Medicare ESRD program quadrupled between 1974 and 1981[22] and has continued to increase by 11.1% per year.[15]

There have been significant technical advances in treatment by dialysis and transplantation in recent years, but the total number of patients on dialysis has increased greatly in proportion to the number of patients who have received a kidney transplant. Whereas the number of patients transplanted is primarily related to the availability of donor organs, at least until the advent of cyclosporine, most dialysis patients were not regarded as possible candidates for a cadaver kidney transplant. Thus, in recent years in the United States, approximately 10% of dialysis patients have received a transplant each year, but more than 80% of all patients are being treated by long-term dialysis. The potential for the success of dialysis as a long-term treatment is evidenced by the fact that there are now a large number of patients in the United States and elsewhere who have survived more than 10 years on dialysis, and the longest survivor is now in his 25th year on hemodialysis.

Unfortunately, in the past, the protagonists of dialysis and of transplantation have tended to emphasize their favored forms of treatment over those of the other, and not always in the patients' best interests. Clearly what is required, at a time when patients are entering into their third decade on treatment with either dialysis or transplantation, is an integrated approach to the treatment of ESRD in which patients may be treated not only by transplantation but also by other available modalities of dialysis, depending upon the patient's needs at a given point in time. In order to achieve this, it is important that transplant surgeons work closely with their nephrologist counterparts to provide the best treatment for the individual patient. The problem of lack of dialogue between nephrologists and transplant surgeons so poignantly commented upon by a physician–patient in 1972 should by now have been eliminated.[11]

HEMODIALYSIS

History

The term *dialysis* was first used by Thomas Graham in the 1860s to describe the separation of crystalloids from colloids in solution by diffusion through a semipermeable membrane.[33] Fifty years later,

Abel, Rowntree, and Turner[1] developed what they called an "artificial kidney," which was used for experiments on the dialysis of both endogenous and exogenous substances from the blood of animals. Their plans to use this technique in humans were prevented by the outbreak of World War I, which interfered with the importation from Hungary of the leeches from which they extracted the anticoagulant hirudin. Consequently, the first human dialysis was performed by Haas in 1924,[35] but it was not until the early 1940s that the first modern artificial kidney was developed by Kolff in the Netherlands.[43]

Following World War II, a number of different artificial kidneys were developed in Europe, Canada, and the United States and were increasingly used throughout the 1950s for the treatment of patients with acute renal failure. However, the long-term treatment of chronic renal failure was not practicable because of the need for repeated cut-downs to obtain vascular access for dialysis. It was the invention of the Teflon arteriovenous shunt by Scribner and co-workers[60] at the University of Washington in 1960 that first made possible the continuing long-term treatment of patients with ESRD. This sparked interest in improving the technique of dialysis and related technology and in re-examining the management of patients with chronic renal failure. These developments, together with introduction of the arteriovenous fistula for blood access by Brescia and associates[10] in 1965, made possible the large-scale implementation of dialysis. Readers interested in the history and development of hemodialysis are referred to the detailed account by Drukker.[18]

Physiology

The principle of hemodialysis is based on the diffusion of accumulated uremic toxins across a semipermeable membrane from high concentrations in the blood to lower concentrations in the dialysis fluid (dialysate). Hemodialysis requires a blood flow of 150 ml/min to 300 ml/min through the artificial kidney. The blood flows on one side of a semipermeable membrane made from cellulose acetate, regenerated cellulose (Cuprophan), or a variety of synthetic membranes.[66] A dialysate flow of 200 ml/min to 500 ml/min on the other side of the membrane maintains the diffusion gradient responsible for removal of uremic toxins. Transfer of water is dependent upon membrane permeability and the transmembrane hydrostatic pressure; the latter can be controlled either by increasing the pressure in the blood compartment of the artificial kidney or, more commonly, by exerting a negative pressure on the

dialysate compartment. The usual dialysis membrane surface area is between 0.6m² and 1.8m², and the membrane may be arranged in the form of parallel plates, a coiled tube, or, as most commonly used today, in hollow fibers through which the blood passes and around which the dialysate flows. The dialysate is usually prepared from treated tap water mixed with a solute concentrate by means of a proportioning system. The typical dialysate composition is 135 mEq/liter to 145 mEq/liter of sodium, 0 to 2.0 mEq/liter of potassium, 3 mEq/liter to 3.5 mEq/liter of calcium, 0.5 mEq/liter to 1.0 mEq/liter of magnesium, 0 to 200 mg/dl of glucose, and either 36 mEq/liter to 40 mEq/liter of acetate or 30 mEq/liter to 35 mEq/liter of bicarbonate, the remainder of the anion being chloride. The proportioning system is equipped with various monitors and alarms so that the dialysis can be carried out safely without the need for constant staff supervision.[21] For most patients, dialysis is performed three times per week for 2.5 to 5 hours, either in an outpatient facility or in the patient's home.

Complications of Hemodialysis

Hemodialysis, properly carried out, is a safe procedure. The death rate from technical or human error is said to be only about one in 75,000 treatments,[29] equivalent to one death every 480 years for a patient dialyzing three times per week. Nevertheless, complications do occur during hemodialysis, some of which may be life threatening. The most common complications include the occurrence of episodes of hypotension, cramps, nausea, and malaise during the course of dialysis,[16] usually associated with short dialysis, removal of a large volume of ultrafiltrate, or the use of an acetate-containing dialysate in conjunction with a large surface area dialyzer.

Hypotension occurs in as many as 25% of hemodialyses,[61] and its occurrence is usually related to rapid fluid removal or hemorrhage. Other contributing factors include change in osmolality, accumulation of acetate, and the presence of autonomic neuropathy. Hypotension resulting from blood loss is treated by transfusion; otherwise, hypotension can be treated by infusion of saline, slowing the blood flow rate, or changing the dialyzer to one of lesser efficiency. The frequency of hypotension can generally be reduced by attention to the details of the dialysis process and by use of a dialysate with a sodium content of 140 mEq/liter.[38] Muscle cramps are often related in time to the occurrence of hypotension and may be severe, particularly in older patients. These, too, may be relieved by use of a higher dialysate sodium concentration (140 mEq/liter) or intravenous injection of hypertonic saline or dextrose.[52] Quinine sulfate by mouth has been used as a precautionary measure.[41]

Another less common cause of symptoms during hemodialysis is the disequilibrium syndrome. This is also secondary to rapid solute removal, resulting in "reverse urea" shift because of slower clearance of urea from the cerebrospinal fluid, leading to cerebral edema,[42] and can be avoided by using less efficient dialysis of shorter duration in patients with extreme degrees of uremia. The disequilibrium syndrome is associated with nausea, vomiting, and headache and may lead to seizures and death. It is not a major problem for stable patients on chronic maintenance dialysis, although it must be distinguished from subdural hematoma, which may also occur in hemodialysis patients. Subdural hematoma should always be considered when focal neurologic signs occur in a dialysis patient,[47] and tomographic scans may be required to confirm the diagnosis.

During hemodialysis, the patient is always at some risk from air embolism because of the extracorporeal blood circuit and because of the use of a blood pump.[72] Symptoms include shortness of breath, cough, tightness in the chest, and loss of consciousness. Prevention by care during dialysis and the use of an air detection alarm is vital. If air embolism occurs, infusion of air must be stopped by clamping the venous return line and switching off the pump, the patient should be turned on the left side with head and chest down, and oxygen should be given. Use of a decompression chamber may be helpful in serious cases.

Fever occurring during hemodialysis may be related to contamination of the equipment, to the occurrence of endotoxemia, or may be due to infection, the most common site being in association with vascular access.[44] Other infections may also be of importance in dialysis patients. In the past, viral hepatitis was a serious risk in dialysis facilities, causing deaths in both patients and staff. Now, with attention to precautionary techniques and the recent availability of a vaccine against hepatitis B, this is usually no longer a major problem.[14] Nevertheless, non-A, non-B hepatitis also occurs in dialysis patients and remains a potential hazard, particularly as it may result in chronic hepatitis.[31] The risk associated with the dialysis of patients who have antibodies to HIV remains uncertain but is probably small, although dialysis patients may have been exposed to this virus as a result of transfusions or intravenous drug abuse. The degree to which such patients should be isolated remains to be defined.[27]

Hemorrhage is always a potential problem for dialysis patients, particularly during hemodialysis when the patient is heparinized. Bleeding may occur into the gastrointestinal tract, brain, pericardium, pleura, peritoneal space, skin, and elsewhere. The risk of bleeding during dialysis may be minimized by use of a lower dose of heparin or by use of regional heparinization. Blood loss may also occur during hemodialysis owing to separation of lines or membrane rupture.

The role played by acetate in the dialysate in producing symptoms during hemodialysis has been studied recently. Acetate was first used to replace bicarbonate in dialysate in 1964 in order to allow preparation of concentrate for use with proportioning systems. Problems began to arise with acetate with the development of large surface area, high efficiency dialyzers—use of which can result in a large acetate load to the patient and a significant loss of bicarbonate across the dialyzer.[57] This can result in worsening of the metabolic acidosis during dialysis. Some patients are unable to tolerate these events and develop headaches, vomiting, nausea, cramps, and hypotension. For many patients, symptoms during dialysis may be reduced by use of bicarbonate rather than acetate in the dialysate.[32]

Many other problems may be associated with hemodialysis, including electrolyte problems associated with improperly prepared dialysate, hemolysis owing to presence of copper or other metals in the dialysate, overheating of the dialysate, or the presence of nitrates or chloramines in the dialysate. Recently, aluminum accumulation has been shown to be associated with the development of both dialysis dementia and osteomalacia.[4]

PERITONEAL DIALYSIS

Peritoneal dialysis as a treatment for chronic renal failure has been available since the early 1960s. For the two preceding decades, peritoneal dialysis was used quite frequently as a method of treatment for acute renal failure, but because of problems in obtaining repeated peritoneal access and the high risk of developing peritonitis, it was not used for the treatment of patients with chronic renal failure. Development of the indwelling Tenckhoff catheter[69] and of a reverse osmosis proportioning system for producing peritoneal dialysate made long-term intermittent peritoneal dialysis a feasible treatment in the early 1970s.[68] More recently, the development of CAPD and CCPD using an automatic cycler have extended the use of peritoneal dialysis much more widely, even as, at the same time, the limitations of long-term intermittent peritoneal dialysis in patients who have lost their residual renal function have become evident.[3]

The peritoneal membrane has a surface area of between 1 m² and 2 m², and solute removal occurs by diffusion from the blood in the peritoneal capillaries to a dialyzing solution infused into the peritoneal space.[56] Solutes with molecular weights of up to 30,000 daltons may cross the peritoneal membrane, and the middle molecule hypothesis was based on the idea that this ability of the peritoneal membrane to transport larger molecules may be the reason why peritoneal dialysis patients do not develop neuropathy and other serious complications, even though they are not as well dialyzed from a biochemical point of view as are patients on hemodialysis.[5] Solute removal with peritoneal dialysis depends upon dialysate flow rate, temperature, *p*H, and osmolality, and fluid removal is achieved by using a dialysate of a higher dextrose content. Dextrose is poorly absorbed across the peritoneal membrane and therefore creates an osmotic gradient for fluid removal.[37] Peritoneal dialysate, unlike the dialysate used for hemodialysis, must be sterile.

Intermittent Peritoneal Dialysis

Intermittent peritoneal dialysis (IPD) is generally carried out using a machine to deliver the sterile dialysate to the peritoneal cavity through a permanently implanted silastic catheter.[69] After a suitable dwell time, the fluid is removed by a pump or by siphonage to a container for spent dialysate or to a drain. The simpler piece of equipment now generally used for peritoneal dialysis is the cycler. This operates by gravity and feeds sterile peritoneal dialysate from a number of bags through an octopus head of plastic tubing to a heater chamber, then into the patient's peritoneal cavity for a preset dwell time, and finally draining the cavity automatically and repeating the cycle.[17] The second type of equipment, which is no longer manufactured in the United States, depends upon reverse osmosis, a process that uses hydrostatic pressure to overcome osmotic pressure and results in the flow of pure water through a semipermeable membrane. This sterile, pyrogen-free water is then mixed with sterile concentrate by a proportioning pump to produce peritoneal dialysate, which is pumped into the peritoneal cavity.[68] Timers are used to preset the duration of inflow, dwell time, and outflow time. Although the reverse osmosis equipment is much more complex and expensive than the cycler, the supplies required for each dialysis are much less expensive.

The main long-term problems with IPD are the eventual occurrence of underdialysis as the patient's residual renal function declines and a mortality rate that is higher than that with long-term hemodialysis.[3]

Continuous Ambulatory Peritoneal Dialysis

Continuous ambulatory peritoneal dialysis (CAPD) is a form of home peritoneal dialysis in which the patient dialyzes continuously by infusing 2 liters of sterile dialysate from a flexible plastic bag into the peritoneal cavity. The bag is then rolled and carried in a pocket or belt during the dwell time of 4 to 6 hours or overnight. During the dwell time, the patient can be ambulant and carry on normal activities. At the end of the dwell time, the dialysate is drained into the empty bag, which is then detached and replaced by a fresh bag, which is used to refill the peritoneal cavity. The process of drainage, disconnection/connection, and infusion takes about 45 minutes.[55] CAPD is simple to do, does not require the assistance of a second person, allows the patient mobility, does not require the use of a machine, and is well tolerated by many patients. Its problems are its continuous nature, 7 days weekly, and the risk of peritonitis. The latter occurs on average at a rate of 1.4 episodes per patient-year,[67] and repeated episodes of peritonitis may lead to technique failure and a need for the patient to switch to hemodialysis. The cumulative probability of transferring from CAPD within 2 years of starting this treatment is about 34%.[67]

Continuous Cycling Peritoneal Dialysis

Continuous cycling peritoneal dialysis (CCPD) is a combination of IPD and CAPD in which a patient uses a machine (cycler or reverse osmosis equipment) to perform peritoneal dialysis overnight, each night, while sleeping.[17] Prior to disconnection in the morning, 2 liters of fresh dialysate is instilled into the peritoneal cavity, and this remains in place until connection for the next dialysis that evening. This technique reduces the number of connections compared with CAPD, and so may lessen the risk of peritonitis. It also eliminates the need to make bag changes during the day.

Complications of Peritoneal Dialysis

Complications associated with peritoneal dialysis include mechanical problems, infections, metabolic effects, and cardiovascular and pulmonary problems.

Mechanical complications include the occurrence of pain in the rectum or bladder area resulting from malposition of the catheter or pain in the shoulder referred from the diaphragm and associated with abdominal distention from air or excess dialysate. Bleeding may occur into the peritoneal cavity, but despite appearances, this is usually not a serious problem. Leakage of dialysate can occur, particularly around the catheter, and subcutaneous dissection with dialysate can occur when one of the catheter holes is outside the peritoneal cavity or with leakage through the peritoneum into the muscles and subcutaneous tissues. The most serious mechanical complication is bowel perforation. The risk of this can be minimized by careful attention to detail during insertion of the peritoneal catheter.

Peritonitis remains the single most important complication with all forms of peritoneal dialysis. The incidence rate varies in different programs, but with IPD, the frequency should not be more than about one episode per 24 months of treatment. The latest data on CAPD suggests a peritonitis rate of 1.4 to 1.5 episodes per patient-year of treatment, and, for CCPD, 1.3 to 1.4 episodes per patient-year of treatment.[67] Bacteria can gain entry into the peritoneal cavity either through the lumen of the catheter or by way of the catheter tract. Use of meticulous sterile technique during connections and disconnections is vital. Peritonitis usually presents with fever, abdominal pain, tenderness, discomfort, and/or cloudy peritoneal fluid on outflow. A specimen of fluid should be sent immediately for gram stain, cell count, and culture, and appropriate antibiotic therapy should be started. Many episodes of peritonitis can be treated by suitably trained patients themselves at home and without admission to the hospital. Infection can also occur along the catheter tract and requires meticulous local care and use of systemic antibiotics. Catheter replacement may be required with resistant episodes of catheter tract infection.

Infection with hepatitis B virus may also be a problem for peritoneal dialysis patients, and such patients should be tested routinely because of the risk associated with the high concentrations of virus that may occur in the peritoneal fluid. Whether the same risk applies to patients who have antibodies to HIV or who have acquired immunodeficiency syndrome (AIDS) remains to be determined.

Pulmonary complications of peritoneal dialysis include pneumonia and atelectasis as a result of abdominal distention and limited respiratory movements. If serious abdominal distention occurs, the volume of the exchange can be reduced. Pleural effusion may occur and is usually right-sided, commonly because of dialysate passing through a diaphragmatic defect. Cardiovascular problems can also occur, particularly in patients with pre-existing cardiac problems who become either severely overdistended or severely volume depleted.

Metabolic problems associated with peritoneal dialysis include protein loss in the dialysate, which may be as much as 9 g to 10 g of protein daily. However, most patients eating a protein intake of 1.2 g/kg body weight/day probably will not have problems with this. Another common problem is hyperglycemia owing to aborption of glucose from the dialysate. This may also be associated with hyperlipidemia and perhaps an increased risk of development of vascular disease.

WHEN TO START TREATMENT

No clear guidelines are available as to when treatment should be started by dialysis or transplantation, and this depends, at least in some countries, upon finances and the availability of facilities and treatment. The pathophysiology and biochemistry of uremia are still not completely defined, but it would seem logical to correct metabolic disturbances as completely and as early as possible. Nevertheless, most patients are started on dialysis only when their creatinine clearance falls to 5 ml/min or less and their serum creatinine is in the range of 12 mg/dl to 15 mg/dl.[7] This is usually preceded by a period of conservative management with a low-protein diet and control of hypertension and hyperphosphatemia by medical measures. Bonomini and associates[9] have suggested that there are advantages in starting dialysis earlier, often without low-protein dietary management, relying only on clinical signs and symptoms. He and co-workers have begun hemodialysis in patients with creatinine clearances of 10 ml/minute to 12 ml/minute, and improved patient survival, reduced frequency of hospitalization, and improved rehabilitation have been claimed to result from this.[9] These results remain to be confirmed by other researchers. Unfortunately, this approach entails the patient becoming dependent upon dialysis at a time when residual renal function is still sufficient to maintain life, and it increases the cost of treatment even when dialysis is performed only twice weekly.[9]

Recent studies have shown that properly conducted conservative care in the predialytic phase with careful dietary management, including protein restriction and possibly supplementation with essential amino acids or ketoacids,[54] phosphate restriction,[51] and control of hypertension[6] may have a significant effect in slowing progression of renal disease as well as in relieving uremic symptoms.

Thus, although there is still not clear definition of when to start treatment, a practical approach would be to suggest that dialysis should be commenced at that point in time when the patient develops symptoms related to uremia and its complications that are not readily controlled by simple conservative measures such as diet and control of hypertension. This would mean that most patients will start dialysis with a creatinine clearance of 5 ml/minute to 7 ml/minute or less, and a serum creatinine of 10 mg/dl or greater. Currently, a major prospective controlled study is underway in the United States to confirm whether strict control of dietary protein intake together with supplementation with essential amino acids and/or ketoacids may delay the need for dialysis without putting patients at risk from malnutrition and other nutritional problems. In the meantime, it is probably better to err on the side of conservatism by starting treatment as previously suggested, rather than postponing this until patients become sick, protein malnourished, and unemployed.

PATIENT SURVIVAL WITH DIALYSIS AND TRANSPLANTATION

Several questions are not completely resolved in the minds of many physicians and patients. These include whether the patient who is being treated with dialysis should be encouraged to undergo transplantation, what the relative risks of dialysis and transplantation are, and, specifically, whether the risk to the patient may be increased following cadaver transplantation. Despite the increased use of patient survival estimates to describe the results of treatment in individual dialysis or transplant programs,

until recently there has been little attention to statistical methods to directly compare patient survival on dialysis with that following transplantation and to compare different programs providing these services. Such comparisons must take into account patient and treatment characteristics that may affect survival and that differ between various treatment groups, such as age and co-morbidity. Use of new statistical techniques, such as the Cox proportional hazards model,[13] permits compensation for these differences by adjusting for the various risk factors present in different patient populations. Many of the comparisons reported in the past compared the survival of a younger group of selected transplanted patients with that of patients treated only by dialysis and failed to take into account differences in the patient populations. The Cox model allows comparison of survival experience of two or more treatment groups while simultaneously adjusting for the different distribution among the groups of other factors (covariates) known to affect survival. An individual weight or coefficient is calculated for each covariate entered into the model, and these coefficients measure the influence of the covariate on survival. Covariates whose values may change over time are termed *time-dependent* and can also be used in the Cox model.

In a recent study in the Northwest Kidney Center program, a comparison was made between patient survival for related donor transplant, cadaver donor transplant, and hemodialysis (without taking into account the time on dialysis of those patients with transplants).[71] Transplantation appeared to be superior to dialysis (Fig. 13-1). However, when the time that the transplanted patient spent on dialysis before transplantation is credited to dialysis survival, this more nearly approaches that of patients treated

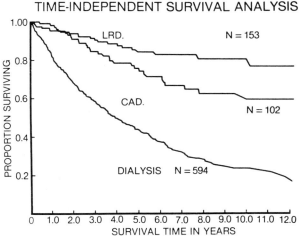

FIGURE 13-1. The probability of survival for 849 patients with primary renal disease receiving transplants from living-related donors (LRD) or cadaveric donors (CAD) or being treated with dialysis only. Estimates were obtained by using the method of Kaplan and Meier. (Reproduced with permission from Vollmer WM, Wahl PW, Blagg CR: Survival with dialysis and transplantation in patients with end-stage renal disease. N Engl J Med 308:1553, 1983.)

TIME-DEPENDENT UNADJUSTED SURVIVAL ANALYSIS

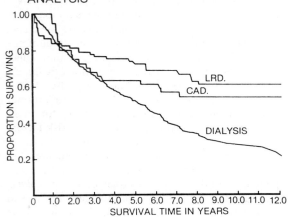

FIGURE 13-2. The probability of survival for 849 patients with primary renal disease, according to transplant classification. Estimates were obtained by using the method of Kaplan and Meier, taking into account the time-dependent nature of the treatment status. (Reproduced with permission from Vollmer WM, Wahl PW, Blagg CR: Survival with dialysis and transplantation in patients with end-stage renal disease. N Engl J Med 308:1553, 1983.)

CAUSE OF RENAL FAILURE

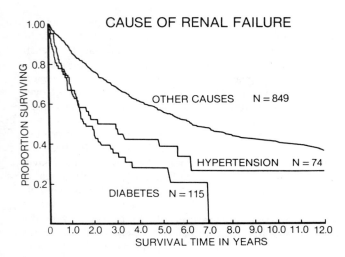

FIGURE 13-3. The probability of survival for 1038 patients, according to the cause of renal failure. Estimates were obtained by using the method of Kaplan and Meier. (Reproduced with permission from Vollmer WM, Wahl PW, Blagg CR: Survival with dialysis and transplantation in patients with end-stage renal disease. N Engl J Med 308:1553, 1983.)

SURVIVAL BASED ON AGE AT ENTRY

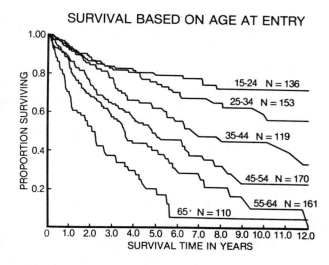

FIGURE 13-4. The probability of survival for 849 patients with primary renal disease, according to age at entry. Estimates were obtained by using the method of Kaplan and Meier. (Reproduced with permission from Vollmer WM, Wahl PW, Blagg CR: Survival with dialysis and transplantation in patients with end-stage renal disease. N Engl J Med 308:1553, 1983.)

by cadaver transplantation (Fig. 13-2). Patient survival also relates to other factors. Survival for patients with renal failure resulting from conditions other than diabetic nephropathy and primary hypertensive disease is similar ($p<0.25$), but that of patients with renal failure owing to diabetes and to primary hypertensive disease is significantly poorer (Fig. 13-3). Sex has no influence on survival in these patients, but age is a major factor in survival (Fig. 13-4), as is the number of associated diseases (Fig. 13-5). The difference between the dialysis and transplantation populations is illustrated by the fact that both age and the number of associated diseases differed significantly ($p<0.001$) between patients treated by living-related donor transplant, cadaver transplant, and dialysis (Table 13-1).

When the Cox proportional hazards model was used to adjust patient survival for age, diagnosis, number of associated diseases, and year of transplantation, no difference in survival was found between patients treated by dialysis and those treated by cadaver transplantation, but survival in patients treated by related donor transplantation was significantly better (Table 13-2). The positive coefficients for age and number of associated diseases reflect decreased survival with larger values for these covariates. The negative coefficient with related donor transplant reflects the improved survival compared with dialysis. For cadaver transplantation, the difference is not significant, and the adjusted time-dependent log-rank statistic is 0.00043 ($p<0.95$), confirming the lack of significant difference. These coefficients can be used to estimate the relative risk of death with the two forms of transplantation compared with dialysis. Table 13-3 shows these risks in 3 columns based on "time-independent (unadjusted)" analysis as in Figure 13-1, with "time-dependent (unadjusted)" analysis as in Figure 13-2, and with "time-dependent (adjusted)" analysis, which takes into account the effects of age, number of associated diseases, and year of entry. Further analysis showed that exclusion of those patients whose graft had failed from the estimation of trans-

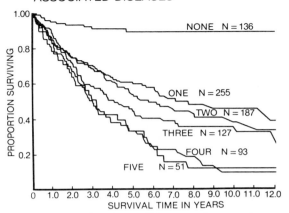

SURVIVAL BASED ON NUMBER OF ASSOCIATED DISEASES

FIGURE 13-5.   *The probability of survival for 849 patients with primary renal disease, according to the number of associated diseases. Estimates were obtained by using the method of Kaplan and Meier. (Reproduced with permission from Vollmer WM, Wahl PW, Blagg CR: Survival with dialysis and transplantation in patients with end-stage renal disease. N Engl J Med 308:1553, 1983.)*

plantation survival had no significant effect on the results. When a subset of 189 patients with either diabetes or primary hypertensive disease as the cause of renal failure was analyzed in the same fashion, the results were similar (Table 13-4). Thus, it would appear that although patient survival with a related donor transplant is better, there is no difference in patient survival following cadaver transplantation or with dialysis, survival being dependent upon factors such as diagnosis, age, and associated diseases. Similar findings have been reported by other investigators.[39] Although the data on which these studies were based were accumulated in the precyclosporine era, cyclosporine appears to have no significant effect on patient survival with transplantation[45]; thus, these conclusions are still likely to be valid.

"Quality hemodialysis" is now considered to

TABLE 13-1   *Comparison of Mean Age and Average Number of Associated Diseases in 849 Patients Treated by Dialysis and Transplantation*

	RELATED DONOR TRANSPLANT	CADAVER DONOR TRANSPLANT	DIALYSIS ONLY
MEAN AGE IN YEARS ± STANDARD ERROR	27 ± 0.845	32 ± 1.200	50 ± 0.631
AVERAGE NUMBER OF ASSOCIATED DISEASES	1.4 ± 0.097	1.4 ± 0.122	2.1 ± 0.056

Patients were Caucasians, aged 15–55 years. Those with renal failure owing to diabetic nephropathy or primary hypertensive disease were excluded.

TABLE 13-2   Survival Analysis With Covariate Adjustment for Patients With Primary Renal Failure

COVARIATES*	COEFFICIENT	STANDARD ERROR	SIGNIFICANCE†
Age at entry	0.3226	0.0467	$p<0.0001$
Number of associated diseases	0.1734	0.0510	$p=0.0003$
Year of entry	0.1297	0.1802	$p=0.2358$
LRD transplant	−0.5988	0.2697	$p=0.0132$
CAD transplant	0.0083	0.2750	$p=0.5120$

* Age at entry, number of associated diseases, and year of entry are standardized as follows: (age—44)/10, (number—2), and (year—1974)/10. LRD = living-related donor, CAD = cadaveric donor. A LRD (or CAD) transplant is assigned a value of 1 if the first transplant was from a living-related (or cadaveric) donor, and a value of 0 otherwise.

† All p values are one-sided.

TABLE 13-3   Relative Risk According to Type of Analysis

TREATMENTS COMPARED*	TYPE OF ANALYSIS		
	Time-Independent (Unadjusted)	Time-Dependent (Unadjusted)	Time-Dependent (Adjusted)†
LRD with dialysis	0.23‡	0.29‡	0.55§
CAD with dialysis	0.53‡	0.58§	1.01
LRD with CAD	0.43‖	0.50§	0.54§

* LRD = living-related donor, CAD = cadaveric donor.

† Adjusted for age, number of associated diseases, and year of entry.

‡ One-sided p value less than 0.001.

§ One-sided p value between 0.01 and 0.05.

‖ One-sided p value between 0.001 and 0.01.

TABLE 13-4   Survival Analysis With Covariate Adjustment for Patients With Diabetes or Hypertension or Both

COVARIATES*	COEFFICIENT	STANDARD ERROR	SIGNIFICANCE†
Age at entry	0.1991	0.0735	$p=0.0034$
Number of associated diseases	0.3112	0.1132	$p=0.0030$
Year of entry	−0.4576	0.4400	$p=0.1150$
LRD transplant	−0.9299	0.5961	$p=0.0600$
CAD transplant	−0.2312	0.5376	$p=0.3400$

* Covariates are defined as in Table 13-2. LRD = living-related donor, CAD = cadaveric donor.

† All p values are one-sided.

be the "gold standard" treatment for patient survival.[50] The prospect for survival with hemodialysis for patients 20 to 40 years of age with primary renal disease, without systemic disease or significant complications, is a potential 7-year survival rate of 90%,[8,64] and many hemodialysis patients around the world have now survived more than 10 years. In our own program, the longest survivor is now in his 25th year on hemodialysis. It appears that survival with CAPD is comparable to that with hemodialysis,[53] but that survival with IPD may be inferior.[3] It is too early to say whether survival with CCPD will be comparable to that with CAPD or more closely resemble that of IPD, but the former appears more likely. Nevertheless, for most patients, the eventual technique failure with all forms of peritoneal dialysis is such that these cannot be considered long-term treatments.[53]

MORBIDITY ASSOCIATED WITH DIALYSIS AND TRANSPLANTATION

Long-term effects and the complications of dialysis and transplantation are more important in determining the ultimate quality of life for the patient than are issues of patient survival.

Hypertension and cardiovascular disease remain the major problems for many dialysis patients and for transplanted patients. Nevertheless, the grim prognosis for accelerated atherosclerosis predicted by Scribner's group[48] in 1974 can be improved dramatically by control of blood pressure.[12,36,49] It has also become increasingly clear that poorly controlled hypertension is the major factor causing progression to end-stage renal failure in patients with primary renal disease, other than progression of the renal disease itself,[6,58] and there is evidence that the diseased kidney is particularly prone to further damage from high blood pressure.[6] Good control of hypertension is important in the management of both dialysis patients and transplanted patients and is probably the most important factor that can be addressed to reduce the risk of complications and death associated with cardiovascular disease in these patients.

Perhaps the major ongoing problem affecting the day-to-day well-being of dialysis patients is what Eady,[20] himself a dialysis patient, has described as "lack of vitality." This presumably relates, at least in part, to the anemia of ESRD as well as to other uremic complications. One of the most exciting recent developments is the synthesis of human erythropoietin by genetic engineering; this is currently being tested in dialysis patients for the first time. Erythropoietin deficiency is the major factor in causing the anemia of patients with ESRD,[2] and if this hormone could be made readily available, the well-being of dialysis patients should be improved considerably. Nevertheless, it is likely that most patients with a well-functioning transplant and relatively normal renal function will feel better than patients on dialysis, particularly if they are receiving corticosteroids as part of their immunosuppressive therapy.

Bone disease was a crippling complication for many of the early dialysis patients, but with a better understanding of the management of renal osteodystrophy with vitamin D analogs and of the role of parathyroidectomy,[65] and with an increasing understanding of the role that aluminum may play in the development of dialysis osteomalacia,[4] it is hoped that renal bone disease will not be a major problem for most patients in the future. At the same

time, it must be remembered that aseptic necrosis has been a frequent complication in many transplanted patients treated with corticosteroids; hip and knee replacements are common in such patients. Again, it is hoped that with development of cyclosporine other new immunosuppressive agents and very low steroid dosage, this too will become much less frequent.

One concern that is frequently ignored is the patient's self-image and appearance. Most dialysis patients are pale and slightly pigmented. Consequently, many patients do not look well. On the other hand, they do not have iatrogenic Cushing's syndrome, the facial characteristics of which, in the past at least, have been distressing, particularly to young female patients who have been transplanted. Other potential problems resulting from corticosteroid therapy include the development of cataracts and the aggravation of bone disease. It is worth remembering that, "The course of untreated Cushing's syndrome is deleterious . . . In general, a patient with untreated Cushing's syndrome has a life expectancy of three to ten years, on average of 5 years,"[46] although presumably life expectancy is better in mildly cushingoid patients.

Finally, there is concern about the development of malignancy in dialysis and transplant patients. After years on dialysis, some patients develop a multicystic disease affecting the kidney,[19] and a percentage of these patients may develop malignancy in association with the cysts.[62] Whether or not other forms of malignancy are more frequent in dialysis patients remains uncertain.[59] In the case of transplantation, recent data from the European Dialysis and Transplant Association confirm that there is a higher incidence of both non-Hodgkin's lymphoma and skin cancer in transplanted patients than in either dialysis patients or the normal population.[73]

REHABILITATION AND QUALITY OF LIFE

From the patient's point of view, perhaps the most important consideration in selecting treatment is the quality of life that can be anticipated. Concern has been expressed about the poor quality of life in many dialysis patients, particularly after publication of the paper by Gutman and colleagues[34] in 1981. A study from the pre-cyclosporine era comparing hemodialysis patients and cadaver transplant recipients found that those with a successful cadaver transplant had greater physical and occupational rehabilitation than did dialysis patients. Nevertheless, on subjective measures, successful transplant and dialysis patients were similar in reporting normal effect, but failed transplant patients had a diminished quality of life.[40]

The recent National Kidney Dialysis and Transplant Study, sponsored by the Health Care Financing Administration, undertook a detailed study of 859 patients on home and center hemodialysis, CAPD, and transplantation.[26] Patients were randomly selected from 10 programs across the United States chosen to represent a typical cross section of dialysis and transplant facilities. Data were gathered from the patients, the facilities and their staff, and from the patients' physicians using a large number of well-tested instruments to measure, among other items, both subjective and objective quality of the patient's life. Because of the problem of comparing patients on the different modalities of treatment, the data were analyzed to take case-mix differences into account. The results showed that in terms of rehabilitation and both subjective and objective measures of quality of life, patients with a successful transplant did better than patients on any form of dialysis. However, those patients with a failed transplant overall had a less satisfactory quality of life than those with functioning transplant or those who were on home hemodialysis. It is hoped that this will change in the future with the improved graft survival rates reported using cyclosporine.[45] Among the dialysis patients, those on home dialysis fared significantly better than those treated by either CAPD or in-center hemodialysis, even when allowances were made to adjust for the differences in patient populations. However, one of the most striking results was that compared to the general population, although all patients had lower quality of life scores, these were not markedly lower, even in the patients treated by in-center hemodialysis, presumably reflecting the ability of patients with ESRD to make a significant readjustment to their circumstances.

COST OF TREATMENT

Not a great deal of reliable information is available to compare the cost of dialysis and transplantation over the long term. Data from the Health Care Financing Administration suggests that for the Medicare ESRD Program, the higher initial cost of transplantation is paid back in about 4 years following a successful transplant. The cost to Medicare of transplantation has to take into account the costs of hospitalizations associated with the transplantation operation, transplant failure, or death. In 1979, the first-year cost to Medicare of a successful transplant was $29,860. If the transplant failed during the year, the cost increased by $12,572, and, if the patient died, the cost increased by $30,819 over the cost of a successful transplant. In the second and third years post-transplantation, if the graft functioned, the cost was $4,074 per year; but, if the graft failed, the cost in the year of failure was $30,189. The cost of dialysis per year to Medicare averaged $21,325.[23]

Krakauer[45] examined the unaudited charges for treatment and the Medicare reimbursement for the first half of 1984 for dialysis patients, and for 1982 and 1983 for transplant patients. The mean charge associated with 1 year of dialysis was $27,125; or, if the patient died during the year, the mean charge was $24,425. However, as the patient would then only have generated dialysis charges for an average of 6 months, the net event cost of death in a dialysis patient was a mean of $9,975. For successful transplantation and the first 60 days of post-transplantation treatment, the mean charge was $33,467, and the 1-year maintenance charges after a successful transplantation totaled $9,367. Graft failure without death during the first year resulted in charges for the year, including transplantation and dialysis, of $65,433, with a net event cost for treatment of the rejection of $9,500. If the patient died within the first year post-transplantation, the total cost for surgery and treatment and death-related charges was $47,500, and the net event charge for the death was $11,300. Actual Medicare reimbursement was less than these charges, because only in-hospital charges are paid in full; physician fees and outpatient charges, including dialysis being paid at 80%, and outpatient drugs are not covered at all. For transplantation using antithymocyte globulin or antilymphocyte globulin, the charges were considerably higher, the mean charge for a successful transplant being $54,100. With cyclosporine, the mean charges for a cadaver transplant and the first 6 months of treatment was $47,700. It was also found that the charges from major transplantation centers can vary by as much as ± $14,000. As far as financial projections based on the improvement in transplant graft survival anticipated with cyclosporine, it appears that these balance the drug's extra cost in 3 years; but, if cyclosporine is used for only 6 months after transplantation, there are savings to the Medicare End-Stage Renal Disease Program. Using these data and assuming a 20% overall graft failure rate, transplantation of 100 patients who survive 3 years is clearly less expensive than 100 patients treated by hemodialysis.

However, in addition to the direct costs of treatment, the effect of improved transplantation results on the number of dialysis patients and also the improved rehabilitation and opportunity for gainful employment following successful transplantation must be taken into account. Krakauer[45] has estimated that as a result of the improved results of transplantation with cyclosporine, by 1991 there will be 9200 patients alive with functioning transplants and 4800 fewer patients on dialysis. Because transplant patients generally are better rehabilitated,[26] he has estimated that this could result in additional aggregate income to patients of between $42 million and $89 million per year. There are also indirect financial benefits to the government such as fewer unemployment benefits and benefits for surviving spouses and families, and increased payment of taxes. Thus, although it is difficult to estimate the overall cost–benefit of transplantation over dialysis, it appears that in the long run, transplantation, at least in the age groups currently transplanted, is somewhat more cost-effective. Unfortunately, no detailed analysis of this is available as yet.

AN INTEGRATED APPROACH TO THE TREATMENT OF PATIENTS WITH END-STAGE RENAL DISEASE

The availability of several different effective treatments for patients with ESRD allows a great deal of flexibility in the approach to management of individual patients. Optimal treatment can best be achieved by integration of the various available treatment modalities. Such integration implies that ''the option to convert from one therapy to another is not prejudiced at any stage, that the treatment options are available in geographical proximity, and that there is close cooperation between the various specialist staff involved. A successfully integrated approach to management minimizes morbidity and mortality and offers each individual the best opportunities for achieving an acceptable quality of life.''[70]

While successful transplantation remains the goal for as many patients as possible, nevertheless, because of age and other complications and the occurrence of preformed antibodies after previous transplantation, it is likely that at least 50% of all patients with ESRD will undergo treatment by dialysis at any given time. Consequently, an essential prerequisite for a good transplantation program is a good dialysis program to support patients prior to transplantation and following graft failure. Such a program should provide both in-center and home

hemodialysis, and peritoneal dialysis, primarily as CAPD and CCPD. In order to encourage independence and the opportunity for rehabilitation, all dialysis patients should be encouraged to consider some form of home dialysis except when a related donor transplant is known to be imminent. If a new patient is a transplant candidate but does not have a willing living-related donor, his or her initial dialysis treatment should be associated with multidisciplinary involvement of staff to provide orientation and education on the various treatment options. If possible, it is advantageous to provide this introduction to dialysis in a separate area.[24] Patients should have all the appropriate treatment options fully explained to them by the nephrologist and should also be seen by a transplant surgeon unless they clearly are not candidates for transplantation.

There must be opportunity for interaction with nursing staff, nutritionists, social workers, financial counselors, vocational rehabilitation counselors, and, if appropriate, psychologists and other staff to assist in the decision on selection of the best treatment. When appropriate, the emphasis should be on some form of self-dialysis in the home, and the patient should be trained for this at the earliest opportunity. A short period of time on home dialysis helps to give the patient confidence that in the event that a subsequent transplant fails, dialysis can be integrated into his or her life successfully. In fact, home dialysis patients are frequently the best candidates for transplantation not only because of the patient selection that has already occurred but also because they have acquired a considerable degree of confidence and independence.

The patient will undoubtedly make his or her selection of treatment with the guidance of the nephrologist; the latter, however, may be biased[30] in terms of preference for a specific mode of treatment, or the facility may be biased against home dialysis and transplantation.[63] Nevertheless, a recent survey of selected younger nephrologists showed that, for themselves, most would prefer home hemodialysis to either cadaver kidney transplantation or CAPD.[28] This too may change with further experience with cyclosporine.

Unfortunately, in the United States, despite the ready availability of funds for both dialysis and transplantation, the true integration of dialysis and transplant programs has not occurred in many areas. In part, this has been because of institutional jealousies and rivalries, and also because of financial incentives to retain patients in dialysis units. These factors may be related to the needs of proprietary dialysis corporations or to nephrologists' fees for providing care to dialysis patients, because, unlike the situation in Great Britain, the United States is not accustomed to the concept of primary, secondary, and tertiary care facilities closely interrelating and working together.

FINAL COMMENT

For patients with ESRD, the primary options are dialysis and transplantation. At this time, for most patients, dialysis in one form or another will play a major role in their lives for the next 20 or more years. To achieve the best survival, quality of life and rehabilitation require the availability of good dialysis programs. Survival also requires that transplant programs work closely with dialysis programs to ensure that patients are treated in such a way that all who might be transplant candidates will have the option of transplantation, that they have a full understanding of the consequences of receiving a transplant or remaining on the most appropriate modality of dialysis, and that the care provided to them be the optimum that can be achieved by a team that includes transplant surgeons and nephrologists working together in the best interests of the patient.

REFERENCES

1. Abel JJ, Rowntree LC, Turner BB: On the removal of diffusible substances from the circulating blood by means of dialysis. Trans Assoc Am Physicians 28:51, 1913
2. Adamson JW, Eschbach J, Finch CA: The kidney and erythropoiesis. Am J Med 44:725, 1968
3. Ahmad S, Gallagher N, Shen F: Intermittent peritoneal dialysis: Status reassessed. Trans Am Soc Artif Intern Organs 25:86, 1979
4. Alfrey AC: The toxicity of the aluminum burden. Semin Nephrol 3:329, 1983
5. Babb AL, Ahmad S, Bergstrom J et al: The middle molecule hypothesis in perspective. Am J Kidney Dis 1:46, 1981
6. Baldwin DS: Chronic glomerulonephritis: Nonimmunologic mechanisms of progressive glomerular damage. Kidney Int 21:109, 1982
7. Berlyne GM, Giovannetti S: When should entry into a regular hemodialysis programme occur? Nephron 16:81, 1976
8. Blagg CR, Wahl PW, Lamers JY: Treatment of chronic renal failure at the Northwest Kidney Center, Seattle, from 1960 to 1982. ASAIO J 6:170, 1983
9. Bonomini V, Feletti C, Scolari MP et al: Benefits of early initiation of dialysis. Kidney Int 28(Suppl)17: S-57, 1985
10. Brescia MJ, Cimino JE, Appel K et al: Chronic hemodialysis using venipuncture and a surgically created arteriovenous fistula. N Engl J Med 275:1089, 1966
11. Calland CH: Iatrogenic problems in end-stage renal failure. N Engl J Med 287:334, 1972
12. Charra B, Calemard E, Cuche M et al: Control of hypertension and prolonged survival on maintenance hemodialysis. Nephron 33:96, 1983
13. Cox DR: Regression models and life tables (with discussion). J R Stat Soc (B) 34:187, 1972
14. Crosnier J, Drueke T, Degos F: The liver in dialyzed and nondialyzed uremics. In Nissenson AR, Fine RN, Gentile DE (eds): Clinical Dialysis, p 351. Norwalk, CT, Appleton-Century-Crofts, 1984
15. The Data Committee of the National Forum of End-Stage Renal Disease Networks: Using end-stage renal disease facility surveys to monitor end-stage renal disease program trends. JAMA 254:1776, 1985
16. DeGoulet P, Proulx J, Aime F et al: Programme Dialyse-Informatique III Doneés epidémiologiques. Stratégies de dialyse et resultats biologiques. J Urol Néphrol 82:1001, 1976
17. Diaz-Buxo JA: Continuous cyclic peritoneal dialysis. In Nolph KD (ed): Peritoneal Dialysis, 2nd ed, p 247. Boston, Martinus Nijhoff, 1985
18. Drukker W: Hemodialysis: A historical review. In Drukker W, Parsons FM, Maher JF (eds): Replacement of Renal Function by Dialysis, 2nd ed, p 3. Boston, Martinus Nijhoff, 1983
19. Dunnill MS, Millard PR, Oliver D: Acquired cystic disease of the kidneys: A hazard of long-term intermittent maintenance haemodialysis. J Clin Pathol 30:868, 1977
20. Eady RAJ: In Giardano C, Friedman EA (eds): Uremia: Pathobiology of Patients Treated for 10 Years or More, p 44. Milan, Wichtig Editorie, 1981
21. Easterling RE: Mechanical aspects of dialysis including dialysate delivery systems and water for dialysate. In Nissenson AR, Fine RN, Gentile DE (eds): Clinical Dialysis, p 53. Norwalk, CT, Appleton-Century-Crofts, 1984
22. Eggers PW, Connerton R, McMullan M: The Medicare experience with end-stage renal disease: Trends in incidence, prevalence, and survival. Health Care Financ Rev 5:69, 1984
23. Eggers PW: Trends in Medicare reimbursement for end-stage renal disease: 1974–1979. Health Care Financ Rev 6:31, 1984
24. Eschbach JW, Seymour M, Potts A et al: A hemodialysis orientation unit. Nephron 33:106, 1983
25. Evans RW, Blagg CR, Bryan FA Jr: Implications for health care policy. A social and demographic profile of hemodialysis patients in the United States. JAMA 245:487, 1981

26. Evans RW, Manninen DL, Garrison LP Jr et al: The quality of life of patients with end-stage renal disease. N Engl J Med 312:553, 1985

27. Favero, MS: Recommended precautions for patients undergoing hemodialysis who have AIDS or non-A, non-B hepatitis. Infect Control 6:301, 1985

28. Friedman EA: Choosing uremia therapy in the mid-1980's. Transplant Proc 17:23, 1985

29. Friedman EA: Controversy in renal disease: Dialysis-induced hypotension. Am J Kidney Dis 2:289, 1982

30. Friedman EA: Physician bias in uremia therapy. Kidney Int 28(Suppl) 17:S-38, 1985

31. Galbraith RM, Dienstag JL, Purcell RH et al: Non-A non-B hepatitis associated with chronic liver disease in a haemodialysis unit. Lancet 1:951, 1979

32. Graefe U, Milutinovich J, Follette WC et al: Less dialysis-induced morbidity and vascular instability with bicarbonate in dialysate. Ann Intern Med 88:332, 1978

33. Graham T: Liquid diffusion applied to analysis. Phil Trans Roy Soc London 151:183, 1861

34. Gutman RA, Stead WW, Robinson RR: Physical activity and employment status of patients on maintenance dialysis. N Engl J Med 304:309, 1981

35. Haas G: Versuche der Blutauswaschung am Lebenden mit Hilfe der Dialyse. Clin Wochenschr 4:13, 1925

36. Haire HM, Sherrard DJ, Scardapane D: Smoking, hypertension, and mortality in a maintenance dialysis population. Cardiovasc Med 3:1163, 1978

37. Henderson L: Ultrafiltration with peritoneal dialysis. In Nolph KD (ed): Peritoneal Dialysis, 2nd ed, p 159. Boston, Martinus Nijhoff, 1985

38. Henrich WL, Woodard TD, McPhaul JJ Jr: The chronic efficacy and safety of high sodium dialysate: Double-blind, crossover study. Am J Kidney Dis 2:349, 1982

39. Hutchinson TA, Thomas DC, Lemieux JC et al: Prognostically controlled comparison of dialysis and renal transplantation. Kidney Int 26:44, 1984

40. Johnson JP, McCauley CR, Copley JB: The quality of life of hemodialysis and transplant patients. Kidney Int 22:286, 1982

41. Kaji DM, Ackad A, Nottage WG et al: Prevention of muscle cramps in haemodialysis patients by quinine sulphate. Lancet 2:66, 1976

42. Kennedy AC: Dialysis disequilibrium syndrome. Electroencephalogr Clin Neurophysiol 29:206, 1970

43. Kolff WJ: First clinical experience with the artificial kidney. Ann Intern Med 62:608, 1965

44. Kolmos HJ, Moller S: The epidemiology of febrile reactions in haemodialysis. Acta Med Scand 203:345, 1978

45. Krakauer H: Technical report on immunosuppressants in renal transplantation. Prepared for the Task Force on Organ Transplantation and the Office of Organ Transplantation, HRSA, PHS, 1985

46. Labhart A: Clinical Endocrinology: Theory and Practice, p 354. New York, Springer-Verlag, 1976

47. Leonard A, Shapiro FL: Subdural hematoma in regularly hemodialyzed patients. Ann Intern Med 82:650, 1975

48. Lindner A, Charra B, Sherrard DJ et al: Accelerated atherosclerosis in prolonged maintenance hemodialysis. N Engl J Med 290:697, 1974

49. Lundin AP, Adler AJ, Feinroth MV et al: Maintenance hemodialysis. Survival beyond the first decade. JAMA 244:38, 1980

50. Lundin AP: Quality hemodialysis: A "gold standard" treatment for survival. Kidney Int 28(Suppl) 17:S-12, 1985

51. Maschio G: Is phosphate more important than protein in lower protein diets? Kidney Int 28(Suppl) 17:S-71, 1985

52. Milutinovich J, Graefe U, Follette WC et al: Effect of hypertonic glucose on the muscular cramps of hemodialysis. Ann Intern Med 90:926, 1979

53. Mion CM, Mourad G, Canaud B et al: Maintenance dialysis: A survey of 17 years' experience in Languedoc-Rouissillon with a comparison of methods in a "standard population." ASAIO J 6:205, 1983

54. Mitch WE: The influence of the diet on the progression of renal insufficiency. Ann Rev Med 35:249, 1984

55. Moncrief JW, Popovich RP: Continuous ambulatory peritoneal dialysis. In Nolph KD (ed): Peritoneal Dialysis, 2nd ed, p 209. Boston, Martinus Nijhoff, 1985

56. Nolph KD, Twardowski ZJ: The peritoneal dialysis system. In Nolph KD (ed): Peritoneal Dialysis, 2nd ed, p 23. Boston, Martinus Nijhoff, 1985

57. Pagel MD, Ahmad S, Vizzo JE et al: Acetate and bicarbonate fluctuations and acetate intolerance during dialysis. Kidney Int 21:513, 1982

58. Parving HH, Andersen AR, Smidt UM et al: Early aggressive antihypertensive treatment reduces rate of decline in kidney function in diabetic nephropathy. Lancet 1:1175, 1983

59. Pateras VR: Malignancy in chronic dialysis patients. Int J Artif Organs 8:301, 1985

60. Quinton W, Dillard D, Scribner BH: Cannulation of blood vessels for prolonged hemodialysis. Trans Am Soc Artif Intern Organs 6:104, 1960

61. Rubin LJ, Gutman RA: Hypotension during hemodialysis. The Kidney 11:21, 1978

62. Ruggenenti P: Acquired renal cystic disease and renal adenocarcinoma in long-term dialysis patients. Int J Artif Organs 8:303, 1985

63. Schmidt RW, Blumenkrantz M, Wiegmann TB: The dilemmas of patient treatment for end-stage renal disease. Am J Kidney Dis 3:37, 1983

64. Shapiro FL, Umen A: Risk factors in hemodialysis patient survival. ASAIO J 6:176, 1983

65. Sherrard DJ: Renal osteodystrophy. Semin Nephrol 6:56, 1986

66. Shinaberger JH, Miller JH, Gardner PW: Characteristics of available hemodialyzers. In Nissenson AR, Fine RN, Gentile DE (eds): Clinical Dialysis, p 99. Norwalk, CT, Appleton-Century-Crofts, 1984

67. Steinberg SM, Cutler SJ, Novak JW et al: Report of the National CAPD Registry of the National Institutes of Health: Characteristics of participants and selected outcome measures for the period January 1, 1981,

through August 31, 1984. Potomac: EMMES Corporation, 1985

68. Tenckhoff H, Meston B, Shilipetar G: A simplified automatic peritoneal dialysis system. Trans Am Soc Artif Intern Organs 18:436, 1972

69. Tenckhoff H, Schechter H: A bacteriologically safe peritonal access device. Trans Am Soc Artif Intern Organs 14:181, 1968

70. Thompson JF, Chapman JR: Dialysis and transplantation. In Morris PJ (ed): Kidney Transplantation, 2nd ed, p 33. Orlando, Grune & Stratton, 1984

71. Vollmer WM, Wahl PW, Blagg CR: Survival with dialysis and transplantation in patients with end-stage renal disease. N Engl J Med 308:1553, 1983

72. Ward NK, Shadforth M, Hill AV et al: Air embolism during haemodialysis. Br Med J 3:74, 1971

73. Wing AJ, Broyer M, Brunner FP et al: Combined report on regular dialysis and transplantation in Europe, XIII, 1982. Proc Eur Dial Transplant Assoc 20:5, 1983

CHAPTER 14

Access for Dialysis

Carl E. Haisch

Access for dialysis is of two types: vascular and peritoneal. Successful long-term hemoaccess has been the major obstacle to successful hemodialysis. The most successful arteriovenous fistula is made between the radial artery and cephalic vein. If the patient does not have suitable vessels for construction of a fistula, a jump graft must be considered. The graft material most commonly used is polytetrafluoroethylene (PTFE). This graft may be placed in various positions in the arm as well as the leg.

Complications of both natural and jump grafts include bleeding, occlusion or threatened occlusion, infection, and hemodynamic problems. Infection is less common with natural than with jump grafts.

The average life span of an external shunt is 7 to 10 months. The Brescia-Cimino fistula has a better patency rate than the shunt and a lower infection rate. The patency rate of the PTFE grafts is between 45% and 80% at 2 years and is related to graft location.

By bathing the peritoneal surface in a dialysate, urea and fluid can be removed from the blood stream. The major advantage is that the patient is not on a machine for dialysis. The major disadvantages are that dialysis must be done daily and there is an incidence of peritonitis. Problems of peritoneal catheters include peritonitis, cuff extrusion, catheter tunnel infection, omental wrapping, and catheter migration out of the pelvis. The average catheter longevity is 80% to 85% at 1 year, with the figure dropping to approximately 60% at 2 years.

HEMODIALYSIS

History

The history of vascular access is closely intertwined with the development of hemodialysis. Dialysis began in the 1800s in the laboratory of a chemist, Thomas Graham; these studies were continued by George Haas. The first human dialysis occurred in 1924 following the technique of Haas in dogs. Kolff, in the early 1940s, constructed a dialysis machine using cellulose tubing. One of his patients had terminal uremia and a blood pressure of 245/150. Surgical cut-downs were necessary for continuous dialysis, but after all sites were used, the patient died. Kolff realized that repeated long-term dialysis in uremic patients was not possible until a method for repeated vascular access was available.[13]

In 1949, an arteriovenous fistula was constructed in a rabbit using silicon glass tubes. This was applied to humans but was unsuccessful because of clotting and infection.[13] In 1960, Quinton, Dillard, and Scribner[41] described a device made of Teflon that made repeated dialysis in uremic patients possible; however, there were still problems with clotting and infection. The construction by Brescia and colleagues[5] of an arteriovenous fistula in a side-to-side configuration between the radial artery and cephalic vein minimized infection and clotting.

There was still the problem of construction of a fistula in a patient who had no cephalic vein. This led to the development by May and associates[32] of a jump graft between the brachial artery and a vein in the forearm using a saphenous vein. In the case of a patient who did not have an adequate saphenous vein, a bovine graft was used. Polytetrafluoroethylene (PTFE) has largely replaced the bovine heterograft.[23]

Indications

All types of vascular access must meet certain requirements: They all require multiple use, a high flow system, and a system that will withstand highly irritating solutions. The most common indication for vascular access is acute or chronic renal failure. Other uses include total parenteral nutrition, particularly in an outpatient setting,[58] chemotherapy,[42] and plasmapheresis.

The ideal system for vascular access would allow immediate use, have high flow, withstand multiple punctures, and have no propensity to infection or thrombosis. None of the currently available techniques answers all these requirements; the limitations are caused primarily by thrombosis and infection.

Types of Angioaccess: External

The earliest successful type of vascular access used was the Scribner shunt (Fig. 14-1).[41] This used a Teflon tip inserted into both the artery and vein with silastic tubing to exit the skin. Upon exiting the skin, the ends were connected, thus allowing continuous blood flow. These shunts were most commonly placed in the forearm, using the radial artery and cephalic vein. In the leg, the posterior tibial artery and saphenous vein have frequently been chosen. The Allen test must be used in the hand to ensure adequate collateral circulation by way of the ulnar artery. At present, the Scribner shunt is rarely selected for vascular access; however, it may be indicated in instances in which other percutaneous forms of access are considered hazardous or are unavailable. The major complications of the Scribner shunt are thrombosis, infection, limitation of activity, bleeding, skin erosion, and dislodgement.

Thrombosis is a major complication, especially if there is injury to the vessel intima. This damage can occur during placement or if the cannula has not been well secured and the tip is free to injure the vessel wall. Thrombosis is most often encountered in patients with small or previously injured

vessels, that is, diabetics, small women, or those with severely atherosclerotic vessels. Infection occurs with a frequency of 1 per 6.9 patient months to 1 per 35 patient months. The most common organism found is *Staphylococcus aureus*. Infection can be prevented by aggressive local catheter care. Dislodgement can result in exsanguination and subsequent death.[9,43] There have also been documented cases of suicide using the external shunt.

The average shunt life span is 7 to 10 months, with a range of 2 to 14 months, most failures being caused by infection or thrombosis.[26,30] Aspirin used in low doses (160 mg/day) will decrease thrombosis from 72% in a placebo group to 32% in an aspirin-treated group over a 5-month period.[22] Coumadin use (prothrombin time 1.5× normal) will also decrease thrombosis rate from 1 per 3.6 months to 1 per 13 months.[9]

External percutaneous catheters can be placed by way of the subclavian vein or the femoral vein. These have the advantages of not damaging vessels for later permanent vascular access and having an infection rate that is one fifth that of external shunts.[11] Femoral catheters are placed using the Seldinger technique and may be used to maintain dialysis for a prolonged period of time. Possible catheter placements are femoral artery and femoral vein, two femoral catheters in the same femoral vein, a catheter in each femoral vein, and a catheter in the femoral vein with a return in a peripheral arm vein. The major disadvantage of the femoral catheters is that they should be removed after each use to prevent infection and thrombosis. The complications of femoral catheter use include ileofemoral thrombosis, local bleeding, retroperitoneal hematoma, or arterial puncture and injury. The incidence of these complications is less than 1%.[29,46]

The subclavian catheter has been used com-

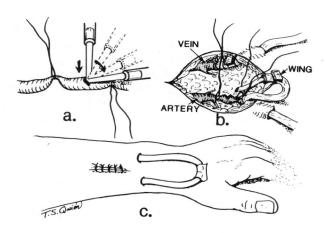

FIGURE 14-1.   *Placement of an external shunt.* (a) *Isolation of the vessel with arteriotomy/venotomy for Teflon tip placement.* (b) *Location of the wings and ties for shunt.* (c) *Closure with shunt in place.*

monly but is still subject to complications, including subclavian vein thrombosis or stenosis, and occasional subclavian vein perforation with resultant death.[10,15] A major advantage of these catheters is they can be left in place for a time and allow patient ambulation.

The Quinton hemocatheter or similar catheters have been used for permanent dialysis. These catheters have either a single or double lumen and are placed into the venous system surgically by way of the internal jugular vein. The catheter tip is placed into the superior portion of the right atrium or adjacent portion of the superior vena cava. The Dacron cuff is placed in the subcutaneous tissue, and the catheter lumens are filled with undiluted heparin. The major advantage is that the patient can be dialyzed immediately. The complications of this technique include outflow obstruction, cuff erosion, infection, limited catheter flow, and subclavian thrombosis.[33,48]

Types of Angioaccess: Internal

Natural veins and arteries have less tendency to thrombose than do prosthetic materials. This is the reason that the Brescia-Cimino fistula was such a major advance over the Scribner and other shunts. It is still considered the gold standard for comparison of new techniques in fistula surgery.[5] Since it uses the radial artery anastomosed to the cephalic vein, an Allen test must be performed prior to surgery to test adequacy of collateral flow from the ulnar artery. The various anatomic considerations include side to side, end vein to side artery, end artery to side vein, and end artery to end vein. The preferred anastomosis is side to side because it allows greater variations in flow and because the length of the anastomosis can be varied. The usual length of anastomosis is 10 mm to 12 mm, which gives a flow of between 300 and 500 ml/minute.[17]

There are other locations and types of fistulas that can be constructed. These are ulnar artery to basilic vein, basilic vein to brachial artery for retrograde flow into the cephalic vein, and cephalic vein to brachial artery at the antecubital fossa.

The patency of natural fistulas varies. The Brescia-Cimino fistula has a patency rate of between 55% and 85% at 2 years.[16,23,40,56] The variability is related to the aggressiveness with which the fistula is constructed. The early failure rate of 10% to 15% is caused by poor blood vessels, venous outflow obstruction, excessive dehydration, or hypotension. The patency rate for the brachiocephalic fistulas is 80%.[16]

Complications of Internal Fistulas

Vascular access problems are the most common cause for hospital admission in chronic dialysis patients. One study indicated that this was the reason for admission in 26% of the cases.[25] It should be noted that difficulties with vascular access are much less frequent in patients with a natural fistula than with a xenograft. Complications may be categorized into four groups: bleeding, occlusion or threatened occlusion, infection, and hemodynamic problems. Bleeding is rare in natural fistulas and is the result of a technical problem such as a broken suture or an unrecognized vessel injury. The most common complication is stenosis at the proximal venous limb (48%), followed by thrombosis (9%), and aneurysms (7%).[34] Thrombosis can be prevented in many instances by careful evaluation by nurses and physicians caring for dialysis patients. An increase in venous resistance, difficulty with cannulation, poor flow, diminished thrill, or an increasingly prominent pulsation are all indications of fistula problems that could lead to thrombosis. Aneurysms can be prevented by making sure that needles for access are placed in multiple places and not continually inserted in the same location. This will prevent vessel wall weakening.[47]

Infection occurs rarely in natural arteriovenous fistulas (less than 3%).[24,56] It occurs much less commonly than in external shunts or bridge-type fistulas. The hemodynamic consequences are usually heart failure, steal syndrome, or venous hypertension. Heart failure can occur in patients with borderline cardiac reserve and a fistula flow rate of more than 500 ml/minute and can be reversed either by Teflon banding of the fistula or by fistula ligation. The arterial steal syndrome is unusual in wrist fistulas (0.25%) but more likely in elbow brachiocephalic fistulas (approximately 30%). The steal is caused by blood taking the path of least resistance into the low-resistance venous system.[21] In the wrist fistula, 30% of the flow is furnished by blood from the hand supplied by the palmar arch. Venous hypertension results in a swollen hand, hyperpigmentation, skin induration, and eventual skin ulceration and is seen much more commonly in side-to-side wrist fistulas than in other types.[21] There is commonly a partial stenosis in the proximal venous end causing blood to flow distally. It is for this reason that distal vein ligation may not always solve the problem but may result in fistula occlusion. Occasionally, a patient will develop neurovascular problems such as pain, weakness, paresthesia, and muscle atrophy. These problems can be reversed by fistula closure if not allowed to progress too far.[31]

Prosthetic Grafts for Vascular Access

As older patients are coming to dialysis and patients are living longer on dialysis, more patients are being evaluated who have no or few veins left for construction of vascular access. This means that some sort of prosthetic material has to be used to construct bridge grafts where no vein and artery can be brought into proximity for a natural fistula. The material to be used should be nonantigenic, resistant to deterioration in the body, easy to handle and suture, minimally thrombogenic and capable of mechanical declotting to re-establish patency and should heal into the body easily, seal after repeated needle puncture, resist infection, and maintain integrity under infected conditions without degeneration or hemorrhage.[45] It was hoped that the saphenous vein would meet these criteria; however, there is extensive dissection required for use and a 50% thrombosis rate at 1 year. Also, the saphenous vein is used for coronary artery bypass grafts; thus, other materials have been tried.[18] A number of other materials have been used, including Dacron and bovine grafts, made from the carotid artery of the cow. The Sparks-Mandril graft, made by putting a prosthetic material into the subcutaneous space, has been abandoned because of problems in making the graft. Dacron has not been used widely. Bovine grafts have a tendency to form aneurysms and to become infected, leading to disintegration and massive hemorrhage.[4]

The most commonly used prosthetic material at present is PTFE. This material meets many of the criteria for an ideal prosthetic material: It is well incorporated into body tissues; forms a neointima, which makes declotting easier than in other prosthetic grafts; and is resistant to degeneration when infection occurs.

Technique of Arteriovenous Jump Grafts

In construction of a jump graft, good arterial inflow and venous outflow are necessary. Venous outflow may be compromised by venous stenosis caused by multiple needle punctures. In tunneling the graft, care must be taken to avoid rotation of the graft or making too sharp a bend in the loop configuration. The graft must be in place long enough before use (2 to 3 weeks) for tissue ingrowth to occur, thus preventing a perigraft hematoma after the initial use.[23]

There are a number of configurations that have been used for graft placement. The overall plan is the same as for natural fistulas, to start as far distal as possible in the nondominant arm. A straight graft has been used between the radial artery at the wrist and the cephalic vein at the elbow (Fig. 14-2A). This has the lowest patency of all the jump grafts because of the low flow through the radial artery. This may be a good configuration if there has been a previous natural arteriovenous fistula in place that has become unusable because of an aneurysm or high flow. A forearm loop between the brachial or preferably ulnar artery just below the elbow and an arm vein at the elbow is a good approach (Fig. 14-2B). Use of the ulnar artery results in a lower incidence of steal syndrome. In the upper arm, a graft can be placed between the brachial artery above the elbow and the axillary vein (Fig. 14-2C). Another configuration is a loop graft between the axillary artery and axillary vein (Fig. 14-2D). Both of these latter configurations can result in a steal syndrome, because large vessels are involved and resistance is low through the graft.

In the lower extremity, two types of grafts have been used: One is a jump between the popliteal artery and saphenous or femoral vein in the groin; the other is a loop between the femoral artery and saphenous vein or femoral vein. Both of the grafts are subject to a high incidence of infection with subsequent high amputation and mortality rates.[35]

In the patient who has used all the sites for vascular access, a few options are available. These configurations include axillary artery to axillary vein across the chest, axillary artery to axillary vein with a loop on the chest, and arterial-to-arterial graft.[20]

Complications

The complications with a jump graft are the same as those for a natural fistula. Bleeding or early hemorrhage occurs from three sources: (1) the anastomosis, (2) the tunnel during placement of the graft, or (3) needle puncture of the graft. The first problem is prevented by attention to detail at the initial surgery. Bleeding in the tunnel is prevented by taking care to avoid vessels as the tunnel is placed and not using systemic heparin. Hemorrhage from the graft is usually caused by tearing the graft when the needle is placed or by using the graft too early after placement.

Thrombosis usually occurs for anatomic reasons, that is, inflow or outflow narrowing.[6] Thrombosis from these causes can be repaired with a bypass of the stenotic area, patch graft, or balloon dilatation.[47] There are several reports of streptokinase dissolution of clot with balloon dilatation of stenotic areas. The results have been mixed.[19,52,57] Infection is a major problem with jump grafts. If a bovine graft is in place, infection can lead to graft breakdown and major hemorrhage.[4] The use of

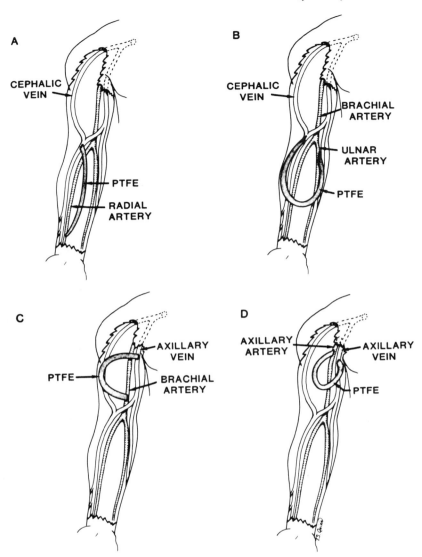

FIGURE 14-2. Most common configurations for upper arm jump grafts.

PTFE has allowed local wound care of an infected graft if the suture line is not involved. The other reasons to remove a PTFE graft are an infected clotted graft and a tunnel infection. These are both likely to eventually involve the suture line. The salvage rate of infected grafts are low, with a success rate of approximately 25%.[3]

The hemodynamic complications of venous hypertension, congestive heart failure, and steal syndrome can all occur as they do in natural fistulas. The use of the rapid taper graft (4 mm to 7 mm by Gore-Tex) has decreased the incidence of the steal syndrome by decreasing the flow rate through the graft.[44]

Patency

The long-term patency of jump grafts is less than that of natural arteriovenous fistulas. PTFE has been noted to have a 12-month patency rate between 45% and 70%. Location of the graft makes a difference in long-term patency according to Munda et al.[36] They showed a 12-month patency of 60% for PTFE graft in the upper arm and a 12-month patency rate of 35% for a forearm graft between the radial artery and cephalic vein. They found the best patency in forearm loops (78% at 12 months).[36] Wilson uses a thigh graft as a first choice and reported an 80% 12-month patency rate. Obviously, patency rate is dependent upon the arterial inflow and outflow in a given location.[55]

Physiology

The physiologic consequence of a fistula depends upon the size of the fistula; this determines the proximal arterial blood flow. Other factors of importance are venous outflow resistance, arterial collaterals, and the peripheral vascular bed. A fistula may have a diastolic flow that is 80% to 90% of the systolic flow. This results in an increased flow through the venous system. One must also keep in mind that the fistula size changes below 20% and above 75% of arterial diameter result in minimal flow changes; however, between these two extremes, fistula size can influence flow markedly. It should be noted that most clinical fistulas are constructed so that the size is greater than the diameter of the artery, allowing for later stenosis.[55]

In a larger functioning fistula, local and systemic alterations occur. There will be a decrease in both systolic and diastolic blood pressures, an increase in cardiac output, an increase in heart rate, an increase in venous pressure, and an increase in blood volume. These are all reversible with fistula closure.[12]

Local changes occur within the vessel walls. The proximal artery and vein will both enlarge significantly and show progressive lengthening. Microscopically, there will be smooth muscle hypertrophy, which will eventually lead to smooth muscle atrophy with aneurysmal dilatation and a tortuous vessel.[55]

Summary

Without vascular access, dialysis would never have been possible. The three major developmental landmarks were (1) the external shunt, (2) the natural wrist fistula, and (3) the jump graft with prosthetic material. These techniques have all been improved and have shown improved patency rates and fewer complications.

PERITONEAL DIALYSIS

History

Peritoneal dialysis would not have been possible without the work of Wegner[54] in 1877 and Starling and Tubby in 1894,[49] who showed that the perito-

neal membrane is semipermeable. The first use of peritoneal dialysis in patients was by Ganter in 1923.[17] In subsequent years, many improvements were made, and, in 1960, the first patient was started on chronic dialysis. The major problem with peritoneal dialysis is how to obtain leak-free access to the peritoneal cavity. Numerous catheters have been used, including rubber and plastic. At present, most catheters are constructed of soft, silicone rubber with Dacron cuffs to prevent infection and to anchor the catheter.[14]

Physiology

The exact surface through which peritoneal dialysis occurs is not known. The visceral peritoneum has a much larger surface area than does the parietal peritoneum; thus, most of the exchange is thought to occur through the visceral peritoneum. Blood flow to the peritoneum is estimated to be between 60 ml/minute and 100 ml/minute.[2] The rates of molecular exchange through the peritoneum are determined by the size of the molecule. B_{12}, a middle-sized molecule, is cleared at a rate of 1008 liters per week in normal kidneys, 30 liters per week in hemodialysis, and 50 liters per week in chronic ambulatory peritoneal dialysis (CAPD). Hemodialysis results in better clearance of small molecules such as urea; the clearances are 604 liters per week for normal kidneys, 135 liters per week for hemodialysis, and 84 liters per week for CAPD. These clearances can be increased by increasing fluid exchange rates, but, to obtain a urea clearance of 40 ml/minute, 18 liters/hour must be exchanged.[37]

The exact role of blood flow in peritoneal dialysis is not known. Vasoconstriction decreases peritoneal clearance, and vasodilatation increases peritoneal clearance. However, peritoneal dialysis still shows a clearance rate of 70% of normal in patients in shock. Therefore, some mechanism other than blood flow must be active.[37]

Indications

There are a number of situations in which peritoneal dialysis is used, including (1) acute renal failure, (2) abdominal placement of chemotherapeutic agents, and (3) when awaiting maturation of vascular access. CAPD can be used in a number of clinical settings. It has been used in patients (1) who want home dialysis, (2) with diabetes, (3) with cardiovascular instability, (4) with no available sites for vascular access, and (5) of the Jehovah's witness faith.[39,51]

The only absolute contraindication is lack of diaphragmatic integrity, which allows dialysis fluid to move into the chest and results in cardiovascular and pulmonary compromise. Relative contraindications are found in patients with (1) a history of low back pain; (2) multiple previous abdominal surgeries causing multiple adhesions, so there is not enough surface area for dialysate diffusion or for catheter placement; (3) a large hernia, (4) a diffuse peritoneal malignancy, (5) a history of respiratory compromise that would be worsened by increasing abdominal volume, or (6) a history of multiple previous catheter infections.[37]

Practical Considerations

A number of catheters are used today for peritoneal dialysis. These include the curled Tenckhoff, single-cuff Tenckhoff, Toronto-Western, column-disc, Vali, and Gore-Tex catheters. For acute dialysis, the single cuff Tenckhoff is the only catheter that can be placed percutaneously. It is placed aseptically below the umbilicus, with the cuff at the fascial level and the tip directed toward the pelvis. The other catheters listed must be placed surgically. The incision is paramedian and placed below the umbilicus. The anterior fascia of the rectus is opened, the muscles are split, and a purse string is placed in the posterior fascia. The catheter is placed through a small fascial defect, which is then closed. The deep Dacron cuff is placed at the posterior fascial level, the anterior fascia is closed, and the catheter is brought out by way of a tunnel through a separate stab wound. The superficial cuff is placed at least an inch from the skin opening. Care must be taken to place the catheter tip in the pelvis and to avoid bowel injury. Fixation of the catheter under direct vision reduces the incidence of nonfunctioning catheters.[8,38]

The electrolyte composition of peritoneal dialysate is similar to that of blood. The major differences are in bicarbonate (blood 25 mEq/liter and dialysate 0), phosphate (blood 2.5 mEq/liter and dialysate 0), lactate (blood 0 and dialysate 45 mEq/liter), and potassium (blood 4 mEq/liter and dialysate 0). Glucose concentrations in the dialysate vary depending upon the amount of ultrafiltration desired. A 1.5% concentration causes little ultrafiltration (200 ml for a 2 liter exchange) contrasted to the 4.5% solution used to treat fluid overload (800 ml for a 2 liter exchange). The usual regimen is 2 liters exchanged four times per day. This is convenient for the patient and allows good flexibility. The major point to be made, however, is that the patient must pay attention to detail to avoid infection.[28]

Complications

Complications can be divided into those of the immediate perioperative period and those that occur after the patient has left the hospital. The major perioperative complications are (1) intraperitoneal bleeding, (2) tunnel bleeding, (3) leakage of dialysis fluid, (4) hollow viscus injury, and (5) ileus. All except ileus, which usually resolves within 24 hours, can be prevented by meticulous attention to technical detail.[37]

The most frequent postoperative complication is peritonitis. This most commonly occurs by means of the lumen of the catheter; however, hematogenous spread from remote sources, transmural spread from the bowel, and contamination by cuffs or catheters also occur.[53] Peritoneal infection occurs approximately once every 6 to 8 months. The most common organisms are gram positive and account for 75% of the infections. Gram-negative organisms are responsible for approximately 20% of the infections. Anaerobes account for up to 3% of infections, with fungus and tuberculosis being uncommon causes.[27,37,53] Treatment is dictated by the particular organism cultured and its sensitivity pattern. When the catheter tunnel is involved, infections can be treated with appropriate antibiotics alone if the cuff is not involved. If the Dacron cuff is involved, the catheter must be removed.[53] The Dacron cuff occasionally becomes infected after extrusion from the skin. This can be resolved by shaving away the infected cuff along with administration of appropriate antibiotics.[28]

Mechanical complications result in poor inflow and outflow of dialysate. These complications may be caused by (1) kinking of the catheter along its track, (2) migration of the catheter out of the pelvis, (3) omental wrapping of the catheter, or (4) occlusion of the catheter lumen with clot or fibrin. Omental wrapping and catheter migration can be prevented by tacking the catheter down into the pelvis. The kinking can be prevented by paying attention to technical detail when the catheter is placed. Fibrin and blood clots can be dissolved using urokinase.[37]

Catheter Longevity

The average catheter longevity is approximately 80% to 85% at 1 year, with the figure dropping to approximately 60% at 2 years.[50] There are data to indicate that the Toronto Western catheter has a significantly better survival rate than the medically inserted Tenckhoff catheters.[28] Catheters placed for the first time had a better survival rate than did those placed subsequently.[28]

Summary

The advantage of peritoneal dialysis is that the patient is not attached to a machine, but there are still problems, including peritonitis, catheter infections, and mechanical problems. Catheter longevity is comparable to the longevity of the jump graft but shorter than that of natural fistula.

REFERENCES

1. Anderson CB, Etheredge EE, Harter HR et al: Local blood flow characteristics of arteriovenous fistulas in the forearm for dialysis. Surg Gynecol Obstet 144:531, 1977

2. Anne S: Transperitoneal exchange. I. Peritoneal blood flow estimated by hydrogen gas clearance. Scand J Gastroenterol 5:99, 1970

3. Bhat DJ, Tellis VA, Kohlberg WI et al: Management of sepsis involving expanded polytetrafluoroethylene grafts for hemodialysis access. Surgery 87:445, 1980

4. Bone GE, Pomajzl MJ: Prospective comparison of polytetrafluoroethylene and bovine grafts for dialysis. J Surg Res 29:223, 1980

5. Brescia MJ, Cimino JE, Appel D et al: Chronic hemodialysis using venipuncture and a surgically created arteriovenous fistula. N Engl J Med 275:1089, 1966

6. Butt KMH, Friedman EA, Kounts SL: Angioaccess. Curr Probl Surg 13:1, 1976

7. Cerilli J, Lembert JG: Technique and results of the construction of arteriovenous fistulas for hemodialysis. Surg Gynecol Obstet 137:922, 1973

8. Cerilli J, Walker J, Bay W: A new technique for placement of catheters for peritoneal dialysis. Surg Gynecol Obstet 156:663, 1983

9. Curtis J, Eastwood J, Smith E et al: Maintenance hemodialysis. Q J Med 38:49, 1969

10. Davis D, Petersen J, Feldman R et al: Subclavian venous stenosis: A complication of subclavian dialysis. JAMA 252:3404, 1984

11. Dorner DB, Stubbs DH, Shadur CA et al: Percutaneous subclavian vein catheter hemodialysis—impact on vascular access surgery. Surgery 91:712, 1982

12. Dow P, Hamilton WF: Handbook of Physiology, Section 2, Circulation, Vol. 3. American Physiological Society, Washington DC, 1965

13. Drukker W: Haemodialysis: A Historical Review. In Drukker W, Parsons FM, Maher JF (eds): Replacement of Renal Function by Dialysis. Boston, Martinus Nijhoff, 1983

14. Drukker W: Peritoneal dialysis: A historical review. In Drukker W, Parsons FM, Maher JF (eds): Replacement of Renal Function by Dialysis. Boston, Martinus Nijhoff, 1983

15. Fine A, Churchill D, Gault H et al: Fatality due to subclavian dialysis catheter. Nephron 129:99, 1981

16. Friedman EA, Bett KMH, Pascua LJ et al: Vascular access update. Trans Am Soc Artif Intern Organs 25:526, 1979

17. Ganter G: Uber die beseitigung giftiger stoffe aus dem blate durch dialyse (On the elimination of toxic substances from the blood by dialysis). MMW 70:1478, 1923 (in German)

18. Girandet RE, Hackett RE, Goodwin NJ et al: Thirteen months experience with the saphenous vein grafts arteriovenous fistula for maintenance hemodialysis. Trans Am Soc Artif Intern Organs 16:285, 1970

19. Gordon DH, Glanz S, Butt KM et al: Treatment of stenotic lesions in dialysis access fistulas and shunts by transluminal angioplasty. Radiology 143:53, 1982

20. Haimov M: Vascular access for hemodialysis—New modifications for the difficult patient. Surgery 92:109, 1982

21. Haimov M, Baez A, Neff M et al: Complications of arteriovenous fistulas for hemodialysis. Arch Surg 110:708, 1975

22. Harten HR, Burch JW, Majerus PW et al: Prevention of thrombosis in patients on hemodialysis by low-dose aspirin. N Engl J Med 301:577, 1979

23. Hertzer NR: Circulatory Access for Hemodialysis. In Rutherford RB (ed): Vascular Surgery. Philadelphia, WB Saunders, 1984

24. Higgins MR, Grace M, Bettcher KB et al: Blood access in hemodialysis. Clin Nephrol 6:473, 1976

25. Hirschman GH, Wolfson M, Mosimann JE et al: Complications of dialysis. Clin Nephrol 15:66, 1981

26. Ishihara AM, Myers CH: Longevity of arterio-venous shunts for hemodialysis. Ann Surg 168:281, 1968

27. Kurtz SB, Wong VH, Anderson CF et al: Continuous ambulatory peritoneal dialysis: Three years' experience at the Mayo Clinic. Mayo Clin Proc 58:633, 1983

28. Khanna R, Oreopoulos DG: Complications of peritoneal dialysis other than peritonitis. In Nolph KD (ed): Peritoneal Dialysis. Boston, Martinus Nijhoff, 1983

29. Kjellstrand CM, Merino GE, Mauer SM et al: Complications of percutaneous femoral vein catheterizations for hemodialysis. Clin Nephrol 4:37, 1975

30. Ku G, Moorhead JF: The present status of hemodialysis. Practitioner 207:622, 1971

31. Matolo N, Kostagiv B, Stevens LE et al: Neurovascular complications of bracheal arteriovenous fistula. Am J Surg 121:716, 1971

32. May J, Tiller D, Johnson J et al: Saphenous-vein arteriovenous fistula in regular dialysis treatment. N Engl J Med 280:770, 1969

33. McGonigle DJ, Schrock LG, Hickman RO: Experience using central venous access for long-term hemodi-

alysis: A new concept. Am J Surg 145:571, 1983

34. Mennes PA, Gilula LA, Anderson CB et al: Complications associated with arteriovenous fistulas in patients undergoing chronic hemodialysis. Arch Intern Med 138:1117, 1978

35. Morgan AP, Knight DC, Tilney NL et al: Femoral triangle sepsis in dialysis patients: Frequency management and outcome. Ann Surg 101:460, 1980

36. Munda R, First MR, Alexander JW et al: Polytetrafluoroethylene graft survival in hemodialysis. JAMA 249:219, 1983

37. Nolph KD: Peritoneal anatomy and transport physiology; and Mrou, CM: Practical use of peritoneal dialysis. In Drukker W, Parsons FM, Maher JF (eds): Replacement of Renal Function by Dialysis. Boston, Martinus Nijhoff, 1983

38. Olcott C, Feldman CA, Coplon NS et al: Continuous ambulatory peritoneal dialysis: Technique of catheter insertion and management of associated surgical complications. Am J Surg 146:98, 1983

39. Oveopoulos DG: Chronic peritoneal dialysis. Clin Nephrol 9:165, 1978

40. Palder SB, Kirkman RL, Whittlemove AD et al: Vascular access for hemodialysis: Patency rates and results of revision. Ann Surg 202:235, 1985

41. Quinton W, Dillard D, Scribner BH: Cannulation of blood vessels for prolonged hemodialysis. Trans Am Soc Artif Intern Organs 6:104, 1960

42. Raaf JH: Vascular access grafts for chemotherapy use in forty patients at M.D. Anderson Hospital. Ann Surg 182:614, 1975

43. Ralston AJ, Harlow GR, Jones DM et al: Infections of Scribner and Brescia arteriovenous shunts. Br Med J 3:408, 1971

44. Rosenthal JJ, Bell DD, Gaspar MR et al: Prevention of high flow problems of arteriovenous grafts. Am J Surg 140:231, 1980

45. Sabanayagam P, Schwartz AB, Soricelli RR et al: A comparative study fo 402 bovine heterografts and 225 reinforced expended PTFE grafts as AVF in the ESRD patient. Trans Am Soc Artif Intern Organs XXVI:88, 1980

46. Sharp KW, Spees EK, Selby LR et al: Diagnosis and management of retroperitoneal hematomas after femoral vein cannulation for hemodialysis. Surgery 95:90, 1984

47. So SKS: Complications of vascular access. In Simmons RL, Finch ME, Ascher NL et al: (eds): Manual of Vascular Access, Organ Donation and Transplantation. New York, Springer-Verlag, 1984

48. So SKS: Venous access for hemodialysis in children: Right atrial cannulation. In Simmons RL, Finch ME, Ascher NL et al: (eds): Manual of Vascular Access, Organ Donation and Transplantation. New York, Springer-Verlag, 1984

49. Starling EH, Tubby EH: On absorption from and secretion into the serous cavities. J Physiol (London) 16:140, 1894

50. Steinberg SM, Cutler SJ, Novak JW et al: Report of the National CAPD Registry of the National Institutes of Health. January, 1984

51. Tenckhoff H: Home peritoneal dialysis. In Massry SG, Sellers AL (eds): Clinical Aspects of Anemia and Dialysis. Springfield, IL, Charles C Thomas, 1976

52. Tortolani EC, Tan AHS, Butchart S: Percutaneous transluminal angioplasty: An ineffective approach to the failing vascular access. Arch Surg 119:221, 1984

53. Vas SI: Peritonitis. In Nolph KD (ed): Peritoneal Dialysis. Boston, Martinus Nijhoff, 1983

54. Wegner G: Chirurgische bermerkungen uber die peritonealhohle mit berucksichtigung der ovariotomie (Surgical considerations regarding the peritoneal cavity with special attention to ovariotomy). Langenbecks Arch Chir 20:51, 1877 (in German)

55. Wilson SE, Owens ML (eds): Vascular Access Surgery. Chicago, Year Book Medical Publishers, 1980

56. Winsett OE, Wolma FT: Complications of vascular access for hemodialysis. South Med J 78:513, 1985

57. Zeit RM, Cope C: Failed hemodialysis shunts: One year of experience with aggressive treatment. Radiology 154:353, 1985

58. Zincke H, Hirsche BL, Amomoo DG et al: The use of bovine carotid grafts for hemodialysis and hyperalimentation. Surg Gynecol Obstet 130:350, 1974

CHAPTER 15

Patient Selection for Renal Transplantation

Alan G. Birtch

Recipient evaluation attempts to quantitate risk factors and identify remediable conditions reducing the risk pretransplantation.

Absolute contraindications to transplantation include incurable malignancy or infection, patient noninterest, and refractory noncompliance. Relative contraindications may include those with advanced age (>65 years), unreconstructable cardiovascular disease, chronic pulmonary disease, or Fabry's disease. Some patients, although at increased risk, may be considered satisfactory candidates following pretransplant preparation (oxalosis, reconstructable cardiovascular disease, unusable lower urinary tracts).

In patients who have significant risk factors with potentially adverse effects on outcome, such as patients younger than 5 years and young diabetics, the advantages of transplantation are thought to outweigh the risk. In some patients, the chance of success may be improved by appropriate timing of the transplant. The risk from posttransplant gastrointestinal disease can be minimized by pretransplant correction of remediable lesions. Immunologic high responders have a reduced graft survival rate and require special attention to maximize their chance of success.

Diseases in which recurrence accounts for 10% or more of graft losses include oxalosis, scleroderma, focal segmental glomerulonephritis, and mesangiocapillary glomerulonephritis types I and II.

Gastrointestinal and psychiatric evaluations are essential, particularly for refractory peptic ulcer diseases, pancreatitis, or diverticulitis, which may require surgical intervention prior to transplantation.

Urologic evaluation attempts to ensure that a functional, infection-free receptacle for urine flow is present for the allograft. Present indications for bilateral nephrectomy include infected kidneys (pyelonephritis, ureteral diversions, or grade III or IV reflux, with pyelonephritis), uncontrollable hypertension, heavy proteinuria, and renal tumors.

Procedures to evaluate infections include chest x-rays, purified protein derivative (PPD), nasal and urine cultures, dental evaluation, and HB_2Ag screening. The extent of the cardiovascular evaluation is dictated by age and disease category, remembering that cardiovascular disease is the second leading cause of death post-transplantation.

Careful pretransplant evaluation, selection, and preparation cannot guarantee success; however, it will minimize the preventable poor outcome.

Identification of the patient suffering from end-stage renal disease (ESRD) who will be best served by becoming a transplant recipient is an important and seemingly straightforward task. The ideal candidate is a young, healthy, cooperative patient whose renal failure is not due to a systemic disease or a disease that has a high potential for recurrence. Such candidates have a normal lower urinary tract and a well-matched willing sibling donor. Such patients make up only a small fraction of the candidate pool, the majority are less than ideal for several reasons.

The background against which the decisions concerning candidacy for transplantation are made is constantly changing. For some patients, the increasing use and acceptance of chronic ambulatory peritoneal dialysis (CAPD) has provided a more attractive alternative to transplantation than was previously available with in-center or home hemodialysis. Donor-specific transfusions, third-party transfusions, and cyclosporine immunosuppression have improved transplant success and lowered transplant mortality and morbidity in most centers. The improved transplant results have led or may lead to relaxation of patient selection criteria in many centers. Unfortunately, the data available at the present time to establish these criteria are largely based on experience accumulated in the azathioprine-prednisone era, and they must be used recognizing this bias and shortcoming.

The risks of transplantation for each patient can be assessed only after a careful work-up and evaluation by the nephrologist and transplant surgical team unless one of the absolute contraindications to transplant is present. Educating the patient about the relative risks and benefits of each available mode of treatment is important so that he or she can be an informed participant in making this decision.

The purpose of this chapter is to provide information, representing current knowledge and some personal preference, that may assist transplant centers in deciding who is best served by the distribution of this limited resource—a kidney transplant.

RECIPIENT SELECTION

General Guidelines

In the assessment of each patient as a transplant candidate, there are a number of obvious considerations that must be taken into account. The patient should have a reasonable life expectancy irrespective of the renal failure and be able to withstand the surgical intervention of the transplant procedure, including possible preparatory operations with a reasonable operative risk. There must be sufficient reserve in each major organ system to tolerate the expected incidence of perioperative stresses and long-term complications secondary to immunosuppression. The availability of a related donor will favorably prejudice the evaluation, because the lower the dosage of immunosuppression required, the lower the incidence of complications and the better the chance for graft and patient survival.

The following sections detail risk factors that may affect a successful outcome for the patient and the transplanted kidney.

Absolute Contraindications

Absolute contraindications include (1) incurable malignancy and infection, (2) informed patient refusal, and (3) refractory noncompliance.

Of patients with an uncured malignancy or an infection that is not and cannot be eradicated, there is an extremely high probability that these conditions will be exacerbated by immunosuppressive medication, and transplantation is unwise.

After being thoroughly appraised of the potential benefits and risks involved in transplantation, some patients will, for religious or emotional reasons, temporarily or permanently decide against this option. Other patients, because of psychiatric disease or mental incapacity, will be unable to comprehend the problems or comply with the requirements for care necessary to allow a reasonable chance of success.

Relative Contraindications

The list of relative contraindications (Table 15-1) includes those factors or conditions that most transplant centers would define as having significantly increased risk, and only under unusual circumstances would they consider patients with these risks to be suitable transplant candidates. Some of these conditions are remediable, and, with appropriate planning and preparation (e.g., construction of ileal or colonic conduit, coronary bypass surgery, or aortoiliac reconstruction), the patient may become an acceptable candidate. Age is not remediable. Patients over age 65 years are rarely transplanted (72 of 12,427)[27] because of the cumulative effects of aging on operative risk, poor tolerance of immunosuppression and its complications, the occurrence of de novo malignancy, and the high incidence of vascular disease. Chronic pulmonary disease increases operative risk and assumes particular importance since pulmonary infections represent the most common serious immunosuppressive complication.

Significant Risk Factors

In addition to the absolute and relative contraindications previously mentioned, a number of other

TABLE 15-1 *Relative Contraindications*

Unusable lower urinary tract*
Chronic cardiac failure*
Aortoiliac disease*
Age > 65 years
Chronic pulmonary disease
Renal disease with high recurrence rate†

* Requires special evaluation and possible surgical intervention pretransplantation.

† See section entitled Recurrence of Original Disease in the Transplant.

TABLE 15-2   *Significant Risk Factors*

Age: < 5 years, > 45 years
Systemic Disease Leading to Renal Failure
   Diabetes
   Amyloidosis
   Fabry's
   Systemic lupus erythematosus
   Scleroderma
Previous Gastrointestinal Disease
   Liver Disease
   Pancreatitis
   Peptic ulcer disease
   Diverticulitis
Obesity and malnutrition
Immunologic high responders
Renal disease with moderate risk of recurrence
Prior malignancy

risk factors have a potentially adverse effect on out-come (Table 15-2). Some of these factors primarily decrease the likelihood of graft success, whereas many also have a negative effect on patient survival.

Age

Patients at both ends of the acceptable age range have a decreased rate of success. Successful transplantation has been reported in the neonate,[10] but those recipients younger than age 5 years have had inferior patient and graft survival[27] owing to an increase in technical vascular problems, donor selection, and rejection.[3,50] Transplantation, however, for the pediatric patient has advantages, allowing more nearly normal growth and development as well as psychological benefits, which make it the treatment of choice. Although collected data suggest a gradual decline in patient and graft survival from age 7 years to age 66 years, a break point for increased risk at the upper end of the age spectrum is present in many series, and, in most series, it occurs at about age 45 years.[27] Much of the detrimental effect in the older recipient accrues from increased patient mortality rather than from allograft loss. In the azathioprine era, patient survival for the 45- to 65-year-old age group receiving cadaver transplants was not significantly better in transplant patients than in dialysis patients.[22,*] This was true even though immunologic responsiveness and thus rejection loss appeared to decrease with advanced age.[40] In this age group, therefore, rehabilitation potential, availability of a related donor, center experience, and patient preference will play dominant roles in patient selection.

   * Birtch AG: ESRD 15, Illinois Transplant Results: Unpublished data, 1983

Systemic Disease as the Cause of Renal Failure

Each of these diseases have nonrenal manifestations that intensify the operative and long-term risks.

Diabetes.   Diabetic patients have increased risk secondary to cardiovascular complications, poor wound healing, and decreased resistance to infection that is accentuated by immunosuppression. Their care is complicated and occasionally compromised by the presence of symptoms and altered physiology caused by neuropathy, retinopathy, gastroparesis, neurogenic bladder dysfunction, and so on.

   Despite considerable improvement in patient and graft survival in diabetic recipients,[17,56] they continue to have a success rate inferior to that achieved in nondiabetics.[11] Although not all agree,[43] transplantation is considered by most programs to be the optimal therapy for the young diabetic patient.

Amyloidosis.   Both primary and secondary amyloidosis affect the heart, liver, gastrointestinal tract, and spleen as well as the kidneys. Patients with renal failure secondary to amyloid deposition have had a higher than average post-transplantation mortality rate (25%–45% at 1 year).[23,25] In some patients, this may be due to heart failure secondary to cardiac amyloid deposition; however, most patients have died of sepsis. Despite the increased risk, transplantation for patients with renal amyloidosis is appropriate in selected cases. A recent report suggests that cyclosporine treatment may produce unusual gastrointestinal and systemic symptoms in the subgroup with familiar Mediterranean fever.[53]

Fabry's.   This disease, resulting from an inborn error in glycosphingolipid metabolism, results in the accumulation of a neutral glycosphingolipid in all tissues, including heart and kidneys. Early reports of renal transplantation reversing the metabolic defect have not been substantiated. Poor wound healing, sepsis, and high mortality have caused skepticism as to whether transplantation is a viable option for these patients.[1,30]

Systemic Lupus Erythematosus.   Since the encouraging report by the Advisory Committee of the ACS/NIH Registry in 1975,[1] systemic lupus erythematosus has not been considered a contraindication to renal transplantation. Transplantation is withheld until the condition is "burnt out," that is, clinically quiescent and anti-DNA titers are absent after discontinuance of steroid therapy; despite this, reactivation of systemic symptoms and rarely renal recurrence have been reported.[2] Patient and graft survival approach the average for other etiologies of renal failure.[32]

Scleroderma. Transplantation experience is limited in this multisystem disease. A recent compilation of the reported experience (10 cases) suggests that the mortality and success rate are acceptable.[44] Extrarenal manifestation may be improved in some patients following transplantation.

Previous Gastrointestinal Disease

Liver Disease. Pre-existing liver disease represents an increased risk since both azathioprine and cyclosporine are potentially hepatotoxic. Advanced cirrhosis is a contraindication to renal transplantation. There is disagreement concerning the magnitude of the risk from pretransplant hepatitis B surface antigenemia (HBsAg). There is, of course, risk to the dialysis and transplant teams as well as to the patient in this situation. There are, however, several points of general agreement: (1) The patient is unlikely to lose HBsAg + status post-transplant and sustains an increased risk of further liver dysfunction and chronic active hepatitis[42]; (2) decrease in long-term patient survival is likely, partially owing to an increased incidence of hepatic failure and infection[19,48]; and (3) lower dosages of immunosuppression are appropriate, and even withdrawal of azathioprine has been advocated in the presence of active hepatitis.[54] There is evidence that it may be inadvisable to transplant HBsAg-positive patients; it may be best to allow them to remain on dialysis until they have converted to HBs antibody (Ab) status.[42] Even then, one report suggests that patients with HBsAb may have reduced graft survival.[24]

Pancreatitis. A past history of pancreatitis is a significant risk factor for the potential transplant recipient. Azathioprine[55] and prednisone[31] have been identified as potential etiologic factors in de novo pancreatitis and may play a role in recurrence following transplantation, frequently with a poor prognosis.[47] Contributing factors such as gallstones, hyperparathyroidism, and alcohol intake should be sought and corrected in order to reduce the risk of recurrence.

Peptic Ulcer Disease. Active peptic ulcer disease is a contraindication to transplantation, and a past history of ulcer disease requires careful evaluation, because a recurrence post-transplantation carries significant mortality.[16] H$_2$ antagonists have decreased the necessity for surgery in many cases, but the dialysis patient with recurrent or refractory ulcer disease despite adequate therapy should undergo corrective surgery before being considered for transplantation. Truncal vagotomy with pyloroplasty or antrectomy remains our procedure of choice.

Diverticulitis. Diverticulitis in the transplant patient is accompanied by a very high morbidity and mortality.[35] The dialysis patient desiring a transplant who has or has had documented diverticulitis should have the involved colon resected before being considered ready for transplantation.

Obesity and Malnutrition

Both obesity and malnutrition have a deleterious effect on wound healing and increase the potential for wound infection in any patient. Since these two wound problems are further adversely affected by uremia and immunosuppression, every effort should be made pretransplantation to correct these conditions in order to minimize the additive risks.

Immunologic High Responders

These patients may be identified either by the presence of a broad antibody reactivity to the screening lymphocyte panel or by their vigorous and early rejection of a previous allograft. The risks and possible remedial actions are covered in detail elsewhere in this book. Graft survival in these patients remains poorer than the mean.[21] A recent report suggests that CAPD patients may have partial restoration of immunologic integrity compared with hemodialysis patients, leading to poorer graft survival with azathioprine and prednisone therapy.[18] This finding has not yet been substantiated.[15]

RECURRENCE OF ORIGINAL DISEASE IN THE TRANSPLANT

Most forms of renal disease except for congenital abnormalities have some tendency to recur in the allograft. There are several problems that make difficult the documentation of and therefore prediction of recurrence in the allograft. First, many patients have inadequate histologic documentation of their original disease; biopsies, when taken, are often performed late in the course. Second, disease present in the donor organ pretransplantation, ischemic injury, rejection, drug toxicity, and de novo glomerulonephritis compound the histologic interpretation of transplant biopsies. Several excellent and detailed reviews focusing on aspects of the problem of recurrence are available (glomerulonephritis[8] and recurrence in the pediatric patient[28]). The frequency and clinical significance of recurrence varies widely. In the following section, these diseases are pragmatically categorized by the likelihood of recurrence affecting the outcome of the allograft (Table 15-3).

Oxalosis

Early results of transplantation in patients with oxalosis were very poor because of deposition of oxalate in the allograft. The ACS/NIH advisory committee in 1975 suggested that "oxalosis is a form of chronic renal failure that is unsuitable for treatment by renal transplantation."[1] However, several recent reports[4,14,20,39,57] and one series of 11 patients[51] have emphasized that by taking appropriate measures pre- and post-transplantation, one can decrease or prevent recurrence and obtain a satisfactory rate of graft survival. Biopsies in these reports documented the presence of oxalate deposition in about half of the cases. With prolonged survival, however, progressive disabling oxalate bone disease may be seen more frequently.[7]

Scleroderma

Only 10 transplants in patients with renal failure secondary to scleroderma have been reported. Two kidneys were lost within 2 to 3 months from recurrent disease.[33] Two patients died, but graft function in the remaining six patients was satisfactory, without evidence of recurrence in several that were biopsied.[44] Nonrenal manifestations of the disease were improved to varying degrees in most of the survivors.

Focal Segmental Glomerulonephritis

This disease recurs in about one quarter of those transplanted, occasionally presenting as heavy proteinuria and the nephrotic syndrome within hours or days of transplantation. Although the course may be protracted and early biopsies may show little change, over half of the recurrences eventually lead to graft failure. Leumann and Briner[28] have summarized the following factors that are thought to place the patient at high risk for recurrence: (1) short clinical course to renal failure (< 3 years, 50% recurrence; > 3 years, 10% to 20%); (2) presence of mesangial proliferation in the native kidney biopsy (50+% recurrence); and (3) age at onset (6 to 20 years, 52%; < 6 years, 16%; > 20 years, low). The high recurrence rate in "A" matched related donor kidneys suggested by Zimmerman[59] is at present unconfirmed.

Mesangiocapillary Glomerulonephritis Type II

The recurrence rate as judged by electron microscopic evidence of intramembranous deposits is very high, whereas clinical signs of recurrence occur less often (25%).[8] The clinical course usually progresses slowly, but eventually results in the loss of 10% to 25% of grafts.[8,28]

TABLE 15-3   *Significant Recurrence in Allograft*

PRIMARY RENAL DISEASE	APPROXIMATE RECURRENCE RATE (%)	APPROXIMATE GRAFT LOSS SECONDARY TO RECURRENCE (%)
Oxaluria		
Pre-1975*	90	60
Post-1975†	40	20
Scleroderma‡	20	20
Focal segmental glomerulonephritis§	25	10–15
Mesangiocapillary		
Glomerulonephritis type II	25 (clinical)	10–25
(dense deposit disease)§	90 (histologic)	
Mesangiocapillary		
Glomerulonephritis type I§	30	10–25
Henoch-Schönlein purpura§	30	5

* Data from ASC/NIH Renal Transplant Registry[1]

† Collected data[4,14,20,39,52,57]

‡ Data from Paul et al[44]

§ Data from Cameron[8] and Leumann and Briner[28]

Mesangiocapillary Glomerulonephritis Type I

Because the histologic findings of recurrence are easily confused with those of rejection,[9] the exact rate of recurrence varies considerably among series. The incidence of histologic recurrence is less than in type II; however, when present, it may be more likely to cause functional impairment and graft loss.[8]

Henoch-Schönlein Purpura

The experience with transplantation for this condition is limited. Recurrence in the allograft occurs with moderate frequency (30%), usually without other clinical evidence of recurrent disease.[8,28] Graft loss from recurrence has been the exception. Since recurrence has been associated with a short disease interval prior to transplantation, it has been suggested that transplantation be preceded by a 12-month interval on dialysis.[29]

Conditions with a Low Incidence of Clinically Significant Recurrence

Many diseases leading to primary renal failure infrequently cause significant graft dysfunction. There are several possible reasons for this. The event causing the primary failure may be transient and may have a low likelihood of being repeated, especially while the patient is on immunosuppressive agents; or the renal damage may occur gradually over many years, rarely becoming clinically significant in the allograft during its life span.

An example of the former case appears to be systemic lupus erythematosus. When transplanted after the disease is quiescent or "burnt out," there is a low likelihood of recurrence—three recurrences in more than four hundred transplants.[28] Experience in Wegner's granulomatosis[26] and polyarteritis nodosa have been limited, but recurrence has been infrequent.[28] In anti-glomerular basement membrane (GBM) nephritis, if the antibody titer is absent for a period of time before transplantation, the recurrence rate has been low (<5%).[8] One transplant has been performed in the presence of antibody using plasmapheresis with a successful outcome.[13]

Patients with Alport's syndrome have had infrequent recurrence in the allograft, but they may have an increased susceptibility to a de novo diffuse crescentric glomerulonephritis.[34] Recurrence of membranous nephropathy has been reported relatively infrequently (except for one series)[36] and de novo disease in the allograft is more common than recurrence.[28]

Diabetes is a good example of a disease with slow progression. Biopsies at 2 years or later after transplantation have demonstrated histologic recurrence in all cases but without evidence of clinical impairment.[5,37] Histologic recurrence is common in amyloidosis (~15%), cystinosis (~100%), and IgA nephropathy (~60%), but progression to clinically significant allograft impairment is rare.

Prior Malignancy

A previous malignancy that has been excised for cure still represents an increased risk because of the potential of immunosuppression affecting the host–tumor interaction, allowing metastasis or recurrence. The biological behavior of each tumor must be considered in gauging the length of disease-free interval necessary to minimize the likelihood of recurrence post-transplantation. Reports from the Transplant Tumor Registry[45,46] have described the recurrences following transplantation for a spectrum of tumors. Nonmelanoma skin cancers and small renal tumors found incidentally at bilateral nephrectomy carry little risk. A 24-month disease-free interval decreases the risk to acceptable levels (<10% recurrence) for most tumors. Exceptions to this are Wilms' tumor and low-grade papillary carcinoma of the thyroid, where 12 months may be adequate; symptomatic renal cell carcinoma, where 48 months is required to decrease recurrences to less than 10%; and breast and colon cancer, melanoma, and soft tissue sarcomas, which have a high recurrence rate even up to 5 years following initial treatment.

PATIENT WORKUP

Evaluation of the individual potential transplant recipient attempts to identify those factors that will determine the operative, technical, and immunosuppressive risks. These risks must be balanced against the likelihood of success and the advantages of a successful allograft.

New immunosuppressive approaches such as random and donor-specific transfusion and cyclosporine have resulted in higher allograft success rates and improvement in patient survival. This is due largely to the occurrence of fewer rejection episodes that require high-dose immunosuppression. These advances have enlarged the pool of patients who can safely be considered for transplantation but do not negate the need for careful pretransplantation evaluation and selection.

The accurate and timely evaluation of the potential transplant candidate requires a cooperative effort between the transplant surgeon and the patient's nephrologists and their team of ancillary personnel (e.g., social worker, dietician, dialysis nurses).

Psychiatric Evaluation

A routine evaluation of each candidate by a psychiatrist familiar with the stresses imposed by dialysis and transplantation is valuable. Patients with a past history of mental illness or drug abuse or those identified as noncompliant by dialysis personnel will require more attention. Although these problems may improve after successful transplantation, most do not and they may be intensified. A successful outcome is highly dependent upon the patients' cooperation and compliance with the immunosuppressive and general regimen. Disqualification on these grounds is occasionally justified.

Gastrointestinal Evaluation

Because there is a high risk of morbidity and mortality from gastrointestinal (GI) disease following transplantation, it is important to search out potential problems and correct any pathology identified while the patient is on dialysis. An upper GI series and gallbladder (GB) sonogram are standard screening procedures in adults in many programs, and cholecystectomy should be performed if cholelithiasis is identified. Patients with peptic ulcer diseases should undergo endoscopy and optimal medical therapy. With the use of histamine$_2$ antagonists, most can be healed. Failure to heal the ulcer or its recurrence, however, justifies operative intervention (truncal vagotomy and pyloroplasty or antrectomy), because post-transplant recurrence is frequent[41] and carries a high morbidity. A history of diverticulitis or its occurrence on dialysis is sufficient indication for elective partial colectomy pretransplantation since diverticulitis post-transplantation is frequently accompanied by free perforation and a high mortality rate.[35] Pancreatitis occurring in the dialysis patient requires a careful work-up to seek out predisposing factors and correction of cholelithiasis, hyperparathyroidism, alcoholism, and so on if present. Since recurrent pancreatitis post-transplantation carries a high morbidity and mortality, a disease-free interval of 6 to 12 months may be justified prior to transplantation but does not guarantee that recurrence will not occur.

Urologic Evaluation

The extent of the urologic evaluation necessary to ensure an optimal drainage system for the allograft and to rule out the presence of urinary tract infec-

tion, malignancy, or bladder dysfunction varies from patient to patient. The minimal evaluation should include a detailed urologic history, urinalysis, and serial urine cultures. In the patient with a history of urinary tract infections, voiding difficulties, diseases with a high incidence of bladder dysfunction, or advanced age in the male (>45 years), a voiding cystourethrogram (VCUG) is indicated. Many centers (our own included) perform a VCUG routinely for all potential recipients, as the incidence of positive findings is substantial and the risk is low.

Post-transplant urinary tract sepsis is frequent,[49] and the clinical significance of residual bladder urine or reflux into the native ureters increases with immunosuppression. In many cases of bladder dysfunction, a usable bladder can be obtained by thorough evaluation and corrective surgery as needed. If this is not possible, the bladder may maintain its reservoir function and intermittent self-catheterization can be used.[52] In some patients, conduit diversion is necessary; in these, a colonic sigmoid loop preparatory to the transplant allows the construction of a nonrefluxing ureteral anastomosis[12,*] and is preferable to an ileal loop.

The indications for bilateral nephrectomy in preparation for transplantation have progressively decreased over the years. The procedure, even in experienced hands, carries significant morbidity and mortality,[58] and the anephric patient is more difficult to manage on dialysis. Most investigators now agree that when indicated, the procedure is more safely performed as a preparatory step at least 4 to 6 weeks pretransplantation rather than at the time of the transplantation. Generally accepted indications for nephrectomy include (1) renin-dependent hypertension that cannot be controlled medically, (2) renal failure resulting from pyelonephritis with persistent bacilluria, (3) Grade III or IV reflux (with bacilluria-absolute/without relative), (4) polycystic kidneys with significant infection or significant hemorrhage (size alone rarely justifies unilateral nephrectomy), (5) heavy proteinuria producing uncontrollable nephrotic syndrome, (6) renal tumors, and (7) kidneys diverted into conduits, sigmoid colon, or by skin ureterostomies. If nephrectomy without full ureterectomy is indicated and the kidney is not large, the posterior operative approach may lesson morbidity and mortality.[38]

Infectious Evaluation

The presence of active infection is an absolute contraindication to proceeding with transplantation;

---

* Texter JH, Birtch AG, Cordray ML: Non refluxing colon conduits in renal transplantation. (unpublished observation)

occult infection is a potential trap. A thorough search for infection should be made in each candidate so that problems can be irradicated before approving the patient for transplantation. Chest x-ray and appropriate sputum cultures plus PPD skin test usually act as a sufficient screen for pulmonary infection. Serial urine cultures may indicate the need for more detailed urinary tract evaluation. Careful dental examination and repair or extraction of carious teeth should be performed. Nasal culture to identify chronic staphylococcal carriers will allow irradication of the carrier state. Meticulous care and observation of CAPD catheters is required to ensure that the catheter is not the site of occult infection at transplantation. Recent peritonitis secondary to CAPD should keep the patient from consideration for 3 to 6 weeks after successful treatment. Dermatologic evaluation and treatment may be helpful to minimize the risk in some patients, particularly diabetics, with chronic skin lesions. All adult female patients should undergo gynecologic examination and Pap smear to rule out occult infection or malignancy.

Screening for HB_2Ag is routine in dialysis centers and identifies patients at risk (see GI risk factors) and alerts the transplant team of the potential for exposure to personnel. Screening for other viruses (herpes simplex, varicella zoster, cytomegalovirus, and Epstein-Barr virus) may be helpful because they may produce clinical infection post-transplantation. These results will not affect transplant candidacy except for patients who are sero-positive for HTLV-III. Concerns that an HTLV-III+ patient would develop clinical acquired immunodeficiency syndrome (AIDS) on immunosuppression seem to justify withholding transplantation at this time.

Cardiovascular Evaluation

Patients with chronic renal failure have a high incidence of early vascular disease, most marked in the uremic diabetic. This may lead to cerebrovascular, coronary, or peripheral vascular complications during dialysis or following transplantation. Evaluation must be tailored for each patient according to age and presence of systemic disease, but, in addition to a careful history and physical examination, the minimum for adults usually includes an electrocardiogram (EKG), cardiac sonogram, and cardiology consult. Signs or symptoms suggesting cerebral or peripheral vascular insufficiency must be thoroughly evaluated and corrected pretransplantation if operable. Braun and associates[6] have documented a high incidence (39%) of significant coronary artery disease (i.e., >70% occlusion) or left ventricular dysfunction in 100 consecutive diabetic transplant evaluations. This suggests that routine angiography may, in this patient group, identify both those with reconstructible lesions and those with unreconstructible double and triple vessel disease who are at an inordinately high risk.

Hypertension must be controlled prior to transplantation and will occasionally require bilateral nephrectomy.

Pulmonary Evaluation

Chest x-ray and routine assessment may be all that is required for most patients in evaluating their pulmonary status. Patients with pulmonary complaints must be thoroughly evaluated with pulmonary function studies and arterial blood gas determinations. Those with minimal reserve may be particularly susceptible to pulmonary infections, which remain common post-transplantation. Patients should be strongly urged to avoid smoking in order to lessen its adverse effects on subsequent pulmonary complications and cardiovascular disease progression.

CONCLUSION

Good patient and graft survival rates can be obtained by transplant centers that choose to transplant only young healthy candidates or primarily patients who have a related donor. In a time when cadaver donor organs and financial resources are relatively finite, this practice may have some defense. However, it does not provide each patient on dialysis with the best opportunity for a successful outcome. Thus all the numerous factors mentioned in this chapter must be weighed, shared with the patients, and used to decide for or against transplantation as the optimal mode of therapy in each case.

REFERENCES

1. Advisory Committee to the Renal Transplant Registry: Renal transplantation in congenital and metabolic diseases. JAMA 232:148, 1975

2. Amend WJC, Vincenti F, Feduska NJ et al: Recurrent systemic lupus erythematosus involving renal allografts. Ann Intern Med 94:444, 1981

3. Arbus GS, Hardy BE, Balfe JW et al: Cadaveric renal transplants in children under 6 years of age. Kidney Int 24 (Suppl 15): S111, 1983

4. Bohannon LL, Norman DJ, Barry J et al: Cadaveric renal transplantation in a patient with primary hyperoxaluria. Transplantation 36:114, 1983

5. Bohman SO, Wilczek H, Jaremko G et al: Recurrence of diabetic nephropathy in human renal allografts: Preliminary report of a biopsy study. Transplant Proc 16:649, 1984

6. Braun WE, Phillips DF, Viat DG et al: Coronary artery disease in 100 diabetics with end-stage renal failure. Transplant Proc 16:603, 1984

7. Breed A, Chesney R, Friedman A et al: Oxalosis-induced bone disease: A complication of transplantation and prolonged survival in primary hyperoxaluria. J Bone Joint Surg 63:310, 1981

8. Cameron JS: Glomerulonephritis in renal transplants. Transplantation 34:237, 1982

9. Cameron JS, Turner DR: Recurrent glomerulonephritis in allografted kidneys. Clin Nephrol 7:47, 1977

10. Campbell DA, Dafoe DC, Roloff DW et al: Cadaver renal transplantation in a 2.2 kilogram neonate. Transplantation 38:197, 1984

11. Cats S, Galton J: Effect of original disease in kidney transplant outcome. In Terasaki PJ (ed): Clinical Kidney Transplants 1985, Chapter 7, p 111. Los Angeles, UCLA Tissue Typing Laboratory, 1985

12. Confer DJ, Banowsky LH: The urological evaluation and management of renal transplant donors and recipients. J Urol 124:305, 1980

13. Cove-Smith JR, McLeod AA, Blamey RW et al: Transplantation, immunosuppression and plasmaphoresis in Goodpasture's syndrome. Clin Nephrol 9:126, 1978

14. David DS, Cheigh JS, Stenzel KH et al: Successful renal transplantation in a patient with primary hyperoxaluria. Transplant Proc 15:2168, 1983

15. Donnelly PK, Henderson R, Stratton A et al: Specific and nonspecific immunoregulatory factors and renal graft survival—a single-center five-year experience. Transplant Proc 17:2277, 1985

16. Feduska NJ, Amend WJC, Vincenti F et al: Peptic ulcer disease in kidney transplant recipients. Am J Surg 148:51, 1984

17. Feduska NJ, Melzer J, Amend W et al: Dramatic improvement in the success rate for renal transplantation in diabetic recipients with donor-specific transfusions. Transplantation 38:704, 1984

18. Guillon PJ, Will EJ, Davison AM et al: CAPD—a risk factor in renal transplantation? Br J Surg 71:878, 1984

19. Hillis WD, Hillis A, Walker WG: Hepatitis B surface antigenemia in renal transplant recipients. JAMA 242:329, 1979

20. Hussey JL: Letter to the editor: Transplantation 36:472, 1983

21. Iwaki Y, Iguro T, Terasaki PI: Effect of sensitization on kidney allografts. In Terasaki PJ (ed): Clinical Kidney Transplants 1985, Chapter 9, p 139. Los Angeles, UCLA Tissue Typing Laboratory, 1985

22. Jacobs C, Broyer M, Brunner FP et al: Combined report on regular dialysis and transplantation in Europe, XI, 1980. Proc Eur Dial Transplant Assoc 18:4, 1981

23. Jacob ET, Siegal B, Bar-Nathan N et al: Improving outlook for renal transplantation in amyloid nephropathy: Transplant Proc 14:41, 1982

24. Jarvinen H, Shofer FS, Burke JF et al: Antibody to hepatitis-B surface antigen and kidney graft survival. Transplant Proc 15:1094, 1983

25. Kennedy CL, Castro JE: Transplantation for renal amyloidosis. Transplantation 24:382, 1977

26. Kuross S, Davin T, Kjellstrand CM: Wegner's granulomatosis with severe renal failure: Clinical course and results of dialysis and transplantation. Clin Nephrol 16:172, 1981

27. Lee PC, Terasaki PI: Effect of age on kidney transplants. In Terasaki PJ (ed): Clinical Kidney Transplants 1985, Chapter 8, p 127. Los Angeles, UCLA Tissue Typing Laboratory, 1985

28. Leumann EP, Briner J: Recurrence of the primary disease in the transplanted kidney. In Fine RN, Gruskin AV (eds): End-Stage Renal Disease in Children, Chapter 37, p 528. Philadelphia, W B Saunders, 184

29. Levy M, Mouossa RA, Habib R et al: Anaphylactoid purpura nephritis and transplantation. Abstract. Kidney Int 22:326, 1982

30. Maizel SE, Simmons RL, Kjellstrand C et al: Ten-year experience in renal transplantation for Fabry's disease. Transplant Proc 13:57, 1981

31. Mallory A, Kern F: Drug-induced pancreatitis: A critical review. Gastroenterology 78:813, 1980

32. Mejia G, Zimmerman SW, Glass NR et al: Renal transplantation in patients with systemic lupus erythematosus. Arch Intern Med 143:2089, 1983

33. Merino GE, Sutherland DER, Kjellstrand CM et al: Renal transplantation for progressive systemic sclerosis with renal failure. Am J Surg 133:745, 1977

34. Millner DS, Pierides AM, Holley KE: Renal transplantation in Alport's syndrome: Anti-glomerular basement membrane glomerulonephritis in the allograft. Mayo Clin Proc 57:35, 1982

35. Misra MK, Pinkus GS, Birtch AG et al: Major colonic diseases complicating renal transplantation. Surgery 73:942, 1973

36. Morzycka M, Croker BP, Seigler HF et al: Evaluation of recurrent glomerulonephritis in kidney allografts. Am J Med 72:588, 1982

37. Najarian JS, Sutherland DER, Simmons RL et al: Ten-year experience with renal transplantation in juvenile onset diabetes. Ann Surg 190:487, 1979

38. Novick AC, Ortenburg J, Baun WE: Reduced morbidity with posterior surgical approach for pretransplant bilateral nephrectomy. Surg Gynecol Obstet 151:773, 1980

39. O'Regan P, Constable AR, Jolkes AM et al: Successful renal transplantation in primary hyperoxaluria. Postgrad Med J 56:288, 1980

40. Ost L, Groth C, Lindholm B et al: Cadaveric renal transplantation in patients of 60 years and above. Transplantation 30:339, 1980

41. Owens ML, Wilson SE, Saltzman R: Gastrointestinal complications after renal transplantation. Arch Surg 111:467, 1976

42. Parfrey PS, Forbes RDC, Hutchinson TA et al: The impact of renal transplantation on the course of hepatitis B liver disease. Transplantation 39:610, 1985

43. Parfrey PS, Hutchinson TA, Harvey C et al: Transplantation versus dialysis in diabetic patients with renal failure. Am J Kidney Dis 5:112, 1985

44. Paul M, Bear RA, Sugar L: Renal transplantation in scleroderma. J Rheumatol 11:406, 1984

45. Penn I: Renal transplantation in patients with preexisting malignancies. Transplant Proc 15:1079, 1983

46. Penn I: Kidney transplantation following treatment of tumors. Transplant Proc 18 (No. 4, suppl 3):16, 1986

47. Penn I, Durst AL, Machado M et al: Acute pancreatitis and hyperamylasemia in renal homograft recipients. Arch Surg 105:167, 1972

48. Pirson Y, Alexandre GPJ, van Yperselee Strihou C: Long-term effect of HBs antigenemia on patient survival after renal transplantation. N Engl J Med 296:194, 1977

49. Ramsey DE, Finch WT, Birtch AG: Urinary tract infections in kidney transplant recipients. Arch Surg 114:1022, 1979

50. Rizzoni G, Malekzadeh MH, Pennisi AJ et al: Renal transplantation in children less than 5 years of age. Arch Dis Child 55:532, 1980

51. Scheinman JI, Najarian JS, Mauer SM: Successful strategies for renal transplantation in primary oxalosis. Kidney Int 25:804, 1984

52. Schneidman RJ, Pulliam JP, Barry JM: Clean, intermittent self-catheterization in renal tranplant recipients. Transplantation 38:312, 1984

53. Siegal B, Zemer D, Pras M: Cyclosporine and familial Mediterranean fever amyloidosis. Transplantation 41:793, 1986

54. Strom TB: Editorial retrospective: Hepatitis B, transfusions, and renal transplantation—five years later. N Engl J Med 307:1141, 1982

55. Sturdevant RAL, Singleton JW, Deren JJ et al: Azathioprine-related pancreatitis in patients with Crohn's disease. Gastroenterology 77:883, 1979

56. Sutherland DER, Morrow CE, Fryd DS et al: Improved patient and primary allograft survival in uremic diabetic recipients. Transplantation 34:319, 1982

57. Whelchel JD, Alison DV, Luke RG et al: Successful renal transplantation in hyperoxaluria. Transplantation 35:161, 1983

58. Yarimizu SN, Susan LP, Straffon RA et al: Mortality and morbidity in pretransplant bilateral nephrectomy. Urology 12:55, 1978

59. Zimmerman CE: Renal transplantation for focal segmental glomerulosclerosis. Transplantation 29:172, 1980

CHAPTER 16

The Living Donor in Kidney Transplantation

William H. Bay   Lee A. Hebert

In 1984, 32% of all renal transplants were from living donors. Living donor grafts are used because they have a greater success rate than cadaveric renal grafts and because living donor kidneys supplement the inadequate supply of available cadaveric kidneys.

The most effective means for identifying living-related donors is to have the prospective recipient ask possible donors. During evaluation of the living-related donor, it is most cost-effective to perform a history, physical examination, nephrologist's urinalysis, and routine laboratory studies before performing tissue typing and crossmatch. The most common reasons for exclusion of prospective donors are the discovery of hypertension, diabetes, heart disease, renal disease, and psychiatric disorders. A family history of diabetes, hereditary nephritis, or lupus nephritis does not exclude an individual from being a live kidney donor; however, special testing must be done, and precautions, particularly informed consent, must be taken.

A review of published reports and a current survey of 5698 live donor transplants demonstrated 1 death for every 1600 donor nephrectomies.

Reports from both animal and human studies have suggested that the renal donor may be at risk to develop focal glomerulosclerosis. However, 10- to 15-year followup studies of kidney donors have demonstrated no evidence for progressive damage in the donor's remaining kidney. Nevertheless, yearly medical evaluations of donors, especially for the presence of hypertension and renal disease, is advised.

JUSTIFICATION

The use of living donors in renal transplantation is widely practiced in the United States. At the present time, virtually all living donors are closely genetically related to the recipients. In the 1960s, prisoners, friends, or family members genetically unrelated to the recipient were also permitted to serve as kidney donors. However, this practice was later abandoned when it was determined that the outcomes in these kidney transplants were not different from kidney transplants using cadaveric donors; that is, it was regarded as unethical to subject living unrelated persons to the risks of kidney donation when the results of such a kidney transplant were not different from those using cadaveric donors. However, with the recent discovery that donor-specific blood transfusion can identify patients who are likely to accept a kidney graft from a specific living donor, the use of nonrelated living donors (usually spouses) has re-emerged in the United States. Preliminary data suggest that living unrelated donor transplants are usually successful.[16] In a large study with nonrelated living donor transplants reported from Brazil and the University of Wisconsin, good results were obtained by administering either donor-specific or donor-nonspecific blood transfusions to the recipient.[23] Ethical guidelines for the use of nonrelated living donors have recently been published by the Council of the Transplant Society[38] and by the American Society of Transplant Surgeons. These guidelines require that nonrelated living donors be considered only when a satisfactory related or when cadaveric donors are not immediately available. In addition, the donor must be "emotionally related" to the recipient, and the donor may not receive payment from the recipient, because the donation of a kidney is a "gift of extraordinary value" and the motives for donation must be altruistic.

Although the use of living donors in renal transplantation is now widely accepted, it is by no means universally accepted. For example, of the 10 largest renal transplant centers in the United States, one center, as a matter of policy, performs no renal transplants using living donors.[52] Furthermore, a recent survey of 148 European renal transplant centers revealed that 22% of the centers believe that living donor transplantation is "ethically unacceptable," and an additional 15% of the centers abandoned the practice because of an adverse experience with the donor.[33] Even in centers where living donor renal transplantation is regularly practiced, it is done so in widely varying degrees. For example, of the 10 largest renal transplant centers in the United States in 1984, living donor transplantation ranged from 4% to 46% (median 24%) of all kidney transplants.[33] For the United States as a whole, 32% of all renal transplants in 1984 involved living donors.[54] European renal transplant centers that use living donors generally use them to a lesser extent than do centers in the United States. For example, in the United Kingdom, the percentage of kidney transplants that involve living donors is only 12%.[52]

The two most commonly given reasons for justifying live donors in kidney transplantation are: (1) Properly selected live donor grafts have a higher success rate than do cadaveric renal grafts, and (2) there is an inadequate supply of kidneys from cadaveric donors. Thus, if it were not for the availability of living kidney donors, many fewer renal failure patients would receive a renal transplant. In addition, living donor transplantation may be scheduled for a specific time. Thus, in many instances, it is possible to schedule renal transplantation just before it is necessary to begin chronic dialysis treatments or at a time when it is not disruptive to the recipient's education or employment.

In this chapter, we will discuss (1) the evaluation of the living donor (based on analysis of our practices and the practices of 12 other large renal transplant centers; these centers represent all those that in 1983 performed 30 or more transplants using living donors);[55] (2) the effect of nephrectomy on the long-term health of the renal donor.

EVALUATION OF THE LIVING DONOR

When to Initiate the Search for Family Donors in a Patient With Progressive Renal Insufficiency

Many patients progress to renal failure under circumstances in which it is not possible to make arrangements for evaluation of family donors prior to the onset of end-stage kidney failure. However, in many other instances, it is entirely possible to evaluate family donors, select the most appropriate donor, and perform the renal transplant before it is necessary to initiate dialysis treatments. In the past, that strategy for the management of end-stage renal failure was seldom used, in large part because of a generally held pessimism concerning the long-term success of renal transplants. Thus, the renal transplant was usually not offered until the patient required dialysis therapy. In that way, the "limited" life of the renal transplant would not be "wasted" by providing additional renal function for the patient before it was absolutely needed. However, current experience is that most renal grafts can be expected to provide excellent long-term function. Thus, it makes relatively little difference if the graft is provided a few months before the actual onset of end-stage kidney failure. This approach is particularly relevant to children in whom dialysis avoidance is advantageous.

Other arguments that have been raised to justify the delay of renal transplantation until the patient had been begun on dialysis include:

1. Dialysis, not transplantation, was the primary therapy for end-stage renal disease (ESRD).
2. If kidney transplantation were performed prior to the institution of dialysis therapy and the kidney transplant were to subsequently fail, it would be an emotionally traumatic event to the patient who had not previously been acclimated to dialysis.
3. Performing renal transplantation in patients in whom the biochemical abnormalities of renal failure had not been controlled by regular dialysis might increase the surgical risk of renal transplantation.

However, because of the excellent results in renal transplantation using living or cadaver donors, it is now generally accepted that renal transplantation should be the primary therapy for chronic renal failure in all patients except those who are unlikely to tolerate renal transplant surgery or immunosuppressive therapy. One cannot justify placing all patients on dialysis so that the few patients whose kidney transplant will eventually fail, will have less psychological trauma as they submit to chronic dialysis treatments for the first time. Finally, the fear that inordinate risks to the recipient would be incurred by providing renal transplantation without first providing dialysis is not supported by experience. In our survey of the 12 largest renal transplant centers performing live donor transplantation, patients are regularly receiving renal transplants without the interposition of dialysis. The percentage of patients in those centers receiving renal transplants without prior dialysis ranged from 5% to 40%, median 15%. In the United States in 1984, 4% of all renal transplants involved patients who did not require dialysis.[54]

In adults, the renal transplant should preferably be performed when patient's serum creatinine is about to reach 10 mg/dl. At this level of renal function, most adult patients are free of important signs or symptoms of uremia. A plot of the reciprocal of the serum creatinine versus time will accurately predict when a specific serum creatinine level will be reached. Extrapolation of that line, by calculation of the slope and intercept of the linear regression calculated from those points, usually provides a reliable estimate of the time at which a specific serum creatinine level will be reached.[35]

Identification of the Living Renal Donor

The manner in which the prospective donor is approached and evaluated has an important bearing on the efficiency with which willing and suitable donors are identified. There are three general ways to approach a prospective donor:

1. *The prospective recipient directly asks an individual (usually a ''blood'' relative).* This is the most common and most effective means for identifying prospective donors. Prospective recipients are more effective in obtaining a family donor if, prior to approaching the family members, the prospective recipient is well informed about the process and prognosis of renal transplantation.
2. *The prospective donors are contacted by an interested family member, usually a parent of the prospective recipient.* If the renal patient has been living at home at the time that the renal failure approaches, the patient's mother usually becomes well informed about the patient's problem. In that situation, the mother may make the initial contact with the prospective family donors. Although worthwhile, it is less effective than the first approach, because it indicates that the relationship between the recipient and prospective donors is not optimum.
3. *Prospective donors are contacted directly by the physician caring for the renal patient.* This is the least common method of identifying prospective donors. It is most likely to be successful when: (a) written material concerning kidney transplantation is available for family members, and (b) the written materials themselves (rather

than the physicians) speak to the issues of whether a given family member should be evaluated as a donor.

Occasionally, without being asked, family members request to be considered as potential donors; however, this occurs infrequently.

Donor Evaluation

The proper sequencing of the evaluation of prospective kidney donors is important in controlling the costs of living donor evaluation. Living donor tissue typing and cross-match have a relatively high cost and a relatively low probability (<5%) of excluding prospective donors. Therefore, it is more cost-effective to perform a history, physical examination, careful urinalysis, and routine laboratory studies as the screening steps after the establishment of ABO blood type compatibility between prospective donor and recipient. The cost of this clinical evaluation is less than $150, and approximately 20% of prospective donors are excluded by this screening step.[49] The most common reasons for exclusion are hypertension, diabetes, heart disease, renal disease, and psychological disease.

There is a recommended sequence for evaluation of living donors (Fig. 16-1). The written information provided to prospective donors may vary from center to center, depending upon the patient population served. Prospective donors, recipients, and some family members should be invited to the teaching sessions. These sessions should supplement the information in the written material given to prospective donors by providing visual presentations (slides, video) on relevant aspects of kidney transplantation. The ABO blood type test is relatively inexpensive and decisive; thus, it is the ideal screening test. Those patients who are ABO blood type compatible should then undergo a history, physical examination, and routine blood and urine tests (Table 16-1). The intravenous pyelogram should not be obtained at the time of this initial visit. Commonly, the intravenous pyelogram is obtained at the time that the blood specimens are obtained for tissue typing and cross-match. If the donor is a man older than 45 years or a woman older than 50 years, we obtain a stress MUGA, particularly if the patient has risk factors for heart disease. Pulmonary function tests are also obtained routinely in smokers. At the conclusion of the donor evaluation, the patient has a renal arteriogram. In some centers, digital subtraction angiography has been substituted for the renal arteriogram.[17]

It is important to document each step of the

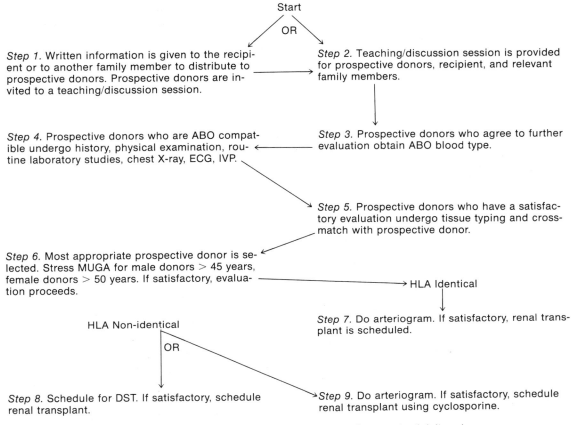

Start

OR

Step 1. Written information is given to the recipient or to another family member to distribute to prospective donors. Prospective donors are invited to a teaching/discussion session.

Step 2. Teaching/discussion session is provided for prospective donors, recipient, and relevant family members.

Step 4. Prospective donors who are ABO compatible undergo history, physical examination, routine laboratory studies, chest X-ray, ECG, IVP.

Step 3. Prospective donors who agree to further evaluation obtain ABO blood type.

Step 5. Prospective donors who have a satisfactory evaluation undergo tissue typing and crossmatch with prospective donor.

Step 6. Most appropriate prospective donor is selected. Stress MUGA for male donors > 45 years, female donors > 50 years. If satisfactory, evaluation proceeds.

HLA Identical

HLA Non-identical

Step 7. Do arteriogram. If satisfactory, renal transplant is scheduled.

OR

Step 8. Schedule for DST. If satisfactory, schedule renal transplant.

Step 9. Do arteriogram. If satisfactory, schedule renal transplant using cyclosporine.

FIGURE 16-1. *Sequence for evaluation of prospective kidney donors. (See text for more detailed discussion for each of the numbered steps.)*

evaluation and to indicate whether the results are satisfactory or unsatisfactory (see Table 16-1). The completed record is then certified by the signature of the physician evaluating the donor and then forwarded to the Transplant Surgery Service. The chance for an error of omission in donor evaluation is substantial because of the large amount of information generated during donor evaluation and because the data are generated at various times during the course of evaluation. By maintaining a single record that documents all relevant aspects of the evaluation, the chance for error is minimized.

Criteria for Exclusion of Persons as Kidney Donors

The criteria suggested for donor exclusion are based on a survey of 11 large transplant centers.

1. *Age less than 18 years or greater than 55 years.* Only under exceptional circumstances are older donors used. The utilization of older donors

raises the issue of patient rights. For example, if after informed consent the person over age 55 still wishes to donate, does the physician have the right to prevent it. Donors younger than 18 years are rarely used, but there are legal procedures for using donors who are younger than the age of majority.[19]

2. *Hypertension.* All the centers surveyed indicated that hypertension in the donor was an exclusion criterion, but a family history of hypertension in the donor was not an exclusion criterion. Patients whose systolic pressure is consistently above 140 and whose diastolic pressure is consistently above 90 or patients who require antihypertensive medications are excluded. However, blood pressures taken in the physician's office frequently substantially overestimate the prevailing blood pressure.[18,28,42] In these patients, ambulatory blood pressure monitoring may establish whether the patient is hypertensive.

TABLE 16-1   Worksheet for the Medical Evaluation of the Prospective Renal Donor

Donor name _____   ABO type _____   Haplo type _____

Recipient name _____   ABO type _____   Disease _____

		Satis-factory	Unsatis-factory
1.	History and physical examination _____		
2.	CBC _____		
3.	Comprehensive battery of blood tests: Na, K, Cl, CO_2, BUN, creatinine, Ca, uric acid, chol, trigly, I phos, T bili, alk phos, LDH, SGOT, SGPT _____		
4.	Two FBS or GTT _____		
5.	Hgb/A1C _____		
6.	Serologic test for syphilis _____		
7.	HBS ag _____		
8.	HBS ab _____		
9.	HBC ab _____		
10.	HTLV-III antibody _____		
11.	24-hour urine: creatinine, protein, calcium, oxalate, cysteine, and uric acid _____		
12.	Urinalysis by nephrologist _____		
13.	Urine culture (if evidence of bacteruria or pyuria) _____		
14.	Pregnancy test _____		
15.	EKG _____		
16.	Chest x-ray _____		
17.	Urine osmolality (after overnight thirst)		
18.	Intravenous pyelogram _____		
19.	TB skin test _____		
20.	Candida skin test _____		
21.	Stress MUGA (>50 yr of age, females; >45 yr of age, males) _____		
22.	Renal arteriogram _____		

Comments:

Approved for assignment to transplant treatment protocol
(physician signature and date) _____

Approved for organ donation
(physican signature and date) _____

Rejected for transplant
(physician signature and date) _____

3. *Diabetes.* Glucose tolerance is assessed by measuring hemoglobin A1C and by measuring fasting blood glucose levels twice. If these values are abnormal, the patient should be excluded from organ donation. Some centers require that donors be tested with the standard 5-hour glucose tolerance test.

4. *History of kidney stone or evidence of kidney stone on x-ray.* A search for the factors that predispose to kidney stone disease is indicated and is done by measuring the 24-hour urinary excretion of calcium, uric acid, oxalate, and cysteine. Several potential donors have been identified who have hypercalciuria and/or hyperoxaluria on normal calcium and oxalate dietary intakes. These persons may be at increased risk to develop renal calculi. If used as donors, they should have prolonged medical follow-up and adjust their diet and fluid intake appropriately.

5. *Abnormal glomerular filtration rate (GFR).* GFR is estimated from the measurement of serum creatinine concentration (minimum of two measurements) and relating that level to body size. For adults who weigh less than 50 kg, the average serum creatine must be 0.9 mg/dl or less (normal range, 0.9 mg/dl–1.3 mg/dl). For adults weighing 50 kg to 80 kg, the average serum creatinine concentration must be 1.2 mg/

dl or less. For well-muscled adults who weigh more than 80 kg, an average serum creatinine level of up to 1.3 mg/kg is acceptable. Because of frequent errors in the collection of 24-hour urine, the measurement of creatinine clearance is not relied upon as a means to evaluate GFR. It is more reliable to estimate GFR from multiple measurements of serum creatinine level and to relate this to body size.

6. *Unexplained microscopic hematuria.* All donor urine sediment should be examined by a nephrologist. Twelve ml of a concentrated urine specimen is centrifuged in a conical tube. The tube contents are entirely decanted, and the sediment is promptly aspirated into a class pipette and placed on a glass slide. Using this rather sensitive technique to identify microscopic hematuria, most normal persons, male and female, will have an average of less than 1 red cell per high-power field. There is a high incidence of identifiable disease in patients with greater numbers of red cells in their urine sediment. Many laboratories regard as normal urine sediments that contain up to 3 red cells per high-power field. However, in our opinion, using those criteria for normal would include patients with significant renal disease. The importance of this is illustrated by the two cases of glomerulonephritis detected after kidney donation in our survey. In one patient, the oversight could have been avoided by the more stringent urine sediment criteria.

7. *Abnormal proteinuria.* Prospective donors must have no evidence of proteinuria on qualitative urinalysis of a concentrated urine specimen ($\geq$1.020 specific gravity) and/or urine osmolality ($\geq$700 mOsm/liter), tested by both dipstick and sulfosalicylic acid, and no abnormal rate of proteinuria in a 24-hour collection of urine. A dipstick may give a false-positive test for protein when the urine is very alkaline (pH 8.0 or greater) or when the urine is very concentrated (specific gravity, 1.028 or greater).[1]

8. *Inability to concentrate the urine to greater than 700 mOsm/liter after an overnight dehydration.* In early tubulointerstitial disease, GFR as estimated by serum creatinine and creatinine clearance may be normal and the urine sediment may be unremarkable. However, these patients may have a conspicuous inability to concentrate the urine. Thus, to exclude patients with significant and potentially progressive tubulointerstitial disease, the donor must be able to provide a well-concentrated urine specimen.

9. *History of any systemic disorder that has impaired general health or can be expected to impair general health in the future.* This is such a broad exclusion criterion that it is not feasible to define it succinctly. However, a stress MUGA for male donors over age 45 years and for female donors over age 50 years, particularly if they have any risk factors for the presence of heart disease is strongly suggested. Pulmonary function tests are conducted in all smokers.

10. *Obesity.* Generally, potential donors who are more than 15% above ideal body weight are advised to lose the excess weight before the kidney transplant will be scheduled.

11. *Prior history of thrombophlebitis or thromboembolic disease.* These patients are excluded because they may be at increased risk to develop pulmonary embolism postoperatively.

12. *Psychiatric disorder.* A formal psychiatric evaluation is usually obtained only if the psychiatric abnormality is suggested by the medical evaluation; however, some programs obtain a routine psychiatric consult on all donors.

13. *A positive HIV antibody test.* The cytopathic human retrovirus, HTLV-III, is associated with the immune deficiency syndrome, AIDS. We recommend screening for AIDS using the following guidelines adapted from recommendations of the American Red Cross.
    a. The HIV antibody test should be performed with the person's informed consent, and the testing results must be kept confidential.
    b. Persons who have a positive HIV antibody test and a confirmatory Western blot test should not be kidney donors.
    c. A strongly reactive and repeated HIV antibody test but a negative Western blot test is probably also a true positive, and the donor should be excluded. A weakly reactive, repeated HIV antibody test and a negative Western blot test usually denotes a false-reactive result, and additional testing is warranted before designating the donor as an HIV positive person.

Occasionally, a person will insist on being a kidney donor even though, in the best judgment of the physicians evaluating the renal donors, he or she is unfit as a donor for medical, psychological, or ethical reasons. In this situation, we recommend that a second evaluation of the donor be undertaken by another transplant center. It is hoped that the second evaluation will definitely resolve the problem. If it does not, it is certainly the right of the prospective donor to seek additional opinions or another center that will perform the transplant.

However, regardless of the prospective donor's search, it is the right of the physician to refuse to use that person as a donor if the physician regards him or her to be an unfit donor.

The following conditions are not reasons for exclusion as a live kidney donor; however, special precautions must be taken.

1. *Family history of adult polycystic kidney disease.* In these families, the prospective donor must be 30 years of age or older. The donor should be studied by both intravenous pyelography and by ultrasound of the kidneys and liver. In addition to no manifestations of polycystic kidney disease, they should have no extra-renal organ manifestation of polycystic kidney disease such as hepatitis or pancreatic cysts or signs of valvular heart disease. Using this guideline, there is less than a 5% chance that polycystic kidney disease will be detected in the future.[37] If these patients proceed to arteriography, the arteriogram is scrutinized for evidence of renal cysts. Several centers obtain an abdominal CAT scan, searching for evidence of cysts in kidney and other splanchnic organs. In the near future, gene analysis may be a valuable tool in detecting future polycystic patients.

2. *Diabetes in both parents of the prospective donor.* In this situation, the probability that the donor will eventually develop glucose intolerance is quite high, perhaps reaching 100%.[20] Thus, great care should be used in considering these patients as prospective kidney donors, and they probably should be rejected as renal donors.

3. *Family history of hereditary nephritis.* Hereditary nephritis usually manifests as microscopic hematuria at an early age. Furthermore, if the disease is progressive, proteinuria is also present at a relatively early age. Indeed, progressive renal disease rarely develops in a patient with hereditary glomerulonephritis, who, at 25 years or older, was free of proteinuria. Thus, in a family with hereditary nephritis in whom the donor is age 25 years or older and there is no evidence of renal disease on repeated urinalyses done by a nephrologist, that person is an acceptable donor if all other donor criteria are met. In most centers surveyed, it was simply stated that the donors must be free of the disease. Donors were often required to sign a statement that the physicians would not be responsible if, in the future, the donor developed progressive glomerulonephritis.

4. *A family history of systemic lupus erythematosus*

(SLE). There is an increased frequency of autoimmune disease in relatives of patients with SLE.[30] However, a family history of SLE should not be a contraindication to kidney donation unless lupus or a lupus-like syndrome is present in the donor.

THE SURGICAL RISK TO THE LIVE KIDNEY DONOR

There are at least 16 published reports* that review the surgical mortality of living kidney donors. Of the 2495 donors described in these reports, three died from events that were thought to be related to the surgical procedure: one of hepatitis 1 month after nephrectomy, one with myocardial infarction, and one with a pulmonary embolus. Thus, the mortality rate of donor nephrectomy from these combined series is 0.1%. There was also a 1.8% major complication rate that included pulmonary embolus, severe infection with sepsis, renal failure, hepatitis, or myocardial infarction. In a survey of the 12 largest renal transplant centers performing living donor transplantation who collectively performed 5698 living donor transplants, two donor deaths related to donor nephrectomy were reported, with an overall surgical mortality rate of 0.04%. Thus, when the data from the published reports and combined survey are combined, the mortality risk of live kidney donation is about 1 death per 1600 donors.

To place this risk in perspective, it is necessary to compare it to other common human activities that may result in loss of life. For example, in the state of Ohio with a population of 10.7 million, there are approximately 1700 vehicular/pedestrian deaths each year. Assuming that all 10.7 million people in Ohio travel in vehicles and/or are pedestrians, the average yearly mortality rate for this type of activity is approximately 1/6500. Thus, the renal donor incurs as much risk of dying from donating a kidney as the average Ohio citizen does from dying of a vehicular/pedestrian accident for each four years of residence in Ohio. Donating a kidney is, of course, a once-in-a-lifetime risk. However, the risk of dying from a vehicular/pedestrian accident is a continuing risk. Thus, the cumulative risk of traveling in vehicles and/or being a pedestrian in Ohio far exceeds the risk of donating a kidney.

---

* References 8, 12, 14, 15, 22, 24, 31, 34, 41, 43, 47, 50, 51, 53, 57, and 58

Long-Term Risk to the Kidney Donor

Recent studies in experimental animals and in humans indicate that as renal mass is progressively reduced, there is an increase in glomerular hydrostatic pressure, perfusion rate, and hypertrophy of the remaining glomeruli.[10] Studies in the rat have shown that with a severe reduction in renal mass (5/6 nephrectomy model), progressive glomerulosclerosis develops, apparently because of the concomitant "glomerular hypertension."[10] The evidence that it is the glomerular hypertension that causes the progressive glomerulosclerosis in the 5/6 nephrectomized rat rests on the observations that therapy with low protein diets[36] or angiotensin-converting inhibitors,[3] both of which reduce glomerular hydrostatic pressure, arrest or slow the rate of progression to renal failure. These observations may be relevant to the renal donor because of the sustained increase in renal blood the GFR per nephron that develops in the donor after nephrectomy.

Concern for the long-term effect of renal donation has also been raised by reports showing that patients with unilateral renal agenesis can develop focal glomerulosclerosis and progressive failure of their solitary kidney.[26] Central to the argument that the renal donor may be susceptible to progressive glomerulosclerosis is the assumption that the presence of only one normal kidney can cause a sufficient degree of glomerular hypertension to result in glomerulosclerosis. However, in contrast to rats subjected to 5/6 nephrectomy, dogs subjected to 75% nephrectomy did not develop progressive renal failure during a 4-year evaluation.[44] Also, patients with a solitary kidney and unilateral renal agenesis who do develop progressive renal disease often have had bilateral disease that was unrecognized. Indeed, one theory suggests that renal agenesis is the result of vesicoureteral reflux in utero.[4] Thus, it is possible that in patients with renal agenesis and focal glomerulosclerosis, vesicoureteral reflux may have been bilateral, but more severe on the side with the renal agenesis. Thus, patients with unilateral renal agenesis who develop progressive renal failure may have had bilateral renal disease and a greater decrease in total nephrons than originally believed.

Other studies examining the long-term effects of a solitary kidney do not suggest that patients with a single normal kidney are at increased risk to develop progressive renal failure. In a series of 24 adult patients, 7 developed proteinuria 2 to 7 years after nephrectomy, but all had proteinuria less than 1.5 gm/24 hours. Six of the 7 proteinuric patients were followed for 5 to 18 years and maintained normal serum creatinine levels. All were normotensive.[60] In another report of 27 infants and children who had unilateral nephrectomy,[45] none developed abnormal proteinuria. After a mean follow-up of 23 years, the creatinine clearance averaged 74.3% of normal, a value comparable to that seen in the early postnephrectomy period. None of these patients had clinically important hypertension. Finally, in an autopsy study of 10 adult nephrectomized patients who died 8 to 46 years after nephrectomy, none had evidence of focal glomerulosclerosis in their solitary kidney.[26]

Followup Studies in Renal Donors

In recent years, there have been numerous reports of follow-up studies of renal function and blood pressure levels in renal donors.[2,5,9,13,21,29,39,40,48,56,59] The results of four studies[2,21,48,56] with a minimum follow-up of 10 years is summarized in Table 16-2 and Figure 16-2. Renal donors evaluated 10 to 15 years after elective nephrectomy had an average increase in proteinuria of 100 mg/24 hours to 200 mg/24 hours, which exceeded the prenephrectomy proteinuria and age-matched controls. Few patients had proteinuria greater than 500 mg/24 hours. In patients who had greater than 1 gm of proteinuria, most appeared to have acquired renal disease for reasons independent of renal donation. Thus, proteinuria observed in renal donors occurs in a minority of donors, is generally mild, appears to be nonprogressive, and, interestingly, is mainly nonalbumic protein.[7,56] This suggests that the proteinuria is nonglomerular in origin and may not reflect glomerular injury.

There is probably no increased likelihood of developing hypertension after renal organ donation, although male donors may have a slightly increased tendency to hypertension.[2,21,59] Similarly, there is no trend for mean serum creatinine to increase over time (see Fig. 16-2). However, substantial losses of GFR could be occurring in these patients that is not reflected in an increase in serum creatinine or decrease in creatinine clearance because of a compensatory increase in tubular secretion of creatinine.[6,46] However, such an interpretation is not supported by the data available on simultaneous inulin and creatinine clearance in renal donors followed sequentially. That is, a progressive increase in the ratio of creatinine clearance to inulin clearance has not been observed in renal donors followed up to 4 years.[9] Furthermore, the trend line described by the reciprocal of the serum creatinine versus time was not found to be different postnephrectomy compared

TABLE 16-2   *Published Long-term (>10 years) Follow-up Studies in Renal Donors*

	AUTHORS				TOTAL OR AVERAGE
	Vincenti et al[56]	Hakim et at[21]	Smith et al[48]	Anderson et al[2]	
Number of patients	20	52	40	100	212
Number of males	7	29	20	48	104
Number of females	13	23	20	52	108
Mean follow-up (yr)	15.8	12.9	11.8	12.6	12.8
% Hypertensive diastolics >90 mm Hg	15%	48%	15%	19%	25%
% Males	NA	62%	10%	19%	30%
% Females	NA	30%	20%	19%	22%
% Proteinuria >150 mg/24 hr	20%	25%	20%	13%	17%
% Males	NA	31%	NA	13%	18%
% Females	NA	17%	NA	13%	15%
% Proteinuria 500–999 mg/24 hr	0	8%	NA	2%	4%
% Males	0	10%	NA	2%	5%
% Females	0	4%	NA	2%	3%
% Proteinuria >1 gm/24-hr	0	2%	NA	1%	1%
% Males	0	3%	NA	2%	2%
% Females	0	0%	NA	0%	0%
Mean serum creatinine (mg/dl)	1.16	1.25	1.29	1.20	1.23
Males	NA	1.30	NA	1.31	1.31
Females	NA	1.18	NA	1.09	1.12
Renal disease*	1	1	0	2	4

* Number of patients who developed an identifiable renal disease after kidney donation.

with prenephrectomy levels in a large number of patients followed for 5 years.[48] In renal donors, pregnancy, a state known to be accompanied by sustained increases in GFR and renal blood flow per nephron, does not adversely affect renal function.[56]

In summary, proteinuria develops in some renal donors. However, the proteinuria is mild, appears to be nonprogressive and may not represent proteinuria owing to glomerular injury. Hypertension also develops in some renal donors, usually men; however, it probably does not occur with an overall increased frequency. Finally, there is no evidence that progressive renal injury develops in the solitary kidney of renal donors.

Recommendations for Advice to Renal Donors Regarding Management of Their Renal Status

Based on current evidence, we suggest that the following represents prudent advice to prospective renal donors:

1. Careful long-term studies of renal donors have not revealed evidence that removing one kidney causes progressive harm to the other kidney. However, it remains a theoretical possibility that damage to the remaining kidney could occur. If damage to the kidney occurs, certain treatments may be effective. Thus, careful follow-up is advised. Yearly examinations seem appropriate and should include an assessment for the presence of hypertension and renal disease. Routine laboratory studies should include serum creatinine, 24-hour urine for protein and creatinine, and a urinalysis.

2. Avoidance of a high protein intake (>1 gm/kg/day) is recommended. The theoretical advantages are:
   a. There is evidence that patients on reduced dietary protein intakes tend to have lower blood pressure levels than patients on higher protein diets.[25]
   b. There is an abundance of evidence that, in patients with a greater than 50% reduction in the number of functioning nephrons, dietary protein restriction may stabilize the function of those nephrons.[27]
   c. Meat proteins are a major source of cholesterol; thus, reducing the amount of meat proteins in the diet may diminish the risk factors for atherosclerotic cardiovascular disease.
   d. A high-protein intake can increase urinary calcium excretion,[32] and this may increase the risk for urolithiasis.

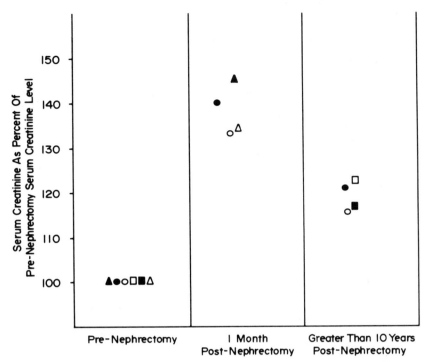

FIGURE 16-2. *Changes in serum creatinine levels of renal donors before and after donor nephrectomy. Values were obtained 1 month after nephrectomy and more than 10 years but less than 15 years after nephrectomy. Serum creatinine levels are expressed as a percentage of pre-nephrectomy values. The symbols are as follows: ● ref 2, ○ ref 56, ■ ref 48, □ ref 21, ▲ ref 9 and △ ref 29*

ACKNOWLEDGMENTS

We thank the following centers for completing a survey of their experience with living-related donors:

University of Minnesota Hospital, Minneapolis, Minnesota

St Vincent Medical Center, Los Angeles, California

University of California at San Francisco, California

Oregon Health Sciences University, Portland, Oregon

University of Texas, Medical Branch, Galveston, Texas

University of Wisconsin Hospital, Madison, Wisconsin

University of Alabama Hospital, Birmingham, Alabama

Vanderbilt University Hospital, Nashville, Tennessee

Shands Teaching Hospital and Clinics, Gainesville, Florida

University of Pennsylvania Hospital, Philadelphia, Pennsylvania

Hermann Hospital, Houston, Texas

Ohio State University Hospital, Columbus, Ohio

REFERENCES

1. Abuelo JG: Proteinuria: Diagnostic principles and procedures. Ann Intern Med 98:186, 1983
2. Anderson CF, Velosa JA, Frohnert PP et al: The risks of unilateral nephrectomy: Status of kidney donors 10 to 20 years postoperatively. Mayo Clin Proc 60:367, 1985
3. Anderson S, Meyer TW, Rennke HG: Control of glomerular hypertension limits glomerular injury in rats

with reduced renal mass. J Clin Invest 76:612, 1985

4. Arant BS Jr, Sotelo-Avila C, Bernstein J: Segmental "hypoplasia" of the kidney (ASK-UPMARK). J Pediatr 95:931, 1979

5. Aurell M, Ewald J: The use of living donors. Glomerular filtration rate during the first year after donor nephrectomy. Scand J Urol Nephrol (Suppl) 64:137, 1981

6. Bauer JH, Brooks CS, Burch RN: Clinical appraisal of creatinine clearance as a measurement of glomerular filtration rate. Am J Kidney Dis p 337, 1982

7. Bertolatus JA, Friedlander MA, Scheidt C: Urinary albumin excretion after donor nephrectomy. Am J Kidney Dis 5:165, 1985

8. Blohme I, Gabel H, Brynger H: The living donor in renal transplantation. Scand J Urol Nephrol Suppl 65:143, 1981

9. Boner G, Shelp WD, Newton M et al: Factors influencing the increase in glomerular filtration rate in the remaining kidney of transplant donors. Am J Med 55:169, 1973

10. Brenner BM: Hemodynamically mediated glomerular injury and the progressive nature of kidney disease. Kidney Int 23:647, 1983

11. Buszta C, Steinmuller DR, Novick AC et al: Pregnancy after donor nephrectomy. Transplantation 40:651, 1985

12. Connor WT, VanBuren CT, Floyd M et al: Anterior extraperitoneal donor nephrectomy. J Urol 126:443, 1981

13. Davison JM, Uldali PR, Walls J: Renal function studies after nephrectomy in renal donors. Br Med J 1:1050, 1976

14. Diethelm AG, Sterling WA, Alchete JS: Retrospective analysis of 100 consecutive patients undergoing related living donor renal transplantation. Ann Surg 183:502, 1976

15. Eklund B, Eklund P, Lindfors O et al: Living donor nephrectomy: Surgical aspects. Scand J Urol Nephrol Suppl 64:157, 1981

16. Feduska NJ: Non-related transplantation: Should living donors be used? Abstract, p 89, National Meeting of The American Society of Nephrology, New Orleans, LA, December, 1985

17. Flechner SM, Sandler CM, Houston GK et al: 100 living-related kidney donor evaluations using digital subtraction angiography. Transplantation 40:675, 1985

18. Floras JS, Jones JV, Hassan MO et al: Cuff and ambulatory blood pressure in subjects with essential hypertension. Lancet p 107, July 18, 1981

19. Fost N: Children as renal donors. N Engl J Med 296:363, 1977

20. Goto Y, Kakizaki M, Toyota T: Heredity of diabetes mellitus. In Melish JS, Hanna J, Baba S (eds): Genetic Environmental Interaction in Diabetes Mellitus, p 18–29. Amsterdam, Excerpta Medica, 1982

21. Hakim RM, Goldszer RC, Brenner BM: Hypertension and proteinuria: Long-term sequelae of uninephrectomy in humans. Kidney Int 25:930, 1984

22. Harrison JH, Bennett AH: The familial living donor in renal transplantation. J Urol 118:166, 1977

23. Hoette M, Tavora E, Mocelin A et al: Living non-related kidney donors (LNR) for transplantation. Abstract, p 281A, National Meeting of The American Society of Nephrology, New Orleans, LA, December, 1985

24. Jacobs SC, McLaughlin AP, Halasz NH: Live donor nephrectomy. Urology 5:175, 1975

25. Kaplan NM: Use of non-drug therapy in treating hypertension. Am J Med Suppl 77:96–101, 1984

26. Kiprov DD, Colvin RB, McCluskey T: Focal and segmental glomerulosclerosis and proteinuria associated with unilateral renal agenesis. Lab Invest 46:275, 1982

27. Klahr SL, Beurkert J, Purkerson ML: Role of dietary factors in the progression of chronic renal disease. Kidney Int 24:579, 1983

28. Kleinert HD, Harshfield GA, Pickering TG et al: What is the value of home blood pressure measurement in patients with mild hypertension? Hypertension 6:574, 1984

29. Krohn AG, Ogden DA, Holmes JH: Renal function in 29 healthy adults before and after nephrectomy. JAMA 196:110, 1966

30. Lahita RG, Chiorazzi N, Gibofsky A et al: Familial systemic lupus erythematosus in males. Arthritis Rheum 26:39, 1983

31. Leary FJ, Deweerd JH: Living donor nephrectomy. J Urol 109:947, 1973

32. Linkswiler HM, Joyce CL, Anand CR: Calcium retention of young adult males as affected by level of protein and calcium intake. Trans NY Acad Sci 36:330, 1974

33. Living related kidney donors. Lancet, p 696. September 25, 1982

34. McLoughlin MG: Related living donor nephrectomy. J Urol 111:304, 1976

35. Mavrelis P, Hebert LA, Lemann J Jr et al: Method for detecting a progressive renal disorder superimposed on a preexisting progressive renal disorder. Am J Kidney Dis 1:172, 1981

36. Meyer TW, Anderson S, Brenner BM: Dietary protein intake and progressive glomerular sclerosis: The role of capillary hypertension and hyperperfusion in the progression of renal disease. Ann Intern Med 98:832, 1983

37. Milutinovic J, Fialkow P, Phillips LA et al: Autosomal dominant polycystic kidney disease: Early diagnosis and data for genetic counselling. Lancet, p 1203, June 7, 1980

38. Morris PJ, Tilney NL et al: Commercialization in transplantation: The problems and some guidelines for practice. Lancet, p 715, September 28, 1975

39. Ogden DA: Consequences of renal donation in man. Am J Kidney Dis 2:501, 1983

40. Pabico RC, McKenna BA, Freeman RB: Renal func-

tion before and after unilateral nephrectomy in renal donors. Kidney Int 8:166, 1975

41. Penn I, Halgrimson CG, Ogden D et al: Use of living donors in kidney transplantation in man. Arch Surg 101:226, 1970

42. Perloff D, Sokolow M, Cowan R: The prognostic value of ambulatory blood pressures. JAMA 249:2792, 1983

43. Ringden O, Friman L, Lundgren G et al: Living related kidney donors: Complications and long-term renal function. Transplantation 25:221, 1978

44. Robertson JL, Goldschmidt M, Kronfeld DS et al: Long-term renal responses to high dietary protein in dogs with 75% nephrectomy. Kidney Int 29:511, 1986

45. Robitaille P, Mongeau J-G, Lortie L et al: Long-term follow-up of patients who underwent unilateral nephrectomy in childhood. Lancet, p 1297, June 8, 1985

46. Shemesh O, Golbetz H, Kriss JP et al: Limitations of creatinine as a filtration marker in glomerulopathic patients. Kidney Int 28:830, 1985

47. Smith MJV: Living kidney donors. J Urol 110:158, 1973

48. Smith S, Laprad P, Grantham J: Long-term effect of uninephrectomy on serum creatinine concentration and arterial blood pressure. Am J Kidney Dis 6:143, 1985

49. Spanos PK, Simmons RL, Kjellstrand CM et al: Screening potential related transplant donors for renal disease. Lancet, p 645, April 13, 1974

50. Spanos PK, Simmons RL, Lampe E et al: Complications of related kidney donation. Surgery 776:741, 1974

51. Thomson NM, Scott DF, Marshall VC et al: Living related renal transplantation: Experience in 22 cases. Aust NZ J Surg 49:608, 1979

52. Top 10 U.S. Transplant Centers for 1984. Contemporary Dialysis & Nephrology, September, 1985

53. Uehling DT, Malek GH, Wear JB: Complications of donor nephrectomy. J Urol 111:745, 1974

54. The U.S. ESRD Program: Selected 1984 Statistics. Contemporary Dialysis & Nephrology, December, 1985

55. The U.S. ESRD Program: Selected 1983 Statistics. Contemporary Dialysis & Nephrology, December, 1984

56. Vincenti F, Amend WJC Jr, Kaysen G et al: Long-term renal function in kidney donors. Sustained compensatory hyperfiltration with no adverse effects. Transplantation 36:626, 1983

57. Weiland D, Sutherland DER, Chavers B et al: Information on 628 living-related kidney donors at a single institution, with long-term follow-up in 472 cases. Transplant Proc 16:5, 1984

58. Weinstein SH, Navarre RJ Jr, Loening SA et al: Experience with live donor nephrectomy. J Urol 124:321, 1980

59. Williams S, Jorkasky D: Long-term effects of kidney donation: A sibling study. Abstract. Annual Meeting, The American Society of Nephrology, Washington, DC, December, 1984

60. Zucchelli P, Cagnoli L, Casanova S et al: Facial glomerulosclerosis in patients with unilateral nephrectomy. Kidney Int 24:649, 1983

CHAPTER 17

Operative Technique for Living-Related Kidney Donors

Thomas L. Marchioro

The technique described here for removal of kidneys from volunteer living-related donors for renal homotransplantation has been in continuous use with only minor modifications since it was first described by the author and his colleagues.[3]

DONOR PREPARATION

Appropriate consent must be obtained from prospective donors. ABO and histocompatibility should be established first, along with a negative white cell crossmatch. Other immunologic studies may be done if desired, but the aforementioned studies represent the minimum necessary to proceed.

Complete history and physical examination with chest film, electrocardiogram, and blood chemical screen follows. Renal function is then assessed with three creatinine clearances, standard urinalyses, and urine cultures. These are followed by excretory urography. Finally, a flush aortogram is done to assess vascular anatomy. We do not use digital subtraction angiography because of its lack of detail and the possibility of overlooking additional renal arteries. If the donor passes all these tests, he or she is accepted for nephrectomy. Our experience over 24 years with more than 400 donors indicates that there will be zero operative risk, less than 2% postoperative complications, almost all of which are minor wound infections, and no significant long-term morbidity resulting from the nephrectomy. This is in keeping with others' experience.[1]

On the evening before the proposed donor nephrectomy, 1,000 ml of 5% dextrose in lactated Ringer's solution is given, followed by 500 ml of 5% dextrose in water over a period of 10 to 12 hours. Approximately 45 minutes prior to being taken to the operating room, 12.5 g of mannitol is given to the donor to ensure a diuresis at the time that anesthesia is induced.[3]

OPERATIVE TECHNIQUE

An inlying urinary catheter is placed. Depending upon the vascular anatomy as demonstrated by the aortogram, a decision has been made to take either the right or the left kidney. For either right or left nephrectomy, a flank approach is used. The technique to be described will be that for right nephrectomy. Where details differ on the left, they will be discussed as appropriate.

The patient is positioned so that the costal arch is over the kidney rest (Fig. 17-1A). The upper body is rotated toward the left, elevating the right shoulder approximately 60 degrees from the table. The kidney rest is then raised. The incision is made in such a manner that it parallels the 11th rib and runs inferomedially paralleling the border of the rectus abdominus (Fig. 17-1A).

The rib is resected subperiosteally after dividing the external oblique muscle (Fig. 17-1B). We use rib resection principally because of the security of the closure that can be obtained and not for any particular additional exposure. Once the rib is removed, incision in its bed gives access to the perinephric space. This permits the surgeon to put two fingers into this space and gently push the peritoneum away. The overlying internal oblique and transversus abdominus muscles are lifted up on the fingers and cut (Fig. 17-1B). The peritoneum is then swept off the posterior musculature, beginning at the psoas major muscle inferiorly. A large retractor is placed.

Gerota's fascia is opened longitudinally exposing the perinephric fat (Fig. 17-1B). The perinephric fat is entered, identifying the true capsule of the kidney. It is a simple matter to free the perinephric fat from the convex border of the kidney from pole to pole. Occasionally, patients will have had prior injuries to their kidneys from contact sports or heavy labor. In such patients, there will be a reasonably

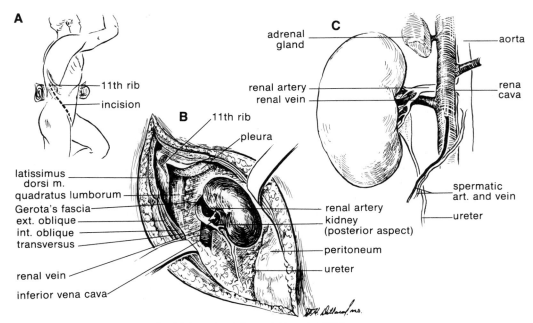

FIGURE 17-1.   Technical details of living-related donor right nephrectomy.

dense adherence of the capsule of the kidney to the perinephric fat. This can pose some difficulties, but, with care and patience, the perinephric fat can be freed from the renal capsule.

The relationship of the upper pole of the kidney to the adrenal gland on the right differs from that on the left side. As shown somewhat simplistically in Figure 17-1C, the adrenal on the right is truly suprarenal and is held by its attachment to the liver anteriorly. It is rare to see more than the tip of the gland on the right if dissection is kept on the true capsule of the kidney. On the left, however, the gland crowds the renal artery and vein medially and must be carefully separated from these structures.

Once the upper pole is freed, the renal vein–vena caval junction is exposed, care being taken not to injure the gonadal vein (Fig. 17-1C). On the left side, both gonadal and adrenal veins are identified, ligated, and divided to provide additional length. If the adrenal has not been mobilized, the gland does not develop venous congestion.

Next, the renal artery is identified. It is usually posterior and just cephalad to the vein but may be directly behind it. If additional length of artery is desired on the right, dissection behind the vena cava can be done, but this is best left until the ureter has been freed.

After identifying the artery and the renal vein–venal caval junction on the right or where the vein crosses the aorta on the left, attention is directed to

the ureter, which is exposed in its inferior course as it crosses the iliac vessels (Fig. 17-1B). If the ureter is taken inferior to the arterial supply deriving from the internal iliac artery, this vessel must be individually identified, ligated, and divided prior to transecting the ureter. As dissection of the ureter proceeds proximally, a triangle is formed by distracting the ureter laterally away from the vena cava on the right or the aorta on the left. Dissection should be done adjacent to the vena cava or aorta to minimize the possibility of damage to the blood supply to the drainage system.

Occasionally a double renal vein is encountered. These are almost always posteriorly placed, inferior to the artery, and are generally smaller than the larger anterior vein. On the right, the structure is best ligated and divided after test clamping with a vascular clamp to ensure absence of venous hypertension in the kidney. The venous drainage of the kidney intercommunicates within the organ, and ligation of one vein has never in our experience caused venous hypertension.

On the left, the posterior vein may be larger than the anterior branch, and, in a very few instances, it may be the only venous drainage. Since the posterior vein passes retroaortically, it is best divided at an appropriate site to the left of this structure. Far more often, on the left side, one encounters one or more large "lumbar" veins, which arise on the posterior inferior aspect of the renal vein and, closely apposed to the aortic wall, pass behind this structure. Not uncommonly, these vessels branch shortly after they leave the renal vein. Care must be taken to clearly identify these structures and any of their branches so that they may be securely ligated prior to division.

Once the artery, vein, and ureter have been completely freed, the kidney is ready for removal (Fig. 17-1B). At any point during the dissection, it may be wise to give the donor patient infusions of mannitol or Lasix or both. It is our policy to do this if the kidney appears to be somewhat soft. In any event, we always infuse mannitol, 12.5 g intravenously, prior to placing the clamps on the renal artery and vein. This gives maximal diuresis at the time of the removal, thus enhancing subsequent function in the recipient.

For vascular control, we use vascular clamps placed centrally on the renal vessels. An appropriate clamp is placed as far centrally as possible on the renal artery, and, immediately thereafter, a clamp is placed on the vena cava just beyond the junction with the renal vein. On the left, the venous clamp is placed over the aorta. Transection is accomplished, leaving approximately 3-mm to 5-mm cuffs on each structure, thus permitting adequate control of the vessels by vascular suture.

Once the kidney has been removed from the wound, it is immediately perfused with chilled electrolyte solution. We continue to use the lactated Ringer's solution containing procaine and heparin as originally described.[1] If nephrectomy has been carefully performed, the organ washes out immediately. We make a deliberate point of infusing at least 300 ml to be certain that the kidney is essentially bloodless, heparinized, and adequately cooled.

Once the kidney has been removed, the vessels are closed—the vena cava with a running figure-of-eight suture of Prolene, and double ligature of the artery. On the left side, the renal artery usually has been transected within 0.5 cm of the aorta. For this reason, the stump is closed with a running figure-of-eight vascular suture. It is imperative that the left renal vein be transected as far centrally as possible to eliminate a "stump" that could form a clot with

its attendant risk of pulmonary embolism. The wound is then closed. If a pneumothorax has occurred, closure is accomplished by apposing the diaphragm to the periosteum of the rib bed and aspirating the pleural space by a catheter placed through a pursestring suture.

Postoperative care is routine. Most donors are able to take fluids on the morning after the operation and are alimenting by the second postoperative day. Most leave the hospital before the sixth postoperative day.

The availability of kidneys from living-related donors continues to be important in renal transplantation because of superior allograft survival rates, particularly with HLA-identical combinations, and insufficient cadaveric organs to meet current needs. However, the use of kidneys from living-related donors involves a major ethical dilemma. Such procedures would be justified only if the surgical mortality and morbidity are extremely low and the long-term well-being of donors is not jeopardized. The living-related donor nephrectomy has been demonstrated to be a relatively safe procedure, although postoperative complications do occur. The complication rate has been reported from other centers to range from 15% to 56%.[2,4,5] However, most of these complications are minor, with no significant consequences thereafter. Spanos et al[4] reported a total complication rate of 28.2% in 287 healthy donors, including a 3.1% incidence of wound complications, an 8.7% incidence of lower urinary tract infection, and a 15% incidence of minor intrathoracic complications. Serious complications occurred in 4 patients (1.4%), including one case of pulmonary embolism and one case of deep thrombophlebitis. One patient developed glomerulonephritis 9 months after the donation, and another developed hemolytic-uremic syndrome 3 weeks following nephrectomy. All these patients recovered after proper treatment and no death occurred in this series.[4] Similar results have been confirmed by other researchers. Mortality following living-related donor nephrectomy is rare, although fatalities have been reported.[5]

REFERENCES

1. Anderson CF, Velosa JA, Frohnert PP et al: The risks of unilateral nephrectomy: Status of kidney donors 10 to 20 years postoperatively. Mayo Clin Proc 60:367, 1985
2. Farrell RM, Stubenbord WT, Riggio RR et al: Living renal donor nephrectomy: Evaluation of 135 cases. J Urol 110:639, 1973
3. Marchioro TL, Brittain RS, Hemann G et al: Use of living donors for renal homotransplantation. Arch Surg 88:711, 1964
4. Spanos PK, Simmons RL, Lempe E et al: Complications of related kidney donation. Surgery 76:741, 1974
5. Uehling DT, Wear JB: Complications of donor nephrectomy. J Urol 111:745, 1974

CHAPTER 18

Cadaver Kidney Organ Procurement

Neil Lempert

The shortage of organ donors has become an increasing problem for transplant centers. The advent of cyclosporine has increased the success of renal transplants, thereby compounding the already critical problem of organ donation.[21] The reduction of the federal speed limit and the increased use of seat belts have reduced the number of car accidents and fatal head injuries, resulting in further limitation of the availability of potential donors.[20]

The problem of kidney procurement is exacerbated by the increasing number of people receiving dialysis treatment, which increases by more than 6000 annually. Although the rate of transplantation has increased substantially, the number of people on dialysis will double within 10 years if a further increase in kidney transplantation does not occur.[4] Clearly there is a need to find solutions to the everincreasing need for organ donors.

CAUSES OF DONOR KIDNEY SHORTAGE

The shortage of organs for transplantation is of multiple causation. The Centers for Disease Control (CDC) estimates that there are 27,000 deaths per year under circumstances permitting easy retrieval of organs for transplantation.[38,48] The House Energy and Commerce Committee has recognized that organ procurement agencies have not been able to meet the growing need for donor placement created by scientific advances that have greatly increased the success of transplantations. This committee filed a report arguing for appropriate legislation:

Organs for transplantation must be obtained from patients who have tragically suffered from head injury. Many experts believe that there are over 20,000 such tragedies in the nation each year. However, fewer than 15 percent of these patients actually donate organs. The low organ donation rate is largely attributed to the lack of organization in the nation's organ procurement efforts. While those now involved in organ procurement activities work very hard, many areas of the nation do not have a strong, effective organ procurement "organization."[16]

Since the shortage of donors is obviously not due to a lack of suitable donors, the cause must lie elsewhere. The major cause is directly attributable to a failure to properly identify donors, obtain consent to donate, and retrieve organs from the supply of suitable donors.[17,48] Part of the problem is ignorance; there is a general lack of knowledge about the whole donor process on the part of both the public and the medical community.[21] Accompanying this lack of knowledge are clouds of misconceptions and fear about the issue. Basically, the public supports the idea of organ transplantation, but the thought of actually donating elicits a less enthusiastic response. The reason for the failure to obtain sufficient organs is, thus, a combination of negative public attitudes and an inefficient procurement system.[15,20,39]

One of the basic problems is the public's failure to will their organs. Nearly 94% of the population has heard of organ donation and transplantation, but only 19% of these people have willed their organs by carrying a signed donor card.[20] Since the number of willed donors is obviously insufficient, the responsibility of locating enough suitable donors is placed on the medical community and, more specifically, the procurement centers. To help rectify the problem, a Uniform Anatomical Gift Act has been enacted in all 50 states. This legislates that donor cards (which have been incorporated on some state's driver's licenses) that are signed by the holder and two witnesses are a legal instrument permitting physicians to remove organs after death is declared. However, this system has failed to generate sufficient donors to meet the growing need.[17,48] Although the number of donors obtained through donor cards is not large, the system does seem to prompt the discussion of possible donation within families. Discussing organ donation and how important it is to donate before a tragedy occurs is extremely important.[40,48] It is still the practice to not use a donor if the family objects, even if the potential donor has signed a donor card. This practice is not legally necessary but is used to avoid conflict and controversy.

Misconceptions and misunderstandings are a frustrating problem surrounding the organ shortage. The family of a brain-dead patient may refuse to donate an organ from the patient because they believe that there is hope of recovery or for religious reasons. However, whether or not a family eventually gives consent frequently depends upon how the subject of donation is presented. A compassionate approach to donation is an extremely important aspect of the donor retrieval process.[48] Equivocation on the part of the physician in declaring death while artificial ventilation is maintained will undoubtedly cause the family to withhold consent. If a physician tries to diminish the seriousness of a patient's condition in order to ease the pain of the family when death is declared, the family may refuse consent. While trying to comfort the family in a grievous time, the doctor may actually cause them to cling to the false hope of a miracle. Some people simply refuse to donate because of old superstitions and mistrust of the medical community.[48]

There are six major reasons why people do not donate their organs.[38]

1. Hastiness of organ retrieval and a feeling that declaration of death and immediate subsequent removal of organs interferes with the family's expression of grief
2. Mutilation
3. Fatalism and superstition
4. Religion
5. Age (people believe that they are too old to donate)
6. The thought never occurred to them

Misconceptions about liability also inhibit physician participation. With the increased number of lawsuits, physicians are hesitant to cooperate in the donation process. A request for help in procuring an organ is frequently ignored.[16] In addition to the fear of litigation, some physicians believe that organ donation is an added burden to their busy sched-

ules. Unfortunately, the procurement agencies are left with the never-ending task of educating medical practitioners and the public concerning the critical need for organs for transplantation[16] and providing the necessary informational system that a successful organ procurement program demands.

The problems faced by organ procurement facilities have not gone unnoticed. Several publicized cases of people in dire need of transplants have attuned the media to organ transplantation. There is growing awareness of the shortage of organ donors created by the media that has touched the political world—even President Ronald Reagan. Surgeon General C. Everett Koop held a workshop in 1983 to address the problems facing organ transplantation. He suggested that the American Hospital Association (AHA) and the Federation of American Hospitals (FAH) should require all member hospitals to institute policies to improve relations with procurement agencies. Koop also recommended that state health departments and the Joint Commission on Accreditation of Hospitals incorporate policies to determine potential donors and referral procedures into their certification process. A system that has already been established is the 24-hour hotline of the United Network for Organ Sharing (UNOS) Organization (telephone number, (1-800-24-DONOR or 1-800-24-ALERT). This is an information and referral service for doctors and nurses who are not affiliated with an organ procurement program.

REQUIRED REQUEST LAW

A new law has been enacted in many states, and recently on a federal basis, that has the potential to reduce the shortage of organ donors. This law requires hospitals to ask the family of a deceased patient for a donation of organs and tissue if the deceased is a suitable candidate for organ donation. A suitable candidate for donation would meet all the medical criteria of the screening process for potential donors. A patient is acceptable if the organs or tissues are useful not only for transplantation but also for research and educational purposes. In general, the law states the hierarchy of people to whom the request must be directed as follows: spouse, son/daughter over 21 years of age, a parent, brother/sister over 21 years of age, guardian of person of decedent death. Usually the request is not required if the hospital has previous knowledge of the decedent's or family's objection to such a donation. Also, if donation is contrary to a religious belief, the request is not mandatory.[26,29]

At present (December 1986), 28 states have

passed required request legislation during this calendar year. Two of the 30 states, New York[25] and Kentucky, have levied penalties for noncompliance. Nine states have incorporated an immunity from criminal prosecution clause in their laws. There has been approximately a 50% increase in donor referrals in those states that have enacted some type of required request law.

The required request system has the potential to increase organ procurement greatly, but there is still room for improvement. Lack of coordination, unclear policies, and vague lines of responsibility are major inhibiting factors. There is need for an active network of procurement agencies that would establish contacts over an increased area. Cooperation between these agencies would enhance the possibility of a successful transplantation.[39,47]

With the advent of the required request law, the necessity of providing an active organ procurement group is apparent. Organ procurement groups with in-service programs at multiple local hospitals are a necessity for the growth of the donor program. These in-service programs provide an organized, systematic approach to the education of local hospital nurses, physicians, and ancillary personnel. On a local level, the culmination of the required request law and local in-service programs has doubled cadaver harvesting during the past year.[18]

BRAIN DEATH

One of the obstacles faced by organ transplantation agencies is determining when a potential donor is dead and when the procurement process may proceed. From antiquity to the recent past, the heart was believed to be the central organ of the body. Therefore, with this organ's failure, the body would die. The determination of death was based on the definition:

The cessation of life, the ceasing to exist: defined by physicians as a total stoppage of the circulation of the blood, and a cessation of the animal and vital functions consequent thereupon, such as respiration, pulsation, etc.[36]

This quote from Black's Law Dictionary served as a definition for many years but has become obsolete. The advent of new technology has made apparent the need for a new definition.[37] If resuscitative efforts are only partially successful, a patient's heart may beat, but irreversible brain damage may have occurred. According to the old definition of death, these patients would have been "alive" because their hearts were beating. With the use of a ventilator and other supportive equipment, these "brain dead" patients can maintain circulatory function for days or months.[36]

The controversy created by this new technology centers around the definition of death applied to patients who are sustained on life support systems. Is a person technically alive if even one brain cell is active, or is the total death of the brain, including the brain stem important? Some say death is the irreversible loss of the capacity for consciousness and the irreversible loss of the capacity to breath. These functions depend upon cortical and brain stem function. Therefore, in this perspective, brain death requires both cortical and brain stem death.[31]

Using this definition of death, a patient on a ventilator who has lost the ability to breathe spontaneously and is unresponsive would therefore be considered dead. Fortunately, some guidelines have been established to aid in the determination of brain death. These guidelines have firm criteria defined, so, when fulfilled, death can be determined and support systems can be removed with the confidence that recovery is totally impossible.[6-8]

Contemporary descriptions and guidelines of brain death began in 1959 when a theory called *coma depasse* was written by Mollaret and Goulin.[22] Coma depasse was observed in patients with massive brain injuries who were being maintained by artificial respiration. These patients were unresponsive to external stimuli; disintegration of internal homeostatic mechanisms had occurred, and their EEG patterns were flat. From these observations, Mollaret and Goulin concluded that the patient was dead, but they failed to discuss a definition of death.

Since the theory of coma depasse, there have been more than 30 different groups of criteria for brain death proposed;[4] two are of special interest. The first is the Harvard Criteria for Brain Death. The Harvard Criteria were published by the Ad Hoc Committee of the Harvard Medical School in a paper titled, "A Definition of Irreversible Coma." In the paper, "irreversible coma" was stated as synonymous to "brain death syndrome." The criteria are as stated below:[36]

1. Unreceptivity and unresponsivity
2. Absence of spontaneous muscular movement or respiration
3. Absence of reflexes
4. Flat EEG

Unreceptivity and unresponsivity are determined by the absence of response to even painful external stimuli. A response of any level would include a groan, withdrawal of limb, or the quickening of respiration. The second criterion, absence of motion, refers to respiration, with special attention to any muscular movement or spontaneous breathing. If the patient was breathing with the aid of a ventilator, natural breathing could be observed by turning off the machine for intervals of 3 minutes. The fulfillment of the third criterion would be confirmed by the absence of pupillary responses, ocular movement, postural activity, swallowing, and vocalization. The EEG was used as a reinforcement of the other tests and was to be administered in intervals of at least 10 minutes. In the original report, the EEG was used as a confirmation of the previous tests, but 1 year later, a second report was published stating that the EEG was not essential.[30,32] Repetition of the entire process 24 hours later was also required. This repetition was to confirm that none of the clinical observations had changed. If the requirements had been met and no changes had occurred, the respirator could be removed, but only after death was formally declared.

The Harvard Criteria were very helpful in the search for guidelines to determine death, but as new knowledge was gathered, the guidelines needed to be refined. In November 1976, the Conference of Royal Colleges and Faculties of the United Kingdom endorsed a paper, "The Diagnosis of Brain Death," which has become known as the "UK Code." This paper outlined specific preconditions that must be fulfilled and certain exclusions that must be made if brain death is to be considered. This process was entirely clinical and an EEG was not required.[6,32]

The following is an outline of the UK Code:

1. Preconditions
   • comatose patient on ventilator
   • positive diagnosis of irremedial structural brain damage
2. Exclusions
   • hypothermia
   • severe metabolic or endocrine disturbances
3. Tests
   • absent brain stem reflexes
   • persistent apnea

To verify that the patient was in a coma and the condition was not drug related, it is necessary to obtain a detailed history and drug screen and allow sufficient time to eliminate the possibility of a persistent drug.[3,4] There could be very severe abnormalities detected in either the serum electrolytes, acid–base balance, or blood glucose concentration. If these abnormalities are detected, the patient would not be considered brain dead.[6] Under the UK Code, the following are the tests to confirm brain death:[7, 8]

1. Absent brainstem reflexes
   • pupils are fixed
   • absent corneal reflexes
   • absent vestibulocular reflexes
   • absent cranial nerve responses
   • absent motor responses within the cranial nerve distribution tested by adequate somatic stimulation
   • absent gag reflex
2. Apnea
   • measured by blood gases

Repetition of these tests was advisable if the diagnosis of brain death was not certain. Twenty-four hours between tests was suggested, but this interval is flexible, based on medical judgment. The use of an EEG was not necessary, and the decision to remove the life support system would be considered only after fulfilling the requirements previously stated. The consultation of a fellow physician was advised if there was any uncertainty in determining brain death. The UK Code has received wide acceptance.[3,4] In an addendum to the original report, it stated that "brain death represents the stage at which a patient becomes truly dead, because by then all functions of the brain have permanently and irreversibly ceased." In conclusion, the UK Code states that brain death signifies the patient's death regardless of the function of organs maintained by artificial means.[7] Since the publication of the UK Code, the work on brain death has not ceased. In 1981, more than half of the states had passed statutes that declared death on the basis of "irreversible cessation of all functions of the brain."[37] However these "definition of death" statutes were inconsistent and vague. The slight differences in terminology and form of each state's statute has created substantial confusion in the medical community.[49]

In an effort to clear the confusion surrounding the determination of death, the Uniform Definition of Death Act (UDDA) has been proposed.[37] Endorsed by the American Bar Association, the American Medical Association, The National Conference of Commissioners on Uniform State Laws, and the President's Commission for the Study of Ethical Problems in Medicine and Biomedical and Behavioral Research, the UDDA is stated that. . . . "An individual who has sustained either irreversible cessation of circulatory and respiratory functions, or irreversible cessation of all functions of the entire brain, including the brain stem, is dead. A determination of death must be made in accordance with accepted medical standards." This statement concerning accepted medical standards was added because the guidelines will have to change as new discoveries are made in the medical community.[35]

DONOR MANAGEMENT

Initially, a physician, nurse, or physician's associate should recognize a potential donor early enough to properly identify the donor and minimize organ damage. The local transplantation coordinator and, in some instances, the 24-hour toll-free lines for multiple organ donation (1-800-24-DONOR or 1-800-24-ALERT) and kidney donation (1-800-446-2726) will give advice if a local coordinator is not available. This input includes medical advice for maintenance of the donor, donor assessment, and proper affirmation and documentation of brain death. It is important to note when the legal time of death (i.e., brain death) is pronounced and certified.

Clearly, complicated conditions of drug and metabolic intoxication, hypothermia and shock and of young children demand that special precautions be maintained when applying neurologic criteria to the determination of irreversible brain death.

The evaluation and management of the cadaver donor becomes a reality at the time of the pronouncement of death. In general, cadaveric donors are young adults who have succumbed to cerebral vascular problems or fatal head injuries. An occasional patient with anoxic brain injury secondary to cardiac arrest or other forms of hypoxia may also be presented for donor evaluation. The established criteria for renal donation have included:

1. Age—6 months to 65 years
2. Absence of acute or chronic renal disease
3. No evidence of generalized sepsis—active or transmissible
4. No history of malignant neoplasms except for those primary cancer tumors confined to the central nervous system
5. Absence of significant diabetes mellitus
6. Acceptable renal function and urinalysis
7. Absence of peritoneal contamination

Using pediatric donors involves specialized technical problems with variable results. Early studies in 1979 indicated that pediatric donors of any age gave equivalent survival rates compared with adult donors.[12] However, with pediatric donors between 0 and 5 years of age, there appears to be a high incidence of primary nonfunction of the donor kidney. When kidneys with primary nonfunction were eliminated, the graft survival rate was greatly improved. Kidneys in the 0 to 2-year age group demand careful surgical techniques of harvesting, preservation, and transplantation,[13,34,53] and results may still not be optimal.[52] Kidneys from 2- to 5-year-old or older donors can be transplanted into adult recipients without an increase in acute tubular necrosis (ATN) or improved allograft survival.[9] Similarly, donors in the 6th decade of life have a similar higher rate of graft loss attributed to a high incidence of primary nonfunction.[11] In this group, however, careful evaluation and selection can provide an additional source of usable kidneys.[27]

Systemic or generalized abdominal sepsis precludes a potential donor from further consideration. However, donors with pneumonia or even bacteriuria resulting from catheter drainage of the bladder are often acceptable.[28]

Viral diseases in the donor are always of concern to the transplant surgeon because of the possible transfer to the recipient. Acquired immune deficiency syndrome (AIDS), hepatitis,[19] encephalitis, and Guillain-Barré syndrome therefore contraindicate organ donation. Kidneys from patients with Reye's syndrome,[10] however, have proved to be free of transmittable infection and function well in the host. In certain isolated instances, prior treatment for systemic infections in the donor with subsequent negative blood cultures and gram stains may permit donor utilization. For instance, a patient with previously treated meningococcemia has been harvested and the kidneys successfully transplanted. Meningococcus is unusual in that it is extremely sensitive to the cold. Therefore, when lymph nodes and kidneys are exposed to 7°C, the organisms uniformly die, thus rendering the lymph nodes safe for tissue typing and the kidneys free for transplantation.[18]

The cardinal points of renal donor management include the maintenance of excellent urine output with vigorous intravenous fluid replacement, central line placement for monitoring, and maintenance of an adequate blood pressure with the use of intravenous dopamine or Isuprel and the avoidance of Aramine or Levophed. Even high-dose dopamine has been shown to be detrimental in cadaver donor management.[54] The presence of diabetes insipidus requires treatment with aqueous Pitressin, 20 units in 500 ml fluid intravenously, to maintain urine output at 300 ml/hour to 500 ml/hour. Occasionally, diabetes mellitus may be present in the terminal patient and should be treated with intravenous insulin. In fact, mild diabetes mellitus is not considered a contraindication to organ donation, and one report suggests that pathologic changes in a diabetic kidney will reverse when placed in a nondiabetic recipient.[1] However, essentially normal renal function should be present in the diabetic donor under consideration for donation.

TECHNIQUE FOR DONOR NEPHRECTOMY

Prior to the time of bilateral nephrectomy, the donor chart is carefully checked for permissions and authorizations for postmortem examination. The need for postmortem examination to ascertain that the donor is free of both communicable or malignant disease cannot be overemphasized.[33] Even certain primary brain tumors, such as medulloblastoma, in pediatric patients have been known to metastasize.

The general principles of cadaver donor nephrectomy include optimal management of the donor, careful identification of the renal vasculature, and meticulous avoidance of interruption of the blood supply to the ureter. The assurance that disruption of the intima of the renal arteries is avoided can be accomplished by gentle dissection and particular care at the time of renal artery cannulation if individual arteries are cannulated. The principle of en bloc dissection and excision will allow for identification of multiple renal arteries, in particular a lower polar artery to the ureter. The avoidance of stripping the ureters or carrying the dissection of the ureter into the hilum will help to preserve the blood supply to the ureter. Similarly, the avoidance of excessive stretching or tension on the renal vessels will avoid intimal disruption.[2]

In the operating room, large volumes of fluids, diuretic agents, and mannitol are used to ensure a brisk diuresis.[24] Cardiovascular monitoring and the use of vasoactive agents may also be indicated to preserve blood pressure, reduce vasospasm, and promote renal blood flow and diuresis.[14]

When only the kidneys are to be removed, bilateral nephrectomy can be undertaken through a xiphoid to pubis incision with bilateral extensions. Frequently, it is expedient to also divide the sternum to ensure adequate exposure. The preference for most transplant surgeons includes en bloc removal of both kidneys with a segment of the aorta vena cava and both ureters. With this technique, the renal arteries need not be identified until the en bloc specimen is removed, at which time a careful dissection can easily be performed. Initially, exploration of the abdomen will include a careful estimation of the presence of any important pathology,

including infection or carcinoma. A record should be kept of the initial findings and recorded in the chart for the pathologist's use. The initial dissection includes mobilizing the right colon and small bowel over to the ligament of Treitz, with division of the inferior mesenteric vein. The colon and small bowel can then be retracted superiorly and to the left. The duodenum and pancreas are also retracted superiorly, and the proximal aorta and vena cava are isolated. If only the kidneys are removed, the celiac axis and superior mesenteric artery are ligated (Fig. 18-1). In liver excision for transplantation, the celiac axis and superior mesenteric artery are preserved. Tapes are then placed around the proximal vena cava (above the entrance of the right renal vein) and aorta (above the celiac axis).

Following the proximal dissection, the distal dissection is completed, freeing up long segments of ureters and then the distal aorta and vena cava. The flushing cannulas are inserted into the aorta and vena cava either through the iliac artery or directly into the aorta (Fig. 18-2). A cannula is also placed in the vena cava to allow egress of cooling fluid. Heparin (10,000 units) is given intravenously prior to cross clamping of the blood supply to the kidneys. The en bloc of kidneys, ureters, vena cava, and aorta is then removed, starting from the distal area and dissecting proximally. One has a choice of ligating the lumbar vessels or simply dividing them when the initial hypothermic flush is completed and the en bloc excision is undertaken. The kidneys are then freed up in the general fashion by incising through Gerota's fascia, care being taken not to strip the kidneys of their capsule or including all the perinephric fat, Gerota's fascia, and the adrenal glands with the specimen. When the kidneys and ureters are adequately isolated with special care being maintained not to dissect the ureters into the hilum of the kidneys, the en bloc dissection can then be completed in a relatively leisurely manner, providing that the kidneys are noted to be cold and well perfused. The kidneys are flushed during the dissection with several liters of Ringer's lactate containing 10,000 units of heparin per liter. Other researchers have added mannitol as well as other medications into the perfusate (see chapter concerning preservation). Following initial flushing with ice cold Ringer's lactate, the kidneys should be pale and cold; they are then flushed with a preservative solution if they are to be stored on ice. Observation that the kidneys have flushed poorly indicates the likelihood of ischemia and vasoconstriction and resulting acute ATN or cortical necrosis. Once free from the donor, the kidneys can be separated if they

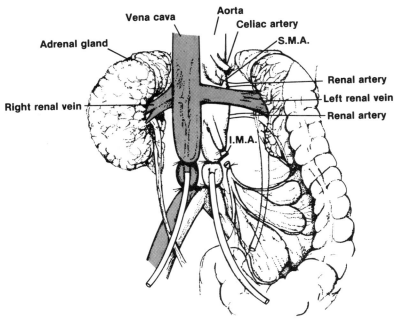

FIGURE 18-1.   *Ligation of the celiac axis and superior mesenteric artery.*

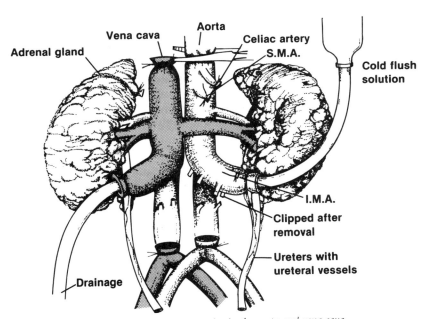

FIGURE 18-2.   *Placement of flushing cannulas in the aorta and vena cava.*

are to be stored on ice (Fig. 18-3), or they can be perfused through an intact aorta for storage by pulsatile perfusion.

If the donor undergoes cardiac arrest[42], a large-bore catheter is quickly inserted in the femoral ar-

tery, and voluminous amounts of ice cold Ringer's lactate with heparin (10,000 units/liter) are infused. The femoral vein is also cannulated to allow egress of blood and flushing solution. It is imperative that the kidneys be removed in this emergent technique

CHAPTER 19

Kidney Preservation by Perfusion

James H. Southard   Folkert O. Belzer

Continuous hypothermic perfusion of the kidney is a practical clinical method for organ preservation. The method utilizes a preservation machine designed to deliver perfusate to the organs at low flow and low pressure while maintaining the temperature of the perfusate and organ at 6°C to 10°C. Continuous perfusion supplies the organ with nutrients and oxygen and removes end products of metabolism. Many perfusion fluids have been shown to satisfactorily preserve the viability of the organ for 48 to 72 hours.

The essential components of successful perfusion perservation appear to be (1) hypothermia, (2) a colloid such as albumin to prevent tissue edema, (3) an osmolality of about 300 mOsm/liter obtained with electrolytes, hydrogen ion buffers, and other metabolites, and (4) low perfusion pressure (20 mm Hg–40 mm Hg).

Perfusate design must take into account metabolic needs but must also compensate for the detrimental effects of hypothermia on metabolism, such as (1) hypothermic-induced inhibition of the membrane-bound ion pumps (Na-pump) and loss of volume regulation, (2) loss of energy stores (ATP), (3) increased leakiness of cell membranes, and (4) ultrastructural changes in the kidney. Swelling in glomerular endothelial cells and loss of integrity of the endothelial epithelial (podocyte) cells result from perfusion and appear after 72 hours of preservation.

With the advent of cyclosporine, it has been increasingly necessary to transplant organs with minimal damage. Cyclosporine appears to be more toxic to organs with delayed graft function. Thus, there is a continual need to improve preservation techniques for the kidney to ensure immediate graft function. In the future, it may be possible to use longer term preservation (a week or more) to alter the immunogenicity of the organ and reduce the need for continual high-dose immunosuppression.

Kidneys were first clinically preserved by continuous perfusion during the late 1960s. Since then, perfusion preservation has greatly contributed to making kidney transplantation a relatively routine operation that is performed in more than 200 transplant centers in the United States and in many centers in Europe. During the 1970s, simple cold storage was increasingly used to preserve kidneys, but, in recent years, there has been a resurgence of interest in perfusion preservation. This renewed interest is partly a result of the increased use of Cyclosporine A for immunosuppression and the accompanying evidence that Cyclosporine A can induce nephrotoxicity,[49,88] especially in poorly preserved or damaged organs. In their efforts to secure

minimally damaged organs, to continue making transplant surgery semielective, and to increasingly share organs, a growing number of transplant centers are reconsidering continuous perfusion for renal preservation.

Preservation by continuous hypothermic perfusion offers both advantages and disadvantages relative to simple cold storage. Advantages include (1) extension of preservation time (72 hours vs. about 30 hours); (2) preservation of organs damaged by warm ischemia, (3) support of metabolism by regulating various processes and products (nutrient supply, osmotic and oncotic factors, O_2 availability, oxidation-reduction control, pH regulation, the removal of metabolic end products) and by adding potentially beneficial agents (e.g., superoxide anion scavengers) to the organ; (4) elimination of vasospasm; (5) thorough washout of blood and blood elements; (6) analyses of flow characteristics and perfusion-pressure changes as aids to monitoring the physiologic status of the organ;; (7) monitoring of rates of enzyme release from the organ as indications of cell damage; (8) regeneration of function in a damaged organ; (9) potential for decreasing the antigenicity of an organ; and (10) reduced incidence of delayed renal function after transplantation.

Disadvantages include (1) expense of preservation equipment and trained personnel; (2) possibility of technical failure (machine malfunction); (3) removal of cell constituents important for renal function; and (4) physical disruption of kidney architecture, especially the vascular system.

The quality of kidney preservation depends upon the quality of the organ before it is harvested. Kidneys damaged before they are harvested are more likely to function poorly during preservation and after transplantation. Once the kidney is removed from the body, irreversible cell death begins. Preservation retards this process but does not prevent it. A damaged organ will therefore undergo irreversible cell death more rapidly than an optimally harvested organ. The most likely method of preventing complete cell death is cryopreservation (at $-70°C$ to $-140°C$), but a suitable technique has yet to be developed. Even effective cryopreservation, however, will necessitate perfusion to introduce preservative agents into the kidney and to remove these agents before transplantation. Finally, the key to preservation is hypothermia, and an understanding of how hypothermia affects the physiology, biochemistry, and ultrastructure of the kidney is essential to improving current preservation techniques.

FLUSHING

A harvested kidney is flushed through the cannulated renal artery to remove blood and induce cooling. Fluids used for flushing typically include heparinized saline, Collins' solution, or lactated Ringer's solution. The fluid container is suspended 60 cm to 100 cm above the kidney, which is flushed with 200 ml to 500 ml of fluid or until it becomes blanched. Some studies suggest that large-volume flushing[13] and rapid cooling[45] are detrimental to renal function after preservation and transplantation. Rapid cooling is reported to induce renal vasospasm[34] and the loss of glycolytic enzyme activity.[35] Normothermic flushing has been reported to prevent vasoconstric-tion and to facilitate subsequent hypothermic flushing.[29]

Wusteman and associates[90] developed a flushing fluid that greatly improved the removal of blood from both fresh and kidneys damaged from ischemia. These investigators maintain that trapped erythrocytes become less flexible as they remain in the vasculature as ATP reserves are consumed. The hyperosmolar (400 mOsm/liter) fluid used in their study contained 50 g/liter of dextran-40, and high concentrations of magnesium (67 mEq/liter) and glucose (167 mmol/liter). Dextran improved the removal of blood only in kidneys damaged from ischemia.

PERFUSION MECHANICS

The mechanical systems for continuous perfusion are based on either a pulsatile or a continuous-delivery (roller) pump. As the names imply, pulsatile pumps deliver an intermittent flow of fluid, and roller pumps deliver a constant flow. The pulses are usually set at 60 per minute. The systolic pressure is initially set at 8 kPa (60 mm Hg), which usually results in a dyastolic pressure of 1.07 to 1.87 kPa (8 mm Hg–14 mm Hg). Perfusion pressure decreases to 5.33 kPa (40 mm Hg) during about the first hour of perfusion and remains constant for as long as 3 days. An increasing perfusion pressure usually signifies a damaged kidney and often results in poor post-transplantation function.[5,7] The exact cause of the rise in pressure is not known but is usually attributed to cell swelling. In our experience, a 3-day rise in perfusion pressure correlates well with poor preservation in the autotransplant model. The absence of a rise in pressure, however, does not necessarily indicate excellent preservation quality.

Kidneys damaged from ischemia usually have higher vascular resistance than freshly harvested organs.[32] In addition, organs exposed to hypotension can undergo vasoconstriction because of circulating catecholamines. Pretreating the donor with alpha-adrenergic blockers[87] has been shown to increase the renal cortical perfusion of damaged kidneys; Dibenzyline is used in our clinical transplantation unit.

In general, perfusion pressure should be as low as possible to avoid mechanically induced renal damage. Denuded basement membranes and a severely disrupted endothelium can occur in kidneys perfused at high pressures (8 kPa [60 mm Hg].)[20] The damage was decreased with lower perfusion pressure (4 kPa [30 mm Hg]) and higher colloid osmotic pressure (COP). Griffiths and colleagues[37] also found abnormal characteristics in kidneys perfused at high pressures and suggested that 2.8 kPa to 4.8 kPa (22 mm Hg–36 mm Hg) produced adequate perfusion. An examination of the relationship between perfusion pressure (pulsatile), fluid flow rate, change in kidney mass, and kidney function after transplantation indicates that a pressure of 2.67 kPa to 4.00 kPa (20 mm Hg–30 mm Hg) yields the smallest mass gain and the best postoperative renal function and is therefore, optimal.[39] The optimal flow rate seems to be 0.8 ml/min at an O_2 tension of 18.7 kPa (140 mm Hg).

Pulsatile flow has the advantage over continuous flow of exposing the vasculature to a transient high pressure that can reduce vasospasm and facilitate the removal of trapped blood products. Continuous pulsation may induce structural damage, however.[77] The debate over the relative benefits of pulsatile and continuous flow has not been fully resolved. In short-term perfusion experiments (24 to 48 hours), there appears to be little difference in post-transplantation function[1,38,54,65,83] when pulsatile and continuous techniques are compared. However, cold-stored (nonperfused) kidneys are often fully viable after 48 hours of preservation; thus, this period is not adequate to resolve the controversy.

OXYGEN

In addition to the pumping mechanism, perfusion machines include membrane oxygenators that use air, pure oxygen (O_2), or a mixture of O_2 and CO_2. The hypothermally induced depression of tissue metabolism eliminates the need for O_2-carrying compounds or cells, and the O_2 dissolved in the perfusate is adequate to support the energy demands of the kidney. Oxygen tensions provided by air (pO_2 = 16.0 kPa to 20.0 kPa [120 mm Hg–150 mm Hg]) and O_2 (pO_2 = 59.85 kPa to 86.45 kPa [450 mm Hg–650 mm Hg]) are much greater than required to support hypothermic metabolism. In fact, rabbit kidneys preserved 48 hours[64] and dog kidneys preserved 72 hours[8] were successfully transplanted when N_2 (pO_2 = 1.33 kPa to 2.67 kPa [10 mm Hg–20 mm Hg]) was used. Although O_2 may not be necessary for renal preservation under ideal conditions, it may be necessary for regenerating function in kidneys damaged by warm ischemia.[66] In this study, post-transplantation serum creatinines were significantly improved when damaged kidneys were perfused with O_2 (pO_2 = 86.45 kPa [650 mm Hg]). Understanding the role of O_2 in preservation quality

is complicated by the recent observation that kidneys cold stored are persufflated with O_2 were fully viable, but without O_2, they were less viable.[68] The role of O_2 apparently was not related to the stimulation of ATP synthesis, either during preservation or after normothermic reflow. It has been argued that excess O_2 during preservation could induce the generation of cytotoxic O_2-derived free radicals.[15,62] This response has been difficult to demonstrate experimentally, and O_2-induced tissue damage more likely occurs during reperfusion at normothermia.

TEMPERATURE

Hypothermia is the key to successful preservation, and the most commonly used temperature range for perfusion is 6°C to 10°C. At this temperature, metabolism is reduced by 90% to 95%,[52] thereby minimizing the need for a continual supply of substrates, nutrients, and so on. The optimal temperature for perfusion has not been systematically determined, in part because of the interrelationships among temperature, perfusion pressure, perfusate composition, O_2 tension, viscosity, and flow rates—all of which may affect the outcome. Higher temperatures may be more suitable for renal preservation[78] when all other relevant factors are changed to accommodate temperature effects on renal metabolism. Higher perfusion temperatures may necessitate the use of different oxidizable substrates (among other additives) not currently used in perfusates. Because of the large number of variables that must be considered in such a study, investigations are limited.

Perfusion machines also include perfusion chambers, a bubble trap, a temperature probe, and a pressure transducer. Currently, the only commercially available preservation machine (Waters Inc., Minneapolis, MN) uses pulsatile perfusion and a membrane oxygenator. The Gambro system, manufactured in Sweden and used primarily in Europe, is no longer produced, although the disposable sterile cassettes are still available for already existing machines. This machine used a roller pump for perfusion. The Belzer system (Belzer L1-400) was the first machine designed for kidney preservation and is no longer commercially available. We have designed a stainless steel cassette that replaces the disposable cassettes. These new cassettes are reusable and are shown in place in a Belzer L1-400 portable perfusion machine in Figure 19-1. A recently developed machine (AED Corp., Grosse Point, MI) uses a roller pump and a thermoelectric

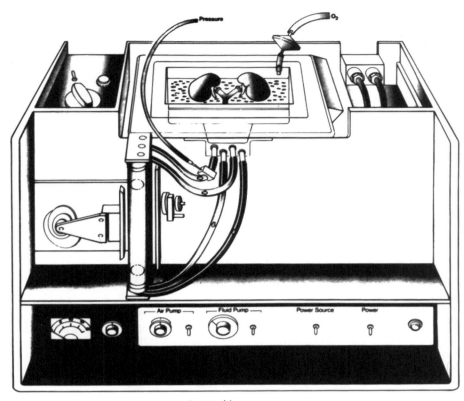

FIGURE 19-1. *Belzer L1-400 Preservation Machine.*

cooling unit, but it has not yet received adequate experimental testing.

PERFUSATES

The development of perfusates for renal preservation has held the attention of experimenters for many years. This interest is based on the idea that the composition of the perfusate is a critical determinant of successful preservation.

The successful 3-day preservation reported by Belzer and colleagues[6] depended upon modifying the plasma by cryoprecipitating the lipoproteins and subsequently removing them with ultrafiltration. Lipoproteins were implicated as the cause of increased perfusion pressure because they were trapped in the capillaries during perfusion.[7] Cryoprecipitated plasma (CPP) quickly became widely used for clinically preserving kidneys. But because CPP is difficult to prepare, lacks shelf stability, poses potential immunologic complications,[31] and is subject to hepatitis contamination, other investigators tried to develop simpler perfusates. Claes and Blohme[23] dem-

onstrated that a human-serum albumin (HSA)-containing perfusate could preserve kidneys for as long as 3 days. Similar results were reported for a plasma protein fraction (PPF) perfusate[46] and for a silica-gel fractionated plasma solution.[82] The components of these perfusates are shown in Table 19-1. A clinical, prospective trial comparing CPP, HSA, and PPF perfusates showed that they were equally effective.[22]

Recently, excellent 3-day preservation of dog kidneys was reported using a new perfusate containing HSA and a number of other agents not normally present in saline-based perfusates.[9] The perfusate was developed from laboratory studies on how several agents affect renal metabolism at 10°C. Chloride anions were replaced with gluconate anions (which have a higher relative molecular mass) to suppress hypothermally induced cell swelling. Adenosine and phosphate were included to stimulate energy metabolism in the hypothermally perfused organ.[75] The concentration of K was increased to 25 mmol/liter to suppress the hypothermally induced efflux of K from the cell. Glutathione was added to counteract the tendency of perfused kid-

TABLE 19-1   Composition of Common Perfusion Solution

SUBSTANCES(mM)	CPP	PPF	SGF	MSGF	HSA
Na$^+$	145	130	140	145	150
K$^+$	7	15	4.1	20	5
Mg^{2+}	5	6	5	16	5
Ca^{2+}	3.5	4.4	3.5	—	0
Cl$^-$	95	105	100	—	155
HCO$_3^-$	5	13	5.0	—	0
PO$_4^-$	—	—	—	—	0
Glucose	17	8.3	17	56	0
Mannitol	0	2.0	0	—	0
Protein (g/dl)	4.5	3.7	5.1	10.0	4.5
Antibiotics	+	+	+	+	+
Hydrocortisone (mg)	100	250	100	100	100
Insulin (unit)	80	100	40	40	80
*p*H	7.4	7.4	7.4	7.4	7.2
mOsm/liter	290	280	300	430–470	300

Abbreviations: CPP = cryoprecipitated plasma; PPF = plasma protein fraction; SGF = silica gel fraction of plasma; MSGF = modified slice gel; HSA = human serum albumin containing perfusate

neys to lose this component of the cell. The composition of the perfusate is shown in Table 19-2. This perfusate has had clinical use since 1982, with excellent results both in our hospital[11] and in another transplant center.[57] Human serum albumin (MW = 69,000) is a common colloid for kidney preservation solutions. However, the HSA can be replaced by hydroxyethyl starch (HES) (MW av = 250,000) and, in the laboratory, is as effective as the HSA-containing perfusate (Fig. 19-2). These results are comparable, or slightly better, than those obtained in the past with the CPP perfusate.

PRINCIPLES OF KIDNEY PRESERVATION

Continuous hypothermic perfusion is designed to continuously supply the organ with metabolites and remove the potentially toxic end products of metabolism. Hypothermia (6°C–10°C) significantly reduces metabolic rate and is the primary reason why preserved organs remain viable. Although metabolism continues at about 10% of the normal (normothermic) rate during hypothermia, the rates of different enzyme catalysis reactions are differently affected by reduced temperature. The rate-controlling steps at normothermia therefore may not be the same at hypothermia. Furthermore, membrane-bound enzymes are usually more affected by low temperatures than are soluble enzyme systems. This difference is apparently due to the temperature-induced decrease in membrane fluidity, which is related to the effect of temperature on the physical state of the membrane-bound lipids. A primary ex-

TABLE 19-2   Composition of Gluconate-Based Perfusate

SUBSTANCE	CONCENTRATION (mM)
Sodium gluconate	80
KH$_2$PO$_4$	25
Glucose	10
Glutathione	3
Magnesium gluconate	5
HEPES	10
CaCl$_2$	1.5
Adenosine	5
Phenol red (mg/liter)	12
Hydrocortisone (mg/liter)	12
Insulin (units/liter)	80
Penicillin (units)	200,000
Mannitol	20
Colloids*	
Human serum albumin (g/liter)	37.5
or	
Hydroxyethyl starch (g/liter)	50

* The perfusate used in the clinic contains albumin; the one used in the laboratory contains hydroxyethyl starch.
Final values: NA$^+$ = 130–135 mM; K$^+$ = 25 mM; *p*H = 7.4 (adjusted with NaOH); mOsm/liter = 130–320

ample is the hypothermic effect on the activity of the membrane-bound ion-transport system (i.e., the Na pump).[56,89]

Tissue swelling is another consideration in preservation, and there are two forms associated with hypothermic kidney perfusion. One is the actual swelling of cells; the other is the increase in the volume of interstitial spaces. Kidneys undergo a 20% to 40% increase in mass during hypothermic

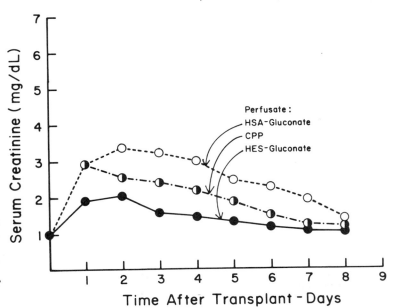

FIGURE 19-2. Serum creatinine values in dogs after transplantation with kidney preserved for 72 hours. Three perfusates were tested: (1) HSA: -Gluconate = A gluconate-adenosine = PO₄ perfusate; (2) CPP = cryoprecipitated plasma; (3) HES-gluconate = same as number 1 but with hydroxyethyl starch (5 g/dl) as the colloid. Kidneys were perfused for 72 hours and transplanted (autotransplant), followed by immediate contralateral nephrectomy. Six kidneys were used for each group.

perfusion—an increase caused by water in the cells, the interstitial spaces, and the dilated tubules. The interstitial edema results from an imbalance between the colloid osmotic pressure and the perfusion pressure (hydrostatic pressure). Albumin produces about 0.667 kPa (5 mm Hg) of oncotic pressure per gram. At albumin concentrations commonly used for preservation (3.5 g/dl–5.0 g/dl), the colloidal oncotic pressure is equivalent to 2.27 kPa to 3.33 kPa (17 mm Hg–25 mm Hg). Mean perfusion pressure is 1.07 kPa to 1.87 kPa (8 mm Hg–14 mm Hg), with a systolic pressure of 5.33 kPa (40 mm Hg). Based on mean pressure, albumin concentrations are sufficient to prevent fluid movement into the interstitial space. However, albumin can leak from the vascular space and increase tissue edema.

Cell swelling results from a decrease in the activity of the Na pump, and possibly from hypothermic effects on the permeability of the cell membrane. Potassium leaks out of the cell; the exchanged Na does not cause a change in the intracellular osmolality and does not induce cell swelling. However, the inefficient pumping of electrolytes causes a decrease in the membrane potential. Chlorine anions are thus free to enter the cell down a concentration gradient and to maintain electroneutrality; Na enters the cell. The increase in Na and Cl causes an increase in osmolality, which in turn results in the influx of water and thus causes cell swelling. Cell swelling alone is tolerated by the cell,

at least for a short time. However, swelling can stretch the membrane and cause intracellular components necessary for cell metabolism to leak from the cell. Amino acids,[55] glutathione,[14] free fatty acids,[67,71] coenzymes,[70] and intracellular enzymes leak from perfused kidneys. Localized cell swelling in the kidney is possible, and swelling in endothelial cells may be more pronounced than in parenchymal cells. Swollen endothelial cells have been seen in electron micrographs of preserved kidneys and may be responsible for the loss of endothelial integrity associated with preservation. Perfusion-induced cell swelling can be suppressed by impermeants such as mannitol, sucrose, phosphate, sulfate, and gluconate. The use of uncharged compounds, such as mannitol, requires hyperosmolar conditions that may be detrimental to the function of the organ when it is reperfused. The use of monovalent impermeant anions allows the design of an iso-osmotic perfusate.

ADENINE NUCLEOTIDE METABOLISM

Adenine nucleotide metabolism is altered during hypothermic preservation, with a resultant loss of ATP.[4,25,27,74] The cell membrane is permeable to the breakdown products of ATP (adenosine, inosine, and hypoxanthine), which are flushed from the kidney during perfusion (Fig. 19-3).[16,17] This loss of ATP does not appear to result from an uncoupling

METABOLISM OF ADENOSINE

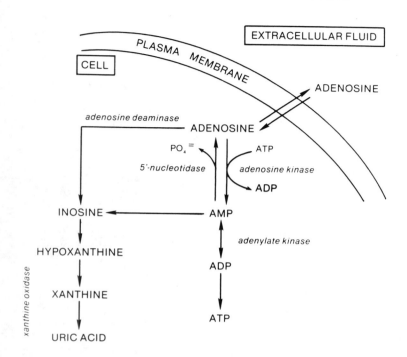

FIGURE 19-3.   *Catabolic pathway for adenine neucleotides.*

of mitochrondria[78] but, instead, from the effect of hypothermia on adenine nucleotide translocase, which limits the rate of ATP synthesis. As a consequence, ADP accumulates in the cell and is metabolized to AMP by adenylate kinase. The AMP is further catabolized to oxypurines. The loss of ATP poses two problems for renal metabolism: (1) the lack of energy during preservation, and (2) the lack of energy during reperfusion. Although there have been attempts to correlate the extent of ATP loss with kidney viability,[4,18,76] no convincing relationship has been demonstrated. It is possible to show that renal function is improved by maintaining the ATP concentration during preservation;[74,76] however, this maneuver does not improve transplantation results. It is likely, therefore, that multiple lesions are responsible for poor renal function after preservation and that they all need to be corrected at the same time to improve function after transplantation.

SUBSTRATE REQUIREMENTS

Mitochondrial respiration is reduced by hypothermia, but the oxidative reactions necessary for the generation of ATP continue to occur. The kidney therefore needs a supply of O_2 and oxidizable substrates. Oxygen consumption, at five different experimental pressures, remains relatively constant at about 1 µg/(g·min) over a 72-hour perfusion period.[39] This constancy is probably related to the low rates of glomerular filtration and Na reabsorption that occur at the low perfusion pressures of renal preservation. At hypothermia, the O_2 requirement of the kidney is about 0.05 µmol/(g·min). At 10°C the O_2 content of a perfusate is about 0.4 µmol/ml when equilibrated with air at a partial pressure of 20 kPa (150 mm Hg). Therefore, a flow rate of 1 ml/(g·min) would supply the kidney with about eight times the O_2 required for sustaining oxidative metabolism. At normothermia, the kidney metabolizes primarily fatty acids and glucose. At 10°C, the kidney metabolizes primarily short-chain fatty acids, such as octanoate[43,44] and ketone bodies.[43] The importance of free fatty acids for preservation is not clear, and contradictory results have been reported.[40,72] A doubled concentration of free fatty acids in normal serum albumin causes an uncoupling of mitochondrial oxidative phosphorylation and poor preservation.[24] However, 3-day preservation is possible without adding any oxidizable substrate to the perfusate, an observation that suggests that the kidney uses endogenously stored metabolites to support respiration.[42] The finding that perfused kidneys lose phospholipids[43,73] and free fatty acids also indicates that endogenous lipid metabolism fuels respiration. The activation of phospholipid degradation during preservation could produce changes in the membrane-bound phospholipids and damage the membrane. Phospholipase activation occurs in ischemic organs[21] and can be prevented with drugs, such as chlorpromazine.[59] Glucose is apparently metabolized very slowly in hypothermally perfused kidneys and may not be a necessary ingredient of perfusates. But cellular glucose may be important for metabolism during the beginning of normothermic reperfusion.

MAINTENANCE OF A NORMAL INTRACELLULAR COMPOSITION

Maintaining the internal environment of the cell is essential for maintaining the viability of the cell. Several essential metabolites, including carbohydrates, amino acids, proteins, lipids, cofactors, metal ions, and various organic compounds, are sequestered within the cell or subcellular compartments. The cell expends considerable energy maintaining the concentrations and ratios of these elements that are necessary for normal cell functions. Continuous hypothermic perfusion causes a disequilibrium in cellular reaction rates and changes the properties of cellular membranes; consequently, it alters the "interior milieu." The selective permeability and ionic pumps of the cell membrane largely determine the intracellular composition of the cell. Both of these membrane functions are altered at low temperatures. Thus, it might be expected that hypothermic perfusion would dramatically alter the internal composition of the cell. There is some evidence to support this hypothesis, but, clearly, more work is needed.

Potassium (K) is lost from the cell during continuous perfusion because the Na pump is suppressed.[56] The rate at which K leaks from the cell can be substantially reduced by increasing the external concentration of K from 15 mmol/liter to 25 mmol/liter.[47] This increase results in some suppression of the efflux of K during organ perfusion. The effects of perfusion on the efflux of only a few other metabolites have been studied. Glutathione is rapidly released from normothermally perfused kidneys,[14] and probably from hypothermic kidneys as well. Amino acids,[55] lipids,[67,71] cholesterol,[48] and coenzyme A[70] are also depleted from the tissue during perfusion. Krebs[50] suggested that the optimal perfusion of organs necessitates the smallest possible

volume of perfusate, because the tendency to disrupt the equilibration of important metabolites is reduced under these conditions.

Studies on the efflux of enzymes from the cell provide additional evidence for the efflux of metabolites from the kidney. Lysosomal enzymes and lactic dehydrogenase (LDH) are more active in the perfusate during perfusion.[6,63,78] The amount of LDH released from the kidney during perfusion ranges from about 50 mU to 400 mU/(ml·day). Kidneys exposed to warm ischemia show a greater tendency to release LDH during perfusion. Efforts to correlate viability with the release of LDH have been unsuccessful.

Maintaining an ideal intracellular *p*H should be easier during perfusion than during simple cold storage, because the perfusate can be buffered with phosphate, bicarbonate-CO_2, or buffers such as TRIS and HEPES. The ideal *p*H for renal preservation appears to be somewhat higher than that for normal physiologic function (*p*H 7.5).[19]

ULTRASTRUCTURE OF THE PERFUSED KIDNEY

The relationship between ultrastructural changes in the kidney and damage from perfusion preservation is not entirely clear. Perfusion-induced mechanical damage to the organ may be one factor limiting excellent, long-term preservation. Of particular concern is the effect of perfusion on the vascular endothelium. A disruption of the endothelial lining of the vasculature can cause the formation of blood clots, suppress reflow to the organ, and lead to renal failure. The importance of keeping the endothelium intact was recognized early in the history of preservation research,[33] and perfusates must be designed to protect the endothelium.

There have been few attempts to explain the relationship between perfusion damage and ultrastructural changes in the kidney. Electron microscopy biopsies of allografts 1 hour after transplantation from kidneys preserved by pulsatile perfusion show evidence of endothelial cell damage, including breaks in the lining, areas of complete endothelial denudation, and bared areas of the basement membrane.[41] Damage is less severe in kidneys preserved by simple cold storage. High perfusion pressure or low levels of colloids causes severe endothelial disruption.[20] Cold-stored kidneys do not show the glomerular changes seen in perfused kidneys, but all kidneys show evidence of damage to the proximal tubules. The normal appearance of perfused kidneys 3 months after transplantation is evidence for the

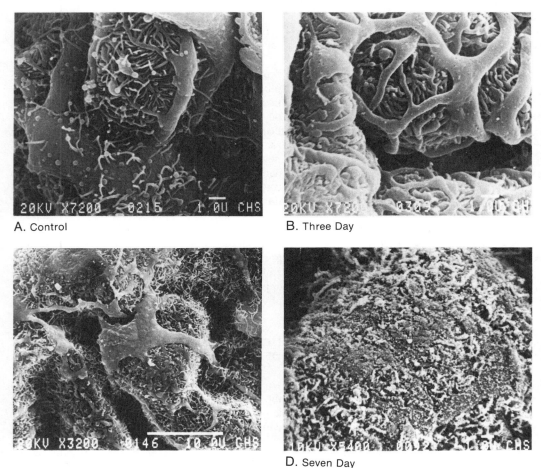

A. Control   B. Three Day

D. Seven Day

FIGURE 19-4.   *Effect of perfusion preservation on the surface morphology of dog kidney glomerular epithelial cells (podocytes). Dog kidneys were perfused for 0 to 7 days with a perfusate containing hydroxyethyl
starch. Following preservation, the kidneys were perfused, fixed with glutaraldehyde and processed for scanning electron microscopy. (A) Freshly harvested kidney (mag = 7200×, bar = microns); (B) Three-day
perfused kidney at a pressure of 40 mm Hg (systolic); (C) Five-day perfused kidney (mag = 3200×); (D)
Seven-day perfused kidney (mag = 5400×). The podocyte structure (cell body, primary to tertiary foot processes) appears normal after 3 days of preservation. After 5 days of preservation, the foot processes no longer
appear to interdigitate around the glomerular vessels, although they appear to be intact. By 7 days, the
podocytes have lost their characteristic shape and show many blebs and an amorphus character.*

repair of perfusion-induced damage.[69] Morphologic
studies of kidneys preserved for 7 days show some
beading of the endothelium, but endothelial cells
formed a continuous layer over the basement membrane of the glomerulus.[58] The epithelium shows
retracted foot processes, and the tertiary foot processes have villous extensions into Bowman's space.
However, the glomerular damage seen in pretransplant biopsies is similar for both cold-stored and
perfused kidneys.[53] However, kidneys perfused for
60 hours have tubular necrosis, fused glomerular
epithelial foot processes, and bulbous projections on
the glomerular endothelium.[30] Cold storage and
perfusion for as long as 7 days clearly affect the
ultrastructure of canine kidneys.[77] The major ultrastructural damage found in perfused kidneys is confined to the glomerular epithelial cells and appears
most severe after 5 to 7 days of perfusion (Fig.
19-4). Cold-stored kidneys show no such damage
(Fig. 19-5). It is known that kidneys cold stored for
7 days are nonviable, yet the architecture of the
podocyte appear well preserved. This suggests that
metabolic damage, by itself, does not induce major
changes in the surface morphology of the kidney.

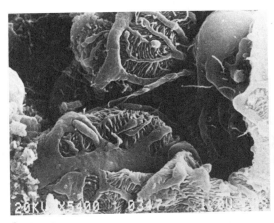

A. One Day

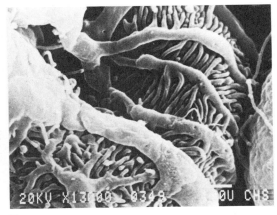

B. Three Day

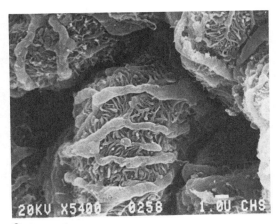

C. Seven Day

FIGURE 19-5.   Effect of cold storage on the surface morphology of dog kidney glomerular epithelial cells (podocytes). Dog kidneys were cold stored for 1 to 7 days in Collins' solution; this was followed by vascular flushout with glutaraldehyde. Notice that even after 7 days of preservation, the podocytes still retain a normal-appearing architecture.

Therefore, the combination of metabolic damage and perfusion pressure must be responsible for the architectural changes. Preliminary studies in our laboratory indicate that on reperfusion of cold-stored kidney, changes in the morphology of the podocyte occur that are similar to those seen in Figure 19-4C and D.

The surface morphology of kidneys perfused or cold stored for up to 7 days is shown in Figures 19-6 and 19-7. The endothelium remains intact for up to 5 days of perfusion and 3 days of cold storage. Prolongation of the preservation then causes endothelial cell swelling and widening of the fenestrations. These changes may account for the increased tendency for blood clot formation or reperfusion of kidneys perfused for long periods of time.

FUTURE OF KIDNEY PERFUSION

Kidneys are fully viable after 3 days of perfusion, although the serum creatinine of the recipient is usually elevated for at least a week after transplantation. The renal damage induced by perfusion preservation is usually fully reversible, however. Many permutations of preservation methods, perfusate compositions, and so on have been tried, in our laboratory and in others, without consistent improvement in either the quality of function or the duration of preservation. There is an ongoing need for research to minimize kidney damage during preservation and to extend preservation time to 7 days or more. The development of long-term preservation will open new research into methods of

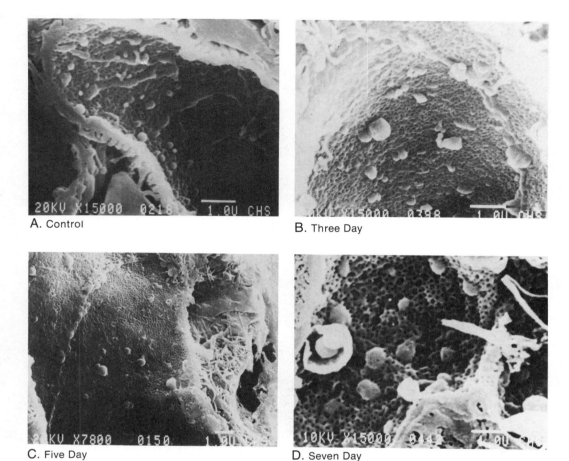

A. Control   B. Three Day   C. Five Day   D. Seven Day

FIGURE 19-6.   Effect of perfusion preservation on the morphology of kidney glomerular endothelium. Dog kidneys were perfused as described in Figure 19-4. The endothelial fenestrations appear similar to control kidneys (A) after 3-day (B) and 5-day (C) preservation. By the seventh day (D), the endothelium shows evidence of disruption, including swelling and widening of the endothelial fenestrations.

modifying the immunogenicity of the organ and of reducing the need for continual immunosuppression therapy, which remains a major problem for transplant recipients.

LIVER PRESERVATION

Preservation of the liver has not been as successful as preservation of the kidney. Recent successes obtained clinically with liver transplantation have placed renewed emphasis on the development of techniques that will increase the safe time of preservation. Unlike the kidney, the liver must function almost immediately after transplantation and, therefore, must undergo minimal damage during preservation. Currently, the safe period of preservation is only 6 to 8 hours. This limits the number of livers available to a transplant center, makes the surgery an emergency procedure often performed late at night, and requires two surgical teams, one for the harvest and one for the transplant. Preservation periods of 24 hours or greater would increase the number of livers available, make the surgery semi-elective, and provide time for prospective tissue crossmatching.

Cold storage is the method currently used to preserve the liver clinically. Starzl's group[12] in Pittsburgh uses a Collins' solution and Calne's group[86] in Cambridge, England uses a PPF solution. Attempts to extend the preservation time beyond 6 to 8 hours by cold storage have been disappointing; only limited success has been obtained with 24-hour preservation in the dog model.[51,60] Perfusion

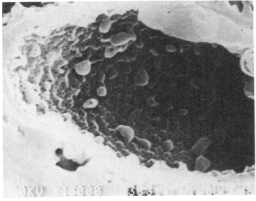

A. One Day

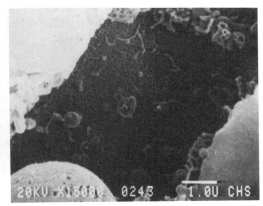

B. Three Day

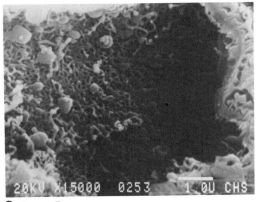

C. Seven Day

FIGURE 19-7. *Effect of cold storage on the morphology of kidney glomerular endothelium. Dog kidneys were cold stored as described in Figure 19-5. The endothelium appears relatively intact up to 3 days of cold storage but shows signs of swelling and widening of the fenestrations after 3 days.*

preservation has also not been particularly successful. Belzer and associates[10] obtained successful 10-hour preservation using cryoprecipitated plasma as the perfusate, but all pigs died with excessive bleeding with livers preserved for 17 to 18 hours. Other attempts, using perfusates similar to kidney preservation solutions, have also not been consistently successful.[80] Although perfusion preservation of the liver is more difficult than simple cold storage, a number of reports suggest that for longer-term storage, this method may be required.[28,36]

Because liver transplantation has become clinically successful with 1-year graft survival of 60% to 80%, there is renewed interest in its preservation methods. In the near future, methods should be developed that are clinically applicable and that yield successful 24-hour or more preservation.

HEART PRESERVATION

The heart, like the liver, has little time to regain function following preservation. Thus, for successful heart preservation, little or no preservation damage can be tolerated. With an increasing number of transplant centers performing heart transplants, the need for a reliable preservation method for 24 hours is obvious. Simple cold storage is the method of choice for clinical heart preservation.[2] This method allows about 5 to 7 hours of storage. Many attempts to increase preservation times by cold storage[81] have not met with much success. Perfusion preservation methods have resulted in successful 24-hour preservation in the orthotopic and heterotopic dog model.[26] The perfusion solutions resemble those developed for the kidney. However, these methods have not been developed for clinical testing because of the question of reliability of the quality of preservation.

PANCREAS PRESERVATION

Transplantation of the pancreas to reverse the consequences of diabetes is increasing in popularity owing to increased graft survival. The whole or segmental pancreas is preserved by simple cold storage using Collins' kidney preservation solution. The limit to preservation is about 6 hours. Pancreatic islet cells (beta-cells) appear to be quite tolerant to cold storage, and they can even be successfully frozen and thawed. Recently, successful 72-hour preservation of the pancreas has been reported with dogs surviving in a normoglycemic state for at least 4 to 6 months.[84] The solution used was a modification of the Belzer kidney perfusion solution and was designed primarily to prevent reperfusion edema of the transplanted pancreas.[85] A large–molecular weight anion (lactobionate) was used in combination with raffinose and K as the major cation. This solution is currently undergoing clinical testing in our center. This method of simple cold storage appears adequate for pancreas preservation.

CLINICAL UTILIZATION OF PERFUSED ORGANS

The kidney is currently the only organ clinically perfused prior to transplantation. In the early 1970s, the number of transplant centers that used perfusion preservation far outnumbered those that used simple cold storage. This changed, however, in the late 1970s, and about two thirds of the transplant centers used simple cold storage. This was due, in part,

to studies that showed no advantage to perfusion versus cold storage[61] in clinical transplantation. Also, most centers were transplanting kidneys within 24 hours of harvest. Furthermore, perfusion techniques were considered cumbersome and not convenient for transporting kidneys between centers. Thus, with the formation of large networks for kidney sharing, a simple transportation system was desired, such as provided by simple cold storage.

Perfusion preservation may, however, be regaining popularity. This is due to the recognition that perfusion is less damaging to initial renal function than cold storage, and this fact is important when cyclosporine is used for immunosuppression. The nephrotoxicity of cyclosporine appears exacerbated in damaged organs.[44] Additionally, development of a new perfusion fluid,[35] which yields excellent clinical results,[11] has also stimulated other centers to renew use of perfusion preservation.[3, 57]

Most kidneys are transplanted within 24 hours, and, in our center, the average perfusion time is about 36 hours. Kidneys have been transplanted in our center with up to 60 hours of perfusion with results equal to those perfused for shorter times. Acute tubular necrosis or delayed graft function results are variable between centers and range from less than 12% (in our center) to 40%. Barry and co-workers[3] reported an 89% dialysis rate in patients receiving kidneys preserved for 48 hours by cold storage and 30% for 24-hour cold storage. Nonutilization rates are also variable; in our center, it is only about 1%. Furthermore, many of our kidneys are harvested from non–heart-beating cadavers with warm ischemic times on average 25 minutes. These kidneys are perfused an average of 36 hours with no increase in delayed graft function or the need for postoperative dialysis when compared with kidneys harvested from ideal donors.

REFERENCES

1. Abouna CN, Pashly DH, Grensburg JM et al: Kidney preservation by hypothermic perfusion with albumin versus plasma and with pulsatile versus nonpulsatile flow. Br J Surg 61:555, 1974
2. Angell WW, Shumway NE: Resuscitative storage of the cadaver heart transplant. Surg Forum 17:224, 1966
3. Barry JM, Fischer S, Lieberman C et al: Successful human kidney preservation by intracellular electrolyte flush followed by cold storage for more than 48 hours. J Urol 129:473–474, 1983
4. Beck TA: Machine versus cold storage preservation

and TAN versus the energy charge as a prediction of graft function post-transplant.
5. Belzer FO, Ashby BS, Downes GL: Lactic and dehydrogenase as an index of future function of cadaveric kidneys during isolated perfusion. Surg Forum 19:105–106, 1968
6. Belzer FO, Ashby BS, Dumphy JE: 24-hour and 72-hour preservation of canine kidneys. Lancet 2:536–539, 1967
7. Belzer FO, Ashby BS, Huang JJ et al: Etiology of rising perfusion pressure in isolated organ perfusion. Ann Surg 168:383–391, 1968

8. Belzer FO, Hoffmann RM, Southard JH: Aerobic and anaerobic preservation of kidneys. In Pegg DE, Jacobsen IA, Halasz NA (eds): Organ Preservation Basic and Applied Aspects, pp 253–260. Lancaster, Boston, The Hague, MTP Press, 1982

9. Belzer FO, Hoffmann RM, Southard JH: A new perfusate for kidney preservation. Transplantation 33:322–323, 1982

10. Belzer FO, May RE, Berry A et al: Short-term preservation of porcine liver. J Surg Res 10:55–61, 1970

11. Belzer FO, Sollinger HW, Glass NR et al: Beneficial effects of adenosine and phosphate in kidney preservation. Transplantation 36:633–635, 1984

12. Benichou J, Halgrimson CG, Starzl TE: Canine and human liver preservation for 6 to 18 hours by cold infusion. Transplantation 24:406, 1977

13. Bradley JW, Zalnerailis BP, Franklin C et al: The effect of initial flushing solutions on kidney preservation. Dial Transplant 13:706–709, 1984

14. Brezis M, Rosen S, Silva P et al: Selective glutathione depletion on function and structure of the isolated perfused rat kidney. Kidney Int 24:178–184, 1983

15. Bry WI, Collins GM, Halasz NA et al: Improved function of perfused rabbit kidneys by prevention of oxidative injury. Transplantation 38:579–583, 1984

16. Buhl MR, Jorgensen S: Breakdown of 5' adenine nucleotides in ischemic renal cortex estimated by oxypurine excretion during perfusion. Scand J Clin Lab Invest 35:211–217, 1975

17. Buhl MR, Kemp G, Kemp E: Hypoxanthine excretion during preservation of rabbit kidneys for transplantation. Transplantation 21:460–465, 1976

18. Calman KC: The prediction of organ viability: 2. Testing an hypothesis. Cryobiology 11:7–12, 1974

19. Carter JN, White FN, Collins GM et al: Studies of the ideal [H$^+$] for perfusional preservation. Transplantation 30:409–410, 1980

20. Cerra FB, Raza S, Andres GA et al: The endothelial damage of pulsatile renal preservation and its relationship to perfusion pressure and colloid osmotic pressure. Surgery 81:534–540, 1977

21. Chien KR, Abrams J, Serrone A et al: Accelerated phospholipid degradation and associated membrane dysfunction in irreversible, ischemic liver cell injury. J Biol Chem 253:4809–4817, 1978

22. Cho SI, Bradley JW, Garoroy MR et al: Prospective controlled trial of cryoprecipitated plasma, plasma protein fraction and serum albumin solution for kidney preservation. Br J Surg 141:440–445, 1981

23. Claes G, Blohme I: Experimental and clinical results of continuous albumin perfusion of kidneys. In Pegg DE (ed): Organ Preservation II, pp 51–57. Edinburgh, London, New York, Churchill Livingstone, 1973

24. Cohen GL, Burdett K, Hunt L et al: Uncoupling of oxidative phosphorylation by octanoic acid during 5-day hypothermic kidney preservation. Cryobiology 21:699–700, 1984

25. Collste H, Bergstrom J, Hultman E et al: ATP in the cortex of canine kidneys undergoing hypothermic storage. Life Sci 10:1204–1206, 1971

26. Cooper DRC, Wicomb WW, Rose AG et al: Orthotopic allotransplantation and autotransplantation of the baboon heart following 24-hour storage by a portable hypothermic perfusion system. Cryobiology 20:385–394, 1983

27. Cunarro JA, Johnson WA, Uehling DT et al: Metabolic consequences of low-temperature kidney preservation. J Lab Clin Invest 88:873–884, 1976

28. D'Alessandro A, Southard JH, Kalayoglu M et al: Comparison of cold storage and perfusion of dog livers on function of tissue slices. Cryobiology 23:161–167, 1986

29. Das S, Maggio AJ, Sacks SA et al: Effects of preliminary normothermic flushing on hypothermic renal preservation. Urology 15:505–508, 1979

30. Evans AP, Gattone VH II, Fila RS et al: Glomerular endothelial injury related to renal perfusion: A scanning electron microscopic study. Transplantation 35:436–440, 1983

31. Filo RS, Dickson LG, Suba EA et al: Immunologic injury induced by ex vivo perfusion of canine renal autografts. Surgery 76:88–100, 1974

32. Flax SW, Webster JG, Updike SJ et al: Renal perfusion dynamics during perfusion. Ann Biomed Eng 6:68–77, 1978

33. Folkman J: Foreword. In Norman JC (ed): Organ Perfusion and Preservation, p 31. New York, Appleton-Century-Croft, 1968

34. Fonteles MC, Karow AM: Vascular alpha-adrenotropic response to the isolated rabbit kidney at hypothermia. Arch Int Pharmacodyn Ther 227:195, 1976

35. Francanlla A, Brown JH, Fore R et al: Preservation of organs for transplantation. Evidence of detrimental effect of rapid cooling. Eur Surg Res 5:384–389, 1973

36. Fuller BJ, Attenburrow VD: The effects of hypothermic storage of liver by continuous perfusion and simple portal flushing on hepatic protein synthesis and urea production in the rat. In Pegg DE, Jacobsen IA (eds): Organ Preservation II, pp 278–291. Edinburgh, Churchill Livingstone, 1979

37. Griffiths GJ, Kormano M, Morris T: Relationship of perfusion pressure to the microcirculation of the preserved canine kidney. Invest Radiol 12:338–347, 1977

38. Grundman R, Pitschi H, Berr F: Nonpulsatile vs pulsatile canine kidney perfusion. Surgery 75:178–182, 1974

39. Grundman R, Rabb M, Meuse E et al: Analysis of the optimal perfusion pressure and flow rate of the renal vascular resistance and oxygen consumption in the hypothermic perfused kidney. Surgery 77:451–461, 1975

40. Halasz NA, Collins GM: Fatty acid utilization during perfusion. Transplantation 23:354–355, 1975

41. Hill GS, Light JA, Perloff LJ: Perfusion-related injury in renal transplantation. Surgery 79:440–447, 1976

42. Hoffmann RM, Southard JH, Lutz MF et al: 72-hour preservation of dog kidneys using a purely synthetic perfusate containing hydroxyethyl starch. Arch Surg 118:919–921, 1983

43. Huang JS, Downes GL, Belzer FO: Utilization of fatty acids in perfused hypothermic dog kidneys. J Lipid Res 12:622–625, 1971

44. Jablonski P, Harrison C, Howden B et al: Cyclosporine and the ischemic rat kidney. Transplantation 41:147–151, 1986

45. Jacobsen IA, Chemnitz S, Kemp E et al: The effect of cooling rate during perfusion on function and morphology of rabbit kidney grafts. Scand J Urol Nephrol (Suppl) 54:90–92, 1980

46. Johnson RWG, Anderson M, Fear CTG et al: Evaluation of a new perfusate solution for kidney preservation. Transplantation 13:270–275, 1972

47. Johnson RWG, Anderson M, Taylor RMR et al: The assessment of renal injury prior to transplantation. In Pegg DE (ed): Organ Preservation, pp 191–207. Edinburgh, London, New York, Churchill Livingstone, 1973

48. Kleist H, Jonsson O, Lunstam S et al: Metabolism in the hypothermically perfused kidney: Utilization of mevalonate in the human and in the dog kidney. Eur Surg Res 14:236–244, 1982

49. Klintmalm G, Bohman S-O, Sundelin B et al: Interstitial fibrosis in renal allografts after 12–46 months of cyclosporin treatment: Beneficial effects of low doses in early post-transplantation period. Lancet 2:950, 1984

50. Krebs HA: Metabolic requirements of isolated organs. Transplant Proc 6:1237–1239, 1974

51. Lambotte L, Pontegnie-Intase S, Otte JB et al: The effect of isoproterenol and Collins' solution on the preservation of canine livers with simple cooling. Transplant Proc 6:301, 1974

52. Levy MN: Oxygen consumption and blood flow in the hypothermic, perfused kidney. Am J Physiol 197:111–114, 1959

53. Limas C, Spector D, Wright JR: Histologic changes in preserved cadaveric renal transplants. Am J Pathol 88:403–427, 1977

54. Lokkegaard H, Gyrd-Hansen N, Hansen RI et al: Kidney preservation with pulsatile and nonpulsatile hypothermic serum perfusion. Acta Med Scand 188:245–255, 1970

55. Lundstam S, Jagenburg R, Jonsson O et al: Metabolism in the hypothermically perfused dog kidney. Utilization and production of amino acids. Eur Surg Res 9:191–205, 1977

56. Martin DR, Scott DF, Downes GL et al: Primary cause of unsuccessful liver and heart preservation: Cold sensitivity of the ATPase system. Ann Surg 175:111–117, 1972

57. McCabe R, Lin J, Cooke L et al: Short-term kidney preservation. To perfuse or not to perfuse with the new Belzer perfusate. Proc EDTA-ERA 21:1027–1031, 1984

58. Menz LJ, Codd JE, Jellinek M et al: Ultrastructural observations in canine kidneys perfused hypothermically for 7 days in a comparative study of three preservation solutions. Cryobiology 19:407–427, 1982

59. Mittnacht S Jr, Sherman SC, Farber JL: Reversal of ischemic mitochondrial dysfunction. J Biol Chem 254:9871–9878, 1979

60. Monden M, Fortner JG: Twenty-four and 48 hour canine liver preservation by simple hypothermia with prostaglandin. Ann Surg 196:38–42, 1982

61. Opelz G, Terasaki PI: Advantage of cold storage over machine perfusion for preservation of cadaver kidneys. Transplantation 33:64–68, 1982

62. Parks DA, Buckley GB, Granger DN: Role of oxygen-free radicals in shock, ischemia, and organ preservation. Surgery 94:428–432, 1983

63. Pavlock GS, Southard JH, Starling JR et al: Lysosomal enzyme release in hypothermically perfused dog kidneys. Cryobiology 21:521–528, 1984

64. Pegg DE, Green CJ, Foreman J: Renal preservation by hypothermic perfusion. 2. The influence of oxygenator design and oxygen tension. Cryobiology 11:238–247, 1974

65. Pegg DE, Green CJ: Renal preservation by hypothermic perfusion. III. The lack of influence of pulsatile flow. Cryobiology 13:161–167, 1976

66. Pegg DE, Wusteman MC, Foreman J: Metabolism of normal and ischemically injured rabbit kidneys during perfusion for 48 hours at 10°C. Transplantation 32:437–443, 1981

67. Pettersson S, Claes G, Schersten T: Fatty acid and glucose utilization during continuous hypothermic perfusion of dog kidneys. Eur Surg Res 6:79–86, 1974

68. Rolles K, Foreman J, Pegg DE: Preservation of ischemically injured canine kidneys by retrograde oxygen persufflation. Transplantation 38:102–106, 1984

69. Skaaring P, Bierring F, Hefnal J et al: Ultrastructure of the glomerular filtration membrane of autotransplanted canine kidneys stored for 24 hours. Cryobiology 12:224–230, 1975

70. Skrede S, Lange G, Slattelid O et al: Coenzyme A in dog kidneys during hypothermic perfusion. Cryobiology 20:290–297, 1983

71. Skrede S, Slaattelid O: Fatty acid metabolism during hypothermic perfusion of the isolated dog kidney. Scand J Clin Lab Invest 39:765–771, 1979

72. Slaattelid O, Flatmark A, Skrede S: The importance of perfusate content of free fatty acids for dog kidneys preservation. Scand J Clin Lab Invest 36:240–245, 1976

73. Southard JH, Ametani MS, Lutz MF et al: Effects of hypothermic perfusion of kidneys on tissue and mitochondrial phospholipids. Cryobiology 21:20–24, 1984

74. Southard JH, Kunyoshi M, Lutz MF et al: Comparison of the effect of 3 and 5 day hypothermic perfusion on metabolism on tissue slices. Cryobiology 21:285–295, 1984

75. Southard JH, Lutz MF, Ametani MS et al: Stimulation of ATP synthesis in hypothermically perfused dog kidneys by adenosine and PO_4. Cryobiology 21:13–19, 1984

76. Southard JH, Rice MJ, Belzer FO: Preservation of renal function by adenosine stimulated ATP synthesis

in hypothermically perfused dog kidneys. Cryobiology 22:237–242, 1985

77. Southard JH, Scott GA, Lewandowski P et al: Time-dependent changes in the ultrastructure and the glomerulus of hypothermically perfused dog kidneys. Transplant Proc 1985

78. Southard JH, Senzig KA, Belzer FO: Effect of hypothermia on canine kidney mitochondria. Cryobiology 17:540–548, 1980

79. Starling JR, Rudolph LE, Ferguson W et al: Benefits of methyl prednisolone in the isolated perfused organ. Arch Surg 177:566–573, 1973

80. Tamaki T, Kamada N, Pegg DE: Hypothermic preservation of the rat liver assessed by orthotopic transplantation: A comparison of flush solutions. Transplantation 41:396–398, 1986

81. Toledo-Pereyra LH: Heart Preservation. In Toledo-Pereyra LH (ed): Basic Concepts in Organ Procurement, Perfusion, and Preservation for Transplantation, pp 301–316. New York, Academic Press, 1982

82. Toledo-Pereyra LH, Condie RM, Malmberg R et al: A fibrinogen-free perfusate for preservation of kidneys for one hundred and twenty hours. Surg Gynecol Obstet 138:901–905, 1974

83. Toledo-Pereyra LH, Wolberg HW, Nargarian JS: Reas-

sessment of non-pulsatile flow for renal hypothermic perfusion. Transplantation 16:385–388, 1975

84. Wahlberg JA, Love R, Landegaard L et al: 72-hour preservation of the canine pancreas. Transplantation 43:5–8, 1987

85. Wahlberg JA, Southard JH, Belzer FO: Development of a cold storage solution for pancreas preservation. Cryobiology 23:477–482, 1986

86. Wall WJ, Calne RY, Hebertson BM et al: Simple hypothermic preservation for transporting human livers long distances for transplantation. Transplantation 23:210, 1977

87. Weber TR, Freier DT, Salles CA et al: Effect of phentolamine on perfusate flow characteristics during renal preservation. J Surg Res 21:21–25, 1976

88. Weinberg JM: Issues in the pathophysiology of nephrotoxic renal tubular cell injury pertinent to understanding cyclosporine nephrotoxicity. Transplant Proc 17(Suppl):81, 1985

89. Willis JS, Li NM: Cold resistance of Na-K-ATPase of renal cortex of the hamster, a hibernating mammal. Am J Physiol 217:321–326, 1969

90. Wusteman MC, Jacobson IA, Pegg DE: A new solution for initial perfusion of transplanted kidneys. Scand J Urol Nephrol 12:281–286, 1978

CHAPTER 20

Kidney Preservation by Cold Storage

Geoffrey M. Collins

Cooling to ice temperatures substantially increases organ tolerance for ischemia by reducing metabolic rate (20–50×). At the same time, however, this effect inactivates energy-requiring processes necessary for maintaining the normal intracellular environment and cell volume. As a result, the full potential of cold storage can only be achieved by the use of specialized intracellular-type flush solutions that have been designed to control cell swelling and the loss of intracellular cations. For the most part, they share some common features, using (1) potassium and magnesium as their principal cations, (2) impermeant solute to prevent cell swelling, and (3) good buffering to limit ischemic acidosis. Cardioplegic solutions are preferred for ice storage of the heart because of the detrimental effects of high levels of potassium with this organ.

Since metabolism continues, albeit at low levels, even at 0°C, the duration of storage attainable by simple cooling is limited. Improvements will require exploration of new approaches such as prevention of free radical injury or provision of oxygenation by vascular persufflation.

All methods for organ preservation in use today depend upon hypothermic depression of metabolism.[73] Whereas ice storage relies on this factor alone, other techniques attempt to support metabolism during preservation either by the use of continuous perfusion or by oxygenation through persufflation of the vascular system or ambient hyperbaria. Despite years of research, it has proved very difficult to prolong viable organ preservation beyond 2 to 3 days by any method. It would seem likely, therefore, that true long-term organ banking must await a solution to the problem of organ freezing.

SURFACE COOLING

At normothermic temperature, ischemia results in complete loss of renal viability after only 1 to 2 hours.[26,37] On the other hand, surface cooling of the kidney to less than 6°C has been shown to result in good preservation for periods of 6 to 8 hours with deterioration after 12 hours.[22,46] However, under optimal conditions, life-sustaining function has been possible even after 24 hours of storage.[23] Evi-

dently, an approximately 12-fold increase in resistance to ischemia can be achieved by simple ice immersion. Although the magnitude of this effect is substantial, it appears to fall short of the extent of metabolic suppression produced by cooling, 20 to 50× at 0°C.[14,97] This relative failure of ice immersion to reach its full theoretical potential may be explained by two considerations. First, surface cooling is an inefficient method for reducing the core temperature of a large kidney,[65] which would therefore be exposed to the damaging effect of several minutes of warm ischemia.[57,110] Second, cooling itself has an adverse effect on cell physiology, producing swelling and exchange of intra- for extracellular ions.[77] An attempt to minimize these effects was the stimulus for the development of specialized flush solutions for hypothermic storage.

It has usually been assumed that cooling should be accomplished as rapidly as possible. However, rapid cooling of the kidney resulted in loss of glycolytic enzyme activity, and rapidly cooled rabbit kidneys functioned poorly when compared with those flushed at room temperature.[50,62] Clearly, cooling rates achieved by immersion and flushing are related to the size of the organ. Thus, rabbit renal cortex can be cooled to 5°C within 5 minutes of immersion in iced saline,[22] whereas the human kidney cools by only a few degrees in the same time period.[65] Since damage from rapid cooling has not yet been reported for large animal kidneys, it seems likely that sufficiently rapid cooling rates are not normally attained with large organs.

FLUSH SOLUTIONS

When first used, flushing of cadaveric kidneys was intended to facilitate rapid cooling and to eliminate blood from the vascular compartment. As it happens, a brief flush as distinct from continuous perfusion, has proved to be only partially effective (approximately 60%) at expelling red cells from the kidney.[30,66] Even so, it may be of some importance since red cells become increasingly rigid with depletion of their ATP stores and might therefore lead to persistent vascular obstruction during the reflow phase.[83]

The importance of the chemical composition of flush solutions was not appreciated prior to the publication by Keeler and colleagues in 1966.[64] They perfused rat kidneys with a solution containing 0.9% sodium chloride at 0°C and found a 50% loss of tissue potassium within 30 minutes and a 15% loss of magnesium over 3 hours. There was a concurrent 73% gain in water and 172% gain in sodium. Postulating that kidney damage might result from these ionic exchanges, Keeler perfused dog kidneys with solutions containing elevated concentrations of potassium and magnesium. In a small series of experiments, they found the optimal concentrations of these ions to be 150 mEq/liter and 50 mEq/liter, respectively. Subsequently, others[75] confirmed Keeler's findings while investigating continuous low-flow perfusion. The use of an extracellular-type solution uniformly yielded nonviable kidneys, whereas a simulated intracellular fluid was highly successful.

Prompted by these findings, experiments were begun to evaluate an intracellular type of flush solution,[23] the composition of which is shown in Table 20-1. The basic formula was very similar to that described by Martin and associates[75]; however, it contained a higher concentration of magnesium sulfate since Keeler had postulated that depletion of magnesium was the most important factor in the production of cell damage. However, magnesium sulfate was effective in prolonging the tolerance of the dog heart to 3 hours of normothermic ischemia.[114]

In our original study, dog kidneys were successfully preserved for 30 hours.[23] Subsequently, these findings have been extended to 72-hour canine kidney storage,[27] and numerous studies have confirmed the value of this type of flush solution for the storage of rabbit, pig, dog, and human kidneys for up to 96 hours.[40,55,68,102] Although the efficacy of this method is well established, the optimal composition of flush solutions and their precise mode of action remain somewhat controversial. The value of the pharmacologic additives in C4 is now rather questionable[25,113]; therefore, the simpler C2 rather than C4 is now used as the standard solution for hypothermic organ storage.

NEW FLUSH SOLUTIONS

Since the importance of the composition of flush solutions was first appreciated, many new formulations have been proposed.[29,41,94,96,109] Although they differ from C2 in many respects, there is a general underlying theme. In addition, novel suggestions such as inclusion of protein[8,109] and substitution of deuterium oxide for water have been tested.[45] Supporting data have been presented by the proponents of each, but there is no general agreement as to whether any of them should replace C2 in clinical practice. The inability to reach a consensus has been hampered by the lack of studies in which all variables in perfusate composition have been analyzed in a systemic fashion and by the fact that both the animal species and the model used to compare flush solutions can influence the results.[29,89]

With the exception of phosphate-buffered sucrose,[21] all these flush solutions contain high potassium levels as well as impermeant solutes and buffering, and it is these features that distinguish them from extracellular-type solutions such as Ringer's lactate. These common properties suggest the following possible explanations for their mode of ac-

TABLE 20-1 Composition of Collins Flush Solution

CONSTITUENTS	mM/L
Na	10
K	115
Mg	30
Cl	15
HCO₃	10
PO₄	57.5
SO₄	30
Glucose	139
Osmolarity	320 mOsm/L

tion: (1) conservation of cell energy substrates as a result of unloading the cell membrane ionic pump by minimizing the transmembrane cation gradients; (2) control of cell swelling as a result of the content of poorly permeant anions and nonelectrolytes; and (3) avoidance of any adverse effects produced by changes in intracellular ion content.

CONSERVATION OF CELL ENERGY

A substantial proportion of the energy derived from respiration is used to support membrane active transport mechanisms, principally extrusion of sodium ions.[71,116] This is reflected in the level of cell respiration being geared to the concentration of sodium in the environment.[10] Thus, lowering the extracellular sodium content of 10 mM/liter (the concentration present in C2 solution) can be expected to reduce the level of kidney cortical-slice respiration by one third.[87] Since significant levels of active transport persist even at 0°C,[15,69] the prospect of additional energy conservation by manipulation of perfusate composition is a theoretical possibility.[42] Thus, Shumakov and colleagues[99] reported that the amount of lactic acid in the washout solution after 24-hour kidney storage was three times as high for a kidney preserved in saline as for one preserved with an intracellular type of solution. Higher levels of adenine nucleotide have been found after storage with Collins' solution than with Ringer's lactate.[26,34] It must be admitted, however, that the significance of changes in adenine nucleotide levels in the pathogenesis of ischemic injury is somewhat questionable.[28,42]

PREVENTION OF CELL SWELLING

Under normal conditions, the stability of cell volume is maintained by the active extrusion of sodium ions, which establishes a Donnan's equilibrium, balancing that of the intracellular protein anions.[63] When the sodium pump is slowed by hypoxia, cold, or metabolic inhibitors, sodium ions enter the cell and other ions diffuse down their electrochemical gradients so that the protein Donnan effect becomes dominant, resulting in swelling of the cell and intracellular organelles.[48,63,71] The extent of these effects, in response to cold stress, depends upon the sensitivity of the sodium pump to hypothermic depression. This varies with the organ, the kidney appearing to be more resistant than either the liver or the heart,[76] and with the particular animal species studied. Regarding the latter, the sodium pump of hibernating animals tends to be especially cold re-

sistant.[119] The marked temperature sensitivity of the membrane adenosine triphosphatase of vascular endothelium[5] is of particular significance for whole-organ preservation since swelling of these cells could contribute to the "no reflow" phenomenon.[48,53]

Preventing cell swelling in ice storage of organs is important. Canine kidney preservation experiments conducted in order to determine which flush solution composition would best maintain the normal tissue electrolye content and cell morphology during storage at 4°C indicated that when Ringer's lactate was used, there was an immediate 50% increase in cell water, reaching 100% by 48 hours.[1] The concentrations of sodium and chloride each increased threefold, whereas the level of potassium went down by a similar factor. Addition of 200 mM glucose to the Ringer's lactate, rendering it hypertonic, almost completely prevented the gain in tissue water and somewhat reduced the increases in sodium and chloride but had no effect on the loss of potassium ions from the cells. When a solution was used containing potassium chloride and made hyperosmolar with glucose, intracellular sodium and potassium levels remained close to normal, but cell swelling still occurred because of an influx of freely diffusible chloride ions. However, this could be prevented by substituting sulfate, a less permeant anion, for chloride in this solution.

Ringer's lactate can be used for organ storage provided that it contains a poorly permeant nonelectrolyte for the prevention of cell swelling.[39,83] This is basically in agreement with our own finding of satisfactory, if not optimal, 48-hour renal preservation using a solution containing sodium as the principal cation together with impermeant solute.[24,25] Both Pegg and Downes have postulated that prevention of cell swelling is the flush solution's only important action, arguing that (1) all "intracellular" solutions contain impermeant anions and nonelectrolytes, (2) tissue water measurements made on stored kidneys show a correlation between maintenance of control levels and efficacy of the flush solution, and (3) the effectiveness of sodium-based solutions can be enhanced simply by adding impermeant solute. It is necessary to point out, however, that there are inconsistencies in the data upon which some of these conclusions are based.[31] Although control of cell swelling appears to be important in the author's opinion, it is not the only factor in the action of flush solutions for hypothermic kidney storage.

Emphasis on the prevention of cell swelling has led to the development of several hypertonic flush solutions.[94,96,109] The hyperosmolar solution described by Acquatella and co-workers[1] was later tested by Schloerb and associates[98] for 48-hour canine kidney preservation with indifferent results; only 25% of the kidneys provided life-sustaining function. Increasing the osmolarity of the C2 solution to 430 mOsm/liter using mannitol, Sacks and colleagues[96] produced successful 72-hour canine kidney preservation for the first time using ice storage. However, this period of preservation can be achieved with the C2 solution, which has an osmolarity of only 320 mOsm/liter.[27] It is possible that marked hyperosmolarity is beneficial only with kidneys exposed to a period of warm ischemia prior to preservation,[56,57] whereas such solutions may be of no benefit or even detrimental with fresh kidney storage.[19,21,25,27,61]

MAINTENANCE OF NORMAL IONIC COMPOSITION AND *p*H

The importance of attempting to maintain the normal intracellular ionic composition during hypothermic storage has been challenged.[39,83] Ionic losses in the cold ought to be reversed upon rewarming,[117] and any advantage conferred by increased amounts of intracellular cations in these solutions is questionable. Flushing with high potassium solutions lacking impermeant solutes has been shown to cause cell swelling and to be harmful.[54,108] Although this effect may be explained by the unrestricted entry of potassium chloride into the cell with accompanying swelling, it is more difficult to understand the findings of Pegg and Gallant[82] and Green and Pegg.[55] These investigators compared two hyperosmolar solutions, WF2 and WF4, and found that although cell swelling was better controlled by the high potassium WF4, renal function was superior after preservation with the WF2 solution, which contained only 4 mEq/liter of potassium and 140 mEq/liter of sodium chloride. The authors concluded that the high potassium concentration in WF4 was harmful. It is noteworthy, however, that the C4 solution containing 115 mEq/liter of potassium yielded the best results after 24- and 48-hour kidney storage. It seems likely, therefore, that if a flush solution contains high levels of potassium, the latter needs to be balanced by appreciable concentrations of impermeant anions so as to counteract the tendency for the potassium to enter the cells and reach damaging levels. Our own data support the use of high potassium, high magnesium solutions, although the type of impermeant anion, whether phosphate, citrate, or sulfate, did not seem to matter.[25,27]

Two components of flush solutions that are most controversial at the present time are magnesium and citrate. Some researchers have reported magnesium to be beneficial,[61,93] whereas others have found it to be of no value,[40,55] apart from an osmotic effect.[39] The theoretical advantages of its inclusion in flush solutions are its action as a metabolic inhibitor,[114] vasodilator,[72] and preserver of intracellular potassium[55] and its ability to inhibit the rigidizing effect on calcium binding to the membrane of ATP-depleted red cells.[83] On the other hand, magnesium tends to form a precipitate with phosphate anions.[115] Fortunately, this has not precluded successful kidney preservation with magnesium-containing solutions. In fact, a cooperative clinical trial demonstrated that the magnesium-containing C2 solution yielded a lower rate of ATN than with the magnesium-free Euro-Collins' solution.[31]

There continues to be disagreement as to the relative merits of citrate versus phosphate as the principal anion in flush solutions.[8,27,94,100,109] It was originally thought that citrate might have some special metabolic properties.[95] However, substitution of a nonmetabolizable analog, tricarballylate, gave equal results provided that the reduced buffering power of this substance was compensated by the addition of 10mM Hepes buffer to the solution.[61]

There are two aspects to the control of *p*H that are relevant to a discussion of hypothermic organ preservation—namely, determination of its optimal value for storage at 0°C, and the need to prevent tissue acidosis by inclusion of buffers in flush solutions. The published data dealing with the ideal *p*H for hypothermic organ storage are confusing. It is clear that acidosis develops rapidly during normothermic ischemia[58] and that the magnitude of this *p*H shift is much reduced by cooling.[36] The conventional viewpoint is that this acidosis is damaging[51,110] and that buffering in a flush solution is advantageous.[12,61] On the other hand, Calman and Bell[17] found the optimal *p*H for hypothermic rat heart preservation to be 7, which is closer to the value chosen empirically for Collins' solution for kidney preservation (7.0–7.2). Likewise, tumor cells and rat renal cortex exposed to normothermic ischemia survived longer at *p*H 5.6 to 6.5 than at 7.4.[84] The decline in cellular *p*H during ischemia is self-limiting, owing to the fact that the key regulatory glycolytic enzyme, phosphofructokinase, is inhibited below a *p*H of 6.7[11]

SUPPORT OF RESPIRATION

In an attempt to provide for cell respiration without continuous perfusion, a number of workers have tried to supplement ice storage with the delivery of oxygen to the tissue in a hyperbaric environment or by gaseous persufflation through the vascular system. Kidney preservation by hyperbaric oxygen, in combination with simple hypothermia has been generally abandoned, since the results on the whole have been inferior to those attained by continuous perfusion or ice storage at atmospheric pressures.[22,60] By contrast, delivery of oxygen to the tissues by gaseous persufflation shows considerable promise as a supplement to ice storage. For instance, kidneys preserved by an initial flush with C2 were persufflated through the renal vein with oxygen at a pressure of 50 mm Hg to 60 mm Hg.[44] Bubbles of gas were allowed to escape through puncture sites in the renal capsular veins. Kidney function after 24-hour preservation was superior to control ice-stored or perfused kidneys. Oxygen persufflation was particularly effective in the case of ischemically injured kidneys. These findings have been confirmed but equally good results can be obtained with gas pressures as low as 10 mm Hg.[95]

NEW CONCEPTS IN ORGAN PRESERVATION–FREE RADICAL INJURY

Despite extensive study, the results obtained using ice storage or continuous hypothermic perfusion today are essentially no better than when the methods were first described in the late 1960s. Fundamentally, it has been assumed that ice storage is limited by the finite reduction in metabolism resulting from cooling to 0°C, and organ perfusion is limited by an inability to support metabolism indefinitely with synthetic perfusates under hypothermic conditions.

Recently, however, a new concept has emerged that promises to alter this situation. This is the recognition of oxygen-derived free radical injury following organ ischemia.[78] It is postulated that much of the damage sustained by an ischemic organ occurs not during the period of hypoxia, but rather following restoration of the circulation when molecular oxygen is reintroduced into the tissues. The proposed mechanism is as follows: Hypoxia leads to degradation of high-energy phosphate with the accumulation of hypoxanthine. At the same time, calcium enters the cell and activates a Ca-dependent protease, which catalyzes the conversion of the normally harmless xanthine dehydrogenase into the enzyme xanthine oxidase. Once the circulation is restored, the latter vigorously catalyzes conversion of hypoxanthine to xanthine with the liberation of oxygen free radicals. This burst of superoxide radical and hydrogen peroxide oxidizes the cellular components, producing serious damage. This concept

rather nicely explains how agents capable of interfering with this chain of events can protect organs from a reperfusion injury following normothermic ischemia or ice storage. These agents include allopurinol, which inhibits xanthine oxidase;[80] calmodulin inhibitors such as trifluoperazine, which block calcium entry into cells,[2] and superoxide dismutase or other chemical agents that scavenge free radicals.[67] The situation with hypothermic organ perfusion using oxygenated perfusates is similar, although, in this case, the organ is exposed not only to reperfusion oxidative injury but also to the ravages of free radical damage during in vitro perfusion itself.

Perfusional preservation can be much improved by including antioxidants (ascorbic acid and glutathione), chemical free radical scavaging agents (glycerol, propylene glycol, or polyethylene glycol), and superoxide dismutase in the perfusate.* Glycerol has similarly been found to be highly beneficial in a perfusate for cardiac preservation.[118]

CLINICAL APPLICATION OF COLD STORAGE

In clinical cadaveric organ transplantation, many factors other than the intrinsic efficacy of the preservation method affect function. These include the deleterious effects of brain death,[35] the details of donor management,[9,74,79] the technique of organ procurement,[52] the experience and skill of the surgical team, the state of hydration of the recipient at the time of reimplantation,[18,106] and the effects of nephrotoxic immunosuppressive agents such as cyclosporine.[47] The dominance of these extraneous factors is illustrated by the difficulty in demonstrating a clear-cut relationship between the incidence of acute tubular necrosis (ATN) and the duration of storage.[30,92,102] In fact, histologic study shows that many of the kidneys destined to suffer ATN after transplantation have pre-existing damage detectable at the time of procurement.[91]

At the present time, cold storage and perfusional preservation would appear to be equally effective for preserving human cadaveric kidneys,[81] with ATN rates in the range of 20% to 40% or even lower in some centers.[92] Under these circumstances, the simplicity, low cost, and suitability for air transport have persuaded an increasing number of centers to switch to the cold storage method.[85] However, since storage times attainable by simple

---

* References 7, 13, 20, 32, and 33

hypothermia are necessarily limited by the finite reduction of metabolism at 0°C, it seems likely that in the long term, this trend will be reversed by advances in methods for organ perfusion.

OTHER ORGANS

The general principles previously outlined for hypothermic renal preservation also apply to ice storage of other transplantable organs. However, unlike kidney transplantation in which ATN is tolerable, although undesirable, inadequate immediate function of a transplanted heart or liver is essentially lethal unless a replacement organ can be quickly found. The lack of a support system during recovery from ischemic injury comparable to dialysis has led to a very conservative approach to clinical preservation of extrarenal organs, relying on simplicity, portability, and minimal storage times. As a result, flush cooling and ice storage is currently the method of choice, despite its limitation to approximately 4 hours for the heart,[105] 10 hours for the liver,[16] and 24 hours for the pancreas.[103]

Flush solutions of intracellular type have been used experimentally to preserve the liver,[6,70] pancreas,[3,38,107] lung,[86] and heart.[101] The repertoire includes Collins' solution, Sacks' solution, Ross citrate solution, modified silica gel plasma fraction, and other plasma-based solutions. As with the kidney, control of cell swelling, intracellular ion content, and buffering are the essential features. All solutions contain impermeant anions and nonelectrolytes as well as supranormal levels of potassium and often magnesium. The Cambridge plasma protein fraction used for liver preservation is an exception to these general concepts, containing only 20 mM potassium and virtually no impermeant solute.[112] It has, however, been found to be inferior to typical "intracellular" solutions experimentally.[104] It seems likely that, as with the kidney, the very short period of preservation used for extrarenal transplants in clinical practice is likely to obscure all but major differences in efficacy among the various flush solutions.

It has been suggested that the pancreas poses a particularly severe test of flush preservation because of a marked tendency to tissue edema, although Toledo-Pereyra and colleagues[107] have successfully stored this organ for 72 hours using modified silica gel fraction. Wahlberg and associates[111] have recently reported excellent preservation for 72 hours by the use of a flush solution containing carefully selected impermeant solutes of larger molecular weight than have been used previously. They found from tissue slice studies that solutes usually considered to be impermeant did indeed enter the cell. Thus, swelling was progressively reduced as the molecular size of the nonelectrolyte was increased from mannitol, to sucrose, to raffinose, and the large anion lactobionate proved better than gluconate, which in turn was better than phosphate in this regard. This rigorous approach to prevention of cell swelling warrants further evaluation as a basis for a general purpose flush solution suitable for all organs.

The general principles governing the composition of flush solutions for myocardial preservation would also appear to be comparable to the kidney. Bayliss and Maloney[4] found that dog hearts flushed with a solution having sodium and potassium content of 30 mEq/L and 130 mEq/L, respectively, and an osmolarity of 350 mOsm/liter beat vigorously and maintained arterial pressure on a parabiotic circuit after 24-hour storage at 0°C. Others have confirmed the efficacy of intracellular-type solutions for 24-hour heart storage provided that the osmolarity of the solution has not been too high.[88,101] However, these experimental data have been largely ignored in clinical practice. Rather, cardiothoracic surgeons have preferred to rely on a very short period of ice storage using cardioplegic solutions developed for producing cardiac arrest during open heart surgery. These solutions generally have relatively low potassium levels and other constituents chosen to minimize the entry of calcium into the myocardium.[49,59,90]

In general, it can be said that the methods in use today for preservation of extrarenal organs are only barely adequate to allow time for transportation between donor and recipient centers. Better methods are sorely needed to alleviate the sense of haste surrounding the transplant process.

REFERENCES

1. Acquatella H, Gonzales MP, Morales JM et al: Ionic and histological changes in the kidney after perfusion and storage for transplantation. Use of high Na vs. high K containing solutions. Transplantation 14:480–489, 1972

2. Anaise D, Bachvaroff RJ, Sato K et al: Enhanced resistance to the effects of hypothermic ischemia in the preserved canine kidney. Transplantation 38: 570–574, 1984

3. Baumgartner D, Sutherland DER, Hect JE et al: Cold

storage of segmental canine pancreatic grafts for 24 hours. J Surg Res 29:248–257, 1980

4. Bayliss CE, Maloney JV: Shelf storage of excised hearts by manipulation of transmembrane gradients. Surg Forum 21:194, 1970

5. Belzer FO, Hoffman R, Huang J et al: Endothelial damage in perfused dog kidney and cold sensitivity of vascular Na-K-ATPase. Cryobiology 9:457–460, 1972

6. Benichou J, Halgrimsom CG, Starzl TE et al: Canine and human liver preservation for 6 to 18 hours by cold infusion. Transplantation 24:407–411, 1977

7. Bennett JF, Bry WI, Collins GM et al: Protection against free radical damage during kidney perfusion. Cryobiology 21:703, 1984

8. Besarab A, Martin GB, Mead T et al: Effect of plasma proteins and buffers in flushing solutions on rat kidney preservation by cold storage. Transplantation 37:239–245, 1984

9. Blaine EM, Tallman PD, Frolicher D et al: Vasopressin supplementation in a porcine model of brain-dead potential organ donors. Transplantation 38:459–464, 1984

10. Blond DM, Whittam R: The regulation of kidney respiration by sodium and potassium. Biochem J 92:158–167, 1964

11. Bock PE, Frieden C: pH-induced cold lability of rabbit skeletal muscle phosphofructokinase. Biochemistry 13:4191–4196, 1974

12. Bore PJ, Sehr PA, Chan L et al: The importance of pH in renal preservation. Transplant Proc 13:707–708, 1981

13. Bry WI, Collins GM, Halasz NA et al: Improved function of perfused rabbit kidneys by prevention of oxidative injury. Transplantation 38:579–583, 1984

14. Buhl MR, Jorgensen S: Breakdown of 5' adenine nucleotides in ischemic renal cortex estimated by oxypurine excretion during perfusion. Scand J Clin Lab Invest 35:211–217, 1975

15. Burg MB, Orloff J: Active cation transport by kidney tubules at 0°C. Am J Physiol 207:983–998, 1964

16. Busuttil RW: Liver transplantation today. Ann Intern Med 104:377–389, 1986

17. Calman KC, Bell PRF: Experimental organ preservation. Transplant Proc 3:647–649, 1970

18. Carlier M, Squifflet JP, Pirson Y et al: Confirmation of the crucial role of the recipient's maximal hydration on early diuresis of the human cadaver renal allograft. Transplantation 36:455–456, 1983

19. Chatterjee SN, Berne TV: Failure of 48 hours of cold storage of canine kidneys using Sacks' solution. Transplantation 19:441–442, 1975

20. Codd JE, Jellinek M, Garvin PJ et al: Redox maintenance in restoration of organ viability. J Surg Res 22:585–592, 1977

21. Coffey AK, Andrews PM: Ultrastructure of kidney preservation: Varying the amount of an effective osmotic agent in isotonic and hypertonic preservation solution. Transplantation 35:136–143, 1983

22. Collins GM, Shugarman MB, Novom S et al: Kidney preservation for transplantation. 12-hour storage in rabbits. Transplant Proc 1:801–807, 1969

23. Collins GM, Bravo-Sugarman MB, Terasaki PI: Kidney preservation for transportation. Initial perfusion and 30 hours' ice storage. Lancet 2:1219–1222, 1969

24. Collins GM, Harley LCJ, Clunie GJA: Kidney preservation for transportation. Experimental analysis of optimal perfusate composition. Br J Surg 59:187–189, 1972

25. Collins GM, Halasz NA: Forty-eight hour ice storage of kidneys: Importance of cation content. Surgery 79:432–435, 1976

26. Collins GM, Taft P, Green RD et al: Adenine nucleotide levels in preserved and ischemically injured canine kidneys. World J Surg 1:237–243, 1977

27. Collins GM, Green RD, Halasz NA: Importance of anion content and osmolarity in flush solutions for 48- to 72-hour hypothermic kidney storage. Cryobiology 16:217–220, 1979

28. Collins GM: Adenine nucleotide levels and recovery of function after renal ischemic injury. Transplantation 31:295–296, 1981

29. Collins GM, Halasz NA: A species difference in the efficacy of two intracellular flush solutions. Transplantation 33:324, 1982

30. Collins GM, Peterson T, Wicomb WN et al: Experimental observation on the mode of action of "intracellular" flush solutions. J Surg Res 36:1–8, 1984

31. Collins GM, Barry JM, Maxwell JG et al: The value of magnesium in flush solutions for human cadaveric kidney preservation. J Urol 131:220–222, 1984

32. Collins GM, Wicomb WN, Halasz NA: Beneficial effect of low concentrations of cryoprotective agents on short-term rabbit kidney perfusion. Cryobiology 21:246–249, 1984

33. Collins GM, Bry WI, Halasz NA: Optimal redox electrode potential for 24-hour rabbit kidney perfusion. J Surg Res 39:246–250, 1985

34. Collste H: Preservation of kidneys for transplantation. Acta Chir Scand (Suppl) 425:31–39, 1972

35. Cooper DKC, Wicomb WN, Lanza RP et al: Barnard effects of brain death and hypothermic perfusion storage on donor heart function. Transplant Proc 17:231–232, 1985

36. Couch NP, Maginn RR, Middleton MK et al: Effects of ischemic interval and temperature on renal surface hydrogen ion concentration. Surg Gynecol Obstet 125:521–528, 1967

37. Craddock GN: Species differences in response to renal ischemia. Arch Surg 111:582–584, 1976

38. deGruyl J, Westbroek DL, MacDicken I et al: Cryoprecipitated plasma perfusion preservation and cold storage preservation of duct-ligated pancreatic allografts. Br J Surg 64:490–495, 1977

39. Downes G, Hoffman R, Huang J et al: Mechanism of action of washout solutions for kidney preservation. Transplantation 16:46–53, 1973

40. Dreikorn K, Horsch R, Rohl L: 48- to 96-hour pres-

ervation of canine kidneys by initial perfusion and hypothermic storage using Euro-Collins' solution. Eur Urol 6:221–224, 1980

41. Fahy GM, Hornblower M, Williams H: An improved perfusate for hypothermic renal preservation. 1. Initial in vitro optimization based on tissue electrolyte transport. Cryobiology 16:618, 1979

42. Farber E: ATP and cell integrity. Fed Proc 32:1534–1539, 1973

43. Fernando AR, Griffiths JR, O'Donoghue EPN et al: Enhanced preservation of the ischemic kidney with inosine. Lancet 1:555–557, 1976

44. Fischer JH, Czerniak A, Hauer U et al: A new simple method for optimal storage of ischemically damaged kidneys. Transplantation 25:43–49, 1978

45. Fischer JH, Knupper P, Beyer M: Flush solution 2, a new concept for one-to-three-day hypothermic renal storage preservation: Functional recovery after preservation in Euro-Collins', Collins' C2, hypertonic citrate, and F2 solution. Transplantation 39:122–126, 1985

46. Fisher ER, Copeland C, Fisher B: Correlation of ultrastructure and function following hypothermic preservation of canine kidneys. Lab Invest 17:99–119, 1967

47. Flechner SM, Payne WD, Van Buren C et al: The effect of cyclosporine on early graft function in human renal transplantation. Transplantation 36:268–272, 1983

48. Flores J: The role of cell swelling in ischemic renal damage and the protective effect of hypertonic solute. J Clin Invest 51:118–126, 1972

49. Follette D, Mulder DG, Maloney JV et al: Advantages of blood cardioplegia over continuous coronary perfusion or intermittent ischemia. J Thorac Cardiovasc Surg 76:604–619, 1978

50. Francavilla A, Brown TH, Fiore R et al: Preservation of organs for transplantation. Evidence of detrimental effect of rapid cooling. Eur Surg Res 5:384–389, 1973

51. Fry DE, Ratcliffe DJ, Yates JR: The effects of acidosis on canine hepatic and renal oxidative phosphorylation. Surgery 88:269–273, 1980

52. Garvin PJ, Buttorff JD, Morgan R et al: In situ cold perfusion of kidneys for transplantation. An experimental and clinical evaluation. Arch Surg 115:180–182, 1980

53. Glaumann B, Trump BF: Studies on the pathogenesis of ischemic cell injury. 3. Morphological changes of the proximal pars recta tubules of the rat kidney made ischemic in vivo. Virchows Arch (Cell Pathol) 19:303–323, 1975

54. Gordon EE, Maier DM: Effect of ionic environment on metabolism and structure of rat kidney slices. Am J Physiol 207:71–76, 1964

55. Green CJ, Pegg DE: Mechanism of action of "intracellular" renal preservation solutions. World J Surg 3:115–120, 1979

56. Grundmann R, Strumper R, Kurten K et al: Nieren-konservierung durch hypotherme lagerung nac Collins und Sacks: Der einfluu von 0-30 min warmer ischamie auf die erreichbare konservierungszeit. Lagenbecks Arch Surg 346:11–24, 1978

57. Halasz NA, Collins GM: Forty-eight hour kidney preservation. A comparison of flushing and ice storage with perfusion. Arch Surg 111:175–177, 1976

58. Hardie IR, Clunie GJ, Collins GM: Evaluation of simple methods for assessing renal ischemic injury. Surg Gynecol Obstet 136:43–46, 1973

59. Hearse DJ, Stewart DA, Braimbridge MV: Cellular protection during myocardial ischemia: The development and characterization of a procedure for the induction of reversible ischemic arrest. Circulation 54:193–202, 1976

60. Hendry WF, Struthers NW, Duguid WP et al: Twenty-Four-hour storage of kidneys. Lancet 1:1221–1225, 1968

61. Jablonski P, Howden B, Marshall V et al: Evaluation of citrate flushing solution using the isolated perfused rat kidney. Transplantation 30:239–243, 1980

62. Jacobsen IA, Kemp E, Buhl MR: An adverse effect of rapid cooling in kidney preservation. Transplantation 27:135, 1979

63. Jamison RL: The role of cellular swelling in the pathogenesis of organ ischemia. West J Med 120:205–218, 1974

64. Keeler R, Swinney J, Taylor RMR et al: The problem of renal preservation. Br J Urol 38:653–655, 1966

65. Kerr WK: Renal hypothermia. J Urol 81:236–242, 1960

66. Kerstein MD, Bergentz S-E, Lewis DH: Clearance of red blood cells from the cadaver kidney: A study of colloidal perfusing solutions. Ann Surg 171:347–351, 1970

67. Koyama I, Bulkley GB, Williams GM et al: The role of oxygen free radicals in mediating the reperfusion injury of cold preserved ischemic kidneys. Transplantation 40:590–595, 1985

68. Kreis H, Lacombe M, Ciancioni C et al: 48-hour kidney preservation (initial perfusion with potassium and magnesium—rich solution). Rev Eur Etudes Clin Biol 17:192–196, 1972

69. Lambotte L: Persistence of active and passive ionic transport during low temperature liver preservation. Surgery 73:8–14, 1973

70. Lambotte L, Pontegnie-Istace S, Otte JB et al: The effects of isoproterenol and Collins' solution on the preservation of canine livers with simple cooling. Transplant Proc 6:301–303, 1974

71. Leaf A: Maintenance of concentration gradients and regulation of cell volume. Ann NY Acad Sci 72:396–404, 1959

72. Levowitz BS: Magnesium ion blockade of regional vasoconstriction. Ann Surg 172:33–44, 1970

73. Levy MN: Oxygen consumption and blood flow in the hypothermic, perfused kidney. Am J Physiol 197:1111–1114, 1959

74. Lokkegaard H, Nerstrom B: Clinical experiences with

preservation of necrokidneys. The effect of treatment with chlorpromazine and the use of a perfusate which mimics the intracellular ion composition. Acta Med Scand 194:5–11, 1973

75. Martin DC, Smith G, Fareed DO: Experimental renal preservation. J Urol 103:681–685, 1970

76. Martin DR, Scott DF, Downes GL et al: Primary cause of unsuccessful liver and heart preservation: Cold sensitivity of the ATPase system. Ann Surg 175:111–117, 1972

77. Mason J, Beck F, Dorge A et al: Intracellular electrolyte composition following renal ischemia. Kidney Int 20:61–70, 1981

78. McCord JM: Oxygen-derived free radicals in postischemic tissue injury. N Engl J Med 312:159–163, 1985

79. Najarian JS, Gulyassy PP, Stoney RJ et al: Protection of the donor kidney during homotransplantation. Ann Surg 164:398–417, 1966

80. Nordstrom GG, Seeman T, Hasselgren PO: Beneficial effect of allopurinol in liver ischemia. Surgery 97:679–683, 1985

81. Opelz G, Terasaki PI: Advantage of cold storage over machine perfusion for preservation of cadaveric kidneys. Transplantation 33:64–68, 1982

82. Pegg DE, Gallant M: Water and electrolyte contents and extracellular space of rabbit kidneys after perfusion and storage for 24 hours at 4°C. Cryobiology 14:568–574, 1977

83. Pegg DE: An approach to hypothermic renal preservation. Cryobiology 15:1–17, 1978

84. Penttilla A, Trump BF: Extra cellular acidosis protects Ehrlich ascites tumor cells and rat renal cortex against anoxic injury. Science 185:277–278, 1974

85. Perdue ST, Terasaki PI, Cats S et al: Kidney transplantation trends from the UCLA Registry data, 1975–1982. Transplantation 36:658–665, 1983

86. Pinsker K, Montefusco C, Yipintsoi T et al: Total in vivo functional adequacy of canine lung autografts after 24-hour preservation. Transplant Proc 11:599–606, 1979

87. Reichmann K, Hardie IR, Clunie GJ et al: In vitro analysis of the cation content of solutions for kidney storage. Cryobiology 9:296–299, 1972

88. Reitz BA, Brady WR, Hickey PA et al: Protection of heart for 24 hours with intracellular (high K+) solution and hypothermia. Surg Forum 25:149, 1974

89. Rice MJ, Southard JH, Hoffman RM et al: Effects of hypothermic kidney preservation on the isolated perfused kidney: A comparison of reperfusion methods. Cryobiology 22:161–167, 1985

90. Rich TL, Brady AJ: Potassium contracture and utilization of high-energy phosphates in rabbit heart. Am J Physiol 226:105–113, 1974

91. Rohr MS: Renal allograft acute tubular necrosis. II. A light and electron microscopic study of biopsies taken at procurement and after revascularization. Ann Surg 197:663–671, 1983

92. Rosenthal JT, Herman JB, Taylor RJ: Comparison of pulsatile machine perfusion with cold storage for cadaver kidney preservation. Transplantation 37:425–426, 1984

93. Ross H, Werther M: Kidney preservation. Lancet 1:867, 1974

94. Ross H, Marshall VC, Escott ML: 72-hour canine kidney preservation without continuous perfusion. Transplantation 21:498–501, 1976

95. Ross H, Escott ML: Gaseous oxygen perfusion of the renal vessels as an adjunct in kidney preservation. Transplantation 28:362–364, 1979

96. Sacks SA, Petritsch PH, Kaufman JJ: Canine kidney preservation using a new perfusate. Lancet 1:1024–1028, 1973

97. Schirmer HKA, Walton KN: The effect of hypothermia upon respiration and anaerobic glycolysis of dog kidney. Invest Urol 1:604–609, 1964

98. Schloerb PR, Postel J, Moritz ED et al: Hypothermic storage of the canine kidney for 48 hours in a low chloride solution. Surg Gynecol Obstet 141:545–548, 1975

99. Shumakov VI, Onishchenko NA, Stengold ES: Clinical experience of kidney storage by non-perfusion technique for periods up to 58 hr. Trans Am Soc Artif Intern Organs 20:545–549, 1974

100. Southard JH, Rice MJ, Ametani MS et al: Effects of short-term hypothermic perfusion and cold storage on function of the isolated-perfused dog kidney. Cryobiology 22:147–155, 1985

101. Spray TL, Watson DC, Roberts WC: Morphology of canine hearts after 24 hours' preservation and orthotopic transplantation. J Thorac Cardiovasc Surg 73:880–886, 1977

102. Squifflet JP, Pirson Y, Gianello P et al: Safe preservation of human renal cadaver transplants by Euro-Collins' solution up to 50 hours. Transplant Proc 13:693–696, 1981

103. Sutherland DER: Current status of clinical pancreas and islet transplantation with comments on the need for and application of cryogenic and other preservation techniques. Cryobiology 20:245–255, 1983

104. Tamaki T, Kamada N, Pegg DE: Hypothermic preservation of the rat liver assessed by orthotopic transplantation: A comparison of flush solutions. Transplantation 41:396–397, 1986

105. Thomas FT, Szentpetery SS, Mammana RE et al: Long-distance transportation of human hearts for transplantation. Ann Thorac Surg 26:344–350, 1978

106. Tiggeler RGWL, Berden JHM, Hoitsma AJ et al: Prevention of acute tubular necrosis in cadaveric kidney transplantation by combined use of mannitol and moderate hydration. Ann Surg 201:246–251, 1985

107. Toledo-Pereyra LH, Bock G, Schneider A et al: Pancreas preservation with TP-IV: A hyperosmolar colloid solution. Cryobiology 22:40–46, 1985

108. Trump BF, Ginn FL: Studies of cellular injury in isolated flounder tubules. Cellular swelling in high potassium media. Lab Invest 18:341–351, 1968

109. Vij D, Toledo-Pereyra LH: Failure of hypertonic citrate solution to preserve canine renal transplants af-

ter 24 hours of hypothermic storage. Transplantation 29:90, 1980

110. Vogt MT, Farber E: On the molecular pathology of ischemic renal cell death. Am J Pathol 53:1–26, 1968

111. Wahlberg JA, Love R, Landegaard L et al: Seventy-two hour preservation of the canine pancreas. Transplantation 43:5–8, 1987

112. Wall WJ, Calne RY, Herbertson BM et al: Simple hypothermic preservation for transporting human livers long distances for transplantation. Transplantation 23:210–218, 1977

113. Watkins GM, Prentiss NA, Couch NP: Tissue and organ preservation: Successful 24-hour kidney preservation with simplified hyperosmolar hyperkalemic perfusate. Transplant Proc 3:612–615, 1971

114. Webb WR, Dodds RP, Unal MO et al: Suspended animation of the heart with metabolic inhibitors. Effect of magnesium sulfate or fluoride and adrenochrome in rats. Ann Surg 164:343–350, 1966

115. Welch LT, Flanigan WJ: Kidney preservation. Lancet 2:1444–1445, 1973

116. Whittam R, Willis JS: Ion movements and oxygen consumption in kidney cortex slices. J Physiol 168:158–177, 1963

117. Whittembury G: Sodium extrusion and potassium uptake in guinea pig kidney cortex slices. J Gen Physiol 48:699–717, 1965

118. Wicomb WN, Cooper DKC, Novitzky D et al: Cardiac transplantation following storage of the donor heart by a portable hypothermic perfusion system. Ann Thorac Surg 37:243–268, 1984

119. Willis JS: Characteristics of ion transport in kidney cortex of mammalian hibernators. J Gen Physiol 49:1221–1239, 1966

CHAPTER 21

Multiple Organ Procurement

R. Patrick Wood   Byers W. Shaw, Jr.

The increasing demand for solid organs for transplantation requires that all individuals involved in organ procurement become familiar with the intricacies of the multiple organ procurement process. Multiple organ procurement, as described in this chapter, involves a coordinated effort among a number of highly trained professionals in order to obtain donor organs of optimal quality.

This process begins with the organ procurement coordinator who identifies, evaluates, and helps manage potential multiple organ donors. The coordinator works closely with colleagues at the institutions that will be harvesting the various organs to coordinate the arrival of the various procurement groups at the donor hospital. During the procurement procedure, the coordinator is able to make a more precise estimate of the time that will be required to complete the donor procedure and return to the various recipient hospitals. The precise timing is imperative if the cold ischemia time of the various organs is to be minimized. With the majority of extrarenal organs, the recipient operation will have to begin prior to the arrival of the organs at the recipient hospitals. Most transplant surgeons believe that it is optimal to keep cold ischemia time to a minimum for each organ. But, in addition, each center sets an upper limit on the acceptable cold ischemia time, and an organ kept cold beyond this limit is felt to be unusable. These limits, which vary from program to program, are roughly 48 hours for cold-preserved nonperfused kidneys, 8 to 10 hours for livers, 4 to 24 hours for pancreas, 3 to 4 hours for hearts, and less than 1 hour for heart–lungs and single lungs.

An anesthesiologist who is both knowledgeable about the types of physiological support required by multiple organ donors and who is also well-informed about particular recovery procedures to be undertaken is invaluable in ensuring the optimal quality of the donor organs. The anesthesiologist is responsible for maintaining the donor in optimal physiological condition throughout the recovery procedure. The surgeons participating in the recovery procedure are thus obliged to discuss the procedure thoroughly with the participating anesthesiologist in order to ensure that the appropriate fluids and drugs are administered at the appropriate times.

Finally, all surgeons participating in multiple organ recoveries bring with them their own expertise and technique for the harvest of that particular organ. As the number of centers performing solid organ transplants continues to expand rapidly, all organ recovery teams will need to develop mutually agreeable working relationships with teams from an increasing number of new centers. In this new era of organ transplantation, lack of understanding, lack of communication, or unwillingness to cooperate should never be allowed to threaten the functional quality of any donor organ. To this end, before a recovery procedure begins, a brief conference between surgeons and coordinators from the participating organ recovery teams should allow the formulation of a step-by-step plan that is agreeable to everyone present.

The primary limiting factor in the expansion of solid organ transplantation today is the availability of suitable donor organs. Two recent surveys demonstrated an increased public awareness about solid organ transplantation. These studies showed that between 50% and 70% of people surveyed would donate their own organs or the organs of a loved one.[8,15] In a recent report from Pittsburgh,[44] 82% of families were willing to donate the organs of a loved one when offered this option.

On the other hand, retrospective reviews of the causes of in-hospital deaths have estimated that as

TABLE 21-1   *United States Transplant Statistics 1985**

| ORGAN | CASES PERFORMED/YEAR | | | |
	1983	1984	NUMBER WAITING	POTENTIAL BENEFIT
Cornea	21,500	23,500	3,500	250,000
Kidney	6,112	6,730	12,000	25,000
Heart	280	400	100	14,000
Liver	168	308	330	5,000
Pancreas	61	87	50	10,000
Heart–lung	13	17	50	1,000

* modified from The American Council on Transplantation, July–August, 1985.

many as 20,000 to 30,000 of these deaths occurred under circumstances that provide for the option of organ donation. Yet organs are actually recovered from fewer than 10% to 25% of these potential organ donors.[3,4,6,16] This indicates that in addition to continuing to educate the public about the need for donor organs, a much greater educational effort must be directed toward physicians and other medical personnel. Table 21-1 shows that despite the increased number of transplants performed in the last several years, a huge segment of the population continues to be denied transplantation simply because of the shortage of donor organs.[15] At present, 27 states have adopted laws that require hospitals to offer the option of organ donation to the family of any person dying in the hospital. The effectiveness of such laws in increasing the number of organs available for transplantation remains to be seen.

From this analysis, two facts seem obvious. First, everyone in the field must do a much better job of identifying and recovering potential organs for transplantation. Second, each cadaveric donor must be considered as a potential multiple organ donor.

Each transplantation center has its own set of criteria for evaluating potential donor organs. When a potential organ donor is identified, the responsibility of the local transplantation group or, more specifically, the local or regional organ procurement agency is to attempt to identify potential recipients for the various organs. The local procurement officer is also responsible for contacting transplant centers with potential recipients for the organs and for coordinating the arrival of the procurement teams who will be recovering the various organs. In many centers, the organ procurement coordinator will also help manage the donor after brain death has been declared, making sure that all necessary consultations, laboratory tests, and appropriate consents have been obtained.

DONOR SELECTION

A general set of criteria that will fulfill most centers' requirements for multiple organ donors are listed in Table 21-2. Table 21-3 gives a breakdown of general age ranges for different donor organs. The most stringent criteria are those for heart–lung donors. Each of the other organ systems have specific but somewhat less stringent criteria. These criteria are only guidelines, and each donor is evaluated with a view toward the particular circumstances surrounding that donor and the specific requirements (such as the urgency of need) of a center's recipients at that particular point in time.

ANESTHESIA

For the most part, multiple organ donors require greater intraoperative anesthesia support than kidney donors. Multiple organ procurement takes a variable period of time (2–4 hours), involves greater blood and fluid replacement, and requires the administration of a variety of drugs. The majority of organ donors have suffered catastrophic neurologic injury that often results in the loss of a significant number of the body's regulatory functions.[16] Because most donors will lack the capacity for thermoregulation and because of the wide exposure required during the procedure, rapid cooling of the donor may occur prematurely. Thus, the donor's core temperature should be monitored with either a rectal or esophageal temperature probe. The procurement team should attempt to maintain the donor's core temperature above 35°C to avoid cardiac arrhythmias. Placing a heating blanket on the operating table before beginning the procedure and the use of a heated humidifier in the ventilator circuit are both useful measures for maintaining the donor's core temperature.

Many donors will be profoundly volume de-

TABLE 21-2   General Criteria for Multiple Organ Donors

1. Age varies with organ
2. No history of pre-existing disease in that organ*
3. No history of cancer except skin or primary brain*
4. Absence of sepsis, hepatitis, AIDS*
5. No recent history of IV drug abuse*
6. No prolonged episodes of hypotension or asystole*
7. Limits for vasopressors vary with organ*
8. ABO compatible with recipient*
9. No evidence of DIC*
10. Donor size compatible with recipient[†,‡,§]
11. No infiltrate on chest x-ray[†,‡]
12. $PO_2 > 250$ mm Hg,[†] or > 70 mm Hg[‡,§,‖,¶] on FiO_2 of 1.00
13. Normal EKG, normal cardiac exam[†,‡]
14. LFTs within normal range[§]
15. Coagulation studies within normal range[§]
16. BUN, creatinine within normal range[‖]
17. UA normal for circumstances of the donor[‖]

---

* All organs
† Heart–lung
‡ Heart
§ Liver
‖ Kidney
¶ Pancreas

TABLE 21-3   Age Ranges for Organ Donors

ORGAN	AGE RANGE
Heart–lung	10–40 yr
Heart	15–45 yr, female
	15–40 yr, male
Lung	8–40 yr
Liver	Newborn–50 yr
Kidney	1–60 yr
Pancreas	8–40 yr

pleted as a result of the treatment for their head injury and will also have massive urinary outputs secondary to diabetes insipidus as a direct result of their head injury. Frequent balancing of fluid infusions with fluid losses is needed to avoid profound hypovolemia. Systemic Pitressin infusion in these donors may provide a margin of safety by markedly reducing urinary losses, although injudicious use may cause pulmonary edema, and the prolonged use of high doses of this agent carries the potential danger of compromising tissue perfusion, especially to the liver.

Hemodynamic stability must be maintained throughout the donor procedure, especially in heart and heart–lung donors. A central venous (CV) catheter, or, ideally, a pulmonary artery (PA) catheter is required to regulate the donor's fluid balance. An arterial catheter provides constant, on-line measurements of arterial blood pressure (BP) as well as ready access for arterial blood gas (ABG) determinations. Both the PA (or CV) and arterial catheters should be placed in the upper extremity, since both the inferior vena cava and aorta will eventually be ligated during the procurement procedure.

The donor should have at least one large-bore intravenous line in the upper extremity for rapid fluid and blood administration. Ideally, blood products should be infused to maintain a near normal coagulation profile and a hemoglobin above 10 gm/dl. With sufficient fluid resuscitation in the operating room, donors that required vasopressor support in the intensive care unit may prove much easier to manage. In general, when pharmacologic support of the donor BP is required, dopamine in doses that are either dopaminergic or inotropic should be tried before resorting to doses that are clearly vasoconstrictive (>15 mcg/kg/min). Without adequate fluid resuscitation, the use of vasopressors in an effort to maintain a certain BP may seriously compromise tissue perfusion and thus jeopardize the functional quality of the organs that are to be procured.

Table 21-4 is a checklist that summarizes measures taken to ensure that the donor is maintained in optimal condition throughout the procurement procedure. The anesthesiologist may be requested to administer a variety of medications throughout the procedure, including muscle relaxants, steroids, diuretics, and alpha blocking agents. Anesthesia support is continued throughout the procurement procedure until the preservation solution is infused just prior to organ removal.

THE SURGICAL PROCEDURES

During multiple organ recoveries, as many as four separate surgical teams may be involved in the recovery of the various organs. Each team is concerned with its own particular organ and with its own protocols for the procedure. Complete cooperation among all the teams is essential to ensure the quality of all the organs recovered. To accomplish this, the involved surgeons must discuss the proposed procedure thoroughly before it begins. This will ensure that each understands and agrees with the others' plans. Because the critical nationwide shortage of all transplantable organs demands that the number of donors that provide multiple organs increases, all surgeons involved in organ procurement must be familiar with the standard procedures for the procurement of other organs.[17,22,33,36,38,40,41]

In addition to cooperation among themselves, all surgical recovery teams must ensure that the procurement is carried out as expediently as possible

TABLE 21-4 Checklist for Operating Room

1. Heating blanket on table
2. Esophageal or rectal temperature probe in place
3. CVP line or PA catheter in place and monitored
4. Large-bore IV and arterial line in upper extremity
5. Foley catheter, urimeter in place
6. Blood, in room, checked and ready for transfusion
7. Drugs to be given ready in OR
8. Check baseline ABG
9. Ensure recovery teams have discussed procedure
10. Discuss procedure with anesthesiologist
11. Contact various recipient hospitals when organs inspected and determined to be adequate

and with minimal stress and inconvenience to the donor hospital. Multiple organ recovery can be carried out in any hospital that is capable of performing routine major surgical procedures. Each recovery team is responsible for bringing with them any specialized equipment that may not be available at the donor hospital. As an example, the authors' liver transplantation group brings special chest and abdominal retractors, all necessary infusion cannulas and solutions, as well as a Lebsche knife and mallet. All other equipment is usually available in the donor hospital.

Incision

No matter which combination of organs is to be recovered, the standard incision is made in the midline from the suprasternal notch to the pubis. Liberal use of the electrocautery on the coagulating current provides for maximal hemostasis. To avoid injuring the bowel, the peritoneum is opened over the liver in the cephalad portion of the abdominal incision (Fig. 21-1).

A quick inspection of the abdomen is carried out after the abdominal portion of incision is completed and the falciform ligament is ligated and divided. If no contraindications to proceeding with the recovery are identified, the midline sternotomy is completed in the standard fashion after ensuring that the heart is freed from the undersurface of the sternum. As the sternal retractor is opened, both pleural spaces are opened to ensure that the donor does not develop a tension pneumothorax. In addition, a short segment of diaphragm is freed from the inner thoracic cage to prevent tearing during the opening of the retractors, and a thorough inspection of all organs to be recovered is carried out.

Heart, Liver, and Kidney Recovery

At present, the most common triple organ procurement involves the recovery of the heart, liver, and kidneys.[22,32,33] Bone, skin, and corneas may also be procured with any of the various combinations of organ recoveries.[5,17,43] The techniques described for the recovery of these organs are easily adaptable to any variation of combined procurement. Table 21-5 provides a step-by-step outline of the various stages of the procurement procedure.

The initial liver dissection is carried out first. The gallbladder is freed from any peritoneal attachments. A finger is inserted into the foramen of Winslow to palpate for an aberrant right hepatic artery. This artery, which arises from the superior mesenteric artery (SMA) in 17% of patients, runs posterior to the portal vein.[24] If the right hepatic artery arises from the SMA, it must be traced back to its junction with the main SMA and meticulously preserved.[10,27] A second arterial anomaly, a branch to the left lateral segment arising from the left gastric artery, must also be identified and, if present, preserved. This branch is located in the gastrohepatic ligament under the left lateral segment. The common bile duct (CBD) is freed-up and divided at the level of the duodenum. The gallbladder then is opened, and normal saline is used to flush out both the gallbladder and CBD to prevent autolysis of the biliary endothelium. The cut end of the CBD is inspected. If two lumens are present, the cystic duct lumen is identified by the leakage of the gallbladder irrigation fluid from this lumen. This has obvious importance during the biliary reconstruction of the donor liver. The biliary reconstruction of the donor liver (either choledochocholedocotomy or Roux-en-Y choledochojejunostomy) will be carried out to the lumen of the common bile duct. The donor gallbladder is routinely removed at the completion of the transplantation procedure. The areolar tissue over the remaining hilar structures is ligated and divided. Care is taken throughout the procedure to ligate all tissue on the donor side of the dissection to prevent bleeding following revascularization of the liver.

The gastroduodenal artery and right gastric artery (if present) are identified, ligated, and divided. Whenever a branch of the hepatic artery is ligated, care must be taken to ligate it well away from the main vessel to prevent an intimal dissection in the main hepatic artery. The location of the hepatic artery is relatively constant, running between a lymph node located on the medial aspect of the hilum and the superior edge of the pancreas. The areolar tissue between the artery and the pancreas is divided, keeping well away from the artery to avoid causing spasm in the vessel. In addition, the coronary vein will require ligation and division during this dissection. The splenic and left gastric arteries (if no anomalous branch to the liver is present) are iden-

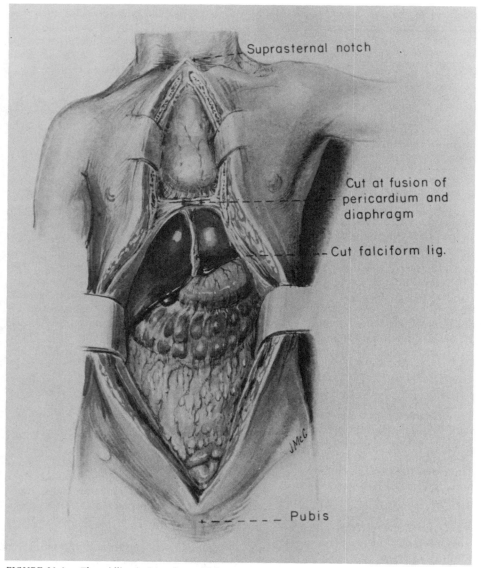

Suprasternal notch

Cut at fusion of
pericardium and
diaphragm

Cut falciform lig.

Pubis

FIGURE 21-1.   The midline incision for multiple organ procurement from suprasternal notch to pubis. (Reproduced with permission of the author and publisher from Starzl TE et al: A flexible procedure for multiple cadaveric organ procurement. Surg Gynecol Obstet 158: 223–230, 1984.)

tified, ligated, and divided, again keeping well away from the main celiac trunk.

Attention is then turned back to the hilum, where the portal vein is freed, as are its splenic and superior mesenteric branches. Following ligation of the distal splenic vein, a cannula is placed into the portal vein by way of the proximal splenic vein (Fig. 21-2). A very slow infusion of iced Ringer's lactate is begun. Although this pre-cooling step is omitted by some procurement groups, the authors believe

that, as originally described by Starzl,[32] it provides initial cooling of the liver while it still has an arterial supply. This is probably more important in adult- than pediatric-sized organs in enhancing core cool- ing of the organ.

While a slow pre-cooling is continued, the left triangular ligament is divided, and the supraceliac aorta is freed from the diaphragmatic crus and en- circled with an umbilical tape. The abdominal aorta is mobilized at the iliac bifurcation as is the inferior

TABLE 21-5   Outline of Heart, Liver, and Kidney Recovery

INITIAL LIVER DISSECTION

1. Free gallbladder from peritoneal attachments
2. Identify the blood supply to the liver, checking for left gastric branch to left lobe and for SMA branch to right lobe
3. Divide common bile duct at the duodenum, flush by way of gallbladder
4. Trace common hepatic artery to celiac axis, ligate right gastric and gastroduodenal arteries
5. Divide splenic and left gastric arteries*
6. Free splenic vein and SMV and cannulate portal vein
7. Encircle supraceliac aorta
8. Free and encircle distal aorta and vena cava

INITIAL HEART DISSECTION

1. Open pericardium, tack-up
2. Free aorta and vena cava from PA
3. Place cardioplegia needle after heparinization

INITIAL KIDNEY DISSECTION

1. Mobilize right colon
2. Free ureters, divide, and culture
3. Identify, ligate, and divide SMA†
4. Minimal freeing up of kidneys

PRE-COOL STEPS

1. Heparinize patient 3 mg/kg (100 U/kg–400 U/kg)
2. Ligate distal aorta and vena cava and cannulate
3. Ligate SMV, increase rate of pre-cool
4. Pre-cool until donor temperature 28°–31°C or arrhythmia develops
5. Staple SVC, clamp infrainnominate aorta
6. Start cardioplegia, clamp supraceliac aorta
7. Start aortic flush, change portal flush to Euro-Collins' or other solution
8. Discontinue anesthesia support

FINAL HEART DISSECTION

1. Divide IVC at right atrium
2. Divide left pulmonary vein

3. Divide main pulmonary artery at bifurcation
4. SVC divided proximal to the staple line
5. Right pulmonary veins divided
6. Left atrium freed from pericardium
7. Aortic clamp removed and aorta stapled and divided
8. Heart removed, prepared for implantation and packaged

FINAL LIVER DISSECTION

1. Aortic flush continues until 0.5 liter–1.5 liter infused
2. Slow portal flush after 0.5 liter–1.0 liter infused
3. Identify proximal end of SMA, crossclamp aorta at orifice of SMA
4. Continue kidneys flush with Euro-Collins' or other preservation solution
5. Divide aorta between aortic cross-clamps
6. Divide vena cava above renal veins
7. Free suprahepatic vena cava from diaphragm
8. Remove liver with wide cuff of diaphragm
9. Free liver from retroperitoneal attachments
10. Package liver on back table
11. After kidneys removed:
    a. Iliac artery and vein harvested for grafts
    b. Lymph nodes and piece of spleen removed for matching

FINAL RENAL DISSECTION

1. Aorta and vena cava divided below cannulas
2. Assistant holds up ureters and aortic and vena caval cannulas
3. Dissecting on vertebral column, kidneys removed enbloc
4. Kidneys separated on the back table, packaged individually
5. Lymph nodes and piece of spleen removed for matching

---

* Only if no left gastric branch to liver
† Only if no SMA branch to liver

---

vena cava (IVC). Both are encircled with two umbilical tapes, taking care to avoid injuring the lumbar branches. The right colon is completely mobilized up to the SMA, and the tissue over the infrahepatic vena cava is divided until both the renal veins are identified. As the dissection of the aorta is carried proximally, the inferior mesenteric artery is ligated and divided, and the left renal vein is identified. The SMA is dissected free from its ganglion and encircled with two heavy silk ties.

The preliminary heart and kidney dissections are carried out next.

The heart team begins its dissection by opening the pericardium and tacking it up to the sternal border.[6,11,17,22,30,33,37,41] The PA is freed from the aorta, and the superior vena cava (SVC) is freed from the PA.

The nephrectomy team may perform the preliminary kidney dissection next. However, if desired, the entire renal dissection may be completed after the liver has been harvested.[6,7,14,17,22,25,33,41] In either case, the ureters are mobilized, taking care to preserve their blood supply. They are divided at the bladder and cultured. The kidneys are gently freed from their retroperitoneal attachments until they are mobilized.

Before the infusion of the preservation solutions, the final steps occur in rapid succession. The donor is heparinized with 3 mg/kg of heparin (usually 100 U/kg–400 U/kg). The distal aorta and vena

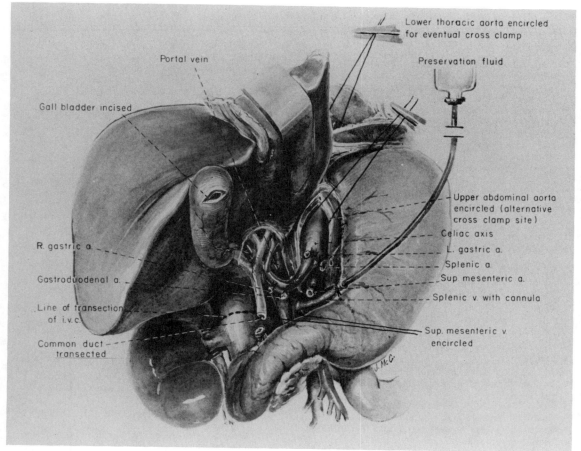

FIGURE 21-2.   *Preliminary dissection for hepatectomy. Note that the common bile duct is divided and that the gall bladder is opened. The splenic vein is cannulated in preparation for precooling. The hepatic artery is exposed, and the left gastric and splenic arteries have been ligated and divided. The supraceliac aorta is encircled with an umbilical tape. The dotted line indicates the site at which the inferior vena cava (IVC) will be transected. (Reproduced with permission of the author and publisher from Starzl TE et al: A flexible procedure for multiple cadaveric organ procurement. Surg Gynecol Obstet 158: 223–230, 1984.)*

cava are ligated at their bifurcations, and both are cannulated. The clamped aortic cannula is connected to tubing from a bottle containing preservation solution, and the clamped IVC cannula is attached to an empty urinary drainage bag (Fig. 21-3). The cardiac team cannulates the aorta and attaches the clamped cannula to a cardioplegia solution (Fig. 21-4). The PA or CV catheter is removed from the great veins. The SMA is ligated and divided, and the superior mesenteric vein (SMV) ligated.

At this point, if the donor's cardiovascular status has remained satisfactory, the pre-cool infusion rate of the Ringer's lactate into the portal vein is increased, and the warming blanket is turned off.

In many cases, the donor's core temperature can be lowered to below 30°C without cardiac arrythmias developing. This may involve the infusion of upward of 2 liters to 4 liters of cold solution in adult donors. As volume is infused rapidly, care must be taken to drain off blood through the vena cava cannula to avoid central venous hypertension. This can be facilitated by monitoring both the CVP and arterial pressures, both of which change rapidly with alterations in blood volume.

During this stage, the cardiac surgeon monitors the action of the heart. He has the option of interrupting the pre-cooling at any time that he deems appropriate. Most stable donors will easily tolerate core temperature lowering to at least 30°C.

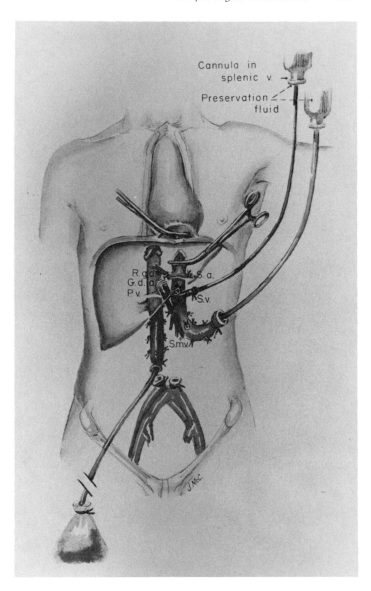

FIGURE 21-3.   *The preliminary dissection of all organs is complete, and cannulas are placed in the distal aorta and inferior vena cava (IVC) in preparation for the in situ flushing of the liver and kidneys with preservation solution (see text for details). (Reproduced with permission of the author and publisher from Starzl TE at al: A flexible procedure for multiple cadaveric organ procurement. Surg Gynecol Obstet 158: 223–230, 1984.)*

In any case, when it is deemed necessary to discontinue pre-cooling, a number of maneuvers are performed simultaneously.

The cardiac surgeon staples the superior vena cava 2 cm proximal to its junction with the right atrium (RA). He then clamps the ascending aorta just proximal to the innominate artery and begins the rapid infusion of cold cardioplegia solution through the previously placed catheter. At the moment that all of this is occurring, the liver surgeon opens the IVC cannula to exsanguinate the donor, clamps the supraceliac aorta, and immediately opens the flush of cold preservation solution

through the distal abdominal aorta. The cardiac surgeon may elect to open the IVC in the chest in order to decompress the heart rather than rely on exsanguination through the distal IVC cannula. Anesthesia support is discontinued when the heart arrests.

The cardiac team now rapidly completes the removal of the arrested heart.[6,11,17,22,33,37,41] If not done previously, the IVC is divided at the atrium (leaving as much cava length as possible for the liver team), and blood and preservation fluid are aspirated from the pericardium. The left pulmonary veins are divided at the pericardium, and the main

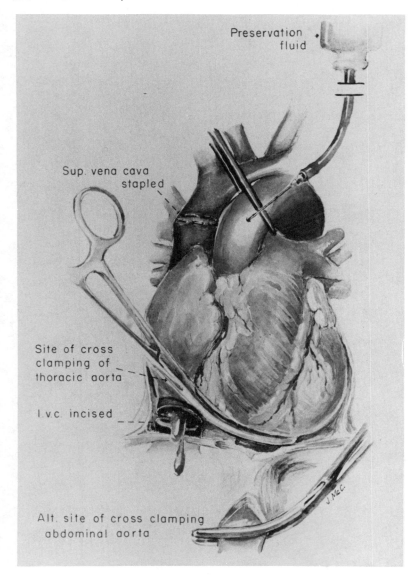

Preservation fluid

Sup. vena cava stapled

Site of cross clamping of thoracic aorta

l.v.c. incised

Alt. site of cross clamping abdominal aorta

J.McC.

FIGURE 21-4.   Cardiectomy is completed as described in the text. Note that the descending aorta may be clamped either in the chest or just proximal to the celiac axis in the abdomen. (Reproduced with permission of the author and publisher from Starzl TE et al: A flexible procedure for multiple cadaveric organ procurement. Surg Gynecol Obstet 158: 223–230, 1984.)

pulmonary artery is divided at the bifurcation. The SVC is divided proximal to the line of staples, and the right pulmonary veins are transected at the pericardium. The posterior attachments of the left atrium to the pericardium are divided as the heart is lifted in a cephalad direction. The aorta is stapled at the level of the crossclamp and divided distal to the staple line. Many surgeons leave the cannula in situ to allow continued infusion of cold preservation solution while the heart is being sewn into the recipient.

The heart is removed and immediately immersed in cold crystalloid solution. In preparation for implantation, the left atrium is opened through the orifices of the pulmonary veins and the right atrium by incising through the vena caval openings. The heart is placed in a sterile container with cold crystalloid solution and then placed in an ice chest for transport.

While the heart is being removed, the liver and kidneys are being flushed with cold preservation solution. The portal vein cannula is switched from Ringer's lactate to preservation solution as soon as the aortic infusion is begun. The venous effluent is drained both by the IVC cannula and the transected inferior vena cava in the chest. The aorta is flushed with 1 liter to 2 liters and the portal vein with 500 ml to 1000 ml of preservation solution.

The liver surgeon then identifies the aortic stump of the SMA and, after ensuring that the renal arteries are safe, places a second aortic crossclamp at the level of the SMA orifice. This allows for the continued perfusion of the kidneys while the liver is removed. After application of this second aortic clamp, the liver is removed rapidly by first dividing the aorta between the aortic crossclamps and freeing this segment of the aorta (which contains the celiac axis) from its retroperitoneal attachments. Care must be taken to maintian the dissection well away from the celiac trunk in order to avoid inadvertent injury to this vessel. The suprahepatic vena cava is freed, taking a wide cuff of diaphragm that will be removed prior to implantation of the donor liver. The SMV and splenic vein are divided between the previously placed ligatures, and the infrahepatic vena cava is divided just above the renal veins. The liver is then lifted cephalad, and, taking care to protect the major vascular structures, the posterior attachments are divided, maintaining the plane of dissection within the muscle fibers of the diaphragmatic crus.

The liver is taken to the back table where it is placed in two plastic bags with preservation solution and packed in an ice chest.

The renal recovery team now removes the kidneys.[6,7,14,22,25,29,33,41,48] The aorta and vena cava are divided below the cannulas, and, with an assistant holding up the previously divided ureters along with the vena caval and aortic cannulas, the posterior aspects of these vessels are rapidly dissected free from the retroperitoneum, keeping the scissors on the spinous ligament. In this way, the kidneys are removed rapidly with little or no chance of injury. The kidneys are separated on the back table and packaged individually.

The majority of centers no longer machine perfuse the kidneys.[2] However, if the kidneys are to be machine perfused, the kidney team normally would have done a more extensive dissection of the kidneys[18,19] earlier in the procedure with meticulous ligation of all branches of the aorta. The kidneys can be removed individually or en bloc and separated on the back table and then placed on machine perfusion (Figs. 21-5 and 21-6).

After the kidneys have been removed, the iliac arteries and veins are harvested by the liver team from the bifurcation to the inguinal ligament. These will be used to provide vascular grafts if they are required during implantation of the liver.[34] In addition, lymph nodes are removed for the kidney, liver, and heart teams. These nodes are used for

prospective crossmatching with kidney (and in some centers heart or pancreas) recipients and retrospective crossmatching with the liver recipient.

Starzl[36] has described a modification of the above technique for the recovery of multiple organs which is particularly applicable in hemodynamically unstable donors that may not tolerate a long operative procedure. This "rapid flush technique" involves the placement of the aortic and vena caval cannulae as described above as the initial step in the procedure. After these cannulae have been placed, the cardiac team completes its initial dissection, arrests the heart, and performs the cardiectomy as described above. While the cardiectomy is being performed, the supraceliac aorta is cross-clamped, and the abdominal viscera are flushed with up to 15 liters of 4° C solution. The remaining dissection of the liver, pancreas, and kidneys is then carried out in a bloodless field after the organs have been cooled. While some centers have adopted this technique as the routine donor procedure, most procurement groups reserve the procedure only for hemodynamically unstable donors.

Pancreas Recovery

The pancreas can be removed either as a segmental graft, or the entire pancreas and spleen can be removed together. If a segmental pancreas graft is to be removed, this can be accomplished with any combination of organs.[13,17,40,42] However, if a total pancreaticoduodenal transplantation is to be carried out, the pancreas graft will need to include both the SMA and the celiac axis (to provide the gastroduodenal, pancreaticoduodenal, and splenic arteries). This normally will preclude liver donation, because the liver transplant team invariably requires that the entire celiac axis be included intact with the liver graft. However, it is now possible to use the entire pancreas and liver with a technique applied in one of our cases and in a series of cases described in detail in the chapter on pancreas transplantation.

In our case, the entire celiac axis was left intact with the donor liver. The splenic and gastroduodenal arteries of the pancreas graft were reconstructed with an iliac artery graft from the donor. The internal iliac branch of the artery graft was anastomosed end-to-end with the splenic artery of the pancreas graft and the external iliac with the gastroduodenal artery. The common end of the iliac artery graft was then anastomosed end-to-side with the recipient's external iliac artery, as was a Carrel patch of donor aorta, which contained the opening of the SMA. Most of the length of the portal vein

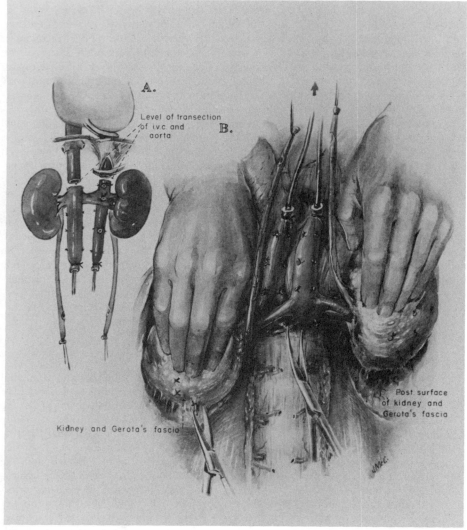

FIGURE 21-5.   *The kidneys are removed* en bloc. *They can then be divided on the back table (see Fig. 21-6) and either machine perfused or stored in ice. (Reproduced with permission of the author and publisher from Starzl TE et al: A flexible procedure for multiple cadaveric organ procurement. Surg Gynecol Obstet 158: 223–230, 1984.)*

(PV) was left with the liver graft. In order to obtain adequate length on the pancreas graft, a segment of donor common iliac vein was sewn end-to-end to the stump of PV. This was then sewn end-to-side with the recipient external iliac vein at the time of transplantation. All these reconstructive preparations were done on the back table with the graft immersed in slush solution. Greater experience with this technique may ultimately open the door to this particular combined procurement procedure.

The incision is made as previously described,

and the lesser sac is entered through the gastrocolic ligament. The spleen is mobilized by division of the lienophrenic and lienocolic ligaments. Using the spleen as a handle, the tail of the pancreas is freed from the retroperitoneum. The dissection is carried medially until the SMA is visualized as it emerges from under the pancreas.

The surgeon now has several options for removing the segmental pancreas graft. If the liver is to be procured, the liver surgeon can offer the option of an in situ flush of the pancreas by leaving the

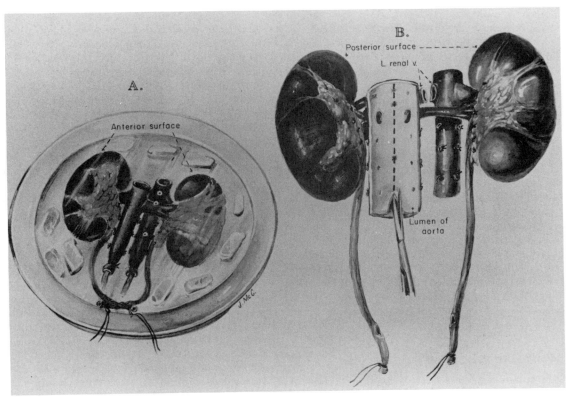

FIGURE 21-6.   *The kidneys are separated on the back table after* en bloc *removal. Dividing the aorta longitudinally along its posterior wall between the lumbar ostia facilitates the identification of aberrant renal arteries. (Reproduced with permission of the author and publisher from Starzl TE et al: A flexible procedure for multiple cadaveric organ procurement. Surg Gynecol Obstet 158: 223–230, 1984.)*

splenic artery intact on the celiac axis and cannulating the portal vein through the inferior mesenteric branch rather than through the splenic vein. Then the pancreas can be perfused with cold preservation fluid in situ, along with the other organs when the aortic flush is started. At the time that the splenic vein is divided and the final portal flush of the liver is begun, the pancreatic end of the vein should be left open to allow blood and fluid to escape. This is necessary to prevent venous engorgement of the pancreas during the flushing process. After the aortic flush is completed, the pancreas is removed either independently or in combination with the liver and separated, as described below, on the back table.

If an in situ flush of the pancreas is not desired, the segmental graft can be removed just after the liver surgeon has completed the dissection of the celiac axis and before the pre-cooling is begun. To accomplish this, the pancreas surgeon divides the splenic artery at its origin from the celiac axis and the splenic vein at its junction with the SMV. At the

same time, the portal vein cannula can be inserted into the hepatic end of the splenic vein as described previously. Next, the pancreas is divided at its neck, the distal splenic vessels are ligated and divided, and the spleen is removed. The segmental pancreas graft is placed in iced saline, the splenic artery is cannulated, and the pancreas is flushed with the preservation solution of choice.

After either method of procurement, the pancreas is stored in the same solution with which it was flushed and then packaged in an ice chest. The remainder of the dissection of the liver, heart, and kidneys is identical with that previously described.

If the total pancreas is to be transplanted, the initial incision and the initial dissection are performed as just described.[23,35] The left gastric branch of the celiac axis is ligated and divided, and the hepatic artery is traced to its gastroduodenal branch. The hepatic artery is ligated distal to the gastroduodenal artery, and the proximal duodenum is mobilized until the superior mesenteric vessels are identified. These are ligated and divided as they emerge from under the pancreas. The proximal and distal duodenum are divided with the stapler.

The whole pancreas can then be perfused in situ as described previously or removed and flushed out on the back table. Once the in situ flush is completed, the aorta is dissected retrograde as described before except that the SMA is left intact. If possible, a clamp is placed on the aorta between the SMA and the renal arteries to allow continued in situ perfusion of the kidneys while the pancreas is removed. The aortic segment removed with the pancreas contains the orifices of both the SMA and the celiac axis. This allows for the anastomosis of a Carrel patch containing both of these arteries to the side of the recipient's iliac artery. In addition, the portal vein is dissected high up into the hepatic hilum to allow as much length as possible for later anastomosis end-to-side to the recipient's iliac vein. Usually the pancreas is removed with the spleen attached, and the entire unit is placed in the same solution as used for flushing and packed in an ice chest. The kidneys are removed as described previously.

Heart–Lung Recovery

The techniques described for heart–lung harvest limit the organs that can be procured simultaneously.[6,12,17–19] At present, most centers are reluctant to harvest the liver or the pancreas from a heart–lung donor because of the added length of time for dissection of these other organs and the potential for added blood loss and donor instability with resultant injury to the lungs. Most centers require that the heart–lung donor be transported to the institution where the transplant will take place, and many harvest the heart–lung complex on cardiopulmonary bypass. This is because of the limited time that the heart–lung complex can be stored. (The University of Pittsburgh has recently reported promising results with a system for the transportation of the heart–lung complex with extended preservation times.[39] The technique involves maintaining a normothermic, heart-beating, and ventilated preparation during transport. Although experience with the technique has been limited, they report adequate preservation up to 3 hours after removal from the donor.)

For all these reasons, the kidneys are usually the only additional organs recovered from these donors. However, since the donor is often cooled to 4°C while on cardiopulmonary bypass, the liver or pancreas, in addition to the kidneys, should be suitable for transplantation. Starzl[31] has achieved successful transplantation of liver grafts harvested in this way.

The liver or pancreas and kidney teams may be allowed to perform their initial dissection prior to the institution of cardiopulmonary bypass. Alternatively, all the dissection can be done while the donor is on cardiopulmonary bypass (by way of the femoral artery and femoral vein) and after the heart–lung complex has been removed. In the latter instance, the abdominal procurement teams can perform in situ flushes of their organs with preservation fluid as soon as the cardiac team is out of the way and after any initial dissection of the abdominal organs has been completed. If the donor core temperature is not cooled down to the cytoprotective level while on cardiopulmonary bypass, the abdominal teams must be ready to perform in situ flushing by way of a distal abdominal aortic cannula, just as described previously, the moment that the aorta is interrupted in the chest.

The actual dissection of the heart–lungs is straightforward. The cardiac team begins by first freeing the aorta from the pulmonary artery at the level of the innominate artery. The inferior pulmonary ligaments are divided bilaterally. The trachea is freed into the neck, well above the carina. Once the dissection is complete, a large-bore needle or cannula is inserted into the ascending aorta for infusion of cardioplegia solution. The infrainnominate aorta is clamped, and, immediately, the infusion of the cardioplegia is begun by the aortic root cannula. The superior and inferior vena cavae are divided, and blood and fluid are allowed to escape from the graft. If the abdominal organs are to be procured, the IVC must be clamped just above the diaphragm to avoid sudden exsanguination of the cadaver.

To complete the removal of the heart and lungs as a unit, the aorta is stapled proximal to the clamp and divided between the clamp and the staple line. The trachea is divided just above the carina, and the heart–lung complex is lifted out of the chest. The organs can be placed in preservative solution with or without inflation of the lungs. The complex is reimplanted as soon as possible.

The remainder of the multiple organ recovery is carried out much as described previously. Because the donor core temperature has been lowered to 4°C to 6°C on bypass, the need for the initial precooling step is eliminated. The abdominal teams complete the dissection of their various organs, including ligation of various arteries (such as the IMA, SMA, and distal femoral arteries), which supply nonessential organs. In addition, the proximal aorta can be reclamped just below the diaphragm to avoid loss of preservative into the chest. Then, to complete the perfusion of the abdominal organs, the surgeon simply uses the femoral artery cannula (used for return of blood from the bypass machine) to flush the abdominal aorta with preservative solution. The abdominal organs are then removed as previously described.

Single Lung Recovery

Because the time that lungs may be preserved is extremely limited, the majority of single-lung harvests occur in the institution in which the lung is to be procured.[6,9,17,45–47] When a single lung is harvested, the heart usually cannot be taken simultaneously because of the need for generous left atrial and pulmonary artery cuffs for the lung graft. However, all other organs can be harvested by the techniques previously described.

After the initial dissection of the other organs, attention is turned to the left lung. The inferior pulmonary ligament is divided. After freeing the left pulmonary artery to the level of the first branch, the avascular plane between the left mainstem bronchus and the left atrium is bluntly dissected. The visceral pleura is divided posteriorly. At this time, the patient is heparinized and cannulas are placed in the abdominal aorta and inferior vena cava. The aortic crossclamp is placed at the appropriate level, depending upon the other organs to be recovered, and the infusion by the aortic cannula is begun. At the same time, the left pulmonary artery is divided as proximally as possible between clamps. The left lung is inflated, and the left mainstem bronchus is clamped proximal to the left upper lobe bronchus. The lung thus remains inflated. After the bronchial arteries are ligated and divided, the left atrium is divided in order to provide a generous cuff of atrium, which includes the left inferior and superior pulmonary veins. The pulmonary artery is cannulated, and the solution of choice is infused until the effluent from the pulmonary veins is clear and the lung is blanched and cold. The pulmonary artery and left atrial cuff are clamped. The lung may either be stored inflated or uninflated in a preservative solution and is reimplanted as soon as possible.

After the lung is removed, the remaining organs are recovered as previously described.

CONCLUSION

With the huge demand for organs for transplantation, all organ donors must be viewed as potential multiorgan donors. The recovery of multiple organs from a single donor requires cooperation of all participating teams. However, the techniques described allow for each organ to be protected while the other organs are procured. The authors stress the use of in situ flushing techniques because warm ischemia to any of the organs can be eliminated. Anatomic considerations are the only factors limiting which organs can be recovered simultaneously. A number of studies support the concept that organs recovered from multiple organ donors function at least as well as those procured from a single organ donor.[20,21,26,28,29] When success is obtained with the clinical transplantation of other solid organs, such as the small intestine, these organs can be procured simultaneously, with only minor modifications of technique.

REFERENCES

1. Action Items of Note. Published by the American Council on Transplantation, July–August, 1985
2. Barry JM, Metcalfe JB, Farnsworth MA et al: Comparison of intracellular flushing and cold storage to machine perfusion for human kidney preservation. J Urol 123:14–16, 1980
3. Bart KJ, Macon EJ, Humphries AL et al: Increasing the supply of cadaveric kidneys for transplantation. Transplantation 31:383–387, 1981
4. Bart KJ, Macon EJ, Whittier RJ et al: Cadaveric kidneys for transplantation: A paradox of shortage in the face of plenty. Transplantation 31:379–382, 1981
5. Bondoc CC, Burke JF: Clinical experience with viable frozen human skin and a frozen skin bank. Ann Surg 174:371–382, 1971
6. Cederna J, Toledo-Pereyra LH: Multiple organ harvesting; Selection, maintenance, surgical techniques. Contemp Surg 25:15–26, 1984
7. Colberg JE: En bloc excision of cadaver kidneys for transplantation. Arch Surg 115:1238–1241, 1980
8. Council on Scientific Affairs of the American Medical Association. Organ Donor Recruitment. JAMA 246(19):2157, 1981
9. Crane R, Torres M, Hagstran JWC et al: Twenty-four hour preservation and transplantation of the lung without function impairment. Surg Forum 26:111–113, 1975
10. Gordon RD, Shaw BW Jr, Iwatsuki S et al: A simplified technique for revascularization of homografts of the liver with a variant right hepatic artery from the superior mesenteric artery. Surg Gynecol Obstet 160:475–476, 1985
11. Hardesty RL, Griffith BP, Trento A et al: Multiple cadaveric organ procurement for transplantation with emphasis on the heart. Surgical Rounds 6:18–34, 1985

12. Jamieson SW, Reitz BA, Oyer PE et al: Combined heart and lung transplantation. Lancet 1:1130–1132, 1983

13. Land W, Landgraf R (eds): Segmental pancreatic transplantation. International workshop. Horm Metab Res [Suppl] 13:1–104, 1983

14. Linke CA, Linke CL, Fridd CW: Cadaver kidney retrieval for transplantation. Surgical Rounds 11:19–26, 1984

15. Manninen DL, Evans RW: Public attitudes and behavior regarding organ donation. JAMA 253:3111–3115, 1985

16. Montefusco CM, Mollenkopf FP, Kamholz SL et al: Maintenance protocol for potential organ donors in multiple organ procurement. Hosp Phys 3:9–14, 1984

17. Montefusco CM, Veith FJ: Organ selection and preservation for transplantation. Hosp Phys 1:98–101, 2:29–33, 1985

18. Reitz BA, Pennock JL, Shumway NE et al: Simplified operative method for heart and lung transplantation. J Surg Res 31:1–5, 1981

19. Reitz BA, Wallwork JL, Hunt SA et al: Heart–lung transplantation: Successful therapy for patients with pulmonary vascular disease. N Engl J Med 306:557–564, 1982

20. Rolles K, Calne RY, McMaster P: Technique of organ removal and fate of kidney graft from liver donors. Transplantation 28:44–46, 1979

21. Rosenthal JT, Denny D, Hakala T: Results from a single procurement center. J Urol 129:111–113, 1983

22. Rosenthal JT, Shaw BW Jr, Hardesty RL et al: Principles of multiple organ procurement from cadaver donors. Ann Surg 198:617–621, 1983

23. Schneider A, Toledo-Pereyra LH: Simultaneous transplantation of the kidney and pancreas for end-stage diabetic nephropathy. Surg Gynecol Obstet 158:286–289, 1984

24. Schwartz ST: Liver. In Schwartz SI (ed): Principles of Surgery, 5th ed, pp 1257–1305. New York, McGraw-Hill, 1984

25. Schweizer R, Sutphin BA, Bartus SA: In situ cadaver kidney perfusion. Transplantation 32:482–487, 1981

26. Shaw BW Jr, Hakala T, Rosenthal JT et al: Combination donor hepatectomy and nephrectomy and early functional results. Surg Gynecol Obstet 155:321–325, 1982

27. Shaw BW Jr, Iwatsuki S, Starzl TE: Alternative methods of hepatic graft arterialization. Surg Gynecol Obstet 159:490–494, 1984

28. Shaw BW Jr, Rosenthal JT, Griffith BP et al: Early function of heart, liver and kidney allografts following combined procurement. Transplant Proc 16:238–242, 1984

29. Shaw BW Jr, Rosenthal JT, Griffith BP et al: Techniques for combined procurement of hearts and kidneys with satisfactory early function of renal allografts. Surg Gynecol Obstet 157:261–264, 1983

30. Shumway NE, Stinson EB: Two decades of experimental and clinical orthotopic homotransplantation of the heart. Perspect Biol Med 22:81–88, 1979

31. Starzl TE: Personal communication

32. Starzl TE: Experience in hepatic transplantation. Philadelphia, WB Saunders, Philadelphia, 1969

33. Starzl TE, Hakala T, Shaw BW Jr et al: A flexible procedure for multiple cadaveric organ procurement. Surg Gynecol Obstet 158:223–230, 1984

34. Starzl TE, Halgrimson CG, Koep LJ et al: Vascular homografts from cadaveric organ donors. Surg Gynecol Obstet 149:737, 1979

35. Starzl TE, Iwatsuki S, Shaw BW Jr et al: Pancreaticoduodenal transplantation in humans. Surg Gynecol Obstet 159:265–272, 1984

36. Starzl TE, Shaw BW Jr, Iwatsuki S et al: Orthotopic liver transplantation in 1984. Transplant Proc 27:250–258, 1985

37. Stinson EB, Dong E, Iben AB et al: Cardiac transplantation in man: Surgical aspects. Am J Surg 118:182–187, 1969

38. Taylor RJ, Rosenthal JT, Hakala T: Combined cadaveric hepatic and renal organ procurement in infants; techniques for salvage of all organs. Arch Surg 120:1084–1085, 1985

39. Teodori MF, Stevenson NC, Ladowski JS et al: Autoperfusion heart–lung preparation for preservation in heart–lung transplantation. Surg Forum 36:311–313, 1985

40. Toledo-Pereyra LH: Multiple organ harvesting for transplantation. Surg Gynecol Obstet 158:573–576, 1984

41. Toledo-Pereyra LH: Organ harvesting. In Toledo-Pereyra LH (ed): Basic Concepts in Organ Procurement, Perfusion, and Preservation for Transplantation, pp 57–72. New York, Academic Press, 1982

42. Toledo-Pereyra LH, Mittal VK: Segmental pancreatic transplantation: Donor and recipient operation. Arch Surg 117:505–508, 1982

43. Van Horn DL: Cornea. In Karow AM Jr, Pegg DE (eds): Organ Preservation for Transplantation, pp 428–429. New York, Marcel Dekker, 1981

44. Van Thiel DH, Shade RR, Hakala TR et al: Liver procurement for orthotopic transplantation: An analysis of the Pittsburgh experience. Hepatology 4:665–715, 1984

45. Veith FJ, Crane R, Torres M et al: Effective preservation and transplantation of lung transplants. J Thorac Cardiovasc Surg 72:97–105, 1976

46. Veith FJ, Kamholz S, Mollenkopf FP et al: Lung transplantation 1983. Transplantation 35:271–278, 1983

47. Veith FJ, Richards K: Improved techniques for canine lung transplantation. Ann Surg 171:553–558, 1970

48. Zeichner WD, Toledo-Pereyra LH, MacKenzie GH et al: Cadaveric nephrectomy: Procurement harvesting, preservation. Contemp Surg 22:53–62, 1983

CHAPTER 22

Technical Aspects of Renal Transplantation

H. M. Lee

Iliac vessels are dissected free with careful ligation of the lymphatic vessels overlying them to minimize a lymph leak. Dissection of the entire length of the iliac arteries, including the hypogastric artery, and the entire length of the iliac veins, with the ligation and division of the internal iliac vein, makes it easy to perform the torsion free end-to-end arterial anastomosis and short renal vein anastomosis.

The renal artery is anastomosed either to the hypogastric artery end-to-end, or an end-to-side anastomosis to the external iliac artery is done. The renal vein is anastomosed to the external iliac vein end-to-side.

There are many variations in the technique to reconstruct the ureterovesical continuity. Two techniques are most commonly practiced: (1) classical ureteroneocystostomy, and (2) extravesical ureteroneocystostomy, the Lich and Gregoir technique.

Variations of the operation for (1) multiple arteries, (2) pediatric age recipients, and (3) a small pediatric kidney as a donor organ are also described briefly.

Surgical technique for human renal transplantation became fairly well standarized in the early 1960s.[11,17,23,33,34,50] Although the general principles of the operative technique are not different from that of general surgery, some emphasis should be placed on hemostasis and aseptic technique.[16,44,46] The transplant recipients are generally uremic and will undergo immunosuppressive therapy. They are often nutritionally depleted. These underlying conditions make the recipient more prone to bleeding and more vulnerable to infection and poor wound healing. The operative techniques require vascular anastomosis and careful opening and handling of the urinary tract. One cannot overemphasize the importance of meticulous hemostasis, aseptic technique, and gentle handling of the tissues to prevent surgical complications.

The transplanted kidney is placed in the retroperitoneal space in either the right or left pelvic fossa, regardless of the original side of the donor kidney. Most surgeons would prefer the right-side approach with the left donor kidney. The placement of the left kidney on the right pelvic fossa leaves the renal pelvis and ureter ventrally and superficially exposed, making them easier to approach if one needs to do ureteropelvic anastomosis or ureteroureteral anastomosis at a subsequent time. In the left-side approach, the sigmoid colon is close to the kidney and the iliac veins lie deeper. Consequently, in old patients, diagnosis and treatment of sigmoid diverticulitis may be more difficult.[46]

Preparation of the Recipient

It is preferable to prepare the recipient through optimal nutritional support; adequate dialysis; and treatment and removal of the sources of infection. If necessary, gastrointestinal tract evaluation and treatment, possibly including peptic ulcer surgery and resection of colonic diverticulitis, evaluation of hepatitis, and cardiac evaluation and treatment, including coronary artery surgery,[16,46] should be conducted. However, increased experience and the improved diagnostic and therapeutic regimens available in recent years have made many of the rigidly practiced old preparatory procedures, such as routine bilateral nephrectomy of the native kidney, prophylactic peptic ulcer surgery, and resection of the sigmoid colon with diverticulae, less imperative.[46] Bilateral nephrectomy of the native kidney is now practiced only for uncontrollable hypertension despite an adequate medical regimen on dialysis, or for kidney infections. We also perform a complete ureterectomy with nephrectomy for reflux when there is a history of infection. Indications for bilateral nephrectomy for certain immunologic nephropathy remain controversial. Infrequently, it may become necessary to remove the large polycystic kidney to create the space for the transplanted kidney. The native kidney may be removed through a midline incision or a subcostal incision or through a posterior approach. A splenectomy may be performed for hypersplenism to improve leukopenia so that one may use myelosuppressive and immunosuppressive agents more effectively.

We use a left subcostal incision, crossing over the midline slightly for the staged elective pretransplant bilateral nephrectomy. This incision can also be used when the bilateral nephrectomy is performed at the same time as the transplant. Some surgeons recommend a posterior approach for its simplicity and low morbidity.[36] One should be aware of a possible closed-space, retroperitoneal infection when using this approach in the infected kidney. The posterior approach here is essentially the same as that in a bilateral adrenectomy. A long midline incision is used for a bilateral nephrectomy combined with a complete ureterectomy.

Use of Prophylactic (Perioperative) Antibiotics

Infection remains one of the most serious complications of the early and late period after transplantation. Besides meticulous care to prevent hematoma-related wound infections and an aseptic and gentle operative technique, the perioperative use of antibiotics is widely accepted as an effective method of reducing wound infection.[46]

Antibiotics should be based on the experience of the microbiology laboratory of each center and the organisms found in the urinary tract. The general practice is to use a short-term, high-dose, broad-spectrum antibiotic regimen (such as cefoxitin) to cover staphylococcus and gram-negative bacilli.

Immediate Preoperative Preparation

All the potential sources of infection such as teeth, skin, and the bladder should be checked and treated.

If necessary, the patient should undergo a short hemodialysis to control fluid overload or electrolyte problems, particularly hyperkalemia, before surgery. A repeat cytotoxic crossmatch with fresh serum should be performed against the donor lymphocytes. If the skin is to be shaved, this should be done just before surgery to avoid skin infection. An indwelling catheter should be inserted with a gentle and strictly aseptic technique. One should instill antibiotics or an antiseptic solution into the bladder to minimize bacterial contamination of the wound at the later ureteral implantation.[5,11,16,17,23,33,34,36,46,50]

THE INCISION

A curvilineal incision in the right lower quadrant of the abdomen is most commonly used (Fig. 22-1).[17,44] This incision should start at the anterior axillary line 3 cm to 4 cm above the iliac crest, coming down 4 cm to 5 cm above and parallel to the inguinal ligament, reaching the midline just above the pubic spine. This incision can be carried up to the costal margin to increase the exposure, as in the case of a child receiving an adult kidney.

The aponeurosis of the external oblique muscle is divided in the direction of its fiber, and the muscle is split at the lateral corner of the incision. Medially, this is carried into the rectus sheath for a centimeter or more to facilitate later exposure of the bladder. The internal oblique and transverse abdominis muscles are divided as a unit in line with the skin incision. This is best done by starting at the medial corner of the portion of the fascia just lateral to the rectus, then incising the underlying, thin transversalis fascia, with care being taken not to cut the underlying peritoneum. Usually there is enough properitoneal fat separating the peritoneum from the transversalis fascia. One can insinuate the finger through this incision into the properitoneal space, separating the peritoneum from the transversalis fascia. It is easy to divide the internal oblique and transverse abdominis muscles simultaneously with electrocautery or knife.

The spermatic cord in the male is often not divided.[17,46] Even though some early descriptions of the operative technique suggest the division of the cord for better exposure of the field or for the prevention of ureteral obstruction, it is often unnecessary. The round ligament in the female is usually divided.

The inferior epigastric vessels are ligated and divided. The epigastric artery may be preserved if possibly needed for anastomosis with a donor organ that has multiple arteries. The peritoneum is re-

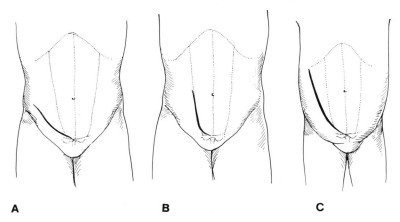

FIGURE 22-1.   *Incision. (A) adult;*
(B) ''J'' incision; (C) child.   **A**   **B**   **C**

tracted upward from the psoas muscles and iliac vessels. Adequate space for the transplant kidney is created in the iliac fossa with gentle, blunt dissection.

Some surgeons use a J-shaped incision.[5] The short limb of the incision starts at the midline a little above the pubic symphysis, extending laterally, while the long limb of the incision, following the lateral border of the rectus sheath, reaches up to the level of the umbilicus. Deeper incision and dissection remain extraperitoneal.

DISSECTION OF THE ILIAC VESSELS

The iliac vessels are dissected ligating the overlying tissue and lymphatics to lessen lymph leak.

We dissect the entire external iliac artery, the common iliac artery, and the hypogastric artery. The dissection of almost the entire length of the common and external iliac artery gives greater technical ease and a less angular curve to the hypogastric artery–renal artery anastomosis, without adding undue difficulty. The hypogastric artery is dissected down to its bifurcation. Unless one plans to use the bifurcation for anastomosis to the multiple arteries of the donor organ, the hypogastric artery is ligated just proximal to the bifurcation, thereby saving this potential collateral connection. (Ligating the hypergastric artery distal to the bifurcation does provide increased length and also increases the safety of the distal ligature.)

The iliac vein is dissected in a similar fashion, starting inferiorly. The entire length of the external and common iliac veins is dissected free. Usually there are one large and two small tributaries that must be ligated and divided. This procedure should be done carefully, because these tributaries are short

and disappear into the sacrum. This dissection of the iliac veins allows maximal mobility, enabling easy venous anastomosis, preventing the kinking of veins, and avoiding the propagation of pelvic vein thrombosis into the iliac veins.[17,43]

Some surgeons prefer to limit the dissection of vessels to the hypogastric artery and the portion of the vein to be used for the anastomosis (Fig. 22-2).[5] There is an increasing trend to anastomosing the renal artery to the side of the external iliac artery and not using the hypergastric. This greatly simplifies the procedure, avoids dissection deep in the pelvis, and bypasses a region of high frequency atherosclerosis (hypogastric artery origin).

REVASCULARIZATION

The cadaver kidney should be inspected at this point, particularly the anatomy of the renal vessels. If the kidney has multiple renal arteries, bench surgery may be required at this time.[35,46]

The arterial anastomosis can be done first. This requires technical finesse, and, by placing the kidney into the intended position with the arterial anastomosis, the site of venous anastomosis on the iliac vein can be better selected.

Some surgeons perform the venous anastomosis first,[5,16,43,44] presumably because it is deeper and more difficult. If the entire length of the iliac vein is not dissected free and the right kidney with a short vein on the ipsilateral side is used, venous anastomosis may be more difficult.

The most commonly practiced arterial anastomosis is the end-to-end anastomosis of the renal artery to the hypogastric artery in front of the external iliac artery (Fig. 22-3). If the hypogastric artery is not deemed suitable because of its size or

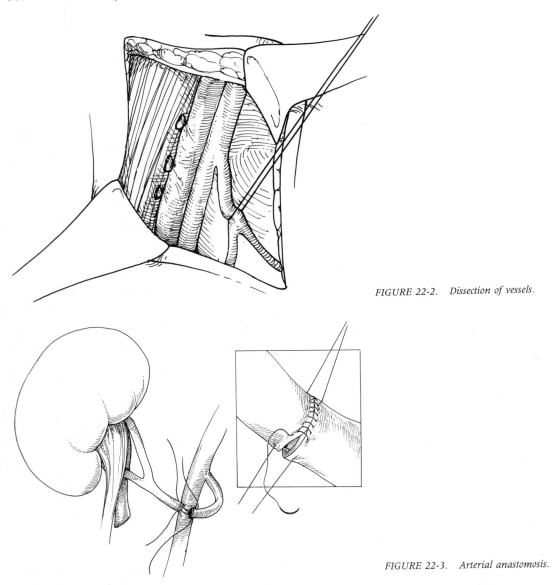

FIGURE 22-2.   *Dissection of vessels.*

FIGURE 22-3.   *Arterial anastomosis.*

atherosclerosis, one may use the end-to-side anastomosis to the iliac artery. In the case of multiple renal arteries of the donor kidney or a second transplant, the end-to-side anastomosis may be the preferred choice. The end-to-side arterial anastomosis may be better because of fewer problems with kinking and size discrepancy of the vessels.[5]

Just before receiving the donor kidney, the hypogastric artery is doubly ligated with 2-0 silk suture just proximal to the bifurcation. The origin of the hypogastric artery or both the common and external iliac arteries are clamped with a gentle vascular

clamp such as a bulldog clamp. Then the hypogastric artery is divided, and the lumen is irrigated with heparinized saline. If the hypogastric artery is significantly atherosclerotic, the endarterectomy may be performed by gently everting the entire length of the hypogastric artery. One should be careful not to initiate the dissection of the wall of the external iliac artery at the site where the hypogastric artery branches off.

Stay sutures are placed superiorly and inferiorly on the cut end of the hypogastric artery where it curves in front of the external iliac artery. At each corner, we use a 6-0 monofilament double-armed suture, 32 inches long, as an everting mattress suture. One may gently dilate each artery with a hemostat to compensate for the size discrepancy.

The donor renal artery is sutured to the hypogastric artery, using the two-corner stay sutures placed previously, and the suture is tied. The anastomosis is performed by starting the medial row first with continuous over-and-over everting sutures, which are tied to the stay suture at the inferior corner and carried over to the lateral row to complete. Heparin saline flush is used to remove any debris just before the completion of the anastomosis sutures.

For the end-to-side anastomosis, a small rim of aorta may make the anastomosis easier. In the case of children who receive a small kidney that is expected to grow along with the patient, interrupted sutures in one half the circumference should be used. Rarely is it necessary to endarterectomize the

wall of the iliac artery, and it is never necessary to give heparin systemically.[46]

Approximately 10% to 20% of kidneys will have multiple renal arteries. When there are two renal arteries, there is usually one main renal artery and a smaller, but significantly sized artery, or one main renal artery with one very small polar artery at either the upper or lower pole. The lower polar artery is considered more important than the upper because of its contribution to the ureteral blood supply. Either the upper or lower polar artery, if not reconstructed, can cause segmental parenchymal infarct resulting in a calyceal fistula.[35,46] If it is very small, the upper polar artery can be ligated without a significant problem. A variety of techniques have been described to deal with the problem of multiple renal arteries, some of which are shown in Figure 22-4.

The classical technique is the aortic "patch" technique, described by Carrell and Guthrie.[7,8] This

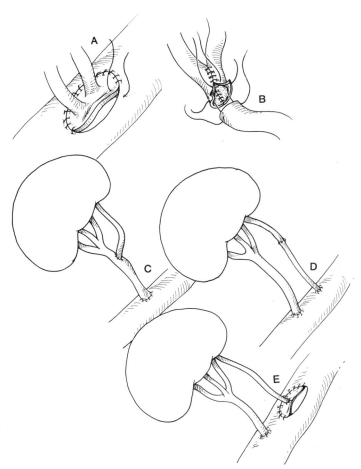

FIGURE 22-4.   Multiple artery anastomosis. (A) "Carrell Patch''; (B) "Double Barrell''; (C) polar artery to main renal artery; (D) saphenous vein bridge; (E) saphenous vein patch.

is the simplest and most effective technique in cadaver donor kidney transplant. Other techniques include (1) the use of the two branches of the hypogastric artery; (2) double-barrel anastomosis, in which two renal arteries of fairly equal size are made into a single trunk and anastomosed to the hypogastric artery[50]; (3) anastomosis of one renal artery to the hypogastric artery and the other to the side of either the common or external iliac artery; (4) end-to-end anastomosis of the inferior epigastric artery to the lower polar artery; (5) the use of the saphenous vein bridge; and (6) the use of the vein patch to form a Carrell patch for the smaller artery in end-to-side anastomosis.[1,32,35] With the advent of microvascular surgery techniques combined with the extracorporeal method of bench surgery, the small polar artery may be anastomosed to the main renal artery end-to-side, using magnifying glasses or an operative microscope.[35,46] One may use 7-0 or smaller monofilament interrupted sutures. Bench surgery can be used for more complex reconstruction of multiple arteries into a single main trunk for simple artery anastomosis to lessen the warm ischemia time.

After the completion of the arterial anastomosis, the iliac vein is isolated between two vascular clamps, one of which is applied inferiorly, just above the inguinal ligament, and the other superiorly, high up in the common iliac vein, placing the vein lateral to the iliac artery.* The kidney is placed into the iliac fossa in the intended position, and the renal vein is allowed to lie comfortably against the iliac vein. This localizes the best site for venous anastomosis on the iliac vein.[17] The iliac vein is picked up with the forceps, and an ellipse is cut from the iliac vein, comparable to the length of the renal vein. After flushing the lumen of the vein with heparin saline solution, the stay sutures are placed at the superior and inferior corners of the venotomy opening using 5-0 monofilament sutures. The correct length of the renal vein is visually estimated, and any redundancy is trimmed. The stay sutures are placed through the superior and inferior angles of the renal vein and tied. One lateral wall stay suture is now placed at the midpoint of the lateral wall, triangulating the venotomy opening to prevent the inadvertent catching of the opposite wall during the anastomosis.

Starting from the superior corner, the medial (anterior) row of the venous anastomosis is completed with an everting running suture. This is tied to the inferior stay suture, care being taken not to create a pursestring effect. The kidney is now reflected medially, exposing the lateral (posterior) row of the anastomosis. The everting running suture is continued from the inferior stay suture and completed by tying at the superior stay suture. The renal vein wall is rather thin in some cases, particularly the posterior wall of the right renal vein. Gentle handling of the vein and avoidance of excessive traction of the kidney will help to prevent tearing of the vein wall during the anastomosis. Leaving a 3-mm to 4-mm cuff of vena cava from the cadaver donor makes this anastomosis much easier.

In the case of a double renal vein, it seems that single-vein anastomosis is sufficient to drain the entire kidney.[5] In rare situations, if these two veins are equal in size and small, one may have difficulty with venous hypertension if only one vein is anastomosed.[1] Therefore, both veins should be anastomosed.

At the completion of the venous anastomosis, all the vascular occlusive clamps are removed in quick succession—the superior venous clamp, inferior venous clamp, and arterial bulldog clamp, respectively.* The kidney should regain its normal pink color and turgor. It is important at this time to ensure an adequate circulating blood volume and hydration. With the routine use of effective dialysis treatment, the recipient is often at the optimal "dry weight" and underhydrated. Infusion of an adequate volume of fluids and blood can be monitored through a central venous line. Mannitol (12.5 g–25 g) and furosemide (20 mg–40 mg for the living donor transplant, 100 mg–500 mg for the cadaver donor transplant) are also administered to ensure the initiation of diuresis of the cold-preserved kidney. Most small leaks of the anastomosis suture line stop in a short time with simple pressure.

When the kidney is placed on the ipsilateral side, particularly the right kidney to the right iliac fossa, one may place the kidney head down, with the ureter gently looping back to the bladder. This places the renal collecting system anteriorly, making future repair of the collecting system easy.[16,46] However, the advantages of this are minimal, as the incidence of urinary tract problems requiring reoperation is less than 1%.

---

*It should be noted that many surgeons only dissect free the external iliac vein; the venous anastomosis can be readily accomplished with this approach.

*The vascular anastomosis can be "pretested" by placing small clamps on the renal artery and vein before releasing the iliac vessel clamps.

REESTABLISHMENT OF THE URINARY TRACT

After the completion of the vascular anastomoses, the kidney is placed in the iliac fossa in the most "comfortable" position, without undue kinking of the vessels, and the continuity of the urinary tract is re-established. A variety of techniques have been described, such as ureteroneocystostomy, uretero-ureterostomy, pyeloureterostomy and pyelopyelostomy. Several factors determine which technique is best for a given case: the length and condition of the donor ureter, the condition of the recipient ureter and bladder, and the familiarity of the surgeon with the technique. Currently, two variations of ureteroneocystostomy have gained wide usage. The variation that is a modification of the Politano–Leadbetter and Paquin techniques is the classical approach.[24,37–39,44,49]

Ureteroneocystostomy produces an effective antireflux mechanism with minimal immediate and future urinary complications. It may be somewhat complicated and difficult, requiring more technical experience and finesse. It also requires a fairly large opening of the bladder, making it less desirable for an infected bladder or a bladder scarred from previous surgery or repeated infections, with a marginal blood supply.

The anterior wall of the bladder is opened near the dome slightly lateral to the midline. Care should be taken to minimize the damage to the blood supply to the bladder wall by gentle handling, minimal dissection, and careful use of electrocautery. The bladder opening should be wide enough to allow the exposure of the trigone area and ipsilateral ureteral orifice with the help of the retractors. The point just lateral to the ureteral orifice and another point about 1 cm to 1.5 cm lateral to this point are picked up with atraumatic forceps. An incision is made into the mucosal ridge created between these forceps. Using the tip of a right-angle clamp, a submucosal tunnel, about 1 cm wide and 2 cm long, is created in the superior-lateral direction. After completing the creation of a submucosal tunnel, a retractor inside the bladder is removed with a right-angle clamp still in the tunnel. The tip of this right-angle clamp is pushed against the lateral bladder wall, then through the wall. It may be necessary to cut sharply over the tip of the clamp to push through. By spreading the clamp, a wide opening is created. The opening through the muscle layer should be as wide or wider than the submucosal tunnel to prevent the stenosis of the ureter in the tunnel.

In male patients, the ureter is brought under the spermatic cord through the opening in the bladder wall and submucosal tunnel. The ureter should be a comfortable length, not short enough to create tension and not long enough to kink. The ureter is handled gently so that its blood supply will not be damaged. The redundant portion of the ureter is partially divided laterally, and a small incision, about 2 mm, is made in the longitudinal axis of the ureter as a part of the fishmouth incision at the lateral corner. The superior-lateral corner of the fishmouth is sutured to the superior-lateral corner of the bladder mucosal opening, using 4-0 or 5-0 chromic catgut, through the full thickness of the ureter and mucosa of the bladder. Once this corner suture is tied, acting as a stay suture, the remaining redundant segment of the ureter is removed. Another fishmouth incision is made at the medial corner of the ureter in a similar manner as described. The medial and lateral corner sutures of the inferior flap are placed next, including the trigone muscles in the stitch. This anchors the ureter securely and tilts the new ureteral opening downward. Finally, a suture for the medial corner of the superior flap is placed. These are not watertight closures. Unless the opening of the bladder mucosa is much larger than the ureteral fishmouth opening, no additional sutures are necessary. No attempt is made to create the "cuff" or "nipple" of the ureter opening.[39] Adequacy of the ureteral opening is tested with the tip of a right-angle clamp. No ureteral stent is left in place (Fig. 22-5).

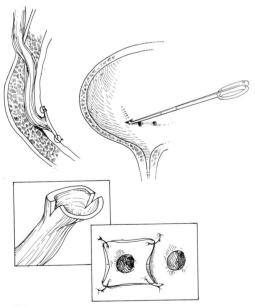

FIGURE 22-5. Ureteroneocystostomy.

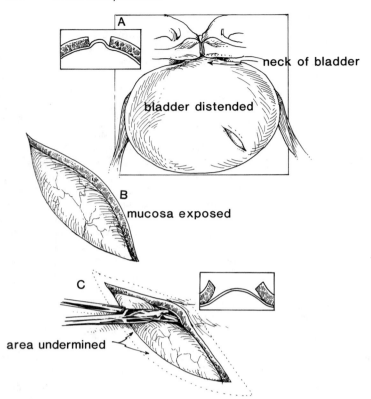

A

neck of bladder

bladder distended

B
mucosa exposed

C

area undermined

FIGURE 22-6.   *Extravesical ureteroneocystostomy.*

The bladder is irrigated with neomycin solution to clear any blood clots. One may instill topical thrombin solution if the mucosal surface is oozy. The cystostomy is closed in two layers. The first layer closure includes mucosa and muscle, using a continuous 2-0 plain catgut suture. This suture should include a large bite to avoid strangulation necrosis of the suture line and should be watertight. The second layer closure includes perivesical tissue and muscle, using a 2-0 chromic catgut interrupted suture in the manner of the Lembert suture. Both corners are reinforced and inverted by the Marshall U-stitch. A fixation suture of the ureter at the entry into the lateral wall of the bladder is not necessary and may damage the blood supply of the ureter. An indwelling catheter, the largest "comfortable" size, is used for the decompression of the bladder. It is removed on the fifth postoperative day.

The other technique to implant the ureter in the bladder that has gained popularity in recent years because of its simplicity is the extravesical ureteroneocystostomy (Figs. 22-6 and 22-7).* This

* References 2, 5, 6, 14, 22, 27, 31, and 40

technique is a modification of the antireflux procedure described by Lich and associates[25] and Gregoir and colleagues.[15] It is fairly simple and requires only a small opening in the bladder. It requires a shorter length of ureter than that for the ureteroneocystostomy previously described.[30] The bladder is distended with approximately 300 ml of neomycin or Betadine (povidone-iodine) solution. This is usually done when the indwelling catheter is inserted. At the dome, a portion of the anterolateral wall of the bladder is exposed. A 3-cm to 4-cm longitudinal incision toward the bladder neck is made in the muscle wall until mucosa bulges into the incision. The mucosa is carefully freed by undermining the muscle 1 cm on each side of the incision. The proper and comfortable length of the ureter is selected, and the excess is removed. The distal end of the ureter is spatulated with a 1.5-cm longitudinal incision. A 1.5-cm incision is made into the bulging mucosa at the distal end of the myotomy. A stay suture of 4-0 chromic catgut is placed through the v tip of the ureter and the full thickness of the bladder and is tied. One may place another stay suture at the proximal corner of the mucosal incision of the bladder and at the apex of the spatulating incision of the

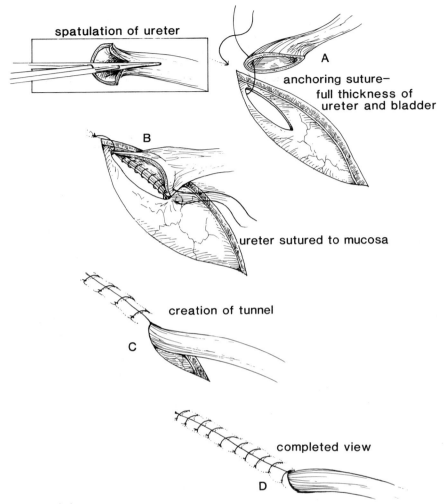

FIGURE 22-7. *Extravesical ureteroneocystostomy.*

ureter with 4-0 chromic catgut. The ureter is anastomosed to the opening of the bladder mucosa with a simple running suture of 4-0 chromic catgut (or 6-0 monofilament suture). The muscle layer is closed over the ureter with a 2-0 chromic catgut interrupted suture, snugly but not tightly, to create a submucosal tunnel, 2 cm to 3 cm long, to prevent reflux. Care should be taken not to obstruct the ureter with the last stitch at the proximal corner of the myotomy.[14] We do not use a ureteral stent; however, some use a ureteral stent routinely for a few days. Although this technique has certain advantages, such as (1) a small opening into the bladder, (2) reducing the risk of contamination and cystostomy leaks, and (3) the shorter length of ureter required, reducing the risk of inadequate blood supply to the ureter tip, particularly in the cadaver

donor kidney, it is not advised for a bladder with a thin or scarred wall.[30] Earlier, there was some concern that this was not as effective an antireflux measure as the Politano–Leadbetter modification. Recent reports suggest that this may not be the case.[47,48]

Ureteroureterostomy continues to be the technique preferred by Hamburger's group[16] and by others when ureteroneocystostomy is not feasible and/or the recipient ureter can be used. They cite simplicity with minimal risk of infection. Anastomosis leak is acknowledged to be a particular complication. Use of microvascular surgery technique with magnifying loops and synthetic monofilament suture is recommended to decrease the incidence of such leaks.[16] The donor ureter is divided a short distance, 2 cm to 3 cm, from the ureteropelvic junction, and a 1.5-cm longitudinal cut is made on the medial side to spatulate it. The recipient ureter is dissected with just enough length to reach the donor ureter without tension so as not to disturb the blood supply. A 1.5-cm cut is also made at the end of the recipient ureter to spatulate and meet the end of the donor. The anastomosis is made with a simple, continuous, 6-0 monofilament, synthetic suture after placing the stay sutures at each corner of the anastomosis. The ureteral stent is not left in place.

Pyeloureterostomy is a modification of the ureteroureterostomy. Proponents claim some advantages to this procedure: (1) an ensured blood supply to the donor renal pelvis, (2) a large anastomosis stoma to prevent ureteral obstruction or stenosis, and (3) avoidance of the risk of contamination from the bladder opening. However, immediate leaks appear to be more common, and any leak or complication is more difficult to manage. This technique should be used only for the repair of late ureteropelvic stenosis.

A double collecting system may be handled in two different ways. In one technique, the double ureters are joined at the distal end by spatulating and suturing them together with fine chromic catgut. Then this common stoma is used for ureteroneocystostomy.[39] Each ureter may be separately implanted in the bladder using an extravesical or intravesical approach. In another technique, the renal pelves are joined, after removing the ureters at the ureteropelvic junction, in the same manner used for joining double renal arteries in double-barrel anastomosis. The common stoma is then used for ureteropyelostomy.

With the broadening indication of renal transplant for a variety of end-stage renal diseases, the ileal conduit has been used as a substitute bladder in the group of patients who do not have a functioning bladder. Even though there are relatively few reports in the literature, a number of long-term survivors have been reported.*[9,13]

The construction of the conduit follows the technique described by Bricker.[3] The conduit is constructed 1 month to 1.5 months prior to the projected transplant to ensure adequate healing. The length of the conduit should be as short as possible (10 cm–12 cm). The stoma of the conduit can be constructed on either the right or left side, and the kidney is transplanted on the contralateral side; the transplant can be intraperitoneal or extraperitoneal. The renal pelvis or ureter is anastomosed to the

---

*Because of the advantages of sterile intermittent catheterization, a conduit is now rarely indicated except in patients without a bladder.

conduit using the two-layer technique, first using 5-0 chromic catgut interrupted sutures for the mucosa-to-ureter layer and, second, reinforcing the serosal layer with 5-0 silk sutures. The opening of the peritoneum is closed loosely around the proximal end of the conduit with a 2-0 or 3-0 chromic catgut suture.[19,28]

CAPSULOTOMY, BIOPSY, DRAINAGE, AND WOUND CLOSURE

After completion of revascularization and re-establishment of the urinary tract, a capsulotomy may be performed.[17] Some researchers have suggested that the capsulotomy predisposes to spontaneous rupture of the kidney. However, we have never seen a rupture of the kidney attributable to the capsulotomy. The renal capsule is split at its convex surface from pole to pole with a knife under a hemostat guide. It is not stripped away from the line of capsulotomy; a metal clip is applied to the upper pole, midpoint, and lower pole of the capsule for later radiologic identification. A small biopsy can be taken from the posterior lower pole of the kidney for base line reference. Hemostasis of the biopsy site is obtained by a 2-0 chromic suture with a fat pad. The wound is inspected carefully for hemostasis and irrigated with a neomycin solution. The incision is closed in layers. The internal oblique and transverse abdominis muscles with transversalis fascia are closed together using 1-0 chromic catgut running sutures. The external oblique muscle and apponeurosis is closed with 2-0 monofilament synthetic interrupted sutures.

PEDIATRIC TRANSPLANTATION

Kidney transplantation in children is essentially the same as in the adult if the child is of adequate size with a body weight of more than 20 kg.[4,29] Vessel anastomosis would be higher to the aorta or common iliac artery and vena cava or common iliac vein. We have used the same extraperitoneal approach in children weighing as little as 15 kg. In smaller children who receive "normal"-size adult kidneys, the transabdominal approach is required.[45] The kidney is placed in the retroperitoneal position after reflecting the cecum and ascending colon to the left. The renal artery and vein are anastomosed to the side of the aorta and vena cava or common iliac vessels. The ureter is brought retroperitoneally and implanted in the bladder.[43] The cecum and ascending colon are placed back over the kidney. Although not usually necessary, an adult kidney will fit into the abdominal cavity of an infant less than 1 year of age. A kidney from a small child can be transplanted into an adult and function adequately.[12,18,20,41] If the donor is 1 year old or older, a single kidney with an aorta and vena cava patch can be used with the routine procedure. If the recipient and donor both are children and an aorta patch is not used, anastomosis of vessels should be done with interrupted sutures in at least half the circumference to allow future growth. Pediatric kidneys have been transplanted en bloc of two kidneys

into children and adults.[10,21,26,42] Indications for this technique are controversial because a single kidney may be sufficient for adequate function. Donor kidneys are removed with a segment of aorta and vena cava. The cranial ends of these vessels are oversewn. The caudal end of the donor aorta and vena cava are anastomosed to the side of the common iliac vessels. The ureters are separately implanted in the bladder. To prevent the axis rotation or kinking of renal vessels, the superior poles of the kidneys are sutured to the side of the aorta. The ureters can be short to reach the bladder.

REFERENCES

1. Belzar FO, Schweizer RT, Kountz SL: Management of multiple vessels in renal transplantation. Transplant Proc 4:639, 1972

2. Briand O, Nussaume O, Cohen G et al: Reimplantation uretero-vesicale technique derivee du procede de Loch et Gregoive. Nouv Presse Med 11:2779, 1982

3. Bricker EM: Bladder substitution after pelvic evisceration. Surg Clin North Am 3:1511, 1950

4. Broyer M, Gagnadoux MF, Beurton D et al: Transplantation in children: Technical aspects, drug therapy and problems related to primary renal disease. Proc EDTA 18:313, 1981

5. Calne RY: Color Atlas of Renal Transplantation. Oradell, NJ, Medical Economics Books, 1984

6. Campos FG Jr, Goes GM, Campos FJG: Extravesical meteral implantation in kidney transplantation. Urology 111:304, 1974

7. Carrell A, Guthrie CC: Anastomosis of blood vessels by the patching method and transplantation of the kidney. JAMA 47:1648, 1906

8. Carrell A, Guthrie CC: Transplantation of blood vessels and organs. Br Med J 2:1796, 1906

9. Castro JE, Mustapha N, Mee AD et al: Ileal urinary diversion in patients with renal transplants. Br J Urol 47:603, 1975

10. Dreikorn K, Rohl L, Horsch R: The use of double renal transplants from pediatric cadaver donors. Br J Urol 49:361, 1977

11. Dubost CH, Oeconomos N, Vaysse J et al: Note preliminaire sur l'etude des fonetions renales de rains greffes chez chamme. Bulletins et Memorires de la Societe Medicale des Hopitanx de Paris 67:105, 1951

12. Fine RN, Brennan LP, Edelbrode HH et al: Use of pediatric cadaver kidneys for homotransplantation in children. JAMA 210:477, 1969

13. Firlit CF, Merkel FV: The application of ileal conduits in pediatric renal transplantation. J Mol 118:647, 1977

14. Fjeldborg O, Kim CH: Ureteral complication in human renal transplantation. Mol Int 27:417, 1972

15. Gregoir W, Van Regemorter G: Le reflux vesico-meteral congenital. Urol Int 18:122, 1964

16. Hamburger J, Crosnier J, Bach J-F et al: Renal Transplantation, Theory and Practice, 3rd ed. Baltimore/London, Williams & Wilkins, 1981

17. Hume DM, Magee JH, Kauffman HM Jr et al: Renal homotransplantation in man in modified recipients. Ann Surg 158:608, 1963

18. Iitaka K, Martin LW, Cox JA et al: Transplantation of cadaver kidneys from ancephalic donors. J Pediatr 93:216, 1978

19. Kelly WD, Morkel FK, Markland C: Ileal urinary diversion in conjunction with renal homotransplantation. Lancet i:222, 1966

20. King LR, Gerbie AG, Idviss FS et al: Human renal transplantation with kidney grafts from the newborn. Invest Urol 8:622, 1971

21. Kinne DW, Spanos PK, Deshazo MM et al: Double renal transplants from pediatric donors to adult recipients. Am J Surg 127:292, 1974

22. Konnak JW, Herwig KR, Finkbeiner A et al: Extravesical meteroneocystostomy in 170 renal transplant patients. J Urol 113:299, 1975

23. Kuss R, Teinturier J, Milliez P: Quelques essais de greffos du rein chez l'homme. Mem Acad Chir 77:755, 1951

24. Libertino JA, Rote AR, Zimman L: Ureteral reconstruction in renal transplantation. Urology 12:641, 1978

25. Lich R Jr, Howerton LW, Davis LA: Recurrent urosepsis in children. J Urol 86:554, 1961

26. Lindstrom BL, Ahonen J: The use of both kidneys obtained from pediatric donors as en bloc transplants into adult recipients. Scand J Urol Nephrol 29:71, 1975

27. MacKinnon KJ, Oliver JA, Morehouse DD et al: Cadaver renal transplantation: Emphasis on urological aspects. J Urol 99:486, 1968

28. Markland C, Kelly WD, Buselmeier T et al: Renal transplantation into ileal conduits. Transplant Proc 4:629, 1972

29. Martin LW, McEnery PT, Rosenkrantz JG et al: Renal homotransplantation in children. J Pediatr Surg 14:571, 1979

30. McDonald JC, Rohr MS, Frentz GD: External uretero-neocystostomy and ureteroureterostomy in renal transplantation. Ann Surg 190:663, 1979

31. Mehta SN, Kennedy JA, Loughridge WGG et al: Urological complication in 119 consecutive renal transplants. Br J Urol 51:184, 1979

32. Merkel FK, Straus AK, Andersen O et al: Microvascular techniques for polar artery reconstruction in kidney transplants. Surgery 79:253, 1976

33. Merrill JP, Murray JE, Harrison JH et al: Successful homotransplantation of the human kidney between identical twins. JAMA 160:277, 1956

34. Murray JE, Harrison JH: Surgical management of fifty patients with kidney transplants including eighteen pairs of twins. Am J Surg 105:205, 1963

35. Novick AC, Magnusson M, Braun WE: Multiple artery renal transplantation: Emphasis on extracorporeal methods of donor arterial reconstruction. J Urol 122:731, 1979

36. Novick AC, Ortenburg J, Braun WE: Reduced morbidity with posterior surgical approach for pretransplant bilateral nephrectomy. Surg Gynecol Obstet 151:773, 1980

37. Paquin AJ Jr: Ureterovesical anastomosis: The description and evaluation of a technique. J Urol 82:573, 1959

38. Politano VA, Leadbetter WF: An operative technique for the correction of vesicoureteral reflux. J Urol 79:932, 1958

39. Prout GR Jr, Hume DM, Lee HM et al: Some urological aspects of 93 consecutive renal homotransplants in modified recipients. J Urol 97:409, 1967

40. Robson AJ, Calne RY: Complication of urinary drainage following renal transplantation. Br J Urol 43:586, 1971

41. Salvatierra O, Belzer FO: Pediatric cadaver kidneys: Their use in renal transplantation. Arch Surg 110:181, 1975

42. Schneider JR, Sutherland DER, Simmons RL et al: Long-term success with double pediatric cadaver donor renal transplants. Ann Surg, April 1985

43. Simmons RL, Kjellstrand C-M, Najarian JS: Technique, complication and results. In Najarian JS, Simmons RL (eds): Transplantation. Philadelphia, Lea & Febiger, 1972

44. Starzl TE: Experience in Renal Transplantation. Philadelphia, WB Saunders, 1964

45. Starzl TE, Mardioro TL, Morgan WW et al: A technique for use of adult renal homografts in children. Surg Gynecol Obstet 119:106, 1964

46. Tilney NL, Lazarus JM: Surgical Care of the Patient with Renal Failure. Philadelphia, WB Saunders, 1982

47. Van Caugh PJ, Michel L, Squifflet JP et al: Letters to the editor: Re-evaluation of anterior extravesical meteroneocystostomy in kidney transplantation. J Urol 128:153, 1982

48. Wasnik RJ, Butt KMH, Laungani G et al: Evaluation of anterior extravesical ureteroneocystostomy in kidney transplantation. J Urol 126:306, 1981

49. Weil R III, Simmons RL, Tallent MB et al: Prevention of urological complication after kidney transplantation. Ann Surg 174:154, 1971

50. Woodruff MFA, Robson JS, Ross JA et al: Transplantation of a kidney from an identical twin. Lancet 1:1245, 1961

CHAPTER 23

Pediatric Renal Transplantation

Jeremiah G. Turcotte   Darrell A. Campbell, Jr.   Donald C. Dafoe
Robert M. Merion   Aileen B. Sedman   Leslie L. Rocher
John W. Konnak   Robert C. Kelch

Renal transplantation is the treatment of choice for most children with end-stage renal disease. Some diseases such as focal segmental glomerulosclerosis, dense intramembranous deposit disease, hemolytic uremic syndrome, and primary oxalosis may cause severe damage to the transplanted kidney with recurrence, but are not absolute contraindications to transplantation. Severe mental retardation, most cancers, persistent sepsis, and complete thrombosis of the vena cava and iliac veins are important contraindications.

With the onset of end-stage renal insufficiency at an early age, as much as 12 inches of growth may be lost. Intermittent hemodialysis or intermittent peritoneal dialysis have not permitted normal growth to occur. If transplantation is performed under the age of 7 years and if steroid immunosuppression can be reduced to a minimum, accelerated catch-up growth has been observed. Pretransplant chronic ambulatory peritoneal dialysis is preferred, because there is less blood loss, fewer blood transfusions, better control of hypertension, fewer episodes of disequilibrium syndrome, and more liberal fluid and diet restrictions.

Adult kidneys can be implanted into small children, but it is preferable to use an appropriate-size kidney when available. Kidneys from donors as young as 1 year of age are suitable.

Routine pediatric immunizations are updated, and it is also desirable to immunize against the influenza virus and hepatitis B virus when indicated. Hypertension can be a major problem in children, both in the pretransplant period as well as immediately post-transplantation.

All patients undergo voiding cystourethrography, and those with significant urologic histories should be evaluated with cystoscopy, upper urinary tract, and cystometric studies. Anatomic urinary tract abnormalities are seen more often in children than in adults. Surgical procedures to correct any bladder, urethral, or ureteropelvic abnormalities may be necessary.

For immunosuppression, the trend is to use a triple drug program combining low doses of cyclosporine, azathioprine, and steroids with the rationale of avoiding the long-term toxic side-effect of any single drug.

In children under 20 kg, the renal artery of the graft is implanted into the side of the distal aorta, and the renal vein is implanted into the side of the inferior vena cava rather than using the iliac vessels. When the vascular clamps are removed intraoperatively, special precaution must be taken to avoid hypotension, hyperkalemia, and acidosis, because a large kidney implanted in a small child may sequester a significant proportion of the child's blood volume. Postoperatively, fluid and electrolytes must be monitored every 15 minutes; a large kidney can easily excrete the equivalent of an infant's blood volume in 1 hour.

Results with HLA-identical grafts approach 100%. HLA semi-identical grafts also have a good survival rate (93% for approximately 5 years) if donor-specific transfusions have been used. Cadaveric grafts have a 5-year survival rate of approximately 50%.

INTRODUCTION

The development of renal failure in a child is a progressive debilitating process that taxes the endurance of the patient, the family, and the physician. Life becomes a series of bewildering disappointments and frightening medical treatments for the affected child.

Recent advances in dialysis and transplantation have dramatically changed this scenario.[11,16,55] Both modalities now complement each other, with dialysis safely supporting the child through the initial phases of end-stage renal disease (ESRD) until circumstances can be optimized for transplantation. This chapter summarizes the specialized discipline of pediatric renal transplantation, with particular emphasis on those considerations germaine to the pediatric age group.

Etiology and Indications

The reported incidence of ESRD in children varies from 0.5 to 5.5 per million per year, depending upon the age group included and the source of survey information.[13] The average annual incidence for children younger than 16 years of age is 2 to 3 per million.[31]

The etiology of renal failure and the likelihood of recurrent disease in the transplanted kidney are summarized in Table 23-1. With diseases in which recurrence usually does not significantly injure the allograft, transplantation is not contraindicated. Even when frequency and severity are much more significant, transplantation may be preferred to other management options. Cadaveric organ donors rather than volunteer donors are often preferred in these circumstances.

Focal segmental glomerulosclerosis is more likely to recur if there is mesangial proliferation and if the child is older than 6 years of age (Table 23-1).[5,44] Patients with Henoch-Schönlein purpura, hemolytic-uremic syndrome, and antiglomerular basement membrane nephritis should be transplanted when their disease is quiescent for several months.[44] Kidney transplantation may be used in patients with cystinosis or oxalosis, but it does not relieve the bone disease or other systemic manifestations associated with these inborn errors of metabolism. Only selected patients with primary hyperoxaluria (Type I) should receive transplants.[57] These patients should be treated with special diets and medications to prevent or minimize the effects of recurrence.[28,44] Leumann and associates[29] recommend daily dialysis in the peritransplant period. Najarian and colleagues[36] noted that recurrence of

disease is now the major cause of transplant loss with mismatched related kidneys. In their experience, hemolytic-uremic syndrome, focal segmental glomerulosclerosis in children with steroid-resistant nephrotic syndrome, primary oxalosis, and dense intramembranous deposit disease (Type II membranoproliferative glomerulonephritis) were the causes of transplant loss.[36]

Several conditions temporarily or permanently preclude transplantation. Severe mental retardation, most cancers, persistent sepsis, and complete thrombosis of the vena cava and iliac veins are commonly encountered contraindications. After a disease-free interval of 1 to 2 years, transplantation in children who have undergone bilateral nephrectomy for Wilms' tumors may be undertaken. Exceptions are sometimes made for other solid organ cancers such as hepatoblastoma after an extended cancer-free interval. Chronic infection such as chronic osteomyelitis can often be eliminated in preparation for transplantation. With pelvic vein thrombosis, successful transplantation can be accomplished when a patent distal external iliac vein with good venous run-off persists.

Growth, Cognitive Function, and Age

The most rapid periods of growth for children are the first two years of life and during the onset of puberty. The cause of growth retardation is multifactorial and includes protein and calorie deprivation, renal osteodystrophy, aluminum toxicity, insulin resistance, acidosis, impaired somatomedin activity, and glucocorticoid administration.[20] With the onset of chronic renal insufficiency at an early age, as much as 12 inches of growth may be lost. Catch-up or accelerated growth to within normal percentiles has been observed when transplantation is performed up to age 7 years, but not after that time.[2,13,19,42] When the epiphyses have closed, additional bone growth is not possible, and little growth occurs after a bone age of 12 has been reached.[16] Neither peritoneal nor hemodialysis have been successful in permitting normal growth. High doses of corticosteroids, sometimes required for immunosuppression following renal transplantation, also retard growth.

Central nervous system development is also impaired in infants with severe renal insufficiency. Malnutrition and deposition of calcium or aluminum are some of the associated etiologic factors. Studies of identical twins discordant for ESRD strongly suggest that the earlier the onset and the longer the duration of renal insufficiency, the more severe the impairment of cognitive function, espe-

TABLE 23-1 *Etiology of Chronic Renal Failure in Children and Likelihood of Recurrence Rate in a Kidney Transplant*

DISEASES	RECURRENCE RATE
GLOMERULAR	
Focal segmental glomerulosclerosis*	Moderate
Membranoproliferative glomerulonephritis*	Moderate
Membranous glomerulonephropathy*	Moderate
Rapidly progressive glomerulonephritis	Moderate
Henoch-Schönlein glomerulonephritis	High
IgA nephropathy	High
Shunt nephritis	Rare
Lupus nephritis	Rare
Dense deposit disease	Very high
Hereditary nephritis	Rare
Crescentic glomerulonephritis (idiopathic)	Moderate
CONGENITAL STRUCTURAL ABNORMALITIES	
Hypo/dysplasia	None
Obstructive uropathy	None
Oligomeganephronia	None
Reflux nephropathy	None
HEREDITARY NEPHROPATHIES	
Alport's syndrome	None
Cystinosis	Rare
Polycystic disease	None
Oxalosis*	Very high
Medullary cystic disease	Unknown
VASCULAR NEPHROPATHIES AND MALIGNANCY	
Hemolytic-uremic syndrome	Low
Renal venous thrombosis*	Low
Bilateral Wilm's tumor*	High
Renal arterial occlusion*	Rare

* When the disease recurs, the damage to the kidney is usually severe.
Note: Data compiled from references[5,9,11,12,14,15,20,28,29,35,36,43,51,55,56]

cially learning and problem-solving skills.[10] Successful transplantation may halt this progression of impaired cognitive function.[41]

The potential for achieving accelerated growth and avoiding mental retardation, osteodystrophy, and other complications suggests that transplantation should be recommended at an early age.[47] The introduction of the immunosuppressant cyclosporine may permit steroid administration to be reduced and thus enhance the growth permissive effect of transplantation. These potential advantages must be balanced against the recognition that many centers report poor long-term results with younger children. Enough information has been accumulated to suggest that good success can be achieved in centers experienced with pediatric renal transplantation in children older than 2 years of age, especially if a related donor is used (see Tables 23-5 and 23-6). Although results with related donors are superior, in some cases a logical strategy is to initially use a cadaveric graft for very young children and hold an available related graft in reserve in case the cadaveric graft fails. Transplantation is recommended for most children with ESRD who are older than 2 years of age and selected children younger than age 2 years.[6]

Dialysis and Vascular Access

There is no absolute requirement to begin chronic dialysis prior to transplantation, and, in some cases, it is possible to avoid chronic dialysis completely. Indications for pretransplantation dialysis are, as in the adult, hyperkalemia, volume overload, acidosis, intractable hypertension, and symptoms such as nausea and vomiting. Rapid restoration of normal renal function after a transplant brings about a precipitous decrease in concentration of blood urea nitrogen, creatinine, and other molecules and a rapid correction of acidosis. With rapid changes in fluid and electrolyte balance, children may have symptoms similar to those encountered in the dialysis disequilibrium syndrome, including convulsions and coma.[20] If children have not been dialyzed prior to transplantation and are very uremic, prophylactic anticonvulsant therapy is recommended for the first 2 postoperative weeks. If phenobarbital or Dilantin is administered, the cyclosporine dosage must usually be increased substantially to compensate for increased hepatic degradation of cyclosporine through the cytochrome P-450 system.

In recent years, peritoneal or chronic ambulatory peritoneal dialysis (CAPD) is used to prepare or maintain most children prior to transplantation. This mode of dialysis is well tolerated and avoids the problems of multiple needle punctures and establishing and maintaining vascular access.[20] With peritoneal dialysis, there is less blood loss, fewer blood transfusions, better control of hypertension, fewer episodes of the disequilibrium syndrome, and more liberal fluid and diet restrictions. Hypertriglyceridemia secondary to glucose absorption is one disadvantage of peritoneal dialysis. The peritoneal catheter is placed on the side opposite the planned transplant site and can be left in place postoperatively if dialysis is required. Chronic hemodialysis can be accomplished successfully even in children smaller than 20 kg, but, frequently, multiple operations are necessary to revise or fashion new vascular access sites. A 5-year actuarial survival of 95% for 81 children undergoing hemodialysis was reported by the Boston Children's Hospital Medical Center group.[3] Most groups report lower survivals, such as the 66% 5-year actuarial survival reported by the European Dialysis and Transplant Association.[3,4]

When hemodialysis is desired, the choice of vascular access site depends upon the child's size.[46] For those under 15 kg to 20 kg, the brachial artery and brachial, antecubital, or low axillary vein or the femoral vessels can be used for placement of external plastic shunts. For larger children, an internal radial arteriovenous fistula is preferred, or external shunts can usually be inserted at the wrist or ankle. Prosthetic bridge grafts can also be used in children who weigh more than 15 kg. Dialysis can also be accomplished through single-vessel access.[49] A Hickman or Broviac catheter is inserted into the right atrium through the subclavian or jugular veins. This method is especially helpful as a temporary method of dialysis in the perinatal or perioperative period if peritoneal dialysis is contraindicated. Sometimes such a central catheter is placed preoperatively for monitoring and to facilitate blood drawing or administration of fluid and medications.

DONORS

The use of immediate family blood relatives for kidney donation offers several advantages, including a lower incidence of acute postoperative tubular necrosis, fewer episodes of acute rejection, less immunosuppression, and better patient and graft survival. In addition, the waiting time for a kidney is usually much shorter. Parents are frequently highly motivated donors and are the most common source of related kidneys. Siblings, with the exception of identical twins, are usually not used as donors until they are 18 years old, the legal age of consent. Identical twin donors should be old enough to understand the potential risks before being asked to donate; this usually means that they be at least 10 years old.

Cadaveric kidneys can also be used with good success in pediatric patients. The improved immunosuppression obtained with pretransplantation blood transfusions and cyclosporine have greatly improved results with unrelated donors. A good histocompatibility match may be of more importance to pediatric patients, because these allografts must function for long periods of time, and the improved results with better matches are usually not apparent until 5 or 10 years after transplantation.

The indications and contraindications to donation and the evaluation of cadaveric and related donors for pediatric transplantation are the same as for adult transplantation except for kidney size considerations.[31] An adult kidney can be successfully transplanted into an infant as small as 5 kg.[32,33,52] However, it is preferable to use small adult or pediatric kidneys of a size appropriate to the recipient when available. A related donor with the smaller kidney may be selected rather than an otherwise equivalent relative. Because of the shortage of pediatric donors, kidneys from cadaveric donors younger than 16 years of age should be given to children preferentially.

There is a high degree of positive correlation between the success of maternal donor kidney transplantation and sibling 1-haplotype HLA-matched donor kidney transplantation with a history of breast feeding of the recipient.[7,24] Breast feeding may be "nature's first donor-specific transfusion." The mechanism is presumed to be the result of absorption of maternal antigen from the breast milk through the gut by the infant who will later be a kidney recipient. The effect is somewhat nonspecific, since a correlation was found when siblings as well as mothers were used as donors. A significant difference was found for both graft survival and number of rejection episodes. For instance, 1-year graft survival in breast-fed recipients was 81% compared with 61% for non–breast-fed maternal-offspring transplants. When 1-haplotype-matched sibling transplants were compared, the 5-year graft survival was 79% when both donor and recipient were breast-fed versus 30% when neither donor nor recipient were breast-fed.

RECIPIENT PREPARATION FOR TRANSPLANTATION

The general health of the child should be returned to the most optimal condition possible prior to transplantation. Some patients with long-standing uremia are severely malnourished. Vigorous dialysis combined with tube feeding may be necessary. All active or potential sites of infection are eliminated, and most operations necessary to eradicate infection or correct congenital anomalies are performed prior to transplantation. The evaluation of the recipient is similar to that in an adult and includes hepatitis B antigen and antibody tests and cytomegalovirus serum antibody titers. All routine pediatric immunizations are updated. If hepatitis studies are negative, immunization against hepatitis B virus should be accomplished. Immunization against cytomegalovirus and varicella are under development and should be considered for use when available. Pretransplantation dialysis is not always necessary, and many of the complications of chronic uremia can be avoided in a few patients with an available donor by early transplantation. An optimal antihypertensive regimen should be established prior to transplantation. Several peritransplant factors, such as volume load, renin release by a relatively large renal graft, and the hypertension associated with cyclosporine administration, may make hypertension a serious post-transplantation complication. Pretransplant bilateral nephrectomy is indicated for uncontrolled renin-mediated hypertension not responsive to dialysis or medical management. Routine recipient nephrectomy, splenectomy, thymectomy, or parathyroidectomy are not indicated.

Children frequently have urinary tract abnormalities that need correction prior to transplantation.[44] The surgical goals are to sterilize the urinary system, correct any bladder or urethral abnormalities so that the bladder can be used as a conduit, and correct any upper tract abnormalities to eliminate chronic pyelonephritis and preserve recipient kidneys when possible. Recipient kidneys are a source of vitamin D and erythropoietin and facilitate dialysis management if they continue to excrete significant volumes of water despite otherwise poor

clearance. Recipient nephrectomy is indicated only for persistent infection, uncontrolled renin-mediated hypertension, renal tumors, or, occasionally, when a polycystic kidney bleeds or is large enough to cause symptoms or anatomically interfere with the planned transplant. Recipient nephrectomy can be performed expeditiously by the posterior retroperitoneal approach through the flank or 12th rib bed with the patient in the prone position; this permits resumption of peritoneal dialysis immediately after operation and is usually less of a physiologic shock to the patient than the transabdominal approach.

All patients should undergo voiding cystourethrography, and those with significant urologic histories should be evaluated with cystoscopy, upper urinary tract studies, and cystometric studies as indicated. Urethral valves, ureteropelvic and ureterovesical obstruction, urethroceles, and bladder diverticula are all lesions that can be repaired prior to transplantation.

The storage capacity of the bladder should be determined. Some patients, especially those with defunctionalized bladders, may have small-capacity nondistensible bladders. However, even the smallest of bladders has a remarkable ability to expand. If the patient has an adequate urethra and normal neuromuscular function, a bladder augmentation procedure such as cecal cystoplasty, performed prior to transplantation, can be considered. Construction of an ileal loop conduit as a first stage prior to transplantation with implantation of the allograft ureter into the loop at the time of transplantation is also a very successful option and can be used in children with neurogenic bladders and uncorrectable vesicle neck or urethral obstruction. Some groups prefer colon to ileal conduits, but we have not had experience with this procedure in transplant patients. Repeated clean bladder catheterization by the patient is another option.

IMMUNOSUPPRESSION

More than 70 independent studies document that preoperative blood transfusions improve graft function rates. This beneficial effect has been observed in both adults and children, with random and donor-specific transfusions and with cadaveric and 1-haplotype-mismatched related grafts.[39] A few groups have used preoperative transfusions with haplotype identical related grafts. There is a progressive improvement in cadaveric graft survival with increasing numbers of transfusions. The optimal number seems to be five transfusions, since the

TABLE 23-2   Dosage Schedule for Immunosuppressive Drugs Used in Pediatric Transplantation at the University of Michigan

DRUGS	PRETRANSPLANT	POST-TRANSPLANT
Cyclosporin A Adjust dosage to 200 ng/ml trough by HPLC; 100–150 ng/ml after day 60	5 mg/kg IV over 6 hr	2.5 mg/kg IV b.i.d until eating, then 8 mg/kg b.i.d.
Prednisolone or predni- sone	1.5 mg/kg IM on call to OR	0.75 mg/kg b.i.d orally initially taper to 0.5 mg/kg orally by day 30. Then taper to 0.1 mg/ kg q.d. or q.o.d.
Azathioprine Adjust depending upon WBC, RBC, and plate- lets	3 mg/kg daily on days −2 and −1	3 mg/kg orally daily on days 0–10; taper slowly to 1 mg/kg if stable

beneficial effect begins to plateau when this number is exceeded. Preoperative random transfusions are preferred for all cadaveric transplants and donor-specific transfusions for 1-haplotype-mismatched related grafts, with a high stimulation index in mixed lymphocyte culture rather than rely entirely upon the improved immunosuppressive potential of cyclosporine. There is not convincing evidence that the use of cyclosporine is equivalent to or obviates the need for preoperative transfusions, and the long-term nephrotoxic side effects of cyclosporine are unknown. Five transfusions of approximately 2.5 ml/kg of packed red blood cells are given every 2 to 3 weeks prior to transplantation. Infants should be monitored for possible volume overload and hyperkalemia. Azathioprine, 1 mg/kg, is begun 1 to 5 days before the first transfusion and continued until transplantation to decrease sensitization. The dose is reduced if leukopenia, thrombocytopenia, or anemia develop. Patients should be monitored with periodic hematology surveys and for the development of cytotoxic antibody or a positive transplant crossmatch with a related donor. The transplant team at the University of California in San Francisco reported a 93% actuarial kidney survival at 6 years for 50 children receiving donor-specific transfusions. Most of these children had highly reactive mixed lymphocyte cultures with their donors.[39]

The immunosuppressive drug protocols used in children for the prevention and treatment of rejection are similar to those used in adults. A few differences are noteworthy. In small children, using surface area results in a higher dosage than using body weight. This partially explains why groups basing dosages on weight have observed that higher doses of cyclosporine per kilogram are often needed in children to maintain the same blood level com-

TABLE 23-3   Immunosuppression Protocols Dependent Upon Donor Relationship, HLA Matching, and MLC Stimulation Used at The University of Michigan

DONOR SOURCE	PROTOCOL
Cadaver	RT, CYA, PRED
HLA-Identical sibling	AZA, PRED
HLA Semi-identical sibling or par- ent-child with low MLC stimula- tion	CYA, PRED
HLA Semi-identical sibling or par- ent-child with high MLC stimu- lation	DST, AZA, PRED

Abbreviations: RT = random transfusions; CYA = cyclosporine; PRED = prednisone; AZA = azathioprine; DST = donor-specific transfusions; MLC = mixed lymphocyte culture; HLA = human lymphocyte antigen. The schedules for each drug are listed in Table 23-2.

pared with adults.[18,21,50] Hirsutism seems to occur more regularly in children as a side-effect of cyclosporine. Growth is not impaired by cyclosporine, and Knight and associates[22] from Australia suggested that cyclosporine might even have a growth-stimulating effect. In children, a greater effort is made to reduce steroid dosage to the lowest level possible to avoid growth retardation and appetite stimulation. Obesity can become a serious physical and psychological problem. Antithymocyte globulin and antilymphoblast globulin can be used as in adults, but, in small children, they are usually administered through a central venous catheter.[17,26,30] There is less experience with monoclonal antibody preparations, but good results have been reported with OKT3 (Ortho Pharmaceutical Corporation, Raritan, NJ).[27] For maintenance therapy, the trend is to use triple drug regimens of cyclosporine, aza-

TABLE 23-4 Treatment of Rejection

DRUGS	AMOUNT AND PERIOD OF ADMINISTRATION	USES
Methylprednisolone pulses	15 mg/kg IV daily or q.o.d. for 3 or 4 doses	In the early post-transplant period, the steroid taper is temporarily discontinued
ATGAM	15 mg/kg IV for 14 days	For rejection resistant to 3 or 4 steroid pulses
MALG	20 mg/kg IV for 14 days	Use like ATGAM
OKT3	5 mg IV for 10–14 days 2.5 mg IV under 30 kg	Reserve for resistant rejection

Abbreviations: ATGAM = Antithymocyte globulin, Upjohn Company, Kalamazoo, MI; MALG = Minnesota antilymphoblast globulin, University of Minnesota, Minneapolis, MN; OKT3 = anti-T$_3$ monoclonal antibody, Ortho Pharmaceutical Company, Raritan, NJ

thioprine, and steroids, with the strategy of using low dosages of each individual drug to avoid chronic dose-related side-effects.[45] When managing acute rejection, so-called rescue protocols with antithymocyte and/or monoclonal antibody are commonly used if the rejection episode does not promptly reverse with steroid pulse therapy.[38,54] The protocols currently used at the University of Michigan are outlined in Tables 23-2 to 23-4.

SURGICAL TECHNIQUE AND PERIOPERATIVE MANAGEMENT

Preoperative preparation is similar to that in an adult. The largest size Foley catheter that will fit comfortably is inserted, and a urine culture and sensitivity are obtained. Central venous and arterial lines are placed, usually in the operating room. In infants, a Broviac or Hickman catheter can be used as a central venous line and is left in place for blood drawing and antithymocyte globulin administration after transplantation. If a permanent peritoneal dialysis catheter is present, this should be left in place and can be used postoperatively for dialysis. Children are very sensitive to fluid shifts intraoperatively, and dehydration should be corrected before operation. With related transplants, cephazolin is used as a prophylactic antibiotic and is discontinued 24 hours after operation. With cadaveric transplants, either gentamicin and nafcillin or vancomycin are used prophylactically and continued until the culture reports from the donor kidney vein are available. Appropriate antibiotics are continued for another 10 days if the vein culture report is positive. With cadaveric transplantation, up to 25% of either the vein or urine cultures will be positive. Culturing the donor artery or ureter does not add new information. During the operation, core temperature is monitored carefully with a rectal or esophageal probe.

In infants, a lower abdominal curvilinear transplant incision is used and extended medially and toward the costal margin as necessary, depending upon the relative size of the donor kidney. The peritoneum is dissected widely from both the retroperitoneum and the anterior abdominal wall. The peritoneum may need to be dissected behind the right lobe of the liver to accommodate a large kidney. Many groups use a vertical midline incision and a transabdominal approach for transplants in infants.[33] The kidney is then placed into a retroperitoneal pocket or remains free in the abdomen. The retroperitoneal approach is quite feasible and has several advantages. Peritoneal dialysis can be instituted in the immediate postoperative period if necessary. Ureteral leaks or abscesses can be managed with a retroperitoneal drain without soiling the abdominal cavity. Adhesion of bowel to the kidney is avoided, and percutaneous renal biopsy is facilitated.

In children under 20 kg, the side of the distal aorta and inferior vena cava rather than the iliac vessels are usually used for the vascular anastamoses (Fig. 23-1). A Carrel patch allows the use of a continuous suture without concern about future relative renal artery stenosis as the child grows. If a Carrel patch is not possible, interrupted sutures are recommended. Venous outflow must be adequate, especially with a large donor kidney in a small child, and this almost always requires an end-to-side anastamosis to the vena cava. Heparin is administered prior to placing the vascular clamps and is reversed with protamine after the clamps are released. A Lich external ureteroneocystostomy is preferred for the ureteral anastamosis,[25] and in almost one thousand of these anastamoses, there has been a very low complication rate. The advantages compared with

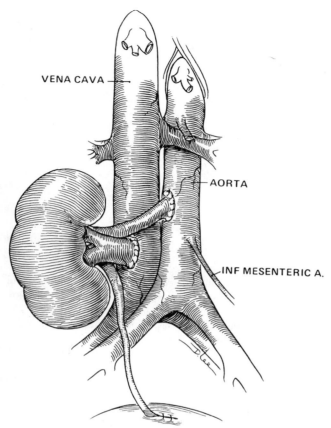

VENA CAVA

AORTA

INF MESENTERIC A.

FIGURE 23-1.   Most common technique used for kidney transplantation in pediatric patients at the University of Michigan. Often a more generous end-to-side Carrel patch of donor aorta or spatulated renal artery than illustrated is used for the arterial anastomosis. Note the external ureteroneocystostomy.

the Leadbetter–Politano technique are technical simplicity, avoidance of the anterior cystotomy incision, and fewer clots in the bladder, which can be a problem when only a small catheter can be inserted into the bladder.

Special precautions need to be taken when the vascular clamps are released to avoid hypotension, hyperkalemia, and acidosis. Revascularization of a large kidney in a child will suddenly sequester a significant proportion of the child's blood volume in the new kidney. Reactive hyperemia and vasodilation of the lower extremities with sequestration of more blood volume will occur as a result of having had the aorta clamped. The blood being released from the legs can be acidotic and hyperkalemic. The child should be volume loaded until the central venous pressure rises to 14 cm of water just prior to releasing the vascular clamps. One mEq/kg of sodium bicarbonate is given intravenously. The aortic clamp is released very slowly with intermittent finger compression. Usually a rapid infusion of intravenous fluid is necessary to avoid hypotension. Serum potassium and *p*H are monitored. An intra-

venous drip containing glucose and insulin may also be administered during the clamp release period.

When closing the abdominal wound in infants, special precautions must be taken to avoid kinking the renal vessels because of the frequent size discrepancy between the large donor kidney and the small recipient. Torsion or kinking of vessels can occur whether the kidney has been implanted retroperitoneally or transabdominally. Before tying the last few abdominal wall sutures, the blood flow should be checked with a Doppler probe placed on the surface of the kidney. In a few instances, we have closed only the skin and subcutaneous tissue immediately over the kidney placed in the retroperitoneal position under a transverse curvilinear incision.

Postoperatively, fluid and electrolytes must be monitored and replaced more frequently than in adults, that is, every 15 minutes. A large kidney can easily excrete the equivalent of an infant's blood volume in 1 hour. Hypertension can be severe and must be treated promptly to avoid encephalopathy and convulsions. Hyperglycemia occurs more often in children than in an adult and can cause a significant osmolar diuresis. If large quantities of intravenous fluids are required to replace urine output, non-glucose containing solutions should be used. Serum concentrations of calcium, phosphorus, and magnesium should be monitored closely, especially if urine output is high.

RESULTS

The major variables influencing results are related versus cadaveric donors, HLA match within the living-related donor group, the use of preoperative blood transfusions or cyclosporine, and children younger than 2 or 3 years versus older children.

Tables 23-5 and 23-6 summarize results from the literature.[1,2,8,23,30,34,36,37,39,40,52,53]

The results with HLA-identical sibling grafts are excellent. The University of Minnesota reported 100% patient and graft survival at 5 years for 16 HLA-identical sibling grafts.[36] With HLA semi-identical donors, results are also excellent if donor-specific transfusions are used. The University of California at San Francisco (UCSF) reported a 93% actuarial graft survival rate at 5 years using donor-specific transfusions.[39] Our own results in 18 patients, most of whom were semi-identical and did not receive either donor-specific transfusions or cyclosporine were 100% patient survival and 78% graft survival at 1 year.[52] There is less experience with cyclosporine, but the University of Minnesota

TABLE 23-5   Results of Living Related Transplantation in Children

| | | PERCENT ACTUARIAL SURVIVAL | | | |
| | | One-Year | | Five-Year | |
	NUMBER	Patient	Graft	Patient	Graft
HLA IDENTICAL					
U. Minnesota	16	100	100	100	100
HLA SEMI-IDENTICAL					
U. Minnesota	210	95	84	85	64
UCSF with DSTs	37	—	97	—	93
ALL LIVING RELATED					
UCSF	60	87	—	89	71
Boston Children's	82	92	—	92	—
U. Michigan	18	100	78	—	—
LESS THAN 2 OR 3 YEARS OF AGE					
U. Minnesota	44	92	88	—	67
U. Michigan	2	100	100	—	—

Abbreviations: UCSF = University of California at San Francisco
Note: Data compiled from references [1,2,8,23,30,34,36,37,39,40,52,53]

TABLE 23-6   Results of Cadaveric Transplantation in Children

| | | PERCENT ACTUARIAL SURVIVAL | | | |
| | | One-Year | | Five-Year | |
	NUMBER	Patient	Graft	Patient	Graft
ALL CADAVERIC					
U. Minnesota	78	95	72	84	54
UCSF	85	72	—	70	43
Boston Children's	36	88	—	85	—
U. Michigan	15	93	53	—	—
LESS THAN 2 OR 3 YEARS OF AGE					
U. of Minnesota	4	100	—		
U. Michigan	6	83	50		

Note: Data compiled from references [1,2,8,23,30,34,36,37,39,40,52,53]

reported no graft loss from rejection in a small series on a low-dose cyclosporine regimen. At 10 years, Minnesota reported 100% patient and graft survival with 16 HLA-identical transplants, and San Francisco reported a 55% graft function rate for 60 related transplants.[36,40] In children younger than 2 years, good results can also be obtained with semi-identical related grafts. The largest experience is that of Minnesota, which reported an 88% 1-year and 67% 5-year actuarial graft survival in children between 0.5 and 1 year of age.[36]

Results with cadaveric transplantation have been good in terms of patient survival but have met with only moderate success in long-term graft function.[36,40] Minnesota reported a 5- and 10-year patient survival rate of 84% and 73%, respectively, but the 5-year graft survival rate was only 54%. UCSF reported a 5-year graft survival rate of 43%, and the University of Toronto reported a 10-year graft function rate of 59% in 78 cadaveric allografts.

There is only limited experience with cadaveric grafts in infants; at Michigan, in six patients younger than 2 years of age, there was an 83% 1-year patient survival rate and a 50% graft function rate with cadaveric grafts.[52] Again, in most current reports, the majority of patients have not been treated with cyclosporine or pretransplant blood transfusions. In addition, results with retransplantation have improved with experience.[48]

In addition to survival, transplantation has the advantage of permitting growth and preventing the progression of neurologic damage compared with chronic dialysis. CAPD may be more beneficial in preventing growth and neurologic complications than intermittent peritoneal or hemodialysis. With children younger than 2 years of age, transplantation is less successful, and, as a result, there is controversy as to whether transplantation or CAPD is preferred. However, for most children older than 2 years, there is no doubt that with the introduction of cyclosporine, pretransplant blood transfusions, and antilymphocyte antibody, that "transplantation is the only reasonable choice."[11]

REFERENCES

1. Arbus GS, Galiwango J, DeMaria JE et al: The first 10 years of the dialysis-transplantation program at The Hospital for Sick Children, Toronto. 2. Transplantation and complications of chronic renal failure. Can Med Assoc J 122:659–664, 1980
2. Arbus GS, Hardy BE, Balfe JW et al: Cadaveric renal transplants in children under 6 years of age. Kidney Int 24 (Suppl 15):S111–S115, 1983
3. Avner E, Harmon W, Grupe W et al: Mortality of chronic hemodialysis and renal transplantation in pediatric end-stage renal disease. Pediatrics 67(3): 412–416, 1981
4. Broyer M, Donckerwolcke RA, Brunner FP et al: Combined report on regular dialysis and transplantation of children in Europe. Proc Eur Dial Transplant Assoc XII 20:79–108, 1983
5. Cameron JS: Glomerulonephritis in renal transplants. Transplantation 34:237–245, 1982
6. Campbell DA Jr, Dafoe DC, Roloff DW et al: Cadaveric renal transplantation in a 2.2 kilogram neonate. Transplantation 38(2):197–198, 1984
7. Campbell DA Jr, Lorber MI, Sweeton JC et al: Maternal donor-related renal transplants: Influence of breast feeding on reactivity to the allograft. Transplant Proc Vol XV 1:906, 1983
8. Conley S, Flechner S, Rose G et al: Use of cyclosporine in pediatric renal transplant recipients. J Pediatr 106(1): 45–49, 1985
9. Eddy A, Sibley R, Mauer SM et al: Renal allograft failure due to recurrent dense intramembranous deposit disease. Clin Nephrol 21:305–313, 1984
10. Fennell R, Rasbury W, Fennell E et al: Effects of kidney transplantation on cognitive performance in a pediatric population. Pediatrics 74(2): 273–278, 1984
11. Fine RN: For children, renal transplantation is the only realistic choice. Kid Intern 28 (Suppl 17): S-15, 1985
12. Folman R, Arbue GS, Churchill B et al: Recurrence of the hemolytic uremic syndrome in a 3 1/2 year old child, 4 months after second renal transplantation. Clin Nephrol 10:121–127, 1978
13. Gradus D, Ettenger R: Renal transplantation in children. Pediatr Clin North Am 29(4):1013–1038, 1982
14. Habib R, Hebert D, Gagnadoux MF et al: Transplantation in idiopathic nephrosis. Transplant Proc 14:489–495, 1982
15. Hebert D, Sibley RK, Mauer SM: Recurrence of hemolytic uremic syndrome in renal transplant recipients: Scope of the problem. Kidney Int 30:S-51–58, 1986
16. Herrin J: Pediatric renal transplantation. Nephrology Forum. Kidney Int 18:519–529, 1980
17. Hoyer P, Offner G, Brodehl J: Acute rejection episodes after renal transplantation in children. Clin Nephrol 19(2):61–66, 1983
18. Hoyer P, Ofener G, Wonigeit K et al: Dosage of Cyclosporin A in children with renal transplants. Clin Nephrol 22(2):68–71, 1984

19. Ingelfinger J, Grupe W, Harmon W et al: Growth acceleration following renal transplantation in children less than 7 years of age. Pediatrics 68(2):255–259, 1981

20. Kaskel F, Feld L, Schoeneman M: Renal replacement therapy in infants and children. Adv Pediatr 32:197–268, 1985

21. Klare B, Walter J, Hahn H et al: Cyclosporin in renal transplantation in children. Lancet 2:692, 1984

22. Knight J, Roy L, Sheil A: Catch-up growth in children with successful renal transplants immunosuppressed with cyclosporin alone. Lancet 1:159–160, 1985

23. Kohaut E, Whelchel J, Waldo F et al: Living-related donor renal transplantation in children presenting with end-stage renal disease in the first month of life. Transplantation 40(6):725–726, 1985

24. Kois WE, Campbell DA Jr, Lorber MI et al: Influence of breast-feeding on subsequent reactivity to a related renal allograft. J Surg Res 37:89–93, 1984

25. Konnak JW, Herwig KR, Finkbeiner A et al: Extravesical ureteroneocystostomy in 170 renal transplant patients. J Urol 113:299–301, 1975

26. Leichter H, Ettenger R, Jordan S et al: Short-course antithymocyte globulin for treatment of renal transplant rejection in children. Transplantation 41(1):133–135, 1986

27. Leone M, Funnell B, Jenkins R et al: Monoclonal antibody for reversal of acute renal allograft rejection in pediatric patients. Transplantation 40(5):574–577, 1985

28. Leuman E, Briner J: Recurrence of the primary disease in the transplanted kidney. In Fine R, Gruskin A (eds): Treatment of End-Stage Renal Disease in Children, pp 528–540. Philadelphia, WB Saunders, 1984

29. Leumann EP, Wegmann W, Largiadre F: Prolonged survival after renal transplantation in primary hyperoxaluria of childhood. Clin Nephrol 9:29–34, 1978

30. Lum C, Fryd D, Najarian J: Kidney transplantation in children zero to 10 years of age. Curr Surg 27–29, 1986

31. Lum C, Wassner S, Martin D: Current thinking in transplantation in infants and children. Pediatr Clin North Am 32(5):1203–1232, 1985

32. Miller L, Bock G, Lum C et al: Transplantation of the adult kidney into the very small child: Long-term outcome. J Pediatr 100(5):675–680, 1982

33. Miller L, Lum C, Bock G et al: Transplantation of the adult kidney into the very small child. Technical considerations. Am J Surg 145, 1983

34. Moel D, Butt K: Renal transplantation in children less than 2 years of age. J Pediatr 99(4):535–539, 1981

35. Morgan JM, Hartley MJ, Miller AC et al: Successful renal transplantation in hyperoxaluria. Arch Surg 109:430–433, 1974

36. Najarian J, So S, Simmons R et al: The outcome of 304 primary renal transplants in children (1968–1985). Ann Surg 204(3):246–258, 1986

37. Nevins TE, Knaak M, So SKS et al: Preliminary results of low dose cyclosporine A in pediatric renal transplantation. Int J Pediatr Nephrol 7(2):91–94, 1986

38. Orta-Sibu N, Chantler C, Bewick M et al: Comparison of high-dose intravenous methylprednisolone with low-dose oral prednisolone in acute renal allograft rejection in children. Br Med J 285:258–260, 1982

39. Potter D, Garavjoy Hopper S, Terasak P et al: Effect of donor-specific transfusions on renal transplantation in children. Pediatrics 76(3):402–405, 1985

40. Potter D, Holliday M, Piel C et al: Treatment of end-stage renal disease in children: A 15-year experience. Kidney Int 18:103–109, 1980

41. Rasbury W, Fennell R, Morris M: Cognitive functioning of children with end-stage renal disease before and after successful transplantation. J Pediatr 102(4):589–592, 1983

42. Rizzoni G, Malekzadeh M, Pennisi A et al: Renal transplantation in children less than 5 years of age. Arch Dis Child 55:532–536, 1980

43. Scheinman JI, Najarian JS, Mauer SM: Successful strategies for renal transplantation in primary oxalosis. Kidney Int 24:804–811, 1984

44. Sheldon C, Najarian J, Mauer S: Pediatric renal transplantation. Surg Clin North Am 65(6):1589–1621, 1985

45. Simmons RL, Canafax DM, Fryd DS, et al: New immunosuppressive drug combinations for mismatched related and cadaveric renal transplantation. Transplant Proc XVIII:2(Suppl) 1:76–81, 1986

46. Simmons RL, Najarian JS: Kidney transplantation. In Simmons RL, Finck ME, Ascher NL et al (eds): Manual of Vascular Access Organ Donation and Transplantation, pp 292–328. New York, Springer-Verlag, 1984

47. So SKS, Chang PN, Najarian JS et al: Renal transplantation in infants: The impact on growth and development. (submitted for publication)

48. So SKS, Simmons R, Fryd D et al: Improved results of multiple renal transplantation in children. Surgery 98(4):729–738, 1985

49. So SKS, Mahan JD Jr, Mauer SM et al: Hickman catheter for pediatric hemodialysis—a 3-year experience. Trans Am Soc Artif Intern Organs 30:619–623, 1984

50. Starzl T, Iwatsuki S, Malatack J et al: Liver and kidney transplantation in children receiving Cyclosporin A and steroids. J Pediatr 100(5):681–686, 1982

51. Striegel JE, Sibley RK, Fryd DS et al: Recurrence of focal segmental glomerulosclerosis in children with steroid resistant nephrotic syndrome following renal transplantation. Kidney Int 29:S-44–50, 1986

52. Tagge EP, Campbell DA Jr, Dafoe DC et al: Pediatric renal transplantation with an emphasis on the prognosis of patients with chronic renal insufficiency since infancy. Surgery (accepted for publication)

53. Trompeter R, Haycock G, Bewick M et al: Renal transplantation in very young children. Lancet 1:373–375, 1983

54. Turcotte JG, Feduska NJ, Carpenter EW et al: Rejection crises in human renal transplant recipients. Control with high dose methylprednisolone therapy. Arch Surg 105:230–236, 1972

55. Umeyama T, Hasegawa A, Ogawa O et al: Rehabilitation of pediatric renal allograft recipients: The present status and the problems. Transplant Proc XVI(6): 1984

56. Van Buren D, Van Buren CT, Flechner SM et al: De novo hemolytic uremic syndrome in renal transplant recipients immunosuppressed with cyclosporine. Surgery 98:54–62, 1985

57. Welchel JD, Alison DV, Luke RG et al: Successful transplantation in hyperoxaluria. Transplantation 35:161–164, 1983

CHAPTER 24

Management of the Adult Renal Transplant Patient

G. James Cerilli

Marked improvements in the results of kidney transplantation have decreased first-year mortality to less than 5% accompanied by a significant improvement in graft survival. The significant cost advantages to transplantation, coupled with the advantages of better rehabilitation and quality of life, make it the treatment of choice for patients with end-stage renal disease (ESRD). Children and highly sensitized patients are usually given priority. With the exception of a positive crossmatch on current sera, the immunologic contraindications to transplantation are decreasing rapidly.

Bilateral nephrectomy or vagotomy and pyloroplasty for ulcer disease are rarely performed prior to surgery. Splenectomy was once thought to have a beneficial effect but is now used only for persistent severe leukopenia. It is almost always possible to use the patient's own bladder to implant the ureter, and ileal conduits are almost never indicated except in patients with prior cystectomies. The evidence appears strong that donor-specific transfusions with living-related and living-unrelated transplantation and random transfusions both for living-related and cadaveric donors improve graft survival. Unfortunately, there is a small but cumulative incidence of sensitization from such transfusion protocols. Cyclosporine is decreasing the impact of transfusion on graft survival.

The role of tissue typing in transplantation remains controversial. However, it is relevant in living-related donor transplantation to identify the HLA-identical sibling combinations. Its relevance in cadaver transplantation results is smaller and appears to be decreasing as immunosuppression improves. Pretransplant sensitization to a variety of antigens, both histocompatibility or tissue specific, appears of increasing importance in the etiology of graft loss. Intraoperative hypotension usually has a specific cause, such as low circulating blood volume, excessive anesthesia, or low cardiac output. Recognition of the cause is essential if proper management is to be instituted.

Postoperatively, urinary output should be prompt with living-related donors, and acute tubular necrosis (ATN) should be rare; the dialysis rate following cadaveric transplantation should not exceed 15% to 20%. A variety of immunosuppressive protocols are used throughout the country, but the trend is toward triple therapy with cyclosporine, Imuran, and prednisone. Rejection is usually treated with Solu-medrol and possibly ATG or OKT3 monoclonal antibody, depending upon the patient's response. Excessive steroid or immunosuppressive dosages result only in an excessive mortality rate with a relatively small yield in improved graft survival.

Following transplantation, patients have a higher degree of rehabilitation than do patients maintained on hemodialysis. Most patients who experience irreversible transplant rejection want a second kidney transplant, although the graft success rate for retransplantation is not quite as good as it is with the initial transplantation, particularly if the patient has become significantly sensitized.

Ethical issues include (1) What represents the fairest distribution of transplantable organs? (2) Should living-related donors be used? (3) Should transplanted organs be considered marketable? (4) Should kidneys procured in the United States be used only in U.S. citizens?

The goal of this chapter is to provide a sequential approach for the management of an adult patient undergoing renal transplantation. It is based on the author's personal performance of more than 700 renal transplants and the management of several hundred others. It will, of necessity, include some topics that are discussed in much greater detail in other chapters, but it is hoped that this chapter will provide an easily readable summary of an overall management plan for the adult renal transplant patient.

BACKGROUND FOR TRANSPLANTATION

Almost all patients who present for renal transplantation have been on chronic dialysis. Both modalities of therapy have had significant improvements in their results during the past several years, but this is particularly so for transplantation.[37] During the past 5 to 6 years, the 1-year mortality rate following renal transplantation has dropped to approximately 5%, with a marked improvement in graft survival that attracts increasing numbers of end-stage renal disease (ESRD) patients. Most importantly, the knowledge that quality of life and rehabilitation are markedly enhanced following successful transplantation attracts most patients to transplantation. With fewer patients returning to hemodialysis as the result of rejected grafts and transplant complications, this source of discouragement and negative input for potential transplant candidates has diminished.

With the onset of the Medicare financial coverage for the treatment of ESRD in 1972, the cost of transplantation or dialysis has been of less concern to patients with ESRD. Currently, transplantation is more cost-effective than is dialysis. The average first-year cost using a living-related donor is approximately $28,000 (hospital and physician), and a cadaver transplant costs approximately $32,000. The average first-year cost following transplantation is approximately $5,000, diminishing to about $1,000 per year when the patient attains stable function. In-center hemodialysis costs about $25,000 per year, and peritoneal dialysis costs between $15,000 and $20,000 per year (dialysis and hospitalization); these costs continue until the patient dies or is transplanted. Thus, there is little question that over a 3- to 5-year period, there are significant cost advantages with transplantation, particularly since a higher percentage of successfully transplanted patients is capable of working, paying taxes, and supporting themselves.

SELECTION AND EXCLUSION OF PATIENTS

With the current shortage of kidneys, the tranplant surgeon must, unfortunately, prioritize patients for transplantation. All children should be promptly transplanted, whereas those patients in the upper age group, that is, over 60 to 65 years of age, can, in most instances, be well managed on chronic dialysis. Patients doing poorly on dialysis or highly sensitized patients (sera reactive to a high percentage of a random panel of lymphocytes) should receive priority if a donor kidney with a negative crossmatch with current sera is available. With these exceptions, a kidney is usually given to the patient who has either been waiting the longest or who has the best HLA match. It is still unknown whether the time on dialysis pretransplant, exclusive of transfusion effect, affects subsequent graft success.[3]

Contraindictions to transplantation either on a clinical or immunologic basis are decreasing, and, in fact, there are currently few absolute contraindications. A patient with another life-threatening disease process such as recurrent carcinoma or HIV infection is not a transplant candidate. Also, a patient who has rapidly (less than 6 months) rejected two prior transplants, particularly if the second transplant used a living-related donor, is considered a very poor candidate for a third transplant because the current results of such transplantation are poor. If the supply of available kidneys suitable for transplantation was to increase, it is hoped that it would no longer be necessary to exclude any patient from an opportunity for a renal transplant.

DONOR SELECTION

Xenografts

Cross-species transplantation of kidneys, livers, and hearts has been attempted in humans, pioneered by the work of Reetsma and Starzl. However, clinical trials have been unsuccessful, and although a rare xenograft transplant has functioned for several weeks, most have rejected within a few days. At this time, there are no laboratory or clinical data to support the current use of xenografts for transplantation. It is hoped that further research in the pathogenesis of rejection and an ability to modify preexistent sensitization will make this possible in the future, but the lack of clinical and laboratory success currently make further clinical trials inappropriate at this time (1987).

Living-Related Donors

The main justifications for the utilization of living-related donors are that graft survival with living-related donors is still better than that obtained with cadaveric donors,[2] and there is a shortage of cadaveric donors. Also, a highly sensitized patient is more likely to have a sibling (particularly HLA-identical) with a negative lymphocytotoxicity crossmatch than a random cadaver donor. The utilization of living-related donors also allows more prompt transplantation, thus avoiding some of the complications of dialysis. When the supply of cadaveric organs is adequate and the results from cadaveric transplantation more closely approximate those of living-related donors, living-related donor transplantation will be unjustified.

Living, Nonrelated Donors

During the 1960s, a few living, nonrelated donors were used for renal transplantation. These cases documented the fact that much of the poor graft function seen immediately following cadaveric transplantation was secondary to acute tubular necrosis (ATN) and not to rejection. However, as the graft survival with living, nonrelated donors approximated that of a cadaveric donor, living, nonrelated donation was discontinued. There has been a recent increase in the utilization of living, nonrelated donors giving donor-specific transfusions to the recipient. Whereas the earlier reports with living, nonrelated donors and donor-specific transfusions suggested that graft survival would not be improved, more recent results by Sollinger[32a] and others indicate that living, nonrelated donors combined with donor-specific transfusions are yielding graft survivals equal to those observed with living-related donors and donor-specific transfusions. If this observation is confirmed, in those instances in which there is a documentable emotional relationship between the living, nonrelated donor (husband/wife, extremely close friend), the utilization of living, nonrelated donors may be ethically acceptable.

Cadaveric Donors

Cadaveric sources constitute approximately 60% to 70% of kidney donors. There is still an inadequate supply of such donors, particularly of the O blood type. Only about 20% of potential cadaveric donors are used in the United States, but it is hoped that continued public and physician education and the implementation of such legislation as "required request" will improve the supply of cadaveric organs. The discipline of transplantation is totally dependent upon an adequate supply of cadaveric organs, which is in turn dependent upon meticulous adherence to the principles of brain death, informed consent, appropriate utilization of such organs, and public trust.

PRETRANSPLANT PREPARATION OF THE RECIPIENT

Optimal results in transplantation depend upon proper preparation of the patient for transplantation, which includes (1) the loss of excess wieght, and (2) the discontinuance of smoking to lessen pulmonary complications and the risk of carcinoma in patients on immunosuppression. Infections located at hemodialysis shunt sites or chronic ambulatory peritoneal dialysis (CAPD) catheters should be treated. Skin infections (often staphylococcus or fungus) at the site of the transplant incision must be controlled to minimize the likelihood of wound infection. Pulmonary infections, whether bacterial, tuberculosis, or fungus, must also be treated and stabilized prior to transplantation, and the patient must be kept on the appropriate antibiotics following transplantation. Patients with coronary artery disease manifested by either persistent angina despite medical therapy, left main coronary artery disease with ventricular injury, or three-vessel disease should be strongly considered for pretransplant coronary bypass surgery or coronary angioplasty. Patients presumably cured of a prior cancer are not excluded from transplantation, because there is little evidence that immunosuppression increases the recurrence rate of carcinoma.[11,34] Therefore, patients who have had a bilateral nephrectomy for renal carcinoma are transplant candidates if they have been tumor-free for a minimum of 2 years.

ROLE OF ADJUVANT SURGERY IN PRETRANSPLANT PREPARATION

Although there are isolated reports to the contrary, there is little evidence indicating that retention of the patient's native kidneys is detrimental to the recipient except in a few extremely well-defined circumstances.[30] When hypertension is impossible to control despite aggressive medical management, pretransplant bilateral nephrectomy is indicated. Similarly, patients with chronic pyelonephritis with continued infection of the urinary tract, particularly those with ureteric obstruction, should undergo pre-transplant bilateral nephrectomy. However, the presence of only ureteral reflux and dilatation in the absence of urinary tract infection is not an indication for bilateral nephrectomy. Despite the enormous size of polycystic kidneys, they need not be removed unless the patient has had frequent documented bouts of pyelonephritis and infected cysts. The unnecessary removal of kidneys is harmful to the potential recipient, because it aggravates anemia while on hemodialysis. This requires an increased number of blood transfusions, which can cause sensitization and possibly jeopardize the likelihood of receiving a successful transplant. Also, fluid and electrolyte management are easier if the hemodialyzed patient produces even small amounts of urine.

Recipient splenectomy requires, in most instances, a pretransplant operation and increases the incidence of post-transplant sepsis. Although Pneumovax and long-term prophylactic antibiotic use decrease the long-term incidence of post-splenectomy sepsis, nevertheless, it is higher than in the nonsplenectomized transplant population. This is particularly true for children and adolescents, where acute fulminant deaths occur in the splenectomized recipient.[9] Therefore, splenectomy is rarely indicated for the initial transplant, particularly since the advent of cyclosporine therapy.[35]

For many years, it was customary in some centers to perform vagotomy and pyloroplasty prior to transplantation in those patients who had a history of duodenal ulcer. This is no longer indicated, because H-2 inhibitors and aggressive antacid therapy coupled with more judicious use of the corticosteroids have essentially eliminated the problem of post-transplant upper gastrointestinal hemorrhage and perforated duodenal ulcer. Appropriate antacid therapy requires the utilization of 20 ml to 30 ml of antacids orally every 1 to 2 hours for the first 2 to 3 weeks following transplantation. Antacid dosage can then be decreased concomitant with steroid dose. Antacids given every 4 hours are essentially useless.

UROLOGIC EVALUATION OF THE TRANSPLANT RECIPIENT

Anatomic urologic problems should usually be corrected prior to transplantation. These include symptomatic prostatic hypertrophy, urethral valves, or urethral strictures. Patients with any history of difficulty in voiding should undergo pretransplant cystoscopy and cystourethrogram. It is rarely necessary to create an ileal conduit for urinary drainage in

transplant recipients. Patients with bladder dysfunction secondary to chronic pyelonephritis and cystitis resulting in a small scarred bladder can still use their own bladder.[6] Bladder size will gradually return to normal, and bladder function will be adequate with the implantation of a new kidney and ureter. Similarly, patients with a neurologic bladder and little ability to empty the bladder are best treated with intermittent bladder catheterization than with the creation of an ileal conduit. The complications of an ileal conduit, including reflux, chronic pyelonephritis, and obstruction of the ureteric implantation site, exceed the problems of clean intermittent bladder catheterization.[32] Therefore, ileal conduits should be essentially confined to those rare patients who have had a prior cystectomy.

ROLE OF TRANSFUSION IN THE PREOPERATIVE PREPARATION

Often, patients on dialysis develop severe fatigue or angina when anemia becomes profound. This requires the frequent use of transfusions, which may induce significant sensitization in about 25% of patients who receive five or more third-party transfusions. Because about 40% to 50% of the sensitized patients on cadaveric transplant waiting lists have become sensitized from blood transfusions, this is clearly a clinically important problem. Although sensitization secondary to transfusions does not appear to be as deleterious a risk factor for graft survival as sensitization secondary to a rejected graft, it nevertheless often leads to a delay in transplantation because of the difficulty in finding a suitable donor.[23] Patients sensitized to less than 30% of a random panel of lymphocytes will usually wait a minimum of 2 years for a suitable cadaveric kidney in contrast to a less than 6 month wait for patients who are nonsensitized. There is recent evidence that concentrating on the public specificities of the alloantibodies rather than private specificities may optimize the identification of a potential crossmatch compatible donor.[10]

Whereas recipient sensitization secondary to a rejected graft is probably not preventable, that secondary to transfusions may be preventable in many instances. Administering immunosuppression simultaneously with third-party transfusions, or, secondly, treating the blood with specific anti-donor antiserum as suggested by Terness and Opelz[39] may decrease the incidence of sensitization as it has with donor-specific transfusions.[27] Thirdly, using blood that is compatible with the recipient for public specificities might decrease the incidence of sensitization. An improvement in the organ supply would decrease sensitization secondary to blood transfusions by permitting earlier cadaveric renal transplantation. Sensitization of patients with a living-related donor is less frequent, because they are promptly transplanted. The use of stored blood or fresh blood with concomitant recipient immunosuppression has markedly decreased the incidence of sensitization secondary to donor-specific transfusions (from 35% to 10%) without apparently decreasing the beneficial effect on graft survival that such transfusions have produced.

OVERVIEW OF IMMUNOLOGIC ANALYSIS IN PRETRANSPLANT PREPARATION

The immunologic aspects of transplantation are discussed in detail elsewhere in this book. However, an overview summarizing those aspects that have clinical relevance is appropriate here.

Transplantation across the ABO barrier is still immunologically contraindicated except under special circumstances. With ABO incompatibility, the presence of the AB antigens on the vascular endothelial cell (VEC) usually leads to immediate graft loss unless (a) the recipient is immunologically manipulated or (b) A_2 kidneys transplanted to O recipients. Alexandre and colleagues[1] in Belgium have successfully transplanted recipients of living-related donors across the ABO barrier by the appropriate combination of plasmapheresis, donor-specific platelet transfusions, immunosuppression, splenectomy, and treatment with donor type A or B antigens. This important clinical accomplishment, as well as the observation that, in some instances, HLA antibody can be removed and its resynthesis can be inhibited, supports the possibility that it may be possible to overcome exogenously induced HLA sensitization secondary to transfusions or prior transplantation.[36]

The relevance on graft outcome of matching for the Class I and Class II loci remains controversial in cadaveric transplantation; however, matching for Class I and Class II antigens is relevant and important with related donors. A recipient with an HLA-identical, living-related donor should undergo prompt transplantation using relatively small doses of immunosuppression (Imuran, corticosteroids). Graft survival in this group approximates 90%; however, 10% do reject secondary to an immunologic response of the recipient to antigens not on the membranes of the lymphocyte such as the VEC-specific antigens. Approximately 80% of patients

who reject an HLA-identical transplant are sensitized to a VEC-specific antigen system, indicating that VEC antigens are potent immunogens that can lead to graft rejection despite HLA identity. (See Chapter 11—Tissue-Specific Antigens.)

The degree of HLA antigen disparity now seems irrelevant to graft outcome with non-HLA-identical, living-related donors. The transplantation of either single- or double-haplotype mismatches with donor-specific transfusions has yielded graft survival comparable to an HLA-identical transplant. In cadaveric transplantation, the clinical significance of tissue matching is still controversial despite 20 years of study. Patients who are well matched (no mismatched antigens) for Class I and II antigens do somewhat better (about 10%), particularly as time post-transplant increases.[31] The greatest beneficial effect of matching is seen with second transplants and in those combinations with no mismatched antigens; graft survival appears much less influenced by the number of mismatched antigens.[38] Interestingly, graft survivals were identical in centers from the European Dialysis and Transplant Association that place strong clinical importance on HLA matching compared with centers that place little or no importance on matching.[18] While cyclosporine does not seem to have completely eliminated the beneficial effects of matching, it appears that as immunosuppressant therapy improves, the clinical relevance of matching in cadaveric recipients seems to be decreasing.[17,26] Therefore, currently, cadaveric kidneys are transplanted, attempting to give a patient the best possible match but never denying a patient needing a transplant because a good match is not available.

The clinical relevance of pretransplant sensitization is being increasingly recognized and understood. The presence of antibody in recipient current sera to donor T cell antigens detected by a standard NIH crossmatching technique will usually be associated with hyperacute rejection. However, patients who have positive crossmatches on historical sera (older than 6 months) but who have negative crossmatches on current sera have graft survivals almost equal to those without any antibody, particularly if such sensitization was secondary to blood transfusions and not prior transplantation. Thus, the etiology and evolution of recipient anti-HLA antibody is extremely important to graft outcome. Antibody to the B cell antigens of the donor, if they are detectable only at 4°C, are probably not clinically relevant, whereas those detected at room temperature or 37°C are associated with a poorer graft survival.[25] Importantly, it is now well documented that it is possible to hyperacutely reject a kidney in the ab-

Screening Required to Absolutely Minimize
Graft Loss From Pre-Sensitization

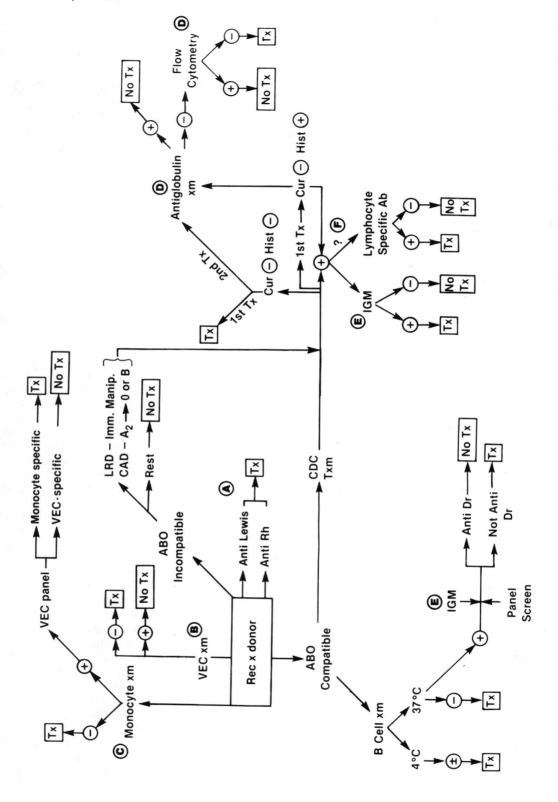

FIGURE 24-1. *If the goal is to absolutely minimize graft loss due to presensitization, a complex system of screening is currently required. (A) Unless recipient auto-Lewis titers are very high, Lewis incompatibility does not appear important. (B) There is recent evidence that use of donor vascular endothelium as an antibody target increases the detection of recipient sensitization. (Cerilli et al: Presented at American Society of Transplant Surgeons, 1987) (C) See Chapter 11—Tissue-Specific Antigens. (D) Antiglobulin and flow cytometry are most useful for retransplantation to detect low levels of antibody. (E) Antibody of the IgG class does not appear as immunologically detrimental to graft survival as IGG. (F) A small percentage of ⊕ CDC lymphocyte crossmatches may be secondary to antibody directed against lymphocyte-restricted antigens and thus not transplant-relevant. The risk factor for graft loss varies significantly for the different types of presensitization. Improving immunosuppression may decrease the clinical relevance of some forms of presensitization.*

sence of any sensitization to donor T cell or B cell antigens (HLA). Hyperacute rejection of both transplanted kidneys and hearts has been documented in recipients with positive monocyte crossmatches to the donor in the absence of any anti-donor T or B cell sensitization. A positive monocyte crossmatch represents in the recipient sensitization to a VEC antigen system that is shared, in most instances, between the monocyte and the VEC.[7] Therefore, preoperative immunologic analysis should include ABO typing, typing for Class I and Class II antigens (particularly in living-related donors), and T and B cell and monocyte crossmatches to exclude recipient sensitization to donor histocompatibility and VEC antigens. A more thorough discussion of these issues is presented elsewhere in this book, but the complexity of in vitro analysis for sensitization is reflected in Figure 24-1A.

IMMEDIATE PREOPERATIVE PREPARATION OF THE RECIPIENT

Excellent dialysis is available throughout most of this country; therefore, almost all patients come to surgery carefully prepared. However, particularly with cadaveric transplantation, metabolic abnormalities can be present pretransplantation, especially volume overload, hyperkalemia, or acidosis. Patients with a symptomatic volume overload should be dialyzed prior to transplantation, after other causes of heart failure, such as cardiac tamponade and recent myocardial infarction have been ruled out. Pretransplant electrolyte abnormalities are more frequently present than are volume abnormalities. Hyperkalemia (K > 6.5 mEq/liter) may be present, particularly in the noncompliant patient who has not been dialyzed for several days. Whereas patients with ESRD often maintain an elevated serum potassium, any patient with a serum potassium greater than 6.5 mEq/liter should be dialyzed prior to transplantation, particularly if ATN is expected. Children, particularly anephric children, are susceptible to a rapidly progressive hyperkalemia when they are transfused prior to trans-

plantation or if they are treated pretransplant with corticosteroids. Chronic peritoneal dialysis may be associated with volume depletion, requiring volume replacement either prior to or during the operative procedure. Clotting abnormalities are unusual with adequate dialysis and are usually correctible by fresh frozen plasma or cryoprecipitated plasma.

SURGICAL PROCEDURE

Details of the surgical transplant operation are discussed elsewhere in this book, but, based on more than 700 personally performed renal transplants, some aspects deserve emphasis here. Skin preparation should be thorough, and sterile technique must be meticulous throughout the operation. The wound should be irrigated with an antibiotic solution at the conclusion of the procedure, and hemostasis to avoid even a small hematoma must be extremely meticulous. By careful adherence to such principles, wound infections should almost never occur in renal transplant recipients. Most wound infections are derived from organisms within the recipient's bladder.[20] Therefore, careful irrigation of the bladder and the installation of an antibiotic solution at the beginning of the procedure is indicated and will aid in decreasing the magnitude of bacterial contamination. In the author's experience, no kidney has ever been lost because of wound infection, and there has not been a wound infection requiring therapy in the last 500 cases. It is easier to place all transplant kidneys on the right side of the recipient, anastomosing the renal vein to the external iliac vein and the renal artery to the side of the external iliac artery; heparinization of the recipient is unnecessary. This minimizes dissection within the pelvis, which may increase the likelihood of a postoperative lymphocele. In addition, the external iliac artery is less likely to subsequently become involved with atherosclerosis than is the internal iliac artery. During the anastomosis, particularly with small cadaveric kidneys, the kidney should be kept cold by surface cooling. The ureteral implantation can be accomplished by several techniques, but a ureteroneocystostomy using only four plain catgut sutures at the anastomosis is extremely satisfactory. The urologic aspects of the operation are best performed by the transplant surgeon in order to conserve time and expense and to consolidate post-transplant responsibility. With the advent of the certification of training programs in transplant surgery by the American Society of Transplant Surgeons, all transplant surgeons should be adequately trained in handling the urologic and vascular aspects of the transplant procedure. The wound should be carefully closed in layers with no drainage, and the total operating time required for almost all patients is about 2 hours. The adherence to these principles should result in an extremely low technical complication rate (Table 24-1).

MANAGEMENT OF SPECIFIC OPERATIVE PROBLEMS

Hypotension

Hypotension during the operative procedure usually has very specific and identifiable causes that must be corrected. Patients with ESRD may be sensitive to the customary dosage of anesthetic agents. Decreasing the amount of inhalation or intravenous anesthesia being used will often return blood pressure to normal. Hypotension may also be secondary to volume depletion, particularly in those patients who have been recently dialyzed or patients on CAPD. This usually responds promptly to the intravenous infusion of 500 ml to 1000 ml of fresh frozen plasma or normal saline. The sudden release from the kidney of a preservation solution with a high potassium content can cause an acute arrhythmia and hypotension in a patient with hyperkalemia. The slow release of the vascular clamps or immediate preoperative dialysis will eliminate this complication. Except in children or patients with severe cardiac disease, it is usually not necessary to monitor central venous pressure or pulmonary artery wedge pressure.

TABLE 24-1 *Operation complication rates— author's experience of recent 250 consecutive cases*

COMPLICATIONS	PERCENT
Ureteral anastomotic obstruction	<0.5
Ureteral fistula	<0.5
Bladder fistula	0
Wound infection	0
Arterial stenosis	<0.5
Venous thrombosus	0
Lymphoceles	1.2

Hemorrhage

Coagulation defects are rarely the cause of significant intraoperative hemorrhage. Rarely, however, patients appear to bleed more than usual, and the clots seen are soft and mushy. The utilization of fresh frozen plasma and sometimes platelets will correct this. Most often bleeding in excess of 250 ml to 300 ml during a transplant procedure is from the anastomosis or from an unligated vessel in the kidney hilum such as a posterior branch of the renal vein. It is always possible to get complete hemostasis, and the incision should never be closed without complete hemostasis.

Metabolic Complications

In those patients in whom hyperkalemia, hyperglycemia, or acidosis was present prior to surgery, the intraoperative assessment of potassium concentrations, glucose levels, and acid-base balance is indicated. These complications should be appropriately treated by the judicious use of intravenous insulin or bicarbonate during surgery. Mild acidosis will rapidlly correct itself with the successful functioning of a transplanted organ. However, particularly in diabetics, the acid-base balance should be checked during surgery and in the recovery room.

A Poorly or Nonperfused Kidney

Normally upon re-establishment of vascular perfusion, the kidney should promptly become pink and firm and transected vessels on its surface and in the hilum or ureter should bleed a bright red blood. This is particularly true with living-related donors or with cadaveric kidneys that were transplanted under ideal circumstances. Failure to obtain good perfusion or, particularly, the loss of adequate perfusion after a few minutes is indicative of a serious problem that must be diagnosed and appropriately treated if possible. The causes of a "blue," poorly perfused kidney include (1) position of the kidney, (2) a technical vascular complication, (3) immunologic causes, (4) excessive ischemia with ATN, (5) hypotension, (6) a storage perfusion error, or (7) other factors. When a kidney appears poorly perfused, its position should first be assessed to be sure that it has not become twisted 180 degrees on its hilum, resulting in an occlusion of the vein and/ or artery. Occasionally, in the absence of twisting, the adequacy of kidney perfusion will be position-dependent. This may be due to a kinking of the artery secondary to excessive arterial length. In such circumstances, the kidney must be positioned laterally or, preferably, the arterial anastomosis should be redone. If the problem is not positional, the anastomoses must be checked for patency. If the renal vein pressure is significantly greater than that in the external iliac vein, the venous anastomosis should be partially opened and its patency evaluated. If the pulse in the iliac artery is significantly better than that in the renal artery, the arterial anastomosis should be redone. Vasoconstriction with secondary poor perfusion of the kidney, ultimately resulting in acute tubular necrosis, can have several causes: (1) excessive warm ischemia, (2) a cold nonperfused preservation time in excess of 24 hours, (3) prolonged hypotension of the donor, (4) significantly compromised renal function in the donor (creatinine above 4.0 mg/liter), or (5) difficulty in performing the vascular anastomosis in the recipient. Vasoconstriction as a cause for poor perfusion is a difficult diagnosis to make intraoperatively, and other causes for poor perfusion must be excluded prior to accepting it as a reasonable probability.

Systemic hypotension can cause intraoperative kidney transplant hypoperfusion. A blood pressure in the range of 110 to 120 systolic may represent hypotension and may be associated with vasoconstriction in patients who are accustomed to systolic blood pressures of 180 to 190 mm Hg. Correction of volume deficits and a decrease in the levels of anesthesia usually relieve the hypotension and improve kidney perfusion. An unrecognized aortic or proximal iliac stenosis from atherosclerosis can be the cause of regional hypotension. However, such vascular stenosis should be assessed prior to graft implantation by the careful examination of the iliac and femoral pulses.

Preservation errors can cause a poorly perfused kidney following transplantation. These errors include (1) failure to keep the kidney cold during preservation, (2) preservation with a plasma solution unknowingly containing cytotoxic antibody to donor histocompatibility antigens,[12] and (3) the use of an erroneous preservation solution. Such occurrences, although rare, must be recognized. The temporary interruption of pulsatile perfusion or even the transient infusion of air into the vasculature of the kidney usually does not cause significant renal injury.

If adequate perfusion initially occurred and if other causes of poor perfusion have been excluded, a poorly perfusing kidney often has an immunologic etiology. Its usual cause is the presence in the recipient of a nonidentified antibody directed at antigen systems located on the donor VEC. The most obvious of these is the naturally occurring anti-A and anti-B antibodies, and the AB blood groups should be rechecked to exclude this etiology. Anti-Rh antibody present in the recipient is not detrimental to graft function, because the Rh antigens are not located on the vascular endothelium. Current lymphocytotoxic crossmatching techniques that involve extended incubation and careful preparation of donor T cells and B cells have progressively decreased the incidence of hyperacute rejection secondary to anti-HLA antibody present in the recipient. The antiglobulin crossmatch technique and flow cytometry are further increasing the sensitivity of antibody detection, but antibody detected only by such methods does not appear to be associated with hyperacute rejection. However, standard lymphocyte crossmatching techniques do not detect the presence in the recipient of antibody directed against donor VEC antigens, and such antibody has been associated with hyperacute rejection.

The confirmation of hyperacute rejection in the operating room is often difficult. The classic pathologic picture of hyperacute rejection with (1) infiltration of polymorphonuclear cells in the glomerulus and around peritubular capillaries, (2) platelet and fibrin deposition in the glomeruli, and (3) the deposition of immunoglobulin on the VEC does not always promptly occur. Polymorphonuclear cells in the peritubular capillaries are often found earlier in hyperacute rejection than those in the glomeruli, and because they are rarely found normally in the peritubular capillaries, their presence in that location is highly supportive of the diagnosis of hyperacute rejection. However, hyperacute rejection can be difficult to diagnose using frozen section biopsies taken immediately after its presumed occurrence. Any treatment of hyperacute rejection once it has occurred will be unsuccessful. Heparin, anticomplement factors (i.e., cobra venom), plasmapheresis, thoracic duct drainage, or Fab2 fragments specific for donor antigens will not ameliorate hyperacute rejection.[13] Therefore, if the kidney has minimal cortical perfusion and other causes of hypoperfusion have been excluded, the kidney should be removed. In contrast, a kidney that is hypoperfused because of vasoconstriction or ATN should not be removed, because it will usually establish adequate function.

GENERAL POSTOPERATIVE MANAGEMENT

Most wound infections are secondary to bacterial organisms in the bladder; therefore, transplant patients should be given antibiotics (usually a broad-spectrum cephalosporin) beginning prior to transplantation and continuing for about 3 days. Recipient isolation except for profound leukopenia or infection is unnecessary, because immunosuppression levels are currently much more appropriate. Prompt ambulation is encouraged, and nasogastric de-compression is usually discontinued within 24 hours. Antibiotic ointment should be placed around the urethral meatus daily, and the Foley catheter should be carefully monitored for obstruction and irrigated under sterile conditions if occluded by a clot. Catheter drainage for 3 to 4 days postopera-tively is routine, but, in those instances in which very early removal has been necessary, no bladder fistulae have occurred in the author's experience. Postoperative hematuria is usually transient, and, when it persists, removing the catheter often im-proves the hematuria significantly. A gortex graft or external shunt will frequently clot post-transplant upon the restoration of normal clotting and normal blood pressure. A CAPD catheter can be electively removed as an outpatient when renal function is stabilized. A regular diet is started by postoperative Day 2 or Day 3 with no protein restriction if the patient does not require dialysis. If the patient is significantly hypertensive, salt restriction should be instituted, approximately 2 g/day to 4 g/day of salt. Diabetic patients on steroids will require careful monitoring of their glucose postoperatively, usually with blood sugars measured every 4 to 6 hours and covered with regular insulin. As steroid dosage is reduced, insulin requirements will decrease.

MANAGEMENT OF FLUIDS

Essentially all recipients of a living-related donor kidney will have urine output begin during the op-erative procedure or shortly thereafter. There should be no ATN following living-related donor transplan-tation, and any significant delay in onset of urinary output is usually indicative of a technical or im-munologic problem. In cadaveric transplantation during the last 3 years, fewer than 10% of our patients have required dialysis following transplan-tation, and urinary output in almost all instances has begun during the operative procedure. How-ever, we have recently noted an increase in the incidence of ATN with the utilization of cold storage and multiple organ harvest, particularly when large volumes of flush cooling solutions are used in the donor. In centers using a large percentage of shared or "shipped" kidneys with longer storage periods, the post-transplant dialysis rate can be as high as 35%. There is some evidence that the incidence of graft rejection is higher in patients with ATN, pos-sibly secondary to the immunologic stimulus of an-tigens shed because of the tubular necrosis.[14] Some patients will have a large diuresis (500 ml/hr–1000 ml/hr) following transplantation, particularly if they

have a significant volume overload or are hypergly-cemic. It is important not to "chase" the urinary output but rather to replace a decreasing percentage of urinary volume with higher urinary output (e.g., replace 90% of a urinary output of 150 ml/hr, but replace 50% of a urinary output of greater than 500 ml/hr). If urinary output is below 50 ml/hr, it is replaced with an equal volume, assuming that the patient has ATN with oliguric renal failure. Several different electrolyte solutions can be successfully used post-transplant, but a simple protocol that re-quires little monitoring of serum electrolytes in-volves alternating 5% dextrose 0.45 normal saline solution (NSS) with 5% dextrose/NSS. If the patient is diabetic, solutions containing less glucose should be used. Potassium replacement is usually not ini-tially necessary except in patients with a large di-uresis. After 24 hours, in almost all patients, the urinary output will be appropriate for their weight and renal function, and fluid replacement can be changed to 5% dextrose/0.2 NSS at about 125 ml/hr.

The etiology of post-transplant oliguria or an-uria must be diagnosed, because it usually requires therapy. The most common cause is the occlusion of the catheter from blood clot, which must be cor-rected by sterile irrigations. Children and diabetic patients should be closely observed for volume de-pletion following transplantation. A low central ve-nous pressure with tachycardia usually indicates in-adequate blood volume, requiring replacement therapy. In cadaveric transplantation, the most fre-quent cause of postoperative oliguria is ATN sec-ondary to injury to the donor kidney during the terminal phases of the donor's illness or during kid-ney procurement. ATN may be present despite an initial adequate urinary output. In these instances, the serum creatinine will change very little, and urinary output will often decrease later as oliguric renal failure develops. The delayed onset of oliguria may occasionally represent accelerated rejection; however, in most instances, with careful cross-matching techniques, it reflects ATN. With severe oliguria or especially anuria, a technical etiology must be excluded. A renal flow scan will document the adequacy of blood flow to the kidney. Ureteric patency can be evaluated by ultrasound imaging and assessing dilatation of the ureter and/or the renal pelvis. If the information is not conclusive, an antigrade pylogram will provide definitive infor-mation. Retrograde visualization of the recently im-planted ureter through the bladder is extremely dif-ficult and usually a waste of time. Any external compression of the renal hilum by hematoma or acute lymphocele causing decreased renal blood flow or ureteric obstruction can also be evaluated by ultrasound imaging. In such instances, the patient is usually experiencing severe wound pain, and emergency wound exploration is indicated to prevent venous thrombosis. Occasionally, a patient has normal urinary output for several days post-transplantation and then has the acute onset of marked oliguria. Flow scans appear normal, and severe dehydration is absent. Some of these patients respond to additional fluids and high-dose intravenous diuretics, which should be tried prior to exploring the patient in search of a technical etiology for the oliguria.

IMMUNOSUPPRESSION

The immunosuppressive management of patients has improved dramatically during the last 4 to 5 years as new protocols of immunosuppressive management have been initiated.[4] The ideal immunosuppressive regimen should (1) have minimal toxicity with adequate immunosuppression, (2) avoid duplication in mechanisms of drug action, (3) require simple in vitro monitoring of toxicity or effectiveness, and (4) minimize or eliminate steroid utilization. Ultimately, the optimal regimen would achieve allograft survival not by toxic drugs that indiscriminately suppress the immune response but by achieving immunologic unresponsiveness only to the immunologically relevant antigens of the transplanted organ. Significant progress has been made toward achieving many of these goals.

Prior to the late 1970s, immunosuppression consisted of azathioprine (Imuran), prophylactic steroids in high dosages, prophylactic antithymocyte globulin (ATG), and frequently splenectomy. This approach was associated with a 2-year cadaver graft survival of approximately 50% and a significant morbidity and mortality (15%–25%) primarily from the complications of the high steroid and ATG dosages. It was not unusual for patients to receive 10 g to 20 g of Solu-medrol to treat a rejection episode, which led to a high incidence of sepsis, gastrointestinal hemorrhage, hypertension, diabetes, and so on. Recently, the use of donor-specific transfusions or cyclosporine plus the most important recognition that corticosteroids can be used effectively in a low dose has led to a much more rational application of immunosuppressive therapy. Although there are several different protocols currently being used successfully in clinical transplantation, we have adopted the following approach.

Recipients with an HLA-identical living-related donor are promptly transplanted and treated with low doses of Imuran (1.5 mg/kg–2 mg/kg) and low-dose steroids. Low-dose steroids entail an initial dose of approximately 30 mg of prednisone per day, dropping rapidly to 10 mg/day to 15 mg/day within 1 to 2 months if renal function is stable (Fig. 24-2). Recipients with a non-HLA-identical living-related donor receive donor-specific transfusions using either stored blood or fresh blood plus simultaneous administration of Imuran (0.75 mg/kg/day–1.0 mg/kg/day). The post-transplant immunosuppression is similar to an HLA-identical sibling transplant. Using this approach, our living-related donor graft survival is 89% at 2 years. The current lack of data on the long-term adverse effects of cyclosporine therapy and the reported lack of improved results with cyclosporine do not warrant, in the author's opinion, its use at this time in living-related donors when graft survivals approximating 90% can be obtained with Imuran and low-dose steroids. In patients receiving a cadaveric transplant, cyclosporine should be used in low doses (3 mg/kg/day–5 mg/kg/day) combined with Imuran (0.75 mg/kg–1.0 mg/kg) and low-dose corticosteroids (30 mg of prednisone per day decreasing to 10 mg by Days 30 to 45). Whole blood levels of cyclosporine are very carefully monitored (initially daily and then 1 to 3 times per week) and kept at 250 ng/ml to 350 ng/ml (RIA method). Renal biopsy has not proved useful in our center for reliably differentiating early rejection from cyclosporine toxicity. By maintaining whole blood levels of Cyclosporin A at 250 ng/ml to 350 ng/ml, conversion to azathioprine has rarely been necessary because of nephrotoxicity, although such conversion can be accomplished with a low risk of rejection and graft loss.[24] Therefore, post-transplant rises in creatinine in our center are almost always secondary to rejection; this protocol is associated with only a 14% graft loss from immunologic causes at 1 year in our center. Immunosuppressive therapy must be indefinitely maintained, because the total cessation of immunosuppression will ultimately result in graft loss. However, the need to maintain immunosuppression in patients with excellent renal function several years post-transplantation was questioned in a study by Campos and associates[5] of 39 recipients in whom azathioprine was discontinued; graft survival was 57% compared with 63% in a matched control group with a mean follow-up of 32 months.

DIAGNOSIS OF REJECTION

Hyperacute rejection, which is primarily antibody mediated, has been discussed earlier in this chapter.

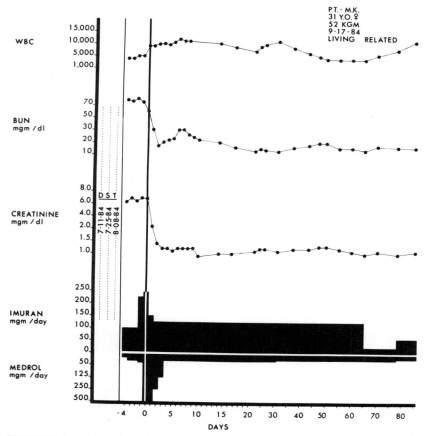

FIGURE 24-2. *Living-related donor with donor-specific transfusion. The patient was treated with Imuran and low-dose steroids. Leukopenia required temporary decrease of Imuran.*

Accelerated rejection, which occurs within the first few days after transplantation, probably occurs in patients with low levels of undetected humeral sensitization to HLA or VEC antigens. Intraoperative renal biopsies that assess the deposition of immunoglobulin in the kidney are not helpful in predicting the development of accelerated rejection.[8] As immunosuppression has become increasingly effective, acute rejection episodes are delayed and milder but can occur at any time post-transplant. Any fever within the first 3 weeks post-transplant should be considered as graft rejection until otherwise diagnosed. It is often low-grade and associated with mild hypertension, weight gain, and increase in kidney size and tenderness. Urinary output falls, creatinine clearance decreases, and serum creatinine rises. A large decrease in platelet count is indicative of a severe rejection process and ominous prognosis.

A large number of in vitro tests, such as monitoring urinary neopterin levels and inhibition of macrophage migration have been used to aid in the

diagnosis of rejection, but their cost and lack of specificity have discouraged their widespread application.[21,40] Renal biopsy reveals edema, cellular infiltrates with lymphocytes, and mononuclear cells. These are often grouped around capillaries early in the rejection process. Glomeruli initially appear relatively normal. While there is no conclusive evidence that a delay of a few hours or even 1 or 2 days in diagnosing most rejection episodes influences its reversibility, nevertheless, prompt therapy is indicated to avoid the conversion of acute rejection into the stage of vascular thrombosis and necrosis. Rejection must be distinguished from other causes of renal failure, particularly obstruction of the arterial, venous, or ureteric anastomosis, or cyclosporine toxicity. A renal scan using DTPA (diethylenetriamine penta-acetic acid) will provide evidence as to the adequacy of the vascular input to the kidney based on the rapidity with which the radioactive material gets into the kidney and the rate at which it clears the kidney. Delays in input are suggestive of arterial obstruction, but a kidney that is significantly edematous from rejection will also have a slow arterial input phase. An arteriogram is usually necessary for the definitive diagnosis of renal artery stenosis. Normally, DTPA is excreted promptly into the bladder, and a dilated ureter from obstruction or a ureteric leak can be visualized. An ultrasound will help diagnose ureteric obstruction and detect a perirenal lymphocele or hematoma that can occlude the ureter or renal vein. Imaging of the transplanted kidney by nuclear magnetic resonance shows promise for distinguishing rejection from ATN and cyclosporine toxicity.[15]

The patient with a slowly rising creatinine months to years post-transplant is usually undergoing chronic rejection, although other causes of renal failure such as ureteric obstruction and arterial stenosis must be excluded. Unlike acute or accelerated rejection, these kidneys are usually nontender and small and are not associated with fever. Ultrasound and renal scan will usually reveal a kidney that is decreased in size and has diminished blood flow. A biopsy shows the classic picture of chronic rejection with interstitial fibrosis, small islands of mononuclear infiltrate, but, most importantly, the narrowed "onion-skinned" appearance of the small arteries and the progressive hyalinization of the glomeruli. This form of rejection is extremely difficult to treat, although there is some evidence that Persantine and aspirin may decrease the rapidity of the chronic rejection process. It is important to distinguish chronic rejection from an acute rejection episode that can occasionally occur months or years after the transplant, because acute rejection episodes are susceptible to steroid or ATG therapy. Biopsy can be extremely helpful in these instances.[28] Patients with chronic rejection rarely need a transplant nephrectomy, because these kidneys are small and fibrotic and are not associated with the toxic manifestations of rejection, infection, or rupture of the transplanted organ.

In contrast, those kidneys that reject within the first 1 or 2 months following transplantation usually require transplant nephrectomy. The earlier a transplant nephrectomy is performed, the lower the morbidity; an absence of blood flow on renal scan is an indication for prompt nephrectomy. The kidney is removed extraperitoneally through the prior transplant incision by clamping and oversewing the entire hilum except for the ureter. Removal of the ureter from the bladder is not necessary, and it need only be divided and tied. Meticulous hemostasis is important to avoid hematoma and subsequent sepsis. The procedure requires 30 to 45 minutes and should be associated with less than a 0.5% wound infection rate. All immunosuppression therapy, including steroids, should be immediately and completely stopped following nephrectomy. In more than 150 transplant nephrectomies performed over an 18-year period, corticosteroids needed to be resumed in only one instance because of mild postural hypotension, weakness, and low-grade fever. The continuation of steroid therapy following transplant nephrectomy unnecessarily subjects patients to the continued risk of steroid toxicity, particularly infection.

TREATMENT OF REJECTION EPISODES

There are multiple protocols for treating acute rejection, most of which are equally effective. The following is the procedure currently used by the author.

Upon the diagnosis of rejection, 250 mg of Solu-medrol is given daily for 3 to 6 days. If renal function improves, this is continued for about three more doses on an alternating day basis. If a minimal response occurs (creatinine does not begin to fall or stabilize), the patient is begun on intravenous antilymphocyte globulin (ALG) (7.5 mg/kg–10 mg/kg) for 10 to 21 days, depending upon the response (Fig. 24-3). With ALG therapy, the white blood cell (WBC) and/or platelet count occasionally falls and Imuran dosage should be decreased or discontinued (Fig. 24-4). Recently OKT3 has been used to treat rejection episodes that recur following ALG therapy. The success rate in these steroid–ALG failures has been less than 30%. OKT3 has recently been used to "cover" highly sensitized patients who are experiencing ATN following cadaveric transplant. No rejection episodes have occurred in two highly cytotoxic (plasma renin activity [PRA] > 90%) patients who have rejected two prior transplants and were treated with OKT3 post-transplant for 10 to 16 days followed by cyclosporine therapy.

The recurrence of a third rejection episode during the first several weeks post-transplant usually results in total graft rejection, particularly if the serum creatinine level did not become normal between rejection episodes or if the interval between the second and third episodes of rejection was brief.[22] Plasmapheresis, heparinization, graft irradiation, and plasma leukopheresis have been reported to be effective sporadically but must be considered of unproven efficacy.

Chronic rejection does not respond to this approach. In our experience, switching the patient from Imuran and prednisone to cyclosporine and prednisone has, in several instances, resulted in stabilization and even improvement of renal function

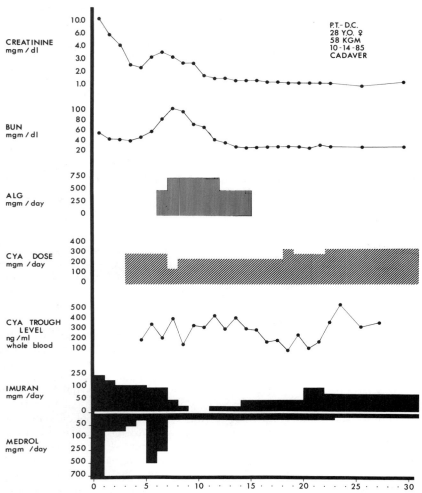

FIGURE 24-3.   *Rejection episode responded quickly to brief course of Solu-medrol followed by antilymphocyte globulin (ALG). Maintenance steroid dose of 10 mg/day was achieved by Day 23.*

and the preservation of graft function when total chronic rejection had seemed inevitable.

SPECIAL PROBLEMS

Pregnancy

Successful term pregnancies are extremely uncommon in the patient on chronic dialysis, whether it be hemodialysis or chronic peritoneal dialysis. However, a patient should be informed that her ability to conceive can rapidly return after a successful transplant, and, if pregnancy is not desired, appropriate contraceptive measures should be undertaken. There is no evidence that birth control pills

interfere with Imuran or steroid effectiveness, but they do influence cyclosporine blood levels, presumably by inhibiting hepatic microsomal enzymes.[29] There is little evidence that Imuran or steroids are associated with an increased incidence of fetal anomalies. Very high dosages of cyclosporine in mice have been reported to be associated with fetotoxicity, but no similar correlation has been reported to date in human pregnancies. There is a somewhat higher incidence of premature deliveries and smaller babies with Imuran and steroids, but the incidence of spontaneous abortion is not significantly affected. Patients can deliver either vaginally or by cesarean section, but cesarean section is frequently used. Immunosuppressive therapy should be restarted promptly after delivery, particularly the

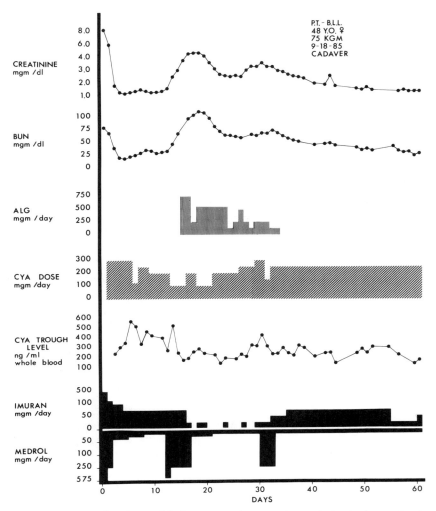

FIGURE 24-4.   *Antilymphocyte globulin (ALG) and Imuran therapy had to be decreased and then discontinued because of severe leukopenia (not shown).*

reinstitution of cyclosporine. However, there does not appear to be an increased incidence of graft loss associated with pregnancy.

Retransplantation

Most patients who lose a kidney graft from rejection desire retransplantation, particularly if the graft rejected months or years after the initial transplantation. If there are minimal toxic manifestations of immunosuppression, retransplantation can be promptly performed. However, if leukopenia or the toxic effects of steroids (e.g., cushioned appearance, thin skin, diabetes) are present, a delay is indicated. Unless otherwise indicated, it is not necessary to remove the initial transplant, because the second transplant kidney is placed on the contralateral side. Although controversial, overall, the results of retransplantation are poorer than those of primary transplantation. This is particularly true if (1) the first kidney was from a living-related donor and the retransplant must involve a cadaveric donor (2) significant sensitization has occurred (PRA > 50%), and (3) the first transplant rejected within 6 months.[33] Most patients who reject a graft will develop anti-HLA antibody, and essentially all patients develop anti-VEC antibody; thus, the immunologic screening for retransplantation should include monocyte crossmatching. Retransplantation of the patient sensitized from a previous transplant is difficult if he or she has greater than a 50% reactivity to a random lymphocyte panel. Multicenter cooperative programs to improve the likelihood of obtaining a nonreactive donor can increase the transplantation rate of sensitized patients, but a national program has yet to be developed.[19] The formation of large regional sharing programs for the purpose of transplanting sensitized patients is essential if these patients are to be successfully transplanted.

Immunosuppression of these patients is usually similar to that of the first transplant, but, if cyclosporine was not used initially, it should be used with the second transplant. There is some evidence that splenectomy may improve the results of secondary transplants, but splenectomy appears most useful in those patients with persistent leukopenia in whom it is intended that Imuran or ATG be used as immunosuppressive therapy.[16]

EXPECTATION OF TRANSPLANTATION

The results of transplantation are covered in great detail in another section of this book. However, the author's personal experience with the most recent 250 consecutive renal transplants reflects a patient mortality with living-related donors of 2%, and with cadaver donors of 5% during the first post-transplant year. Graft survival for all living-related donors at 2 years has been 89%, with the graft survival of HLA-identical and either 1- or 2-haplotype-mismatched familial donors using donor-specific transfusions being approximately the same. In the last 500 consecutive transplants, only one kidney has been lost for technical reasons—a small child receiving an adult kidney that resulted in kinking of the arterial inflow. In the same 500 cases, no kidney grafts have been lost from wound infection. The 1-year actuarial cadaver graft survival rate at the Albany Medical Center using the triple drug therapy is 84% at 1 year in 102 consecutive cadaveric transplants if patients dying (myocardial infarction, insulin overdose) with normal renal function are excluded.

ETHICS IN TRANSPLANTATION

The success of clinical transplantation depends completely upon public trust, both from the point of view of the indications for transplantation and, most importantly, in the ability to obtain organs for transplantation. Dialysis is an acceptable method of treating chronic ESRD. For patients to abandon an adequate form of therapy and undertake a major operative procedure, they must be confident that the clinical discipline of transplantation is conducted in an ethical fashion and, in particular, that informed consent is thorough and honest.

Donor procurement has created several ethical issues, and the shortage of organs places enormous pressure on the ethical standards of the procurement system. The medical criteria for brain death must always be strictly followed. The public must have total confidence that the interests of the donor are in no way compromised by his or her willingness to consider donating organs for transplantation. On this issue, there can be no compromise and no hesitation in severely reprimanding and punishing any proven violation of the concept of brain death. The use of living donors is generating increasing concern in the field of clinical transplantation. No major operative procedure, including that of live donor organ donation, can be conducted without morbidity and, occasionally, a death. There must be fully informed consent to the living donor and assurance that there are no familial pressures being exerted on the potential donor. Similarly, there must be no financial remunerations to the donor in excess of reasonable expenses.

The successful application of the concept of donor-specific transfusions to mismatched familial donors has initiated an interest in living-nonrelated donors for transplantation. This has created the possibility of the sale of organs by persons desirous of financial gain in exchange for a kidney. The sale of organs involves many ethical issues, but the process is to be condemned and is currently against recent legislation passed by the federal government. However, the use of living-nonrelated donors may be acceptable in specific circumstances, particularly in cases in which there is a strong and confirmed emotional relationship between the potential donor and the recipient. Such a situation might be husband and wife or two very close friends who may be dependent upon each other. Careful monitoring of the use of living-nonrelated donors must be conducted to ensure that there is no abuse with such donors.

REFERENCES

1. Alexandre GP, Squifflet JP, DeBruyere M et al: Splenectomy as a prerequisite for successful human ABO-incompatible renal transplantation. Transplant Proc 17:138, 1985

2. Belzer FO, Glass NR, Miller DT et al: Should the advisability of live donor renal transplantation be reappraised? Dialysis Transplant 13:26, 1984

3. Berthoux FE, Genin C, Guerin C et al: Influences of duration of dialysis on cadaver kidney graft survival in a one-center prospective analysis. Transplant Proc 17:2799, 1985

4. Borel JF, Feurer C, Magnee C et al: Effects of the new anti-lymphocytic peptide Cyclosporin A in animals. Immunology 32:1017, 1977

5. Campos H, Kreis HA, Rioux P et al: Azathioprine withdrawal in renal transplant recipients. Transplantation 38:29, 1984

6. Cerilli J, Anderson GW, Evans WE et al: Renal transplantation in patients with urinary tract abnormalities. Surgery 79:248, 1978

7. Cerilli J, Brasile L, Galouzis T et al: The vascular endothelial cell antigen system. Transplantation 39:286, 1985

8. Cerilli J, Holliday JE, Wilson CB et al: The clinical significance of the one hour biopsy in renal transplantation. Transplantation 26:291, 1978

9. Cerilli J, Jones L: A reappraisal of the role of splenectomy in children receiving renal allografts. Surgery 82:510, 1977

10. Delmonico FL, Fuller A, Cosimi AB et al: New approaches to donor crossmatching and successful transplantation of highly sensitized patients. Transplantation 36:629, 1983

11. Evans DB, Calne RY: Renal transplantation in patients with carcinoma. Br Med J 4:134, 1974

12. Filo RS, Dickson LG, Suba EA et al: Immunologic injury induced by ex vivo perfusion of canine renal allografts. Surgery 76:88, 1974

13. Fish JC, Flye MW, Williams A et al: Inability of thoracic duct drainage to prevent hyperacute rejection. Transplantation 36:134, 1983

14. Hall BM, Duggin GG, Philips J et al: Increased expression of HLA-Dr antigens on renal tubular cells in renal transplants: Relevance to the rejection response. Lancet 2:247, 1984

15. Jordan ML, Novick AC, Geisinger M et al: Imaging of the transplant kidney with nuclear magnetic resonance. Transplant Proc 17:32, 1985

16. Kauffman HM, Swanson MK, McGregor WR et al: Splenectomy in renal transplantation. Surg Gynecol Obstet 139:33, 1974

17. Krakauer H, Spees EK, Vaughn WK et al: Assessment of prognostic factors and projection of outcomes in renal transplantation. Transplantation 36:372, 1983

18. Kramer P, Broyer M, Brunner FP et al: Combined report on regular dialysis and transplantation in Europe, XII, 1981. Proc Eur Dial Transplant Assoc 19:4, 1982

19. LeFor WM, Tardif GN, Niblack GD et al: Use of seopf regional crossmatch trays to share kidneys for sensitized patients. Transplantation 40:637, 1985

20. Lobo PI, Rudolf LE, Krieger JN: Wound infections in renal transplant recipients—A complication of urinary tract infections during allograft malfunction. Surgery 92:491, 1982

21. Margreiter R, Fuchs D, Hauser A et al: Neopteria as a new biochemical marker for diagnosis of allograft rejection. Transplantation 36:650, 1983

22. Matas AJ, Simmons RL, Kjellstrand CM et al: When should the third renal transplant rejection episode be treated? Ann Surg 186:104, 1977

23. Moore SB, Sterioff S, Pierides AM et al: Transfusion-induced alloimmunization in patients awaiting renal allografts. Vox Sang 47:354, 1984

24. Morris PJ, French ME, Dunnill MS et al: A controlled trial of cyclosporine in renal transplantation with conversion to azathioprine and prednisolone after three months. Transplantation 36:273, 1983

25. Morrow CE, Sutherland DER, Fryd DS et al: Renal allograft survival in patients with positive B cell crossmatch to their donor. Ann Surg 199:75, 1984

26. Opelz G: Correlation of HLA matching with kidney graft survival in patients with or without cyclosporine treatment. Transplantation 40:240, 1985

27. Raftery MJ, Lang CJ, Schwar G et al: Prevention of sensitization resulting from third-party transfusion. Transplant Proc 17:2499, 1985

28. Rao KV, Rose JK: Incidence, histological pattern, and clinical outcome of rejection episodes occurring in the late post-transplant period. Transplantation 40:631, 1985

29. Ross WB, Roberts D, Griffin PJ et al: Lancet 330, 1986

30. Sanfilippo F, Vaughn WK, Spees EK: The association of pretransplant native nephrectomy with decreased renal allograft rejection. Transplantation 37:256, 1984

31. Sanfilippo F, Vaughn WK, Spees EK et al: Benefits of HLA-A and HLA-B matching on graft and patient outcome after cadaveric-donor renal transplantation. N Engl J Med 311:358, 1984

32. Shneidman RJ, Pulliam JP, Barry JM: Clean intermittent self-catheterization in renal transplant recipients. Transplantation 38:312, 1984

32a. Sollinger HW, Kalayoglu M, Belzer FO: Use of the donor specific transfusion protocol in living unrelated donor–recipient combinations (abstr). American Surgical Association, April 1986, p 39

33. Spees EK, Vaughn WK, McDonald JC et al: Why do secondary cadaveric renal transplants succeed? Results of SEOP Foundation Prospective Study 1977–1982. J Urol 129:484, 1983

34. Spees EK, Light JA, Smith EJ et al: Transplantation in patients with a history of renal cell carcinoma: Long-term results and clinical considerations. Surgery 91:282, 1982

35. Sutherland DE, Fryd DS, So SKS et al: Long-term effect of splenectomy versus no splenectomy in renal transplant patients. Transplantation 38:619, 1984

36. Taube DH, Cameron JS, Ogg CS et al: Renal transplantation after removal and prevention of resynthesis of HLA antibodies. Lancet 1:824, 1984

37. Terasaki PI, Perdue ST, Sasaki N et al: Improving success rates of kidney transplantation. JAMA 250:1065, 1983

38. Terasaki PI, Toyotome A, Mickey MR et al: Patient, graft, and functional survival rates: An overview. In Terasaki PI (ed): Clinical Kidney Transplants 1985, p 1. Los Angeles, UCLA Tissue Typing Laboratory, 1985

39. Terness P, Opelz G: Suppression of antibody response to transfusions in rats by preconditioning with antibody-coated cells. Transplantation 40:389, 1985

40. Turnipseed WD, Cerilli J: An immunologic study of renal allograft rejection using the direct macrophage inhibition test. Transplantation 20:414, 1975

CHAPTER 25

The Role of Immune Evaluation in Transplantation

Ronald H. Kerman   Barry D. Kahan

To circumvent untoward loss to hyperacute or accelerated allograft rejection, it is necessary to include immunologic considerations when determining a patient's appropriateness for transplantation.

Testing for recipient/anti-donor reactivity should include (1) matching recipient and donor for ABO antigens; (2) matching recipient and donor for HLA-A, -B and -DR antigens; and (3) assessing for the presence of recipient/anti-donor complement–dependent and/or lymphocyte–dependent antibodies as well as lymphocyte-mediated cytotoxicity and, in the case of living-related donor pretransplantation, performance of a mixed lymphocyte culture (MLC). The clinical significance of the results must be weighed against the immunosuppressive therapy.

Nonspecific immune considerations may be more relevant than the histocompatibility factors in assessing graft outcome. The extent that the preoperative immune responder status and/or blood transfusion history can influence graft outcome is also related to whether patients receive azathioprine or cyclosporine therapy.

Post-transplant, both donor-specific and nonspecific parameters may be used to define the emerging alloimmune dynamics of the graft. Even though they are not prognostic or diagnostic of rejection, nonspecific parameters appear to be more informative than donor-specific assays. In addition to evaluation of peripheral blood immune vectors, intragraft immune vector analysis by either needle biopsy or fine-needle aspiration cytology has proved to be beneficial.

Finally, postoperative assessment of recipient accommodation (by assessing altered immune response status and changing host/anti-donor alloresponsiveness) may allow discrimination of recipient hyporesponsiveness. Delineation of postoperative recipient hyporesponders could allow for individualization of postoperative medications. Therefore, routine immune monitoring may be therapeutically appropriate.

THE ALLOGRAFT RESPONSE

The most common cause of allograft loss is immune destruction resulting from a complex process of humoral and/or cellular mechanisms acting alone or in concert with one another.[6,9,110] The concept of immune monitoring evolved from the notion that the immune vectors responsible for graft destruction and loss could be identified and evaluated.[14,54,78,103] The allograft response follows activation of helper T cells by Class II major histocompatibility complex (MHC) antigens, such as HLA-DR, that stimulate the release of a macrophage stimulant resulting in the formation of receptors for insulin, transferrin, interleukin 1 (IL-1), and interleukin 2 (IL-2). Cytotoxic T-lymphocytes, stimulated by Class I HLA antigens (HLA-A, -B, and -C) develop IL-2 receptors. Subsequently, stimulated macrophages and other accessory cells release IL-1, which stimulates the release of IL-2. IL-2 interacts with specific IL-2 receptors expressed on activated helper and cytotoxic T cells. This interaction stimulates both the initiation of DNA synthesis and clonal proliferation of IL-2 receptor–bearing cells. IL-2 also causes release of gamma-interferon as well as release of B cell growth factor, which stimulates the proliferation of antigen-activated B cells. Allograft destruction and rejection results from the cytodestructive effects caused by antibody-activated macrophages and cytotoxic T cells.[74]

IMMUNE REJECTION

Several types of rejection have been defined clinically following the allograft response.[76] Hyperacute rejection occurs in the first 24 hours after transplantation and is always antibody mediated. It is seen in a recipient presensitized against donor histocompatibility or the transplant-relevant ABO antigens. Accelerated rejection occurs in the first 5 days and is considered to be the equivalent of a second set reaction in the experimental animal. This type of rejection may be mediated by cells and/or antibody. Acute rejection usually occurs in the first few weeks and is a primary immune response of host versus graft, primarily mediated by T cells. Finally, chronic rejection occurs at any time later following transplantation and is associated with an insidious decline in renal function, accompanied by typical vascular changes in the graft that are primarily due to humoral rejection mechanisms but may also result from low-grade cellular attack.

PRETRANSPLANT IMMUNE CONSIDERATIONS

Preoperative immune evaluation, therefore, needs to test for recipient anti-donor reactivity (to avoid hyperacute and accelerated rejection) as well as recipient-nonspecific immunocompetence (to delineate immunologically high-risk recipients who are likely to lose their allografts in the early postoperative period).[48,55,57,58,82] Pretransplant immune considerations include (1) matching donor and recipient for ABO antigens (because most persons have natural antibodies to these antigens and transplantation across a major ABO mismatch produces vigorous hyperacute rejection); (2) matching donor and recipient for HLA-A, -B, -C and -DR antigens; (3) testing for recipient anti-donor presensitization; (4) assessing recipient nonspecific immunocompetence; and (5) quantitating pretransplant blood transfusions.

One must keep in mind that the clinical relevance of pretransplant immune considerations almost certainly relates to the postoperative immunosuppressive regimen used. Azathioprine (Aza) and prednisone (Pred) have been the backbone of immunosuppression in renal transplantation for 20 years, however, with allograft and patient survival results reflective of the impact (on this regimen) of HLA incompatibilities, lack of blood transfusions, and recipients' strong immune responder status.[48,58,82] The use of cyclosporine (CsA) and Pred as immunosuppression in renal transplantation has altered the impact of these considerations, as a result most probably of CsA interfering with the activation sequence of lymphocytes and more effectively blocking humoral and cellular effector mechanisms that participate in rejection.[48,55,58,66,74]

Histcompatibility

The allograft recipient's response to graft antigens is the most crucial response in determining the fate of the transplant. It is generally accepted that the HLA antigens of the human 6th chromosome are the major histocompatibilty antigens in humans, including HLA-A, -B, -C, -DR, -DP, and -DQ.[3] Matching completely for HLA-A, -B, and -DR antigens has been shown to be influential on the outcome of kidney graft survival.[86] The roles of other molecules encoded in the HLA system, such as HLA-DP and HLA-DQ, in determining graft outcome have not been fully analyzed. The influence of the HLA complex on graft outcome is most evident in transplants from living-related donors. Because of the close linkage of the genes in the complex, they are inherited as a block. In transplants between HLA-identical siblings, graft survival is better than 90%, whereas if only 1 haplotype is shared, graft survival is 70% when Aza–Pred is used. Because of the polymorphism of the HLA loci, the chances of completely matching graft HLA antigens between unrelated persons is extremely low. The role of matching in cadaver (CAD) transplantation has had a more uncertain relationship than that in living-related donors (LRD). Although controversy has raged for many years, there is now a consensus of opinion that well-matched recipients/donors for HLA-A and -B antigens result in a 10% to 15% improved graft survival in cadaver recipients treated with Aza–Pred. This is also true when matching for the HLA-DR antigens.[82] In our studies, well-matched Aza–Pred patients (<2A, B, and 0–1 DR mismatches) compared with poorly matched recipients (>2A, B, and 2DR mismatches) had significantly better graft survival of 73% versus 38% ($p < 0.02$), thus confirming the advantage in matching for HLA in Aza–Pred recipients. Initial studies of CsA-treated recipients failed to confirm this same advantage; however, more recent data allow for the correlation of HLA-B and -DR matching with improved renal function (nadir and 30-day serum creatinine) as well as HLA-A matching associated with reduced rejection episodes in CsA-treated recipients.[47,48] Recent international multicenter analysis, however, tends to support the concept that matching for HLA improves graft survival, even in CsA-treated recipients.[86]

In addition to affecting CAD recipient outcome, analysis of our HLA-identical recipients also confirms a benefit of CsA therapy to this group.[27] The 3- to 5-year graft survival for CsA-treated HLA-identical recipients was significantly better when compared with comparable Aza–Pred recipients, 96% versus 76% ($p < 0.02$). Moreover, there were fewer rejection episodes per patient and fewer graft losses owing to rejection.

Donor-Specific Presensitization

Prior exposure to transplantation antigens can lead to sensitization, which results in the development of cytotoxic antibodies or sensitized T cells against HLA antigens. Antibody sensitization to HLA antigens can be detected by screening for these cytotoxic antibodies. Between 30% and 90% of patients on dialysis develop lymphocytotoxic antibodies as a result of blood transfusions, pregnancies, a previous failed graft or viral infections.[118] A renal transplant performed in the presence of a positive visual lymphocytotoxic crossmatch usually resulted in hyperacute or accelerated rejection.[69,90,125] Therefore, the performance of a crossmatch test before transplantation was considered mandatory, and it was accepted dogma that transplantation was contraindicated in the presence of a positive crossmatch. However, recent analysis of the various components of the crossmatch test (visual assessment of a standard complement-dependent antibody [CDA], generated microlymphocytotoxicity assay) has better defined the relevance of the target cells used and the temperature at which immunoglobulins are reactive.[117] Antibodies detected in the standard visually assessed crossmatch could be directed against HLA-A, -B, and -C antigens (T cells), HLA-DR antigens (B cells), and autoreactive antigens. Therefore, a positive standard crossmatch could reflect antibody reactivity to donor T or B cells or to an autologous antigen. In a retrospective study, Ettenger and associates[22] found that successful transplantation could be achieved with a positive crossmatch if the antibodies reacted only with the B and not the T cells of the donor. At the same time, there were reports that if a positive crossmatch against the donor's unseparated lymphocytes was due to an antibody that also reacted with the patient's own lymphocytes (autoantibody), a successful transplant could result.[17]

Detection of host presensitization by standard visual assessment (dye exclusion) of the microlymphocytotoxicity assay may be too insensitive to detect minimal reactivity, and it may not measure other immune vectors, such as lymphocyte-dependent antibody (LDA, non-complement-dependent antibody that may be reactive in antibody-dependent cell cytotoxicity graft destruction) or lymphocyte-mediated T cell cytotoxicity (LMC) by chromium-release (^{51}Cr-release) assays.[31,33,55,64,65] There are, in fact, several reports of the benefit of detecting anti-donor LDA and/or LMC in the presence of a negative standard visual crossmatch.[31,33,55,64,65,67,110] Our own studies suggest that when Aza–Pred patients present with a negative visual crossmatch but positive ^{51}Cr-release assay, the majority of grafts were lost.[55,64,65,67] However, in the presence of CsA–Pred therapy, comparable patients enjoyed successful allograft survival.[55] In addition to the ^{51}Cr-release assays, indirect immunofluorescence may be a sensitive and practical assay to detect antibody bound to cell surface antigens. Garovoy and colleagues[32] reported that automated cytofluorography could be used to detect antibodies selective for B cells or T cells, even when potentiated crossmatches (antiglobulin) failed to detect them. Although sensitivity is improved with the use of the flow cytometry methodology, it remains to be proved whether the weakly bound cell surface antibodies detected in this manner play a role in allograft rejection or graft loss.[67]

As stated earlier, formation of antibodies to HLA antigens can occur following transfusions, viral illness, pregnancies, and previously failed allografts. Patients with a high percentage of reactive antibody (PRA) to HLA antigens in their sera (highly sensitized patients) are difficult to crossmatch negatively against a potential donor allograft. These patients are passed over when considering recipients for transplantation. As discussed previously, sera displaying a positive crossmatch may not be deleterious to the graft outcome (depending upon the antibody specificity). Cardella and colleagues[7] took this concept even further when they questioned the validity of not transplanting a patient whose historic serum sample was positive but whose current serum sample was negative in a donor crossmatch. This group reported successful graft outcome in these patients. Other reports soon followed with similar results.[77,96,100] Since CsA-treated patients with a positive ^{51}Cr-release assay crossmatch had good graft survival, we questioned whether patients whose historic serum displayed positive donor crossmatches could be successfully transplanted using CsA–Pred. Our results showed that primary allograft recipients (but not retransplant recipients) whose historic but not current serum displayed a positive donor crossmatch could be successfully transplanted.[55]

It has been well recognized that lymphocytes

do not present the only relevant antigens in transplantation. There have been reports concerning the detection of antibodies to vascular endothelium or peripheral blood monocytes that are distinct from HLA-A, -B, -C, and -DR antibodies. These antibodies can be detected by immunofluorescence and are reactive with either monocyte antigens or vascular endothelium.[4,8,11] These antibodies have been associated with early graft loss in HLA-identical donor–recipient transplants.[4,8,11]

Finally, the use of well-matched LRD for renal transplantation has been associated with excellent allograft survival and diminished recipient morbidity and mortality when using Aza–Pred immunosuppression.[82] HLA-identical LRD transplants generally enjoy a smooth postoperative course with excellent prospects for long-term graft function. However, this is not true for all HLA-nonidentical LRD recipients. A clear difference in allograft survival is seen for haploidentical donor–recipient pairs displaying marked recipient lymphocyte stimulation in mixed lymphocyte culture (MLC) reactions. One-year graft survival is 57% when donor-specific MLC stimulation is greater than 6.5, compared with 81% ($p < 0.01$) when the MLC is nonstimulatory.[63] Therefore, the MLC stimulatory reaction reflects a high-risk immune parameter found in the majority (60%–80%) of potential LRD.[26] One approach to improving this clinical problem was to treat the recipients with deliberate donor blood transfusions. If the recipient did not display antibody development toward donor alloantigens, transplantation was carried out resulting in a 90% 1-year graft survival. The disadvantage of this approach has been that 30% of the potential recipients become sensitized to their prospective donors, as evidenced by the formation of anti-donor T and B cell antibodies.[53,97] A second approach at improving graft survival in these immunologically high-risk patients was to treat them with CsA–Pred postoperatively. Flechner and co-workers[26] reported that haploidentical LRD recipients, with donors who caused proliferative MLC responses, enjoyed a graft survival of 92% at 1 year. No patients were preoperatively dropped from receiving a transplant because of sensitization (as in the donor-specific blood transfusion protocol). Therefore, CsA–Pred therapy offers a viable alternative to these high-risk recipients.

Assessment of Nonspecific Immune Competence

Of the factors other than histocompatibility that influence the outcome of allograft survival, the recipient's immunocompetence may be the most relevant. The concept that a given host may have a genetically inherited capacity for immune responsiveness toward specific antigens (strong responder compared to weak or nonresponder) was first demonstrated in animal models.[124] Moreover, clinical studies also support this concept of a system of immune response genes being operative in humans. Data from cancer patients show a correlation between pretreatment immunocompetence and prognosis. Patients with strong pretherapy immunocompetence have good prognosis, whereas those with weak immunocompetence, have a poor prognosis.[43] This concept is relevant to transplantation in that some patients may display a strong and vigorous alloantigen responsiveness, whereas others display a weak responsiveness. This display of a pretransplant strong immune responsiveness can be useful in delineating immunologically high-risk recipients (as in haploidentical LRD recipients with highly proliferative donor MLC reactions). Similarly, it also allowed for discrimination of weak immune responders. Pretransplant knowledge of immune responder status could influence the choice of posttransplant immunosuppression.[25,26,48,59,118]

Since the original reports of Opelz and associates,[88] it has been conventionally accepted that responder or nonresponder status was related to whether a person developed lymphocytotoxic antibodies following a blood transfusion, wherein nonresponders tended to retain their histoincompatible grafts. Since this report, many have delineated immune competence by assessing cellular immune responsiveness, including tests of primary and delayed cutaneous hypersensitivity, T cell enumeration by rosettes or T cell subsets, and spontaneous, mitogen, or alloantigen in vitro lymphocyte responsiveness.[14,54,79,109] There is, in fact, ample evidence to support the concept that renal failure alters cell-mediated immunity, including reduced capacity to elicit delayed cutaneous hypersensitivity to either microbial skin test antigens or dinitrochlorobenzene (DNCB), reduction in T cells, and altered T cell subset ratios as well as poor mitogen and alloantigen (MLC) responsiveness.[14,44,48,54,58,63,78,108]

Patient pretransplant nonspecific immune responsiveness has been correlated with graft survival in many studies. Most chronic renal failure patients on maintenance dialysis tend to have absolute lymphopenia; furthermore, when assessing pretransplant microbial skin test responses, many have reduced responses, whereas only a minority of patients are totally anergic, and these patients do not seem to have significantly better graft survival rates than positive reactors.[8] In contrast to the un-revealing nature of assessing secondary cutaneous hypersensitivity, Rolley and colleagues[95] reported that primary in vivo sensitization to DNCB was informative regarding graft survival. Patients who were anergic to DNCB displayed better allograft survival rates than those who were DNCB-reactive (78% vs. 29%). Moreover, a small subgroup of patients who demonstrated a rapid irritant response displayed an even poorer 1-year graft survival rate of 20%. Although some transplant centers have confirmed that delayed hypersensitivity skin response to DNCB in humans is negatively correlated with graft survival, some investigators have observed that this may be associated with pretransplant blood transfusions.[8,95,122]

The peripheral blood lymphocytes of many patients awaiting transplant display a diminished blastogenic response to mitogens.[119] A very low preoperative response has been correlated with good subsequent graft survival in some, but not all, studies.[107,116,119] Measurement of spontaneous blastogenesis was more informative than mitogen-induced blastogenesis. Patients with weak spontaneous blastogenesis had a graft survival rate of 76% versus 41% ($p < 0.01$) for patients with strong blastogenesis.[9]

The overall nonspecific status of T cell–mediated immunity in chronic renal failure patients can be assessed by enumeration of two T cell populations (total T and active T cells) based on their ability to bind sheep red blood cells in a rosette configuration as well as T cell subsets (enumerated by using murine monoclonal antibodies and flow cytometry).[57,61,65,133] Active T cells are recognized as a subpopulation of the total T cell population with immune surveillance properties that more closely reflect cell-mediated immunity.[57,61,62,65,133] The total T cell response has been variable in its correlation to graft survival; however, low numbers of active T cells correlated with good graft survival, whereas high numbers of active T cells were associated with a poor prognosis.[58,62,63]

In our transplant center studies, we have chosen to put together a battery of pretransplant nonspecific immune assays, including total T, active T, T-helper (T_H), T-suppressor (T_S) cell enumerations, spontaneous blastogenesis (SB), mitogen responsiveness, panel mixed lymphocyte culture (PMLC), and cutaneous hypersensitivity skin testing of both primary (DNCB) and recall (microbial) antigens.[58,62,63] We found that the majority (about 75%) of end-stage renal disease (ESRD) patients present as strong immune responders, whereas about 25%

present as weak immune responders. Strong responder immune parameters that correlated with poor allograft survival included active T cells ($> 36.5\%$), spontaneous blastogenesis ($> 14,600$ cpm), panel MLC (> 10.0 SI), and $T_H:T_S$ ratios (> 1.0).[62,63] Strong responder patients treated with Aza–Pred displayed only a 39% 1-year cadaveric graft survival rate, compared with 72% in weak responders.[58,62] Immune responder status was not influenced by HLA matching, and both strong and weak groups had comparable donor–recipient matching for HLA-A, -B, -C, and -DR antigens. The pretransplant delineation of a patient's immune response status, irrespective of HLA matching, will be important when considering individualization of post-transplant immunosuppressive management. For example, in our own series, strong immune responder recipients of cadaveric donor allografts, when treated with anti-thymocyte globulin (ATG), displayed graft survival rates comparable to weak immune responders treated with Aza–Pred.[58] Moreover, the impact of identifiable pretransplant strong immune indices on graft survival was diminished in allograft recipients treated with CsA–Pred.[25–27, 48,55,58]

Blood Transfusion

Until the early 1970s, no one was particularly concerned when a dialysis patient received a transfusion because his or her hematocrit had dropped below a certain level. In 1971, Terasaki and associates[112] reported poor graft survival for patients with lymphocytotoxic antibodies. Since production of these antibodies could result from transfusions, physicians became more cautious about transfusing their patients. This increased the number of untransfused allograft recipients and was paralleled by a gradual decrease in overall graft success rates. Nontransfused recipients had a poor graft success rate compared with all transfused recipients (whether they developed antibodies to HLA antigens, responders, or not at all).[87,88] Since then, most transplant centers have confirmed the beneficial effect of transfusions on graft survival in all transplant recipient categories, including cadaveric, haplo- and HLA-identical LRDs.[85] Little has been decided about the optimal number of transfusions, the proper blood component producing the prolonged graft success, the time that should elapse between the last transfusion and transplantation, or the appropriate age of the transfused blood. Moreover, little is known about the mechanism affecting prolongation of allograft survival, although preferred mechanisms include selection of responders, induction of tolerance to HLA alloantigens, production of antibodies favorable to allograft survival, and/or altered host immunologic responsiveness as a result of the increased T or non-T suppressor/regulator cells.[29,52,67,68,85,91,104,120,123]

Results of studies from our transplant center suggest that pretransplant transfusions improved Aza–Pred allograft survival.[68] Moreover, transfusions probably play a central role in establishing immune responder status. Patients receiving more than five transfusions were (1) weak immune responders with a T_H:T_S ratio of less than 1.0, with high nonspecific adherent mononuclear cell suppressor activity.[68] Patients receiving fewer than five transfusions tended to be strong immune responders, with T_H:T_S ratios greater than 1.0, with little or no nonspecific suppressor cell activity.[68] This reduced immune responder status in highly transfused recipients was comparable to that seen by Watson and co-workers[122] for DNCB reactivity and Fischer and colleagues[29] for T cell cytotoxicity and MLC activity. Serial evaluation of immunocompetence could afford a dynamic measure of the immune response following blood transfusion conditioning. Since we had previously demonstrated the reproducibility of serial immune evaluation tests in untransfused hemodialysis patients, we then serially followed transfused patients.[59,67,68] We demonstrated a conversion from a strong to a weak immune responder status following repeated third-party blood transfusions. We also demonstrated that a portion of this effect was due to the emergence of a nonspecific suppressor cell detected by the capacity to inhibit a third-party mixed leukocyte response (MLR).[1,67,68]

The aforementioned transfusion effect benefiting graft survival and affecting immune responder status was studied in patients treated with Aza–Pred. Clearly, pretransplant blood transfusion conditioning improves survival. However, with the improvement in overall graft survival following the use of CsA–Pred, will transfusion conditioning still be necessary and effective? Our own early results suggested a benefit to transfusions in CsA–Pred-treated recipients of cadaveric donor allografts.[46] However, CsA-Pred–treated HLA-identical and haploidentical LRD transplant recipients could be transplanted successfully without transfusions.[25–27] A more recent review of the transfusion data showed only a correlation of transfused cadaveric donor allograft recipients with lower nadir and 1-month serum creatinines compared with recipients with few or no transfusions but not survival.[47] Opelz,[86] reported that CsA-treated recipients enjoyed improved graft survival compared with conventionally treated re-

cipients. However, he continues to report a benefit to transfusions even with CsA-treated recipients.[86] Not all current reports agree with this interpretation. Lundgren and associates[75] recently reported that whereas matching for HLA-DR reduced the frequency of rejection episodes, neither matching for HLA or pretransplant blood transfusions influenced patient and graft survival rates.

POST-TRANSPLANT IMMUNE EVALUATION

The diagnosis of renal allograft rejection is usually based on the appearance of signs, symptoms, and/or altered biochemical indices suggesting reduced renal function. These presenting manifestations may be later-occurring events in an immunologically mediated rejection process. Early diagnosis of graft injury could permit immediate therapeutic intervention with resolution of the injury process and prolonged allograft survival.[16] Immunologic monitoring of the allograft recipient may allow detection of immune events leading to renal allograft damage.[109] Moreover, serial evaluation of immune parameters, coupled with clinical indices, could allow for discrimination between drug-induced toxicity and/or immune injury leading to graft loss. In a similar manner to pretransplant considerations, assays used for immunologic monitoring after transplantation include those that reflect specific host anti-donor immunity and those that reflect nonspecific host immunologic activation.

Most monitoring techniques use peripheral blood elements to study the cells or serum of the recipient at intervals following transplantation. Use of peripheral blood vectors is open to criticism because (1) in vitro assays may not reflect in vivo conditions of rejection; (2) the assays are labor intensive, and the frequency of testing must reflect the rapid change in immune status; (3) a single test is unlikely to reflect all rejections, because they are mediated by antibody and/or cellular mechanisms directed against a variety of antigens (kidney parenchyma, lymphocytes, and endothelial cells); (4) assays may be in vitro positive at a time of clinical stability; and (5) intragraft sequestration of immune vectors may render them inaccessible for peripheral monitoring.

There is little doubt, however, that by the regular use of combined sensitive monitoring techniques, immune changes can be detected in advance of functional graft deterioration.[14,54,78,108] There is no doubt that monitoring techniques have made a significant contribution to better understanding the mechanisms of transplant rejection. The use of monoclonal antibodies to identify lymphocyte populations and the development of the fine-needle aspiration biopsy procedure have rekindled interest in immune monitoring.

DONOR-SPECIFIC REACTIVITY

Using donor lymphocytes as targets, investigators have looked for humoral and cellular host antidonor post-transplant reactivity. Attempts to correlate the results of donor-specific reactivity with rejection have been varied; therefore, clinically significant interpretations of the results have been controversial. Early studies suggested that a positive complement-dependent antibody (CDA) test (against ^{51}Cr-labeled targets) correlated with rejection and/or compromised prognosis.[9,30,111,119] Development of these antibodies often occurred prior to biochemical evidence of allograft compromise. CDA antibodies could be directed against T or B cell targets or both. Donor-specific anti–B cell antibodies have been associated with rejection and were often found in serum collected during acute or sustained rejection periods but not during quiescent periods.[30] Many investigators were unable to confirm these types of results and, moreover, did not detect CDA until after the allograft was removed.[119] Additionally, the CDA often remained positive long after the rejection episode was resolved.[111] The lymphocyte-dependent antibody (LDA) assay is very sensitive to antibodies directed against cell surface antigens. LDA was associated with acute rejections but not with stable quiescent periods.[30] Other reports suggested that rather than being associated with graft destruction, LDA was associated with immunologic enhancement.[70,111] Since antibody mechanisms of rejection are not amenable to high-dose steroid therapy, more attention was directed toward treatable cellular events. Stiller and co-workers[111] reported that the T cell cytotoxicity (LMC) test was the best predictor of rejection episodes. The LMC test, however, is subject to numerous technical variables, including incubation time, target pretreatment, and assessment of ^{51}Cr release. Nevertheless, the LMC appeared to display fewer false-negative results than the CDA.[70,111] Finally, alloantigen-stimulated lymphocyte proliferation could be serially monitored by donor-specific MLC.[44,111] A fall in circulating MLC cells was attributed to entrapment of immunoreactive cells in the graft or alteration of cell kinetics. Miller and associates[79] reported that the primed lymphocyte test (PLT, measuring secondary or memory MLC responsiveness) was more diagnostic of rejection; however, the length of time to perform the assay (3 days) precluded clinical application.

In our own studies of donor-specific post-transplant reactivity in Aza–Pred patients, we tested for CDA, LDA, and T cell cytotoxic activity versus[51] Cr-labeled target cells. We were unable to significantly correlate positive assays with rejection.[63] Moreover, CsA–Pred-treated recipients experienced significantly fewer rejection episodes per patient (1.8 vs. 0.67; $p < 0.05$) as well as fewer donor-specific immune events per patient (56 vs. 19; $p < 0.01$).[50] Although donor-specific assays should theoretically provide the most discriminating information about the mechanism of allograft rejection, these tests, at present, are of limited utility.

NONSPECIFIC IMMUNE REACTIVITY

Serial evaluations of nonspecific immune parameters following transplantation appear to be superior to host-specific anti-donor assays in delineating immune events leading to rejection. They are easier to perform, require less blood volume, and do not require donor targets (a limitation of donor-specific assays). Moreover, nonspecific assays do not depend upon identification of the specific donor antigens or of immunologic mechanisms.

Nonspecific immune assays that have been reported include (1) T cell enumeration by sheep red blood cell rosetting techniques (total T and active T-RFC), (2) T cell subsets (T_H and T_S), (3) spontaneous blastogenesis (SB, measuring leukocyte cellular metabolic activity), and (4) lymphokine production.

Several investigators have reported on the measurement of T-RFC for the purpose of predicting allograft rejection. Measurement of the total T-RFC did not correlate with clinical immune status.[60,63] Total T cells were of no value in controlling Aza–Pred or ATG allograft therapy or predicting rejections.[2,102,113] Whereas some investigators found increased total T cells in rejection, others could not confirm this.[2,5,61,113] The total T cell (by RFC) has also been found to be variable in several other studies.[61,132,133] In contradistinction, the active T cell does correlate closely with patient clinical immune status[62,63,116,132,133] and has been reported to decrease in conjunction with clinical alloimmune events and rejection.[60,61] Serial monitoring of active T cell kinetics were discriminative of immunity and rejection in both Aza–Pred and CsA–Pred recipients.[57,60]

Methods for estimating T cells by rosetting techniques have now been superceded by the use of monoclonal antibodies to identify lymphocyte subpopulations. Since the description of the two major functional subsets of T cells in humans, defined by antisera against heterologous membrane determinants, both the development and production of monoclonal antibodies against these and other determinants have progressed rapidly.[23,71,94] Cells with T_H and T_S phenotypes have antagonistic roles in amplifying or suppressing T cell proliferative and cytotoxic responses and antibody production by B cells. These subsets show proliferative and cytotoxic responses to autologous viral-infected cells and alloantigens. T_H cell responses are restricted by HLA Class II antigens on the stimulator or target cells, whereas T_S cells are restricted by HLA Class I antigens.

With the introduction of these monoclonal antibodies, studies were initiated to evaluate the significance of subset dynamics in disease. Subsets have proved useful in characterizing lymphoid neoplasms and changes in autoimmunity and suggesting mechanisms of other diseases.[71] Initial reports in renal allograft recipients suggested a correlation between subset activity and clinical events.[16,20] Acute cellular rejection is usually associated with a normal or high T_H:T_S ratio. Increases in the T_H:T_S ratio just before or at the onset were correlated to kidney allograft rejection in Aza–Pred as well as CsA–Pred-treated recipients.[16,20,21,57] However, all reports do not agree with these findings.[10,121] Analysis of our center's data revealed a correlation between increased T_H:T_S ratio and rejection, with a reversal following clinical resolution.[57] Moreover, the T_H:T_S ratio data may help in discriminating between CsA-induced nephrotoxicity or immune injury. Increased T_H:T_S ratios significantly correlated with the occurrence of rejection ($p < 0.001$). In the absence of rejection, if a patient is nephrotoxic, no significant increased ratios occur ($p > 0.5$). However, since increased ratios occur with rejection, when nephrotoxicity occurs concomitantly with rejection, increased T_H:T_S ratios are uninformative ($p > 0.5$). A low T_H:T_S ratio (<1.0) was rarely associated with rejection; however, a clear correlation has been shown between low post-transplant T_H:T_S ratios and viral infections (especially cytomegalovirus, CMV), sometimes concomitant with glomerulopathy.[15]

The use of currently available T_H and T_S reagents has not afforded a reliable predictive index of rejection, but rather confirms the ongoing immune events. Monoclonal antibodies produced to other cell types or different lymphocyte activation receptors may allow for better correlation of lymphocyte subsets and clinical events. For example, increases in circulating monocyte levels have been reported to precede rejection levels.[10,106] More recently, newer monoclonals delineating the inducer of the T_H cells and the inducer of the T_S cells have been reported.[81] With the use of two-color fluorescence and double-labeling methodologies, more discriminative studies will be performed to help dissect the role of these subsets in renal allotransplantation.

Although not a measure of peripheral blood activity, there has been interest in monitoring posttransplant urinary sediments. The occurrence of lymphocyturia or a sharp increase in pre-existing lymphocyturia has been found in relation to immunologic rejection.[28,51,72,83,98] In many cases, it was noted that significant lymphocyturia preceded other clinical signs of rejection and the increase in serum creatinine.[28,51,72,83] Moreover, in a recent report, the results appeared comparable to those achieved with fine-needle aspiration cytology.[98] Monitoring urinary sediments in the early posttransplant period could prove useful in the early detection of interstitial rejection and in differentiating interstitial rejection from other causes of renal function impairment (CsA toxicity).

In addition to enumeration of cell types, nonspecific immune responsiveness of allograft recipients can also be evaluated by following leukocyte metabolic activity (spontaneous or mitogen induced) as measured by ^{3}H-thymidine incorporation reflecting increased DNA or RNA synthesis. Most studies report increased spontaneous blastogenic activity prior to or concomitant with clinical signs of rejection.[42,57,60,62,119] Increased spontaneous blastogenesis will occur during infections as well as subclinical immune rejection episodes.[60,79] Enhanced lymphoproliferation following PHA stimulation was variably reported to correlate with rejection.[107,114] Serial measurement of the nonspecific immune parameters, including active T cells, spontaneous blastogenesis, and T cell subsets, can provide enormous information about postoperative immunity.[49,57] No single parameter alone significantly reflected immune events; however, T_H:T_S cells and spontaneous blastogenesis, active T and spontaneous blastogenesis, or active T and T_H:T_S cells in combinations all significantly reflected immune activation and correlated with rejection episodes.

Complex events associated with the allograft response lead to an activation of specific effector T-lymphocytes mediating allograft rejection.* Lymphokines, including IL-1, IL-2, and gamma-inter-

---

* References 6, 9, 14, 54, 74, 78, 108, and 110

feron are produced and released following T cell alloantigen activation.[84] A future direction of immune monitoring research will be to assess the clinical relevance of quantitating levels of these and other lymphokines. A recent report assessed the ability of peripheral blood lymphocytes (PBL) from CsA-treated allograft recipients to generate IL-2 after mitogenic stimulation.[134] PBL from CsA-treated allograft recipients displayed reduced generation of IL-2 compared with that of normal persons, dialysis patients, or Aza–Pred-treated recipients. PBL were also studied from patients just prior to initiation of high-dose steroid therapy for rejection. All but one patient (6 of 7) undergoing clinically diagnosed rejection displayed high uninhibited generation of IL-2; however, following steroid boluses, the patients displayed profound inhibition of their IL-2 generation.

Activated T cell release of gamma-interferon leads to activation of a macrophage enzyme, guanosine trisphospate–specific cyclohydrolase, which results in increased synthesis and release of neopterin.[101,126] Neopterin is a small, stable molecule that easily penetrates tissue compartments and can represent a marker molecule reflecting endogenous production of interferon. Increased neopterin blood levels have been reported prior to serum creatine changes antecedent to rejection.[101] Moreover, severe unrelenting rejection episodes were characterized by continually high neopterin levels. Further investigations of both IL-2 and interferon, or neopterins, may lead to a more quantitative understanding of the early immune activation events preceding rejection.

Finally, nonspecific humoral factors, including immunoglobulin production, complement levels, and circulating antigen–antibody complexes, have been evaluated during the post-transplant period.[44,105] In summary, these nonspecific humoral factors have failed to provide reliable diagnostic indicators for the onset of rejection.

IN SITU ALLOGRAFT MONITORING

The diagnosis of renal allograft rejection poses several differential diagnostic problems, most of which focus on the graft. As discussed previously, attempts to evaluate intragraft events from either peripheral blood or urine specimens constitute the majority of efforts to immunologically monitor rejection. Few of these methods have yielded sensitive or specific indices to predict rejection. Analysis of the peripheral blood represents the pathway that not only the immune cells and humoral elements take toward the graft but also the infectious agents as well as all the drugs being administered to the patient. Therefore, it is not unexpected to be faced with difficulty and imprecision in delineating events from the periphery. In contrast, the needle biopsy remains the only reliable method for assessing intragraft cellular and humoral insults leading to rejection. Since active T cells and MLC-responsive T cells mediating rejection may be sequestered in the graft, recent monitoring studies examined cells infiltrating renal transplants.[60,61,79] A decreased $T_H:T_S$ ratio was observed in the kidney biopsy specimen compared with that in the peripheral blood in both Aza–Pred and CsA–Pred patients experiencing rejection.[37,93,99] This reduced intragraft $T_H:T_S$ ratio was due primarily to a predominant graft infiltration of T cytotoxic cell phenotype.[99] However, needle biopsies are seldom done repeatedly primarily because of the risk of bleeding. A less traumatic approach for intragraft assessment was the development and refinement of transplant aspiration cytology using the technique of fine-needle aspiration biopsy.

Fine-needle aspiration biopsy (FNAB) is performed by obtaining one or more 10 µl to 50 µl aspiration specimens from the allograft, as well as a peripheral blood specimen from the fingertip. Both specimens are processed onto microscope slides by using a cytocentrifuge and are then stained with standard reagents such as May Grunwald-Giemsa (MGG) stain, or immunochemical techniques can be used with monoclonal antibodies to obtain a more precise identification of the infiltrating cells.[38,129] This procedure can be performed daily without danger to the graft or graft recipient and represents a useful tool for serial sampling of the renal parenchyma and infiltrating cells.[89] A total corrected cell increment is obtained by subtracting the peripheral blood cells contaminating the graft FNAB as determined from the peripheral smear obtained from the fingertip stick. The degree of inflammation in the FNAB and a concomitantly obtained needle biopsy have been closely correlated.[40] In addition to graft parenchymal cells, the following inflammatory cell types are found either by MGG staining or monoclonal antibodies: lymphoblasts (representing primarily T-blasts), plasmablasts (representing primarily B-blasts), plasma cells at different levels of maturation, activated lymphocytes, large granular lymphocytes, which include natural killer (NK) cell population and tissue macrophages in varying stages of morphologic maturation.[39] In most cases, acute rejection follows a distinct pattern characterized by the number of monocytes and lymphocytes increasing in the graft, with lymphoblasts, plasmablasts, and plasma cells being seen in situ.

Usually, the inflammation subsides, and the blast cells disappear from the graft at the same time that the antirejection therapy is given. However, if the number of blast cells increases, still more lymphocytes are seen in the FNAB, and a rapid maturation of monocytes into macrophages occurs; this, then, is the hallmark of prolonged and irreversible rejection. Analysis of the FNAB with monoclonal antibodies revealed decreased $T_H:T_S$ ratio owing primarily to an increasing T cytotoxic cell population present at rejection.[121,130]

Future studies of infiltrating cells delineated by aspiration cytology will be concerned with associating the functional capacity of these cells and the incidence of rejection. This approach will then address the question of whether those cells observed cytologically are mediating rejection.

ALLOGRAFT ACCOMMODATION AND LONG-TERM SURVIVAL

In Aza–Pred-treated allograft recipients, rejections and graft losses usually occur in the first 3 to 6 months post-transplantation. In CsA–Pred-treated allograft recipients, the majority (77%) of rejections occur by post-transplant Day 60, and the overall graft loss is 12%.[49] This implies that the patients who have successfully kept their allografts have done so because of the successful immunosuppression mediated by Aza–Pred or CsA–Pred and/or the establishment of an immunoregulatory mechanism potentiating recipient anti-donor hyporesponsiveness. Immunologic monitoring techniques have until now reported on features associated with poor prognosis, that is, positive LMC or CDA post-transplant assays. However, negative anti-donor test results do not guarantee that the graft will be permanently accepted. Immune monitoring then could detect the emergence of recipient hyporesponsiveness associated with prolonged allograft survival.

Transplantation tolerance or recipient hyporesponsiveness may result from various mechanisms, including serum blocking factors and/or immunoregulatory cells.[19,35,80,103,120,123] It was originally believed that MLC inhibition by recipient serum indicated the presence of enhancing antibodies that could account for prolonged survival; however, these same antibodies were identified in the serum of rejecting patients as well as during quiescence.[128] Anti-idiotypic antibodies conferring immunologic hyporesponsiveness were suggested to account for the capacity of sera from polytransfused patients to block a donor-specific MLC.[103] Unfortunately, putative anti-idiotypic reagents as well as B cold, anti-

Fab, and anti-Fc antibodies never offered consistent or reliable indices of unresponsiveness.[49]

On the other hand, patient unresponsiveness owing to cellular mechanisms appears to be more consistent and demonstrative of immunoregulatory processes. Suppressor cells have been reported in several experimental models of transplantation that are highly different from one another.[18,41,131] Several groups have reported on suppressor cell systems in transplant recipients that accounted for the observed recipient unresponsiveness.[12,13,24,36,73,92,115,127] Most of these reports dealt with emerging unresponsiveness delineated by cell-mediated lymphocytotoxicity (CML) and/or MLC hyporesponsiveness in patients who were long-term Aza–Pred-immunosuppressed recipients. The mechanism of action of CsA has been attributed to inhibition of helper T cells and the possible amplification of suppressor T cells.[45] Therefore, in CsA-treated allograft recipients, suppressor cell mechanisms should be present and could account for the dramatically improved graft survival possibly owing to recipient hyporesponsiveness.

Our center recently reviewed the post-transplant in vitro immune responses in CsA–Pred-treated recipients of a primary cadaveric renal allograft.[56] This report is unique in that we focused on the early post-transplant period to delineate immunoregulatory mechanisms. A dramatic shift in $T_H:T_S$ ratio occurs in the early post-transplant period (first 0–30 days) following CsA therapy, wherein 68% of the recipients present with a weak $T_H:T_S$ ratio of less than 1.0 compared with 19% of the recipients who present with this ratio before transplantation. Analysis of these patients at 1 year revealed that those with an early $T_H:T_S$ ratio of less than 1.0 displayed a lower serum creatinine of 1.8 ± 0.7 mg/dl compared with 2.3 ± 0.6 mg/dl for patients with early post-transplant $T_H:T_S$ ratios greater than 1.0 in spite of equal mean CsA doses and serum levels. Fewer rejection episodes and/or immune graft losses occurred in patients with early $T_H:T_S$ ratios of less than 1.0 compared with patients with $T_H:T_S$ ratios greater than 1.0. Interestingly, patients with early post-transplant $T_H:T_S$ ratios of less than 1.0 displayed a donor hyporesponsiveness (as assessed by MLC testing), with a post-transplant to pretransplant donor MLC ratio of 0.58 ± 0.21 compared with 1.1 ± 0.32 ($p < 0.05$) for recipients with $T_H:T_S$ ratios greater than 1.0.

Patients were also tested for the presence of suppressor cells (inhibition of donor-specific or third-party MLC), including both T cell and monocyte suppressors. In the early post-transplant period (0.5–14 months), we observed that 46% of the recipients tested displayed T suppressor cell activity.

Moreover, 75% of those tested also displayed adherent monocyte nonspecific suppressor activity. Patients displaying any suppressor cell activity (T cell or monocyte) experienced fewer rejection episodes than did patients without suppressor activity. Finally, the benefit from matching donor and recipient HLA-DR antigens for improved survival may result from the lack of MHC Class-II (HLA-DR) antigen presentation to stimulate helper T cells and the preferential presentation of MHC Class I antigens to stimulate suppressor cells.[34] In our study, a significant association between matching donor and recipient for HLA-DR antigens and recipient display of T suppressor cell activity was observed.

Since we had evidence for immunoregulatory mechanisms in CsA-treated cadaveric recipients, we also evaluated living-related transplant recipients. Using changes in MLC response to either donor or third-party MLC assays, Flechner and associates[25] were able to delineate haploidentical living-related hyporesponding recipients. When pre- and post-transplant MLC responses to either donor or third-party MLCs were evaluated, several patients displayed a donor MLC hyporesponsiveness, but not, however, in third-party MLC. These hyporesponsive recipients had their drug immunosuppression individualized, and, subsequently, steroid therapy was withdrawn. These patients displayed both decreased MLC and CML reactivity.[24]

Postoperative immune monitoring may, therefore, be quite useful to delineate immune activity in the early post-transplant period, that is, altered $T_H:T_S$ ratios from pre- to post-transplantation. Moreover, these data can suggest which patients may have converted to weak immune responders displaying donor hyporesponsiveness, who, if followed for 12 months without changed immune responsiveness, could be candidates for individualized immunosuppression and CsA-monodrug therapy.[25]

SUMMARY

Immunologic monitoring remains one of the most controversial areas in clinical transplantation. The projected promise of following donor-specific immunity to delineate immune reactivity, rejection, and/or allograft loss has not resulted in any of these assays being predictive or diagnostic. However, use of nonspecific immune assays to follow altered immune response status has been more successful in revealing the changing immune picture. Understanding of altered post-transplant responsiveness (decreased $T_H:T_S$ ratios and displayed donor and panel MLC hyporesponsiveness) may allow for individualization of post-transplant immunosuppression.

REFERENCES

1. Agostino GJ, Kahan BD, Kerman RH: Suppression of mixed leucocyte culture using leucocytes from normal individuals, uremic patients and allograft recipients. Transplantation 34:367–371, 1982
2. Bishop G, Cosimi AB, Voynow NK et al: Effect of immunosuppressive therapy for renal allografts on the number of circulating sheep red blood cell rosetting assays. Transplantation 20:123–129, 1975
3. Bodmer WF: The HLA system. In Albert ED, Bauer MD, Mayr WR (eds): Histocompatibility Testing 1984, pg 11. New York, Springer-Verlag, 1985
4. Brasile L, Rodman E, Sheild C et al: The association of antivascular endothelial cell antibody with hyperacute rejection. Surgery 99:637–640, 1986
5. Buckingham JM, Ritts RE, Woods JE et al: An assessment of cell mediated immunity in acute allograft rejection in man. Mayo Clin Proc 52:101–105, 1977
6. Bush GJ, Schamberg JF, Moretz RC et al: Four patterns of human renal allograft rejection. Transplant Proc 9:37–42, 1977
7. Cardella CJ, Nicholson MJ, Falk JA et al: Successful renal transplantation in patients with T-cell reactivity to donor. Lancet 2:1240–1243, 1982
8. Carpenter CB, Milford EL: Immunological monitoring before transplantation. In Morris PJ (ed): Kidney Transplantation, 2nd ed, pp 181–197. New York, Grune & Stratton, 1984
9. Carpenter CB, Morris PJ: Immunologic monitoring of transplant patients. Transplant Proc 11:1153–1157, 1979
10. Carter NP, Cullen PR, Thompson JF et al: Monitoring lymphocyte subpopulations in renal allograft recipients. Transplant Proc 15:1157–1159, 1983
11. Cerilli J: Current trends in histocompatibility: Clinical relevance versus laboratory phenomena. Am J Surg 151:716–721, 1986
12. Charpentier B, Bach AM, Lang PH et al: Expression of OKT8 antigen and Fc receptors by suppressor cells mediating specific unresponsiveness between recipient and donor in renal allograft tolerant patients. Transplantation 35:495–501, 1983
13. Charpentier B, Lang P, Martin B et al: Evidence for a suppressor cell system in human kidney allograft tolerance. Transplant Proc 13:90–93, 1981
14. Cohen B, Van Rood JJ, Stiller CR (eds): Second International Symposium on Immunological Moni-

toring of The Transplant Recipient. Transplant Proc 13(3): 1981

15. Colvin RB, Cosimi AB, Burton RC et al: Circulating T-cell subsets in 72 human renal allograft recipients: The OKT4/OKT8 cell ratio correlates with reversibility of graft injury and glomerulopathy. Transplant Proc 15:116–119, 1983

16. Cosimi AB, Colvin RB, Burton RC et al: Use of monoclonal antibodies to T-cell subsets for immunologic monitoring and treatment in recipients of renal allografts. New Engl J Med 305:308–314, 1981

17. Cross DE, Greiner R, Whittier FC: Importance of the autocontrol crossmatch in human renal transplantation. Transplantation 21:307–311, 1976

18. Dorsch S, Roser B: Recirculating suppressor T cells in transplantation tolerance. J Exp Med 145, 1144–1156, 1977

19. Dutton RW: Suppressor T cells. Transplant Rev 26:39–64, 1975

20. Ellis TM, Lee HM, Mohanakumar T: Alterations in human regulatory T lymphocyte subpopulations after renal allografting. J Immunol 127:2199–2203, 1981

21. Ellis TM, Mohanakumar T, Muakkassa W et al: Influence of immunosuppressive therapy and blood transfusions on human T-cell subpopulations. Transplant Proc 15:1173–1175, 1983

22. Ettenger RB, Terasaki PI, Opelz G et al: Successful renal allografts across a positive crossmatch for donor B lymphocyte alloantigens. Lancet 2:56–58, 1976

23. Evans RL, Lazarus H, Penta AC et al: Two functionally distinct subpopulations of human T cells that collaborate in the generation of cytotoxic cells responsible for cell mediated lympholysis. J Immunol 120:1423–1428, 1978

24. Flechner SM, Barker CJ, Kerman RH: Donor-specific MLC hyporesponsiveness is associated with decreased in vitro cytotoxicity in cyclosporine treated renal allograft recipients. Transplant Proc 18:750–753, 1986

25. Flechner SM, Kerman RH, Van Buren CT et al: The use of cyclosporine in living-related renal transplantation: Donor-specific hyporesponsiveness and steroid withdrawal. Transplantation 38:685–691, 1984

26. Flechner SM, Kerman RH, Van Buren CT et al: Successful transplantation of cyclosporine treated haploidentical living related renal recipients without blood transfusions. Transplantation 37:73–76, 1984

27. Flechner SM, Kerman RH, Van Buren CT et al: Does cyclosporine improve the results of HLA-identical renal transplantation? Transplant Proc 19:1485–1488, 1987

28. Firlit JP, Dajani F, First MR et al: Value of urine cytology in renal transplantation. Transplantation 26:133–138, 1978

29. Fischer E, Lenhard V, Seifert P et al: Blood transfusion–induced suppression of cellular immunity in man. Human Immunol 3:187–194, 1980

30. Garovoy MR, Carpenter CB: Immunologic monitoring for renal transplantation. In Rose NR, Friedman

H (eds): Manual of Clinical Immunology, pp 1042–1048. Washington DC, American Society for Microbiology, 1980

31. Garovoy MR, Franco V, Zschaeck D et al: Direct lymphocyte mediated cytotoxicity as an assay of presensitization. Lancet 1:573–576, 1973

32. Garovoy MR, Rheinschmidt MA, Bigos M et al: Flow cytometry analysis: A high technology crossmatch technique facilitating transplantation. Transplant Proc 15:1939–1944, 1983

33. Gauliunas P, Suthanthiran M, Busch G et al: Role of humoral presensitization in human renal transplant rejection. Kidney Int 17:638–646, 1980

34. Goeken N: Preferential activation of human suppressor cells in vitro by heat-modified stimulators. Transplant Proc 15:780–783, 1983

35. Gershon RK: A disquisition on suppressor T cells. Transplant Rev 26:170–184, 1975

36. Goulmy E, Persijn G, Blokland E et al: Cell-mediated lympholysis studies in renal allograft recipients. Transplantation 31:210–217, 1981

37. Hancock WW, Thompson NM, Atkins RC: Composition of interstitial cellular infiltrate identified by monoclonal antibodies in renal biopsies of rejecting human renal allografts. Transplantation 35:458–463, 1983

38. Hayry P, Von Willebrand E: Transplant aspiration cytology. Transplantation 38:7–12, 1984

39. Hayry P, Von Willebrand E: Aspiration cytology in monitoring human allografts. In Williams GM, Burdick JF, Solez K (eds): Kidney Transplant Rejection: Diagnosis and Treatment, pp 247–262. New York, Marcel Dekker, 1986

40. Hayry P, Von Willebrand E, Ahonen J et al: Monitoring of organ allograft rejection by transplant aspiration cytology. Ann Clin Res 13:264–287, 1981

41. Hendry WS, Tilney NL, Baldwin WM: Transfer of specific unresponsiveness to organ allografts by thymocytes. J Exp Med 149:1042–1054, 1979

42. Hersh EM, Butler WT, Rossen RD et al: In-vitro studies of the human response to organ allografts. J Immunol 107:571–578, 1971

43. Hersh EM, Mavligit GM, Gutterman JU: Immunological evaluation of malignant disease. JAMA 236:1739–1742, 1976

44. Kahan BD: Immunologic monitoring: Utility and limitations. Transplant Proc 17:1537–1545, 1985

45. Kahan BD: Individualization of cyclosporine therapy using pharmacokinetic and pharmacodynamic parameters. Transplantation 40:457–476, 1985

46. Kahan BD, Kerman RH, Wideman CA et al: Impact of cyclosporine on renal transplant practice at The University of Texas Medical School at Houston. Am J Kidney Dis 5:288–295, 1985

47. Kahan BD, Mickey R, Flechner SM et al: Multivariant analysis of risk factors impacting on immediate and eventual cadaver allograft survival in cyclosporine-treated recipients. Transplantation 43:65–78, 1987

48. Kahan BD, Van Buren C, Flechner S et al: Cyclospo-

rine immunosuppression mitigates immunologic risk factors in renal allotransplantation. Transplant Proc 15:2469–2478, 1983

49. Kahan BD, Van Buren CT, Flechner SM et al: Allograft rejection in renal allograft recipients under cyclosporine–prednisone immunosuppressive therapy. In Williams GM, Burdick JF, Solez K (eds): Kidney Transplant Rejection: Diagnosis and Treatment, pp 411–422. New York, Marcel Dekker, 1986

50. Kahan BD, Van Buren CT, Lin SN et al: Immunopharmacological monitoring of Cyclosporin A-treated recipients of cadaveric kidney allografts. Transplantation 34:36–45, 1982

51. Kauffman HM, Clark RF, Magee JH: Lymphocytes in urine as an aid in the early detection of renal homograft rejection. Surg. Gynecol Obstet 119:25–29, 1964

52. Keown PA, Descamps B: Improved renal allograft survival after blood transfusions: A non-specific erythrocyte-mediated immunoregulatory process? Lancet 1:20–22, 1979

53. Kerman RH: Effect of blood transfusions on renal allograft survival: Immunological considerations. Am J Kidney Dis 2:125–127, 1981

54. Kerman RH (ed): Fourth International Symposium on Immunological Monitoring of the Transplant Patient. Transplant Proc 16(6): 1984

55. Kerman RH, Flechner SM, Van Buren CT et al: Successful transplantation of cyclosporine treated allograft recipients with serologically positive historical, but negative preoperative, donor crossmatches. Transplantation 40:615–619, 1985

56. Kerman RH, Flechner SM, Van Buren CT et al: Immunoregulatory mechanisms in cyclosporine-treated renal allograft recipients. Transplantation 43:205–210, 1987

57. Kerman RH, Flechner SM, Van Buren CT et al: Immunologic monitoring of renal allograft recipients treated with cyclosporine. Transplant Proc 15:2302–2305, 1983

58. Kerman RH, Floyd M, Van Buren CT et al: Improved allograft survival of strong immune responder high risk recipients with adjuvant ATG therapy. Transplantation 30:450–454, 1980

59. Kerman RH, Floyd M, Van Buren CT et al: Serial measurement of nonspecific immune parameters of chronically hemodialyzed renal failure patients. J Clin Immunol 1:163–168, 1981

60. Kerman RH, Floyd M, Van Buren C et al: Correlation of nonspecific immune monitoring with rejection or impaired function of renal allografts. Transplantation 32:16–23, 1981

61. Kerman RH, Geis WP: Total and active T cell kinetics in renal allograft recipients. Surgery 79:398–407, 1976

62. Kerman RH, Ing TS, Hano JE et al: Prognostic significance of the active T-RFC in renal allograft survival. Surgery 82:607–612, 1977

63. Kerman RH, Kahan BD: Immunological evaluation of transplant rejection: Pre- and postoperative indices detecting immune responsiveness. Ann Clin Res 13:244–263, 1981

64. Kerman RH, Payne W, Van Buren CT et al: Detection of host presensitization to donor alloantigens utilizing a comprehensive immune crossmatch. Transplant Proc 15:1815–1816, 1983

65. Kerman R, Smith R, Ezdinli E et al: Unification and technical aspects of total T, active T and B lymphocyte rosette assays. Immunol Commun 5:685–694, 1976

66. Kerman RH, Van Buren CT, Flechner SM et al: Correlation of visual, ^{51}Cr-release and flow cytometry crossmatch results to graft survival. Transplant Proc 16:1430–1433, 1984

67. Kerman RH, Van Buren CT, Payne W et al: Influence of blood transfusions on immune responsiveness. Transplant Proc 14:335–337, 1982

68. Kerman RH, Van Buren CT, Payne W et al: The influence of pretransplant blood transfusions from random donors on immune parameters affecting cadaveric allograft survival. Transplantation 36:50–54, 1983

69. Kissmeyer-Nielsen F, Olson S, Petersen VP et al: Hyperacute rejection in kidney allografts associated with pre-existing humoral antibodies against donor cells. Lancet 1:662–665, 1966

70. Kovithavongs T, Schlaut J, Pazderka V et al: Post transplant immunology monitoring with special consideration of technique and interpretation of LMC. Transplant Proc 10:547–551, 1978

71. Krensky AM, Lanier LL, Engleman EG: Lymphocyte subsets and surface molecules in man. Clin Immunol Rev 4:95–138, 1985

72. Krishna GG, Fellner SK: Lymphocyturia: An important diagnostic and prognostic marker in allograft rejection. Am J Nephrol 2:185–191, 1982

73. Liburd EM, Pazderka V, Kovithavongs T et al: Evidence for suppressor cells and reduced CML induction by the donor in transplant recipients. Transplant Proc 10:557–561, 1978

74. Loertscher R, Abbud-Filho M, Strom TB: Cyclosporine in renal transplantation. In Robinson RR (ed): Nephrology, Vol II, pp 1661–1673. New York, Springer-Verlag, 1984

75. Lundgren G, Albrechtsen D, Flatmark A et al: HLA-matching and pretransplant blood transfusions in cadaveric renal transplantation: A changing picture with cyclosporine. Lancet 2:66–69, 1986

76. Mason DW, Morris PJ: Effector mechanisms in allograft rejection. Ann Rev Immunol 4:119–145, 1986

77. Matas AJ, Nehlsen-Cannarella S, Tellis VA et al: Successful kidney transplantation with current sera—negative/historical sera positive T cell crossmatch. Transplantation 37:111–112, 1984

78. Miller J (ed): Third International Symposium on Immunological Monitoring of The Transplant Patient. Transplant Proc 15(3): 1983

79. Miller J, Lifton J, Wilcox C: The use of second generation assays in pre and post transplant monitoring:

The primed or second-degree MLC. Transplant Proc 10:573–578, 1978

80. Miyajima T, Higuchi H, Kashiwabara H: Anti-idiotypic antibodies in patients with a functioning renal allograft. Nature 283:306–308, 1980

81. Morimoto C, Letvin NL, Distaso JA et al: The isolation and characterization of the human suppressor inducer T cell subset. J Immunol 134:1508–1515, 1985

82. Morris PJ: Renal transplantation: Current status. In Robinson RR (ed): Nephrology, Vol II, pp 1627–1643. New York, Springer-Verlag, 1984

83. Murphy GP, Williams PD, Merrin CE: Diagnostic value of lymphocyturia in renal allograft rejection in man. Urology 2:227–232, 1973

84. Murphy PA: The interleukins. In Williams GM, Burdick JF, Solez K (eds): Kidney Transplant Rejection: Diagnosis and Treatment, pp 55–74. New York, Marcel Dekker, 1986

85. Opelz G: Blood transfusions and renal transplantation. In Morris PJ (ed): Kidney Transplantation, 2nd ed, pp 323–334. New York, Grune & Stratton, 1984

86. Opelz G: Effect of HLA matching, blood transfusions and presensitization in cyclosporine-treated kidney transplant recipients. Transplant Proc 17:2179–2183, 1985

87. Opelz G, Mickey MR, Terasaki PI: Identification of unresponsive kidney transplant recipients. Lancet 1:868–871, 1972

88. Opelz G, Sengar DPS, Mickey MR et al: Effect of blood transfusions on subsequent kidney transplants. Transplant Proc 5:253–259, 1973

89. Pasternack A: Fine needle aspiration biopsy of human renal homografts. Lancet 2:82–84, 1968

90. Patel R, Terasaki PI: Significance of the positive crossmatch test in kidney transplantation. N Engl J Med 280:735–780, 1969

91. Persijn GG, Cohen B, Lansbregen O et al: Retrospective and prospective studies on the effect of blood transfusions in renal transplantation in the Netherlands. Transplantation 28:396–401, 1979

92. Pfeffer P, Thorsby E, Hirschberg H: Donor specific decreased cell mediated cytotoxicity in recipients of well functioning, one HLA haplotype-mismatched kidney allografts. Transplantation 35:156–160, 1983

93. Platt JL, Ferguson RM, Sibley RK et al: Renal interstitial cell populations in cyclosporine nephrotoxicity. Transplantation 36:343–345, 1986

94. Reinherz EL, Kung PC, Goldstein G et al: Separation of functional subsets of human T cells by monoclonal antibody. Proc Natl Acad Sci USA 76:4061–4065, 1979

95. Rolley RT, Wideman DG, Parks LC et al: Monitoring of responsiveness in dialysis-transplant patients by delayed cutaneous hypersensitivity. Transplant Proc 10:505–507, 1978

96. Rosenthal JT, Rabin B, Taylor RJ et al: Positive T-cell crossmatch with stored recipient sera in cadaveric renal transplantation. Transplantation 39:310–311, 1985

97. Salvatierra O, Vincenti F, Amend W et al: Four year experience with donor-specific blood transfusions. Transplant Proc 15:924–931, 1983

98. Sandoz FP, Bielmann D, Mihatsch M et al: Value of urinary sediment in diagnosis of interstitial rejection in renal transplants. Transplantation 41:343–348, 1986

99. Sanfilippo F, Kolbeck PC, Vaughn WK et al: Renal allograft cell infiltrates associated with irreversible rejection. Transplantation 40:679–685, 1985

100. Sanfilippo F, Vaughn WK, Spees EK et al: Cadaver renal transplantation ignoring peak reactive sera in patients with markedly decreasing pretransplant sensitization. Transplantation 38:119–124, 1984

101. Schafer AJ, Daniel V, Dreikorn K et al: Assessment of plasma neopterin in clinical kidney transplantation. Transplantation 41:454–459, 1986

102. Sengar DPS, Rashid A, Harris JE: Post transplant monitoring of renal allograft recipients for T, B and null lymphocyte subpopulations. Clin Exp Immunol 28:123–129, 1977

103. Singal DP, Joseph S: Role of blood transfusions on the induction of antibodies against recognition sites on T-lymphocytes in renal transplant patients. Human Immunol 4:93–108, 1982

104. Smith MD, Williams JD, Coles GA et al: The effect of blood transfusions on T suppressor cells in renal dialysis patients. Transplant Proc 13:181–183, 1981

105. Smith WJ: Monitoring components of the immune system. In Williams GM, Burdick JF, Solez K (eds): Kidney Transplant Rejection: Diagnosis and Treatment, pp 264–281. New York, Marcel Dekker, 1986

106. Smith WJ, Burdick JF, Williams GM: Fluorescent and light microscopic analysis of peripheral blood leucocytes from human renal allograft recipients. Transplant Proc 16:1546–1547, 1984

107. Stenzel KH, Rubin AL, Novogradsky A: Blastogenic response to mitogens: An approach to the study of cell-surface topography in lymphocytes from transplant recipients. Transplant Proc 10:589–591, 1978

108. Stiller CR, Dossettor JB, Sinclair NRS (eds): First International Symposium on Immunologic Monitoring of The Transplant Patient. Transplant Proc 10(2,3): 1978

109. Stiller CR, Keown PA: Immunologic monitoring: Current perspectives and clinical implications. Transplant Proc 13:1699–1711, 1981

110. Stiller CR, Sinclair NRS: Monitoring rejection. Transplant Proc 11:343–349, 1979

111. Stiller CR, Sinclair NRS, Abrahams S et al: Antidonor immune responses in prediction of transplant rejection. N Engl J Med 294:978–982, 1976

112. Terasaki PI, Mickey MR, Kriesler M: Presensitization and kidney transplant failures. Post Grad Med J 47:89–100, 1971

113. Thomas FT, Lee HM, Lower RR et al: Immunological monitoring as a guide to the management of transplant recipients. Surg Clin North Am 59:253–281, 1979

114. Thomas F, Mendez-Picon G, Thomas J et al: Effective

monitoring and modulation of recipient immune reactivity to prevent rejection in early post transplant period. Transplant Proc 10:537–541, 1978

115. Thomas J, Thomas F, Johns C et al: Consideration in immunological monitoring of long-term transplant recipients. Transplant Proc 10:569–572, 1978

116. Thomas F, Thomas J, Mendez G et al: Pretransplant immune monitoring of donor–recipient compatibility. Transplant Proc 10:429–432, 1978

117. Ting A: The lymphocytotoxic crossmatch test in clinical renal transplantation. Transplantation 35:403–407, 1983

118. Ting A, Dick HM: Transplantation in immunology. In Holborow EJ, Reeves WG (eds): Medicine 2nd ed, pp 577–587. New York, Academic Press, 1983

119. Ting A, Williams KA, Morris PJ: Transplantation: Immunological monitoring. Br Med Bull 34:263–270, 1978

120. Van Rood JJ, Balner H, Morris PJ: Blood transfusions and transplantation. Transplantation 26:275–279, 1978

121. Von Willebrand E: OKT4/OKT8 ratio in the blood and in the graft during episodes of human renal allograft rejection. Cell Immunol 77:196–201, 1983

122. Watson MA, Diamandopoulos AA, Briggs JD et al: Endogenous cell mediated immunity, blood transfusions and outcome of renal transplantation. Lancet 1:1323–1326, 1979

123. Werner-Favre C, Jeannet M, Harder F et al: Blood transfusions, cytotoxic antibodies and kidney graft survival. Transplantation 28:343–346, 1979

124. Williams RM, Benacerraf B: Genetic control of thymus derived cell function. J Exp Med 135:1279–1288, 1972

125. Williams GM, Hume D, Hudson RP et al: Hyperacute renal homograft rejection in man. N Engl J Med 279:611–618, 1968

126. Woloszczuk W, Troppmair J, Leiter E et al: Relationship of interferon-gamma and neopterin levels during stimulation with alloantigens in-vivo and in-vitro. Transplantation 41:716–718, 1986

127. Wonigeit K, Pichlmayr R: Post-transplant monitoring of donor specific T cell reactivity at the precursor cell level. Transplant Proc 10:563–567, 1978

128. Wood RFM: Immunological monitoring after transplantation. In Morris PJ (ed): Kidney Transplantation, 2nd ed, pp 383–406. New York, Grune & Stratton, 1984

129. Wood RFM, Bolton EM, Thompson JF et al: Monoclonal antibodies and fine needle aspiration cytology in detecting renal allograft rejection. Lancet 2:278, 1982

130. Wood RFM, Bolton EM, Thompson JF et al: Characterization of cellular infiltrates in renal allografts by fine needle aspiration cytology. A simple technique using double labeling with monoclonal antibodies. Transplant Proc 15:1847–1848, 1983

131. Wood ML, Monaco AP: Suppressor cells in specific unresponsiveness to skin allografts in ALS-treated marrow injected mice. Transplantation 29:196–200, 1980

132. Wybran J: The active T-rosette test: Its significance and use. In Quastel MR (ed): Cell Biology and Immunology of Leucocyte Function, pp 745. New York, Academic Press, 1979

133. Wybran J, Fudenberg HH: Thymus-derived rosette forming cells. N Engl J Med 288:1072–1073, 1973

134. Yoshimura N, Kahan RD: Pharmacodynamic assessment of the in-vivo cyclosporine effect on interleukin-2 production by lymphocytes in kidney transplant recipients. Transplantation 40:661–666, 1985

The Use and Interpretation of Biopsies in the Management of the Post-Transplant Patient

Richard K. Sibley   Dale C. Snover

Histopathologic assessment by way of tissue biopsy is the most reliable and accurate method available to determine the cause of dysfunction of a transplanted organ.

Foremost among the diagnoses involved in solid organ transplantation is that of allograft rejection. In general, rejection of allografted solid organs can be categorized as hyperacute, acute, and chronic. Hyperacute rejection, best documented in the kidney, is characterized pathologically by fibrin and platelet thrombi, polymorphonuclear infiltration, necrotizing arteritis, and eventual parenchymal destruction.

Acute rejection is characterized by a predominantly lymphocytic infiltrate, which is thought to represent an immunologic response against organ-specific target cells, and endothelialitis, the infiltration and attachment of lymphoid cells to the endothelium of arteries and veins.

Chronic rejection is an extension of the acute process with fibrosis and obliterative endarteritis and is irreversible. All forms of rejection involve to a major degree the vascular endothelial cells (VEC). Other causes of dysfunction that must be considered are those of an infectious, technical, or toxic nature, and recurrence of original disease.

Biopsy has proved to be valuable in assessing the efficacy of therapy for rejection, especially in the heart, liver, and kidney where it is possible to perform repeat biopsies. Use of biopsy will prevent overtreatment of suspected rejection while minimizing the chance of organ failure owing to chronic rejection.

Bone marrow transplantation (BMT) differs from solid organ transplantation in that rejection, as well as graft-versus-host disease (GVHD), is a process that differs clinically, pathologically, and pathogenetically; chronic GVHD is not considered a necessarily irreversible process. Hyperacute GVHD is not considered a necessarily irreversible process. Hyperacute GVHD is not a recognized phenomenon.

Acute GVHD primarily affects the skin, gastrointestinal tract, and liver. Chronic GVHD affects a much larger range of tissues, although skin and liver involvement are also common.

Biopsy may be considered the ultimate procedure in the assessment of transplant organ dysfunction. Clinical and laboratory features must be taken into account before an interpretation is rendered, especially with a complicated or difficult case where an unequivocal diagnosis is not possible. Although immunologic monitoring, radiologic studies, serum levels of cyclosporine, needle aspirates, and so on provide useful information, it is the biopsy that provides the most accurate diagnostic and prognostic information and allows the results of therapy to be adequately assessed. The biopsy not only can identify acute rejection but also can delineate cases of irreversible acute and/or chronic rejection, as well as other causes of graft dysfunction such as obstruction of ureters, bile and pancreatic ducts, vascular accidents, recurrent disease, and infectious complications. If the information obtained from a biopsy is to be useful, the biopsy must be obtained prior to the institution of therapy, and the information must rapidly be made available to the primary care physician. Serious complications of biopsy are extremely rare and should not be a consideration unless the patient has clotting abnormalities.

KIDNEY

In the immediate post-transplant period, the most likely cause of renal failure is ischemic tubular damage, but a vascular accident, ureteral obstruction, a urine leak, so-called pump perfusion injury, an adverse reaction to antilymphocyte globulin (ALG) or cyclosporine (CsA), and hyperacute rejection are possible etiologies. Following normalization of renal function, as many as 80% of patients will have at least one episode of elevated creatinine during the first 6 months post-transplantation.[28] Cyclosporine-nephrotoxicity (CsA-NT), acute rejection, infection, and recurrent disease are the usual causes. Late graft dysfunction is usually a sequela of multiple clinical rejection episodes or persistent subclinical low-grade rejection, which may result in either a slow but progressive loss of renal function or a sudden decline of function associated with severe hypertension. Recurrent disease, de novo glomerulonephritis, and chronic obstruction are additional lesions producing late renal failure.

The value of renal biopsy in preventing the overtreatment of putative acute rejection is difficult to prove. However, in three series, 40%[62,120] to 46%[76] of patients who underwent renal biopsy because of putative rejection were found not to have acute rejection, thus altering their management.

Serial fine-needle aspiration biopsy (FNAB) of the graft during the initial months post-transplantation is a sensitive technique in the identification of interstitial inflammatory infiltrates.[3,4,12,16,53] However, lymphoid infiltrates can be found in routine follow-up biopsies at any time post-transplant.[61,108] Some of the latter patients developed clinical signs of acute rejection from a few days to months later, whereas others do not.[61] Thus, treating an infiltrate found in FNAB without clinical signs of rejection may unnecessarily increase the chances of post-transplant infectious complications or lymphoproliferative disorders.

Acute Tubular Necrosis (ATN)

ATN is the major cause of renal failure in the immediate post-transplant period in cadaver transplantation. Cyclosporine may prolong the duration of post-transplant renal failure and thus increase the period of post-transplant dialysis.[71] This adverse ef-

fect has become less of a problem with modification of the immunosuppression regimen designed to prevent it.[13] A renal biopsy is usually not obtained in a patient with clinical post-transplantation ATN unless there has been no improvement in renal function by 2 to 3 weeks post-transplantation or if there is a rise in creatinine following partial resolution of the ATN. The biopsy taken at this time may show features of ATN alone or ATN with superimposed acute rejection. The histology of ischemic tubular damage is variable tubular ectasia with epithelial simplification and loss of brush border (Fig. 26-1); in some cases, coagulation necrosis with sloughing of epithelium into the tubular lumens, regenerative nuclear atypia, and mitoses are evident.[62,96] Interstitial abnormalities are minor, although there may be edema and scattered macrophages. Intratubular and interstitial oxalate crystals are often evident.

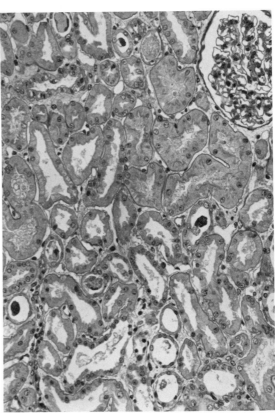

FIGURE 26-1. Acute tubular necrosis. A biopsy was performed on a 33-year-old man who received a cadaver kidney because the serum creatinine did not decrease below 2.8 mg/dl by Day 15 post-transplantation. The biopsy showed foci of tubular ectasia with attenuation of the epithelium but no interstitial inflammatory infiltrate characteristic of ischemic tubular damage (PAS-alcian blue × 190).

With prolonged ATN, more extensive edema, interstitial fibrosis, and tubular atrophy may also be present. These abnormalities can be mimicked or enhanced by acute ureteral obstruction or urinary fistula, septicemia, and drug nephrotoxicity secondary to CsA, amphotericin B, and the aminoglycoside antibiotics. Superimposed acute rejection is indicated by the findings of an interstitial lymphoid infiltrate with tubulitis and edema. Lymphoid infiltrates and tubulitis are not a component of ATN as many suggest.[108]

Mononuclear infiltrates can be found in biopsies in the early post-transplant period in asymptomatic patients. Some of these patients eventually developed clinical rejection, whereas others remained normal. Whether or not these infiltrates represent asymptomatic rejection is unknown.[61]

Hyperacute Rejection and Other Vascular Lesions

Hyperacute rejection occurs as a result of specific anti-donor antibodies to HLA, VEC, ABO antigens in the recipient serum and uniformly results in rapid destruction of the allograft. Hyperacute rejection is usually evident following the vascular anastomosis because of poor function and an abnormal color of the graft. The histologic features of hyperacute rejection are, initially, glomerular and arteriolar thrombosis followed by fibrinoid necrosis of arterioles and massive polymorphonuclear leukocyte exudation. ATN and cortical infarction are found 12 to 36 hours later.[96] If tissue is not examined until the entire graft is infarcted, separation of hyperacute rejection from other causes of renal infarction such as renal artery or venous thrombosis is usually impossible. Only a retrospective search for anti-donor antibodies may identify the etiology of the graft destruction.

There are a number of other causes of glomerular and vascular thrombosis. Thrombosis of glomerular capillaries, and, in some cases, large vessels, occurs (1) in association with recurrent hemolytic-uremic syndrome,[42] (2) as an adverse reaction to ALG,[62] (3) as a reaction to cold-reacting IgM antibodies to red blood cells and lymphocytes,[114] and (4) as an adverse reaction to CsA. There appears to be a higher frequency of large vessel thrombosis in CsA-immunosuppressed patients compared with conventional azathioprine–prednisone immunosuppression.[67] Glomerular thrombotic lesions have also occurred in perfusion-preserved kidneys,[18,56,110] perhaps on the basis of ischemic endothelial damage, and are associated with poor graft survival. Also, nonpolarizable particulate foreign material

may be found in glomeruli and interlobular arteries, associated with fibrin thrombosis and fibrinoid necrosis of the vessel walls. These lesions heal by recanalization or as a cellular proliferative endarteritis; segmental infarction of the graft and hypertension have occurred in several of these patients.

Acute Rejection

Acute rejection most commonly occurs during the first 6 months following transplantation but may occur at any time. Renal biopsy can be important in the diagnosis and management of acute rejection, as the histologic severity of rejection can be used to determine the optimal therapy for the patient—from a simple elevation of steroids to ALG therapy. An acutely or chronically irreversibly damaged kidney can be identified and the patient spared high-dose immunotherapy.[44,62,76,120]

Any structure of the kidney may be damaged in acute rejection. *Acute interstitial* rejection is characterized by focal to diffuse and mild to marked lymphoid and variable macrophage, polymorphonuclear leukocyte, eosinophil and plasma cell infiltrates, edema, hemorrhage, and tubular damage (Fig. 26-2). Lymphoid infiltration of tubular epithelium (tubulitis) is a consistent feature that is usually minor or lacking in chronic rejection, CsA-NT, and recurrent disease. Other tubular lesions include ectasia, epithelial attenuation, and necrosis. It is very important to note that *acute vascular* rejection is evident in most cases of acute rejection. The vascular damage ranges from subendothelial accumulation of lymphocytes (endothelialitis) (Fig. 26-3) in mild cases to necrotizing arteritis with fibrinoid necrosis of the media and thrombosis of the lumen in severe rejection. The latter features are associated with a poor prognosis.[44,62]

The glomeruli in acute rejection may be normal but, more commonly, contain varying numbers of lymphocytes and monocytes within capillary lumens with variable endothelial hypertrophy and hyperplasia.[2] In severe rejection, there may be fibrin thrombosis, necrosis, and infarction.

Immunofluorescent examination, in general, is unrewarding. Granular C3 may be found along tubular basement membranes, and mesangial granular IgM and subendothelial granular IgG and C3 with fibrin may be apparent. The vessels may contain IgM, C3, and fibrin as well as C1q and properdin. Examination of mononuclear cell subpopulations usually reveals an increased ratio of T8/T4 cells.[39–41,52,78] Variable numbers of macrophages are present, as are polymorphonuclear leukocytes, B

cipient disorder characterized by progressive ischemic loss of nephron mass secondary to vascular lesions. It is important to again note the dominance of damage to the vascular endothelium in this form of rejection. Variable tubular atrophy and interstitial fibrosis, and a patchy diffuse, usually intraperitubular capillary mononuclear cell infiltrate are often present. The intralobular and arcuate arteries show intimal fibrosis of variable severity (Fig. 26-4), and juxtaglomerular apparatus hyperplasia is often apparent.[44,62,96] Chronic transplant glomerulopathy may be present. The therapy of superimposed acute rejection may be effective only if the tubules are intact, that is, if moderate to diffuse tubular loss is not evident.

Juxtaglomerular apparatus hyperplasia with little or no tubular loss is found in some patients presenting with hypertension. If the biopsy contains

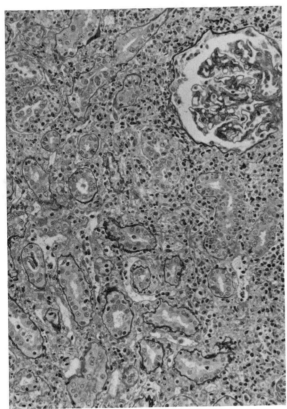

FIGURE 26-2. *Acute rejection. Six weeks post-transplantation, this patient presented with fever and a rising creatinine to 2.8 mg/dl. Biopsy showed an intense mononuclear cell infiltrate in the interstitium with prominent tubulitis and glomerulitis (PAS-alcian blue × 190).*

lymphocytes, and plasma cells. Most of the cells in vascular rejection are cytotoxic/suppressor (T8) lymphocytes and macrophages.

Some patients with biopsy-proven acute rejection do not appear to benefit from antirejection therapy, and repeat biopsy may be necessary to determine whether there is ongoing rejection.[62,96] *Treated rejection* is characterized by the near total absence of the inflammatory cell infiltrate with residual edema and tubular damage, which correlates with renal insufficiency. Blood vessels may show subendothelial foamy macrophages and fibrointimal proliferation, features of resolving acute vascular rejection.

Chronic Rejection

Chronic rejection may occur following an episode of severe acute rejection as early as the first few weeks post-transplantation, but, often, it is an in-

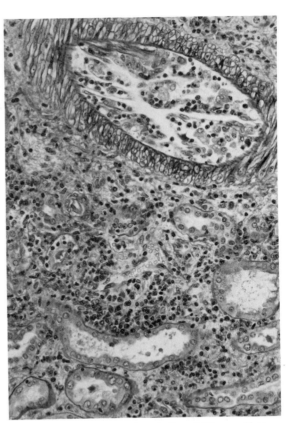

FIGURE 26-3. *Acute vascular rejection. A 24-year-old patient presented with fever and a creatinine rise from 1.1 mg/dl to 2.1 mg/dl. The biopsy demonstrated tubulointerstitial rejection and a prominent endovasculitis characterized by subendothelial mononuclear cell infiltration (PAS-alcian blue × 190).*

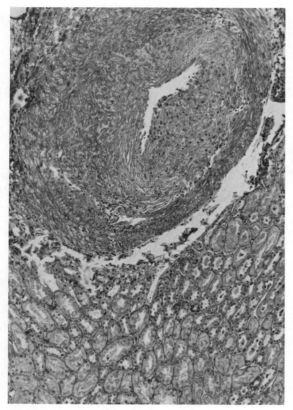

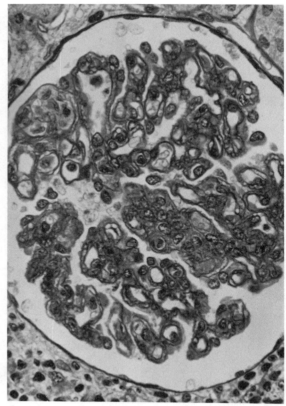

FIGURE 26-4.   *Chronic vascular rejection. This patient presented with hypertension 6 months post-transplantation. The biopsy demonstrated normal glomeruli, tubules, and interstitium as well as interlobular arteries, but the arcuate vessel demonstrated severe proliferative endarteritis as well as low-grade endovasculitis (PAS-alcian blue × 115).*

FIGURE 26-5.   *Chronic transplant glomerulopathy. A 3-year-old boy presented with severe hypertension 1 year post-transplantation. The biopsy showed mild chronic vascular rejection in addition to extensive multicontouring of the capillary walls with little mesangial proliferation or matrix increase (PAS-alcian blue × 480).*

normal intralobular or arcuate arteries and normal glomeruli, angiography is indicated, because the hypertension may be the result of nonimmune renal artery stenosis, which can be surgically corrected. *Chronic transplant glomerulopathy* (CTG) and chronic vascular rejection are, in many cases, caused by endovasculitis and perhaps low-grade humoral injury. The end result is endothelial damage with endothelial basal lamina replication, segmental mesangial interposition, and mild mesangial matrix and cell increase (Fig. 26-5). These features, including the ultrastructural features of electron-lucent finely flocculent subendothelial deposits in a widened subendothelial space help separate CTG from recurrent membranoproliferative glomerulonephritis.[15,45,63,96] Additional glomerular lesions of CTG include segmental sclerosis, global glomerular sclerosis, the formation of Kimmelstiel-Wilson nodules, and

capillary aneurysms.[96] Immunoflourescence may demonstrate subendothelial and mesangial granular deposits of IgM, IgG, C3, properdin, and fibrin, features that are not that different from a recurrent membranoproliferative glomerulonephritis.

Recurrent Disease

Almost any glomerular disease can recur in the transplanted kidney.[11,43,70] Some diseases, such as systemic lupus erythematosus (SLE),[1] recur infrequently, whereas in other diseases, such as dense intramembranous deposit disease,[11,23] recurrence is nearly universal. Recurrent dense intramembranous deposit disease (Fig. 26-6) is usually compatible with long-term graft survival but can be associated with rapid destruction of the graft.[23] Thus, the importance of donor selection becomes apparent. Be-

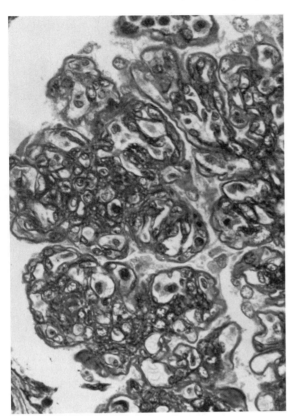

FIGURE 26-6.   *Recurrent disease. A 14-year-old boy underwent renal biopsy because of the development of a nephrotic syndrome 2 years post-transplantation. He had already lost one graft as a result of recurrent dense intramembranous deposit disease. This biopsy showed a membranoproliferative glomerulonephritis characterized by a lobular accentuation, prominent mesangial proliferation, and matrix increase and capillary double contours (PAS-alcian blue × 480).*

cause of the frequency of recurrent disease, it may be reasonable to use only cadaver donors for patients with (1) antiglomerular base membrane nephritis; (2) Alport syndrome, in which de novo antiglomerular base membrane nephritis rarely occurs; (3) membranoproliferative glomerulonephritis with subendothelial deposits; (4) hemolytic uremic syndrome (HUS)[42]; and (5) focal segmental glomerular sclerosis and hyalinosis with mesangial proliferation.[37a,59,112] It should be pointed out that cyclosporine has been associated with a de novo hemolytic uremic syndrome; thus, an immunosuppressive regimen lacking cyclosporine may be indicated in patients whose original disease was HUS.

The frequency and significance of recurrent focal segmental glomerular sclerosis and hyalinosis varies widely in the reported literature. In three of the larger series, the recurrence rate was 30% and 43%.[37a,59,112] In these series, the presence or absence of mesangial proliferation was found to correlate with the incidence of recurrent disease as well as progression to allograft failure. Only 12% of patients with nonproliferative focal segmental glomerular sclerosis lost a kidney because of recurrent disease, whereas 60% of patients with sclerosis and mesangial proliferation lost their grafts from recurrent disease.[112] Mild recurrent diabetes mellitus is commonly found 5 to 10 years after transplantation, which, with progression, may result in Kimmelstiel-Wilson nodules, nephrotic syndrome, and graft failure. The prevention of recurrent oxalosis precludes a serious medical problem, which can be successfully overcome with specific pre- and post-transplant therapy.[89] Any decline in renal function should be followed by renal biopsy in order to rule out early recurrent disease and complications of the high phosphate and magnesium intake. Recurrence of membranous glomerulopathy, Berger's IgA nephropathy, and Henoch-Schönlein purpura is compatible with long-term graft survival, although the patients may have asymptomatic proteinuria and hematuria. Clinical and morphologic manifestations of de novo glomerular disease uncommonly occur in the allograft. Membranous glomerulopathy is the most common form of de novo disease and usually presents with severe proteinuria.[55] Another form of de novo, as well as recurrent disease, is reflux nephropathy–chronic pyelonephritis.[75,96] Acute post-infectious glomerulonephritis with its classic clinical symptoms may also be encountered.

In order to separate de novo and recurrent disease from chronic transplant glomerulopathy, with their often similar clinical manifestations, forms of therapy, and outcome, it is helpful to know what the original disorder was. Ultrastructural and immunofluorescence studies may be a necessity; thus, tissue from all biopsies should be taken so that recurrent or de novo disease and chronic transplant glomerulopathy can be properly identified.

Infection

Renal function may be adversely affected either directly by a bacterial, viral, or fungal infection or secondarily because of septicemia, therapeutic intervention with nephrotoxic drugs, or decrease in immunosuppressive therapy. Cytomegalovirus inclusions associated with interstitial nephritis are rarely encountered in renal biopsies. A more common but less specific abnormality, so-called cytomegalovirus (CMV)-associated glomerulopathy,[80] is

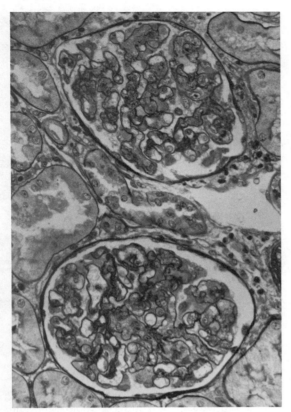

FIGURE 26-7.   *Cytomegalovirus-associated glomerulopathy. This patient developed fever and a rise in creatinine from 1.1 mg/dl to 2.3 mg/dl. Biopsy revealed glomerular capillaries occluded by cytoplasm of hyperplastic and hypertrophic endothelial cells. There was no evidence of interstitial or vascular rejection (PAS-alcian blue × 380).*

characteristic changes include marked dilatation and tortuosity of tubules filled with cellular debris and polymorphonuclear leukocytes, prominent interstitial scarring, and enlarged glomeruli with segmental and global sclerosis.

Cyclosporine

Cyclosporine has added a new dimension not only to the immunosuppressive armamentarium in the prevention of graft rejection but also, because of the unexpected side-effect of nephrotoxicity, to the interpretation of the post-transplant renal biopsy. Whether there are morphologic lesions in the kidney biopsy specific for or associated with CsA is controversial.[26,50,68,69,94,97,117] Renal insufficiency owing to CsA-NT can, in most instances, be recognized and separated from other causes of renal insufficiency.[68,117] In our series, 93% of cases of rejection and CsA-NT were properly identified in a retrospective and prospective multivariant analysis of histologic features.[94,97] Thus our approach is to decide whether the abnormalities are those of classic rejection, recurrent disease, ATN, and so on and if not, whether lesions present in the biopsy could be CsA associated. During the past year, the number of biopsies with features of CsA-NT has been significantly reduced because of utilization of lower doses of CsA.[13] The histologic features of CsA-NT appear to be dependent upon the various immunosuppressive regimens used in different institutions and the duration of the nephrotoxicity. Nephrotoxicity may be either dose dependent or caused by idiosyncratic reaction to the drug. Several histologic abnormalities have been reported in patients with CsA-related renal failure.

Diffuse interstitial fibrosis occurred in cadaver grafts with prolonged ATN where CsA compounded the ischemic damage.[26] The injury can be prevented by lowering the cyclosporine dose or waiting for resolution of the ATN before starting CsA.

"Toxic tubulopathy" usually occurs in the first few months post-transplantation and appears as minor to mild tubular damage in the form of focal ectasia, attenuation of epithelium (see Fig. 26-1), isometric epithelial vacuolization of the straight part of the proximal tubule, foci of dystrophic calcification, and giant mitochondria by electron microscopy.[68] Some cases show inconspicuous lesions even though the creatinine may be as high as 4 mg/dl to 5 mg/dl. Toxic tubulopathy, with or without a minor to mild peritubular capillary infiltrate, is a very common pattern in nephrotoxicity. Vascular lesions, except for arterial hyalinosis in the diabetic population, are usually not apparent. It is claimed that CsA

characterized by glomerular endothelial swelling and hyperplasia with lumen occlusion. (Fig. 26-7). It is found in a low percentage of patients with CMV septicemia. In many instances, the biopsy shows an intense interstitial nephritis inseparable from rejection. These patients can be successfully treated for rejection if they do not have evidence of severe clinical CMV disease. T8/T4 ratios of these infiltrates are exceedingly high compared with the ratios of acute rejection.[39] It is possible that a synergistic action of viral antigen and alloantigen is responsible for the high T8/T4 ratios rather than direct viral damage of the kidney.

The typical morphologic features of acute pyelonephritis are infrequently encountered in post-transplant biopsies.[96] When associated with chronic reflux or obstruction, glomerular and tubulointerstitial lesions identical to those in chronic pyelonephritis–reflux nephropathy are encountered. These

is present in the vacuolated cells in fine-needle aspirates in patients with nephrotoxicity,[122] although we have not been able to confirm this finding in our needle biopsies.

Peritubular capillary infiltration is common in CsA–prednisone immunosuppressed patients and is characterized by minimal to marked mononuclear infiltrates located within the peritubular capillary lumens.[94] Glomerulitis, tubulitis, endovasculitis, and edema, all features characteristic of acute rejection, are absent. Treatment with increased prednisone dosage has little effect on the abnormal creatinine levels, whereas reduction of CsA is efficacious. T8/T4 ratios are nearly normal or only slightly altered compared with classic acute rejection.[78] Lesions commonly found in patients with intraperitubular capillary mononuclear cells include "toxic tubulopathy" and, in some late biopsies, vascular lesions thought to be associated with CsA. This is especially true in patients with repeated episodes of clinical nephrotoxicity.

CsA-arteriopathy (CsA-AA) is a frequent finding in cyclosporine-immunosuppressed patients months to years post-transplantation.[68] The afferent arterioles and the interlobular arteries show a replacement of the media with a hyaline-like material (Fig. 26-8). Some pericytes appear to have lost their nuclei, with karyorrhexic debris being present in the wall, or show anisonucleosis (Fig. 26-9). CsA-AA may be difficult to differentiate from the hyalinosis of diabetes, a problem for centers in which large numbers of diabetics are transplanted. CsA-AA can usually be differentiated from hyalinosis because of the less homogeneous character and pericyte anisonucleosis in CsA-AA. Ultrastructural study, also, convincingly demonstrates the myocyte loss in CsA-AA, whereas myocytes are usually normal in diabetic hyalinosis.[68] Immunofluorescence studies do not differentiate diabetic hyalinosis from CsA-AA, in that IgM, C3, and fibrin are seen in both processes.

Mihatsch and associates[68] found the arteriopathy in 16% of 255 biopsies. Taube and colleagues[117] identified it in 62% of 65 biopsies, in association with acute rejection in 49%, and nephrotoxicity in 80%. We attempted to differentiate CsA-AA from hyalinosis in a blinded fashion in a review of 474 CsA biopsies and 470 azathioprine biopsies. In the CsA patients, CsA-AA was found in 52% of the nephrotoxicity cases and 6% of acute rejection cases, whereas hyalinosis occurred in 15% of acute rejection and 38% of "other." In the azathioprine patients, hyalinosis was found in 26% of the biopsies, and "CsA-AA" was associated with acute rejection in 4% of the biopsies. We have also seen two

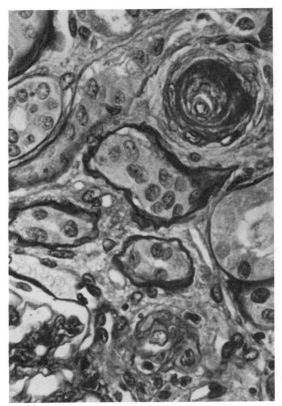

FIGURE 26-8. *Cyclosporine arteriopathy. A 38-year-old woman 18 months post-transplantation had a creatinine rise from 2.5 mg/dl to 4.2 mg/dl. She had previously experienced multiple episodes of nephrotoxicity. The lumen of this vessel was compromised, and the media was partially replaced by fibrinoid-like material. Elsewhere, there were strips of tubular atrophy and inflammation (PAS-alcian blue × 280).*

with glomerular and vessel lesions identical to those of the HUS. Sommer and associates[109] reported similar lesions in a large number of patients. Interestingly, rabbits with acute serum sickness develop glomerular capillary thrombosis when given CsA,[72] and the spontaneously hypertensive rat also has a predilection for HUS-like lesions after receiving CsA.[99]

The long-term consequences of CsA-AA appear to be medial scarring, fibrointimal proliferation, and ischemic cortical atrophy identical to those of benign arterial nephrosclerosis.

Focal or striped cortical fibrosis is the result of prolonged small-vessel vasoconstriction with resultant strips of tubular atrophy, interstitial fibrosis, and inflammation (Fig. 26-10). Early biopsies in CsA-NT include strips of tubular damage characterized by a fine widening of the interstitium and epithelial attenuation, which may be the initial ischemic effect

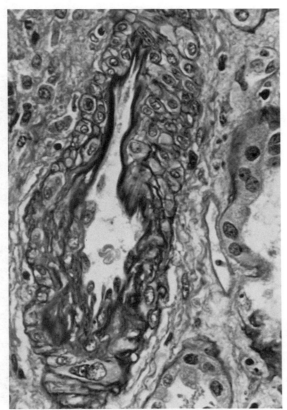

FIGURE 26-9. Cyclosporine arteriopathy. The vessels in this patient with a history of nephrotoxicity demonstrated thickened walls with anisonucleosis as well as nuclear disarray and foci of fibrinoid material in the media. There was also focal tubular atrophy and chronic inflammation in the interstitium (PAS-alcian blue × 260).

of the small-vessel vasoconstriction. It is possible, however, that high-dose CsA can induce tubular injury.[115,125]

It appears that patients can have both CsA-NT and acute rejection as a cause of renal dysfunction.[94] This is especially evident in patients with very high creatinine but only minimal evidence of rejection in the biopsy, for example, minimal endovasculitis and infiltrates that are usually asymptomatic. Decreased CsA doses result in normalization of creatinine levels in these patients—proof that the patient has asymptomatic rejection and CsA-NT.

CsA-NT probably is largely the result of renal ischemia induced by vascular lesions with the zonal tubular damage. Experimental models suggest the same, with increased renal vascular resistance and decreased renal blood flow and glomerular filtration rates (GFR).[46,74,115] In cardiac allograft recipients,

renal plasma flow and mean GFR are also reduced. Moran and co-workers[69] suggested that this is caused by a low glomerular capillary ultrafiltration capacity secondary to CsA directly damaging the glomeruli, or as a consequence of CsA damage of tubules and interstitium.

HEART

Endomyocardial biopsy is the gold standard in the diagnosis of rejection and is extremely important in the management of the cardiac allograft recipient. Right ventricular endomyocardial biopsies can be performed safely on an outpatient basis using the technique developed by Caves and associates[14] and modified by Mason.[60] The endomyocardial biopsy

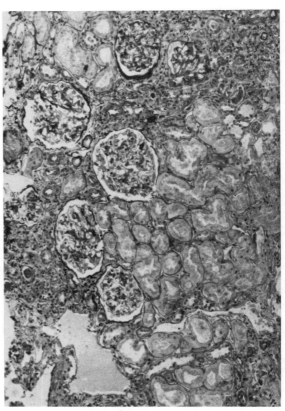

FIGURE 26-10. Chronic cyclosporine nephrotoxicity. A 31-year-old woman presented with a rise of creatinine to 2.3 mg/dl. She received a cadaver kidney 3½ years previously. The biopsy showed alternating zones of tubular atrophy, interstitial inflammation, and fibrosis with normal tubules and glomeruli. Small vessels showed changes of cyclosporine arteriopathy (PAS-alcian blue × 150).

is usually obtained at weekly intervals during the first 6 to 8 weeks, followed by monthly intervals until the sixth month, and thereafter every 3 months to 1 year.

Hyperacute Rejection

Hyperacute rejection of the heart does occur and is characterized by the presence of myocytolysis, capillary congestion with red blood cells, and IgM and fibrinogen in arterials.[36]

Acute Rejection

Prior to the utilization of CsA in cardiac transplantation, criteria for the diagnosis of acute rejection were well established by Billingham.[8,9] Mild rejection was characterized by perivascular and subendocardial infiltrates of pyroninophilic lymphocytes with interstitial edema. Extension of these lymphoid cells into the interstitium with early focal myocytolysis characterized moderate rejection, whereas interstitial hemorrhage, vascular and myocyte necrosis, and polymorphonuclear leukocyte infiltrate indicated severe rejection.

Patients immunosuppressed with CsA frequently have mixed inflammatory and sometimes mononuclear cell infiltrates in the graft that are not associated with clinical signs of rejection and are still present in biopsies taken following the institution of antirejection therapy. These infiltrates do not represent acute rejection; new criteria were established for the diagnosis of rejection, including the presence of myocyte necrosis.[8,19] This appears to be the case in patients receiving CsA, azathioprine, and prednisone as immunotherapy. However, most researchers use the original criteria with some modification for the diagnosis of acute rejection in CsA-immunosuppressed recipients.[34,79,95] The major criteria are a diffuse or intense multifocal interstitial lymphoid infiltrate in all the biopsy fragments in mild rejection, a diffuse infiltrate of greater intensity in moderate acute rejection (Fig. 26-11), and the addition of myocyte necrosis and polymorphonuclear infiltrate in severe rejection. If the infiltrate is minimal and diffuse or mild and multifocal, a repeat biopsy 2 to 3 days later is needed to determine whether the infiltrates are static or have increased in intensity, and thus represent acute rejection.

Based on these criteria, a diagnosis of acute rejection was made in 33 of 800 endomyocardial biopsies from 18 of 78 cardiac transplants at the University of Minnesota between 1978 and 1986. The intensity was mild in 19, moderate in 11, and

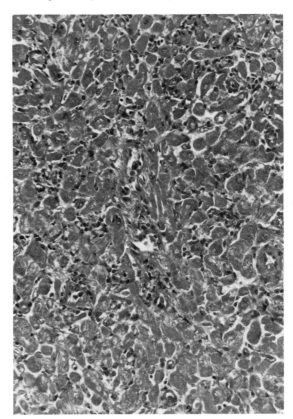

FIGURE 26-11.   *Acute rejection. At 9 months post-transplantation, this 34-year-old man developed decreased voltage on electrocardiogram and an increase in heart size. A biopsy showed a diffuse mild to moderate mononuclear cell infiltrate through all the fragments of the endomyocardial biopsy (hematoxylin and eosin × 190).*

severe in 3. Seven of the biopsies with rejection represented ongoing rejection in repeat biopsies performed to determine the response to antirejection therapy.

Immunofluorescence studies appear to be of little benefit in the diagnosis of acute rejection.[8,34] The mononuclear cell subpopulations of acute rejection in azathioprine-immunosuppressed recipients is similar to that seen in renal transplants with high T8/T4 ratios.[82,124] However, both of these studies fail to show any difference between T8/T4 ratios in rejection and nonrejection in CsA-immunosuppressed patients.

Ongoing and Treated Rejection

The management of patients with biopsy-proved acute rejection includes repeat biopsy 3 to 5 days after institution of therapy to ascertain the effect of antirejection therapy. Ongoing rejection is characterized by nonresolution or even increased intensity of the lymphoid infiltrates. A marked reduction in the lymphoid infiltrate with karyorrhexic debris, residual edema, and macrophage and plasma cell infiltrates is evidence of successful antirejection therapy.[8,9,34,95]

Vascular Rejection

Evidence of acute and chronic vascular rejection is rarely, if ever, present in the endomyocardial biopsy.[79] At autopsy, however, in patients dying of rejection, the main coronary artery and large intramyocardial arteries may show varying degrees of acute and/or chronic rejection identical to that seen in other transplanted organs. These abnormalities include endothelialitis, necrotizing arteritis, and fibrinoid necrosis in acute rejection, and fibrointimal onion-skinning, medial scarring, and collections of foamy macrophages in chronic rejection. These vascular abnormalities have been termed *accelerated graft atherosclerosis*[35,47] but represent vascular rejection and should be recognized as such.[79,95] Five of six Minnesota patients dying as a result of rejection had acute and/or chronic vascular rejection of varying severity. Each of those patients had biopsy-proven and clinical episodes of acute rejection. The importance of the vascular endothelium in the pathogenesis of rejection should again be noted.

Nonrejection Pathology (Table 26-1)

Only a minority of endomyocardial biopsies show features of acute rejection. Recognition of nonrejection pathology is therefore imperative so that infec-

TABLE 26-1 *Nonrejection Pathology Found in 680 Endomyocardial Biopsies*

Previous biopsy site—71%
    Inflammation—61%
    Granulation tissue/organizing thrombus—14%
    Fibrosis—89%
    Nodular subendocardial lymphoid infiltrates—8%
Mononuclear infiltrate—59%
    Focal—80%
    Multifocal—11%
    Diffuse—9%
    Minimal—85%
    Mild—15%
Normal—16%
Perimyocyte fibrosis—5%
Microinfarction—4%

tious complications of overtreatment can be prevented. The significance of many minor infiltrates is uncertain. It is possible that they represent low-grade, nonprogressive forms of rejection or merely a nonspecific inflammatory response to previous myocardial damage.

Biopsy Site Damage

The majority of morphologic abnormalities are caused by damage to the endo- and myocardium because of previous biopsy.[34,79,95] Granulation tissue, organizing thrombus, and necrotic myocytes may be present at the recent biopsy site, and fibrous scars with inflammation may exist at old sites. A polymorphic inflammatory infiltrate is often evident at or adjacent to the biopsy site. Perivascular and interstitial infiltrates with edema and/or fibrosis are commonly present some distance from the biopsy site and can be confused with acute rejection (Fig. 26-12). Examination of different levels through the biopsy often reveals the biopsy site, and, unless tissue fragments show evidence of rejection, that is, a diffuse inflammatory infiltrate of lymphocytes, a diagnosis of rejection should not be made (Fig. 26-13). A helpful clue to the identification of a biopsy site is the finding of myocytes running at an angle rather than parallel to the endocardium. Nodular, well-defined subendocardial lymphoid infiltrates, which may be massive at times, should not be confused with acute rejection or malignant lymphoma. These infiltrates are infrequently found in CsA-immunosuppressed patients.[8,34,95]

Myocyte Necrosis

Foci of myocyte necrosis, subsequent granulation tissue, and small scars secondary to peritransplant ischemic damage may be found in the first several weeks post-transplantation. A prominent infiltrate of pigment-laden histiocytes, polymorphonuclear neutrophilic and eosinophilic leukoctyes, small lymphocytes, and plasma cells with variable edema may be encountered, especially in the clinically symptomatic patient. These abnormalities resolve with time. Myocyte necrosis also occurs at recent biopsy sites and is present in severe acute rejection.

Perimyocyte Fibrosis

An additional feature found in CsA recipients is a fine perimyocyte fibrosis.[8,34,36] This finding is often preceded by or is contiguous with parallel zones of interstitial edema and a mild mononuclear cell infiltrate,[79,95] which probably is the result of biopsy damage and the effect of CsA upon healing response.

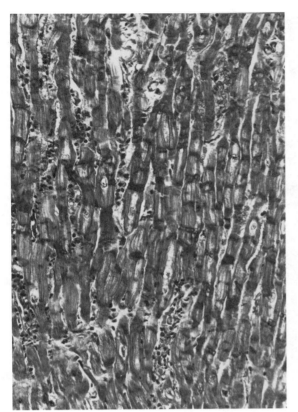

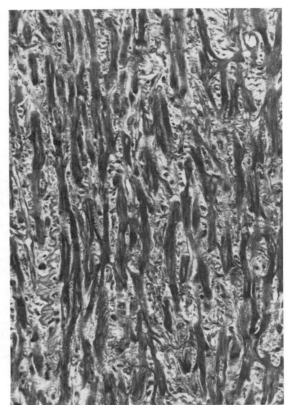

FIGURE 26-12. *Biopsy site. This cardiac transplant patient had undergone multiple previous endomyocardial biopsies. She has never had a clinical episode of acute rejection. Focal mononuclear infiltrates either at the endomyocardium, in the perivascular spaces, or amongst myocardial cells are commonly apparent in patients on cyclosporine immunosuppression. They are usually related to previous biopsy damage (hematoxylin and eosin × 190).*

FIGURE 26-13. *Biopsy site damage. Another feature found in or adjacent to a biopsy site is parallel arrays of myocytes separated by a mildly inflamed and prominently edematous interstitium (hematoxylin and eosin × 190).*

Infections

Not all inflammatory infiltrates represent acute rejection; thus, biopsies should be examined for the presence of infectious organisms. Toxoplasma,[9,79] CMV, and coccidioidomycosis[9] have been found in myocardial biopsies. Myocardial Aspergillus with extensive myocardial infarction at autopsy has been reported in four cases.[95] Endomyocardial biopsy in one of our patients demonstrated a diffuse, myocardial infiltrate of large immunoblast-like cells, which were mistakenly interpreted as rejection. This patient and one other patient had diffuse myocardial infiltrates of atypical cells not only in the heart but in most organs at autopsy and represented atypical lymphoproliferative infiltrates secondary to systemic viral infection.[31,95]

HEART–LUNG

A diagnosis of acute and chronic rejection in the heart in heart–lung transplantation is identical to that in the heart transplant alone.[57,128] Criteria for the recognition of pulmonary rejection have not been completely established. There has been an inordinate number of pulmonary infections in heart–lung transplant recipients compared with that in other transplanted organ recipients, perhaps because of loss of the cough reflex, decreased mucociliary clearance, bronchial mucosal ischemia, and impairment of lymphatic drainage. Peribronchial lymphoid infiltrates and high number of polymorphonuclear leukocytes have been found in a few patients thought to have acute rejection.[37] Chronic rejection may cause airway obliteration secondary to bronchiolitis obliterans. Peribronchial inflammation, arterial and venous fibrointimal hyperplasia, that is, chronic vascular rejection, and interstitial fibrosis are additional lesions found in biopsies or at autopsy.[10,128]

LIVER

Although it was originally reported that the liver was a "privileged" organ resistant to rejection,[127] it has become apparent that liver allograft rejection is a common phenomenon.[20,105] The reason for the earlier reports may have to do with the fact that the major target of liver rejection is the biliary ductal tree, not the hepatic parenchyma, a situation that results in the ability of the organ to withstand a relatively long period of rejection before organ failure occurs. In our experience, acute rejection occurs in approximately 80% of patients who survive the immediate post-transplant period. Other investigators have reported an incidence of 25% to 36%,[20,126] and, at one center, approximately 16% of liver recipients undergo retransplantation because of failure of the first graft owing to rejection.[20] In our experience, the incidence of liver failure as a result of rejection is much lower than this, probably because of liberal use of biopsy to detect and treat early rejection.

It appears that the liberal use of biopsy to document rejection before beginning treatment is the only way to avoid unnecessary immunosuppression when rejection is not present and, at the same time, avoid the problem of liver failure owing to chronic rejection. Several studies have shown the value of frequent biopsy in the management of the liver-transplanted patient.[105,126] Many centers make frequent use of the so-called protocol biopsy, that is, biopsy taken at specific intervals post-transplantation instead of only at the time of clinical evidence of liver disease. The value of such protocol biopsies is illustrated by two cases in which there was biopsy-proven rejection at times when liver function did not indicate a problem that would have triggered a biopsy.

We have performed more than 270 biopsies complicated by four minor bleeding episodes (none requiring surgery) and three pneumothoraces. Other investigators have reported similar low morbidity.[24,126] Using biopsy-directed immunosuppression in our last 60 transplant patients, there has been one significant fungal infection and only three patients have developed chronic rejection requiring consideration of retransplantation. This is in contrast to the treatment of acute rejection predominately on the basis of clinical findings without biopsy at Pittsburgh, where an incidence of "significant" fungal infections of nearly 42% and a

retransplantation rate for rejection of more than 16% has been reported.[20,123]

A biopsy should be obtained at the time of transplantation and at weekly intervals for at least the first 2 or 3 weeks. Biopsies should also be taken as directed by the clinical situation. Because routine laboratory studies such as bilirubin, transaminase, and alkaline phosphatase have not proved useful in the diagnosis of rejection or in the assessment of efficacy of antirejection therapy, biopsy remains the only way to confirm or rule out the diagnosis and determine the cause of the liver dysfunction.[30,90] If rejection is detected, biopsies should be taken at approximately weekly intervals to assess efficacy of therapy. As in any clinical situation, routine contraindications to biopsy such as uncorrectable thrombocytopenia are evaluated before biopsy is undertaken.

As with other organs, liver allograft rejection can be subdivided into hyperacute, acute, and chronic types, based on histologic parameters. Whereas the existence and criteria for acute and chronic rejection have been well characterized, hyperacute rejection remains a controversial entity.

Effect of the Transplantation Process on Liver Histology

It is not surprising that removal, storage, and transport of a liver will result in histologic changes. Study of biopsies taken at the time of transplantation ("time zero biopsies") show a mild degree of hepatocellular swelling and rarefaction of the cytoplasm as an almost universal finding.[105] This may be accompanied by a mild degree of sinusoidal polymorphonuclear infiltration, that is, "surgical hepatitis." The swelling generally resolves within a week of transplantation. Resolution occurs by periportal regeneration, so residual damage persists longest in the centrilobular region.

Hyperacute Rejection

Hyperacute rejection of the liver does occur. In two patients who expired early in their post-transplant course of hyperacute rejection, the pathology was characterized by a massive polymorphonuclear infiltrate, severe bile duct damage, arteritis, hepatocellular damage, and infarction of probable ischemic etiology. Both patients developed clinical evidence of liver dysfunction in the first day post-transplant.

The fact that the liver in these patients did not cause death immediately following insertion of the liver, as is the case with hyperacute rejection in other organs, is probably the same reason that acute rejection does not manifest itself as quickly in the liver. The tremendous reserve of the liver allows some degree of function despite destruction of a large part of the parenchyma. Also, the large mass of the liver can possibly "absorb" pre-existing antibody more effectively, leaving less residual injury.

Acute Rejection

Acute rejection is defined as rejection that is at a stage of potential reversibility with appropriate therapy. It is most likely a cell-mediated process, because it is characterized by an intense inflammatory infiltrate.

Acute rejection is characterized by a triad of portal inflammatory infiltration, damage to the bile duct epithelium in conjunction with lymphocytic infiltration of the bile ducts, and central and/or portal vein endothelialitis (Fig. 26-14).[105] Other features less commonly evident include arteritis and

hepatocellular necrosis. Not surprisingly, cholestasis is also commonly found.

The portal infiltrate in untreated rejection is composed predominantly of small lymphocytes, with lesser numbers of neutrophils and eosinophils in most cases. The role of these latter cells in the rejection process is not certain, but, in rare cases, either cell type may predominate, leading to differential diagnostic problems with biliary obstruction or drug hypersensitivity, respectively. Plasma cells are rare in early acute rejection. The infiltrate varies in intensity with the severity of rejection and is patchy in mild rejection, with virtually all portal areas involved in severe rejection. Spillover into the adjacent parenchyma may be present, and, in occasional cases, true piecemeal necrosis can be identified.

With antirejection treatment, the character of the portal infiltrate is altered. In some cases, the infiltrate will completely resolve within a week of

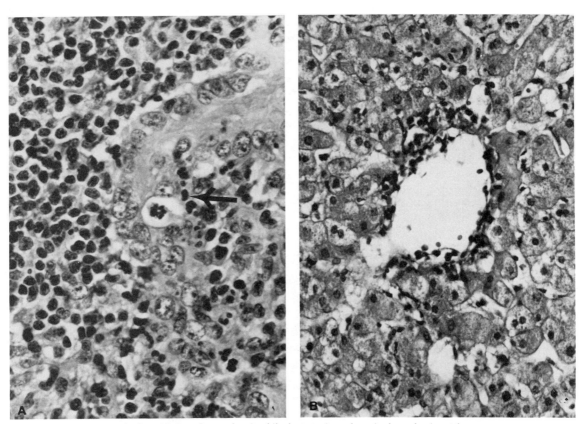

FIGURE 26-14.   *Acute rejection. (A) Portal area showing bile duct atypia and a mixed, predominantely lymphocytic infiltrate. The bile duct contains a mitosis, and several inflammatory cells are seen within the wall (arrow; hematoxylin and eosin × 480). (B) Central vein showing lymphocytes attached to the endothelium (endothelialitis) (hematoxylin and eosin × 256).*

therapy. More commonly, however, the first several weeks post-therapy are characterized by a predominance of neutrophils, presumably because of a selective action of common therapeutic regimens to remove the lymphocyte population, exposing the neutrophils. This histologic finding should not cause diagnostic problems if the previous course of the patient is known, but, if the first biopsy is taken after initiation of therapy, a misdiagnosis of obstructive liver disease can be made. This appears to be an especially difficult problem for a group of patients with so-called prolonged rejection. This subset of patients, most of whom seem to be undertreated for a variety of reasons, show fibrosis and bile duct proliferation in addition to the infiltrate. In most of these patients, the fibrosis will resolve and the liver function will return to normal if adequately treated.[105]

The bile duct damage of rejection consists of nuclear pleomorphism, stratification of cells, cytoplasmic vacuolation, dropout of individual cells, loss of the duct lumen, and/or eventual loss of entire ducts. The interlobular ducts are most prominently involved. The damage is invariably accompanied by the interposition of small lymphocytes between the epithelial cells, frequently accompanied by neutrophils, either in the wall or lumen of the duct. In severe cases, the ducts may be impossible to identify on hematoxylin and eosin-stained sections; in these cases, the trichrome stain is an invaluable aid to the identification of the ducts. As mentioned previously, bile duct and ductular proliferation may be seen, particularly after partial treatment.

Although portal inflammation and bile duct damage are invariably present in acute rejection, the third member of the triad, endothelialitis, is less uniformly present. It consists of the attachment of lymphocytes to the endothelium of central or portal veins. Lymphocytes may be seen both luminally and abluminally and frequently lift the endothelium off the underlying basement membrane. In very severe cases, the entire lumen of the vessel may be filled with cells, making identification of the portal vein particularly difficult. This vascular occlusion may be responsible for areas of parenchymal infarct that are sometimes seen. In the central areas, the infiltrate may involve surrounding parenchyma, occasionally in association with focal necrosis.

Arteritis is sometimes seen in needle biopsies of acute rejection and is possibly more common than realized if wedge biopsies or resection specimens are examined.[20] If present, it may indicate a more severe form of rejection.

Other common findings in acute rejection biopsies include cholestasis and central ballooning de-generation. The cholestasis is not surprising in view of the bile duct damage that is present. Cholestasis is also seen in many nonrejecting post-transplant liver biopsies and may result from sepsis, obstruction, drug toxicity, or perhaps even from the post-transplant regenerative process itself.[105] The central ballooning that is frequently seen is nonspecific. In many cases, it represents residual ischemic damage caused by the transplant procedure, which usually resolves within 2 weeks of the transplant.

Endothelialitis appears to be the most specific feature of the diagnosis of rejection. Bile duct damage and portal inflammation are more sensitive but less specific features. The diagnosis is certain if all three features of the triad are present. In the absence of endothelialitis, other causes of bile duct damage should be considered, including viral and drug-induced hepatitis and obstructive liver disease, particularly if of a low-grade chronic variety.[105] Acute viral hepatitis can usually be differentiated by its more prominent lobular involvement and less severe bile duct damage. Drug hypersensitivity is usually accompanied by an eosinophilia, although large numbers of eosinophils occasionally occur in rejection as well. In the latter case, hypersensitivity must be ruled out on clinical grounds. Low-grade obstruction has not been a major problem in our experience but, if suspected, may be ruled out by appropriate radiologic examinations.

In situ identification of T cell subsets shows that, as with kidney, T8 cells predominate in acute rejection.[93,100] However, in CsA-immunosuppressed patients, we have been unable to distinguish the infiltrates of rejection from those of nonrejection on this basis. Examination of serial biopsies has shown that with antirejection therapy, the percentage of T8 cells decreases with a concomitant increase in T4 cells. The use of this method may permit assessment of adequacy of therapy.[100]

Chronic Rejection

Chronic rejection is defined as terminal or end-stage rejection that will lead to organ failure requiring retransplantation if the patient is to survive. As in other organs, the process is characterized by fibro-obliterative endarteritis.[20,105] In addition, the chronically rejected liver can manifest portal fibrosis and loss of bile ducts as primary features (Fig. 26-15).

Obliterative endarteritis in the liver is identical to that seen in other visceral organ transplants. Medium to large arteries are involved. The earliest manifestation appears to be the accumulation of foamy histiocytes in a subendothelial location with eventual subintimal fibrosis and occlusion. The re-

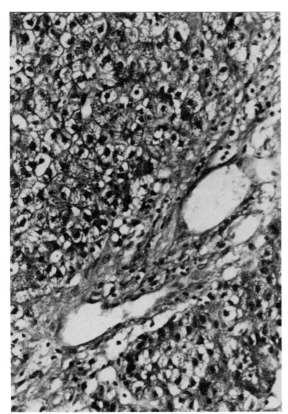

FIGURE 26-15. *Chronic rejection 377 days post-transplantation. This portal tract contains no bile duct and only scant inflammation (hematoxylin and eosin × 190).*

lationship of vasculitis in the acute stage to eventual development of chronic rejection has not been studied in a large number of cases; however, patients with early arteritis are more likely to develop chronic rejection.

In addition to endarteritis, chronic rejection may result in cirrhosis. However, not all livers showing fibrosis post-transplant will develop cirrhosis or chronic rejection. In other words, fibrosis is not synonymous with chronic rejection. Many cases of prolonged rejection will eventually return to normal architecture if adequately treated. The fibrosis of chronic rejection is portal and sharply demarcated from the adjacent parenchyma. The inflammatory response in chronic rejection varies. Usually it is lymphocytic and is scant or nonexistent after the bile ducts have been destroyed. The lack of inflammation probably results from the removal of the major antigenic target, the bile duct. This hypothesis is supported by the fact that in cases with patchy loss of bile ducts, the tracts with ducts have inflam-

mation, whereas those with no ducts lack inflammation. Although loss of bile ducts usually occurs in chronic disease, their destruction in acute rejection is not indicative of irreversible rejection, because regeneration of the bile ducts does occur.

A major problem in the diagnosis of chronic rejection occurs because arteries of a size affected by chronic rejection are rarely found in needle biopsies of liver. In the absence of such arteries, the diagnosis can be suggested by the presence of centrilobular ballooning degeneration with necrosis (Fig. 26-16). Although such central damage is not diagnostic of chronic rejection, taken in the context of a patient with previous acute rejection, inflammatory portal changes and/or paucity of bile ducts, it can be assumed to be due to chronic rejection. Obviously, in the early post-transplant period, ischemia owing to technical problems with the arterial or portal venous anastomoses will produce identical changes. This is most likely in the late period

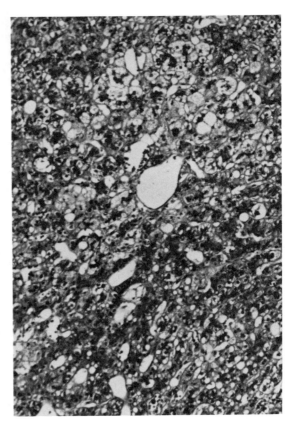

FIGURE 26-16. *Chronic rejection. The central area is showing ischemic changes in the form of ballooning and dropout of cells secondary to vascular rejection (hematoxylin and eosin × 100).*

in a patient with previous rejection. Needless to say, a biopsy showing cirrhosis in similar circumstances can be assumed to represent chronic rejection.

Grading of Acute Liver Rejection

A grading system for rejection must provide the clinician with information regarding the necessity for treatment, the type of treatment to use, and the expected outcome of treatment. Biopsies showing a mild inflammatory infiltrate with focal duct damage involving less than 50% of the bile ducts but without endothelialitis are "consistent with" rejection but not diagnositc. The clinician may elect to treat for rejection if indicated by the clinical circumstances or may wait for the liver to declare itself. Any liver showing bile duct damage with an inflammatory infiltrate *and* endothelialitis is diagnositc of rejection and may be graded as mild or moderate based on the intensity of the infiltrate, diffuseness of the process, and the percentage of bile ducts damaged. In general, if bile duct damage is less than 50%, the process is considered mild, whereas greater than 50% involvement is considered moderate. In cases without endothelialitis, a diagnosis of rejection may be made if greater than 50% of the bile ducts are damaged, lymphocytes are present in some of the damaged ducts, there is a predominately lymphocytic infiltrate, and hepatocellular inflammation and necrosis are not prominent. A diagnosis of severe rejection is made if the criteria for rejection are met and arteritis, central ischemic damage, or paucity of bile ducts is noted.

Recurrence of Original Disease Following Transplantation

There is clear evidence that hepatocellular malignancies and viral hepatitis B recur in most cases following transplantation.[17,111] For this reason, these patients are considered poor candidates for transplant.

Recurrence of other disease, most particularly primary biliary cirrhosis (PBC), is more difficult to ascertain. The recurrence of PBC has been reported, and although the histologic features of PBC are very similar to those of rejection, the clinical features in those patients support the interpretation of recurrent disease.[73]

PANCREAS

Segmental and whole pancreas transplantation for the treatment of diabetes mellitus has recently be-

come feasible because of improved surgical techniques and immunosuppressive regimens for the prevention of rejection.[116] Identification of the cause of pancreatic graft failure is difficult because tissues have thus far been obtained only by means of a laparotomy or autopsy. Loss of function is usually attributed to rejection on clinical grounds alone or to graft infarction secondary to vascular thrombosis, but viral infection, chronic pancreatitis owing to duct obstruction, and recurrent disease can be the cause of graft dysfunction in many patients with putative acute rejection. Furthermore, entirely normal grafts have been found in some biopsies, and the cause of the spontaneously reversible, short-term dysfunction was never determined. In an analysis of 61 wedge or needle biopsies, 61 pancreatectomies, and 7 autopsies from 100 pancreas transplants, the following abnormalities were noted.[97a]

Rejection

A diagnosis of acute and/or chronic rejection was made in 36 of the grafts. The morphologic criteria of acute and chronic rejection of the pancreas are similar to those used in other transplanted organs. The presence of a mononuclear cell infiltrate within the pancreatic parenchyma with endovasculitis is a characteristic feature. The finding of a polymorphonuclear leukocyte and eosinophil infiltrate with acinar necrosis, in addition to lymphoid infiltrates, is a feature of severe acute rejection. As in other organs, endothelialitis and/or fibrinoid necrosis of arteries, present in 27 of the cases, were most useful in the diagnosis of acute rejection (Fig. 26-17). Perivascular, periductular, and perilobular inflammation with fibrosis is a common feature in normally functioning grafts removed because of intra-abdominal infectious complications, hemorrhage, or ascites and cannot be used as evidence for rejection. Similar findings can also be found with partial duct obstruction. The cause of hyperglycemia in acute rejection is not anatomically always evident, because, in most cases, immunoperoxidase staining of the islets reveals normal numbers of beta cells. Although the islets may be entirely normal by light and electron microscopy as well as immunohistochemically in acute rejection, 14 of the cases had a minimal to mild lymphoid infiltrate within the islets. Some of the beta cells appeared to be degranulated in these cases, but, in most instances, normal numbers of beta cells were present.

The major finding in chronic rejection is an obliterative fibrointimal proliferative endarteritis, which is often associated with extensive graft infarction. Graft infarction can also be the result of

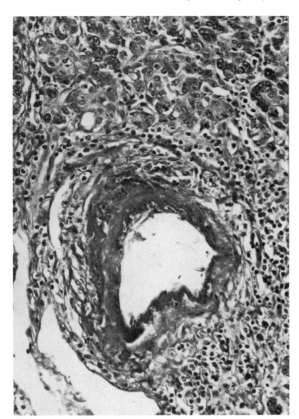

FIGURE 26-17.   Acute rejection. This patient presented with fever and hyperglycemia. A wedge biopsy was performed and revealed an infiltrate of lymphocytes within the exocrine pancreas and fibrinoid necrosis of vessel walls (hematoxylin and eosin × 190).

severe acute vascular rejection with thrombosis and is usually associated with sudden and irreversible loss of function. In some cases of chronic rejection, the islets show a prominent reduction in all islet cell constituents. The immune response of rejection appears to result in the destruction of the islet cells.

A diagnosis of acute or chronic rejection is very difficult in grafts implanted following injection of the pancreatic duct with foreign materials such as prolamine and silastic. These substances cause extensive inflammation and destruction of the exocrine pancreas, with eventual fibrosis of the gland. A search for evidence of acute or chronic vascular lesions of rejection is the best way of identifying a rejection process in these grafts.

Vascular Thrombosis

A major complication in pancreas transplantation accounting for the sudden loss of graft function is arterial and/or venous thrombosis.[116] An explanation for this phenomenon is the abnormal hemodynamics relative to the larger splenic and smaller pancreatic vessels. The end result is graft infarction. Recanalized veins and arteries within the graft are common findings in pancreas biopsies and pancreatectomies. Distal thrombosis of the splenic vessels commonly occurs and is of no significance to graft function.

Infection

Intra-abdominal bacterial infections led to the removal of seven histologically normal grafts. Pancreatic samples from 13 patients revealed evidence of CMV infection. Viral inclusions were found in the islets of 2 patients and involved the exocrine pancreas in 11 patients. Only 2 of the patients had clinical symptoms suggestive of CMV infection prior to the biopsy or pancreatectomy. Two cases were particularly interesting. Both patients experienced severe gastrointestinal hemorrhage, which appeared to be pancreatic in origin. The resected specimens demonstrated CMV infestation of the small intestinal mucosa at the anastomotic site, resulting in necrosis and ulceration. The pathogenesis of the hemorrhage appears to be similar to that of CMV colitis.[29]

Chronic Pancreatitis

Partial or even severe duct obstruction may occur as a late surgical complication at the implantation anastomotic site. Perilobular inflammation and fibrosis as well as duct ectasia with periductal edema and fibrosis reminiscent of large duct obstruction of the liver are found in biopsies of grafts known to have partial duct obstruction. A more extensive and destructive process of the exocrine pancreas occurs in grafts injected with silastic or prolamine (Fig. 26-18).[21,22,33,54] Initially, there is an acute and, secondarily, a chronic pancreatitis that result in near-total destruction of the exocrine pancreas. An intense foreign body giant cell reaction also occurs in silastic duct–injected grafts. The identification of acute rejection is very difficult in these cases, and evidence of vascular rejection must be searched for.

Although these grafts may function for several years following exocrine destruction, function is often ultimately lost. Only 7 of 39 duct-injected grafts at Minnesota were functioning at 3 years post-transplantation. The cause of late graft loss may be on the basis of chronic rejection, but, in many cases, it is the result of the chronic pancreatitis per se. The islets are entrapped in fibrotic tissue, are of variable

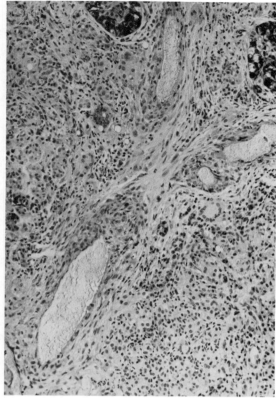

FIGURE 26-18.   *Sialastic damage. The extravasated sialastic has incited a foreign body giant cell reaction as well as a moderate inflammatory infiltrate in the acinar tissues. The islets contain a near-normal number of beta cells (insulin, peroxidase-antiperoxidase method × 190).*

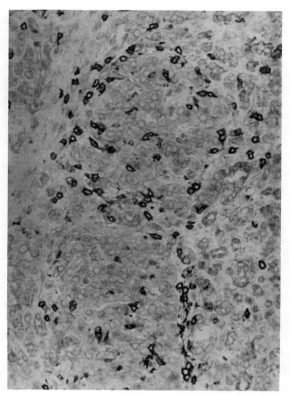

FIGURE 26-19.   *Recurrent diabetes. This 36-year-old woman received an isograft that functioned normally for approximately 3 months but developed increasing graft dysfunction thereafter. Biopsy revealed a prominent isletitis. Later biopsies revealed selective destruction of beta cells and resolution of the inflammation (OKT8-killer suppressor T-lymphocytes; peroxidase-antiperoxidase method × 190).*

size and shape, and have increased numbers of alpha cells and decreased numbers of beta cells similar to that seen in patients developing diabetes mellitus on the basis of chronic pancreatitis.[51] In some cases, there can be an impressive loss not only of beta cells but also of other islet constituents, which may be ischemic or rejection in origin.

Recurrent Disease

Nine patients, four receiving isografts (identical twin transplants) and five receiving allografts from HLA-identical siblings or parent, appear to have developed recurrent disease.[97a] Biopsy in three of the isografts revealed an intense mononuclear cell infiltrate within the islets in biopsies obtained when initial graft dysfunction appeared without evidence of exocrine or vascular rejection (Fig. 26-19). Late biopsies, when there was no further evidence of graft function, showed resolution of the isletitis, and

the islets were devoid of all beta cells, being identical to those of their native pancreas.[98] The process appeared to be mediated by T-lymphocytes, with the majority being cytotoxic/suppressor (T8) lymphocytes.

BONE MARROW TRANSPLANTATION

Graft-Versus-Host Disease (GVHD)

GVHD following bone marrow transplantation (BMT) is generally thought of as the converse of allograft rejection. Instead of the host rejecting the graft, the graft "rejects" the host. A number of organs can be affected by the process. However, all organs are not affected equally, and this disparity of involvement had led to the conclusion that there are two distinct types of GVHD, acute and chronic. Although initially defined on the arbitrary basis of occurrence before or after Day 100 post-transplant,[92,119] it has become clear that there are differences in organ involvement and histologic features between the acute and chronic diseases that have led to the conclusion that acute and chronic disease probably have different pathogenetic mechanisms and, thus, are two separate diseases.[77,92,103] This is in distinction to the situation in other organ rejection where it appears that chronic disease is a result of the same process that produced acute rejection.

Acute Graft-Versus-Host Disease

Acute GVHD was originally defined as GVHD occurring in the first 100 days post-transplant. It is characterized clinically by the triad of a skin rash, diarrhea, and liver function abnormalities.[85,119] Whereas in classical disease, all three organs are involved, many cases will be isolated to one or two organs, with skin involvement being the most common. Whether the lung is a target for acute GVHD is not clear, but interstitial lung disease that clinically corresponds to bouts of acute GVHD can respond to anti-GVHD therapy. Although lymphocytic bronchitis was reported to be characteristic of pulmonary GVHD, this is probably not true.[7,38]

The histologic hallmark of acute GVHD is the finding of single necrotic epithelial cells in the basal layer of the skin, in the crypts of the intestine or stomach, and in the bile ducts of the liver. These dead cells are usually associated with a mild lymphocytic infiltrate. In most cases, the findings of GVHD are not absolutely specific; however, when taken in context, an accurate diagnosis can be made.

Skin.   Acute GVHD of the skin usually presents as a maculopapular rash, frequently beginning on the palms and soles, face, or trunk, with eventual extension onto the extremities.[85] In mild cases, flaky desquamation of the corneal layer ensues prior to resolution, but, in severe disease, life-threatening full-thickness sloughing may occur. In some cases, a picture of toxic epidermal necrolysis (TEN) simulating the Stevens-Johnson syndrome may be seen. Biopsy may not be able to distinguish TEN owing to GVHD from that owing to sulfa antibiotics.

Cutaneous acute GVHD is characterized by basal layer hydropic degeneration and single necrotic (dyskeratotic) cells with attached lymphocytes (so-called satellitosis; Fig. 26-20). Basal hydropic degeneration alone is not diagnostic of GVHD, despite its designation as "grade 1" GVHD (Table 26-2).[84] If accompanied by dyskeratotic cells, it is considered Grade 2. Formation of small subepidermal vesicles and total desquamation are considered Grades 3 and 4 disease, respectively. TEN is also a Grade 4 lesion, even if desquamation has not occurred.

Cytoreductive therapy can produce skin changes virtually identical to GVHD.[84,118] These effects disappear by 21 days post-transplant, although, in some cases, the changes may persist longer. Biopsies taken before Day 21 post-transplant may be

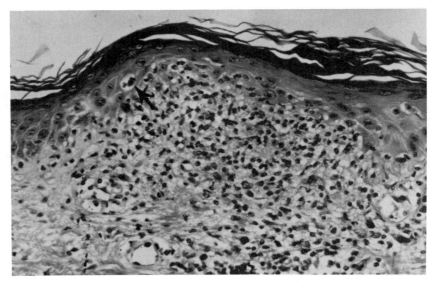

FIGURE 26-20.   Acute cutaneous graft-versus-host disease (GVHD). A lymphocytic infiltrate encroaches on the epidermis with degeneration of the basal layer and occasional dyskeratotic cells (arrow; *hematoxylin and eosin* × 480).

TABLE 26-2   Histologic Grading of Acute GVHD

GRADE	SKIN	RECTUM	LIVER
1	Basal layer degeneration alone	Single cell necrosis without crypt destruction	< 25% damaged bile ducts
2	Grade 1 plus dyskeratotic cells	Grade 1 plus crypt destruction involving no more than 2 contiguous crypts	25%–50% damaged bile ducts
3	Subepidermal vesicle formation	Loss of more than 2 contiguous crypts	50%–70% damage bile ducts
4	Desquamation or toxic epidermal necrolysis	Denudation of mucosa	> 75% damaged bile ducts

inadequate to distinguish GVHD from cytoreductive effect in a definitive manner. However, several features will allow a preference for one or the other etiology. First, cytoreductive damage tends to be uniform and diffuse in distribution, whereas GVHD is usually patchy in the early stage. Second, since the effects of cytoreduction are actually in a regressing phase when observed, one frequently sees dyskerototic cells and atypia without evidence of active destruction, as evidenced by basal layer degeneration. Therefore, if a biopsy has the criteria for Grade 2 GVHD but does not have basal layer degeneration, it is probably a regressing process. In the first weeks after transplant, these findings should suggest cytoreduction as the etiologic event.

Drug toxicity and viral infection may simulate GVHD at any time after transplantation. Bactrim, a drug used almost universally as a prophylaxis for pneumocystis, has been associated with both a lichenoid drug eruption and TEN and should be considered a potential cause of skin rash, especially if other organs are not involved by a GVHD-like process. We have seen two cases of disseminated CMV in which skin biopsy shows changes characteristic of Grade 2 GVHD. Other organs did not support the GVHD diagnosis, and CMV inclusions were identified in the dermis at autopsy.[107]

Gastrointestinal Tract. There are two major manifestations of acute GVHD in the gastrointestinal tract, diarrhea and upper GI pain, nausea and vomiting.[85,86,107] Clinically, the major differential diagnosis for gastrointestinal GVHD is that of infectious disease.

Although the diarrhea associated with GVHD is probably of upper GI origin, rectal biopsy is frequently used to diagnose acute gastrointestinal GVHD.[25,86] The diagnostic feature is the single necrotic cell consisting of a collection of karyorrhexic debris in a clear space in the area of regeneration of the mucosa, the so-called exploding crypt cell (Fig. 26-21). The necrosis occurs predominantly in the crypt of the small and large intestine and in the neck region of the stomach. Cells resembling the exploding crypt cell are frequently seen on the surface of the colorectum, probably as a result of preparative enema, and should be ignored. In addition, occasional apoptotic cells are a normal constituent of the gastrointestinal tract and should not lead to a diagnosis of GVHD. In general, the diagnosis can be made if the dead cells are abundant enough to be seen at medium power. If one needs to search at high power to find one dead cell, GVHD is probably not the diagnosis.

Other less specific changes may accompany the single dead cells in GVHD, including crypt abscesses, a minimal inflammatory infiltrate in the lamina propria, and, with more severe disease, loss of entire crypts. GVHD has been graded on the basis of number of missing crypts. A modification of the Seattle system is detailed in Table 26-2.

As in the skin, cytoreductive therapy and viral infections produce changes histologically identical to GVHD.[25,102] For this reason, biopsy in the first 21 days post-transplant is not diagnostic of GVHD, although a negative biopsy is useful in ruling out the diagnosis. CMV infection of the gastrointestinal tract can also produce the exploding crypt cell[102]; thus, GVHD can neither be diagnosed nor excluded in a gastrointestinal biopsy that contain CMV inclusions. Other infectious diseases such as cryptosporidiosis and pseudomembranous colitis may be recognized on rectal biopsy; these diseases do not simulate GVHD histologically.[58] Changes identical to those of GVHD are also seen in biopsies from children with severe T cell deficiency.[104] In these children, biopsy taken just prior to transplant will provide a useful comparison for later biopsies.

Although the rectal biopsy is easier to perform than the upper GI biopsy, upper GI symptoms often

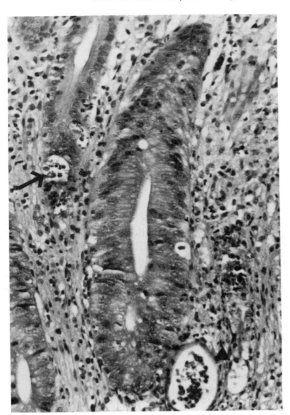

FIGURE 26-21. *Acute rectal graft-versus-host disease (GVHD). An "exploding crypt cell" (arrow) and crypt abscess (arrowhead) are characteristic of GVHD (hematoxylin and eosin × 192).*

predominate; thus, if the rectal biopsy is negative, biopsy of the duodenum and stomach are necessary to establish the etiology of the symptoms.[107] Esophageal biopsy is of limited use in the diagnosis of GVHD but will detect herpes or CMV esophagitis, other common causes of upper GI symptoms.

Liver. The liver is perhaps the least biopsied organ for the diagnosis of GVHD, because the risk of biopsy is considerable in patients with thrombocytopenia. Causes of liver dysfunction include infection (both specifically in the liver as well as generalized sepsis), drug reactions, obstructive liver disease, hyperalimentation, and GVHD. When a liver biopsy is performed, it is as important to rule out other causes of liver diseases as it is to make a firm diagnosis of GVHD, since these patients usually have a diagnosis of GVHD of another organ and frequently have the features of GVHD modified by immunosuppressive GVHD therapy at the time that the biopsy is performed.

GVHD in the liver is predominantly a bile duct destructive lesion, with hepatocellular involvement being variable.[5,6,88,101,106] The bile duct damage is identical to that seen in liver transplant rejection, but, because of the immunologic status of these patients, inflammation is much less intense, usually consisting of a few lymphocytes within the bile duct wall. Endothelialitis may also be seen in GVHD, although it is much less common and more subtle owing to the generalized paucity of inflammatory cells available for mobilization. Hepatocellular damage, when present, consists of ballooning degeneration, focal necrosis, and acidophil bodies, similar to viral hepatitis. Thus, when significant hepatocellular necrosis is present, the possibility of viral hepatitis is difficult to exclude, since some bile duct damage can be seen in viral hepatitis. As a general rule, GVHD is characterized by extensive bile duct damage with mild hepatocellular involvement, whereas acute hepatitis has minimal bile duct damage with predominate hepatocellular destruction. Hepatic GVHD has been graded by the degree of bile duct damage (Grades 1 to 4 representing quartiles of bile duct loss) but has not been shown to serve any purpose other than giving some estimate of the certainty of the diagnosis.

Infection of either bacterial, viral, fungal, or protozoal origin may affect the liver. Liver involvement in bacterial infection usually takes the form of so-called cholestasis of sepsis, a bland cholestatic process without actual destruction or even invasion of the liver by the organism.[129] Occasionally, bacterial abscesses may be seen. Fungal abscesses can be detected by liver biopsy, although they are much more commonly identified at autopsy. Occasionally, a protozoan such as toxoplasmosis will involve the liver. Among the viruses, the more unusual virions of the herpes group are common, and hepatitis A,B, or non-A,non-B may also occur. The herpesviruses produce characteristic histologic findings that should not cause problems in the differential diagnosis of GVHD. Herpes simplex and varicella zoster produce random areas of discrete confluent necrosis with eosinophilic ground-glass nuclear inclusions in the adjacent hepatocytes. CMV may produce confluent necrosis but more commonly is recognized by the characteristic amphophilic to basophilic nuclear inclusions with a surrounding halo, with small amphophilic cytoplasmic inclusions without extensive necrosis. CMV may be seen in any cell type but are most often seen in hepatocytes that are surrounded by neutrophils, making them easily identifiable at low power (Fig. 26-22).[121] When doubt occurs regarding the presence of inclusions, the immunoperoxidase method may be used to confirm

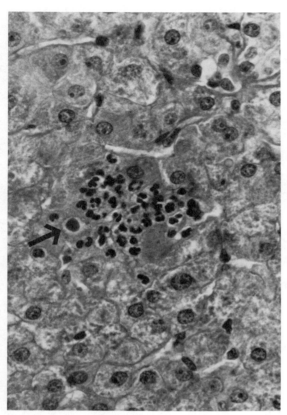

FIGURE 26-22.   Cytomegalovirus hepatitis. An intranuclear inclusion (arrow) *is surrounded by polymorphonuclear cells (hematoxylin and eosin × 480).*

the diagnosis.[29] Adenovirus has been reported to cause extensive bile duct damage. At present, there is no readily available antibody for immunohistochemical detection of adenovirus, and the inclusions are not usually definitive, so culture is necessary to make the diagnosis.

A variety of drug reactions may involve the liver, and bile duct damage as a component of drug toxicity is quite common. We have seen cases of probable Bactrim toxicity that mimicked GVHD except for the presence of abundant eosinophils, which should alert one to the possibility of a drug reaction.

At the present time, there are no data to indicate that cytoreductive therapy causes changes in the liver simulating GVHD. However, the number of biopsies taken in the first 20 days post-transplant are limited. Cytoreductive therapy with a variety of chemotherapeutic agents and radiation therapy has, however, been linked to development of veno-occlusive disease (VOD).[6,91] VOD consists of the oc-

clusion of the central hepatic veins by a fibrotic process resulting in central congestion, hepatocellular necrosis, and ascites. In some centers, the reported incidence is as high as 20% of all transplants done for malignancy; in our experience, it is considerably lower, perhaps owing to differences in diagnostic criteria.[64,65] Biopsy is considered hazardous in these patients because of the potential problem of bleeding; thus, the diagnosis is made on the basis of ascites, liver function abnormalities, and/or hepatosplenomegaly without other cause. These are not specific findings and may be simulated by nodular regenerative hyperplasia (NRH), the diffuse involvement of the liver by nodules of regenerating hepatocytes without fibrosis.[113] NRH seems to be the result of a variety of hepatic insults, with corticosteroids being the most common putative agent. While NRH may present with hepatosplenomegaly, ascites, and liver function abnormalities, it is usually a self-limited process. The abnormalities are milder than in cases of documented VOD and may account for reported cases of nonfatal VOD. If the changes of VOD are present in a liver biopsy, the differential diagnosis of congestive liver disease must be taken into consideration, including heart failure and the Budd-Chiari syndrome.[91]

Chronic GVHD

Chronic GVHD was originally defined by its occurrence more than 100 days post-transplant, but this distinction is artificial because it may occur before Day 100. Chronic GVHD is better defined by its characteristic pattern of organ involvement and histologic changes. Whereas acute GVHD is limited in its organ involvement, the pattern of organ involvement in chronic GVHD is much wider.[92] Acute GVHD can be thought of as a predominantly epithelial destructive phenomenon, whereas chronic GVHD is predominantly a fibrosing process with or without significant epithelial destruction.

Although acute and chronic GVHD appear to be separate processes, approximately 70% of chronic GVHD is preceded by one or more bouts of acute GVHD; the remaining 30% of cases have no history of prior acute GVHD. It is probable that prior tissue damage provides the stimulus for the development of chronic disease. This is best exemplified in the skin, where chronic GVHD has been reported to follow the distribution of sun exposure, of prior measles exanthem, and of tight fitting garments, all possible sources of tissue injury.[27,85]

Skin.   Chronic GVHD of the skin is classified as generalized or localized, based on extent of involvement.[85] The early form of generalized disease presents as an erythematous rash or as hyperkaratotic papules similar to lichen planus. The skin lesions, which are frequently accompanied by lichenoid lesions of the oral mucosa and nail changes, histologically resemble lichen planus and/or lupus erythematosus. The features include hyperkeratosis, basal cell degeneration, a lymphoid inflammatory response with exocytosis, and fibrosis of the papillary dermis with inflammatory involvement of adnexal structures. The intensity of the inflammatory response, involvement of adnexa, and fibrosis distinguish chronic from acute GVHD. The mucosal lesions are also similar to lichen planus, although the inflammatory response may be less intense.

In the later stages, fibrosis becomes the predominant feature. It begins in the papillary dermis, which helps to distinguish chronic GVHD from scleroderma. Eventually, the entire dermis and subcutaneous tissue are involved, resulting in a "hidebound" appearance to the skin. The epidermis becomes atrophic, inflammation is minimal, and, at this stage, the disease grossly resembles scleroderma (Fig. 26-23). In addition to the fibrosis, there may be pigmentary incontinence resulting in alternating hypo- and hyperpigmentation. Needless to say, in order to appreciate the complete histologic picture at this stage, a full thickness biopsy rather than a punch biopsy is needed.

The localized form of chronic GVHD resembles localized scleroderma or may have small patches of hyperpigmentation. The mouth and nails are usually not involved. Histologically, there is hyalinization and fibrosis of the reticular dermis, with little or no involvement of the upper dermis or epidermis. The localized form remains localized or undergoes remission rather than progressing to the more generalized form.

Liver. As with acute GVHD, the clinical and laboratory findings of chronic hepatic GVHD are nonspecific. The differential diagnosis is the same as for acute disease except that VOD is not a major consideration.

Chronic GVHD is characterized by marked bile duct damage and a dense portal inflammatory infiltrate, predominantly lymphocytic and plasmacellular. Both features are more prominent than in acute disease.[106] Hepatocellular damage is minimal and may consist of focal necrosis, although piecemeal necrosis is more common. With the exception of the more extensive bile duct damage, there is little to distinguish chronic active hepatitis of viral origin from chronic GVHD. However, patients will rarely have chronic GVHD limited to the liver; thus, the clinical situation will help determine the etiology.

Cirrhosis is a rare complication of GVHD. More common is the paucity of bile duct syndrome with near-total destruction of the interlobular bile ducts and minimal inflammation, a situation similar to that found in chronic liver transplant rejection. Obliterative endarteritis of the type seen in chronic liver

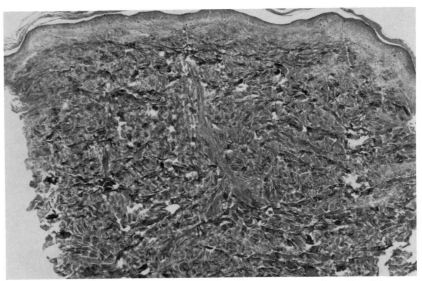

FIGURE 26-23.   *Chronic cutaneous graft-versus-host disease (GVHD). The epidermis is atrophic, and the dermis is heavily collagenized with destruction of adnexal structures (hematoxylin and eosin × 30).*

transplant rejection does not appear to be a feature of chronic hepatic GVHD.

Salivary and Lacrimal Glands.   Involvement of the salivary and lacrimal glands by chronic GVHD is a common problem and leads to the sicca syndrome.[87] Biopsy of lip or buccal mucosa containing minor salivary glands reveals a lymphocytic infiltrate with destruction of acinar and duct epithelium and eventual fibrosis (Fig. 26-24). These findings are identical to those seen in Sjögren's syndrome. In the diagnosis of chronic GVHD, the lip or buccal biopsy may provide information that obviates the need for more invasive biopsies.

Gastrointestinal Tract.   Symptomatic involvement of the gastrointestinal tract by chronic GVHD is much less common than in acute GVHD. Epithelial destruction in the form of single-cell necrosis rarely occurs in patients who have chronic GVHD.[107] Fibrosis of the submucosa and subserosa is the characteristic picture. This results in dysphagia secondary to esophageal involvement and occasionally malabsorption with areas of stricture of the small and large bowel.[66] Because the pathology lies in the submucosa, endoscopic biopsies of the gastrointestinal tract are of little value in the diagnosis of chronic GVHD.

Lung.   Involvement of the lung by GVHD is a controversial subject. An early report of lymphocytic bronchitis as a specific feature of GVHD has not been supported by other studies.[7,38] Obstructive bronchiolitis has been reported as a manifestation of chronic GVHD.[48,81,83] In some of these cases, viral infection appeared to be an inducing factor, with the offending agent being adenovirus, a virus with proclivity to involve the tracheobronchial tree. It appears that in some cases, the obstructive lesion represents chronic GVHD targeted to the bronchi in the same manner that cutaneous chronic GVHD has been limited to areas of measles exanthem.

Other Organs.   Both heart and kidney have been reported to show fibrosing arteritis as a manifestation of chronic GVHD, a process said to resemble scleroderma of these organs.[32] Lymph nodes have been reported to show evidence of depletion in chronic GVHD, a feature that correlates somewhat with the increased prevalence of infection in patients suffering from the disease.[92] That this actually represents an attack on the lymphoid tissue seems unlikely, since it is of donor origin. It may be secondary phenomenon.

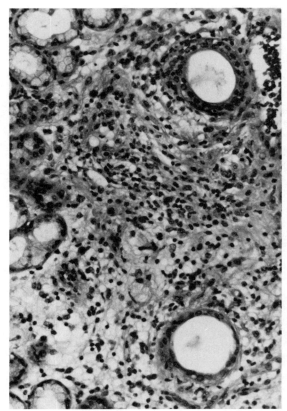

FIGURE 26-24.   *Chronic graft-versus-host disease (GVHD) of minor salivary gland. The acinar tissue has been focally destroyed by a lymphocytic infiltrate. This Sjögren-like picture is typical of chronic GVHD (hematoxylin and eosin × 190).*

Summary of Histologic Features of Rejection/GVHD

The histologic features of rejection as well as chronic GVHD result from a cellular and/or humorally mediated immune response directed against specific HLA antigens and thus bear certain similarities regardless of organ involved. Although the target for acute GVHD is not known, many of the features of this process are similar to those just mentioned.

Hyperacute rejection is characterized by a predominantly polymorphonuclear infiltrate in association with immunoglobulin deposition and arteritis and fibrin thrombi with associated ischemic tissue damage. It has not been identified in lung or pancreas transplantation, although it would be expected to occur in these organs. It has also not been seen as a manifestation of GVHD, although since the process is dependent upon preformed antibodies against the target, it would not be expected to occur under these circumstances.

Acute rejection, as well as acute GVHD, is characterized by a predominately lymphocytic infiltrate with damage to vascular endothelium as well as selected epithelial or mesenchymal target cells, including the tubules of the kidney, bile ducts of the liver, acinar and ductal structures of the pancreas, myocytes of the heart, bronchioles of the lung, and keratinocytes of the skin and gastrointestinal epi-thelial cells in the case of GVHD. Arteritis may be seen and, in general, indicates a more severe grade of rejection.

Chronic rejection, as well as chronic GVHD, is characterized by fibrosing endarteritis with parenchymal destruction and fibrosis. By definition, chronic rejection is an irreversible process, although the same is not necessarily true of chronic GVHD.

REFERENCES

1. Amend WJC, Vincenti F, Feduska NJ et al: Recurrent systemic lupus erythematosus involving renal allografts. Ann Intern Med 94:444, 1981

2. Axelsen RA, Seymour AE, Mathew TH et al: Glomerular transplant rejection: A distinctive pattern of early graft damage. Clin Nephrol 23:1, 1985

3. Baumgartner D, Burger HR, Binswanger U et al: Routine fine needle aspiration biopsy adds clinically relevant information for evaluation and treatment of renal transplant recipients with primary oliguria. Transplant Proc 17:2080, 1985

4. Belitsky P, Campbell J, Gupta R: Serial biopsy controlled evaluation of fine needle aspiration in renal allograft rejection. Lab Invest 53:580, 1985

5. Bernuau D, Gisselbrecht C, Devergie A et al: Histological and ultrastructural appearance of the liver during graft-versus-host disease complicating bone marrow transplantation. Transplantation 29:236, 1980

6. Beschorner WE, Pino J, Boitnott JK et al: Pathology of liver with bone marrow transplantation: Effects of busulfan, carmustine, acute graft-versus-host disease and cytomegalovirus infection. Am J Pathol 99:369, 1980

7. Beschorner WE, Saral R, Hutchins GM et al: Lymphocytic bronchitis associated with graft-versus-host disease in recipients of bone marrow transplants. N Engl J Med 299:1030, 1978

8. Billingham ME: Diagnosis of cardiac rejection by endomyocardial biopsy. Heart Transplant 1:25, 1982

9. Billingham ME: Some recent advances in cardiac pathology. Hum Pathol 10:367, 1979

10. Burke CM, Morris AJR, Dawkins KD et al: Late airflow obstruction in heart-lung transplantation recipients. Heart Transplant 4:437, 1985

11. Cameron JS: Glomerulonephritis in renal transplants. Transplantation 34:237, 1982

12. Campos H, Droz D, Debure A et al: Fine needle aspiration biopsy in the follow-up of kidney transplant recipients. Transplant Proc 17:2077, 1985

13. Canafax DM, Torres A, Fryd DS et al: The effects of delayed function on recipients of cadaver renal allografts: A study of 158 patients randomized to cyclosporine or ALG-azathioprine. Transplantation 41:177, 1986

14. Caves PK, Stinson EB, Graham AF et al: Percutaneous transvenous endomyocardial biopsy. JAMA 225:288, 1973

15. Cheigh JS, Mouradian J, Susin M et al: Kidney transplant nephrotic syndrome: Relationship between allograft histopathology and natural course. Kidney Int 18:358, 1980

16. Cooksey G, Reeve RS, Wenham PW et al: Comparison of fine needle aspiration cytology with histology in the diagnosis of renal allograft rejection. In Kreis H, Droz D (eds): Renal Transplant Cytology. Milano, Wichtig Editore, 1984

17. Corman JL, Putnam CW, Iwatsuki S et al: Liver allograft: Its use in chronic active hepatitis with macronodular cirrhosis, hepatitis B surface antigen. Arch Surg 114:75, 1979

18. Curtis JJ, Bhathena D, Lucas BA et al: "Hyperacute rejection" due to perfusion injury. Clin Nephrol 7:120, 1976

19. Dawkins KD, Oldershaw PJ, Billingham ME et al: Changes in diastolic function as a noninvasive marker of cardiac allograft rejection. Heart Transplant 3:287, 1984

20. Demetris AJ, Lasky S, Van Thiel DH et al: Pathology of hepatic transplantation. A review of 62 adult allograft recipients immunosuppressed with a cyclosporine/steroid regimen. Am J Pathol 118:151, 1985

21. Dubernard J-M, Traeger J, Bosi E et al: Transplantation for the treatment of insulin-dependent diabetes: Clinical experience with polymer-obstructed pancreatic grafts using neoprene. World J Surg 8:262, 1984

22. Dubernard J-M, Traeger J, Touraine JL et al: Rejection of human pancreatic allografts. Transplant Proc 12:103, 1980

23. Eddy A, Sibley R, Mauer SM et al: Renal allograft failure due to recurrent dense intramembranous deposit disease. Clin Nephrol 21:305, 1984

24. Eggink HF, Hofstee N, Gips CH et al: Histopathology of serial graft biopsies from liver transplant recipients. Am J Pathol 114:18, 1984

25. Epstein RJ, McDonald GB, Sale GE et al: The diagnostic accuracy of the rectal biopsy in acute graft-versus-host disease: A prospective study of thirteen patients. Gastroenterology 78:764, 1980

26. Farnsworth A, Hall BM, Ng ABP et al: Renal biopsy

morphology in renal transplantation. Am J Surg Pathol 8:243, 1984

27. Fenyk JR, Smith LM, Warkentin PI et al: Sclerodermatous graft-versus-host disease limited to an area of measles exanthem. Lancer 1:472, 1978

28. Ferguson RM, Sommer BG: Cyclosporine in renal transplantation: A single institutional experience. Am J Kidney Dis 5:296, 1985

29. Foucar E, Mukai K, Foucar K et al: Colon ulceration in lethal cytomegalovirus infection. Am J Clin Pathol 76:788, 1981

30. Freese D, Ascher N, Bloomer J et al: The role of liver biopsy in the accurate evaluation of post-liver transplant patients. Gastroenterology 86:1318, 1984

31. Frizzera G, Hanto DW, Gajl-Peczalska KJ et al: Polymorphic diffuse B-cell hyperplasias and lymphomas in renal transplant recipients. Cancer Res 41:4262, 1981

32. Furst DE, Clements PJ, Graze P et al: A syndrome resembling progressive systemic sclerosis after bone marrow transplantation: A model for scleroderma? Arthritis Rheum 22:904, 1979

33. Gokel JM: Simultaneous pancreas and kidney transplantation in man—graft morphology. Horm Metab Res (Suppl) 13:76, 1983

34. Gokel JM, Reichart B, Struck E: Human cardiac transplantation—evaluation of morphological changes in serial endomyocardial biopsies. Pathol Res Pract 179:354, 1985

35. Griepp RB, Stinson EB, Bieber CP et al: Control of graft arteriosclerosis in human heart transplant recipients. Surgery 81:262, 1977

36. Griffith BP, Hardesty RL, Deeb GM et al: Cardiac transplantation with Cyclosporin A and prednisone. Ann Surg 196:324, 1982

37. Gryzan S, Paradis IL, Hardesty RL et al: Bronchoalveolar lavage in heart–lung transplantation. Heart Transplant 4:414, 1985

37a. Habib R, Hebert D, Gagnadoux MF et al: Transplantation in idiopathic nephrosis. Transplant Proc 14:489, 1982

38. Hackman RC, Sale GE: Large airway inflammation as a possible manifestation of a pulmonary graft-versus-host reaction in bone marrow allograft recipients. Lab Invest 44:27A, 1981

39. Hall BM, Bishop GA, Farnsworth A et al: Identification of the cellular subpopulations infiltrating rejecting cadaver renal allografts. Preponderance of the T4 subset of T cells. Transplantation 37:564, 1984

40. Hammer C, Land W, Stadler J et al: Lymphocyte subclasses in rejecting kidney grafts detected by monoclonal antibodies. Transplant Proc 15:356, 1983

41. Hancock WW, Thomson NM, Atkins RC: Monoclonal antibody analysis of interstitial cell infiltrate during human renal allograft rejection. Transplant Proc 15:352, 1983

42. Hebert D, Sibley RK, Mauer SM: Recurrence of hemolytic uremic syndrome in renal transplant recipients. Kidney Int 30:S51, 1986

43. Honkanen E, Tornroth T, Pettersson E et al: Glomerulonephritis in renal allografts: Results of 18 years of transplantations. Clin Nephrol 21:210, 1984

44. Hsu AC, Arbus GS, Noriega E et al: Renal allograft biopsy: A satisfactory adjunct for predicting renal function after graft rejection. Clin Nephrol 5:260, 1976

45. Hsu H-C, Suzuki Y, Churg J et al: Ultrastructure of transplant glomerulopathy. Histopathology 4:351, 1980

46. Humes HD, Jackson NM, O'Connor RP et al: Pathogenetic mechanisms of nephrotoxicity: Insights into cyclosporine nephrotoxicity. Transplant Proc 17:51, 1985

47. Jamieson SW, Oyer P, Baldwin J et al: Heart transplantation for end-stage ischemic heart disease: The Stanford experience. Heart Transplant 3:224, 1984

48. Johnson FL, Stokes DC, Ruggiero M et al: Chronic obstructive airway disease after bone marrow transplantation. J Pediatr 105:370, 1984

49. Kjellstrand CM, Casali RE, Simmons RL et al: Etiology and prognosis in acute post-transplant renal failure. Am J Med 61:190, 1976

50. Klintmalm G, Sundelin B, Bohman S-O et al: Interstitial fibrosis in renal allografts after 12 to 46 months of cyclosporine treatment: Beneficial effect of low doses in early post-transplantation period. Lancet 2:950, 1984

51. Kloppel G, Bommer G, Commandeur G et al: The endocrine pancreas in chronic pancreatitis. Virchows Arch A 377:157, 1978

52. Kolbeck PC, Tatum AH, Sanfilippo F: Relationships among the histologic pattern, intensity, and phenotypes of T cells infiltrating renal allografts. Transplantation 38:709, 1984

53. Koller C, Hammer C, Gokel JM et al: Correlation between core biopsy and aspiration cytology. Transplant Proc 16:1298, 1984

54. Land W, Gebhardt Ch, Gall FP et al: Pancreatic duct obstruction with prolamine solution. Transplant Proc 12:72, 1980

55. Levy M, Charpenteir B, le group cooperlif de transplantation de l'lle de France: De novo membranous glomerulonephritis in renal allograft. Report of 19 cases in 1550 transplant recipients. Trans Proc 15:1099, 1983

56. Limas C, Spector D, Wright JR: Histologic changes in preserved cadaveric renal transplants. Am J Pathol 88:403, 1977

57. Macoviak JA, Oyer PE, Stinson EB et al: Four-year experience with cyclosporine for heart and heart-lung transplantation. Transplant Proc 17:97, 1985

58. Manivel C, Filipovich A, Snover DC: Cryptosporidiosis as a cause of diarrhea following bone marrow transplantation. Dis Colon Rectum 28:741, 1985

59. Maizel SE, Sibley RK, Horstman JP et al: Incidence and significance of recurrent focal segmental glomerulosclerosis in renal allograft recipients. Transplantation 32:512, 1981

60. Mason JW: Techniques for right and left ventricular endomyocardial biopsy. Am J Cardiol 41:887, 1978

61. Matas AJ, Sibley R, Mauer SM et al: Pre-discharge, post-transplant kidney biopsy does not predict rejection. J Surg Res 32:269, 1982

62. Matas AJ, Sibley R, Mauer SM et al: The value of needle renal allograft biopsy. 1. A retrospective study of biopsies performed during putative rejection episodes. Ann Surg 197:226, 1983

63. Mathew TH, Mathews DC, Hobbs JB et al: Glomerular lesions after renal transplantation. Am J Med 59:177, 1975

64. McDonald GB, Sharma P, Matthews DE et al: Venoocclusive disease of the liver after bone marrow transplantation: Diagnosis, incidence, and predisposing factors. Hepatology 4:116, 1984

65. McDonald GB, Sharma P, Matthews DE et al: The clinical course of 53 patients with venoocclusive disease of the liver after marrow transplantation. Transplantation 39:603, 1985

66. McDonald GB, Sullivan KM, Schuffler MD et al: Esophageal abnormalities in chronic graft-versus-host disease in humans. Gastroenterology 80:914, 1981

67. Merion RM, Calne RY: Allograft renal vein thrombosis. Transplant Proc 17:1746, 1985

68. Mihatsch MJ, Thiel G, Basler V et al: Morphological patterns in cyclosporine-treated renal transplant recipients. Transplant Proc 17:101, 1985

69. Moran M, Tomlanovich S, Myers BD: Cyclosporine-induced chronic nephropathy in human recipients of cardiac allografts. Transplant Proc 17:185, 1985

70. Morzycka M, Croker BP, Siegler HF et al: Evaluation of recurrent glomerulonephritis in kidney allografts. Am J Med 72:588, 1982

71. Najarian JS, Fryd DS, Strand M et al: A single institution, randomized, prospective trial of cyclosporine versus azathioprine-antilymphocyte globulin for immunosuppression in renal allograft recipients. Ann Surg 201:142, 1985

72. Neild GH, Ivory K, Williams DG: Glomerular thrombosis and cortical infarction in cyclosporine-treated rabbits with acute serum sickness. Br J Exp Pathol 65:133, 1984

73. Neuberger J, Portmann B, Macdougall BR et al: Recurrence of primary biliary cirrhosis after liver transplantation. N Engl J Med 306:1, 1982

74. Paller MS, Murray BM: Renal dysfunction in animal models of cyclosporine toxicity. Transplant Proc 17:155, 1985

75. Palmer JM, Chatterjee SN: Urologic complications in renal transplantation. Surg Clin North Am 58:305, 1978

76. Parfrey PS, Kuo YL, Hanley JA et al: The diagnostic and prognostic value of renal allograft biopsy. Transplantation 38:586, 1984

77. Parkman R, Rappaport J, Rosen F: Human graft versus host disease. J Invest Dermatol 74:276, 1980

78. Platt JL, Ferguson RM, Sibley RK et al: Renal interstitial cell populations in cyclosporine nephrotoxicity.

79. Pomerance A, Stovin PGI: Heart transplant pathology: The British experience. J Clin Pathol 38:146, 1985

80. Richardson WP, Colvin RB, Cheeseman SH et al: Glomerulopathy associated with cytomegalovirus viremia in renal allografts. N Engl J Med 305:57, 1981

81. Roco J, Granena A, Rodriguez-Roisin R et al: Fatal airway disease in an adult with chronic graft-versus-host disease. Thorax 37:77, 1982

82. Rose ML, Gracie JA, Fraser A et al: Use of monoclonal antibodies to quantitate T lymphocyte subpopulations in human cardiac allografts. Transplantation 38:230, 1984

83. Rosenberg ME, Vercellotti GM, Snover DC et al: Bronchiolitis obliterans after bone marrow transplantation. Am J Hematol 18:325, 1985

84. Sale GE, Lerner KG, Barker EA et al: The skin biopsy in the diagnosis of acute graft-versus-host disease in man. Am J Pathol 89:621, 1977

85. Sale GE, Shulman HM: The Pathology of Bone Marrow Transplantation. New York, Masson Publishing USA Inc, 1984

86. Sale GE, Shulman HM, McDonald GB et al: Gastrointestinal graft-versus-host disease in man: A clinicopathological study of the rectal biopsy. Am J Surg Pathol 3:291, 1979

87. Sale GE, Shulman HM, Schubert MW et al: Oral and ophthalmic pathology of graft-versus-host disease in man: Predictive value of the lip biopsy. Hum Pathol 12:1022, 1981

88. Sale GE, Storb R, Kolb H: Histopathology of hepatic acute graft-versus-host disease in the dog: A double blind study confirms the specificity of small bile duct lesions. Transplantation 26:103, 1978

89. Scheinman JI, Najarian JS, Mauer SM: Successful strategies for renal transplantation in primary oxalosis. Kidney Int 25:804, 1984

90. Sharp HL, Snover DC, Burke BA et al: The role of clinical evaluation in graft rejection following liver transplantation. In Daum F (ed): Extrahepatic biliary atresia. New York, Marcel Dekker, 1983

91. Shulman HM, McDonald GB, Matthews D et al: An analysis of hepatic venoocclusive disease and centrilobular hepatic degeneration following bone marrow transplantation. Gastroenterolgy 79:1178, 1980

92. Shulman HM, Sullivan KM, Weiden PL et al: Chronic graft-versus-host syndrome in man: A long-term clinicopathologic study of twenty Seattle patients. Am J Med 69:24, 1980

93. Si L, Whiteside TL, Van Thiel DH et al: Lymphocyte subpopulations at the site of piecemeal necrosis in end-stage chronic liver diseases and rejecting liver allografts in cyclosporine treated patients. Lab Invest 50:341, 1984

94. Sibley RK, Ferguson RM, Sutherland DER et al: Morphology of cyclosporine nephrotoxicity and of acute rejection in cyclosporine-prednisone immunosup-

Identification using monoclonal antibodies. Transplantation 36:343, 1983

pressed renal allograft recipients. Transplant Proc 15:2836, 1983

95. Sibley RK, Olivari M-T, Ring WS et al: Endomyocardial biopsy in the cardiac allograft recipient. A review of 570 biopsies. Ann Surg 1986 203:177, 1986

96. Sibley RK, Payne W: Morphologic findings in the renal allograft biopsy. Semin Nephrol 5:294, 1985

97. Sibley RK, Rynasiewicz J, Ferguson RM et al: Morphology of cyclosporine nephrotoxicity and acute rejection in patients immuno-suppressed with cyclosporine and prednisone. Surgery 94:225, 1983

97a. Sibley RK, Sutherland DER: Pancreas transplantation: An immunohistologic and histopathologic examination of 100 grafts. Am J Pathol (in press, 1987)

98. Sibley RK, Sutherland DER, Goetz F et al: Recurrent diabetes mellitus in the pancreas iso- and allograft. Lab Invest 53:132, 1985

99. Siegl H, Ryffel B, Petric R et al: Cyclosporine, the renin-angiotensin-aldosterone system, and renal adverse reactions. Transplant Proc 15:2719, 1983

100. Simonton SC, Snover DC, Platt JF et al: In situ analysis of the inflammatory cell population in liver biopsies following liver transplantation. Lab Invest 52:63A, 1985

101. Slavin RE, Woodruff JM: The pathology of bone marrow transplantation. Pathol Ann 9:291, 1974

102. Snover DC: Mucosal damage simulating acute graft-versus-host reaction in cytomegalovirus colitis. Transplantation 39:669, 1985

103. Snover DC: Acute and chronic graft-versus-host disease: Histopathological evidence for two pathogenetic mechanisms. Hum Pathol 15:202, 1984

104. Snover DC, Filipovich AH, Ramsay NKC et al: Graft-versus-host-disease-like histopathological findings in pre-bone marrow transplantation biopsies of patients with severe T-cell deficiency. Transplantation 39:95, 1985

105. Snover DC, Sibley RK, Freese DK et al: Orthotopic liver transplantation: A pathological study of 63 serial liver biopsies from 17 patients with special reference to the diagnostic features and natural history of rejection. Hepatology 4:1212, 1984

106. Snover DC, Weisdorf SA, Ramsay NK et al: Hepatic graft-versus-host disease: A study of the predictive value of liver biopsy in diagnosis. Hepatology 4:123, 1984

107. Snover DC, Weisdorf SA, Vercellotti GM et al: The histopathology of gastric and small intestinal graft-versus-host disease following allogeneic bone marrow transplantation. Hum Pathol 16:387, 1985

108. Solez K, McGraw DJ, Beschorner WE et al: Reflections on use of the renal biopsy as the "Gold Standard" in distinguishing transplant rejection from cyclosporine nephrotoxicity. Transplant Proc (Suppl 1)17:123, 1985

109. Sommer BG, Innes JT, Whitehurst RM et al: Cyclosporine-associated renal arteriopathy resulting in loss of allograft function. Am J Surg 149:756, 1985

110. Spector D, Limas C, Frost JL et al: Perfusion nephropathy in human transplants. N Engl J Med 295:1217, 1976

111. Starzl TE, Iwatsuki S, Van Thiel DH et al: Evolution of liver transplantation. Hepatology 2:614, 1982

112. Striegel JE, Sibley RK, Fryd DS et al: Recurrence of focal segmental glomerulosclerosis in children with steroid resistant nephrotic syndrome following renal transplantation. Kidney Int 30:S-44, 1986

113. Strohmeyer WF, Ishak KG: Nodular transformation of the liver. Hum Pathol 12:60, 1981

114. Sturgill BC, Lobo PI, Bolton WK: Cold-reacting IgM antibody-induced renal allograft failure. Nephron 36:125, 1984

115. Sullivan BA, Hak LJ, Finn WF: Cyclosporine nephrotoxicity: Studies in laboratory animals. Transplant Proc 17:145, 1985

116. Sutherland DER, Goetz FC, Najaran JS: One hundred pancreas transplants at a single institution. Ann Surg 200:414, 1984

117. Taube D, Neild G, Hobby P et al: A comparison of the clinical, histophatologic, cytologic, and biochemical features of renal transplant rejection, cyclosporine A nephrotoxicity, and stable renal function. Transplant Proc 17:179, 1985

118. Thein SL, Goldman JM, Galton DAG: Acute "graft-versus-host disease" after autografting for chronic granulocytic leukemia in transformation. Ann Intern Med 94:210, 1981

119. Thomas ED, Storb R, Clift RA et al: Bone marrow transplantation. N Engl J Med 292:832, 1975

120. Vangelista A, Frasca GM, Stefoni S et al: Graft biopsy in renal transplantation: Correlation with clinical, immunological, and virological investigations. Kidney Int 23:S-41, 1983

121. Vanstapel M, Desmet VJ: Cytomegalovirus hepatitis: A histological and immunohistochemical study. Appl Pathol 1:41, 1983

122. von Willebrand E, Hayry P: Cyclosporin-A deposits in renal allografts. Lancet 2:189, 2983

123. Wajszczuk CP, Dummer JS, Ho M et al: Fungal infections in liver transplant recipients. Transplantation 40:347, 1985

124. Weintraub M, Masek M, Billingham ME: The lymphocyte subpopulations in cyclosporine-treated human heart rejection. Heart Transplant 4:213, 1985

125. Whiting PH, Thomson AW, Blair JT et al: Experimental Cyclosporin A nephrotoxicity. Br J Exp Pathol 63:88, 1982

126. Williams JW, Peters TG, Vera SR et al: Biopsy-directed immunosuppression following hepatic transplantation in man. Transplantation 39:589, 1985

127. Williams R, Smith M, Shilkin KB et al: Liver transplantaton in man: The frequency of rejection, biliary tract complications and recurrence of malignancy based on an analysis of 26 cases. Gastroenterology 64:1026, 1973

128. Yousem SA, Burke CM, Billingham ME: Pathologic pulmonary alterations in long-term human heart-lung transplantation. Hum Pathol 16:923, 1985

129. Zimmerman HJ, Fang M, Utili R et al: Jaundice due to bacterial infection. Gastroenterology 77:362, 1979

CHAPTER 27

Vascular Complications of Transplantation

Vivian A. Tellis   Arthur J. Matas   Frank J. Veith

Vascular complications of transplantation, reported to be as high as 30%, have diminished markedly. Donor nephrectomy should be done with minimal manipulation, and renal arteries should never be cannulated.

Recipient blood vessels should be adequately mobilized. Ex vivo conversion of multiple to a single artery will minimize warm ischemia, which in turn will reduce the incidence of acute tubular necrosis (ATN). Occlusion of the renal artery, recognized immediately, may be correctable, but delay leads to infarction. Clamp injury to the recipient vessel may require bypass. Small segment infarcts may be ignored, but larger ones lead to urine leaks and sepsis. Venous thrombosis, when diagnosed, can be treated by thrombectomy or anticoagulation, but with a high failure rate.

Renal artery stenosis is the major long-term vascular problem. The incidence rate varies from 1.5% to 12% in hypertensive patients, but up to 28% when routine angiography is done. Diagnosis is by angiography, usually for hypertension, but occasionally because of deteriorating renal function. Stenosis may result from technical errors in donor or recipient operation, disease, or immunologic causes. Correction of severe stenosis can be surgical or by balloon angioplasty, but each carries a risk of loss of kidney. Other complications occasionally occur, such as anastomotic pseudoaneurysms and renal arteriovenous fistulas, which usually result in loss of kidney. The patient's underlying disease, for example, diabetes mellitus, may also be a source of late vascular complications.

Renal transplantation is unique in that it requires the creation of two vascular suture lines in a person who is often anemic and protein deficient and with disordered coagulation parameters. The circumstances are made worse by the fact that these anastomoses are exposed to potentially contaminated urine, and the patient then receives immunosuppressive drugs, which may accentuate problems with healing, infection, and bleeding. What is remarkable, therefore, is not that vascular complications occur, but that the incidence is low. However, as the results of transplantation have improved, more high-risk patients are being transplanted. Thus, increased vigilance must be maintained, because some risk factors such as diabetes, peripheral vascular disease, or age over 50 years may increase the possibility of vascular complications.

In published reports, vascular complications have been noted in up to 30% of transplants;[11,13,22,27] however, the majority of these retrospective reports incorporate the early experience in transplantation, including the use of high-steroid dosage and the unavailability of many of the antibiotics used today. More recently, the Standards Committee of the American Society of Transplant Surgeons reported a 0.1% ± 0.3% incidence of vascular complications in a review of 881 transplants in multiple centers in the United States.[31]

Vascular complications may be arterial or venous, have consequences to the kidney and the host, and may occur as a result of underlying donor or recipient factors or because of the techniques used in harvesting, preservation, and reimplantation of the kidneys. Many complications can be prevented by thoughtful planning and careful technique.

PREVENTION OF COMPLICATIONS

Donor Factors

Infection in potential cadaver donors must be ruled out by review of the patient's course and by obtaining the appropriate cultures. Organs should be cooled in situ, and the kidneys should be removed by en bloc resection to minimize warm ischemia and to reduce the chance of overlooked arterial branches or avulsed venous tributaries.[6,33,37] En bloc resection also permits the maximal possible length of vessel to be made available, rendering the transplant operation easier and therefore safer. After nephrectomy, the vessels should be scrutinized for the presence of atheroma, which may influence the decision to use the kidney or the surgical technique to be used.

Kidneys may be preserved by simple cold storage or by pulsatile perfusion on a machine. Machine preservation requires the insertion of cannulae, which can cause intimal damage at the site of the securing ligature, at the tip of the cannula, and, distally, where the jet of perfusate hits the intima.[23] These problems can be avoided by using a modified "bull-dog" clamp that permits perfusion without cannulation or by cannulating the aorta, which is then used as a conduit.[4,6]

Recipient Factors

Potential recipients should be evaluated by careful physical examination and noninvasive tests for the presence of arterial or venous disease, which may influence the site selected for the transplant or perhaps mandate a prior corrective vascular procedure. If dialysis is unavoidable immediately preceding the transplant, "low-dose" heparin should be used, and the patient should be left in good fluid balance, rather than being depleted.

Perioperative antibiotics that cover common pathogens should be given in order to reduce the risk of sepsis from the transplantation of organs from donors whose cultures at nephrectomy are subsequently reported to be positive.[24] Hemostasis must be meticulous. The iliac artery and vein should be dissected out for an adequate distance to reduce the possibility of distortion of the anastomosis after the kidney is positioned. If the hypogastric artery is to be used, special care must be taken to ensure the absence of plaque at its origin. Plaque can be removed by endarterectomy, but, when it is present, the external iliac artery is probably a better anastomotic site. The latter should also be used in retransplantation when the contralateral hypogastric artery has been previously ligated in order to reduce the possibility of vasculogenic impotence.[2] The site of an external iliac arteriotomy must be planned so that when the kidney is placed in its final position, the renal artery is not distorted or kinked.

Before anastomosis, the kidney should be inspected for unligated blood vessels, tears, and undetected accessory arteries. If the artery has been cannulated, the entire portion that has been in contact with the cannula, not just the ligature site, should be excised.[23,27] If there are multiple vessels, some form of ex vivo anastomosis to fashion a single renal artery should be undertaken if possible.[19] Vascular clamps should be light in weight, and applied with the least amount of pressure necessary to occlude flow. The use of systemic heparin is unnecessary, and its use may lead to troublesome bleeding. Both vascular anastomoses should be performed with careful technique; inversion of adventitia into the venous lumen predisposes to thrombosis, while a careless arterial suture line may result in bleeding, thrombosis, or aneurysm formation. It is better to take a few minutes longer to complete a technically perfect suture line while the kidney is cold than to rush the anastomosis and be forced to reclamp a now warm kidney to correct hemorrhage from anastomotic defects. Special problems may be encountered when blood vessels are abnormally friable. In such instances, the use of Dacron felt pledgets may be necessary. Attempts at anastomosing very short segments of renal vein can result in tearing of the vein in the hilum as a result of excessive tension. We and other investigators have used short segments of autogenous or synthetic grafts to lengthen the vein and prevent such a catastrophe.[12,29] Before extraordinary technical feats are attempted, consideration should be given to the question of whether the risks are justified (such as in a highly cytotoxic recipient) or if the attempt to use a kidney with difficult vessels should be abandoned, in favor of a future, safer procedure.

All measures should be taken to minimize the incidence of acute tubular necrosis (ATN). These include adequate hydration of the donor before and during nephrectomy and of the recipient during the transplant. In addition to volume expansion, the use of loop and osmotic diuretics can also play a role in prevention of ATN.[35,37] If the anastomoses require a prolonged period of ischemia, the temperature of the kidney should be kept low by surface cooling. The patient in ATN usually requires dialysis postoperatively, and the need to use heparin for dialysis increases the risk of postoperative bleeding. In some patients, in spite of preoperative preparation, including adequate dialysis and a normal coagulation profile, troublesome oozing occurs throughout the operation. In such patients, the use of peritoneal dialysis should be considered, and, if the probability of dialysis is high, the peritoneal catheter can be inserted at the time of transplantation.

EARLY COMPLICATIONS

During the operation and in the early postoperative period, the usual manifestations of vascular complications are hemorrhage and occlusion.

Hemorrhage

Intraoperative hemorrhage is usually the result of an anastomotic defect or a missed branch. Management of hemorrhage is self-evident and consists of ligation of the responsible vessel or correction of the defective suture line. Occasionally, the entire anastomosis may have to be taken down and redone; in these instances, the kidney should be flushed and cooled before the anastomosis is begun.

Delayed hemorrhage has been reported up to 107 days after the procedure and may arise from arterial or venous sources, particularly in the presence of a wound infection.[11,22,26,27] Occasionally, exploration for bleeding within hours of operation may reveal an unligated hilar blood vessel or an anastomotic leak that has become apparent only after correction of hypovolemia. One instance has been reported in which a complete disruption of the venous anastomosis was successfully repaired.[22] An unusual, but dramatic, cause of massive hemorrhage is rupture of the kidney. There are numerous possible causes of rupture, some of which can be managed without loss of the kidney.[10]

One of the most common causes of late bleeding is infection, which results in anastomotic disruption and false aneurysm formation. The patient may present with a pulsatile mass but usually becomes hypotensive and complains of severe flank pain. There may be no external evidence of bleeding; occasionally, however, a herald bleed from the wound may precede the catastrophic event. In most series, this complication carries a high mortality.[11,22,26] Nephrectomy is the treatment of choice. If the infection involves an end-to-side anastomosis to

the external iliac artery, the artery should be ligated proximal and distal to the site, and excision of a segment may be required.[3] Attempts at repairing infected arterial suture lines that bleed uniformly eventuate in serious hemorrhage.[11,22,26]

Transplant nephrectomy deserves special mention, because, in many reported series, the mortality of hemorrhage after nephrectomy is as high as 50%, especially if infection had been present.[11,16,26,32] The likelihood of infections after nephrectomy is increased if the patient has had a urinary leak or been subjected to re-exploration in the period preceding the nephrectomy. In our experience, when wounds that had a substantial risk of contamination have been left open and perioperative antibiotics have been used, wound sepsis has been eliminated as a cause of death and serious morbidity.[15] The lesson is clear: Contaminated wounds should be left open or widely drained, and, if infection is suspected in an arterial suture line, the artery should be ligated. While failure to follow such a course leads to fatal bleeding, it has repeatedly been demonstrated that the external iliac artery in most transplanted patients can be ligated without threatening the ipsilateral limb.[3,26,32] In the few patients who later develop claudication, some form of extra-anatomic bypass can be performed.

Occlusion

Arterial occlusion following transplantation may occur as a result of mechanical trauma to the vessels during organ removal and preservation, from technical errors during performance of the anastomoses, or from clamp injury to diseased arteries. If the injury is to the hypogastric artery, the hypogastric artery should be ligated and the renal artery reimplanted into the external iliac artery. If the latter has been used for the anastomosis and the injury occurs distally, the kidney is unaffected, although the patient may require a subsequent bypass for limb ischemia (Fig. 27-1). Clamp injury proximal to the anastomosis presents a more difficult problem, jeopardizing the kidney as well as the limb. Among the choices are endarterectomy and intimal flap repair. In addition, we have been able to salvage a kidney in a patient with proximal clamp injury by replacing the involved segment with a segment of synthetic material and reimplanting the renal artery. Prior to repair, the kidney was flushed with cold Collins' solution after venting and clamping the vein.

Arterial occlusion occurring shortly after the operation almost invariably results in loss of the kidney. When a patient develops anuria in the recovery room and the possibility of arterial occlusion

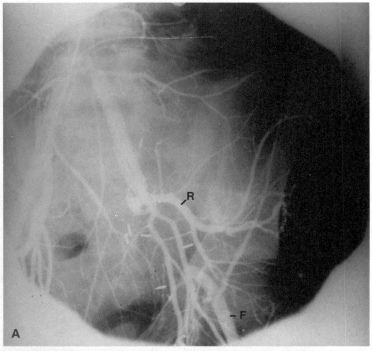

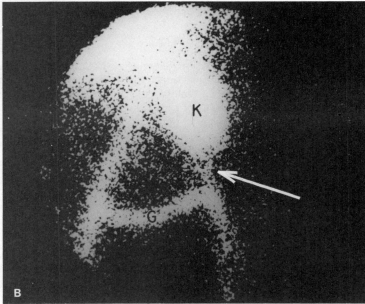

FIGURE 27-1. *(A) Segmental occlusion of distal left external iliac artery demonstrated by right percutaneous transfemoral arteriogram. The renal artery (R) is well perfused, and the femoral artery (F) is reconstituted by collaterals. No treatment is necessary. (B) Radionuclide angiogram showing patent femorofemoral bypass graft (G) done for limb ischemia in another patient following occlusion of external iliac artery (arrow). The kidney (K) continues to be well perfused.*

is seriously entertained, the most expedient approach is to return immediately to the operating room and inspect the anastomosis. Although investigations such as radionuclide scanning or arteriography can help establish the diagnosis, the inevitable delays in arranging and performing such tests only add to the ischemic insult and increase the chances that the kidney will be nonviable. However, there have been reports of successful revascularization of kidneys after ischemic periods of as long as 5.5 hours. Presumably, the occlusion was only partial during some of that time.[25]

Whereas arterial occlusion in the first few hours after surgery is usually a result of technical or mechanical factors, arterial thrombosis that occurs later is often a manifestation of an immunologic process. In addition, there have been recent reports that the administration of cyclosporine has been associated with an increased incidence of unexplained late arterial occlusions.[30] The greater the interval between transplantation and the occurrence of occlusion, the better is the chance that successful revascularization can be surgically achieved, since collateral circulation has had a chance to develop. Several such experiences have been reported from 4 to 50 months after transplantation.[25,34,38] Kidneys that show no evidence of function or those that undergo severe rejection episodes followed by prolonged anuria should be monitored at frequent intervals by radionuclide scanning. At the first sign of total loss of perfusion, nephrectomy should be done before the kidney becomes necrotic.

Segmental infarction occurs when one of several renal arteries or branches is occluded. This may be recognized and accepted at the time of transplantation when the area supplied is small. When a large area is supplied, the resultant loss of substance may include the collecting system and result in a pyelocutaneous fistula.[11] These possibilities should be weighed before the decision is made to use a kidney with multiple arteries. A kidney with an occluded lower polar artery should not be used because of the unacceptably high risk of pelvic or ureteral slough.

Venous occlusion may occur from extrinsic compression or technical error or as an extension of deep venous thrombosis.[7,11,13,22,27] Because the features of venous thrombosis, namely swelling of the kidney and proteinuria, are indistinguishable from those of rejection, the diagnosis is difficult to make. A sudden decrease in urine output associated with proteinuria should raise suspicion. All instances of significant swelling of one or both extremities should be investigated by plethysmography and, if necessary, venography, so that appropriate action can be taken (Fig. 27-2).

Successful venous thrombectomy has been reported, but most cases require nephrectomy.[5,13,22,27] Anticoagulation has been successfully used in cases in which considerable time has elapsed after the transplant.[9] Long-term anticoagulation is necessary to reduce the risk of pulmonary embolism.

DELAYED COMPLICATIONS

Renal Artery Stenosis (RAS)

The major long-term vascular problem following transplantation is renal artery stenosis (RAS). The

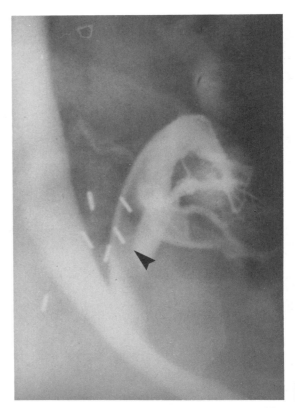

FIGURE 27-2.   *Venogram showing thrombus* (arrow) *within lumen of renal vein.*

possible causes, clinical features, and methods of management of this problem continue to attract interest and controversy. In patients being investigated for hypertension, the incidence has varied between 1% and 16%.[8,13,14,27] However, when routine post-transplantation arteriography is performed, up to a 25% incidence of angiographically detectable RAS is seen (Table 27-1).[17] In one series, 28% of 43 normotensive patients were found to have stenosis on routine digital subtraction angiography (DSA).[8]

The diagnosis of RAS is most commonly suspected when hypertension develops in a previously normotensive person or when hypertension that is already present becomes more difficult to control. Renal function is not necessarily impaired, but, occasionally, RAS may present as a slow deterioration of function, concomitant with hypertension.[14,36] This combination may be mistaken for chronic rejection and left untreated. For example, the patient represented in Figure 27-3 was previously thought to have chronic rejection; however, renal function returned to normal after correction of renal artery stenosis. Before a decision is made to abandon or remove such a kidney, a biopsy should be done; a

TABLE 27-1   *Incidence of Documented Renal Artery Stenosis*

AUTHORS	TYPE OF STUDY	NUMBER OF TRANSPLANTS	NUMBER OF STENOSES	%
Jordan et al[13]	Retrospective	341	17	4.9
Kauffman et al[14]	Retrospective	142	17	12
Palleschi et al[27]	Retrospective	600	9	1.5
Baumgartner et al[1]	Retrospective	779	26	3.3
Tilney et al[36]	Retrospective	914	25	2.7
Lacombe[17]	Retrospective	306	38	12.4
Lacombe[17]	Prospective	100	23	23
Fries et al[8]	Prospective	84*	23	36.5

* 21 angiograms inadequate for evaluation

TABLE 27-2   *Treatment of Renal Artery Stenosis*

	OPERATION		DILATATION	
AUTHORS	No. of Patients	Successful	No. of Patients	Successful
Jordan et al[13]	8	5	4	4
Lacombe[17]	14	10	—	—
Kauffman et al[14]	14	10	3	2
Mollenkopf et al[20]	—	—	17	12
Tilney et al[36]	21	14	5	0
Baumgartner et al[1]	21	21	5	4

histologic picture of well-preserved renal morphology increases the indication for angiography.[36] Conversely, if a kidney shows severe rejection changes, aggressive treatment of RAS is probably not justified.

Whenever the possibility of RAS is considered, an arteriogram should be performed. In some hands, DSA has proved to be an effective method of evaluation for RAS.[8] Digital techniques are relatively noninvasive and cheaper and do not require hospitalization. On the other hand, DSA does not always provide adequate visualization, and a conventional arteriogram may be necessary. In most instances, the site of the stenosis appears to be in the donor artery distal to the anastomosis. Stenosis of the anastomosis itself also occurs, as well as kinks or disease in the recipient artery.[13,14,17,22,36] Occasionally, multiple stenotic sites are noted. We believe that RAS, like other complications, is often preventable. Avoidance of renal artery cannulation, excision of cannulated segments, recognition of occlusive disease in the recipient, and meticulous technique in performing the anastomosis and positioning the kidney will obviate many of the problems. In spite of such precautions, RAS still occurs, sometimes along elongated segments of the donor vessel and, occasionally, at multiple sites (Fig. 27-4A). Among the reasons postulated for such lesions

are immunologic phenomena affecting the donor renal artery and unrecognized trauma to the vessels, with subsequent subintimal fibrosis.[13,14,17,23,36]

The management of stenosis has generated considerable discussion. Because each of the method of correcting stenosis has significant risk to the kidney, most centers first attempt to control hypertension by drug therapy. Only those patients failing medical management undergo angiography and, if necessary, definitive treatment. Severely stenotic lesions, however, must be corrected because of the side-effects of multiple antihypertensive drugs, the loss of renal function, and the risk of sudden occlusion of the artery with loss of the kidney. Two basic approaches are possible: percutaneous transluminal angioplasty (PTA) dilatation and surgical correction (Table 27-2). In experienced hands, PTA can be done with a minimum of risk (Figs. 27-3 and 27-4); however, considerable skill and judgment are required in selecting and positioning the catheter and gauging the amount of pressure to be exerted. Temporary renal dysfunction may occur, and the possibility exists that part or all of the renal circulation may be destroyed. Disruption of the vessel, as well as complications related to the arterial puncture and passage of the catheter, may occur. However, we, as well as other investigators, have reported excellent results with this approach.[1,13,20,38]

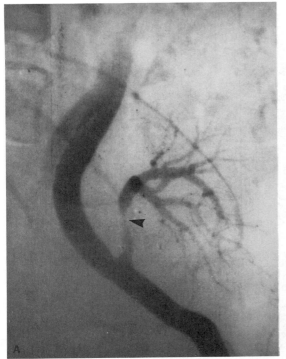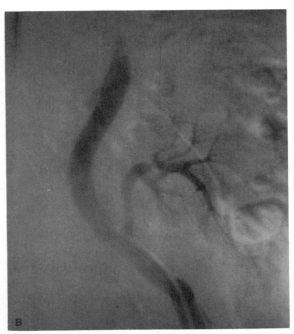

FIGURE 27-3.   Subtraction film from percutaneous transfemoral arteriogram done for hypertension and creatinine rise thought to be due to chronic rejection unresponsive to steroid therapy. (A) Severe stenosis of renal artery (arrow). (B) Following successful PTA, there was complete resolution of stenosis. The patient became normotensive, and the serum creatinine level dropped.

PTA should not be attempted without standby preparations for urgent surgical intervention in case of complications. In most cases, failure of PTA does not preclude surgical correction; however, irreversible damage owing to complications from PTA has been reported.[18]

Reoperation for RAS following transplantation is difficult and poses the hazard of loss of kidney. When the etiology is excessive vessel length or distortion of an anastomosis to the hypogastric artery, the anastomosis can be redone, after excision of the diseased segent. Numerous methods have been used for surgical correction of stenosis, including conversion of an end-to-side anastomosis to an end-to-end anastomosis and vice versa, or the use of autogenous saphenous vein or hypogastric artery grafts for patch angioplasty or bypass. Stenosis of the recipient iliac arteries may require correction.[1,3,27,36] The surgeon operating for correction of RAS must be familiar with all these choices and be prepared to tailor the operation to the patient's needs.

Following either PTA or surgical correction,

long-term treatment with dipyridamole should be administered to protect against a recurrence of the problem.[14] If stenosis recurs, it must be corrected again, and both forms of intervention have been successfully used for recurrent RAS.

It is difficult to select the "best" method of treatment of RAS. Both PTA and operation involve risks and may result in loss of the kidney. A distorted hypogastric anastomosis may be managed better by operation, whereas a segmental stenosis, easily reached through an external iliac anastomosis, may be better suited for PTA. The experience of the institution with regard to the technique is important, as is the nature and location of the lesion itself.

Other Complications

Most vascular disruptions and infections present in the postoperative period with severe hemorrhage. It is possible, however, for such problems to be insidious and present months or years later as an anastomotic pseudoaneurysm causing a pulsatile mass at the transplant or nephrectomy site. When a pseu-

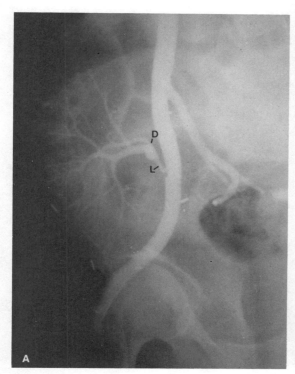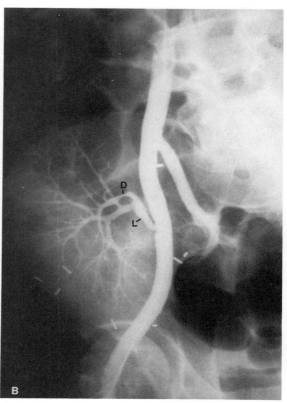

FIGURE 27-4.   Percutaneous transfemoral arteriogram showing long segment stenosis (L) as well as a second lesion in the distal branch (D). (A) Before PTA. (B) After PTA, long segment was significantly improved; distal stenosis shows minimal change.

doaneurysm is found, the possibility of a dormant infection must be strongly considered. We have had a patient present with exsanguinating hemorrhage 3 years after a transplant nephrectomy; the iliac artery was ligated, and the patient is without sequelae 5 years after retransplantation to the opposite side. In another instance, a patient presented with the abrupt onset of anuria 18 months after transplantation, having maintained a creatinine of 1.0 and never having had a rejection episode. At operation, the kidney was normal in appearance but was displaced by a large anastomotic pseudoaneurysm. Transplant nephrectomy and ligation of the external iliac artery were accomplished. The patient required elective femoro-femoral bypass for severe claudication 12 months later. A second transplant was subsequently done, and the patient has good renal function at present. In each of these instances, there had been a septic episode at the time of transplant, with apparent recovery.

Pseudoaneurysm formation may also follow needle biopsy of a transplanted kidney. This procedure can also result in traumatic arteriovenous fistula formation. Diagnosis is accomplished by transfemoral catheter angiography, and successful management has been reported by means of transcatheter embolization of the affected arterial branch.[21]

Finally, one must consider the recipient's underlying disease, which may lead to an inexorable progression of large or small artery stenotic or occlusive disease. These problems are particularly common with juvenile-onset diabetics.[28] Diagnosis can be made by pulse examination and angiography, and appropriate treatment by PTA or vascular surgery can often prevent major amputations.

CONCLUSIONS

Transplantation is a commonly performed operation but has the potential of many complications. Among these are vascular complications, which are relatively uncommon but have serious morbidity and mortality. Attention to detail in donor selection and management, operative technique, kidney preservation, and recipient care can be effective in reducing the incidence of and morbidity from these complications.

REFERENCES

1. Baumgartner D, Keusch G, Retsch M et al: Correction of renal transplant artery stenosis: Early and long-term results. Transplant Proc 16:1308, 1984
2. Billet A, Davis A, Linhardt GE Jr et al: The effects of bilateral renal transplantation on pelvic hemodynamics and sexual function. Surgery 95:415, 1984
3. Blohme I, Brynger H: Emergency ligation of the external iliac artery. Ann Surg 201:505, 1985
4. Cho SI, Bradley JW: New arterial clamp for perfusion preservation of cadaver kidneys. Surgery 87:351, 1980
5. Clarke SD, Kennedy JA, Hewitt JC et al: Successful removal of thrombus from renal vein after renal transplantation. Br Med J 1:154, 1970
6. Colberg JE: En bloc excision of cadaver kidneys for transplantation. Arch Surg 115:1238, 1980
7. Elder R, Schweizer RT: Pelvic lymphocele causing fatal pulmonary embolus in kidney transplant recipient. Transplant Proc 15:2164, 1983
8. Fries D, Tessier J, Charpentier B et al: The value of digital subtraction angiography in early renal transplantation course. Transplant Proc 16:1293, 1984
9. Golden J, Stone RA, Goldberger L: Immune-related renal vein thrombosis in a renal allograft. Ann Intern Med 85:612, 1976
10. Goldman M, De Pauw L, Kinnaert P et al: Renal allograft rupture. Transplantation 32:153, 1981
11. Goldman MH, Tilney NL, Vineyard GC et al: A twenty year survey of arterial complications of renal transplantation. Surg Gynecol Obstet 141:758, 1975
12. Hesse UJ, Grundmann R, Weinand P et al: Prosthetic replacement of the damage renal vein in cadaver kidney transplantation. Transplant Proc 18(3):463, 1986
13. Jordan ML, Cook GT, Cardella CJ: Ten years of experience with vascular complications in renal transplantation. J Urol 128:689, 1982
14. Kauffman HM, Sampson D, Fox PS et al: Prevention of transplant renal artery stenosis. Surgery 81:161, 1977
15. Kohlberg WI, Tellis VA, Bhat DJ et al: Wound infections after transplant nephrectomy. Arch Surg 115:645, 1980
16. Kyriakides GK, Simmons RL, Najarian JS: Wound infections in renal transplant wounds: Pathogenetic and prognostic factors. Ann Surg 182:770, 1975
17. Lacombe M: Arterial stenosis complicating renal allotransplantation in man: A study of 38 cases. Ann Surg 181:283, 1975
18. Majeski J, Munda R: Hazard of percutaneous transluminal dilation in renal transplant arterial stenosis. Arch Surg 116:1225, 1981
19. Mendez R, Mendez RG, Payne JE et al: Management of multiple renal arteries in renal transplantation. Urology III:409, 1974
20. Mollenkopf F, Matas A, Veith FJ et al: Percutaneous transluminal angioplasty for transplant renal artery stenosis. Transplant Proc 15:1089, 1983
21. Moreau JF, Merland JJ, Descamps JM: Post-biopsy false arterial aneurysm of a transplanted kidney: Treatment by bucrylate transcatheter embolization. J Urol 128:116, 1982
22. Nerstrom B, Ladefoged J, Lund FL: Vascular complications in 155 consecutive kidney transplantations. Scand J Urol Nephrol 6:65, 1972
23. Oakes DD, Spees EK Jr, McAllister HA et al: Arterial injury during perfusion preservation: A possible cause of posttransplantation renal artery stenosis. Surgery 89:210, 1981
24. Odenheimer D, Matas A, Tellis V et al: Donor cultures reported positive following renal transplantation—a clinical dilemma. Proceedings of the Second Annual Symposium on Organ Procurement. Transplant Proc 18(3):465, 1986
25. Okiye SE, Zincke H: Renal allograft salvage after prolonged early post-transplant renal artery occlusion. J Urol 129:1216, 1983
26. Owens ML, Wilson SE, Maxwell JG et al: Major arterial hemorrhage after renal transplantation. Transplantation 27:285, 1979
27. Palleschi J, Novick AC, Braun WE et al: Vascular complications of renal transplantation. Urology 16:61, 1980
28. Peters C, Sutherland DER, Simmons RL et al: Patient and graft survival in amputated versus nonamputated diabetic primary renal allograft recipients. Transplantation 32:498, 1981
29. Santiago-Delphin EA, Gonzalez Z: Successful renal vein reconstruction with a polytetrafluoroethylene vascular graft in kidney transplantation. Am J Surg 149:310, 1985
30. Sommer BG, Innes JT, Whitehurst RM et al: Cyclosporine-associated renal arteriopathy resulting in loss of allograft function. Am J Surg 149:756, 1985
31. Standards Committee of the American Society of Transplant Surgeons: Current results and expectations of renal transplantation. JAMA 246:1330, 1981
32. Starnes HF, McWhinnie DL, Bradley JA et al: Delayed major arterial hemorrhage after transplant nephrectomy. Transplant Proc 16:1320, 1984
33. Starzl TE, Hakala TR, Shaw BW Jr et al: A flexible procedure for multiple cadaveric organ procurement. Surg Gynecol Obstet 158:223, 1984

34. Swanson DA, Sullivan MJ: Thromboendarterectomy for anuria 4½ years post-renal transplant: A case report. J Urol 116:799, 1976

35. Tiggeler RGWL, Berden JHM, Hoitsma AJ et al: Prevention of acute tubular necrosis in cadaveric kidney transplantation by the combined use of mannitol and moderate hydration. Ann Surg 201:246, 1985

36. Tilney NL, Rocha A, Strom TB et al: Renal artery stenosis in transplant patients. Ann Surg 199:454, 1984

37. Woods JE, Leary FJ, DeWeerd JH: Renal transplantation without oliguric acute tubular necrosis. Arch Surg 105:427, 1972

38. Zajko AB, McLean GK, Grossman RA et al: Percutaneous transluminal angioplasty and fibrinolytic therapy for renal allograft arterial stenosis and thrombosis. Transplantation 33:447, 1982

CHAPTER 28

Urologic Complications of Renal Transplantation

Alan H. Bennett

Although most urinary bladders are suitable for renal transplantation, there are a significant number of patients who have either congenital or acquired lower tract disease that would complicate the outcome of a successful renal transplantation. Therefore, a simple lower tract urologic investigation, consisting of a voiding cystourethrogram, is recommended for all renal transplantation candidates. If abnormalities are found in either the urethra or the bladder, pretransplantation repair is recommended. For minor problems, especially in the urethra, reparative work can be considered at the time of renal transplantation.

Ureteric fistulas are the most common urologic complication following renal transplantation. Immediate open or percutaneous drainage is indicated. Ureteral obstruction is usually a late complication and can be managed by a variety of open operative and closed percutaneous techniques. Kidney salvage is generally the rule in these cases. Urinary tract infections in the post-transplantation period can often be prevented by early catheter removal and a closed urinary drainage system. Low-dose prophylaxis with urinary antibiotics in the postoperative period is also helpful. The development of hydrocele is related to the practice of spermatic cord ligation. Sexual dysfunction and infertility in the male are commonly recognized as sequelae of chronic renal failure and may persist in spite of successful renal transplantation.

A urologic etiology for chronic renal failure occurs in 15% of cases, with urologic abnormalities being found in 25% of transplant recipients. Most common causes are chronic renal infection and/or nephrolithiasis and long-standing obstructive uropathy, but other conditions such as neurogenic bladder dysfunction or retroperitoneal fibrosis can lead to chronic renal failure.[1,26] Kabler and Cerny[18] reported a 15% incidence of lower tract abnormalities in patients being evaluated urologically prior to transplantation.

PREOPERATIVE PREPARATION

Before performing renal transplantation, a careful history of past urologic conditions or operations must be recorded. For patients with a negative urologic history, the patient should be catheterized for a residual urine and a voiding cystourethrogram (VCUG) should be performed. The catheterized specimen is always cultured. For patients with a history of neurovesical dysfunction and/or diabetes, a cystometrogram and VCUG are performed. Patients with a history of urologic disease are evaluated to ensure that their lower tract is suitable to receive a renal allograft and that no upper tract disease exists that would threaten the prolonged survival of the allograft. Renal size and outline can be adequately assessed with ultrasonography. Cystoscopy and retrograde ureterograms are only necessary if obstructive uropathy is suggested by an abnormal ultrasound examination or a significant post-void residual urine.

UTILIZATION OF ABNORMAL BLADDER

In most cases, the bladder is suitable for transplantation. In the Cleveland Clinic series, there were only seven patients who required a prefashioned ileal or sigmoid conduit.[27] Patients who do not empty the bladder secondary to neurovesical dysfunction can be taught self-intermittent catheterization, and some can also be helped by pharmacologic manipulation. Progressive bladder training can be used to enlarge the small, contracted bladder, which is occasionally found after long periods of defunctionization. Figure 28-1 shows the bladder of a patient after 12 years of nonuse. After 3 months of self-catheterization and gradual hydrodistention, a capacity of 120 ml was achieved, and eventual transplantation was successful. Bladder augmentation can also be considered if hydrodistention fails to expand the bladder sufficiently. Undiversion is a technique that is widely accepted today[16] and should be considered in suitable candidates.[14] Evaluation of the patient with a urinary conduit includes a loop-o-gram to check for loop residual, infection, and the degree of reflux. A catheterization of the urinary bladder should also be performed to ensure that pyocystis does not exist. Better urologic instrumentation (fiberoptic flexible and rigid endoscopes and optical urethrotomes) have made the treatment of urethral strictures much easier. It is unusual to perform an open repair of a short urethral stricture, and urethrotomy, if necessary, can even be performed at the time of transplantation. Ideally, any reparative work on the lower urinary tract should be performed prior to transplantation.

UROLOGIC COMPLICATIONS

Fistula Obstruction

Urologic complications occur in 1% to 15% of renal transplant procedures, depending upon the type of reconstruction and the renal source (i.e., cadaver or living-related).[17,25,32,34] Calyceal fistulas are rare and are usually seen in allografts with multiple arteries.[12] Ureteric fistulas account for up to 60% of urinary leaks and are caused by ischemic injury to the ureter at the time of the harvest, technical problems with the anastomosis itself, or delayed healing secondary to immunosuppression or rejection. Fistulas from the bladder occur either at the neocystostomy entrance or the cystostomy incision and are more common in patients who have had prior bladder surgery.[2,30,37] Diagnosis of a urocutaneous fistula is facilitated by measuring the electrolyte or creatinine content of the fluid or by noting staining of the dressing after an intravenous injection of indigo carmine. When the fistula is internal, other imaging techniques such as cystography, intravenous pyelography, isotope scanning, and ultrasonography will usually confirm the suspected diagnosis. Although fistulas can occur late in the postoperative

period, they usually appear within the first week and, if caused by a technical complication, may be noted within the first few hours of the procedure. Figure 28-2 represents a postoperative intravenous urogram following repair of a ureteric fistula caused by ischemic necrosis of the ureter. The native ureter was anastomosed to the transplant pelvis, and the native kidney was not initially removed. Six months later, the patient presented with flank pain and fever, and pyonephrosis was noted (Fig. 28-3). Delayed nephrectomy was then performed. This case is contrasted to the experience of Baquero and associates,[4] who have not found the need to remove the native kidney after ureteral ligation and use of the native ureter for pyeloureterostomy. In situations in which the native ureter is absent or not usable and the transplant ureter cannot be reanastomosed, a pyelocystostomy can be considered.[6]

Some controversy exists regarding the approach to the urinary leak. Graft loss and successful repair vary widely.[13,28,36] When obstruction accompanies the fistula, percutaneous nephrostomy drainage can be attempted and is often successful. The passage of an antegrade stent has also been reported to be successful as initial and definitive treatment.[7,38] For patients with calyceal or vesical fistulas, simple drainage may effect a successful closure.[35] For the acute ureteric fistula, this author favors early surgical repair in patients who are in good electrolyte balance, are not septic, and have no evidence of obstruction. Usually, reanastomosis of the transplant ureter is possible, and the wound can be closed primarily. The use of an indwelling double J stent may be advised, and a nephrostomy tube is not placed. In the unstable patient, temporizing with a percutaneous nephrostomy can be life- and kidney-saving but will usually only be successful in the dilated transplant kidney. Attempts at catheterization of the transplant ureter by cystoscopic methods is usually difficult unless the ureteroneocystostomy is placed on the floor of the bladder, and this technique for diagnosis and/or treatment has been supplanted by ultrasonography and antegrade techniques.

Obstruction is usually a late complication and most commonly occurs at the ureterovesical anastomotic site. However, ureteric obstruction can be caused by the ureter becoming encased in a fibrotic shell; releasing the ureter from this constricting shell will relieve the obstruction. Also, ischemia, secondary to rejection or poor initial ureteric blood supply, can cause gradual fibrosis and a long-segment ureter usually involving but not limited to the ureteric vessel anastomosis.

The onset of azotemia with other signs and

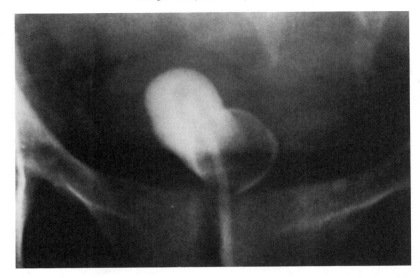

FIGURE 28-1. *This 26-year-old woman had a dysfunctional bladder. A cystogram showed a small contracted bladder with only a 10-ml capacity.*

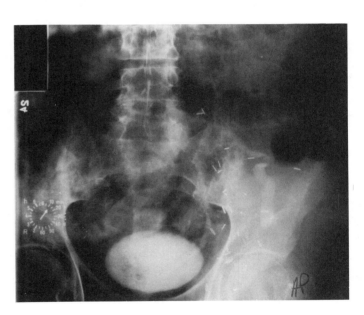

FIGURE 28-2. *Postoperative intravenous urogram following repair of a ureteric fistula.*

symptoms typical of chronic rejection may be a clue of ureteral obstruction. Ultrasonography and radioisotope scans are usually sufficient to make the diagnosis. Initial treatment and confirmation of the diagnosis can also be made by percutaneous antegrade pyelography. Stents can be passed antegrade as well,[21] and balloon dilatation has been tried to treat the ureteral stenosis.[22,24] These techniques are usually only temporizing in nature, and definitive repair is usually necessary. Procedures commonly used include reimplantation of the ureter and ureteropyelostomy with or without native nephrectomy.

URINARY TRACT INFECTION

Acute urinary tract infections occur in up to 75% of renal transplant recipients in spite of preoperative antibiotic prophylaxis.[26] However, the infection becomes persistent in only 10%–15%.[15,20,31] Early catheter removal accompanied by closed urinary drainage and meticulous catheter care should reduce the incidence of urinary tract infection. Also, consideration should be given to low-dose prophylaxis with urinary antibiotics such as sulfamethoxasole, sulfamethoxasole-trimethoprim, or nitrofurantoin in these immunosuppressed patients for the

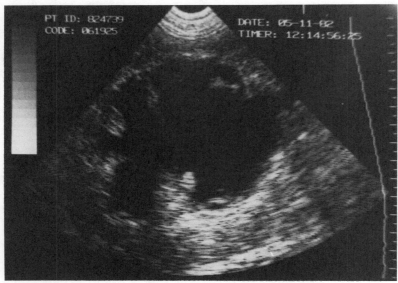

FIGURE 28-3.   Ultrasound study of a patient with a ligated ureter and pyonephrosis 6 months following repair of a ureteric fistula using the native ureter.

first few months post-transplant. Epididymitis occasionally occurs in the transplant recipient and is usually related to prolonged urinary catheter drainage or an active urinary tract infection. Treatment includes appropriate antibiotics, scrotal elevation, and symptomatic relief. However, progression to abscess formation is possible, and open drainage may be necessary if conservative measures fail to control the infection.

HYDROCELE

The incidence of post-transplant hydroceles is directly related to the practice of spermatic cord liga-tion.[29] Although ureteric obstruction by the spermatic cord post-transplantation is rare,[19] cord ligation is still advocated by some transplant surgeons. Avoidance of this procedure will prevent the complication of hydrocele formation, which is often progressive, requiring definitive open repair.

SEXUAL FUNCTION

The detrimental effects of chronic renal failure on sexual function in the male have been recognized for years. In summarizing the literature on the subject, Bailey[3] indicates that 40% of males continue to be impotent in spite of successful transplantation.

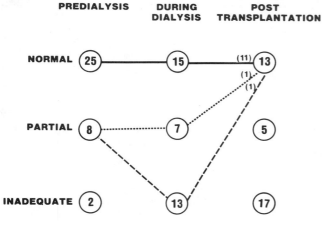

FIGURE 28-4.   Sexual function pre-dialysis, during dialysis, and after successful renal transplantation.

TABLE 28-1 Hormone Levels*

HORMONES		NUMBER OF PATIENTS	NUMBER OF PATIENTS IMPOTENT
FSH	(↑)	7	3
LH	(↑)	10	9
Testosterone	(↓)	14	10
Testosterone	(↑)	2	2
Prolactin	(↑)	2	2
17-Estradiol	(↑)	3	3
Number of patients with 1 or more abnormal tests		26	14

* There were a total of 35 patients in the group.

Salvatierra and co-workers,[33] in a questionnaire analysis, state that 84% of 32 patients with functioning kidneys for more than 3 years had regained the same level of sexual activity that they had experienced prior to the onset of renal failure. A group of 35 patients transplanted at the Albany Medical Center were recently interviewed. Thirty-two of the patients had normal functioning allografts for an average duration of 3.6 years. Of 25 men potent prior to transplantation, 12 became impotent despite successful transplantation (Fig. 28-4). In this group, 75%, were noted to have hormonal abnormalities (Table 28-1). Multiple factors, including an abnormal hormonal milieu, drug therapy, and diabetes account for the high incidence of impotence in transplant recipients. In patients who have had more than one renal transplant, vascular compromise to the penile vascular bed may also be a contributing factor.[8,10] Penile prosthesis placement can certainly be considered and is a practical solution for the impotent transplant recipient. Complications of implantation do not appear to be increased in these patients because of their immunosuppression.

INFERTILITY

The subject of infertility in the transplant recipient has not been carefully studied. There are many reports of pregnancies in transplanted females and transplanted males who have fathered children. It is well known that chronic uremia causes gonadal damage,[11,23] and it has been generally accepted that the abnormal hormonal changes noted in the dialysis patient return to normal after successful transplantation. Abnormal sperm counts in seven male patients who had undergone successful kidney transplantation were noted by Baumgarten and associates.[5] No discernable cause for the oligospermia could be found. Our study of impotence in 35 transplant recipients was also used to assess fertility. Prior to renal transplantation, 26 of the patients were married and 21 (70%) had fathered children. Following transplantation, there were no offspring in the 35 men. Seven patients indicated that they had tried to impregnate their wives for a period of from 2 to 20 years (average 6.4 years). Four of these men had previously fathered children. The hormonal studies were abnormal in six of the seven infertile men, and, of the four who were able to produce a semen specimen, the analysis showed abnormal parameters in all. Four men had an elevated FSH level, often indicative of a defect in spermatogenesis at the testicular level.[9] It is apparent from this selective study and from the few other reports in the literature that fertility potential is impeded in many males who have received a renal allograft.

REFERENCES

1. Advisory Committee to the Renal Transplant Registry; the 13th Report of the Transplant Registry. Transplant Proc 9:9, 1977
2. Anderson EE, Glenn JF, Seigler HF et al: Urologic complications in renal transplantation. J Urol 107:187, 1972
3. Bailey G: Sexual dysfunction in the male patient with chronic renal failure. In Bennett AH (ed): *Management of Male Impotence.* Baltimore, Williams & Wilkins, 1982
4. Baquero A, Ginsberg PC et al: Experience with pyeloureterostomy associated with simple ligation of na-

tive ureter with ipsilateral nephrectomy in renal transplantation. J Urol 133:386, 1985

5. Baumgarten SR, Lindsay GK, Wise GJ: Fertility problems in the renal transplant patient. J Urol 118:991, 1977

6. Bennett AH: Pyelocystostomy in a renal allograft. Am J Surg 125:633, 1973

7. Berger RE, Ansell JS, Tremann JA et al: The use of self-retained ureteral stents in the management of urological complications in renal transplant recipients. J Urol 124:781, 1980

8. Burns JR, Houttuin E et al: Vascular-induced erectile impotence in renal transplant recipients. J Urol 1221:721, 1979

9. Franchimont P, Millet D, Vendrely E et al: The relationship between spermatogenesis and serum gonadotropin levels in azospermia and oligospermia. J Clin Endocrin Metab 34;1003, 1972

10. Gittes RF, Waters WB: Sexual impotency: The overlooked complication of a second renal transplant. J Urol 121:719, 1979

11. Gittes RF, Waters WB: Sexual impotence. J Urol 121:719, 1979

12. Goldman MH, Burleson RL, Tilney NL et al: Calyceal-cutaneous fistulae in renal transplant patients. Ann Surg 184:679, 1976

13. Goldstein I, Cho SI, Olsson CA: Nephrostomy for renal transplant complications. J Urol 126:159, 1981

14. Gonzalez R: Pre-transplant undiversion. Urology Times 13:3, 1985

15. Hamshere RJ, Chisholm GD, Shackman R: Late urinary tract infection after renal transplantation. Lancet 2:7884, 1974

16. Hendren WH: Urinary undiversion and augmentation cystoplasty. In Kelalis, King, Belman (eds): Clinical Pediatric Urology, 2nd ed, Vol One, p 620. Philadelphia, WB Saunders, 1985

17. Hricko GM, Birch AG, Bennett AH et al: Factors responsible for urinary fistula in the renal transplant recipient. Ann Surg 178:609, 1973

18. Kabler RI, Cerny JC: Pre-transplant urologic investigation and treatment of end-stage renal disease. J Urol 129:475, 1983

19. Karmi SA, Dagher FJ, Ramos E et al: Spermatic cord; cause of ureteral obstruction in renal allotransplant recipients. Urology 11:380, 1978

20. Krieger JN, Tapia L, Stubenbord WT et al: Urinary infection in kidney transplantation. Urology 9:130, 1977

21. Lieberman RP, Glass NR, Crummy AB et al: Non-operative percutaneous management of urinary fistulas and strictures in renal transplantation. Surg Gynecol Obstet 155:667, 1982

22. Lieberman SF, Keller FS, Barry JM et al: Percutaneous antegrade transluminal ureteroplasty for renal allograft ureteral stenosis. J Urol 128:122, 1982

23. Lingardh G, Andersson L, Osterman B: Fertility in men after renal transplant. Acta Chir Scand 140:494, 1974

24. List AR, Blohme I, Brynger H et al: Balloon dilatation for ureteral strictures in graft kidneys. Transplantation 35:105, 1983

25. Loughlin KR, Tilney NL, Richie JP: Urologic complications in 718 renal transplant patients. Surgery 95:297, 1984

26. Malkowicz SG, Perloff LJ: Urologic consideration in renal transplantation. Surg Gynecol Obstet 160:579, 1985

27. Novick AC, Braun WE, Magnusson M et al: Current status of renal transplantation at the Cleveland Clinic. J Urol 122:161, 1979

28. Olsson CA, Manneck JA, Schmitt GW et al: Nephrostomy in renal transplantation. Am J Surg 121:467, 1971

29. Penn I, Mackie G, Halgrimson CG et al: Testicular complications following renal transplantation. Ann Surg 176:697, 1972

30. Pfefferman R, Vidne B, Leapman S et al: Urologic complications in renal primary and retransplantation. Am J Surg 131:242, 1976

31. Ramsey DE, Fitch WT, Birch AG: Urinary tract infections in kidney transplant recipients. Arch Surg 114:1022, 1979

32. Sagalowsky AI, Ransler CW, Peters PC et al: Urologic complications in 505 renal transplants with early catheter removal. J Urol 129:929, 1983

33. Salvatierra O, Fortmann JL, Belzen FO: Sexual function in males before and after renal transplantation. Urology 5:64, 1975

34. Salvatierra O Jr, Olcott C, Amend WJ Jr et al: Urologic complications of renal transplantation can be prevented or controlled. J Urol 117:421, 1977

35. Schiff M Jr, McGuire EJ, Webster J: Successful management of caliceal fistulas following renal transplantation. Arch Surg 110:1129, 1975

36. Schiff M Jr, McGuire EJ, Weiss RM et al: Management of urinary fistulas after renal transplantation. J Urol 115:251, 1976

37. Smolev JK, McLoughlin MG, Rolley R et al: The surgical approach to urological complications in renal allograft recipients. J Urol 117:10, 1977

38. Tremann JA, Marchioro TL: Giblons ureteral stent in renal transplant recipients. Urology 9:390, 1977

CHAPTER 29

Development of New Tumors After Transplantation

Israel Penn

Post-transplantation, there is a remarkably high incidence of certain tumors, particularly skin cancers, non-Hodgkin's lymphomas (NHL), Kaposi's sarcoma (KS), in situ carcinomas of the uterine cervix, and carcinomas of the vulva and perineum. The average time of appearance of all tumors after conventional immunosuppressive therapy is 59 months, compared with only 14 months in patients treated with cyclosporine. Since the incidence of cancers increases with the length of follow-up, all transplant recipients must be followed indefinitely.

Skin cancers are 4 to 21 times more common in transplant recipients than in the general population. Unusual features are the young age of the patients, the preponderance of squamous cell carcinomas over basal cell carcinomas, the high incidence of multiple tumors, and the frequency of lymph node metastases. Hodgkin's disease, the most common lymphoma in the general population, is uncommon in transplant patients. NHLs are increased 28- to 49-fold over the general population. Morphologically, reticulum cell sarcomas are the predominant type of NHL. Immunologically, most NHL's arise from B-lymphocytes and have a marked predilection for the brain. Some lesions, mainly in cyclosporine-treated patients, may regress completely following drastic reduction of immunosuppressive therapy.

KS occurs 400 to 500 times more frequently following transplantation than in the general population. In patients with no internal visceral involvement, one fifth may have complete regression of lesions following drastic reduction or cessation of immunosuppressive therapy.

There is a 14-fold increased incidence of in situ carcinomas of the uterine cervix and a 100-fold increase of carcinomas of the vulva and anus.

Reduction or cessation of immunosuppressive therapy has caused complete regression of some KSs and some NHLs but has been disappointing in the treatment of epithelial malignancies. If chemotherapy is used, azathioprine should be reduced to avoid bone marrow depression.

Any state of severe immunodeficiency, whether congenital, acquired (as in AIDS), or iatrogenic (as in organ transplant recipients) is complicated by an increased incidence of certain cancers.[6–8] After transplantation, there is no increase in incidence of the neoplasms commonly seen in the general population, including carcinomas of the lung, prostate, colon and rectum, and female breast and invasive carcinoma of the uterine cervix. Instead, there is a remarkably high incidence of certain tumors.[3–8,12] This chapter is based on data sent to the Cincinnati Transplant Tumor Registry (CTTR) up to December, 1985.

Supported in part by Grant Number 6985 from the Veterans Administration.

INCIDENCE OF MALIGNANCIES

Data obtained by the CTTR from several large transplant centers show a tumor incidence ranging from 1% to 16% of patients, with an average of 4%.[5,6,8] However, this figure underestimates the true incidence, because many patients with short survival times or short lengths of follow-up are included.

AGE AND SEX OF PATIENTS

The neoplasms occurred in a relatively young group of patients whose average age at the time of transplantation was 40 years (range 7 months to 72 years).[5-8] Sixty-four percent of patients were male, and 36% were female, in keeping with the 2:1 ratio of male to female patients who undergo renal transplantation.

TIME OF APPEARANCE OF THE CANCERS

Some malignancies appear at fairly distinct intervals after transplantation. In humans, an interval of 5 to 20 years, or even more, elapses between exposure to many carcinogens and the development of clinical cancer. In contrast, many malignancies appear a relatively short time after transplantation.[3-8] Kaposi's sarcoma (KS) is first to appear at an average of 22 (range 2.5–225.5) months after transplantation. Lymphomas appear at an average of 37 (range 1–154) months after transplantation. Other tumors excluding carcinomas of the vulva and perineum) appear at an average of 62 (range 1–221.5) months following transplantation. Carcinomas of the vulva and perineum appear at the longest interval after transplantation, at an average of 90 (9–215) months.

The average time of appearance of the tumors after conventional immunosuppressive therapy is 59 (range 1–225.5) months. Thus far, the tumors that have occurred in cyclosporine-treated patients (88 persons) have appeared much earlier, at an average of only 14 (range 1–82) months after transplantation.[9] Several of these patients, at the furthest end of the time spectrum, had been switched from conventional therapy to cyclosporine or had received conventional treatment for a first transplant and cyclosporine for a subsequent allograft.

The incidence of cancer increases with the length of follow-up after transplantation. A study of 3846 Australasian renal transplant recipients showed a cancer incidence of 3% at 1 year, 14% at 5 years, and 49% at 14 years.[12] Similarly, in 124 cardiac transplant recipients, the actuarial risk of developing cancer was 2.7 ± 1.9% at 1 year, and 25.6 ± 11.0% at 5 years.[5,6,8] In both studies, the number of long-term survivors at risk for cancer was rather small. Nevertheless, these statistics emphasize the need to follow transplant patients indefinitely.

VARIETIES OF NEW TUMORS

The CTTR has data on 2518 types of cancer that arose in 2353 organ transplant recipients. The patients included 2286 who received kidney, 45 heart, 8 bone marrow, 7 liver, 5 pancreas, and 2 combined heart and lung transplants. The most common types of tumor are indicated in Table 29-1. Several epidemiologic studies confirm the high incidence of certain malignancies. Compared with suitable age-matched controls, there is a four- to sevenfold increase in skin cancer in regions with low sunshine exposure, a 21-fold increase in areas with high sunshine exposure[5,6,8]; a 29-fold increase in lip cancers[1]; a 28- to 49-fold increase in non-Hodgkin's lymphomas (NHL)[3,4]; a 400- to 500-fold increase in KS[2]; a 14-fold increase in carcinoma in situ of the uterine cervix[11]; and a 100-fold increase in carcinomas of the vulva and anus.[1] There are also small increases in carcinomas of the liver and biliary passages, leukemias, and carcinomas of the kidney.[3,4]

Cancer of the Skin and Lips

The skin and lips were the areas affected most; 978 of the 2518 neoplasms (39%) occurred here (Table 29-1). An Australasian study shows that the incidence of skin cancer increases with the length of follow-up. In a series of 3846 renal transplant recipients, 11% had skin cancer at 5 years, 29% at 10 years, and 43% at 14 years.[12]

Skin cancers in transplant patients show several unusual features in comparison with their counterparts in the general population.[5,6,8,12] Basal cell carcinomas (BCCs) outnumber squamous cell carcinomas (SCCs) in the general population, but the reverse is found with the CTTR transplant patients in whom SCCs constitute 52% and BCCs constitute 28%. In the population at-large, nonmelanoma skin cancers occur mostly in people in their 60s or 70s, whereas affected transplant patients' average ages are 30 years younger. The incidence of multiple skin cancers (which were present in at least 417 of 978 patients, 43%) is remarkably high and is comparable to that seen only in patients in the general population residing in areas of abundant sunshine. Several patients each had more than 100 skin tumors. Malignant melanomas constituted 4.8% of the skin cancers in the CTTR in contrast with an incidence of 2.7% in the general population of the United States.[14] This observation is in keeping with an Australasian study showing a fivefold higher incidence of malignant melanoma than in the age-matched general population.[8]

Most skin cancers in the CTTR were of low-grade malignancy, but a significant percentage of squamous cell carcinomas behaved much more aggressively than their counterparts in the general population.[5,6,8,12] Lymph node metastases occurred in 75 patients (8%), 63 of whom has SCCs, 10 of

TABLE 29-1   De Novo Tumors in Organ Transplant Patients

TYPE OF CANCER	NUMBER OF PATIENTS*
Cancers of skin and lips	978
Lymphomas	341†
Carcinomas of uterus	163
Cervix—146	
Body—17	
Carcinomas of the lung	116
Kaposi's sarcoma	93
Carcinomas of colon and rectum	92
Carcinomas of breast	80
Carcinomas of the vulva, perineum, penis, or scrotum	70
Carcinomas of kidney	67
Host kidney—61	
Allograft—6	
Carcinomas of the head and neck (excluding thyroid, parathyroid, and eye)	65
Leukemias	61
Metastatic carcinoma (primary site unknown)	58
Carcinomas of urinary bladder	47
Carcinomas of liver and bile ducts	39
Carcinomas of thyroid	37
Soft tissue sarcomas	32
Cancers of stomach	30
Testicular carcinomas	28
Ovarian cancers	25
Carcinomas of prostate gland	24
Cancers of the pancreas	21
Brain neoplasms	14
Miscellaneous tumors	37
TOTAL	2518

* There were 2353 patients of whom 157 (6.7%) had more than one type of tumor affecting different organs. Eight of these patients each had three different types of cancer.

† One patient had two different types of lymphoma.

whom had malignant melanomas, and 2 of whom had Merkel's cell tumors. Sixty-five patients (7%) died of their skin cancers—42 with SCCs, 21 with malignant melanomas, 1 with BCC, and 1 with Merkel's cell tumor. These findings emphasize a more than 10-fold increase in mortality from SCCs of the skin in Australian renal transplant recipients.[3] The behavior of skin tumors in transplant patients contrasts markedly with that seen in the general population, in whom they cause only 1% to 2% of all cancer deaths, the great majority of which are from malignant melanoma.[13]

Lymphomas

These are the second most common type of tumor seen in transplant patients. They constitute 3% to 4% of all malignancies in the general population but 341 of 2518 cancers (14%) in the CTTR (see Table 29-1). If we exclude nonmelanoma skin neoplasms and in situ carcinomas of the uterine cervix, which are excluded from most cancer statistics, their incidence rises to 20%.

The lymphomas in this series share many features with those encountered in patients with congenital immunodeficiency states and patients with AIDS but are strikingly different from those seen in the general population.[4–6,8] The majority (93%) were NHLs, whereas Hodgkin's disease is the most common lymphoma seen in the community at large. Morphologically, most NHLs were reticulum cell sarcomas (also known as immunoblastomas, large cell lymphomas, or microgliomas). Immunologically, most arose from B-lymphocytes, but a few T cell lymphomas have been encountered. Whereas extranodal involvement was reported in from 24% to 48% of patients in the general population, 75% of NHLs in transplant patients had this distribution. Furthermore, those with extranodal disease were confined to a single organ in 67% of cases, most frequently the brain. In the general population, about 1% of NHLs involve the brain, whereas in transplant patients, 46% affected the central nervous system (CNS), usually the brain, with spinal cord involvement being rare. Brain lesions frequently were multicentric in distribution. Another unusual feature was that in 74% of patients with CNS involvement, the lesions are localized to the brain, whereas in the general population, brain lesions usually were accompanied by involvement of other viscera. The genome of Epstein-Barr virus has been isolated from some NHLs in transplant recipients, congenital immunodeficiency patients, and AIDS victims. It is believed to cause a spectrum of lesions ranging from benign polyclonal B cell hyperplasia on the one hand, to frank monoclonal B cell lymphomas on the other hand.

Forty-six of the NHLs in the CTTR followed immunosuppression with cyclosporine. These differed from those following conventional immunosuppressive therapy in several important respects.[9] In the cyclosporine-related group, they appeared in a remarkably short time after transplantation, at an average of 8.5 (range 1–68) months compared with an average of 41 (range 1–154) months after conventional therapy. The lymphomas more frequently involved lymph nodes than did those in the conventionally treated group and tended to be more widespread. Involvement of the small bowel was proportionally more frequent than that with conventional therapy, whereas brain involvement was rare (in 1 of 46 patients). The cyclosporine-related lymphomas also had a better prognosis in that several underwent partial or complete regression following drastic reduction of immunosuppressive therapy, a hitherto rare happening in conventionally treated patients.

Kaposi's Sarcoma (KS)

KS constituted 93 of the 2518 neoplasms in the CTTR (3.7%) (see Table 29-1). If nonmelanoma skin cancers and in situ carcinomas of the uterine cervix are omitted, KS constitutes 5.3% of tumors in comparison with its incidence in the general population of the United States (before the AIDS epidemic started) of only 0.02% to 0.07% of all cancers. The high frequency of KS in this worldwide collection of patients is comparable to that seen in areas of the world where it has its highest incidence, namely in the rain forest areas of Africa, where it makes up 3% to 9% of all neoplasms.[5–8]

KS was most common in transplant patients who were Jewish, black, or of Mediterranean ancestry.[7] Two thirds of these patients had "benign" KS involving the skin, conjunctiva, or oropharyngolaryngeal mucosa, and one third had the "malignant" variety with involvement of the internal organs, most commonly the gastrointestinal tract and lungs. After treatment, complete remissions occurred in 33 of the 62 patients (53%) with "benign" disease. Seven of the remissions (21%) occurred when the *only* treatment was a drastic reduction of immunosuppressive therapy.[5–8] The other 26 remissions followed surgery, radiotherapy, or chemotherapy. In the malignant group, 5 of the 31 patients (16%) had complete remissions after chemotherapy or radiotherapy together with alteration of immunosuppressive therapy. Twenty-one of the 62 patients with nonvisceral KS died, usually of unrelated causes, whereas 21 of the 31 patients with visceral KS are dead, mostly as a result of their tumors.

KS in transplant patients differs in several respects from that seen in AIDS patients.[8] Visceral disease is less common, lymphadenopathy is rare, and fewer patients die of their neoplasms. In addition, immunosuppression can be reduced with the hope of causing partial or complete remission of the lesions, whereas in AIDS, there is, as yet, no effective means of reversing the unrelenting immunodeficiency state.

Carcinomas of the Uterine Cervix

Carcinomas of the cervix occurred in 146 of the 843 women in the CTTR (17%) (see Table 29-1). At least 79% were in situ lesions.[5,6,8,11] It is advisable that all post-adolescent female patients have regular pelvic examinations and cervical smears to detect such lesions and those involving the vulva and perineum.[5,6,8,10,11]

Carcinomas of the Vulva and Perineum

Carcinomas of the vulva, perineum, scrotum, penis, perianal skin, and anus occurred in 70 patients, 52 women and 18 men (see Table 29-1).[5,6,8,10,11] If nonmelanoma skin cancers and in situ carcinomas of the uterine cervix are excluded, carcinomas of the vulva and perineum constitute 4.0% of tumors in the CTTR, a much higher incidence than in the general population. The patients were surprisingly young compared with persons with similar lesions in the community at large who are mostly in their 60s and 70s. The average age of the women at the time of transplantation was 30 (range 15–55) years and, of the men, 39 (range 25–60) years. In women, there was sometimes a "field effect," with involvement by cancer of the vulva, vagina, uterine cervix, and anus in varying combinations.[5,6,8,10] Several patients had a preceding history of condyloma acuminatum or herpes genitalis, suggesting a viral etiology of these cancers.[10] Small lesions were treated by local excision. More extensive cancers required radical operations such as total vulvectomy and inguinal node dissection, or abdominoperineal resection.[10]

TREATMENT OF CANCERS

In addition to providing conventional therapy of the tumors, we must consider the question of reduction or cessation of immunosuppressive therapy.[5,6,8] It is known that cancers inadvertently transplanted with renal allografts may regress completely, even when widely disseminated, when immunosuppressive therapy is discontinued and tumor-bearing kidney allografts are removed.[5,6] Does such treatment help patients who develop de novo tumors? As previously mentioned, seven cases of KS and several lymphomas regressed following drastic reduction of immunosuppressive therapy. However, the CTTR has rarely received reports of regression of epithelial tumors following such treatment. Nevertheless, one may try to reduce the immunosuppression in a patient with a highly malignant, extensive, or advanced neoplasm in the hope that the immune system may recover and help to eliminate the tumor. However, such treatment carries the risk of allograft rejection. In that event, renal transplant recipients can resume dialysis therapy, but cardiac or hepatic transplant patients are likely to have a fatal outcome.

In those patients requiring cytotoxic therapy for widespread cancers, we must remember that most agents depress the bone marrow.[5,6,8] It is advisable to stop or reduce azathioprine dosage during such therapy to prevent severe bone marrow toxicity. As most cytotoxic agents have immunosuppressive side-effects, satisfactory allograft function may persist for prolonged periods of time. Treatment with prednisone may be continued, because it is an important constituent of many cytotoxic regimens.

POSSIBLE CAUSES OF TUMORS

Space constraints permit only a brief discussion of possible causes of tumors, which probably arise from a complex interplay of several factors. A major possibility is that some alteration in immunity plays a role in their development. For example, the immune surveillance hypothesis suggests that the immune system is able to recognize tumor-specific antigens on neoplastic cells and to destroy early cancers. In the daily course of wear and tear, millions of cells are replaced. A few cells may undergo mutations, some of which may be malignant. The immune system is believed to recognize and destroy such mutant cells before they can develop into overt tumors. A criticism of the immune surveillance theory is that one would expect an increased incidence of all types of malignancies, particularly those that are common in the general population; whereas, in transplant patients, there is a disproportionately increased incidence of only certain neoplasms. Thus, impaired immune surveillance is not the sole explanation of the aforementioned findings.

Another possibility is disturbed immunoregulation. It is known that the immune system has feedback mechanisms that control the amount of lymphoid proliferation that occurs in response to the presence of an antigen. Immunosuppressed states may permit uncontrolled proliferation of lymphoid cells in response to certain antigenic stimuli, such as the presence of a foreign graft, or recurrent or multiple infections.

This leads to another possibility, chronic antigenic stimulation per se acting as an oncogenic stimulus. In experimental animals, repeated administration of antigens has been shown to cause a high incidence of lymphomas. Similarly, transplant patients are subjected to many foreign antigens, including (1) those of the organ graft, which may have been present for years; (2) those from repeated infections; (3) antigens introduced with medications, particularly the foreign proteins of antilymphocyte globulin or monoclonal anti-T cell antibodies. It is possible that some or all of these factors could play a role in causing hyperplasia of lymphoid tissues, which eventually progresses to neoplasia.

Another possibility is that immunosuppressive agents may have a direct oncogenic effect on certain cells. However, we do not have much evidence of this except in patients who have been treated for cancer or other diseases with cyclophosphamide in whom there has been an increased incidence of leukemias and carcinomas of the urinary bladder. It is also possible that some immunosuppressive agents may play a synergistic role with various environmental carcinogens, for example, with tobacco smoke, radiation, or sunlight. In experiments done in our laboratory, hairless mice, which are very prone to develop skin cancers, were treated with various immunosuppressive agents with and without ultraviolet light. We found that the combination of ultraviolet light plus azathioprine caused a higher incidence of neoplasms than either of these agents used alone. If these results can be extrapolated to humans, they may explain the high incidence of skin cancers seen in transplant patients.

Another important possibility is the activation or liberation of oncogenic viruses in immunosuppressed patients. There is much information suggesting that the Epstein-Barr virus may play a role in the development of lymphomas in immunodeficient persons. Papilloma virus may cause carcinomas of the vulva, perineum, uterine cervix, or of other skin areas. Herpes virus may cause carcinomas of the uterine cervix, vulva, lips, or skin. Cytomegalovirus may play a role in causing KS. Hepatitis B virus may cause some hepatocellular cancers that occur in transplant patients.

Under certain circumstances, the immunosuppressive agents may stimulate cellular proliferation. We know that patients given chemotherapy for cancer often have marked depression of all elements of the bone marrow. In some patients, prolonged depression constitutes a preleukemic phase that is subsequently followed by cellular proliferations and the development of a myelocytic or myelomonocytic leukemia. A similar phenomenon may occur in transplant patients, who may first develop an immunosuppressive therapy–induced lymphopenia, which, later, is compensated for by hyperplasia of the lymphoid tissues, which may eventually progress to neoplasia.

One may ask why do not all transplant patients who are heavily immunosuppressed develop cancer? The probable reason is that some patients may be genetically susceptible to develop tumors under certain circumstances. It is known that genetic factors control the person's ability to activate chemical carcinogens, the level of interferon secretion, and the regulation of the immune response.

Transplant patients sometimes receive other treatments that may be oncogenic. Some are given radiation therapy; for example, many bone marrow and some renal transplant recipients receive either total body or total lymphoid irradiation. Dilantin (diphenylhydantoin), which is used to prevent hypertensive encephalopathy in some renal transplant recipients, has been shown to cause pseudolymphomas and even lymphomas.

In summary, there are many factors, acting singly or in combination, that may play a role in the etiology of cancer in transplant patients. Careful investigation is needed to elucidate the causes of the malignancies and how they may relate to similar neoplasms occurring in the general population.

ACKNOWLEDGMENT

The author wishes to thank numerous colleagues, working in transplant centers throughout the world, who have generously contributed data concerning their patients to the Cincinnati Transplant Tumor Registry.

REFERENCES*

1. Blohme I, Brynger H: Malignant disease in renal transplant patients. Transplantation 39:23–25, 1985
2. Harwood AR, Osaba D, Hofstader SL et al: Kaposi's sarcoma in recipients of renal transplants. Am J Med 67:759–765, 1979
3. Kinlen LJ, Sheil AGR, Peto J et al: Collaborative United Kingdom–Australasian study of cancer in patients treated with immunosuppressive drugs. Br Med J 2:1461–1466, 1979
4. Kinlen L: Immunosuppressive therapy and cancer. Cancer Surveys 1:565–583, 1982
5. Penn I: The price of immunotherapy. Curr Probl Surg 18(11):682–751, 1981
6. Penn I: The occurrence of cancer in immune deficiencies. Curr Probl Cancer 6(10):1–64, 1982

* Because of space constraints, an exhaustive list of references could not be included. The work of numerous investigators is cited in the listed references.

7. Penn I: Kaposi's sarcoma in immunosuppressed patients. J Clin Lab Immunol 12:1–10, 1983
8. Penn I: Neoplastic consequences of transplantation and chemotherapy. Cancer Detect Prev (in press)
9. Penn I, First MR: Development and incidence of cancer following cyclosporine therapy. Transplant Proc 18:210–213, 1986
10. Penn I: Cancers of the anogenital region in renal transplant recipients. Analysis of 65 cases. Cancer 58:611–616, 1986
11. Porreco R, Penn I, Droegemueller W et al: Gynecologic malignancies in immunosuppressed organ homograft recipients. Obstet Gynecol 45:359–364, 1975
12. Sheil AGR, Flavel S, Disney APS et al: Cancer development in patients progressing to dialysis and renal transplantation. Transplant Proc 17:1685–1688, 1985
13. Silverberg E: Cancer statistics, 1985. CA 35:19–35, 1985
14. Sober AJ: Diagnosis and management of skin cancer. Cancer 51:2448–2452, 1983

CHAPTER 30

Infection in the Organ Transplant Recipient

Nina E. Tolkoff-Rubin   Robert H. Rubin

Three major factors influence the incidence and severity of infection in transplant patients: (1) the type, intensity, and duration of *immunosuppressive therapy;* (2) the incidence of *technical complications;* and (3) the *epidemiologic exposures* that the patient encounters.

The risk of infection can be best correlated with what is termed the *net state of immunosuppression,* which is determined by the immunosuppressive drugs, the presence of leukopenia, and certain metabolic factors, such as uremia and hyperglycemia. Certain infections themselves (e.g., cytomegalovirus [CMV], Epstein-Barr virus) are immunomodulating and contribute significantly to the net state of immunosuppression. The subgroup of transplant patients at particular risk of opportunistic infection are those with one or more of these viral infections, particularly CMV and non-A, non-B hepatitis.

Certain viruses (herpes group viruses and the hepatitis viruses) produce chronic infection in transplant patients. In addition to the direct infectious disease effects of these viruses and the immunomodulating effects of these viruses, these agents are involved in the pathogenesis of those malignant diseases most commonly observed in transplant patients.

There is a timetable according to which certain infections are expected to occur post-transplant. In the patient who presents at a given time with an infectious disease syndrome such as pneumonia, the timetable can be helpful in generating the appropriate differential diagnosis. When exceptions to the timetable occur, for example, the occurrence of opportunistic infection in the first month post-transplant, this can be an important clue to the existence of an unexpected nosocomial hazard.

Immunosuppressive therapy has a blunting effect on the presenting signs and symptoms of infection. Thus, life-threatening central nervous system (CNS) infection may be present when the only symptom is a headache, or innocent-appearing skin lesions can be clues to metastatic fungal or nocardial infection.

The success of modern transplantation has been the result of a remarkable journey across two major barriers: allograft rejection and life-threatening infection—the former necessitating immunosuppressive manipulation, and the latter resulting from this need for immunosuppression. Despite the successes that have occurred, it is sobering to point out that more than 80% of transplant recipients will have at least one episode of clinical infection in their post-transplant course and that 40% of deaths are due to infection or the combination of infection and rejection.[1,46,50]

There are several challenges to the clinician dealing with the infectious problems of the transplant patient. First, the lifelong need for chronic immunosuppression has multiple general effects: (1) the incidence and severity of acute infections with common pathogens is increased; (2) microorganisms of little pathogenetic significance in the normal host can have life-threatening consequences in this patient population; and (3) chronic infection with certain pathogens, particularly viruses, will cause progressive disease and clinical syndromes unknown in the normal host. Second, the potential sources of infection for the transplant recipient are limitless. These may be grouped into four major categories: (1) the allograft itself; (2) environmental exposures to contaminated air and, to a lesser extent, water; (3) endogenous latent infection reactivated by immunosuppressive therapy; and (4) technical complications that become secondarily infected with a variety of endogenous and exogenous flora. Third, although early diagnosis and aggressive therapy are the keys to successful management of infection in these patients, the physical and radiologic clues to the presence of such infection may be greatly modified by the impaired inflammatory response to microbial invasion engendered by the immunosuppressive therapy being administered. Fourth, the ultimate goal of the clinician is prevention of infection rather than therapy. In particular, the prevention of opportunistic infection of nosocomial origin is of paramount importance.[46,50]

The purpose of this chapter is to outline an approach to the prevention, early recognition, and effective management of infection in the organ transplant patient, concentrating particularly on the renal transplant recipient, for whom the most information is available. Although certain infections relating to technical complications will differ when considering renal, cardiac, and liver transplants, in all other respects these patients are virtually identical in terms of infectious disease risk.

TIMETABLE OF INFECTION IN THE ORGAN TRANSPLANT RECIPIENT

As outlined in the Figure 30-1, infections in the organ transplant recipient do not occur at random but according to an expected "timetable" that is determined by the type, intensity, and duration of immunosuppression administered, technical complications, and environmental exposures. It is particularly useful to divide post-transplant events into three time periods: (1) the first month post-transplant, (2) the period 1 to 6 months post-transplant, and (3) the late period, more than 6 months post-transplant.[46,50]

INFECTION IN THE FIRST MONTH POST-TRANSPLANT

Infections occurring in this time period can be grouped into three categories: (1) those present in the recipient prior to transplant, (2) those conveyed with the allograft, and (3) those bacterial infections of the surgical wound, lungs, urinary tract, and intravenous lines that complicate all forms of surgery, but whose consequences may be greater in the immunocompromised host. It is important to emphasize that infection with such opportunistic pathogens as *Aspergillus, Legionella, Pseudomonas,* or *Nocardia* species should not occur in this time pe-

riod, and, if it does, this is an indication of an unusual exposure, usually owing to excessive hazard in the hospital environment. Experience has taught that a single case of primary infection with such an opportunistic pathogen in this early time period is a clue to an incipient or ongoing nosocomial epidemic. It is also worth emphasizing that the expected lack of opportunistic infection in this first month, at a time when the actual *dosage* of immunosuppressive agents administered is at its highest, is testimony to the fact that *duration* of immunosuppression is a more important determinant of the net state of immunosuppression (and the risk of infection) than the particular dosage being given on a particular day or few days.[46,50]

Impact of Pretransplant Infection

Patients with renal, hepatic, and cardiac failure of a degree that justified organ transplantation are at increased risk of infection even before immunosuppressive therapy is initiated. It is a truism of modern transplantation that such infection should be sought and, whenever possible, eradicated prior to transplantation. Thus, acute pneumonia or bacteremia must be eradicated prior to transplantation.

So-called cold abscesses caused by *Mycobaterium tuberculosis* or *Staphylococcus aureus,* when not detected prior to transplant, have become activated post-transplant, producing miliary or disseminated disease, underlining the need for a careful review of these possibilities prior to transplant. Hepatitis, although causing significant risk for the transplant patient, is not treatable at present, and transplantation usually must be carried out in the face of this form of infection. Of all the treatable infections, the one that must particularly be sought pretransplant is *Strongyloides stercoralis. S. stercoralis* is an intestinal nematode endemic in many areas of the world; it has a complex life cycle.* The most important aspect of this life cycle is that autoinfection commonly occurs, so that although a person may have left an endemic area decades previously, he or she may still harbor this organism. When immunosuppression, as is prescribed for the transplant patient, is administered to a person with asymptomatic *Strongyloides* infections, a disastrous hyperinfection syndrome and/or disseminated strongyloidiasis can occur. The hyperinfection syndrome is an exaggeration of the normal life cycle of the parasite, with major impact

---

* Strongyloidiasis is an increasing problem in transplantation; I have personally seen 10 such cases in the past 18 months. These have occurred in immigrants from Southeast Asia and Central America and residents of the southern United States.

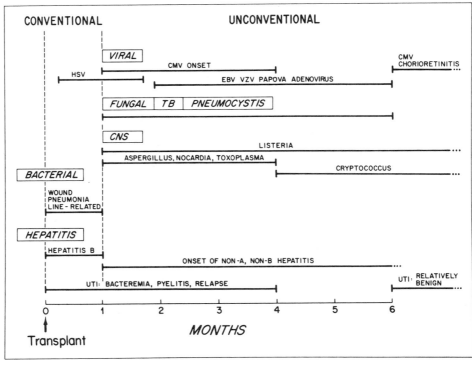

FIGURE 30-1.   *Timetable for the occurrence of infection in the organ transplant recipient. (Reprinted with permission from the American Journal of Medicine from Rubin et al.*[50]*)*

on the gastrointestinal tract (a severe, ulcerating hemorrhagic enterocolitis) and/or lungs, with a hemorrhagic pneumonia commonly noted. Disseminated strongyloidiasis consists of extension of the infection outside its normal domain, with the filariform larvae of this nematode invading all portions of the body. Both of these forms of *Strongyloides* infection are commonly associated with a sustained gram-negative bacteremia or meningitis. Whereas *Strongyloides* infection is relatively easy to treat pretransplant (Thiabendazole, 25 mg/kg twice daily for 3 days; or mebendazole, 200 mg twice daily for 3 days), even prolonged therapy post-transplant is quite difficult. Hence, the emphasis is on screening and prevention prior to onset of immunosuppression. Routine examination of the stools for ova and parasites may not be adequate to rule out a carrier state with *Strongyloides* infection. Examination of purged stool specimens and/or some sampling of the small intestine contents is commonly needed and should be considered in anyone with a past history of residence or exposure to areas of the world endemic for this organism. That is clearly a form of infection that must be prevented rather than treated in its full clinical manifestations.[51,53,54,62]

Infection From the Allograft

The allograft itself can be an important course of infection for the recipient. This is a particularly important consideration when a brain-dead "cadaveric" donor is being used. Although a variety of infections have been conveyed with allografts in the past, the major concerns are described here. *Long-standing infection of the donor, particularly with hepatitis B or HTLV-III (the causative agent of the acquired immunodeficiency syndrome, AIDS), is a major concern.* Acute hepatitis B with potentially disastrous consequences has been well documented to develop in recipients of kidneys from HB$_s$Ag positive donors.[67] Recently, AIDS has been documented to occur in recipients of kidneys from asymptomatic donors who are members of one of the population groups at high risk for AIDS (male homosexuals or bisexuals, intravenous drug abusers, and hemophiliacs) and who possessed antibodies to HTLV-III prior to transplant.[24,37] Because of this, all donors should be tested for hepatitis B and HTLV-III prior to organ donation, and persons who test positive should be disqualified as donors. In addition, because of the present state of HTLV-III antibody testing, it is our belief that unless very special circumstances exist (e.g., the need for an HLA-identical sibling donor for bone marrow transplantation), regardless of the results of HTLV-III serologic testing, no member of the high-risk groups should be used as an organ donor. Thus, HTLV-III testing should be regarded as a means to detect persons who have had an unknown exposure to this agent, rather than to validate the use of persons who have had a high likelihood of exposure to this agent.

Acute infections acquired at the time of terminal care from the indwelling bladder catheters and endotracheal tubes and intravascular lines commonly used in the care of such gravely ill persons are also of major concern. Occult sepsis has contaminated organs taken for transplantation and led to the subsequent disruption of the vascular anastomoses or generalized sepsis, with dire consequences in the recipient. Because of this, we advocate the following guidelines in evaluating potential cadaveric donors:

1. Any potential donor with documented systemic sepsis (i.e., untreated positive blood cultures), systemic viral infection, viral encephalitis, and so on is eliminated from consideration.
2. Even in the absence of symptoms, careful preterminal culturing of the donor (including blood cultures) and of organ perfusates or solutions in which organs are transported should be carried out. Systemic antibiotic therapy is initiated for positive cultures, using shorter duration of therapy (less than 7 days) when only the perfusate or carrying solutions are positive for nonvirulent organisms, and longer durations of therapy (more than 14 days) if blood cultures of the donor are positive or if any of the other cultures yield gram-negative bacilli, *S. aureus,* or *Candida* species—the organisms classically associated with disastrous consequences for the recipient.
3. Certain potential donors are at particularly high risk for occult sepsis and should not be used. These include victims of drowning, burn victims, and patients who have been maintained on a respirator with indwelling lines and catheters for periods of more than 7 days.[26,31,61]

Infection Related to Technical Complications

The most important treatable cause of infection in this time period is wound infection. The most important factor in the prevention of wound sepsis in the transplant recipient is the technical quality of the surgery performed; the incidence of wound sepsis is directly related to the incidence of wound hematoma, urine leak, or lymphocele formation created by the surgery. Other bacterial infections occurring in this time period, namely urinary tract infection, pneumonia, bacteremias, cholangitis, and pleural space infection, are similarly related to technical issues and embody a very important general principle in this population: The immunosuppressed patient tolerates poorly the presence of foreign bodies that bypass local host defenses (e.g., endotracheal tubes, urinary catheters, biliary tree catheters, and plastic intravenous catheters); therefore, these should be used sparingly, removed promptly, and managed with impeccable aseptic technique.[23,46,50]

INFECTION ONE TO SIX MONTHS POST-TRANSPLANT

This is the time period during which transplant patients are at greatest risk of life-threatening infection. There are at least two reasons for this. First, the *duration* of immunosuppressive therapy has now been sufficient so that patients' host defenses are now significantly compromised. The adverse effects of excessive immunosuppression administered in the first few weeks post-transplant will not be felt immediately, but, rather, a few weeks later. This is perhaps the most seductive aspect of antirejection therapy: The rewards for increasing immunosuppressive therapy can be seen quite quickly in terms of improved allograft function; the price is paid weeks later in terms of life-threatening infection. The risk of serious infection unrelated to technical considerations begins to rise significantly 3 weeks following post-transplantation, peaks by 8 weeks, and starts to decrease thereafter.[46,50]

Second, important virus infections (particular herpes group viruses and hepatitis viruses), themselves modulated by the two phenomena that are unique to transplantation—immunosuppressive therapy and allograft rejection—present during this time period. The clinical impact of these viral infections is much greater than that of comparable infections in normal hosts and may be grouped into four general categories:

1. A variety of clinical infectious disease syndromes produced by the virus itself.
2. An immunosuppressed state produced by the virus that is over and above that caused by the immunosuppressive drugs being administered but that contributes significantly to the net immunosuppressed state of the transplant patient and plays an important role in the pathogenesis of opportunistic superinfection owing to *Pneu-*

mocystis carinii, Listeria monocytogenes, fungi, and so on.

3. A form of allograft dysfunction produced by the virus that has a different pathogenesis from that of classic allograft rejection and appears to require a different form of therapy.
4. Malignancy in which viral infection is an important cofactor in its pathogenesis.[46,49,50]

Particularly important in explaining the relatively high rate of opportunistic infection during this time period are the contribution of these viruses (particularly CMV, Epstein-Barr virus, and non-A, non-B hepatitis) to the patient's *net state of immunosuppression.* Experiments with a murine CMV model have illustrated what is believed to be taking place in the human transplant situation: Sublethal murine CMV infection, when combined with otherwise sublethal infection with a variety of bacteria and fungi, causes lethality.[13] Studies in human renal transplant patients have demonstrated that the subgroup of patients at particularly high risk of opportunistic infection are those with viral-induced changes in lymphocyte subsets (see below). Indeed, when opportunistic infection occurs in the absence of significant viral infection (and these lymphocyte changes), this is an important clue to the presence of an excess epidemiologic hazard.[52]

Immunosuppressive therapy, then, has both direct and indirect effects in influencing the occurrence and course of infection—direct, in terms of specific effects on one or another limb of host defense; indirect, in terms of the effects on certain viral infections, which themselves modulate host responsiveness to microbial invasion. Different immunosuppressive agents and regimens appear to have differing effects on the incidence of renal infection. Perhaps the best information in this area comes from studies of CMV infection.[47] Whereas steroids alone have relatively little effect in terms of reactivating or promoting CMV infection, therapy with azathioprine or cyclophosphamide has significant CMV-promoting effects.[10,47] Perhaps the most dramatic CMV-promoting effects are seen with the antilymphocyte antibody treatments.[3,7,27,33] In particular, Cheeseman and associates[7] have reported that when antithymocyte globulin (ATG) was added to conventional azathioprine and prednisone regimens (as has been traditionally prescribed), there was a higher rate of viremia and symptomatic disease in the ATG group, and beneficial effects of prophylactic interferon-alpha therapy were abrogated. Patients at risk for primary CMV infection tolerated antilymphocyte antibody treatment very poorly, with both increased mortality and decreased graft survival. In contrast, patients not at risk for reactivation of CMV infection appear to benefit from such therapy.[48] The adverse effects of antilymphocyte therapy can be diminished by decreasing by 50% or more the dosage of other immunosuppressive agents administered at the same time.[41] A similar, although less detailed experience, has been noted with monoclonal antilymphocyte antibody treatments.[47]

The advent of cyclosporine therapy has added a new consideration to this analysis. Data currently available comparing cyclosporine-based regimens to conventional azathioprine–prednisone regimens would suggest the following: Cyclosporine with or without prednisone therapy and azathioprine–prednisone therapy are associated with similar rates of infection, *provided that no adjunctive antilymphocyte antibody treatment is administered.* However, the cyclosporine group of patients will have an increased graft survival rate. To achieve a graft survival rate comparable to that achieved with cyclosporine-based regimens, antilymphocyte antibody treatment must be added to azathioprine–prednisone regimens, and this is associated with a higher rate of infection. Thus, it would appear that the use of cyclosporine may be associated with a lower incidence of infection for a given rate of allograft survival.[3,30,60]

INFECTION MORE THAN SIX MONTHS POST-TRANSPLANT

An important manifestation of the improved clinical results being achieved with organ transplantation is the fact that increasing attention is now being turned to the long-term results, whereas in years past, virtually all attention was focused on the first 6 to 12 months following the transplant procedure. In the late post-transplant period, infection remains an important concern, with particular groups of patients now being defined with greater or lesser risks of life-threatening infection.[2,3]

First, the majority of patients with functioning allografts and continuing immunosuppression have a remarkably low rate of infectious disease complications provided that their graft function is good, their maintenance immunosuppressive therapy is at a low level, and acute antirejection therapy has not been needed. Thus, of more than 300 long-term renal transplant recipients with a serum creatinine less than 2 mg/dl, daily prednisone dose less than or equal to 15 mg/day, and no evidence of chronic viral infection whom we have followed for periods of up to 10 years, there has been only a single incidence of *Listeria* sepsis, one of cryptococcal meningitis, and one of an isolated cryptococcoma in the lung. Instead, there have been 51 episodes of urinary tract infection treatable as an outpatient (46 in women, only 5 in men), 9 cases of pneumoccoccal pneumonia, 14 cases of influenza (most during community-wide influenza outbreaks), and 2 cases of bacterial sinusitis. Thus, in those patients who are doing well, the risk of opportunistic infection is low, and the pattern of infection observed is similar to that seen in the general community.

Second, a significant minority of patients with less satisfactory results of their transplant remain at high risk for life-threatening opportunistic infection. These patients have common features (1) chronic rejection, (2) higher than usual chronic antirejection therapy, (3) a recurrent need for acute antirejection treatment, and (4) a high incidence of chronic infection with such immunosuppressing viruses as CMV and non-A, non-B hepatitis. Thus, among 100 renal transplant patients more than 6 months posttransplant with a serum creatinine greater than 2 mg/dl, daily prednisone dose greater than or equal to 20 mg/day, and the other characteristics noted, there have been 6 cases of *Listeria* sepsis and/or meningitis, 9 cases of cryptococcal meningitis, 4 cases of disseminated nocardial infection, and 2 cases of invasive aspergillosis, as well as the usual array of community-acquired, more "benign" infections. Management of these patients and prevention of these infections remains difficult. In the case of renal transplantation, it is likely that such patients would be better served by discontinuing immunosuppression and returning the patient to dialysis, allowing him to be retransplanted at a later date. In the case of hepatic and cardiac transplantation, because of the lack of an alternative means· of preserving life, this strategy is not applicable and "preventive retransplantation" is not a satisfactory option. At the present time, close clinical follow-up and assiduous attention to even minor complaints appears to be the best approach.

Third, there is a small group of patients who fall halfway between the two major categories: They are doing well with their transplants (and, hence, resemble the first group of long-term transplant survivors) but have chronic viral infections with late sequelae. The prime examples of this are progressive chorioretinitis resulting from CMV and progressive liver disease resulting from one of the hepatitis viruses (see below). In addition, as outlined in Table 30-1, it is likely that the combination of chronic viral infection, chronic immunosuppression, and other factors (such as sunlight in the case of skin cancers) plays an important role in the relatively high incidence of malignant disease observed in long-term survivors of organ transplantation.

INFECTIONS OF PARTICULAR IMPORTANCE IN THE TRANSPLANT RECIPIENTS

Herpes Virus Group

All four human herpes viruses, CMV, Epstein-Barr virus (EBV), herpes simplex (HSV), and varicella-zoster virus (VZV) are common and clinically important in the transplant patient. Their significance in this patient population is in large part due to three major characteristics:

1. *Latency*—Primary infection with each of these agents results in lifelong dormant infection capable of being reactivated by such factors as immunosuppression and allograft rejection at any point in the future.
2. *Cell-association*—Spread of the virus occurs from

TABLE 30-1   *Virus–Malignancy Associations in the Organ Transplant Recipient**

VIRUSES MOST COMMONLY FOUND IN TRANSPLANT PATIENTS	TYPE OF VIRUS-ASSOCIATED MALIGNANCY
Epstein-Barr virus	B cell lymphoproliferative disease
Cytomegalovirus	Kaposi's sarcoma
Herpes simplex virus	Squamous cell carcinoma of the cervix, uteri, and/or lip
Vericella-zoster virus	?
Hepatitis B	Hepatocellular carcinoma
Non-A, non-B hepatitis	?
Papillomavirus (wart virus)	Squamous cell carcinoma of the skin
Polyomavirus	?
Adenoviruses	?

* Modified from Rubin RH, Tolkoff-Rubin NE: Viral infection in the renal transplant patient. Proc Eur Dial Transplant Assoc 19:513–528, 1982

cell to cell with direct contact between the cells being important, thus rendering neutralizing antibody inefficient and cell-mediated immunity predominant in controlling the infection.

3. *Oncogenicity*—All herpes group viruses must be considered potentially oncogenic.[20]

Cytomegalovirus (CMV)

This virus is the single most important cause of infectious disease morbidity post-transplant, with 60% to 96% of patients demonstrating clinical and/ or laboratory evidence of infection with this agent.[2,20,47,49] There are three epidemiologic patterns of CMV infection in transplant patients, each with differing rates of clinical sequelae.

1. *Primary CMV infection.* In this pattern of CMV infection, the transplant patient has had no previous CMV infection (is CMV-antibody negative pretransplant) and acquires the virus transmitted in latent fashion from a seropositive donor. In the case of kidney and cardiac transplants, it is likely that in more than 80% of instances, the latently infected cells are within the allograft, with the remainder of the cases of primary infection resulting from transfusions of blood products containing latently infected, viable leukocytes. In the case of liver transplantation, in which massive blood requirements are the rule, it is likely that such blood is a more important source of primary CMV infection. Approximately 60% of patients at risk for primary CMV disease (seropositive donor, seronegative recipient) will develop clinically overt infection.[2,20,47,49]

2. *Reactivation CMV infection.* In this pattern, the transplant recipient has previously been infected with CMV (and is seropositive prior to transplant) and reactivates endogenous latent virus post-transplantation. Essentially every patient who is seropositive pretransplantation will reactivate virus post-transplantation, with approximately 20% of these persons becoming clinically ill.[2,20,47,49]

3. *Reinfection CMV infection.* In this pattern, seropositive persons are reinfected by virus latently carried by the allograft from a seropositive donor, and, when immunosuppression is administered, the virus that is reactivated is the donor's virus, not the recipient's endogenous virus. The exact incidence of this reinfection phenomenon is unclear, although it has clearly been shown to occur using molecular virologic techniques to characterize viral isolates.[2,65] Likewise, the clinical significance of reinfection

has still to emerge. However, there are now two studies clearly showing that the clinical outcome of transplanting a kidney from a seropositive donor into a seropositive recipient is significantly worse than transplanting a kidney from a seronegative donor into a seropositive recipient.[12,56]

Clinical Course. With all forms of CMV disease, overt infection begins 1 to 6 months after initiation of immunosuppression, with a peak occurrence 6 to 8 weeks post-transplant in renal and cardiac transplant recipients, and perhaps a few weeks earlier in liver transplant recipients. The latter may be due to the relatively large inoculum administered along with the many blood transfusions given to these patients. Clinical CMV disease has a typical viral prodrome consisting of constitutional symptoms of fever, malaise, and myalgias, closely resembling the mononucleosis syndrome caused by this virus and the closely related EBV in normal persons. In approximately one third of patients who develop fever owing to CMV, a dry, nonproductive cough develops within a few days of the onset of fever. Over several days, increasing respiratory distress may develop, with a typical x-ray picture of a bilateral, peribronchovascular (interstitial) pneumonitis emerging in the periphery of the lower lobes. Occasionally, the x-ray picture may resemble the focal consolidation seen with bacterial or fungal infection.[2,20,27,34,42,47,49,50]

CMV infection in the transplant patient is a systemic infection, and other organ systems frequently manifest the effects of such infection. Small numbers of atypical lymphocytes (less than 10%/ mm^3), leukopenia, and thrombocytopenia occur in 50% or more of symptomatic patients. Approximately one third of persons will have a mild to moderate degree of hepatocellular dysfunction caused by the virus. This event can be quite important in patients receiving liver transplantation, because unless a biopsy is done and reveals the presence of the virus, the clinical episode of hepatic dysfunction can be mistaken for rejection and excessive amounts of immunosuppression can be administered. Thus, during the period of time when acute CMV infection is particularly manifest in these patients (3–6 weeks post-transplant), episodes of hepatic dysfunction should be carefully evaluated with biopsies done on a regular basis to rule out a false diagnosis of hepatic allograft rejection. Additional gastrointestinal system manifestations include ulcerations of the gastrointestinal tract leading to severe hemorrhage—typical CMV inclusions may be seen at these sites of ulceration, and virus can be isolated from these lesions, which are particularly common in the cecum and the remainder of the right colon.[2,20,27,34,42,47,49,50]

In the mid-1970s, prior to the advent of cyclosporine therapy, Simmons and associates[55] described a group of patients with what they termed the *lethal CMV syndrome*. This syndrome was characterized by a desultory onset with initial fever and leukopenia, but progressed rapidly to include severe pulmonary and hepatic disease, central nervous system dysfunction, gastrointestinal hemorrhage, and death, usually due to superinfection or bowel hemorrhage. Such patients are less commonly seen today, but the syndrome can still occur with too intensive immunosuppression administered in a desperate attempt to salvage an allograft.

One manifestation of CMV infection that occurs separately from the acute syndromes that have thus far been defined is a form of severe progressive chorioretinitis, which usually begins 4 to 8 months post-transplant and may occur in persons who had no previous symptoms owing to the virus. Without effective antiviral chemotherapy (see below), this chorioretinitis is usually relentlessly progressive, causing blindness itself or in conjunction with a secondary development of retinal detachment, anterior uveitis, and glaucoma.[2,20,47,49,50]

Even more important than the direct infectious disease effects of CMV infection, is the fact that this virus predisposes to life-threatening superinfection with a variety of microbial agents. As previously noted, infection with CMV is an important contributor to the net state of immunosuppression in a given patient. The most obvious marker for this depression of host defenses is CMV-induced leukopenia. Even more important, however, are the effects of CMV in depressing cell-mediated immunity.[2,20,42,46,47,49,50] In recent years, a marker has emerged for the presence of CMV (and EBV) induced cell-mediated immune depression. This marker is provided by the measurement of T cell subsets (using flow cytometry and monoclonal antibodies that recognize different T cell subsets). Both in normal persons and in transplant recipients, these viruses cause a decrease in the T helper cells and an increase in the T cytotoxic-suppressor cells. If the normal ratio of T helper cells to T suppressor cells is approximately 1.5, CMV-infected transplant patients have ratios of 0.1 to 0.5. There are two major correlates with these viral-induced T cell subset changes: The great majority of opportunistic infections occur in the subset of renal transplant patients with inverted ratios, and CMV-associated allograft injury occurs essentially only in those patients with inverted T cell subsets.[52]

Renal Allograft Rejection. The most controversial aspect of CMV infection in the renal transplant patient is whether the virus is associated with renal allograft dysfunction. Data from two large studies, one from a single institution[12] and one from a multicenter study[48] involving approximately 50 institutions, suggest that particularly when antilymphocyte therapies are administered to patients at risk for primary CMV infection, that such patients are at increased risk for losing their allograft. Richardson and colleagues[39] described a group of patients with allograft dysfunction in association with CMV infection. Their renal biopsies failed to reveal the typical tubulointerstitial changes of rejection and instead showed an unusual glomerular lesion. This glomerulopathy was diffuse and characterized by enlargement or necrosis of endothelial cells and accumulation of mononuclear cells and fibrilar material in glomerular capillaries. The association of this lesion with virus-induced T cell subset changes is consistent with the hypothesis that the virus is involved with the pathogenesis of this lesion. The exact mechanism by which this lesion develops in conjunction with viral infection is not known. Preliminary data suggest that these patients do poorly with increased amounts of immunosuppression conventionally used to treat rejection, that they may improve by decreasing the amount of immunosuppression, and that the incidence of this lesion may be decreased by the administration of prophylactic interferon therapy.

Oncogenic Effect. The possible oncogenicity of CMV has garnered increasing attention in recent years, although direct proof is still lacking. Epidemiologic studies, DNA hybridization studies of tumor tissue, and immunofluorescent demonstration of CMV antigen on tumor cells have all suggested a pathogenetic role for CMV in the development of Kaposi's sarcoma. Particularly provocative is the high incidence of CMV infection in the two populations with the highest occurrence rate for this tumor: patients with the AIDS, and renal transplant patients.[47]

Therapy. The control of CMV infection in the transplant patient has been difficult, to say the least. Prevention of CMV infection may be possible with the administration of prophylactic interferon-alpha[19] or hyperimmune globulin.[57] In addition, efforts are currently underway to develop an attenuated vaccine for this purpose.[36] Until recently, the only approach to the management of the acutely ill patient with CMV infection has been to decrease overall immunosuppression, in particular, to stop cytotoxic drugs and antilymphocyte therapies and attempt to treat any superinfecting pathogens. A new antiviral agent, 9-2-hydroxy-l(hydroxymethyl) ethoxymethyl guanine (DHPG) appears to be the first antiviral agent with sufficient anti-human CMV effects to offer a practical chance for treating patients. Although there is limited experience at present in transplant patients, in the even more challenging AIDS patient with severe CMV disease, this agent has shown a great deal of promise, particularly in patients with progressive CMV chorioretinitis.[28] For the first time, it is not unreasonable to believe that specific antiviral chemotherapy of CMV infection is possible.

Epstein-Barr (EBV) Virus

This virus is almost as common as CMV in transplant patients, with most transplant recipients demonstrating some evidence of EBV reactivation posttransplant. Primary infection has occasionally occurred in pediatric transplant recipients, with a range of clinical syndromes observed, including asymptomatic disease, a mononucleosis-like syndrome, and a rapidly fatal multiorgan lymphoproliferative disease similar to that seen in boys with the X-linked lymphoproliferative disorder that follows EBV infection. The infectious disease consequences of EBV reactivation probably closely resemble those observed with CMV, although because of the ubiquity of CMV, the contributions of EBV to individual patient morbidity may be difficult to discern.[49,50] Much more important are the contributions of EBV to the development of B cell lymphoproliferative disease.

Approximately 10% to 15% of the malignancies observed in organ transplant recipients are a form of lymphoma called *immunoblastic sarcoma* (formerly termed reticulum cell sarcoma), which is characterized by the lymphomatous invasion of the central nervous system, nasopharynx, liver, small bowel, heart, and transplanted kidney. EBV-specific antibody titers, immunofluorescent staining of tumors for the presence of EBV nuclear antigen, and DNA hybridization studies all strongly implicate EBV in the pathogenesis of this tumor.[14–17] The current hypothesis is that in immunologically normal persons who have had previous infection with EBV (and hence are antibody-positive and remain latently infected with this virus), circulating cytotoxic T-lymphocytes specific for EBV-induced antigens on the surface of infected B-lymphocytes serve as an important surveillance mechanism in preventing the outgrowth of virally induced, transformed cells, which are thought to initiate the oncogenic process, which can ultimately result in lymphoproliferative

disease.[5,9,17] In immunosuppressed patients, this surveillance mechanism is impaired, a phenomenon particularly associated with cyclosporine administration[5,9] ever since Calne and associates[6] reported 5 lymphomas occurring among their first 23 patients treated with cyclosporine. Fortunately, more recent experience with cyclosporine suggests that when lower doses are used and blood levels are closely monitored, there is a relatively low incidence of these tumors,[22] and that, at least in the early stages of the tumor when it is still polyclonal in character, regression occurs when the cyclosporine is discontinued and/or acyclovir (an antiviral drug with activity against EBV) is administered.[58] Because of a recent report[4] of a B cell lymphoma developing in a patient treated with relatively low doses of cyclosporine that were meticulously monitored by blood level testing, this remains an area of some concern.

Herpes Simplex Virus (HSV)

Approximately half of all transplant patients develop mucocutaneous lesions as a result of HSV 2 to 5 weeks post-transplant. HSV Type I infection in and around the oral cavity can be quite extensive and is exacerbated by mucosal trauma with nasogastric and/or endotracheal tubes. The former is associated with herpetic esophagitis, and the latter with herpetic bronchopneumonia, which otherwise is quite unusual in organ transplant recipients. Severe anogenital infection, usually caused by HSV Type II, may also occur. At this body site, large coalescing ulcers, often without the classic vesicles associated with HSV infection, may develop. Less commonly, HSV infection can produce zosteriform lesions on the lower back and buttocks or a syndrome known as *eczema herpeticum* (Kaposi's varicelliform eruption) in patients with preceding eczema or other extensive skin damage. HSV infection in organ transplant patients treated with modern immunosuppressive regimens rarely disseminates but is clinically important both for the discomfort it causes and because the break in the mucocutaneous surfaces that ensues may provide a portal of entry for secondary bacterial or candidal invasion.[46,49]

Of all the immunosuppressive regimens, as with the other herpes group viruses, antilymphocyte antibody treatment is particularly associated with severe HSV infection.[7,46,49] Fortunately, the advent of acyclovir therapy (either intravenously at a dose of 5 mg/kg every 8 hours or orally at a dose of 200 mg five times per day in adults with normal renal function) has markedly decreased the morbidity associated with HSV infection in transplant patients.

It should be pointed out, however, that acyclovir therapy may need to be prolonged beyond the usual 5 to 7 days if acute antirejection treatment is ongoing, particularly, if such treatment includes as antilymphocyte antibody.[46,49]

Varicella-Zoster Virus (VZV)

As with the other herpes group viruses, primary infection with this agent may be quite severe. Primary VZV infection in renal transplant patients, as in any immunosuppressed patient, can be a devastating illness characterized by severe pneumonia, gastrointestinal lesions with hemorrhage, central nervous system (CNS) involvement, and disseminated intravascular coagulation. Therefore, a careful check of past chickenpox experience and current exposures is essential, with immediate zoster immune globulin prophylaxis for any significant exposures and institution of acyclovir therapy at the earliest stages of clinical disease.[46,49]

In contrast, reactivation infection (zoster) occurs in approximately 10% of patients between 2 months and 3 years post-transplant. Reactivation VZV infection takes the form of typical, localized dermatomal zoster in the renal transplant patient. Unlike the lymphoma patient, visceral dissemination of VZV in the transplant patient is quite rare, and the routine use of antiviral chemotherapy (e.g., acyclovir, adenosine arabinoside, interferon) is not currently recommended.[46,49]

Hepatitis

Evaluation of episodes of liver dysfunction in organ transplant recipients can be quite difficult. In all these patients, drug toxicity owing to such agents as azathioprine, cyclosporine, alpha-methyl-dopa, isoniazid, and so on, must be considered. Unfortunately, with doses of the agents currently used, it is unusual for hepatic dysfunction in these patients to be due to such drugs. Similarly, CMV and EBV, which commonly cause transient abnormalities in liver function, appear to be rare causes of chronic hepatic dysfunction. Most of the time, in the renal and cardiac transplant recipient, the cause of hepatic dysfunction is infection with a hepatitis virus—hepatitis B, or non-A, non-B hepatitis.[46,49] In the liver transplant patient, the differential diagnosis is rendered particularly difficult by the task of differentiating allograft rejection from these other causes of hepatic dysfunction, particularly viral infection. Given the large amount of blood administered to liver transplant patients, it is likely that a significant proportion of the hepatic dysfunction observed more than 1 month post-transplant is due to one or more of the hepatitis viruses.

Unlike the situation in normal hosts, infection with either hepatitis B or non-A, non-B hepatitis in transplant patients is rarely associated with an acute clinical syndrome. Rather, asymptomatic infection is first detected by the routine measurement of liver function tests, and it is only over the long-term that the consequences of these infections are perceived. Transaminase levels of only one and one half to three times normal over a prolonged period of time have been associated with the subsequent development of end-stage cirrhosis. Similarly, liver biopsies in the first few months or even after years of chronic hepatic dysfunction have been very poor predictors of the clinical outcome in this patient population.[25,32,35,46,49,64]

Hepatitis B is usually acquired prior to transplant from blood transfusions while the patient is undergoing hemodialysis or, rarely, from the allograft if the donor is HB$_s$Ag-positive. In the first 6 to 24 months post-transplant, patients with chronic HB$_s$Ag antigenemia prior to transplant continue to manifest this, there are minimal changes in liver function, and there is no adverse effect on either patient or graft survival. However, beginning 1 to 2 years post-transplant, these patients begin to present with signs and symptoms of far advanced cirrhosis and/or hepatocellular carcinoma.[25,32,35,46,49,64] In fact, actuarial data beginning to accumulate suggest that over time, most successful transplant patients with chronic hepatitis B infection will succumb to one of these effects, provided that no other untoward events occur. In addition, some observers have suggested an increased risk of extrahepatic infection and fatal cardiovascular events in patients with chronic hepatitis B infection.[18,64]

Non-A, non-B hepatitis is probably acquired primarily from blood transfusion. More than 80% of transplant patients who develop non-A, non-B hepatitis post-transplant develop chronic liver disease. It is now apparent that non-A, non-B hepatitis can be a major contributor to the net state of immunosuppression. For example, in the first year post-renal transplantation, there is both an increased incidence of the mortality from extrahepatic infection among patients with non-A, non-B hepatitis. Conversely, the 1-year kidney allograft survival rate in these patients is significantly greater than that for those free of infection.* The other major late manifestation of this chronic hepatitis is the occult development of cirrhosis. After a stable course with only mild abnormalities in liver function observed for many years, patients appear as

---

* This relationship has stimulated some centers to use significantly less immunosuppression in patients with non-A, non-B hepatitis with no adverse effect on graft survival.

long as 10 years post-transplant with ascites, bleeding esophageal varices, spontaneous bacterial peritonitis, and so on; all the manifestations of end-stage liver disease, as a result of their long-standing non-A, non-B hepatitis.[25,46,49,64]

Urinary Tract Infection

Although urinary tract infection and subsequent urosepsis can follow bladder catheterization in any transplant patient, it has a particular impact on the renal transplant recipient. If antimicrobial prophylaxis is not used in renal transplant recipients, urinary tract infection will occur in 35% to 79% of patients.[43,46,50] Even more important, some 60% of all bacteremias in this patient population have been of urinary tract origin.[29] Although the bladder catheter is the presumed portal of entry for the bacteria into the urinary tract, other factors unique to the transplant patient appear to be operative here. In animal models, it has been shown that if kidneys are traumatized, bacteria introduced either into the bladder or into the circulation will lodge in the manipulated kidney. In the transplant patient, it is believed that trauma to the kidney caused by the procurement, perfusion, and implantation procedures and the immunologic injury of rejection predispose similarly to a high rate of pyelonephritis. Presumably, immunosuppressive therapy further exacerbates this problem.[43,46]

Not surprisingly, then, urinary tract infection occurring in the first few months post-renal transplant has a much great clinical impact than urinary tract infection occurring more than 6 months post-transplant. "Early" urinary tract infection is frequently associated with overt pyelonephritis, bacteremia, and a high rate of relapse when treated with a conventional 10- to 14-day course of antibiotics (but is cured with a 6-week course of therapy). In contrast, "late" urinary tract infection is rather benign, can be managed with a conventional 10- to 14-day course of antibiotics, is rarely associated with a bacteremia or requires hospitalization (unless superimposed on some other urinary tract complication), and has an excellent prognosis.[43,46]

Of great importance, it has now been shown that the serious "early" form of urinary tract infection can be essentially eradicated by the use of low-dose antimicrobial prophylaxis during the high-risk period. A single-strength tablet of trimethoprim-sulfamethoxazole (containing 80 mg trimethoprim, 400 mg sulfamethoxazole), 100 mg of trimethoprim, or 250 mg of cinoxacin (and assuredly other agents as well) administered at bedtime has essentially eradicated urinary tract infection in our renal transplant population. Mycostatin is administered

at the same time to minimize mucocutaneous candidal colonization. It is important to note that *this low dosage* of trimethoprim-sulfamethoxazole is not associated with an increased risk of nephrotoxicity in patients receiving cyclosporine therapy.[46,59]

Bacteremia

Bacteremia and candidemia are major causes of morbidity and mortality in the transplant patient. Blood stream invasion with bacteria or *Candida* species can be divided into four major categories: intravenous line-related sepsis, urosepsis, gastrointestinal sepsis, and *Listeria* sepsis.

Intravenous Line-Related Sepsis

As with other seriously ill, hospitalized patients, nosocomial line-related septicemias are not uncommon. The spectrum of organisms is similar in the transplant patient to that observed in other patients—*Staphylococcus epidermidis*, *S. aureus*, aerobic gram-negative rods, and *Candida* species. However, the consequences of such blood stream invasion can be much greater in transplant patients. For example, when candidemia occurs in nonimmunocompromised host as a result of a contaminated central venous line, in more than 95% of patients the only therapy necessary is to remove the contaminated line. In contrast, in immunocompromised patients such as transplant patients, such transient candidemia results in metastatic seeding and the need for systemic antifungal therapy in more than 50% of people.[11] Because of this, the use of intravenous and intra-arterial lines should be kept to a minimum in this patient population; when used, they should be changed frequently; and strict, aseptic technique must be enforced in their use.

Urosepsis

As noted previously, this formerly common cause of microbial blood stream invasion has been greatly minimized in renal transplant patients with the use of low-dose antimicrobial prophylactic programs. Bacterial urosepsis still occasionally appears in patients with some form of anatomic complication that requires prolonged catheterization, repeated manipulation, and so on, emphasizing again the importance of technical perfection in the operative approach to these immunosuppressed patients. One additional form of urosepsis that bears further comment is that due to *Candida*. Candidal pyelonephritis, usually in association with obstruction either at the ureteropelvic junction or ureterovesical junction, owing to the presence of fungal balls, is an occasional cause of disseminated candidiasis in the renal transplant patient. Such infections are most common in diabetes, in patients with poorly functioning bladders, and in those who have had ureteral stents or catheters in place because of technical complications of the transplant. Any transplant patient with candiduria merits both antifungal therapy (low-dose amphotericin plus 5-fluorocytosine being the most effective) and an ultrasonic scan to rule out obstructive uropathy.[46]

Gastrointestinal Sepsis

Traditionally, the two most common causes of sepsis of gastrointestinal origin in transplant patients have been diverticulitis of the rectosigmoid colon and perforation of a gastric or duodenal ulcer. It is important to emphasize that physical and laboratory manifestations of these disastrous abdominal complications in transplant patients may be minimal until late in the course, and an aggressive evaluation of any such patient presenting with abdominal distention, ileus, pain, and/or fever is essential for patient salvage. In contrast to the relative frequency of diverticulitis and ulcer disease in this patient population are the relative rarity of cholecystitis and, even more so, appendicitis.[8]

With the advent of liver transplantation, bacteremias caused by technical complications of the biliary anastomosis and spontaneous bacterial peritonitis in the early postoperative period have been noted. Candidal colonization of the upper gastrointestinal tract of such patients is presumably playing a significant role in the relatively high rate of invasive candidiasis observed in liver transplant patients.[63]

Listeria Sepsis

In renal transplant patients, with the control of both urosepsis and line-related sepsis, *Listeria monocytogenes* has emerged as a major cause of bacteremia; indeed, at our center, it is the leading cause. It is also not an infrequent cause of bacteremia in other transplant patients beginning more than 1 month after successful transplantation. *Listeria* is acquired by the ingestion of the organism (most commonly in contaminated food such as fresh salad materials), followed by subsequent colonization of the gastrointestinal tract, and then blood stream invasion. This organism has a particular tropism for the CNS once it enters the blood stream, causing both a pyogenic meningitis and focal areas of cerebritis (see below).[46,50]

Pneumonia

Infection of the lungs is the most common form of life-threatening infection observed in transplant patients, occurring in as many as 20% of such patients at some point in their course, and accounting for most infectious disease deaths that occur in this group of patients. The key to patient salvage in this circumstance is the rapid diagnosis and prompt institution of effective therapy. Certain clues are useful in attaining these goals: (1) the epidemiologic and clinical settings in which the pulmonary processes are occurring, (2) the rate of progression of the illness, and (3) the pattern of pulmonary abnormality seen on roentgenogram of the chest.[38,46]

The epidemiologic clues useful in evaluating the transplant patient with pneumonia are of three types: (1) the patient's possible remote exposures to mycobacterial or fungal (such as coccidioidomycosis or histoplasmosis) infection, (2) the patient's community or household exposures to persons with such acute respiratory illnesses as influenza, and (3) the patient's possible exposure to endemic or epidemic nosocomial hazards within the hospital environment.[38,46]

The timetable of infection outlined in Figure 30-1 can be of significant help in generating a differential diagnosis. In addition, assessment of the pace at which the pneumonia has developed and progressed can be useful; for example, bacterial pneumonias develop acutely over less than 24 hours, whereas such processes as viral, fungal, or protozoan infections develop subacutely to chronically over days to weeks before they come to clinical attention. When this information is correlated with the appearance of the chest x-ray, the differential diagnosis becomes greatly narrowed (Table 30-2).[38]

Although the intellectual exercise just outlined is helpful in limiting the diagnostic possibilities, it does not lead to the exact diagnosis and therapy that are needed. The next step is to demonstrate the pathogen causing the process. If diagnosis is not immediately apparent on the basis of history, physical examination, and expectorated sputum examination, more invasive techniques are necessary. Unfortunately, such noninvasive techniques as antibody determinations are not useful in this clinical circumstance. A range of procedures is available for the purpose of invasive diagnosis. Choosing the most useful diagnostic technique for the individual patient is the major challenge in this clinical circumstance. The first criterion in making this decision is an assessment of the gravity of the patient's illness: Are you dealing with a therapeutic emergency, or are you dealing with a diagnostic dilemma? If it is a therapeutic emergency, the definitive procedure, open lung biopsy, is carried out as quickly and expeditiously as possible. If the problem is more of a diagnostic dilemma, a lesser procedure is used, knowing that an open lung biopsy might still be used at a later date if needed. The three "interme-

TABLE 30-2   Etiologies of Pneumonitis in the Organ Transplant Recipient Based on the Chest X-Ray and the Rate of Progression of the Illness*

TYPE OF ABNORMALITY ON CHEST X-RAY	ETIOLOGY ACCORDING TO THE RATE OF PROGRESSION OF THE ILLNESS	
	Acute	Chronic
Consolidation	Bacterial (including *Legionella*)	Fungal
	Thromboembolic	Nocardial
	Hemorrhagic (Pulmonary edema)	Tuberculous (Viral, *Pneumocystis*)
Interstitial infiltrate	Pulmonary edema	Viral
	Leukoagglutinin reaction (Bacterial)	*Pneumocystis* (Fungal, nocardial, tuberculous)
Nodular infiltrate	(Bacterial, pulmonary edema)	Fungal
		Nocardial
		Tuberculous (Viral, *Pneumocystis*)

* Modified from Ramsey PG, Rubin RH, Tolkoff-Rubin NE et al: The renal transplant patient with fever and pulmonary infiltrates: Etiology, clinical manifestations and management. Medicine 59:206–222, 1980

Note: An *acute* illness is one that develops, requiring medical attention in a matter of a relatively few hours (less than 24). A *subacute-chronic* process develops over several days to weeks. Note that unusual causes of a process are placed in parentheses.

diate'' procedures that are of greatest use at the present time are transtracheal aspiration, fiberoptic bronchoscopy with bronchopulmonary lavage with or without transbronchial biopsy, and percutaneous needle aspiration. The first of these, transtracheal aspiration, is of particular use in diagnosing acute bacterial pneumonia by providing a sample of lower respiratory secretions uncontaminated by the oral flora. The bronchoscopic procedures are particularly useful in the diagnosis of such diffuse processes as *P. carinii* and CMV infections. Percutaneous needle aspiration is the procedure of choice for focal, particularly cavitary, peripheral, pleural-based, nodular lesions (typically caused by fungi or *Nocardia*).[38,40,44,66]

One final point that bears emphasis when considered pneumonia in the transplant patient is that dual infection and, particularly, superinfection are quite common. Indeed, it is usually the superinfection that causes death, rather than primary infection. Therefore, even if a diagnosis has been proved by a biopsy procedure, the clinician must remain alert to the possibility of additional diagnostic considerations, particularly in the patient who is not responding as expected to appropriate therapy or who has ceased to respond after an initial clinical response to such therapy.[38,40,44,46,66]

Central Nervous System (CNS) Infection

CNS infection occurs in approximately 5% to 10% of organ transplant recipients, thus constituting an important cause of morbidity and mortality in this patient population. There are four major clinical presentations of CNS infection in the transplant patient:

1. Acute meningitis. This is caused by *L. monocytogenes* in approximately 90% of instances.
2. Subacute to chronic meningitis. This is caused by *Cryptococcus neoformans* in more than 90% of instances. In populations in which tuberculosis is endemic or in geographic areas where such systemic mycotic infections as histoplasmosis and coccidioidomycosis are endemic, these may also cause a subacute to chronic meningitis.
3. Focal neurologic dysfunction. This is most commonly caused by *Aspergillus fumigatus* infection, metastatic from a pulmonary or nasal sinus portal of entry. Other, less common causes of focal brain infection are *Nocardia asteroides* (again metastatic from the lung), *Listeria*, and *Toxoplasma gondii*. It should be emphasized that, as in other immunosuppressed patients, the major impact of *T. gondii* in the transplant patient is on the CNS.
4. Progressive dementia. This is due to papovavirus infection (JC virus), causing the condition known as progressive multifocal leukoencephalopathy (PML). In addition to a dementing illness, PML can present with slowly progressive focal neurologic deficits, particularly hemiparesis with and without aphasia, and with seizures.[21,45]

Two clinical points need to be emphasized when considering CNS infection in the transplant patient. The first is that the etiologies of these infections are very different from those causing similar clinical syndromes in the normal host. It is not that the transplant patient is immune to meningococcal or pneumococcal meningitis, it is just that *Listeria* is so much more common. Thus, a broader and a different range of organisms must be considered. Even more important to the clinician is the recognition that this is a particular group of infections in which the anti-inflammatory effects of the immunosuppressive therapy greatly modify the clinical presentation. Thus, only 60% of transplant patients with acute meningitis will have any evidence of meningeal irritation, and, in many of these patients, the findings are quite subtle. Only minor abnormalities in the state of consciousness may be present in florid CNS disease. Thus, the index of suspicion for the clinician must be much greater than that which is normally required. The most reliable combination of clinical findings for suggesting the possibility of important CNS infection is the presence of fever and headache. Any renal transplant patient with an unexplained headache of more than a few hours' duration, especially if fever is present, should undergo careful neurologic examination. If there is no evidence of papilledema or focal neurologic deficit, an immediate lumbar puncture should be carried out, and the fluid should be submitted for routine studies plus measurement of cryptococcal antigen and, possibly, antibody titers for *Histoplasma capsulatum* and *Coccidioides imitis* (if the geographic exposure is appropriate). If papilledema or focal deficits are found on neurologic examination, an immediate computerized axial tomographic (CAT) scan should be performed prior to the lumbar puncture.[21,45]

Dermatologic Infection

Continuing evaluation of the skin and subcutaneous tissue is an important part of the clinical management of the transplant patient. On the one hand, the skin is an important barrier to the invasion of microbial pathogens, and, when this primary barrier is breached in an immunocompromised host, the potential for extensive local and disseminated infection with opportunistic pathogens is great. On the other hand, the skin's rich blood supply provides an opportunity for metastatic spread of infection to the skin from other sources, often providing an early clue to the diagnosis of disseminated infection.[46,48]

Infection of the skin in transplant patients may be divided into four general categories:

1. *Infection originating in the skin and typical of that occurring in immunocompetent persons.* In this category are the typical cellulitic processes caused by gram-positive bacteria, which appear to be both more common and more severe in transplant patients. The major point to be made here is that both fungi, such as *Candida* species and *C. neoformans,* and gram-negative organisms are capable of producing a very similar clinical picture and skin pathology as the more classical, gram-positive cellulitides; thus, the clinician must be alert to a wider differential diagnosis and resort to biopsy much earlier in the disease process.

2. *Extensive involvement of the skin with organisms that usually produce localized or trivial infection in immunocompetent persons.* Prime example of this phenomenon are extensive dermatophyte infections (such "nonvirulent" fungi as *Trichophyton* species and *Fusarium solari*) and the common wart caused by papillomavirus. Both can be extensive, cause disfigurement, and, in the case of the dermatophyte infections, provide a portal of entry for life-threatening superinfection.

3. *Infection originating in the skin caused by opportunistic organisms that rarely produce disease in immunocompetent patients but that may produce localized or disseminated infection in immunocompromised patients.* Skin that has been traumatized by a variety of causes in the transplant patient has proved to be fertile soil for the engraftment of local infection with the fungus *Paecilomyces* and such atypical mycobacteria as *M. marinum* and the algae *Prototheca.* Of even greater concern, is that when skin has been macerated with pressure dressings or damaged in other ways, primary skin invasion with *Aspergillus, Candida,* or *Rhyzopus* species has been documented, with both local and systemically disseminated infection being noted. It is therefore of great importance to protect the skin, particularly in the area around surgical wounds, from the damage that can result in such local, secondary invasion.

4. *Disseminated systemic infection metastatic to the skin from a noncutaneous portal of entry.* In approximately one third of patients with cryptococcal infection, there will be skin lesions present weeks to months prior to the development of CNS disease. Similarly, 10% to 15% of patients with disseminated candidal infection will have the early development of skin lesions; comparable numbers of patients have been observed with skin lesions in the setting of dis-

seminated nocardial and *Aspergillus* infection. Therefore, careful examination of the skin and early biopsy of unexplained skin lesions is important in order to take advantage of this early warning system. It should be emphasized that this is another circumstance in which the al-

tered inflammatory response will tend to minimize the extent of the skin process and tend to underplay the significance of a particular skin lesion. Therefore, an aggressive biopsy approach is necessary.[46,48]

REFERENCES

1. Barnes BA, Bergan J, Braun W et al: The 12th report of the human transplant registry. JAMA 233:787–796, 1975
2. Betts RF: Cytomegalovirus in transplant patients. Prog Med Virol 28:44–64, 1982
3. Bia MJ, Andiman W, Gaudio K et al: Effect of treatment with cyclosporine versus azathioprine on incidence and severity of cytomegalovirus infection post-transplantation. Transplantation 40:610–614, 1985
4. Bia MJ, Flye MW: Immunoblastic lymphoma in a cyclosporine-treated renal transplant recipient. Transplantation 39:673–674, 1985
5. Bird AG, McLachlan SM, Britton S: Cyclosporin A promotes spontaneous outgrowth *in vitro* of Epstein-Barr virus-induced B-cell lines. Nature 289:300–301, 1981
6. Calne RY, Roller K, Thiru S et al: Cyclosporin A initially as the only immunosuppressant in 34 recipients of cadaveric organs: 32 kidneys, 2 pancreas, and 2 livers. Lancer 2:1033–1936, 1979
7. Cheeseman SH, Rubin RH, Stewart JA et al: Controlled clinical trial of prophylactic human leukocyte interferon in renal transplantation. Effect on cytomegalovirus and herpes simplex virus infections. N Engl J Med 300:1345–1349, 1979
8. Cosimi AB: Surgical aspects of infection in the compromised host. In Rubin RH, Young LS (eds): Clinical Approach to Infection in the Compromised Host, 2nd ed. New York, Plenum, (in press)
9. Crawford DH, Sweny P, Edwards JMB et al: Long-term T-cell mediated immunity to Epstein-Barr virus in renal allograft recipients receiving Cyclosporin A. Lancet 1:10–12, 1981
10. Dowling JN, Saslow AR, Armstrong JA et al: Cytomegalovirus infection in patients receiving immunosuppressive therapy for rheumatologic disorders. J Infect Dis 133:399–408, 1976
11. Edwards JE Jr, Lehrer RI, Stiehm ER et al: Severe candidal infections: Clinical perspective, immune defense mechanisms, and current concepts of therapy. Ann Intern Med 89:91–106, 1978
12. Fryd DS, Peterson PK, Ferguson RM et al: Cytomegalovirus as a risk factor in renal transplantation. Transplantation 30:436–439, 1980
13. Hamilton JR, Overall JC Jr, Glasgow LA: Synergistic effect on mortality in mice with murine cytomegalovirus and *Pseudomonas aeruginosa, Staphylococcus aureus,* or *Candida albicans* infections. Infect Immun 14:982–989, 1976

14. Hanto DW, Frizzera G, Gajl-Peczalska K et al: The Epstein-Barr virus (EBV) in the pathogenesis of post-transplant lymphomas. Transplant Proc 13:756–760, 1981
15. Hanto D, Frizzera G, Purtilo DT et al: Clinical spectrum of lymphoproliferative disorders in renal transplant recipients and evidence for the role of Epstein-Barr virus. Cancer Res 41:4253–4261, 1981
16. Hanto DW, Gajl-Peczalska KJ, Frizzera G et al: Epstein-Barr virus (EBV) induced polyclonal and monoclonal B-cell lymphoproliferative diseases occurring after renal transplantation. Clinical, pathologic, and virologic findings and implications for therapy. Ann Surg 198:356–369, 1983
17. Hanto DW, Simmons RL: Lymphoproliferative diseases in immunosuppressed patients. In Morris PJ, Tilney NL (eds): Progress in Transplantation, Vol 1, pp 186–208. Edinburgh, Churchill Livingstone, 1984
18. Hillis WD, Hillis A, Walker WG: Hepatitis B surface antigenemia in renal transplant recipients. JAMA 243:329–332, 1979
19. Hirsch MS, Schooley RT, Cosimi AB et al: Effects of interferon-alpha on cytomegalovirus reactivation in renal-transplant recipients. N Engl J Med 308:1489–1493, 1983
20. Ho M: Cytomegalovirus, Biology and Infection. New York, Plenum, 1982
21. Hooper DC, Pruitt AA, Rubin RH: Central nervous system infection in the chronically immunosuppressed. Medicine 61:166–188, 1982
22. Kahan BD, Van Buren CT, Flechner SM et al: Clinical and experimental studies with cyclosporine in renal transplantation. Surgery 97:125–140, 1985
23. Kyriakides GK, Simmons RL, Najarian JS: Wound infections in renal transplant wounds: Pathogenetic and prognostic factors. Ann Surg 186:770–775, 1975
24. L'Age-Stehr J, Schwarz A, Offerman G et al: HTLV-III infection in kidney transplant recipients. Lancet 2:1361–1362, 1985
25. LaQuaglia MP, Tolkoff-Rubin NE, Dienstag JL et al: Impact of hepatitis on renal transplantation. Transplantation 32:504–507, 1981
26. Majeski JA, Alexander JW, First MR et al: Transplantation of microbially contaminated cadaver kidneys. Arch Surg 117:221–224, 1982
27. Marker SC, Howard RJ, Simmons RL et al: Cytomegalovirus infection: A quantitative prospective study of 320 consecutive renal transplants. Surgery 89:660–671, 1981

28. Masur H: New concepts in the therapy of infections in the acquired immunodeficiency syndrome, p 802. In Fauci AS (moderator): The acquired immunodeficiency syndrome: An update. Ann Intern Med 102:800–813, 1985

29. Myerowitz RL, Medeiros AA, O'Brien TF: Bacterial infection in renal homotransplant recipients; a study of fifty-three bacteremia episodes. Am J Med 53:308–314, 1972

30. Najarian JS, Fryd DS, Strand M et al: A single institution, randomized, prospective trial of cyclosporine versus azathioprine-antithymocyte globulin for immunosuppression in renal allograft recipients. Ann Surg 201:142–157, 1985

31. Nelson PW, Delmonico FL, Tolkoff-Rubin NE et al: Unsuspected donor *Pseudomonas* infection causing arterial disruption after renal transplantation. Transplantation 37:313–315, 1984

32. Parfery PS, Forbes RDC, Hutchinson TA et al: The impact of renal transplantation on the course of hepatitis B liver disease. Transplantation 39:610–615, 1985

33. Pass RF, Reynold DW, Whelchel JD et al: Impaired lymphocyte transformation response to cytomegalovirus and phytohemagglutinin in recipients of renal transplants: Association with antithymocyte globulin. J Infect Dis 143:259–265, 1981

34. Peterson PK, Balfour HH Jr, Marker SC et al: Cytomegalovirus disease in renal allograft recipients: A prospective study of the clinical features, risk factors and impact on renal transplantation. Medicine 59:283–300, 1980

35. Pirson Y, Alexandre GPJ, van Ypersele de Strihou C: Long-term effect of HBs antigenemia on patient survival after renal transplantation. N Engl J Med 296:194–196, 1977

36. Plotkin SA, Smiley ML, Friedman HM et al: Towne vaccine in the prevention of post-transplant CMV disease. Lancet 1:528–530, 1984

37. Prompt CA, Reis MM, Grillo FM et al: Transmission of AIDS virus at renal transplantation. Lancet 2:672, 1985

38. Ramsey PG, Rubin RH, Tolkoff-Rubin NE et al: The renal transplant patient with fever and pulmonary infiltrates: Etiology, clinical manifestations and management. Medicine 59:206–222, 1980

39. Richardson WP, Colvin RB, Cheeseman SH et al: Glomerulopathy associated with cytomegalovirus viremia in renal allografts. N Engl J Med 305:57–63, 1981

40. Rosenow EC III, Wilson WR, Cockerill FR III: Pulmonary disease in the immunocompromised host. Mayo Clin Proc 60:473–487, 1985

41. Rubin RH, Cosimi AB, Hirsch MS et al: Effects of antithymocyte globulin on cytomegalovirus in renal transplant recipients. Transplantation 31:143–145, 1981

42. Rubin RH, Cosimi AB, Tolkoff-Rubin NE et al: Infectious disease syndromes attributable to cytomegalovirus and their significance among renal transplant recipients. Transplantation 24:458–464, 1977

43. Rubin RH, Fang LST, Cosimi AB et al: Usefulness of the antibody-coated bacteria assay in the management of urinary tract infection in the renal transplant recipient. Transplantation 27:18–20, 1979

44. Rubin RH, Greene R: Etiology and management of the compromised patient with fever and pulmonary infiltrates. In Rubin RH, Young LS (eds): Clinical Approach to Infection in the Compromised Host, 2nd ed. New York, Plenum, (in press)

45. Rubin RH, Hooper DC: Central nervous system infection in the compromised host. Med Clin North Am 69:281–296, 1985

46. Rubin RH: Infection in the renal transplant patient. In Rubin RH, Young LS (eds): Clinical Approach to Infection in the Compromised Host, 2nd ed. New York, Plenum, (in press)

47. Rubin RH, Tolkoff-Rubin NE: The problem of cytomegalovirus infection in transplantation. In Morris PJ, Tilney NL (eds): Progress in Transplantation, Vol 1, pp 89–114. Edinburgh, Churchill Livingstone, 1984

48. Rubin RH, Tolkoff-Rubin NE, Oliver D et al: Multicenter seroepidemiologic study of the impact of cytomegalovirus infection on renal transplantation. Transplantation 40:243–249, 1985

49. Rubin RH, Tolkoff-Rubin NE: Viral infection in the renal transplant patient. Proc Eur Dial Transplant Assoc 19:513–528, 1982

50. Rubin RH, Wolfson JS, Cosimi AB et al: Infection in the renal transplant patient. Am J Med 70:405–411, 1981

51. Ruskin J: Parasitic diseases in the compromised host. In Rubin RH, Young LS (eds): Clinical Approach to Infection in the Compromised Host, 2nd ed. New York, Plenum, (in press)

52. Schooley RT, Hirsch MS, Colvin RB et al: Association of herpesvirus infections with T-lymphocyte-subset alterations, glomerulopathy, and opportunistic infections after renal transplantation. N Engl J Med 308:307–313, 1983

53. Scoggin CH, Call NB: Acute respiratory failure due to disseminated strongyloidiasis in a renal transplant recipient. Ann Intern Med 87:456–458, 1977

54. Scowden EB, Schaffner W, Stone WJ: Overwhelming strongyloidiasis: An unappreciated opportunistic infection. Medicine 57:527–544, 1978

55. Simmons RL, Matas AJ, Rattazzi LC et al: Clinical characteristics of the lethal cytomegalovirus infection following renal transplantation. Surgery 82:537–546, 1977

56. Smiley ML, Wlodaver CG, Grossman RA et al: The role of pretransplant immunity in protection from cytomegalovirus disease following renal transplantation. Transplantation 40:157–161, 1985

57. Snydman DR, McIver J, Leszczynski J et al: A pilot trial of a novel cytomegalovirus immune globulin in renal transplant recipients. Transplantation 38:553–557, 1984

58. Starzl TE, Nalesnik MA, Porter KA et al: Reversibility of lymphomas and lymphoproliferative lesions developing under cyclosporin-steroid therapy. Lancet 1:583–587, 1984

59. Tolkoff-Rubin NE, Cosimi AB, Russell PS et al: A

controlled study of trimethoprim-sulfamethoxazole prophylaxis of urinary tract infection in renal transplant recipients. Rev Infect Dis 4:614–618, 1982

60. Tolkoff-Rubin NE, Rubin RH: The impact of cyclosprine therapy on the occurrence of infection in the renal transplant recipient. Transplant Proc 18 (Suppl 1):168–173, 1986

61. Van der Vliet JA, Tidrow G, Koostra G et al: Transplantation of contaminated organs. Br J Surg 67:596–598, 1980

62. Vishwanneth S, Baker RA, Mansheim BJ: *Strongyloides* infection and meningitis in an immunocompromised host. Am J Trop Med Hyg 31:857–858, 1982

63. Wajszczuk CP, Dummer JS, Ho M et al: Fungal infections in liver transplant recipients. Transplantation 40:347–353, 1985

64. Weir MR, Kirkman RL, Strom TB et al: Liver disease in recipients of long-functioning renal allografts. Kidney Int 28:839–844, 1985

65. Wertheim P, Geelen J, van der Noordaa J: Exogenous cytomegalovirus reinfection by renal allograft in seropositive recipients. Lancet (in press)

66. Wilson WR, Cockerill FR III, Rosenow EC III: Pulmonary disease in the immunocompromised host. Mayo Clin Proc 60:610–631, 1985

67. Wolf JL, Perkins HA, Schreeder MT et al: The transplanted kidney as a source of hepatitis B infection. Ann Intern Med 91:412–413, 1979

68. Wolfson JS, Sober AJ, Rubin RH: Dermatologic manifestations of infections in immunocompromised patients. Medicine 64:115–133, 1985

CHAPTER 31

Selected Complications of Renal Transplantation

Alan I. Benvenisty   Mark A. Hardy

Complications of renal transplantation include hypertension, diabetes mellitus, thromboembolic phenomena, several musculoskeletal complications, gastrointestinal complications, hyperparathyroidism, lymphocoeles, and ocular and psychiatric complications.

Hypertension may occur at any time after transplantation, and it may be secondary to chronic rejection, renal artery stenosis, and cyclosporine toxicity. Refractory hypertension mandates angiography. The arterial lesion is usually related to rejection or to a technical problem. Diabetes mellitus is mostly related to high-dose steroid therapy. Thromboembolic phenomena, more common than generally thought, may be increased with the use of cyclosporine.

Avascular necrosis of the femoral heads is the most common orthopedic complication and may not be related to steroid dosage. Hyperparathyroidism usually resolves after a successful transplant; the bony lesion almost never progresses postoperatively.

Pancreatitis and peptic and colonic ulceration/bleeding are the most lethal of the gastrointestinal complications, associated with 50% mortality rates. The role of prophylactic ulcer surgery for recipients with ulcer disease is diminished with the availability of H_2 blockers.

Lymphocele is caused by leaking host lymphatics. Prevention lies in meticulous ligation of divided lymphatics. Large or symptomatic collections should be drained.

Cataracts commonly follow renal transplantation and are related to steroid use. The progression of diabetic retinopathy is not significantly affected by a transplant. The most common psychiatric complication is depression.

The intent of this chapter is to briefly describe complications of renal transplantation not discussed in other sections. It is evident that the major problems associated with renal transplantation are either infectious and/or immunologic. Several specific complications of which the reader needs to be aware are highlighted here.

HYPERTENSION

Hypertension is one of the most common complications of renal transplantation and its incidence rate can be as high as 50%.[4] Several factors in the etiology of post-transplant hypertension must be considered: (1) the status of the native kidneys, (2) the status of allograft function, (3) methods of immunosuppression, and (4) the presence of renal artery stenosis.

The high incidence of hypertension in a series of patients treated with azathioprine and prednisone suggests that the native kidneys do not contribute significantly to post-transplant hypertension. Despite this, some hypertensive patients will respond favorably to native nephrectomy.[41] The association between hypertension occurring after transplantation and decreased long-term graft survival has been noted.[15,19] It is not clear whether such hypertension leads to allograft dysfunction or whether renal dysfunction, usually secondary to chronic rejection or repeated episodes of acute rejection, results in hypertension. The role of corticosteroids in the development of post-transplant hypertension continues to remain uncertain; reduction in steroid doses rarely leads to significant improvement in hypertension. The recent use of cyclosporine as an immunosuppressant has resulted in development of hypertension in recipients of both renal[45] and cardiac[48] allografts.

In patients with hypertension refractory to treatment with antihypertensive medications, the presence of renal artery stenosis (RAS) must be seriously considered. The appearance of a new bruit over the transplant, or alteration of a pre-existing bruit, especially when there is a new onset of hypertension, must also alert the clinician to the possibility of RAS. The incidence of RAS in renal allograft recipients ranges from 3% to 25%,[23,40,68] depending upon the vigor with which the diagnosis is sought.

Percutaneous angiography is diagnostic, and several patterns of RAS have been described. The most common pattern is related to immunologic changes in the artery and is seen just distal to the anastomosis; it is associated with pseudointimal proliferation and no poststenotic dilatation. Changes in the main arterial wall secondary to immunologic damage, even in the absence of rejection in the renal parenchyma, have been suggested. Technical errors, including problems such as inverted adventitia, twisting of the anastomosis, and partial suture closure of the lumen, are obvious causes of RAS that may be occasionally difficult to demonstrate. Injuries to the intima by perfusion cannulae (dissection) and by perfusion injury ("jet effect") may damage the donor artery and eventually result in stenosis. Kinks in the renal artery owing to poor positioning or uncomfortable "lie" of the allograft may also lead to RAS. Such technical complications leading to RAS are usually associated with a poststenotic dilatation. If the diagnosis of RAS is uncertain, captopril, a converting enzyme inhibitor, may be used as a provocative diagnostic agent.[20] It will usually result in an acute deterioration of renal function in those patients who have RAS because of the dependence of the renal blood flow upon the renin–angiotensin system, but it will not have this effect in the absence of RAS.

Surgical correction and percutaneous transluminal dilatation (PTD) are the two alternative methods of treatment of RAS that is not immunologically mediated. Suitable candidates for either procedure will improve if there is no evidence of acute or chronic rejection.[60,68] PTD is relatively safe and has approximately a 76% success rate at 1 month.[46,57] Surgical exploration and repair should be reserved for technically unsuccessful PTDs or for patients with frequent recurrences of RAS after initially successful PTDs. Surgical repair of RAS is best performed by a transperitoneal approach. Optimal treatment includes the use of autogenous vein patch grafts if possible.[23] Other techniques include reimplantation of arteries and/or the use of saphenous vein autografts. A technical success rate of 74% from operative correction can be expected,[51] but the mortality rates are higher than those for PTD, and graft loss has recently been reported to be 10% to 20%, even in the most experienced hands.[51,63]

ACUTE DIABETES MELLITUS FOLLOWING TRANSPLANTATION

Diabetes mellitus following transplantation is thought to occur in 5% to 15% of renal allograft recipients.[28,59] It is usually mild and is frequently responsive to reduction or withdrawal of corticosteroids. It has been suggested that steroids induce the diabetes by producing a relative state of insulin resistance leading to impaired peripheral glucose utilization and increased gluconeogenesis. New onset of diabetes mellitus in transplant recipients is more common in those who have a family history of diabetes.[59] There is a suggestion that certain HLA antigens (A28, DR3, and DR4) are associated with this complication,[22,32] but they are not predictive of development of diabetes. The possibility that islet damage is triggered by a virus has also been considered but never proved. However, patients can develop diabetes mellitus while maintained on cyclosporine despite the recent suggestion by Stiller and associates[66] that this medication can be used in the treatment of Type I diabetes mellitus.

The treatment of this complication depends upon the severity and the form of diabetes. Many patients will be successfully treated by dietary regulation, whereas others will require careful management with insulin. Although there is disagreement about the relationship between the development of acute diabetes mellitus after transplantation and the overall graft and patient outcome, it appears that graft survival in these patients is not affected while the overall patient survival appears decreased.

THROMBOEMBOLIC COMPLICATIONS

Thromboembolic disease following renal transplantation has not been sufficiently emphasized, although it has been reported to occur in 0.6% to 2% of patients.[6,35,43,56] Some patients with renal transplants have decreased platelet aggregation, and others show no postoperative rise in fibrinogen.[43] Despite the fact that most renal transplant recipients are relatively young and therefore at less risk of thromboembolic disease, in one retrospective review of 125 patients, 8.8% developed symptomatic thromboembolic disease within the first year of allografting, and two patients died of pulmonary emboli.[3] Prospective studies using venous plethysmography have shown evidence of deep vein thrombosis without any apparent relation to the location of the transplanted kidney.[6] However, in that series, no pulmonary emboli were detected.

With the increased use of cyclosporine, there may be an associated increase in the incidence and severity of thromboembolic disease. In one recent series of 80 cadaveric allograft recipients, 17 thromboembolic complications occurred in 13 patients, including 10 episodes of pulmonary emboli, 3 episodes of deep vein thromboses, and 1 case of renal vein thrombosis.[69] These complications were associated with increased levels of fibrinogen, antithrombin III, and protein C; the relationship of such changes to the use of cyclosporine is uncertain. Deep vein thrombosis and associated pulmonary emboli should be treated in allograft recipients in the identical way that is used in patients who do not have a renal allograft. Full heparinization should be followed by administration of Coumadin for 3 months for deep vein thrombosis and for 6 months for pulmonary emboli. Patients who have clear contraindications to heparinization or who are bleeding at the time of diagnosis should be seriously considered for placement of a Greenfield filter or for other methods of inferior vena caval interruption despite the presence of a renal allograft attached to one of the iliac veins.

MUSCULOSKELETAL COMPLICATIONS

Avascular osseous necrosis has been a relatively common problem after renal transplantation prior to the "cyclosporine era," occurring in 3% to 4% of patients.[8,34] This most commonly occurs in the femoral heads but may also occur in the femoral condyles, ankles, and humeral heads.[9] Etiology of this problem appears to be related to the use of corticosteroids and may be dose related. It has been suggested that repeated rejection episodes increase the likelihood of an osteonecrotic lesion,[33] but this complication can occur even when low doses of corticosteroids are used.[25] Hypophosphatemia, which leads to increased bone resorption, has also been associated with avascular bone necrosis, but causal relationship has not been established. Conclusive evidence is lacking that hyperparathyroidism of hypercalcemia contributes significantly to the development of avascular necrosis, although its presence has been frequently associated with this complication.

Although the exact etiology of this disorder is not understood, several theories to explain it have emerged. Pressure of intravascular fat globules in nutrient arterioles[38] might cause subsequent ischemic necrosis; microfractures in already osteopenic bone with consequent local disturbance of blood supply have also been implicated.[49] Gradual increase in the pressure of femoral heads and subsequent relief with core decompression have been shown to preserve the blood supply to the bone in experimental models. This approach is currently being used clinically and may prevent the progression of the lesion in the femoral head.[70] Symptoms of avascular bone necrosis usually appear more than 1 year after transplantation, although lesions may be detected earlier by bone scans and even plain bone x-rays. Conservative management of lesions in lower extremities includes non–weight-bearing and non-steroid anti-inflammatory agents. Patients who develop severe disability involving function and/or pain and who are unable to accomplish activities of daily living become candidates for operative intervention. Total hip replacement is frequently necessary in ischemic necrosis of the femoral head. In patient receiving cyclosporine and only small doses of steroids, the incidence of avascular osseous necrosis will hopefully decrease, as appears to be the situation, in preliminary observations.

GASTROINTESTINAL COMPLICATIONS

Pancreatitis

Pancreatitis is a potentially devastating complication following transplantation that occurs in 2% to 7% of renal allograft recipients.[18,27] This complication, associated with the use of corticosteroids, may be precipitated by steroid bolus therapy for rejection and has been related to post-transplant hypercalcemia.[47] The pathogenesis of this complication remains uncertain; its effective treatment is delayed by the use of all immunosuppressants. The early signs and symptoms of acute pancreatitis following transplantation may be subtle, and a high index of suspicion is required for prompt diagnosis. Patients with renal impairment often have mild hyperamylasemia; high levels of serum amylase in the presence of abdominal and back pain are diagnostic. Severe sequelae, including hemorrhagic pancreatitis, abscess, and/or pseudocyst formation, are, unfortunately, relatively common in immunosuppressed patients. Ultrasonography and computed tomographic (CT) scanning should be used to detect such potentially fatal problems. Because of the mortality rate associated with this complication (as high as 53%),[27,58] aggressive treatment should be instituted early. This includes total parenteral nutrition, nasogastric suction, antacid therapy, and careful metabolic monitoring with appropriate corrections, including transfusions. Surgical intervention is indicated only when pancreatic abscess or mature pancreatic pseudocyst exists. Essentials of treatment include prompt reduction in corticosteroid dosage, avoidance of azathioprine, and dose reduction of cyclosporine. The role of cyclosporine in acute pancreatitis remains uncertain. As a potent immunosuppressant, it may delay spontaneous improvement by interfering with host resistance, and its administration should probably cease when the patient shows signs of deterioration. Allograft removal may be necessary if patient recovery is not prompt.[58]

Peptic Ulcer Disease

In a comprehensive review of data from 12 transplant centers, peptic ulcer disease complicated the course in approximately 5% of allograft recipients. Bleeding or perforation, which carried a mortality of approximately 50%, was the presenting symptom in 87% of patients with this complication; mortality was higher in patients with bleeding than in those with perforation..[50] Patients who had known peptic ulcer disease prior to transplantation have done better if they had elective acid-reducing operations, usually vagotomy and pyloroplasty, prior to the time of renal transplantation.[65]

The previously established role of prophylactic surgery for prospective renal allograft recipients[42,50] is currently being re-evaluated with the availability of more efficient antacid therapy. Antacids are recommended for all patients, but especially for those with history of ulcer disease proven by upper GI series and/or gastroscopy. Prophylactic use of cimetidine or another H_2-receptor antagonist has been recommended for those with history of ulcer disease. Randomized controlled studies of the prophylactic use of H_2-receptor antagonists in renal transplant recipients have demonstrated the safety of these agents; no increased incidence of rejection episodes was found in those receiving the drugs, and ulcer incidence was low in both experimental and control groups.[12] Since cimetidine is a potent stimulator of the immune response in vitro, its routine use in all patients has not been recommended. The prophylactic use of antacids has only minor side-effects, and their regular use is urged for at least 6 months following transplantation, with intensification of the dosage regimen during treatment with steroid boosts for rejection.[50]

Colonic Complications

Perforation and lower gastrointestinal hemorrhages are major colorectal complications following renal transplantation.[26] The incidence of hemorrhage is less than 1%, but this complication carries an overall mortality reported as 71% in 15 series of gastrointestinal complications.[67] Colitis of infectious, pseudomembranous, ischemic, or uremic etiology was the main cause for lower gastrointestinal hemorrhage. Prompt diagnosis, usually by colonoscopy, arteriography, and barium examinations is essential to initiate appropriate therapy, which frequently includes withdrawal of immunosuppression or partial colectomy and may require transplant nephrectomy.

Colonic perforation is also a potentially lethal complication following renal transplantation. Although this is a relatively rare complication (11 of 1000 transplants at Cleveland Clinic[17] and 3 of 350 transplants at Columbia Presbyterian Medical Center), the mortality rate from this complication was as high as 88% prior to 1975. At present, mortality is still higher than 30%, even though prompt recognition and operative intervention have led to improved results.

Predisposing factors causing colonic perforation include renal failure itself, frequently associated with constipation, and a resulting high incidence of diverticular disease in young uremic patients. It is not surprising that renal transplant patients are subject to "spontaneous" colon perforations, which are difficult to recognize promptly because they are unexpected in this generally young population. Impaired capacity for healing and tissue weakness in such patients are contributing factors. The possibility of iatrogenic trauma to the colon with retractors must be considered and prevented during the transplant procedure itself. Although no data show a higher incidence of colon perforations in immunosuppressed patients than in nonimmunosuppressed patients, more than half of colon perforations in transplant recipients occur in association with the use of high doses of steroids, either early after transplantation or during treatment of rejection. Diverticulitis is still the leading cause of colonic perforation in renal transplant recipients, especially in those with polycystic kidney disease.[61]

Prompt diagnosis is critical to patient survival. Delay in diagnosis must be minimized when there is masking of symptoms and signs of perforation by steroids and other immunosuppressive agents. The early use of x-rays and CT scans with rectally administered water-soluble contrast agents may be beneficial in defining the problem. Although reduction or discontinuation of immunosuppressive drugs is important in the successful treatment of colon perforations in renal transplant recipients, prompt surgical treatment is most important under the cover of appropriate antibiotics. The mortality rate of colostomy and drainage (60%) was higher than that of resection with exteriorization (46%) in renal transplant patients with perforated diverticulae. Most authors recommend resection or exteriorization of the perforated segment with an end or diverting colostomy with or without a Hartman-type procedure, as appropriate. The recent changes in immunosuppressive regimens and greater awareness of the diagnosis of colonic perforation has resulted in decreasing mortality from this previously fatal complication.

HYPERPARATHYROIDISM

Secondary hyperparathyroidism in patients with end-stage renal disease maintained on dialysis is common and well described.[24] Decreased urinary phosphate excretion and elevated serum phosphate levels in renal failure result in lowering of serum calcium levels. This, in turn, stimulates increased production of parathyroid hormone. Intestinal absorption of calcium is impaired by a decrease in the production by the end-stage kidney of the active vitamin metabolite, 1,25-dihydroxy vitamin D_2, and this decrease in calcium absorption further stimulates increased parathyroid hormone (PTH) release.[11]

Patients with end-stage renal disease who have one or all of the following may require either subtotal parathyroidectomy or total parathyroidectomy with heterotopic autotransplantation of parathyroid tissue: intractable pruritis, metastatic calcifications, and severe renal osteodystrophy.[72] On the other hand, a successful renal allograft will almost always eventually correct secondary hyperparathyroidism and many of its sequelae. In unusual and relatively rare circumstances, secondary hyperparathyroidism may persist after a successful renal allograft.

In 12% to 31% of renal transplant recipients, persistent and rising hypercalcemia may complicate the postoperative course,[24,29,54] especially in children. The large variation in incidence of this complication may be due to variability in the dose of postoperative steroids and/or the use of phosphate supplements that lower serum calcium levels.[2] Approximately 50% to 60% of patients with postoperative hypercalcemia improve within 1 year, while others improve more slowly. In one series,[11] only 6 of 113 patients with postoperative hypercalcemia eventually required partial parathyroidectomy for tertiary hyperparathyroidism. None of these patients had renal deterioration or osteitis fibrosa cystica. Patients with stable hypercalcemia can be safely observed for more than 1 year following transplantation without any operative intervention. If serum calcium levels continue to rise when there is normal renal function, surgical intervention may be indicated to prevent sequelae of hypercalcemia, including calcium precipitation in the kidney and stone formation. Finding of unexpected adenoma is rare, whereas persistent hyperplasia is more common. Although patients with postoperative allograft dysfunction can be demonstrated to have elevated PTH levels,[16] this is usually secondary to impaired renal function rather than a primary parathyroid abnormality. In Garvin and colleagues' series,[29] hypercalcemia did not correlate with deterioration of renal function; careful and prolonged observation of the patients did not appear to adversely affect the ultimate improvement in serum calcium levels.

In conclusion, a policy of expectant observation is recommended in patients with postoperative hypercalcemia following transplantation in order to permit the slow involution of the parathyroid glandular tissue. Parathyroidectomy should be reserved for only those patients whose serum calcium levels continue to rise. Surgical intervention may eventually be indicated in order to prevent severe sequelae of hyperparathyroidism, such as deterioration in bone disease or nephrocalcinosis, which are exceedingly rare in recipients of successful renal allografts.

LYMPHOCELE

A lymphocele is a walled-off collection of lymph that usually originates from an unligated lymphatic. In renal transplantation, a lymphocele lies in the retroperitoneal plane, usually adjacent to the kidney. Its rate of occurrence ranges from 2% to 18%.[10,62] Since the routine use of postoperative ultrasonography, many asymptomatic collections are frequently detected.[31] Occasionally, lymphoceles are related to acute rejection and can cause symptoms primarily by mechanical local compression. Consequent allograft dysfunction is usually related to obstruction of urine flow, which may result from ureteral compression, bladder deformity, and/or paraparenchymal and pelvic pressure. Venous compression may lead to leg edema with compression of external iliac vein and even compression of the vena cava and portal vein.[64] Allograft dysfunction from rejection of cyclosporine toxicity may be confused with symptoms of an enlarging lymphocele.

Routine use of ultrasonography will reliably diagnose a lymphocele and may help in its localization for percutaneous drainage.

Prevention of this complication is based on an understanding of its pathogenesis. Although the donor allograft can produce lymph, with up to 19 times the lymph flow during acute rejection,[52] both lymphangiography[44] and studies using radiolabeled lymph[71] have shown that it is the recipient's perivenous pelvic lymphatics that are the most likely source of lymph that produces a lymphocele. Careful ligation of divided perivenous retroperitoneal lymphatics will significantly lower the incidence of this complication,[13,31,36] which may be troublesome and even dangerous, especially in diabetic patients who have the highest incidence of wound and peritransplant infections.

Lymphoceles should be treated with an initial, even several, simple aspirations. Recurrence with this type of treatment is not uncommon, and the risk of secondary infection is significant. Optimal treatment for recurrent symptomatic lymphoceles is intraperitoneal marsupialization by a transperitoneal midline exploration; this should include excision of a portion of the cyst wall[30,31,36] while carefully avoiding injury to the transplanted ureter. External drainage, with or without marsupialization, is less popular because of the presumed risk of infectious complications.

OCULAR COMPLICATIONS

Several types of ocular complications may occur after renal transplantation. The most common is cataract formation, reported in 23% to 53% of renal transplant recipients,[7,53,55] and absent in matched controls not receiving allografts. Cataracts may develop in patients maintained on as little as 5 mg of prednisolone per day for only 2 months.[21] Patients receiving the highest doses of steroids develop the most severe cataracts. The highest incidence of cataract formation is found in patients followed for several years after renal transplantation, and there is a suggestion that younger patients are more susceptible to this complication than are older patients. Cataracts may be assymetric and are not always bilateral. Treatment of cataracts in patients following renal transplantation is the same as in nontransplanted patients; greater concern about intraocular infection, especially in regard to lens implantations, must be maintained in immunosuppressed patients.

Other ocular problems include cytomegalovirus (CMV) retinitis, which, although relatively uncommon, may be devastating because of its tendency to progress to blindness. Other infectious ocular complications include both viral and fungal inflammations, which require appropriate antibiotic treatment, occasional débridements, and usually reduction of immunosuppression. Immunosuppression needs to be stopped occasionally to prevent progression of the disease to blindness with or without enucleation.

Progression of diabetic retinopathy after successful renal transplantation is influenced unfavorably by hypertension and appears to be unaffected by immunosuppression alone. Repeat laser coagulopathy of the retina in diabetic patients is frequently necessary following, as well as prior to, transplantation. Blindness secondary to diabetic microangiopathy is unfortunately a frequent complication in this rapidly growing subgroup of patients with end-stage renal disease.

PSYCHIATRIC COMPLICATIONS

Many psychological problems arise following renal transplantation that may directly complicate the patient's postoperative course. The newly transplanted kidney must be gradually accepted as the patient's "self." This usually occurs within 1 week of transplantation.[14] In patients with weak sexual identity, serious problems may arise in accepting an organ from a donor of the opposite sex. Major psychiatric sequelae, most commonly depression, occur in 4% to 32% of transplant recipients.[1] Corticosteroids may induce depression, as well as other psychotic episodes, even catatonia. Such changes may present extremely serious management problems, especially during the immediate post-transplantation period.[39] A particular difficulty occurs after transplantation in patients who have a pathologic dependence upon the dialysis unit and its staff when such relationship ceases. The patient may resent, and even try to destroy, the transplant by failing to take the immunosuppressive medications in an attempt to return to the dialysis unit.

Prevention of serious psychiatric problems by careful psychiatric evaluation of potential transplant recipients is the best approach to such complications.[5] Effective psychiatric support of patients following transplantation is most important. Awareness of the interrelationship of various psychotropic medications and immunosuppressive agents, especially cyclosporine, is important if the expected effectiveness of each agent is to be achieved.

The complications described in this chapter have been relatively frequent when conventional immunosuppression with steroids and azathioprine have been used. More recently, with decreased use of corticosteroids in conjunction with cyclosporine, the incidence of some of the complications described here appears to have decreased. Nevertheless, the problems associated with hypertension, thromboembolic disease, ulcer disease, ileocolic complications, diabetes mellitus, ocular problems, tertiary hyperparathyroidism, psychological problems, and even avascular osseous necrosis remain frequent enough and serious enough to deserve a brief description in relation to renal transplantation and immunosuppression.

REFERENCES

1. Abram HS: The psychiatrist, the treatment of chronic renal failure and the prolongation of life III. Am J Psychiatry 128:534–539, 1972
2. Alfey AC, Jenkins D, Groth CG et al: Resolution of hyperparathyroidism, renal osteodystrophy and metastatic calcification after renal homotransplantation. N Engl J Med 279:1349, 1968
3. Arnadottir M, Bergentz SE, Bergquist D et al: Thromboembolic complications after renal transplantation: A retrospective analysis: World J Surg 7:757–761, 1983
4. Bachy C, Alexandre GPJ, van Ypersele et al: Hypertension after renal transplantation. Br Med J 2:1287–1289, 1976
5. Benvenisty AI, Cianci J, Hardy MA: Psychosocial Aspects of Renal Transplantation. Positive Approaches to Living with End-Stage Renal disease: Psychosocial and Thanatologic Aspects. New York, Prager, 1985
6. Bergquist D, Bergentz SE, Bornmyr S et al: Deep vein thrombosis after renal transplantation: A prospective analysis of frequency and risk factors. Eur Surg Res 117:69–74, 1985
7. Berkowitz JS, David DS, Sakai S et al: Ocular complications in renal transplant recipients. Am J Med 55:492–495, 1973
8. Bewick M, Stewart PH, Rudge C et al: Avascular necrosis of bone in patients undergoing renal allotransplantation. Clin Nephrol 5:66, 1976
9. Bradford DS, Szalapski EW, Sutherland DER: Osteonecrosis in the transplant recipient. Surg Gynecol Obstet 159:328–334, 1984
10. Braun W, Banowsky L, Stratton RA et al: Lymphocoeles associated with renal transplantation. Report of 15 cases and review of the literature. Am J Med 57:714, 1974
11. Brunt CM, Wells SA: Surgical treatment of secondary hyperparathyroidism. Ann Chir Gynaecol 72:139–145, 1983
12. Bulseson RC, Kronhaus RJ, Marberger PD et al: Cimetidine, posttransplant peptic ulcer. Complications and renal allograft survival—a clinical and investigational perspective. Arch Surg 117:933–935, 1982
13. Burleson RL, Marberger P: Prevention of lymphocele following renal allotransplantation. J Urol 127:18–19, 1982
14. Castelnuovo-Tedesco P: Ego vicissitudes in response to replacement or loss of body parts. Psychoanal Q 47:381–397, 1978
15. Cheigh JS, Wang J, Fine P et al: Hypertension and decreased graft survival in long term kidney transplant recipients (abstr). Am Soc of Nephrol Washington, DC, 1984
16. Christensen MS, Nielsen HE, Torring S: Hypercalcemia and parathyroid function after renal transplantation. ACTA Med Scand 201:35–39, 1977
17. Church IM, Fazio Vw, Braun WE et al: Perforation of the colon in renal homograft recipients. Am Surg 203:69, 1986
18. Corrodi P, Knoblauch M, Binswanger J et al: Pancreatitis after renal transplantation. Gut 16:285–289, 1975
19. Curtis JJ: Hypertension and kidney transplantation. Am J Kidney Dis 7:181–196, 1986
20. Curtis JJ, Luke RD, Whelchel JD et al: Inhibition of angiotensin-converting enzyme in renal transplant recipients with hypertension. N Engl J Med 308:377–381, 1983
21. David DS, Berkowitz JS: Ocular effects of topical and systemic corticosteroids. Lancet 2:149, 1969
22. David D, Cheigh J, Braun D et al: HLA A28 and steroid induced diabetes in renal transplant patients. JAMA 243:532–533, 1980
23. Dickerman RM, Peters PC, Hull AR et al: Surgical correction of post-transplant renovascular hypertension. Ann Surg 192:639–644, 1980
24. Diethelm AG, Edwards RP, Whelchel JD: The natural history and surgical treatment of hypercalcemia before and after renal transplantation. Surg Gynecol Obstet 154:481–490, 1982
25. Elmstedt E: Avascular bone necrosis in the renal transplant patient. A discriminant analysis of 144 cases. Clin Orthop 158:149–157, 1981
26. Faro RS, Corry RJ: Management of surgical gastrointestinal complications in renal transplant recipients. Arch Surg 114:310–312, 1979
27. Fernandez JA, Rosenberg JC: Post transplantation pancreatitis. Surg Gynecol Obstet 143:795–798, 1976
28. Friedman E, Shyh T, Beyer M et al: Post transplant diabetes in kidney transplant recipients. Am J Nephrol 5:196–202, 1985
29. Garvin PJ, Casteneda M, Linderer R et al: Management of hypercalcemia and hyperparathyroidism after renal transplantation. Arch Surg 120:578–583, 1985
30. Greenberg BM, Perloff LJ, Grossman RA et al: Treatment of lymphocele in renal allograft recipients. Arch Surg 120:501–504, 1985

31. Griffiths A, Fletcher E, Morris P: Lymphocele after renal transplantation. Aust NZ J Surg 49:626–628, 1979

32. Gunnarson R, Arner P, Lundgren G et al: Diabetes mellitus—a more common than believed complication of renal transplantation. Transplant Proc 11:1280–1281, 1979

33. Harrington KD, Murray WR, Kountz SL et al: Avascular necrosis of bone after renal transplantation. J Bone Joint Sug 53A:203, 1971

34. Hawking RM: Avascular necrosis of bone after renal transplantation. N Engl J Med 294:397, 1976

35. Hill R, Dahrling B, Starzl T et al: Death after transplantation. An analysis of sixty cases. Am J Med 42:327, 1967

36. Howard R, Simmons R, Najarian J: Prevention of lymphoceles following renal transplantation. Ann Surg 184:166–168, 1976

37. [Deleted]

38. Jones JP: Alcoholism, hypercortisolism, fat embolism and osseous avascular necrosis. In Zinn WM (ed): Idiopathic Ischemic Necrosis of the Femoral Head in Adults, pp 112–132. Stuttgart, Georg Thieme Verlag, 1971

39. Kemph JP: Renal failure, artificial kidney and kidney transplant. Am J Psychiatry 122:1270, 1966

40. Lacombe M: Arterial stenoses after machine preservation and transplantation of cadaver kidneys. Surgery 86:907, 1978

41. Lifschitz MD, Rios M, Radwin HM et al: Renal failure with post-transplant renin-angiotensin mediated hypertension. Arch Intern Med 138:1409–1444, 1978

42. Linden MM, Kosters W, Rethel R: Prophylactic gastric operations in uremic patients prior to renal transplantation. World J Surg 3:501, 1979

43. Ljungquist V, Bergentz SE, Leondoer L et al: Coagulation and fibrinolysis after renal transplantation. Scand J Urol Nephrol 3:23, 1969

44. Madura JA, Dunbar JD, Cerilli GJ: Perirenal lymphoceles as a complication of renal homotransplantation. Surgery 68:310–313, 1970

45. Merion RM, White DJ, Thirse S et al: Cyclosporine: Five years experience in cadaveric renal transplantation. N Engl J Med 310:699–705, 1984

46. Mollenkopf F, Matas A, Veith FJ et al: Percutaneous transluminal angioplasty for transplant renal artery stenosis. Transplant Proc 15:1089–1091, 1983

47. Murray JE, Wilson RE et al: Five years' experience in renal transplantation with immunosuppressive drugs. Ann Surg 171:309–314, 1968

48. Myers BD, Ross J, Newton L et al: Cyclosporine-associated chronic nephropathy. N Engl J Med 311:699–705, 1084

49. Nielsen HE, Melsen F, Christensen MS: Aseptic necrosis of bone following renal transplantation. Acta Med Scand 202:27, 1977

50. Owens MC, Passano E, Wilson SE et al: Treatment of peptic ulcer disease in the renal transplant patient. Ann Surg 186:19–21, 1979

51. Palleschji J, Novick AC, Braun WE et al: Vascular complications of renal transplantation. Urology 16:61–67, 1980

52. Pedersen DC, Morris B: The role of the lymphatic system in the rejection of homografts: A study of lymph from renal transplants. J Exp Med 131:936–969, 1970

53. Pfefferman R, Gombos GM, Kountz SM: Ocular complications after renal transplantation. Ann Ophthalmol 9:467–473, 1977

54. Pletka PG, Strom TB, Hampers CL: Secondary hyperparathyroidism in human kidney transplant recipients. Nephron 17:371–381, 1976

55. Porter R, Crombie AL, Gardner PS et al: Incidence of ocular complications in patients undergoing renal transplantation. Br Med J 3:133–136, 1972

56. Rao V, Smith E, Alexander W et al:: Thromboembolic disease in renal allograft recipients. What is its clinical significance? Arch Surg 111:1086, 1976

57. Raynaud A, Bedrosian J, Remy P: Percutaneous transluminal angioplasty of renal transplant stenoses. Am J Radiol 146:853–857, 1986

58. Renning JA, Warden GD, Stevens LE et al: Pancreatitis after renal transplantation. Am J Surg 123:293–296, 1972

59. Ruiz JD, Simmons RL, Callender CO et al: Steroid diabetes in renal transplant recipients: Pathogenetic factors and prognosis. Surgery 73:759–765, 1973

60. Sagalowsky AI, Peters PC: Renovascular hypertension following renal transplantation Urol Clin North Am 11:491–502, 1984

61. Scheff RT, Zuckerman A, Herter H et al: Diverticular disease in patients with chronic renal failure due to polycystic kidney disease. Ann Intern Med 92:202–204, 1980

62. Schweizer R, Cho S, Kountz S et al: Lymphoceles following renal transplantation. Arch Surg 104:42, 1972

63. Smith RB, Cosimi AB, Lorden R et al: Diagnosis and management of arterial stenosis causing hypertension after successful renal transplantation. J Urol 115:639–642, 1975

64. Sollinger HW, Glass JR, Belzer FO: Posttransplant lymphocele causing obstruction of the inferior vena cava and portal vein. Transplant Proc 14:440–441, 1982

65. Spanos PK, Simmons RL, Ratlazzi CC et al: Peptic ulcer disease in the transplant recipient. Arch Surg 109:193–199, 1974

66. Stiller C, Laupacis A, Dupre J et al: Cyclosporine for treatment of early type I diabetes; preliminary result. N Engl J Med 308:1226–1227, 1983

67. Stylianos S, Forde K, Benvenisty AI et al: Lower gastrointestinal hemorrhage in renal transplant recipients. Surgery 1987 (in press)

68. Tilney NL, Rocha A, Strom TB et al: Renal artery stenosis in transplant patients. Ann Surg 199:454–460, 1984

69. Vanrentterghem Y, Lerut T, Roels L et al: Thromboembolic complications and hemostatic changes in cyclo-

sporine treated cadaveric kidney allograft recipients. Lancet 1:999–1002, 1985

70. Wang GJ, Duchman SS, Reger SI et al: The effect of core decompression on femoral head blood flow in steroid induced avascular necrosis of the femoral head. J Bone Joint Surg 67:121–124, 1985

71. Ward K, Klingensmith W, Sterioff S et al: The origin of lymphoceles following renal transplantation. Transplantation 25:346–347, 1978

72. Wells SA, Gunnells CJ, Shelburne JD: Transplantation of the parathyroid glands in man: Clinical indications and results. Surgery 78:34, 1975

CHAPTER 32

Results of Kidney Transplantation

G. Melville Williams

Five to 10 years ago, the most important determinant of graft outcome was whether or not the patient received blood transfusions prior to transplantation. Although some studies continue to show a 10% to 15% advantage in 1-year graft outcome for persons receiving cadaver transplants and blood transfusions, this difference has become less notable. More information is clearly needed regarding the 5-year results of transfused and nontransfused cadaver donor recipients treated with cyclosporine (CsA). Donor-specific transfusions remain popular in the treatment of related-living donors. However, many groups are reporting comparable 90% 1-year graft survival rates in one-haplo-type-matched related-living donors treated with CsA. The advantages of earlier transplantation and avoiding the risks of sensitization are real.

Immediate graft function and HLA-matching exert favorable influences on 1-year graft survival. To achieve excellent matches, kidneys must be shared. Sharing increases the likelihood of ischemic injury. Thus, the advantage gained through better matching and sharing may be lost through a greater frequency of delayed graft function.

However, two large series strongly support sharing when there are perfect HLA-A, -B, and -DR matches.

Cyclosporine has improved 1- and 2-year graft survival significantly. Individual centers using multiple immunosuppressive agents during the first week or two following transplantation report 1-year graft survival in excess of 85%. The average 1-year survival rate is 75% and is likely to improve as all centers gain experience with the potent immunosuppressive agents we have available.

The limited data on 4- and 5-year graft survival are encouraging, because they indicate that renal function remains quite stable. However, perfect function remains rare in our experience, and children still fail to develop catch-up growth.

The results of kidney transplantation are determined by a mixture of complex variables. The most significant of these are the center at which the transplant was performed, treatment with cyclosporine, the presence or absence of early graft function, and the source of the donor kidney. There are data supporting an important role for HLA-A, -B, and -DR matching in cadaver transplantation, but there are also data suggesting that this advantage is offset by the length of ischemia time needed to ensure such good matches. The importance of pretransplantation blood transfusions has also become controversial, with some investigators contending that the risks of sensitization and the possibility that the transfusion effect is only short-term mitigate against its docu-mented role in improving 1-year graft function, even in the cyclosporine-treated patient. In this chapter, the current information available on these controversial issues will be presented with the hope of providing a rationale for future management. Before examining current results and predicting future trends, it is always well to gain historical perspective by reviewing the past.

HISTORICAL PERSPECTIVES

From 1963 to 1966, prior to any knowledge of the HLA system, antilymphocyte globulin (ALG), or even the donor–recipient crossmatch, it seems astonishing that the cadaver kidney graft survival rate at the Medical College of Virginia was 38% at 1 year and 32% at 3 years.[33] The concept that rejection crises could be reversed with high doses of prednisone emerged through clinical experience by the Denver team[30] rather than through animal experimentation. This degree of success was achieved with meticulous surgery and scrupulous juggling of Imuran, prednisone, and local irradiation. However, early enthusiasm was dampened by the high mortality rates. Recipients of living-related donor kidneys had a 1-year mortality rate of 25% to 35%, and one half were dead by 18 months. The low therapeutic index of immunosuppresion was expressed well by Marchioro and associates,[18] "In our own institutions [at Denver] the progressively more timid use of azathioprine combined with altered programs of prednisone administration has virtually eliminated the early postoperative deaths from acute bone marrow depression, but at the expense of later diminished function and higher ultimate steroid need in many cases. The eventual mortality has remained relatively fixed with each such adjustment in management."

Pessimism was short lived, however. In the early 1970s, the elucidation of the HLA system promised to select compatible donor–recipient pairs. The group at Duke[31] published excellent results in a series of genotypically similar pairs, and equally good results were expected from the matching of unrelated pairs. The technology of organ preservation offered the ability to deliver compatible kidneys to prospective recipients in other centers. Finally, the immunosuppressive potency of antilymphocyte antibodies offered a means of controlling any "breakthrough" rejection.

Transplantation of the heart electrified the world. Blood transfusions were withheld from prospective recipients to avoid positive crossmatches. Many transplant centers developed kitchen industries, manufacturing antilymphocytic antibodies from their favorite animal species. Sadly, rather than achieving better results, graft survival stabilized and even declined during the mid-1970s. It became clear that the HLA-A and -B system as then defined led to a trivial improvement in graft survival. Paradoxically, withholding blood transfusions led to worse results.[25] Further, although ALG given prophylactically could delay the onset of rejection, it was not the panacea that many researchers had promised. There was always a price to pay for every innovation. Kidney sharing required greater ischemia times. Machine preservation could injure kidneys as well as preserve them. ALG, in addition to reversing rejection, common led to protracted hospitalization and was morbidity associated with cytomegalovirus (CMV) and/or other opportunistic infections. One-year cadaver graft survival fell to 55%.

During this second gloomy period, those involved in transplantation learned that everything related to graft survival was complex and that the real question was why grafts were ever successful. It became obvious that blood transfusions prior to transplantation exerted powerful beneficial effects on graft survival not explained solely by the selection of nonresponders and that antilymphocytic antibodies might better be used in humans to reverse rather than prevent rejection. Most importantly, the understanding and definitions of excessive immunosuppression developed, which resulted in diminishing the mortality from infectious sequelae. While graft survival rates stagnated, patient survival improved throughout this decade, with many centers reporting a 90% 1-year patient survival rate.

At the beginning of the 1980s, it became well recognized that pretransplant transfusions, the use of ALG, transplanting with high-grade HLA matches, and immediate graft function all had important benefits and that secondary transplants, the presence of diabetes, and being non-Caucasian affected results adversely.[16] Results began to improve, and several large multicenter studies reported cadaver graft survival in the range of 60%, with patient survival at 90% at 1 year. The influence of DR matching[32] and of cyclosporine immunosuppression,[4] announced at the Transplantation Society Meeting in 1978 in Rome, reawakened our enthusiasm. Although the current significance of DR matching remains controversial, there is now little question about the importance of cyclosporine. Several multicenter studies have reported 1-year graft survival rates of 70% to 75%. Other major centers using antilymphocyte antibodies or even small doses of Imuran or ALG until renal function is established report 85% 1-year graft survival rates in ABO-matched but HLA randomly matched cadaver graft recipients. These results have led to diminished emphasis on factors that we learned to be important in the past decade.

Is this correct? Or is the field of transplantation about to begin a descent on the roller coaster that has characterized the history of transplantation (Fig. 32-1)? In the pages that follow, factors known to influence results will be examined, with emphasis placed on the most modern studies using cyclosporine as the primary immunosuppressive agent. The fundamental point in this review will be to illustrate the continuing evolution of our understanding of the clinical factors that determine the outcome of kidney transplantation.

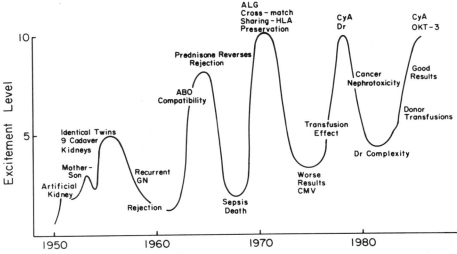

FIGURE 32-1. *The transplantation roller coaster.*

BLOOD TRANSFUSIONS AND OUTCOME

Cadaver Donor

Although reports exist from individual centers providing evidence that cyclosporine overrides the transfusion effect, multicenter studies continue to demonstrate uniformly the significant beneficial effects of transfusions.[6,10,23] At 5 months following transplantation, recipients receiving cyclosporine and no transfusions have graft survival rates varying between 65% and 70%. This contrasts with an 80% graft survival rate achieved in large numbers of patients receiving transfusions. Thus, the magnitude of difference in kidney survival rates between transfused and nontransfused patients continues to be profound at 1 year. As a transplant surgeon wanting to achieve optimal results, it would seem important to implement a purposeful transfusion protocol.

Yet there are two important arguments against this stance. First, purposeful transfusions carry the potential for immunizing some patients, eliminating them as active candidates for transplantation. Because the proportion of patients immunized approximate the proportion benefiting, the greatest good for the greatest number may result from a policy of transfusing only as needed for the symptomatic relief of anemia or for bleeding. Second, in some long-term studies of cadaver graft survival, the transfusion effect was lost with the passage of time.[9,17] The duration of the benefits of blood transfusion cannot be evaluated in cyclosporine-treated patients at 5 years. However, the published actuarial graft survival rates suggest that the maximal transfusion effect is during the early post-transplant period, because the graft survival curves of the transfused and nontransfused patients are closer at 12 months than at 3 or 4 months.

Thus, an issue that seemed very clear 4 years ago is now "muddied," and each transplantation program must make a choice, weighing the clear-cut and significant difference in short-term graft survival with the risks of sensitization, the transmission of viral illness, and the possibility that the gain will be nullified in 5 or 6 years (Fig. 32-2).

Living Donor

Donor-specific transfusion remains popular. In general, there has been a switch away from using three transfusions of fresh blood in order to avoid the 30% sensitization rate that accompanied this protocol. The use of azathioprine during the period of the deliberate transfusions has significantly reduced the rate of sensitization to levels of 5% to 10% with no substantial diminution in graft survival rates.

Several groups, however, have reported equivalent, that is, 85%- to 90%, 1-year graft survival rates in one-haplotype-matched living-related donor pairs treated with cyclosporine. In so doing, one avoids delays in transplantation, the costs of a month and a half of hemodialysis, the logistical difficulties inherent in the transfusion protocol, including the monitoring for donor immunity, and, finally, the real risk of losing the potential kidney donor for the patient. Thus, here again, the transplant surgeon is faced with a choice, and the author

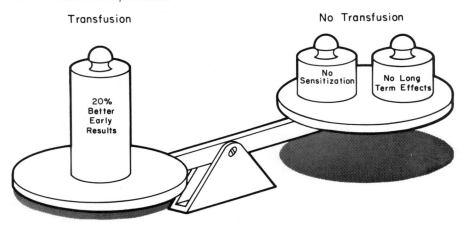

Transfusion   No Transfusion

20%
Better
Early
Results

No
Sensitization

No Long
Term Effects

FIGURE 32-2.   The transfusion dilemma.

believes that the decision should be individualized. Given a patient with a high percentage of reactive antibody but with a negative crossmatch to a prospective living-related donor, cyclosporine offers the best alternative; immunization of this one remaining donor by donor-specific transfusions is a terrible loss. However, since available evidence indicates that donor-specific transfusions exert long-term benefits, a protocol using azathioprine during the transfusion period is logical for the nonsensitized recipient.

Patient survival rates are not greatly influenced by blood transfusions. Certainly, they are not adversely affected, which might be the case if viral infections were imparted through the blood transfusions. In fact, one long-term study that demonstrated the loss of the transfusion effect on graft survival by 6 years continued to show improved patient survival up to 10 years.[13]

HLA MATCHING AND RESULTS

Cadaver Donor Recipients

All collaborative multicenter studies reporting on the influence of HLA matching since 1980 have demonstrated small but significant benefits. Although controversy still exists regarding the relative importance of the various HLA loci in cyclosporine-treated patients, the studies agree that a high-grade AB match or a zero to one antigen mismatch improves cadaver transplant results at 1 year[5,15,22] and that this 10% difference is sustained or becomes wider with the passage of time. However, the impact of matching appears to be decreasing as immunosuppressive regimens become more effective.

The benefits of matching for DR alone remains controversial. It has been found advantageous in multicenter studies and in reports from individual centers in the United States. However, these benefits are disputed by others. It is likely that divergent results are due to technical difficulties still present in assigning the DR antigens accurately.

There is striking agreement in the two largest studies,[19,24] however, reporting that more than 85% of cyclosporine-treated patients enjoyed a 1-year graft survival rate if they were also matched for A, B, and DR antigens. Recipients of zero mismatched A, B, or DR kidneys treated by conventional means now have a 1-year graft survival rate of 75%, which is identical to that of the poorer matched patients treated with cyclosporine. In fact, there is general agreement[5,22] that given any matching category, treatment with cyclosporine increases 1-year graft survival rate by 10%.

Ironically, these results have generally created controversy rather than agreement. With the advent of cyclosporine and the importance of immediate graft function, most centers have ignored matching in favor of transplanting locally procured kidneys, which have a better chance of immediate function (Fig. 32-3). Further, "If poor matches provide results equivalent to my best ones prior to the use of cyclosporine, why not transplant poor matches, avoid delayed function, and discharge the patient promptly?" The desire to transplant the "bird in hand" has been overpowering, and sharing between centers has fallen drastically since the advent of cyclosporine.

However, the evidence from these multicenter studies, which are the only ones providing enough patients for a good analysis at this time, suggests that this approach is shortsighted. For example, the

HLA A,B,& Dr Matching in Patients
Treated with Cyclosporine

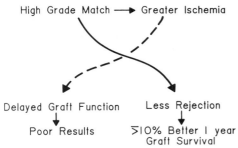

FIGURE 32-3.   HLA A, B, and Dr matching in patients treated with cyclosporine.

collaborative Transplant Study[24] reported a 30% difference in 1-year graft survival between a 2 DR-matched kidney and one that was mismatched for either one or both antigens in recipients immunosuppressed with cyclosporine who received kidneys with cold ischemic times in excess of 36 hours. Paradoxically, the effect of DR matching was less apparent with less ischemia. The conclusion drawn from these studies, which have continued to show a benefit of matching despite protracted ischemia times, is that the advantage of a high match compensates for the disadvantage of protracted cold ischemia. If the 8700 recipients in the United States were to constitute our recipient pool, the likelihood for achieving this six-antigen A, B, DR match has been calculated to occur with one in four cadaver donors, so that one kidney in eight could provide a patient with this substantial advantage.[19] I am forced to conclude that patients will have better results by combining the advantages of good matching and cyclosporine.

Living Donors

Matching within families to identify HLA-identical sibling donors continues to define three subgroups of patients. The sibling pairs sharing identical haplotypes have an outcome that surpasses that of any other type of transplant. The drop-off in graft function after 1 year remains the slowest with a half-life in the neighborhood of 20 years. This group of patients also has the best survival. When rejections occur, they are different histologically from the ordinary acute rejection,[12] and it is in this particular category of patients that pre-existing immunity to another antigen system such as the endothelial

monocyte system may be important. In the future, it is likely that it will be possible to screen for this type of immunity prior to transplantation and avoid rejection, which causes graft failure in 10% of HLA-identical sibling transplants.[7]

A second category of patients share one haplotype in common and are candidates for donor-specific blood transfusions and/or cyclosporine therapy as discussed in the preceding section. One-year graft and patient survival are now nearly equivalent to the better matched pairs. The third group, those sibling pairs that have inherited opposite haplotypes from their parents, may also be considered donors under donor-specific transfusion protocols, as reports from several centers show promising results.

The influence of major histocompatibility complex (MHC) compatibility and outcome is summarized in Figure 32-4. Most centers perform well-matched living-related donor transplants as a first priority, because graft survival exceeds 90% at 1 year and is the most stable after 1 year. The one-haplotype match is the next choice, followed by cadaveric donor transplants. In the future, it may be possible to "reserve" living donor transplants for patients whose only chance of a negative crossmatch is from this source. However, the supply of cadaver donor organs will have to double for this strategy to succeed.

DELAYED GRAFT FUNCTION

Cyclosporine treatment has created a mandate to achieve immediate graft function. In the presence of oligoanuria, hospitalization is prolonged as the ability to monitor and treat acute rejection and/or cyclosporine nephrotoxicity becomes more compli-

Donor Source	Treatment	Graft Survival	
		1 year	5 years
HLA Identical	Aza, Pred	90-95%	80-84%
One Haplotype Identical	Donor Specific Tx Aza, Pred	90%	80-83%
	CyA, Pred	90%	?
No Shared Haplotypes	Donor Specific Tx ALG, Aza, Pred	90%	?
Six Ag Matched Cad	CyA, Pred, + ?	87%	?
2 Dr Ag Matched Cad	CyA, Pred, + ?	85%	?
O-I Mismatch A,B,Cad	CyA, Pred, + ?	80%	?
3-4 Mismatch A,B,Cad	CyA, Pred, + ?	70%	?
O-I Mismatch A,B,Cad	Aza, Pred, + ?	70%	60%

FIGURE 32-4.   Outcome related to donor source and treatment.

cated. Further, there is considerable concern that the ischemic injury and the injury caused by cyclosporine may be additive, such that a significant number of kidneys with early anuria but having the potential for later normal function are damaged irreparably by cyclosporine. Fundamentally, the patient with good early function is discharged healthy at 7 days in contrast to the patient with anuria, who must remain on dialysis and be the subject of scans, magnetic resonance imaging (MRI), and biopsy.

Acute tubular necrosis (ATN) is a major cause of delayed graft function, but it is not the only cause (Fig. 32-5). The reasons for post-transplant oligoanuria are multiple and include kidneys that: (1) originate from unstable donors, (2) are removed improperly, (3) are transplanted improperly, (4) undergo rupture, (5) are preserved improperly, (6) are rejected in hyperacute or accelerated fashion, and (7) are destroyed by cyclosporine nephrotoxicity. Stated another way, every technical miscue and violent rejection are lumped in the group designated as having delayed graft function.

Thus, it is not surprising that patients with delayed graft function fair worse than others. However, the magnitude of the difference in results suggests that reversible renal injury also creates significant adverse effects. In the large series of patients from SEOPF,[27] before cyclosporine, delayed graft function was associated with overall graft losses from all causes ($p < 10^{-5}$), irreversible rejection ($p < 0.001$), and patient death ($p = 0.012$).[27] These differences culminated in a 14% diminution in 1-year graft survival rate and a 12% diminution in 4-year graft survival rates for patients requiring

dialysis in the first week. Even those patients who recovered good graft function at 1 month faired worse than those who do not need dialysis. Similar differences have been observed in patients treated with cyclosporine.[7,24,29]

Accepting that delayed graft function is caused by a potpourri of problems, what can be done to produce early graft function more reliably? One solution has been to perform transplants procured and preserved by a center's own specialized team. Belzer[1] epitimizes this approach and reports immediate function in 84% of the 227 kidneys procured and used at the University of Wisconsin. Eighty-six percent of the kidneys came from local non–heart-beating cadaver donors. The average preservation time was 30 hours, and 94% of the kidneys were functioning at 1 month.

On the other hand, two randomized control studies have been carried out to compare machine and ice preservation.[11,20] In each study, kidneys preserved by a machine had slightly less delayed function (43%, 44%) than those preserved by ice (54%, 57%). In one study, the kidneys preserved by simple cold storage faired slightly better, and, in the other study, the kidneys preserved by machine faired better. Despite excellent intentions, the two studies sited failed to provide convincing evidence of the superiority of either preservation mode despite testing a total of 381 kidneys.

Circumstantial evidence implicates rejection as a major contributing cause of oligoanuria; several studies have shown that good HLA matches improve the chances of early graft function, whereas a high percentage reactive antibody increases the chances of delayed function.[7,24] Another possibility is that a great deal of the injury to the transplant is caused not so much by ischemia in the donor and/or by current preservation techniques but by damage from oxygen-derived free radicals at the time of reperfusion. These extremely toxic molecules can be blocked or dismutated by relatively nontoxic agents. These blocking agents have been very effective in small and large animal models, doubling the function of the treated kidneys compared with that of the untreated control.[14] Thus, it is possible that reperfusion injury should be added to our long list of factors affecting early graft function.

In summary, there are no ready solutions to the problem of delayed graft function. Only a limited number of transplant centers are able to follow the example of Belzer, procuring, preserving, and transplanting as a self-contained unit. Smaller centers with fewer than 100 recipients on their list are commonly able to use less than one half of the kidneys they procure and must share to maintain an efficient

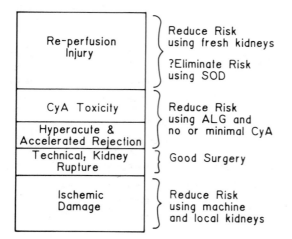

FIGURE 32-5.   *Causes of delayed graft function and prevention.*

operation. Additionally, the methodology of perfusion preservation is difficult, and low rates of anuria are not consistently achieved by other groups using the same technology. Finally, the undisputed major advantage of the six-antigen match achieved through sharing may outweigh the early advantage of immediate function by providing better 5- to 10-year results. Thus, at present, there is a major need for additional laboratory and clinical investigation. In the meantime, surgeons should concentrate on the elimination of technical errors and reduction in ischemic time and make modifications in immunosuppressive therapy to minimize the risk of combined toxic and ischemic injury.

IMMUNOSUPPRESSION

Cyclosporine

Numerous studies have documented the benefits of cyclosporine as a primary immunosuppressive agent in kidney transplantation. In general, cyclosporine in conjunction with prednisone has raised 1-year cadaver graft survival 8% to 15% in most studies.[6,15,23,28] Even under circumstances in which a given center has shown no benefit in 1-year graft survival, patients treated with cyclosporine have left the hospital sooner, have fewer bacterial and viral infections, and are substantially less cushionoid. Almost one half of cadaver donor recipients may be discharged from the hospital 7 to 10 days after their transplant and have minor if any subsequent problems with rejection.

The other half can also be split in half. The patients with the intermediate courses develop elevations in BUN and creatinine, which are resolved fairly easily. Rejection is likely if function deteriorates in the first month, if function deteriorates rapidly, if cyclosporine trough levels are low, and if the biopsy shows vasculitis. Toxicity occurs late, is more indolent, and is frequently associated with high blood levels of drug. To smooth out the clinical course, there is a general tendency to use smaller dosages of cyclosporine and to add modest dosages of azathioprine. At the present time, the results from centers that defer the use of cyclosporine or use it in very low dose until renal function is established are superior to those of centers relying on cyclosporine as the major immunosuppressive agent begun just prior to transplantation. There is experimental evidence that the addition of Imuran to cyclosporine and prednisone contributes to a better therapeutic index.

Our experience is worth citing for some lessons learned. We reasoned that toxicity was related to high peak blood levels and have treated 60 consecutive cadaver transplants by constant intravenous infusion of 4 mg/kg/day of cyclosporine beginning the hour before transplantation. The incidence of delayed graft function was 60%, which was 20% greater than our past experience. There was a significant difference in graft outcome depending upon early function, as one might expect. In fact, five recipients of primary grafts inexplicably never had any renal function, and this rate of primary nonfunction was seven times higher than that experienced in the past. Despite constant intravenous infusion of this low dose, serum levels varied two- to fivefold in the same patient on consecutive days. Our high primary nonfunctioning rate reduced our overall graft survival rate to 73% at 1 year. However, we are persisting with certain details of this protocol, because this regimen proved to be quite immunosuppressive. Of second or third transplants, 16 of 19 were functional at 1 year, despite an 80% incidence of delayed graft function in this group. In our experience, there were no unusual thrombotic episodes, and patient survival was 93% at 1 year.

Kahan and colleagues[13] reported their results using 2 mg/kg/day of cyclosporine by constant intravenous infusion. In this group of patients, there was a higher than usual incidence of renal failure episodes best interpreted as rejection. This combined experience suggests that an intravenous dose of 3 mg/kg/day in combination with Imuran may optimize early immunosuppressive management while providing a greater margin for recovery from renal failure. The same philosophy is being applied by others using antilymphocytic antibodies or all four immunosuppressive agents in modest dose until renal function has been established. We are entering an era of fine-tuning of our potent immunosuppressive drugs.

Approximately one patient in five receiving cyclosporine and prednisone poses a truly difficult problem. These patients present with deteriorating renal function unresponsive to reductions in cyclosporine dosages and/or a course of increased steroid therapy. Biopsies have not been very helpful. The majority will have an interstitial mononuclear cell infiltrate, little if any vasculitis, and unimpressive tubular and vascular changes associated with cyclosporine toxicity. In the absence of findings suggestive of viral illness, including leukopenia, thrombocytopenia, aboration in liver enzyme levels, and fever, a course of therapy with antilymphocytic antibodies has proved to be valuable. Among the antibodies available, the monoclonal antibody OKT3 has proved to be particularly important in this setting.[2,21] It is possible to reduce or eliminate cyclosporine treatment, cover the first and second day febrile reactions associated with OKT3 administration by giving increased amounts of prednisone, and determine by the subsequent clinical course the potential for this particular kidney to regain normal function. If the serum creatinine levels decline from 3 mg/dl to 5 mg/dl to levels under 2 mg/dl within 4 to 5 days of treatment, the prognosis is good and low dosages of cyclosporine, prednisone, and azathioprine are resumed. If the graft was damaged irremediably, the serum creatinine levels do not fall and it is pointless to continue therapy. Thus, in addition to its use in the first week after transplantation to defer rejection and allow for restoration of renal function, antilymphocyte antibodies, particularly OKT3, have proved very useful as agents that "clear the air," reversing rejection, nephrotoxicity, and/or both in this relatively small group of difficult patients.

OTHER FACTORS RELATED TO OUTCOME

The immunologic status of patients on dialysis was an important determinant of graft and patient survival. Patients failing to make a delayed cutaneous hypersensitivity reaction to dinitrochlorobenzene experienced less rejection than those coming to transplantation with delayed hypersensitivity mechanisms intact. However, this difference has been obliterated by current immunosuppressive therapy, and we no longer assay our patients waiting for transplantation.

There continues to be a significant detrimental effect on graft outcome caused by previous transplant rejection and the recipient's ability to form allogeneic antibodies. Persons rejecting more than one previous transplant have a higher risk of rejection than those rejecting just one transplant, and persons having allogeneic antibody to greater than 60% of the lymphocyte panel have a much greater risk of rejection than those with less broadly reactive antibodies. Where cadaver kidneys are in short supply, an argument can be made to limit transplantation to recipients best able to use them, thereby excluding those that had rejected one transplant. Although this point of view may be rational, it is contrary to the patient/doctor contract we traditionally hold. Further, the results of second and third transplants are not so poor as to mitigate against subsequent trials. Results have improved with cyclosporine treatment.[15]

Diabetics and non-Caucasions experienced poorer results, but, in the cyclosporine era, these differences appear to be lessening. Similarly, age was a risk factor that seems to be diminishing in importance. Splenectomy prior to transplantation has been abandoned by the center that principally advocated it in the past.

All multicenter studies have demonstrated variation in results between centers, which is only partially explained by factors known to influence results.[8] Obviously, some of this center variation is related to the proficiency of the surgery and the meticulousness of follow-up care. This type of difference is also reflected in center-to-center variation with other surgical procedures. However, the magnitude of differences never seems to be quite as large as that reported for transplantation. Thus, there must be other factors as yet unknown that remain important determinants of graft outcome. Along this line, we noticed an interesting trend among the patients transplanted at John Hopkins. Prior to cyclosporine, those residing in rural Maryland and Pennsylvania enjoyed a 62% 1-year cadaver graft survival, whereas those residing in the city who were treated by the same surgical team in the same hospital by the same immunosuppressive modalities had only a 46% 1-year cadaver graft survival rate, a significant difference.[3] This difference was not explained by factors of race, exposure to CMV, hepatitis antigen or antibody, age, HLA match, percentage of reactive antibody, primary or secondary transplant, blood transfusions, or diabetes. We were forced to conclude that a "dialysis center effect" existed within a center for inexplicable reasons.

LONG-TERM RESULTS

There are few reports of patient and graft survival 5, 10, and 15 years following transplantation. Those that exist originate from well-established centers but reflect outmoded immunosuppressive practices by today's standards. However, it is worth emphasizing certain points.

First and foremost, there is a clear-cut influence of HLA match in long-term survival. HLA-identical sibling transplants have the lowest rate of long-term decline; one-haplotype-matched transplants have the next lowest rate; and cadaver donor transplants have the sharpest decline. The influence of HLA matching is also seen among the cadaver transplant group, even though the HLA system defined 10 years ago was imperfect. McDonald and co-workers,[17] in their report of 5-year SEOPF experience, found that the HLA match was the strongest determinant of graft survival after 1 year. This report was confirmed and extended by Festenstein and associates.[10] In their study, there was a remarkable difference in 10-year graft survival rate in both transfused and nontransfused patients, depending upon match. Irrespective of transfusion status, those matched for HLA-A and -B antigens enjoyed a 51% 10-year graft survival rate compared with an 18% 10-year graft survival rate in the nontransfused group and a 22% graft survival rate in transfused group sharing none of one antigen. In their study as well as in the report of McDonald's group, the effect of transfusion was early in both the well- and poorly matched group of patients and was sustained only in recipients of cadaveric transplants with middle-degree HLA-A, -B matches. The detrimental influence of pregnancies was noted by Festenstein and co-workers[10] but has not been found in other collaborative studies. Surprisingly, their data also show a beneficial rather than a detrimental effect of the presence of cytotoxic antibodies in 10-year graft survival. The breadth of sensitization and its influence on outcome was not reported.

One feature of transplantation that is difficult to acknowledge is the appreciable loss of graft function with time in all categories of patients transplanted. Although this decline may be slight in the HLA-identical recipient, even here, the half-life of 20 years means that a 20-year-old recipient has only a 50/50 chance of surviving to the age of 40 years with a well-functioning graft. Considering that these patients had no chance of survival 20 years ago, significant strides have been made in transplantation. However, we do not know the long-term influence of many of the variables we consider to be important in improving early results today, particularly the possibility of cumulative cyclosporine nephrotoxicity. However, one surprising feature of cyclosporine therapy is that renal deterioration does not seem to be progressive in renal transplant patients treated long-term with small dosages, whereas it is progressive in patients treated for certain autoimmune diseases and in recipients of cardiac transplants.[26] The reasons for this remain unknown but may have some relationship to denervation of the kidney transplant or dosage.

CONCLUSIONS

Transplantation today is in a rapid state of flux. As we fine-tune our newer immunosuppressive agents, it is likely that this chapter will be of historic interest in 2 or 3 years. Certainly, in 10 or 20 years, our approach is much more likely to be directed toward the specific acceptance of the transplant produced by intense but brief therapy centered just before and shortly after the transplant itself. As we direct our energies into patient care of today, it is wise to remember the lessons of the past. We should not overreact enthusiastically to new discoveries, nor should we despair when the anticipated results are not achieved. Finally, we must aim for the goal of achieving long-term graft acceptance without long-term immunosuppression.

REFERENCES

1. Belzer FO: Perfusion preservation versus cold storage. Transplant Proc 17:1515, 1985
2. Burdick J, Pennington L, Smith W et al: Resetting the immunostat: OKT3 treatment for cyclosporine confusion. Transplant Proc 17:2754, 1985
3. Burdick JF, William GM: What causes center effects in kidney transplantation? Ann Surg 203:311, 1986
4. Calne RY, White DJG, Pentlow BD et al: Cyclosporin A: Preliminary observations in dogs with pancreatic duodenal allografts and patients with cadaveric renal transplants. Transplant Proc 11:860, 1979
5. Cats S: Effect of Cyclosporin A in Kidney Transplantation in Clinical Kidney Transplants, p 217. Los Angeles, UCLA Tissue Typing Laboratory, 1985
6. Cats S, Terasaki P, Perdue S et al: Effect of HLA typing and transfusion on cyclosporine-treated renal allograft recipients. N Engl J Med 311:675, 1984
7. Cerilli J, Brasile L, Galouzis T et al: The vascular endothelial cell antigen system. Transplantation 39:286, 1985
8. Cicciarelli J, Mickey MR, Terasaki PI: Center effect and kidney graft survival. Transplant Proc 17:2803, 1985
9. Fehrman I, Ringdén O, Öst L et al: The long-term effect of pretransplant blood transfusions on cadaveric kidney graft and patient survival rates. Transplant Proc 17:1080, 1985
10. Festenstein H, Doyle P, Holmes J: Pretransplant transfusions, antibody status, sex, and pregnancy in relation to HLA-A, -B matching in London transplant group recipients of cadaver renal transplants. Transplant Proc 17:2273, 1985
11. Halloran P, Aprile M, Robinette M et al: A randomized prospective trial of cold storage versus pulsatile preservation for cadaver kidney preservation. Transplant Proc 17:1471, 1985
12. Hourmant M, Buzelie F, Dubigeon P et al: A new syndrome of hyperacute renal failure in HLA-identical living related and well-matched cadaveric kidney transplantation. Transplant Proc 17:2283, 1985

13. Kahan BD, Lorber MI, Flechner SM et al: Comparison of five cyclosporine-prednisone regimens for induction of immunosuppression in cadaver kidney recipients: A retrospective analysis of 245 cases. Transplant Proc 1986 (in press)

14. Koyama I, Bulkley GB, Williams GM et al: The role of oxygen free radicals in mediating the reperfusion injury of cold-preserved ischemic kidneys. Transplantation 40:590, 1985

15. Kramer NC, Vaughn WK, Bollinger RR et al: Comparison of cyclosporine and conventional immunosuppressive therapy in renal transplantation: A prospective multicenter study. Transplant Proc 17:2196, 1985

16. McDonald JC, Vaughn W, Filo RS et al: Cadaver donor renal transplantation by centers of the Southeastern Organ Procurement Foundation. Ann Surg 193:1, 1981

17. McDonald JC, Vaughn W, Filo RS et al: Cadaver donor renal transplantation by centers of the Southeastern Organ Procurement Foundation. Ann Surg 200:535, 1984

18. Marchioro TL, Terasaki PI, Hutchison DE et al: Renal transplantation at the University of Colorado. Transplantation 5:831–836, 1967

19. Mickey MR, Carnahan B, Tersaki PI: Effectiveness of zero A, B, and DR mismatch for cadaver kidneys. Transplant Proc 17:2222, 1985

20. Mozes MF, Finch WT, Reckard CR et al: Comparison of cold storage and machine perfusion in the preservation of cadaver kidneys: A prospective, randomized study. Transplant Proc 17:1474, 1985

21. Norman DJ, Barry JM, Funnell B et al: OKT3 for treatment of acute and steroid- and ATG-resistant acute rejection in renal allograft transplantation. Transplant proc 17:2744, 1985

22. Opelz G (for the Collaborative Transplant Study): Correlation of HLA matching with kidney graft survival in patients with or without cyclosporine treatment. Transplantation 40:240, 1985

23. Opelz G (for the Collaborative Transplant Study): Effect of HLA matching, blood transfusions, and presensitization in cyclosporine-treated kidney transplant recipients. Transplants Proc 17:2179, 1985

24. Opelz G (for the Collaborative Transplant Study): The influence of ischemic times and HLA-DR matching on cyclosporine-treated cadaver kidney grafts. Transplant Proc 17:1478, 1985

25. Opelz G, Sengar DPS, Mickey MR et al: Effect of blood transfusions on subsequent kidney transplants. Transplant Proc 5:253, 1973

26. Porter GA, Bennett WM: Chronic cyclosporine-associated nephrotoxicity. Transplant Proc 1986 (in press)

27. SanFilipo F, Vaughn WK, Spees EK et al: The detrimental effects of delayed graft function cadaver donor renal transplantation. Transplantation 38:643, 1984

28. Spees EK, Krakauer H, Hodges JF et al: The current experience with cyclosporine in the United States: Cadaver kidney transplantation. Transplant Proc 17:2660, 1985

29. Spees EK, Krakauer H, Hodges JF et al: The current experience with cyclosporine in the United States: The effects of delayed graft function on cadaver kidney graft outcome. Trasplant Proc 17:2821, 1985

30. Starzl TE, Marchioro TL, Waddell WR: The reversal of rejection in human renal homografts with subsequent development of homograft tolerance. Surg Gynecol Obstet 117:385, 1963

31. Stockel DL, Seigler HF, Amos DB et al: Immunogenetics of consanguineous allografts in man. II. Correlation of renal allografting with HLA genotyping. Ann Surg 172:160, 1970

32. van Rood JJ, Persijn GG, van Leeuwen A et al: A new strategy to improve kidney graft survival: The induction of CML nonresponsiveness. Transplant Proc 11:736, 1979

33. William GM, White HJO, Hume DM: Factor influencing the long-term functional success rate of human renal allografts. Transplantation 5:837, 1967

CHAPTER 33

Rehabilitation After Kidney Transplantation

Roberta G. Simmons   Linda Abress   Carol Anderson

Data are presented that (1) compare quality of life among kidney transplant patients, continuous ambulatory peritoneal dialysis (CAPD) patients, and hemodialysis patients, and (2) compare transplant patients on cyclosporine with those on conventional immunosuppression.

The quality of life of transplant patients surpasses that of CAPD or hemodialysis patients, even when "case-mix" factors are carefully controlled. Transplant patients are more likely to be in school or working full-time. Reported sexual functions, at least for males, is superior to that of patients on CAPD or hemodialysis. Results also indicate that prior therapy, in particular, a failed transplant, has an effect on quality of life of dialysis patients. CAPD patients who have experienced no prior course of therapy (neither a failed transplant nor a prior course of hemodialysis) show as high an adjustment as transplant patients, while all other dialysis groups appear considerably less well rehabilitated.

Overall, younger and better-educated patients demonstrate higher quality of life on these end-stage renal disease (ESRD) therapies. Patients for whom the disease is less visible, that is, those who are more satisfied with their appearance, also do better on indicators of quality of life. Also, among CAPD patients, females show significantly better adjustment than do males in terms of physical well-being.

Comparisons of various quality of life indices reveal a distinct advantage for patients on cyclosporine over those on conventional immunosuppression. This difference may be secondary to the lower incidence of infection and rejection episodes with cyclosporine.

When the Medicare End-Stage Renal Disease program was critically reviewed after being in operation for more than 10 years, quality of life was one focus of discussion.[1] The cost of the program is more than 2 billion dollars annually,[6,9,14] and, by 1989, costs are projected to reach 3.2 billion dollars.[14a] In addition, it is also believed that the government will reluctantly agree to cover heart transplants for Medicare beneficiaries.[24,25] It seems appropriate, in light of the strain on Medicare, that policymakers would be concerned about the effects of these treatments on the rehabilitation of the patients.

Studies of the rehabilitation of heart,[5,10,26] pancreas,[36] liver,[12,34,38] and transplant patients are just beginning to be conducted. The work on kidney transplantation is more extensive[8,13,15,19,30,32] and indicates improvement in quality of life post-transplant. While significant side effects occur because of immunosuppression, on average, long-term positive effects have been noted as long as the kidney still functions.[27,28,31] Improvements in quality of life are evident not only among nondiabetic adults but also among higher risk diabetic patients[27,28,31,32] and among persons transplanted as children.[17,18] However, despite these improvements, diabetic patients do not show high quality of life,[27,28] and adolescents exhibit particular difficulties, especially when their appearance is compromised or when kidney rejection is threatened.[18]

Current investigations,[8,15,16,21] including our own, focus on careful quantitative comparisons of quality of life on alternate end-stage renal disease (ESRD) therapies. Our own recent investigations deal first with the comparison of transplant and dialysis patients (continuous ambulatory peritoneal dialysis, CAPD, and hemodialysis) as to quality of life, and second with the comparison of transplant patients on different immunosuppressive regimens.

COMPARISON OF THE QUALITY OF LIFE OF TRANSPLANT VS. DIALYSIS PATIENTS

Method

Subjects

Patients on alternative therapies for ESRD were compared in terms of quality of life. All patients in these studies are nondiabetic, between the ages of 19 and 55 years, and have been on their respective therapies for at least 1 year. In other words, "ideal," low-risk patients were investigated.

Our total sample of recent transplant patients consists of 94 recipients transplanted between 1980 and 1984 at the University of Minnesota and randomized prospectively to either the conventional regimen (antilymphocyte globulin/prednisone/azathioprine) or cyclosporine/prednisone. Patients were measured when they reached 1 year post-transplant. Of these 94 transplant patients, 91 returned questionnaires (a consent rate of 97%); 40 patients assigned to the conventional regimen and 51 to cyclosporine. The comparison groups include the following: (1) a historical control of 82 patients who received transplants at the University of Minnesota between 1970 and 1973 and for whom 5- to 9-year rehabilitation data were available (consent rate, 96%); (2) a large sample of 510 CAPD patients from 185 centers (a consent rate of 83% of eligible patients from these centers. The unique resource that helped secure this large sample was the CAPD Registry, which lists almost all CAPD patients); and (3) a group of 83 in-center hemodialysis patients from eight midwestern centers (consent rate of all eligible patients, 83%).

Findings

The analysis involves (1) overall comparisons among the four groups of ESRD patients (i.e., recent transplant patients, the long-term historical control group of transplant patients, CAPD, and center hemodialysis patients) as to physical well-being, emotional well-being, and social well-being; (2) comparisons of the same four therapy groups, adjusting for case-mix factors; (3) investigations of the effect of a failed transplant as well as of other prior ESRD therapy upon patients' adjustment; (4) attempts to identify those patients who do best within each therapy group; and (5) a comparison of the quality of life of recent transplant patients randomly assigned to either conventional or cyclosporine immunosuppressive therapy.

Overall Comparisons. Our studies[29,30] and those of other investigators[8,15] suggest a higher quality of life for successful transplant patients than for either CAPD or hemodialysis patients.

Vocational rehabilitation is the first aspect of rehabilitation investigated. Among males, findings indicate that vocational rehabilitation is highest among the transplant groups, lowest among center hemodialysis patients, and higher among CAPD patients than among center hemodialysis patients. Table 33-1 provides the proportions of male patients in each group currently working or in school, either full-time or part-time. Among males, only 19% of center hemodialysis patients are at work or school full-time compared with 35% of CAPD patients. However, 64% of current transplant patients and 75% of historical transplant patients are involved in full-time school or work. Data from female ESRD patients are similar, although differences are less

TABLE 33-1 Vocational rehabilitation of male end-stage renal disease patients by treatment group*

	CENTER HEMODIALYSIS (43 Patients)	CAPD (254 Patients)	CURRENT TRANSPLANT (59 Patients)	HISTORICAL TRANSPLANT (40 Patients)
Proportion full-time work or school	19%	35%	64%	75%
Proportion part-time work or school	11%	11%	15%	7%
Proportion not working or in school	70%	54%	20%	18%
	100%	100%	100%	100%

* According to a chi square test, differences between groups are significant, ($p \leq 0.001$).

substantial: 11% of female center hemodialysis patients, 15% of CAPD females, 31% of current transplant females, and 36% of historical transplant females are at work or in school full-time (chi-square test, $p \leq 0.01$).

Other findings from overall comparisons of quality of life are presented in Table 33-2. In order not to overstate statistical significance, F-tests are first run to see whether there is any significant difference among the four therapy groups. If there is a difference, tests comparing particular pairs of therapies can be inspected to see which therapies have a statistical advantage. (See Table 33-2 footnotes.) The data in Table 33-2 clearly reflect statistically

significant differences among therapy groups and, in addition, indicate the advantage that transplant patients perceive regarding their physical well-being, emotional well-being, social well-being, and satisfaction with therapy. On all measures (except hospitalization), the mean scores for the recent transplant group are significantly higher and more favorable than those for either the CAPD group or the center hemodialysis group. For example, on the physical well-being summary measure, transplant patients show high means of 17.55 and 16.95 compared with only 14.64 for CAPD patients and 14.04 for center hemodialysis patients. CAPD patients score higher than center hemodialysis patients on

TABLE 33-2   Relationship of therapy to quality of life

DIMENSION[1]	MEANS (Higher Values Indicate Higher Well-Being, Except for Nights Hospitalized)			
	Center Hemodialysis[2] (83 patients)	CAPD[3] (510 Patients)	Current Transplant[4] (91 Patients)	Historical Transplant[5] (82 Patients)
PHYSICAL WELL-BEING				
Physical Well-Being Summary*	14.04	14.64°	17.55†	16.95
Number of nights hospitalized past 3 months*	3.34	3.90	2.30	—
Health satisfaction*	3.24	3.44°	4.26†	—
EMOTIONAL WELL-BEING				
Self-esteem scale*	3.46ˣˣ	4.37°°°	5.11†	5.46
Happiness scale*	1.94ˣˣˣ	2.33°	3.06†	3.33
Bradburn happiness item**	1.96ˣˣˣˣ	2.07°°	2.26†	2.17
Campbell's Index of Well-Being*	9.77ˣˣˣ	10.51°°	11.70†	—
Index of general affect**	4.72	5.00°°	5.47†	—
Overall life satisfaction*	4.47ˣ	5.07°	5.64†	—
SOCIAL WELL-BEING				
Social Well-Being Summary*	10.12	10.48°	11.93†	12.89§§§
SATTSFACTORY WITH THERAPY				
Therapy Satisfaction Summary*	3.59ˣ	4.59°°	4.85†	4.85

Overall Test of Significance
[1] F-tests of significance from one-way analysis of variance comparing differences *between all groups:*
  * $p \leq 0.001$; ** $p \leq 0.01$; *** $p \leq 0.05$; **** $p \leq 0.10$

Comparisons of Pairs of Therapies—Tests of Significance
[2] Two-tailed T-tests between center hemodialysis and CAPD patients:
  ˣ $p \leq 0.001$; ˣˣ $p \leq 0.01$; ˣˣˣ $p \leq 0.05$; ˣˣˣˣ $p \leq 0.10$

[3] Two-tailed T-tests between CAPD and current transplant patients:
  ° $p \leq 0.001$; °° $p \leq 0.01$; °°° $p \leq 0.05$

[4] Two-tailed T-tests between center hemodialysis and current transplant patients:
  † $p \leq 0.001$; †† $p \leq 0.01$

[5] Two-tailed T-tests between current and historical transplant patients:
  § $p \leq 0.001$; §§ $p < 0.01$

all measures of well-being except frequency of hospitalization (and significantly higher on six of the eleven variables). Although transplantation results have improved greatly over the past decade, there are almost no significant differences between the historical and current transplant groups.

We have also studied the effects of therapy type on family and sexual adjustment. Patients were asked to what extent their health had disrupted family routine and also to rate their satisfaction with sexual activity. In general, family disruption was least among transplant patients and greatest among hemodialysis patients (F-test, $p < 0.0001$). Similarly, among married males, the transplant patients reported highest sexual satisfaction ($p < 0.0001$), although there were no differences among married females across the therapy groups. Differences in family and sexual adjustment persist when statistical controls adjusting for case-mix factors are instituted. (see following section).

Overall Comparisons Adjustment for Case Mix.

Since quality of life differences among therapy groups could be due to initial selection differences rather than to the therapy itself, we have attempted to control background characteristics that differentiate therapy groups. It is, of course, impossible to control all selection differences, just as it is impossible to randomize patients to the different therapies. It is possible, however, to statistically control for those case-mix differences that we know exist. Therefore, the following background differences were controlled: geographic location, race, gender, age, education, marital status, length of illness before treatment, and length of time on current therapy.

Restricting our analysis to only midwestern Caucasian patients and statistically controlling for the remaining background differences with an analysis of covariance, we find (1) that the advantage demonstrated by transplant patients in prior analyses clearly persists, and (2) that the advantage of CAPD patients over center hemodialysis patients is less apparent. On all measures of quality of life, the adjusted means of both groups of transplant patients are higher than the adjusted means of either the center hemodialysis group or the CAPD group. However, where there are significant differences, CAPD patients show an advantage ($p < 0.001$) over center hemodialysis on (1) the physical summary measure, (2) health satisfaction, (3) self-esteem, (4) one happiness measure, (5) therapy satisfaction, and (6) one of the Campbell measures. On the other five measures, either there is no difference or the direction is reversed.

The Effect of a Failed Transplant and of Prior Therapy.

In a study that compared the quality of life of (1) center hemodialysis patients, (2) successfully transplanted cadaveric kidney recipients, and (3) unsuccessfully transplanted cadaveric kidney recipients, Johnson and associates[15] found that patients who returned to dialysis following a failed transplant suffered a diminished level of well-being. Comparing patients who had received only chronic dialysis with those patients who had been unsuccessfully transplanted, these investigators found that the former group of chronic dialysis patients fared much better.[15] Generally, these findings agree with Johnson and colleagues,[15] who report that patients who have experienced a failed transplant suffer negative consequences in terms of quality of life. Johnson and associates[15] and Evans and colleagues[8] indicate that the failed transplant patients should not be ignored when evaluating the success of transplantation as a therapy.

To examine the effect of transplant failure in the current study, we have partitioned our two groups of dialysis patients into five subgroups: (1) patients who have experienced center hemodialysis (Hemo) only; (2) patients who had a failed transplant (TX) prior to center hemodialysis; (3) patients who have experienced CAPD only; (4) patients who had a failed transplant prior to CAPD; and (5) patients who have had a course of hemodialysis prior to CAPD. Case-mix factors were controlled in an analysis of covariance. The results are presented in Table 33-3.

Overall, the findings among the five groups of dialysis patients indicate that CAPD patients who have experienced only CAPD therapy (Table 33-3, column 3) are at an advantage on all measures of quality of life, although differences are not always statistically significant. Not only is it better for a CAPD patient not to have had a failed transplant, it is also better not to have been subject to a prior course of hemodialysis (Table 33-3, column 3 vs column 5). However, when the two largest groups of CAPD patients are compared—those patients with a prior transplant and those patients with a prior course of hemodialysis (Table 33-3 column 4 vs column 5)—all comparisons show the failed transplant group to be the more disadvantaged.

As noted previously, the advantage of CAPD patients over hemodialysis patients is evident for patients who have experienced only one course of therapy (Table 33-3, column 1 vs column 3). Also, patients who have switched from hemodialysis to CAPD perceive a more favorable quality of life than patients who have remained on hemodialysis (Table 33-3, column 1 vs column 5). However, among

TABLE 33-3   *Effect of prior therapy on quality of life of dialysis patients*

| Quality of life Dimension[1] | Midwestern Caucasians Adjusted Means | | | | |
	1 Hemo Only (35 Patients)	2 Hemo with Failed TX (33 Patients)	3 CAPD Only (19 Patients)	4 CAPD with Failed TX (44 Patients)	5 CAPD with Prior Hemo (64 Patients)
PHYSICAL WELL-BEING					
Physical Well-Being Summary	14.72	13.95	15.57	13.82	15.42
Number of nights hospitalized past 3 months	3.57	1.28	.87	4.67	3.55
Health satisfaction***	3.00	3.51	3.94	3.31	3.47
EMOTIONAL WELL-BEING					
Self-esteem scale***	3.42	3.43	5.92	3.54	4.13
Happiness scale***	1.93	1.90	3.01	1.58	2.31
Bradburn happiness item	2.04	2.11	2.09	2.02	2.06
Campbell's Index of Well-Being	10.04	10.08	—[2]	8.99	10.56
Index of general affect***	4.83	4.84	—[2]	4.10	5.05
Overall life satisfaction	4.73	4.76	5.65	4.63	4.80
SOCIAL WELL-BEING					
Social Well-Being Summary****	10.30	10.15	—[2]	8.45	11.07
SATISFACTION WITH THERAPY					
Therapy Satisfaction Summary*	3.82	3.93	4.74	4.55	4.62

[1] F-tests of significance from Analysis of Covariance:
* $p \le 0.001$; ** $p \le 0.01$; *** $p \le 0.05$; **** $p \le 0.10$ all groups, with age, gender, education, marital status, and number of years sick before treatment controlled.

[2] The Ns are too small in this cell to include this variable, owing to missing data.

patients who have experienced a failed transplant (Table 33-3, column 2 vs column 4), CAPD patients are at no advantage over hemodialysis patients, in fact, on most, but not all measures, they are at a disadvantage. Finally, although CAPD patients who have had a failed transplant show poorer quality of life than other CAPD patients, hemodialysis patients with a failed transplant do not differ consistently from patients who have experienced only hemodialysis (Table 33-3, column 1 vs column 2).

We have also examined the effect of a failed transplant upon sexual and family adjustment. Among married male dialysis patients (both center hemodialysis and CAPD), sexual satisfaction is adversely affected by a failed transplant. Similar negative results are found regarding the effect of a failed transplant on male vocational rehabilitation. Comparing male dialysis patients without a prior transplant with dialysis patients who have had a prior transplant, there is a significant difference in the proportion at full-time work or school (36% vs 26%, chi-square test, $p < 0.05$).

It is thus clear that quality of life comparisons among alternate ESRD therapies should take into account the effect or prior courses of therapy. If comparable successful transplant patients are con-

trasted to the five dialysis groups in Table 33-3 (current midwestern Caucasian patients with case-mix factors controlled), successful transplant patients do better than all hemodialysis patients and than CAPD patients with either prior therapy on all measures of quality of life (except for number of nights hospitalized). However, a comparison of successful transplant patients to those who have received only CAPD therapy does not show a consistent advantage for transplant patients. In fact, these CAPD patients score more favorably on number of nights hospitalized (0.87 vs 2.06) and on self-esteem (5.92 vs 4.94), and there is little difference on one of the happiness measures or on "overall life satisfaction." (These means are adjusted by an analysis of covariance for case-mix differences.) However, the small number of cases of patients who experienced only CAPD therapy renders these last conclusions tentative.

Which Patients Do Best.   In general, younger, more educated patients score consistently more favorably on measures of well-being (regression analysis using data from Caucasian patients only). These findings are congruent with Evans and co-workers.[8] Unlike Evans' group, however, we do not find any pattern of negative consequences for non-Caucasian patients when we examine our dialysis groups (two-way analysis of variance). In fact, on many of our measures, non-Caucasian dialysis patients score higher than Caucasian patients.

For each of the three therapies, separate regression equations were run to determine the effects of gender, age, marital status, years of education, years sick before treatment, years on therapy, and (for dialysis patients) history of a failed transplant. These effects were examined for physical well-being, self-esteem, Campbell's Index of well-being, and social well-being. In preliminary analyses, no predictor consistently affected the current transplant group, although CAPD and hemodialysis patients were benefited by a young age and higher education. (It should also be noted that there were hardly any significant differences distinguishing transplant patients with living-related donor transplants from those with cadaveric donor transplants.)

On CAPD, but not on the other therapies, females do significantly better than males in terms of physical well-being ($p < 0.05$). Lindsay and colleagues[20] also report that females show better adjustment than males on CAPD but not on dialysis. They attribute the difference to the lower weight of females and therefore greater ease of water and metabolite clearance. There is also some evidence that satisfaction with one's appearance significantly affects these dimensions of quality of life for patients on all therapies when other predictors are controlled ($p < 0.05$). Our earlier studies of transplanted adults and children[18,32] also indicate that when the disease is visible to others, that is, when a patient's appearance makes him or her appear ill or abnormal, adjustment is compromised. When the disease is perceived as invisible, quality of life along many dimensions improves.

Cyclosporine Versus Conventional Immunosuppression.

Although conventional immunosuppressive therapy (antilymphocyte globulin [ALG]/prednisone/azathioprine) was found in our prior studies of patients transplanted between 1970 and 1973 to favorably affect rehabilitation[32] as well as graft and patient survival rates,[28] patients receiving this regimen reported troubling side-effects and were subject to threatening episodes of rejection and infection. In the current study of patients transplanted between 1980 and 1984 and randomly assigned to either conventional or cyclosporine/prednisone immunosuppression, the effect of alternate regimens on rehabilitation and quality of life was compared.[28a]

As part of a randomized, prospective trial,[3,11,23,27a,33,35,37] a sample of 113 nondiabetic patients ages 19 to 55 years was analyzed (64 patients assigned to cyclosporine and 49 to conventional immunosuppression). Of the randomized transplant recipients, 18 have returned to dialysis, and 6 are now deceased. Of the 64 cyclosporine patients, actuarial graft survival at 1 year is 86%, and patient survival is 95%; of the 49 patients assigned to conventional therapy, actuarial 1-year graft survival is 84%, and patient survival is 98%. (There are no significant differences in either graft or patient survival, chi-square test.)

Survival statistics from other centers are inconsistent. Both the Canadian Multicentre Transplant Study Group[2] and the European Multicentre Trial Group[7] report significantly greater 1-year graft survival among patients treated with cyclosporine; findings from the Canadian study also indicate significantly higher patient survival with the cyclosporine regimen. Cho and associates,[4] Merion and colleagues,[22] Ferguson and associates,[11] Sutherland and co-workers,[35,37] and Najarian and colleagues[23] report no differences in survival between regimens. All studies are not directly comparable, however, since not all are randomized, some are retrospective in nature, and protocols differ.

Because patients on two therapies do not clearly and consistently differ on patient and graft survival, it becomes particularly important to look at any differences in the quality of life between these two groups.

Overall comparisons of the two patient groups at 1 year post-transplant on our various quality of life measures do, in fact, reveal an advantage for patients randomized to the cyclosporine regimen. Table 33-4 provides mean scores for the two groups. On all measures of well-being, cyclosporine-treated patients score higher. Of particular interest are the findings under the dimension of emotional well-being (see Table 33-4). Patients assigned to cyclosporine with reduced doses of steroid medication report greater happiness and life satisfaction, thereby presenting evidence to contradict the notion that transplant patients' reported emotional well-being may be solely due to a "steroid high."

In terms of vocational rehabilitation, the advantage of cyclosporine was not as clear. Because of the small number of cases when the genders are separated, significant differences are either absent or borderline. Cyclosporine does not appear to be an advantage for male vocational rehabilitation (full-time participation in work or school: cyclosporine, 57% vs conventional, 72%; Fisher's exact test, not significant). For women, the direction of difference does favor the cyclosporine group, however (full-

TABLE 33-4   *Relationship of transplant drug regimen to quality of life*

Quality of Life Dimension[1]	MEANS (Higher Values Indicates Higher Well-Being) N = 91	
	Conventional Therapy (40 Patients)	Cyclosporine Therapy (51 Patients)
PHYSICAL WELL-BEING		
Physical Well-Being Summary	16.94	17.96
Health satisfaction*	4.02	4.43
EMOTIONAL WELL-BEING		
Self-esteem scale	5.05	6.04
Happiness scale**	3.47	4.18
Bradburn happiness item*	2.07	2.39
*Campbell's Index of Well-Being**	10.98	12.24
Index of general affect*	5.07	5.77
Overall life satisfaction*	5.32	5.88
SOCIAL WELL-BEING		
Social Well-Being Summary	11.40	12.33
Family summary**	11.92	12.93

One-way analysis of variance: * $p \leq 0.05$; ** $p \leq 0.10$

time participation: cyclosporine, 43% vs conventional, 9%; Fisher's exact test, $p = 0.056$).

The question that arises at this point is why should cyclosporine-treated patients be reporting higher quality of life at 1 year post-transplant? The answer may lie in the incidence of rejection and infection. It has been noted that the incidence of rejection and infection is lower among cyclosporine-treated patients.[3,4,11,33,35,37] In fact, in the current study of patients who have functioning kidneys 1 year post-transplant, 53% of the patients assigned to conventional therapy report having experienced one or more rejection episodes since the transplant, compared with 26% in the cyclosporine-treated group (chi-square test, $p < 0.05$). Similarly, patients in the conventionally treated group report more infection than patients assigned to cyclosporine, although the difference was not significant. Further analysis does, in fact, indicate the importance of rejection and infection in explaining the high quality of life among cyclosporine-treated patients. When mean scores for the two groups of patients are adjusted for rejection and infection incidence in an analysis of covariance, almost all differences are reduced to a level of nonsignificance, although still slightly favoring the cyclosporine-treated patients. Thus, it appears that it is in part because cyclosporine results in fewer episodes of infection and rejection, that patients on this drug therapy show higher quality of life at 1 year post-transplant.

In this study, it was also hypothesized that cyclosporine-treated patients would do better because of fewer side-effects. When asked about medication side-effects, patients in the two regimens did not differ significantly in reports of cushingoid appearance or weight gain, although the cyclosporine-treated group reported more hair growth (chi-square test, $p < 0.001$). Females from both treatment groups reported more weight gain and greater occurrence of cushingoid appearance than did males, demonstrating their greater sensitivity to negative appearance changes (Fisher's exact test, conventional therapy: n.s. and $p \leq 0.10$; cyclosporine therapy: $p \leq 0.05$ in both cases). One should remember that these patients were studied at 1 year post-transplant; it is possible that more dramatic differences in side-effects will become evident at long-term follow-up.

SUMMARY

Our research, as well as that of other investigations, has shown that the quality of life for successful transplant patients surpasses that of patients undergoing alternative therapies. Transplant patients are more likely to be in school or working full-time than are patients on alternative therapeutic regimens. Their sexual function, at least for males, is superior to that of CAPD or hemodialysis patients. Cyclosporine has lessened the incidence of infection and rejection so that transplant patients on cyclosporine show an even higher quality of life than those on other immunosuppressive regimens.

We have attempted to control for case-mix differences among patients on dialysis versus transplantation, although complete control is impossible. When statistical controls are instituted, these advantages of successful transplantation persist. However, one reason that successful transplant patients fare better than CAPD patients may be that the latter are likely to have experienced a prior course of unsatisfactory therapy, either a failed transplant or a course of hemodialysis. Patients who have been treated only with CAPD do not score significantly and consistently worse than successful transplant patients. (These findings have to be considered tentative, however, because of the small number of such CAPD patients.) In any case, in evaluating the quality of life of transplant patients, the investigator must consider the lower adjustment after a failed transplant along with the high levels of rehabilitation after success.

Quality of life remains an ethical issue in transplantation because of the high cost of this technology and the inevitable decisions that will need to be made concerning resource allocation.

REFERENCES

1. Blagg CR: After ten years of the Medicare End-Stage Renal Disease Program. Am J Kidney Dis 3(1):1, 1983
2. Canadian Multicentre Transplant Study Group: A randomized clinical trial of cyclosporine in cadaveric renal transplantation. N Engl J Med 309:809, 1983
3. Canafax DM, Simmons RL, Sutherland DER et al: Early and late effects of two immunosuppressive drug protocols on recipients of renal allografts: Results of the Minnesota randomized trial comparing cyclosporine versus antilymphocyte globulin-azathioprine. Transplant Proc XVIII(2) (suppl) 1:192, 1986
4. Cho SI, Bradley JW, Monaco AP et al: Comparison of kidney transplant survival between patients treated with cyclosporine and those treated with azathioprine and antilymphocyte globulin. Am J Surg 147:518, 1984
5. Christopherson LK, Griepp RB, Stinson EB: Rehabilitation after cardiac transplantation. JAMA 236:2082, 1976
6. Eggers PW, Connerton R, McMullan M: The Medicare experience with end-stage renal disease: Trends in incidence, prevalence, and survival. Health Care Financ Rev 5(3):69, 1984
7. European Multicentre Trial Group: Cyclosporin in cadaveric renal transplantation: One-year follow-up of a multicentre trial. Lancet 2(8357):986, 1983
8. Evans RW, Manninen DL, Garrison Jr LP et al: The quality of life of patients with end-stage renal disease. N Engl J Med 312(9):553, 1985
9. Evans RW, Manninen DL, Hart LG et al: The national kidney dialysis and kidney transplantation study: Selected findings Part III. Contemp Dial Nephrol 6(11):41, 1985
10. Evans RW, Manninen DL, Maier A et al: The quality of life of kidney and heart transplant recipients. Transplant Proc XVII:1579, 1985
11. Ferguson DM, Rynasiewicz JJ, Sutherland DER et al: Cyclosporin A in renal transplantation: A prospective randomized trial. Surgery 92:175, 1982
12. Gaudiani VA, Stinson EB, Alderman E et al: Long-term survival and function after cardiac transplantation. Ann Surg 194:381, 1981
13. Guttmann RD: Medical progress. Renal transplantation (Part 2). N Engl J Med 301:1038, 1979
14. Health Care Financing Administration: End-stage renal disease program medical information system, facility survey tables. Department of Health Services, USA, HCFA, January 1–December 31, 1984
14a. Health Care Financing Administration: Medicare Annual Report. Publication Number 02157. Fiscal Year 1983
15. Johnson JP, McCauley CR, Copley JB: The quality of life of hemodialysis and transplant patients. Kidney Int 22:286, 1982
16. Kaplan De-Nour A, Shanon J. Quality of life of dialysis and transplanted patients. Nephron 25:117, 1980
17. Klein SD, Simmons RG: Chronic disease and childhood development: Kidney disease and transplantation. In RG Simmons (ed): Research in Community and Mental Health, Vol 1, 21. Greenwich, CT, JAI Press, 1979
18. Klein SD, Simmons RG, Anderson CR: Chronic kidney disease and transplantation in childhood and adolescence. In Blum R (ed): Chronic Illness and Disabilities in Childhood and Adolescence. New York, Grune & Stratton, 1984
19. Kutner NG: Predictive criteria in rehabilitation of ESRD patients: Perspectives from rehabilitation medicine. Contemp Dial 4(1):34, 1983
20. Lindsay RM, Oreopoulos DG, Burton H et al: Adaptation to home dialysis: A comparison of continuous ambulatory peritoneal dialysis and hemodialysis, pp 120–130. Procedures of the International Symposium, November 2–3, 1979
21. Matthes DE: Beyond survival. Dial Transplant 9:657, 1980
22. Merion RM, White DJG, Thiru S et al: Cyclosporine: Five Years experience in cadaveric renal transplantation. N Engl J Med 310:148, 1984
23. Najarian JS, Fryd DS, Strand M et al: A single institution, randomized, prospective trial of cyclosporine

versus azathioprine-antilymphocyte globulin for immunosuppression in renal allograft recipients. Ann Surg 201(2):142, 1985

24. Novello AC, Sundwall DN: Current organ transplantation legislation: An update. Transplant Proc 17:1585, 1985

25. Otten AL: Rising success in organ transplants strains hospitals and governments. The Wall Street Journal, September 25, 1985

26. Report from the Council of the British Cardiac Society: Cardiac transplantation in the United Kingdom. Br Heart J 52:679, 1984

27. Simmons RG: Long-term reactions of renal recipients and donors. In NB Levy (ed): Psychonephrology 2. New York, Plenum, 1983

27a. Simmons RG, Abress L, Anderson CR: Quality of life after kidney transplantation: A prospective, randomized comparison of cyclosporine and conventional immunosuppressive therapy. Transplantation (in press)

28. Simmons RG, Anderson CR: Related donors and recipients five to nine years posttransplant. Transplant Proc XIV:9, 1982

29. Simmons RG, Anderson C, Kamstra L: Comparison of quality of life of patients on continuous ambulatory peritoneal dialysis, hemodialysis, and after transplantation. Am J Kidney Dis 4:253, 1984

30. Simmons RG, Anderson CR, Kamstra LK et al: Quality of life and alternate end-stage renal disease therapies. Transplant Proc 17:1577, 1985

31. Simmons RG, Kamstra-Hennen L, Thompson CR: Psycho-social adjustment five to nine years posttransplant. Transplant Proc XIII(1):40, 1981

32. Simmons RG, Klein SD, Simmons RL: Gift of Life: The Effect of Organ Transplantation on Individual, Family, and Societal Dynamics. New Brunswick, Transaction, 1987

33. Simmons RL, Canafax DM, Fryd DS et al: New immunosuppressive drug combinations for mismatched related and cadaveric renal transplantation. Transplant Proc XVIII(2) (Suppl) 1:76, 1986

34. Starzl TE, Koep LJ, Schroter GPJ et al: The quality of life after liver transplantation. Transplant Proc XI:252, 1979

35. Sutherland DER, Fryd DS, Strand MH et al: Results of the Minnesota randomized prospective trial of cyclosporine versus azathioprine-antilymphocyte globulin for immunosuppression in renal allograft recipients. Am J Kidney Dis 5:318, 1985

36. Sutherland DER, Gotz SE, Hess UJ et al: Effect of multivariables on outcomes of pancreas transplant recipients at the University of Minnesota and preliminary observations on the course of preexisting secondary complications of diabetes. In Friedman EA (ed): Diabetic Renal Retinal Syndrome, Vol III: Therapy. New York, Grune & Stratton, 1985

37. Sutherland DER, Strand M, Fryd DS et al: Comparison of azathioprine-antilymphocyte globulin versus cyclosporine in renal transplantation. Am J Kidney Dis 3:456, 1984

38. Wall W, Duff JH, Ghent CN et al: Liver transplantation: The initial experience of a Canadian centre. Can J Surg 28(3):286, 1985

PART FOUR

Other Organ Transplantation

CHAPTER 34

Cardiac Transplantation

Glenn R. Barnhart   Richard R. Lower

Cardiac transplantation is now an accepted alternative for patients with end-stage cardiac disease. Early clinical trials showed that the denervated heart could support the circulation and respond to exercise.

Patients considered for cardiac transplantation are in functional Class IV by NYHA criteria, usually have left ventricular ejection fractions of less than 20%, and either ischemic or idiopathic cardiomyopathy. Absolute contraindications currently include active infection, recent pulmonary infarction, or elevation in pulmonary vascular resistance to greater than 8 Wood units. Relative contraindications include diabetes mellitus, renal or hepatic dysfunction, peripheral vascular disease, and hyperlipidemia.

An acceptable donor should have no history of heart disease or cardiac trauma, have ABO blood group compatibility, and be younger than 35 years of age. Considerations for using a donor of smaller size than the recipient include the urgency for transplantation, the recipient's pulmonary vascular resistance, and the anticipated cold ischemia time.

A cold ischemia time of 3.5 to 4 hours has usually resulted in good recovery of function.

Orthotopic cardiac transplantation is performed through a median sternotomy on cardiopulmonary bypass. Recipient cardiectomy involves dividing the great vessels just above their respective valves and transection of venous return at the mid-atrial level. Once the donor heart has been tailored, left and right atrial anastomoses are performed. Aortic and pulmonary anastomoses complete the operation. Following a brief period of warming, the heart is defibrillated and the patient is slowly weaned from cardiopulmonary bypass. The donor sinus node provides electrical activity for the heart. Denervation does not appear to adversely affect function; autonomic reinnervation has not been demonstrated in human recipients. Ventricular performance is normal at rest and exercise. Cardiac output increases in response to preload and classic Frank-Starling mechanisms. The effects of cardioactive drugs are dependent upon their mechanisms of action in relation to denervation. Rejection graded as moderate or severe usually requires treatment with intravenous methylprednisolone and/or intramuscular RATG.

One- and 5-year survival rates are currently 80% and 50%, respectively. Mortality causes include infection, rejection, graft arteriosclerosis, and malignancy.

Graft arteriosclerosis remains the major cause of patient mortality after the first year and is largely an unsolved problem. The pathogenesis is presumed to have an immunologic basis, although it may occur in recipients never having an identifiable acute rejection. Retransplantation is the only definitive option in patients suffering from end-stage cardiac rejection.

As the number of cardiac transplants increases, the ethical issue of limited donor availability must be addressed. This may require a redefining of recipient criteria so that donor hearts can be used for patients most likely to achieve a good result.

In the almost two decades since the first human heart transplant, those involved in cardiac transplantation have observed the evolution of this new discipline from an experimental procedure to a relatively common, acceptable management of end-stage cardiac disease. The field has grown so much that in 1985, there were 75 centers in the United States reporting cardiac transplant capability. The

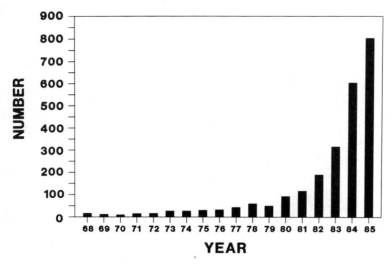

FIGURE 34-1.   *Number of transplants performed per year, recorded by the International Heart Transplant Registry. The 1985 figure represents the total number reported as of February 1986 by 73 centers throughout the world.*

International Heart Transplant Registry records (as of February 1986) 804 transplants performed in 1985. The annual number of cardiac transplants has risen dramatically over the last several years (Fig. 34-1).[42] The increased activity has in part resulted from an improved survival rate, which has now reached 80% at 1 year and is approaching 50% at 5 years. The artificial heart and its role in the treatment of end-stage cardiac disease have further complicated therapeutic decisions and raised many new socioeconomic and ethical issues.

In this chapter, we will summarize the historical aspects of cardiac transplantation, discuss recipient and donor selection, and describe procurement and implantation techniques. We will outline the currently used immunosuppressive agents and discuss their complications and side-effects, discuss rejection and its management, and describe the physiology and function of the transplanted heart. Finally, we will summarize the results of cardiac transplantation and suggest avenues for further investigation to improve patient survival.

HISTORICAL BACKGROUND

The current success in cardiac transplantation reflects the results of years of laboratory investigation. Early investigators needed to deal with certain key issues prior to clinical trials, including (1) a reliable and reproducible technique for transplantation, (2) preservation of the heart during the period of myocardial ischemia, (3) the ability of the denervated heart to support the circulation and respond to the increased physiologic demands of exercise, and (4)

methods for the diagnosis and treatment of rejection.

The first reported experimental investigations of cardiac transplantation were by Alexis Carrel.[12,13] During these experiments, he removed the heart from a small dog and placed it in the neck of a larger dog. Circulation in the heterotopic heart was established by anastomosis of the jugular vein and carotid artery to the aorta, the pulmonary artery, one of the vena cavae, and a pulmonary vein. With some modification, this model remains in use today for research purposes because of easy execution and access to the allograft. Further work by Mann and colleagues[57] refined the techniques of heterotopic transplantation. Additional reports in the 1950s outlined attempts at orthotopic transplantation, but survival could not be maintained longer than several hours.[23,55,63,82,98,99]

The first successful orthotopic canine cardiac transplants were reported by Lower and Shumway[51,52] in 1960. Technical modifications allowed removal of the heart at the mid-atrial level, leaving two atrial cuffs, thereby minimizing the required number of systemic and pulmonary venous anastomoses. This procedure is essentially the same one used today at most centers.

Prolonged survival demonstrated that the denervated heart could effectively support the circulation.[50] Further studies defined the use of the electrocardiogram as a marker for rejection,[49] and it was shown that rejection could be treated successfully with agents such as methylprednisolone, azathioprine, and 6-mercatopurine.[51] These and other laboratory investigations set the stage for initiation of clinical trials.

Hardy and associates[31] reported the first attempted human heart transplant in 1964 when they placed a chimpanzee heart into a 68-year-old patient in cardiogenic shock. The transplanted heart failed shortly after the procedure. The first successful orthotopic cardiac transplant was performed by Barnard[3] in 1967; the patient survived for 17 days but died of pneumonia. In the late 1960s and early 1970s, there was a tremendous surge of interest in transplantation. Early difficulties encountered, such as rejection, infection, and lack of donor availability, resulted in high morbidity and mortality. During the mid-1970s, only a few centers continued clinical trials.

To overcome the problem of limited donor availability, long-distance donor procurement was begun in 1976.[91,96] Extensive laboratory investigation had demonstrated that with topical cooling of the donor heart, periods of up to 4 hours of hypothermic anoxia could be well tolerated. The accuracy of diagnosing rejection was improved in the mid-1970s with the aid of the endomyocardial biopsy,[14] which allowed the periodic assessment of the histology to help direct therapy. Increasing clinical experience in the use of immunosuppressive drugs, intensive surveillance for infection, and improved patient selection have all contributed to a progressively decreasing mortality. The introduction of cyclosporine in the early 1980s has led to a resurgence in the number of patients transplanted.

RECIPIENT CONSIDERATIONS

Recipient selection is a major factor in determining a successful outcome in cardiac transplantation. Many criteria must be considered to identify appropriate candidates.[92] Any patient with end-stage cardiac disease can be considered for cardiac transplantation. Potential candidates are typically in functional Class IV by NYHA criteria and usually have a left ventricular ejection fraction of less than 20%. The majority of these patients have either idiopathic or ischemic cardiomyopathy. Patients with

a history of previous congenital heart defects or rheumatic valvular disease form only a small minority. Those who have undergone previous blood transfusions may have a more favorable prognosis, although they must be evaluated for preformed antibodies.

Although most patients have compensated congestive heart failure at the time of transplantation, certain patients merit urgent consideration because of increasing need for intravenous inotropic support. Intra-aortic balloon counterpulsation, left ventricular assist devices, and artificial heart implantation have all been used to assist cardiac output. Patients with cardiac cachexia, massive edema, ascites, infections, and renal insufficiency present special risks, and the justification for transplantation must be balanced against the limited donor supply so that patients selected are those most likely to achieve a good result. Currently, patients with active infection and significantly elevated pulmonary vascular resistance should be excluded from consideration for cardiac transplantation (Table 34-1). An immunosuppressive regimen, by definition, will alter recipient immune response; thus, active infection would be most difficult to eradicate in the newly transplanted patient.

A pulmonary vascular resistance of greater than 8 Wood units should probably eliminate consideration of orthotopic cardiac transplantation.[92] A resistance of 4 to 8 Wood units makes the decision difficult, because reversible factors such as pulmonary edema can be a cause. A favorable response to pulmonary vasodilators may influence the decision. The newly transplanted heart will usually adjust with time to some elevation of pulmonary vascular resistance, but the risk of refractory right ventricular failure and inability to wean the patient from cardiopulmonary bypass are increased. Recent advances in right and left ventricular assist devices may warrant a re-evaluation of this criterion, although reports of their use show significant mortality.[102]

Age has historically been a dominant factor in predicting a successful outcome. Complications ap-

TABLE 34-1   Contraindications to Cardiac Transplantation

ABSOLUTE	RELATIVE*
1. Active Infection	1. Diabetes mellitus
2. Recent pulmonary infarct	2. Renal or hepatic dysfunction
3. Pulmonary vascular resistance > 8 Wood units	3. Peripheral vascular disease
	4. Hyperlipidemia
	5. History of poor medical compliance

* Factors that alone or in combination may adversely affect survival.

pear to be better tolerated and more easily treated in the younger age groups. Traditionally, the age of 55 years has been the upper limit for the majority of transplant centers. This age limit is currently being re-evaluated by many centers, since overall results have improved in the last several years; our center recently successfully transplanted a 67-year-old patient using only cyclosporine and azathioprine as immunosuppression. The average age of cardiac transplant recipients is 38 years.[42] Early results of transplantation in children are similar to those of adults, but long-term experience is not yet available.[70] As safer immunosuppressive regimens are developed, it is likely that chronologic age will not be as relevant.

Diabetes mellitus constitutes another relative contraindication to cardiac transplantation. If the patient has insulin-dependent diabetes, the use of steroids will render management more difficult. Even patients with diabetes controlled by diet or oral agents may have an increased propensity for the development of infection. With the use of cyclosporine and multimodality immunosuppression allowing for a minimum of steroids, the management of transplant recipients with diabetes will be simplified and results should improve.

Pulmonary infarction is another accepted contraindication to cardiac transplantation. The sites of infarction often become repositories for fungal infection in the cardiac transplant recipient. In any patient who has had a recent pulmonary embolus and/or infarction, radiographic resolution should be demonstrated. The period of time after which cardiac transplantation can be considered safe remains unknown and must be determined according to the factors involved in each case. Any patient sustaining a hemodynamically significant pulmonary embolus should undergo repeated studies of pulmonary vascular resistance prior to cardiac transplantation.

Other factors that may adversely affect the outcome are dysfunction in other organ systems and peripheral vascular disease. Renal and hepatic dysfunction secondary to decreased cardiac output must be distinguished from primary organ dysfunction. With the use of cyclosporine, renal and hepatic function have become particularly important in the recipient's evaluation. We have been reluctant to transplant patients with a preoperative serum creatinine greater than 2 mg/dl, because of the predictable immediate and long-term nephrotoxicity of cyclosporine.[62] Cyclosporine may also cause hepatic dysfunction, although this has been less of a problem. The presence of any form of peripheral vascular disease has the potential for altering the long-term outlook for cardiac transplant recipients. Hyperli-

pidemia should be considered an adverse factor; accelerated graft coronary artery atherosclerosis has been associated with patients who developed this complication.[34]

Psychosocial factors are important in assessing candidacy for cardiac transplantation. The patient's ability to withstand the psychologic impact of transplantation and the complex drug regimens used postoperatively should be thoroughly evaluated. Spouse, family, and friends serve as support for the patient in immediate and long-term handling of problems.

Thus, it can be concluded that recipient selection in cardiac transplantation is a process that must include all members of the cardiac transplant team.

DONOR CONSIDERATIONS

Owing to the recent increase in the number of cardiac transplants being performed, donor availability has become critical. Long-distance procurement introduced in the 1970s[91,96] provided a larger donor pool and decreased the waiting time for recipients. In recent years, the concept of multiorgan procurement has developed so that the majority of cardiac procurements today are done within this context.

Several criteria must be satisfied before a cardiac donor can be accepted. The criteria for brain death, previously outlined by the Harvard Ad Hoc Committee,[75] must be met and permission from the next of kin must be obtained. If the donor has been a trauma victim, one should evaluate the chest x-ray and a two-dimensional echocardiogram to ensure structural integrity of the heart. Cardiac isoenzymes are obtained to rule out a myocardial contusion.

Ideally, a donor should be hemodynamically stable during the evaluation period, and, to achieve this stability, an infusion of dopamine may be required. An adequate circulating volume is provided by blood and colloid administration as required.

There should be no history of any form of heart disease; even a history of an innocent murmur necessitates a two-dimensional echocardiogram. The presence of mitral valve prolapse does not preclude the use of the heart for transplantation, although the natural history of this entity within the transplanted heart is unknown. Age of the donor is an important factor. Any male donor older than 35 years and any female older than 40 years should undergo coronary angiography prior to the use of the heart.

It is customary to satisfy ABO compatibility between donor and recipient, although ABO incompatibility may not invariably result in graft loss. All potential recipients undergo testing in which their serum is crossmatched against a random donor panel of lymphocytes; the result of this crossmatch is expressed as a percent-reactive antibody (PRA). If the PRA is less than 5%, the likelihood of an antibody reaction against the donor heart is low. If the PRA is greater than 5%, donor–recipient pretransplant crossmatching is believed to be necessary, although this complicates the logistics of long-distance procurement. An unmatched HLA-A2 locus may lead to a higher incidence of late graft atherosclerosis,[71] but, currently, we are only able to perform HLA and DR tissue typing, retrospectively. As techniques for long preservation time are developed, prospective donor–recipient tissue typing and lymphocyte serum crossmatching may become of greater importance.

Finally, several considerations are important in determining the ideal donor weight for the recipient. Most recipients have large pericardial spaces capable of accommodating hearts from donors whose weight is 30% more than that of the recipient. Larger hearts will probably perform better in those recipients with significant elevations in pulmonary vascular resistance. The minimal donor heart size for any given recipient is unknown, because cardiac output will increase in response to demand even if a heart smaller than that of the recipient is chosen. In the final determination of matching donor and recipient sizes, one must consider the urgency for transplantation, the pulmonary vascular resistance, and the cold ischemia time.

DONOR HEART PROCUREMENT

The need for donor organs has risen dramatically in the last several years. This need has resulted in a national effort on the part of transplant centers to coordinate procurement activities so that as many organs as possible are used from each donor.[78,87,94]

Multiple organ procurement requires greater time and coordination among operating teams than single organ procurement; thus, anesthesia support is a prerequisite for careful monitoring and replacement of blood, fluid, and electrolyte losses. Hypothermia is a potential problem, because the thoracic and abdominal cavities are widely opened, so body temperature should be monitored. The sequence of multiorgan harvesting requires that cardiectomy be performed last, because circulation must be supporting until other organs are removed. It is important to do a median sternotomy just after laparotomy and prior to any abdominal organ dissection,

allowing the cardiac team quick access to the heart if hemodynamic deterioration occurs, as well as visual inspection of the heart to rule out any structural abnormalities. Exposure in the abdomen is further enhanced by median sternotomy. Events should be coordinated so that if intraportal infusion of cold, lactated Ringer's solution is started, cardiectomy can be performed immediately. In the case of cardiectomy before hepatectomy, care should be taken not to remove too much of the intrapericardial inferior vena cava, since it will be needed more for the liver transplant than for the cardiac transplant.

Cardiectomy is performed with the sternum and pericardium widely opened following administration of intravenous heparin (200 units/kg). It is essential that two suction catheters be available prior to the cardiectomy. The superior vena cava is dissected to the pericardial reflection to gain as much length as possible and is transected 2 cm above the right atrium. Care should be taken not to injure the SA node in the region of the superior vena cava right atrial junction. The inferior vena cava is transected below the right atrium. The heart is allowed to empty. The aorta and pulmonary arteries are transected, leaving the pulmonary artery bifurcation intact. If cardioplegia is used, the aorta is crossclamped prior to the aortic transection, and cardioplegia solution is infused through a 14-gauge catheter. The heart is retracted anteriorly, and each pulmonary vein is transected, completing the cardiectomy. The heart is immersed in cold saline and placed in two concentric bags, each containing iced saline, and the entire collection is surrounded with ice. Cardiectomy should be performed as quickly as possible to minimize warm ischemia time.

Although many centers use potassium cardioplegia prior to cold storage and transport, simple immersion in cold saline has resulted in successful clinical transplants for ischemic periods of up to 5.5 hours (our longest preservation period experienced clinically). Whether potassium cardioplegia provides better protection in these circumstances or whether the high potassium solution that remains in the vessels without washout might be deleterious to the vascular endothelium is not known.

OPERATIVE TECHNIQUE

The technique for orthotopic cardiac transplantation has varied little from the original description in 1960 by Lower and Shumway[52] (Fig. 34-2). Exposure is gained through a median sternotomy and a longitudinal pericardiotomy. If the patient has undergone a previous cardiac surgical procedure, the surgeon

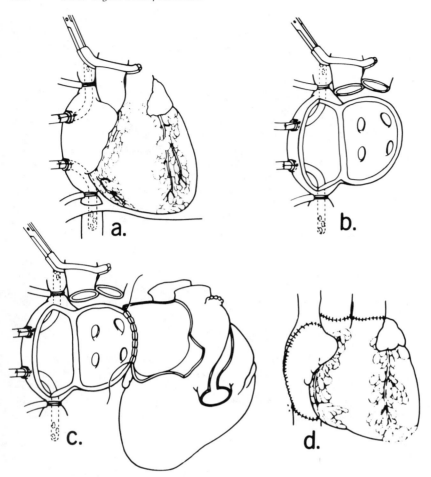

FIGURE 34-2.   *Surgical technique for orthotopic cardiac transplantation. (a) Cardiopulmonary bypass is instituted and the aorta is crossclamped. (b) Recipient cardiectomy is completed, leaving the posterior right and left atrial walls and a ridge of atrial septum. (c) Implantation of the donor heart is begun by anastomosis of its left atrium to the residual left atrial wall of the recipient. (d) The operation is completed by joining the atrial walls, atrial septum, and great vessels.*

may encounter adherence of the right ventricle or bypass graft to the sternum.

After heparinization (3 mg/kg), the aortic cannula is placed in the proximal aortic arch. The superior and inferior vena cavae are cannulated as far laterally as possible in the right atrial wall so that an adequate right atrial cuff will remain following the cardiectomy (Fig. 34-2a). If the patient becomes hemodynamically unstable at any point, partial bypass and systemic cooling is started. If the patient is stable, bypass is begun approximately 15 minutes prior to the anticipated arrival of the donor heart.

Cardiectomy is begun by an incision in the lateral aspect of the right atrium, leaving an adequate cuff of right atrial wall. Upon reaching the inferior aspect of the right atrium, the atriotomy is carried to the level of the tricuspid annulus. Similarly, the incision is carried superiorly to the region of the atrial septum. The aorta and pulmonary artery are transected just cephalad to the aortic and pulmonary valves. The recipient's great vessels just above the valves are then retracted caudally, allowing excellent exposure of the left atrium, which is divided between the appendage and the pulmonary veins. This preserves the relationship between recipient pulmonary veins and recipient arterial remnant. The left atrial incision is continued to the level of the mitral valve annulus. The recipient heart is then lifted anteriorly, and the medial portions of the left and right atrial walls constituting the atrial septum are incised, completing the cardiectomy (Fig. 34-2b). The left and right atrial cuffs are appropriately trimmed, and the recipient coronary sinus is over-sewn where it enters the right atrium. It is helpful to suspend the pulmonary artery and aorta with sutures to facilitate exposure during subsequent anastomoses.

Once the donor heart has arrived, it is placed in a basin of ice cold saline to maintain hypothermia. The superior vena cava of the donor heart is oversewn with a nonabsorbable monofilament suture. The eventual site for the right atrial anastomosis is constructed by extending the inferior vena caval orifice in the direction of the donor heart right atrial appendage. This incision can be later enlarged as needed to fit the recipient right atrium. The left atrial cuff is fashioned by an incision connecting the openings of the four pulmonary veins. The aorta and pulmonary artery are trimmed appropriately to match the respective recipient vessels. The heart should be examined at this time for any unsuspected abnormalities such as an atrial septal defect.

The donor heart is carried to the operating table, and the left atrial anastomosis is started at the level of the left superior pulmonary vein with a 4-0 nonabsorbable monofilament suture (Fig. 34-2c). The anastomosis is performed in a simple running fashion. Quite often there is epicardial fat along the recipient lateral left atrial wall, which should be incorporated in the suture line but should not be allowed to turn into the left atrium to avoid a site for embolization. The left atrial anastomosis is completed by carrying the running suture down the recipient atrial septal remnant.

The right atrial anastomosis is started at the superior medial aspect of the right atrial cuff and continued as a simple running suture. In the region of the atrial septum, the common suture line is used to reinforce the right atrial anastomosis at this level. Before completion of the right atrial anastomosis, a further incision in the donor right atrial appendage can be made to accurately align the two right atrial cuffs.

The pulmonary artery anastomosis is performed next, because exposure is better if this is done prior to the aortic anastomosis (Fig. 34-2d). Simple running suture is used for both the aortic and pulmonary anastomoses. Before declamping the aorta, the lungs are inflated and care is taken to aspirate air from the cardiac chambers and aorta. After the aorta is declamped and coronary perfusion is restored, the heart will often resume spontaneous beating, but, if ventricular fibrillation persists for more than a few

minutes, electrocardioversion is accomplished with 15 to 20 watt-seconds. A temporary pacing wire is placed on the anterior wall of the right ventricle. At this time, the heart is lifted anteriorly to examine the posterior left atrial anastomosis for possible bleeding sites.

Isoproterenol infusion, 1 µg/min is begun for chronotropic support and is used for the first 24 to 48 hours. The patient is slowly weaned from cardiopulmonary bypass over one half to one and one half hours to allow adequate recovery of ventricular function. Occasionally, some donor hearts may require additional inotropic support such as dobutamine or dopamine. Right or left ventricular distention must be avoided, and a vigorous diuresis is advantageous to minimize any increase in pulmonary resistance. A pulmonary artery catheter with mixed venous oxygen saturation capability is positioned in the pulmonary artery to monitor continuous changes in cardiac output and pulmonary artery pressure. When adequate cardiac output is ensured, decannulation is carried out and the heparin is neutralized with protamine. After hemostasis is secured, two chest tubes are placed in the chest cavity for drainage, and the median sternotomy is closed in standard fashion.

ORTHOTOPIC VERSUS HETEROTOPIC TRANSPLANTATION

Although orthotopic transplantation is the preferred method of heart replacement in most centers, heterotopic transplantation has been advocated by some researchers[2,47] as an acceptable alternative, particularly in patients with elevated pulmonary vascular resistance; details of the operative technique have been described elsewhere.[47] In such patients, the retained native right ventricle has already adapted to the increased work load of the abnormal pulmonary vascular bed, whereas the orthotopically transplanted right ventricle may be unable to cope with the high resistance and may fail acutely. Another proposed advantage is that the native heart can augment the circulation during episodes of acute rejection. Moreover, the heterotopically transplanted heart might be removed in the event of irreversible rejection or where reversal of disease in the native heart is anticipated. Finally, some researchers have reported a decreased need for assisted ventilation, intravenous inotropic agents, and cardiac pacing in patients undergoing heterotopic transplantation.[48]

Certain disadvantages to heterotopic heart transplantation exist. Because of the low flow situation and stagnation created in the native heart, the possibility of thromboembolic events is increased[48] and has led to the use of anticoagulants in most heterotopic heart transplants,[47] thus increasing the risk of bleeding complications. Low flow in the native heart also predisposes the patient to bacterial endocarditis as reported by Barnard and co-workers.[2] Furthermore, progression of disease in the native heart may result in disabling angina.[47]

Our experience has led to different conclusions concerning the advantages of heterotopic transplantation. First, with the recently developed immunosuppressive regimens, which include cyclosporine, rejection rarely results in severe hemodynamic deterioration of the orthotopic heart transplant. Thus, there is no need for augmentation of the circulation while acute rejection is being diagnosed and treated. Second, most patients need cardiac transplantation owing to end-stage ischemic or other forms of cardiomyopathy, which is irreversible. Finally, most patients require relatively small and transient amounts of inotropic support and cardiac pacing. Thus, it appears that complete removal of the diseased heart and orthotopic replacement have distinct advantages. It is likely that patients with severe elevation of pulmonary vascular resistance will benefit more from heart–lung transplantation than from heterotopic transplantation.

POSTOPERATIVE MANAGEMENT

Management during the first 48 hours after operation is similar to that of other cardiac surgery patients. Distinctions include the use of a fiberoptic pulmonary artery catheter to monitor continuously pulmonary artery pressure and mixed venous oxygen saturation as an estimate of cardiac output. Most patients will require some inotropic support for the first 24 to 48 hours, such as isoproterenol, dopamine, or dobutamine or ventricular pacing to maintain an adequate cardiac index. Once hemodynamic stability has been achieved, the patient is weaned slowly from inotropic support to avoid any sudden decrease in cardiac output since the denervated heart is especially sensitive to intravenous catecholamines. Any residual elevation of pulmonary vascular resistance may make right heart function precarious. Since the output of the transplanted heart is quite rate-dependent, the chronotropic effect of isoproterenol or pacing is most useful. Factors that may dictate the magnitude and duration of postoperative pharmacologic support include the duration of ischemic time (including cold preservation time), the presence of elevated pulmonary vascular resistance, and a small donor heart size.

To avoid introduction of nosocomial organisms, emphasis is placed on early removal of the endotracheal tube, Foley catheter, and intravascular lines, as well as early discontinuation of prophylactic antibiotics. If more prolonged intravenous infusion of isoproterenol is required for chronotropic effect, this is administered through a peripheral site so that central lines can be removed, thereby reducing the risk of thrombosis and infection. The epicardial pacing wire is usually removed after 1 week.

A strict isolation technique is advocated within the first 48 hours after cardiac transplantation. All personnel who come into contact with the recipient should use mask, gloves, and gown as precautions.

Once extubated, the patient is gradually allowed to increase his activity level. In most cases, the patient is able to sit in a chair 2 days after cardiac transplantation and is able to walk about within the cardiac surgery intensive care unit until conditions permit transfer to a routine care floor. The patient is usually ready for discharge from the hospital within 4 weeks following cardiac transplantation.

IMMUNOSUPPRESSION

The delicate balance between the desired benefit of immune-altering drugs and their adverse effects has constantly challenged transplant surgeons. The struggle for optimal balance continues today, since the ideal immunosuppressive regimen is yet to be defined.

Initially, prednisone and azathioprine were the primary agents available for use in cardiac transplant recipients. Maintenance prednisone doses were high, leading to significant infectious complications, as well as to the late development of cataracts, osteoporosis, and diabetes and the exacerbation of peptic ulcer disease. Anti-thymocyte globulin was later added to the immunosuppressive regimen in the mid-1970s, allowing for some reduction in steroid use.

The addition of cyclosporine in 1980 appears to have had a beneficial impact on morbidity and mortality in cardiac transplant recipients. Early experimental work by Calne and others[9] demonstrated enhanced survival in orthotopic pig heart transplants with the use of cyclosporine. Similar results were found by Jamieson and co-workers[35] in an immunologically mismatched rat model and by Pennock and associates[72] in a primate model. Combining cyclosporine with conventional immunosuppression resulted in an increased infection rate, although this result has not been seen with its clinical use.[4] The adverse effects of cyclosporine continue to require careful monitoring of blood levels to avoid toxicity.

The initial dose of cyclosporine varies, depending primarily upon the patient's preoperative renal status. A loading oral dose of 8 mg/kg to 10 mg/kg is given approximately 3 hours prior to the planned induction of anesthesia, because peak blood levels are achieved 3 to 4 hours following administration.[24] Postoperatively, doses averaging 4 mg/kg to 5 mg/kg are given twice daily to achieve serum trough levels of 200 ng/ml to 400 ng/ml by radioimmunoassay (RIA). High performance liquid chromatography and whole blood RIA are alternative ways used to monitor cyclosporine levels, although no one method has been found to achieve superior results.[30]

During the first week following transplantation, a rise in blood urea nitrogen (BUN) and creatinine may precede or coexist with an oliguric phase. Although this is seen frequently with elevated cyclosporine levels, it may occur with normal or even low levels. When this occurs, the cyclosporine dose should be lowered and the BUN, creatinine, and urine output monitored closely. All renal parameters will usually return to base line in a few days.

After 2 months, if no rejection is present, cyclosporine dosage is adjusted so that serum RIA trough levels are in the 100 mg/ml to 200 mg/ml range, which, it is hoped, will reduce the long-term toxicity of cyclosporine.

The major complications of cyclosporine include nephrotoxicity and hypertension. Whether or not the early renal impairment previously discussed has an association with late renal insufficiency is unknown. Most patients show some renal dysfunction 1 to 2 years following transplantation.[4] Marked renal impairment was found in the early Stanford cyclosporine study; however, this was thought to be dose related.[62] The average serum creatinine in cyclosporine-treated patients at 1 year following transplantation is approximately 2 mg/dl in our center (Fig. 34-3).

Cyclosporine-associated hypertension does not appear to be dose related. Experimental observations of cyclosporine-associated hypertension have demonstrated normalization of cardiac output, maintenance of elevated systemic vascular resistance, and an intense stimulation of the renin–angiotensin–aldosterone system.[86] Hypertension is more prevalent in cyclosporine-treated patients than in conventionally treated patients,[4] and it is often quite refractory to therapy.

Other adverse effects of cyclosporine include neurotoxicity, hirsutism, gingival hyperplasia, and hepatotoxicity.[83] The development of fine tremors is common, and visual hallucinations and psychoses have been reported.[1,66] Seizures occur not infrequently in the first week after transplantation, and the interaction between anticonvulsants and the immunosuppressive drugs should be considered. Hepatotoxicity is a reported side-effect but appears uncommon. Hirsutism and gingival hyperplasia occur

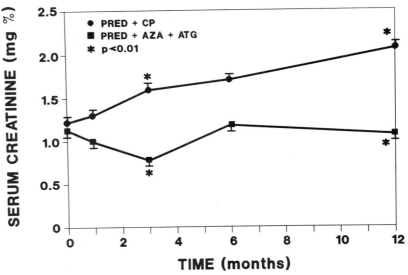

FIGURE 34-3. *Average serum creatinine in patients treated with cyclosporine and prednisone versus conventional immunosuppression. Note the progressive rise in serum creatinine in patients treated with cyclosporine.*

occasionally and may have particularly disturbing cosmetic effects, particularly in pediatric patients.

Methylprednisolone, 500 mg, is given intravenously initially after discontinuing cardiopulmonary bypass and subsequently every 8 hours at a dose of 125 mg for three doses. If prednisone is the only other immunosuppressive drug being used with cyclosporine,[28,29] it is started at 30 mg twice daily and tapered to 20 mg to 30 mg per day during the first 2 months. The rapidity with which it can be tapered is dictated by the presence or absence of rejection.

Our present regimen includes azathioprine 2 mg/kg once daily, in conjunction with cyclosporine, and the dose is adjusted as necessary to avoid leukopenia.

Intramuscular anti-thymocyte globulin, 100 mg is given intramuscularly preoperatively and once daily for 2 days after operation. Further therapy is reserved for rejection that seems resistant to steroid treatment. Adverse effects include pain at the injection site, cellulitis, and an increased susceptibility to viral infection.

Currently, further intravenous steroid administration for the treatment of biopsy-proven rejection (vide infra) and maintenance oral steroids are added only when rejection responds poorly to treatment or when there are multiple recurrences.

Other forms of immunosuppression or antirejection therapy that have been used include anticoagulants,[36] graft irradiation,[26] total lymphoid irradiation with donor bone marrow infusion,[37–39,79] monoclonal antibody, thoracic duct drainage, and plasmapheresis, but their exact therapeutic roles have not been defined.

Preoperative blood transfusions have been associated with improvement in graft survival in cadaveric renal transplants.[67] Experimental[73] and clinical[40] results with this method in cardiac transplant recipients have demonstrated that survival may be enhanced, although further controlled studies are needed to assess its potential value in patients to be treated with cyclosporine.

REJECTION

The diagnosis and treatment of rejection has changed significantly since the early cardiac transplant experience. Patients who were immunosuppressed with azathioprine and steroids frequently developed symptoms of malaise and fatigue during rejection episodes. The physical findings were those of primarily right heart failure, which include a new S_4 gallop, peripheral edema, and jugular venous distention. Serial electrocardiograms showed significant decreases in voltage, which, in the absence of pericardial effusion, led to the presumptive diagnosis of rejection.

Many of these symptoms and physical findings associated with acute rejection may not occur in patients treated with cyclosporine in whom the diagnosis of rejection is made solely on the basis of the biopsy. Thus, all patients undergo endomyocardial biopsies weekly for the first 1 to 2 months to establish the presence or absence of rejection.

The technique of endomyocardial biopsy was introduced in 1962 in a small number of patients with various diagnoses.[81] Caves and associates[14,15] refined the technique using a percutaneous approach for the heart transplant patients (Fig. 34-4), and Mason[58] has reported its efficacy and safety in a large number of patients.

Billingham[7] has established histopathologic criteria for the diagnosis of acute rejection;[7] these findings are summarized in Table 34-2 and are also discussed elsewhere in this book. In most cases, the diagnosis of minimal or mild rejection requires no alteration in immunosuppression. Moderate rejection involves focal myocytolysis and a moderate perivascular, endocardial, or interstitial infiltrate (Fig. 34-5). Severe rejection is defined as myocyte necrosis with interstitial hemorrhage and a prominent neutrophil or histiocytic perivascular and interstitial infiltrate.

Both moderate and severe rejection require additional immunosuppression. Our treatment protocol involves giving either 500 mg or 1000 mg of methylprednisolone intravenously for 3 days for the first or second rejection episode; ATG is added if rejection recurs, and the oral prednisone dose is increased. The majority of rejection episodes will occur within the first 3 months after which host tolerance of the allograft seems to improve. Rejection episodes can, however, occur later in the postoperative period, particularly during changes in immunosuppressive drugs. During treated episodes of rejection, patients are placed in isolation for 24 hours after the last dose of intravenous steroid, and all personnel and visitors follow strict handwashing, mask, and glove precautions.

Although hyperacute rejection has been reported,[100] we have not experienced this complication in more than 180 transplants. The use of antibody screening and, where appropriate, preoperative lymphocyte and monocyte crossmatching should virtually eliminate this catastrophic event. There is evidence that hyperacute cardiac rejection can occur in the absence of any anti-donor HLA antibody and that anti-donor vascular endothelial cell antibody may be responsible.

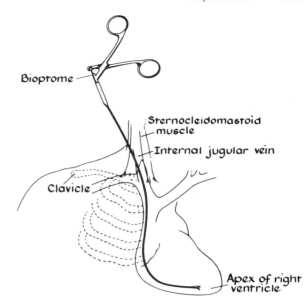

FIGURE 34-4. *Technique of endomyocardial biopsy to determine rejection status of the transplanted heart. Bioptome is passed using percutaneous technique under fluoroscopic guidance to obtain samples of endomyocardium. (Reproduced with permission from Year Book Medical Publishers.)*

Other methods of diagnosing rejection, including radionuclide scanning,[66] M-mode echocardiography,[80] and T cell monitoring[60,68] show some promise. Although these may be helpful in the timing of biopsies, the ultimate treatment decision continues to be based on histopathologic findings.

PHYSIOLOGY AND FUNCTION OF THE TRANSPLANTED HEART

The capacity of the transplanted heart to satisfy the needs of circulation has been well documented. Experimental work demonstrated that function remained adequate for long-term survival in the canine model.[20,49] Relevant physiologic aspects of the cardiac allograft include sinoatrial node function, the effect of denervation, and ventricular performance during rest and exercise.

Donor sinus node function is responsible for electrical activity in the transplanted heart. Although experimental work in dogs demonstrated unequivocal within months after transplantation sympathetic and parasympathetic reinnervation occurred,[20] there has been little or no evidence to date of autonomic reinnervation in human heart trans-

TABLE 34-2   *Endomyocardial Biopsy Grading of Acute Rejection Episodes**

Early rejection (reversible)	Endocardial and interstitial edema
	Scanty perivascular and endocardial infiltrate of pyroninophilic lymphocytes with prominent nucleoli
	Pyroninophilia of endocardial and endothelial cells
Moderate rejection (reversible)	Interstitial, perivascular, and endocardial infiltrate of pyroninophilic lymphocytes with prominent nucleoli
	Early focal myocytolysis
Severe rejection (irreversible or very difficult to reverse)	Interstitial hemorrhage and infiltrate of pyroninophilic lymphocytes and polymorphonuclear leukocytes, vascular and myocyte necrosis
Resolving rejection	Active fibrosis, residual small lymphocytes (nonpyroninophilic), plasma cells, and hemosiderin deposits

* From Billingham ME: Some advances in cardiac pathology. Human Pathol 10:372, 1979. Used with permission.

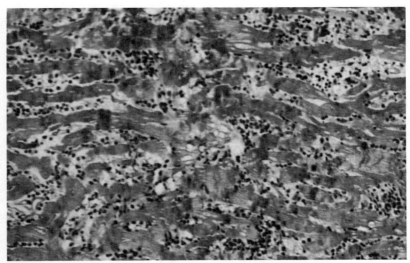

FIGURE 34-5.   *Moderate rejection. Note prominent lymhocytic infiltrate and myocyte necrosis (hematoxylin and eosin ×20).*

plant recipients.[89] Early sinus node dysfunction has been implicated as a sign of poor prognosis,[54] although early sinus node dysfunction can occur in patients without serious sequelae for more than 1 year.[77] Beta receptors remain intact and play a role in response to isoproterenol and norepinephrine infusion.[10]

The effect of deafferentation on the human heart has been studied less extensively. Lower body negative pressure studies demonstrate that the cardiopulmonary baroreflex control is impaired in cardiac transplant recipients.[61] This impairment is not seen in renal transplant patients and, therefore, is not likely caused by the effects of immunosuppression.[90]

Recent studies have shown that cardiac transplant patients may have normal hemodynamics at rest.[84] Left ventricular ejection fraction and segmental wall motion remain normal up to 5 years postoperatively.[22] Ventricular contractile characteristics and reserve also appear to be normal when compared with those of control.[8] Early observations demonstrated the ability of the transplanted heart to increase cardiac output during exercise.[85] It appears that during the early phase of exercise, cardiac output increases in response to augmented preload according to the Frank-Starling mechanism, whereas circulating catecholamines have later inotropic and chronotropic influences.[74] There is an abnormal pattern of cardioacceleration manifested by a higher than normal heart rate at rest, delayed

gradual achievement of maximal heart rate during exercise, and delayed decrease during recovery (Fig. 34-6).[17]

The effects of cardioactive drugs are dependent upon their mechanism of action in relation to denervation. The transplant heart responds normally to norepinephrine, isoproterenol, and propranolol[10]; there is no response to atropine.[11] Intravenous digoxin appears to have little effect on atrioventricular (A-V) conduction in the denervated heart,[25] although orally administered digoxin caused the expected prolongation of the A-V interval.[76] Although beta-blockers should be used with caution in cardiac transplant recipients, their attentuating effects on exercise response are minimal, so they are considered safe for those recipients who develop cyclosporine-associated hypertension.[101]

RESULTS

Since the initiation of clinical cardiac transplantation, improvement in overall care of cardiac surgery patients, additions to immunosuppression such as cyclosporine, and refinements in preservation and long-distance procurement techniques have improved results. Stanford has reported 1-year survival rates of 70% and 5-year survival rates of approximately 50%.[71] Our experience is a 1-year survival rate of 80% and a 5-year survival rate of 50%; our longest living transplant patient has recently cele-

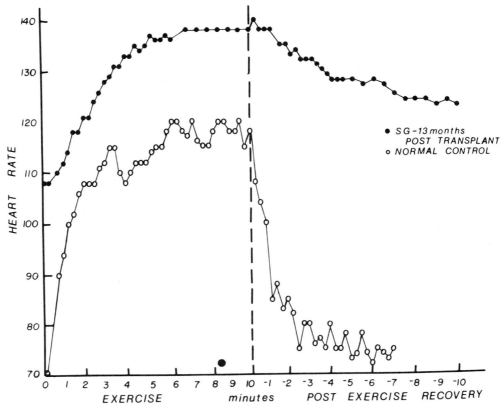

FIGURE 34-6.   *Graph demonstrating response of the transplant heart to exercise. Note higher resting heart rate, delay in maximal heart rate achieved, and delay in decrease to baseline. (Reproduced with permission from the American Journal of Medicine.)*

brated his 15th anniversary. Rehabilitation has generally been excellent with the majority of patients in NYHA Class I,[71] and many are capable of participating in vigorous exercise.[19] Of successful cardiac transplant recipients, 91% have been classified as successfully rehabilitated[16]; more than 90% are able to return to the occupation or activity of their choice.[71]

There are several factors that account for early and late mortality, including, in order of frequency, infection, rejection, graft arteriosclerosis, and malignancy.[71] Since the advent of cyclosporine, acute rejection has become an infrequent cause of death.

Cardiac transplant recipients continue to be at major risk for infection. It appears that cyclosporine may cause an increase in the number of viral infections.[21] Most transplant centers have noted an increase in the incidence of cytomegalovirus. Bacterial and fungal infections are still the most serious infections seen in cardiac transplant recipients.[5] Di-

agnosis must be made early, and treatment must be initiated promptly to eradicate such infections. Avoiding the indiscriminate use of antibiotics may reduce the occurrence of devastating opportunistic infections. The lungs continue to be the most common site of infection[4,56] occurring as pneumonia, empyema, or cavitating lesions from a variety of organisms such as *Aspergillus, Nocardia,* various aerobic and anaerobic organisms,[56] and *Legionella pneumophila.*[18] Diagnostic evaluation includes early bronchoscopy for any patient considered to have a new pulmonary infiltrate. Other important sites of infection include the sternum, the central nervous system, and the urinary tract. Gastrointestinal septic complications occurring in cardiac transplant patients can be difficult to diagnose and result in a high mortality rate.[88]

Although death from acute rejection is now far less common than in the past, repeated treatment of rejection significantly increases the risk of infection. The appropriate timing and frequency of follow-up biopsies to enable detection of late rejection are still uncertain and present logistical problems that emphasize the need for less invasive monitoring techniques.

Graft arteriosclerosis, which is receiving increased attention as more patients survive the initial years,[95] constitutes the major cause of late mortality.[71] This finding was noted in the early experience of both canine and human transplant.[44,93] The exact etiology remains obscure, but it is undoubtedly a form of chronic rejection, although the histopathologic changes are similar to spontaneous atherosclerosis (Fig. 34-7). Repeated or continuous intimal damage from chronic rejection may explain the similarities between graft and spontaneous arteriosclerosis. Chronic immune injury owing to cytotoxic B cell antibodies, or antivascular endothelial cell antibody, as reported in some patients with atherosclerosis,[15] coupled with hypercholesterolemia may be predisposing factors.[34] Attempts to reduce the incidence of this complication have included the use of antiplatelet agents or warfarin and strict attention to serum lipid levels.[6,27]

The diagnosis of graft coronary arteriosclerosis can be suspected in patients with increasing graft dysfunction in the late postoperative period and occasionally can be confirmed by endomyocardial biopsy.[69] Coronary angiography can confirm the diagnosis in many cases[64] but may not identify intramyocardial coronary disease or symmetrically diffuse narrowing.[59] When localized areas of significant narrowing are identified by coronary angiography in accessible areas, balloon angioplasty has occasionally been useful in improving coronary perfusion.[33] This approach to palliation will undoubtedly be used with increasing frequency. Once myocardial failure develops, the decision to proceed with retransplantation is especially difficult in the patient who has diffuse coronary involvement but remains asymptomatic. Sequential orthotopic transplantation is performed in patients with terminal cardiac decompensation, although survival is less favorable than with initial transplantation.[97]

The development of malignancy is a known risk associated with chronic immunosuppression, with an incidence of approximately 10%,[45,46] lymphoma being the most common type. Stanford reported a high incidence of lymphoma in patients treated with high doses of cyclosporine and rabbit anti-thymocyte globulin. Possibly lower cyclosporine doses will reduce the incidence of this complication.

FUTURE DIRECTIONS

Many questions remain unanswered in the field of cardiac transplantation and provide a variety of av-

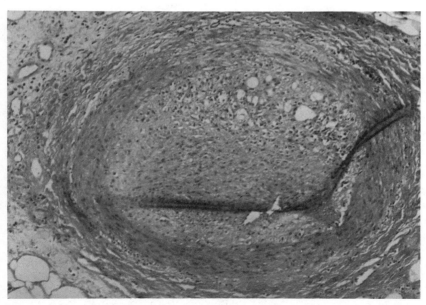

FIGURE 34-7. *Epicardial artery from a cardiac transplant recipient who died suddenly while dancing 18 months after transplantation. Note the intense intimal proliferation causing severe luminal narrowing (hematoxylin and eosin ×25).*

enues for further clinical and experimental research. The most pressing need is for a better understanding of the immunologic mechanisms responsible for the late development of coronary obstructive lesions. A multivariate analysis of various predisposing factors such as hyperlipidemia, hypertension, histocompatibility mismatch, donor age, preservation techniques, and the incidence of acute rejection should improve this understanding. There should also be an intensive ongoing evaluation by collaborating institutions concerning which immunosuppressive regimen results in the lowest incidence of graft coronary arteriosclerosis. Certainly, every effort should be made to reduce or to eliminate hypertension as a complication of cyclosporine therapy and to evaluate whether reduction or elimination of maintenance steroids can reduce the incidence of vascular injury. Whether preoperative histocompatibility matching or other preoperative manipulation of the immune system such as transfusions can play a role in the prevention of graft coronary obstructive disease remains to be determined and could be of utmost importance in improving late survival.

As in all areas of organ transplantation, the avoidance of excessive or of inadequate immunosuppression requires a more precise noninvasive method of determining when the immune system is activated and when it is quiescent in order to reduce the need for frequent biopsies and to alert the clinician to the need for increased immunosuppression before permanent graft damage occurs. Greater sophistication in the monitoring of peripheral T cell subpopulations by monoclonal antibodies offers some promise,[32,41,43] but, as yet, lacks complete predictability. Once the diagnosis of rejection is made, therapy remains largely empirical, and more information is needed about the safest and most effective dosages and duration of therapy with which to treat each rejection episode.

Indeed, all the areas of cardiac transplantation discussed here lend themselves to further investigation. Selection of patients, particularly in regard to age, level of acceptable pulmonary vascular resistance, and deterioration of other organ systems, and the use of mechanical devices should undergo constant reappraisal to establish the best use of the limited donor supply, not only for the best early result but also to provide the best long-term freedom from serious morbidity and mortality. Improved preservation techniques for longer storage periods may become important if histocompatibility matching is shown to have an important bearing on the late development of coronary obstructive lesions.

REFERENCES

1. Atkinson K, Biggs J, Darveniza P et al: Cyclosporine-associated central nervous system toxicity after allogenic bone marrow transplantation. N Engl J Med 310:527, 1984
2. Barnard CN, Barnard MS, Cooper DK et al: The present status of heterotopic cardiac transplantation. J Thorac Cardiovasc Surg 81(3):433–439, 1981
3. Barnard CN: A human cardiac transplant. South Afr Med J 41:1271–1274, 1967
4. Barnhart GR, Hastillo A, Goldman MH et al: Prospective, randomized trial of pretransfusion/azathioprine/prednisone versus cyclosporine/prednisone immunosuppression in cardiac transplantation: Preliminary results. Circulation 72:227–230, 1985
5. Baumgartner WA, Reitz BA, Oyer PE et al: Cardiac homotransplantation. Current Problems in Surgery. Chicago, Year Book Medical Publishers, 1979
6. Becker DM, Markakis M, Sension M et al: Hyperlipidemia and hypertension following heart transplantation: Potential causes of coronary atherosclerosis. J Am Coll Cardiol 7(2A):9, 1986
7. Billingham ME: Some recent advances in cardiac pathology. Hum Pathol 10:367–368, 1979
8. Borow KM, Newman A, Arensman FW et al: Left ventricular contractility and contractile reserve in humans after cardiac transplantation. Circulation 71(5):866–872, 1985
9. Calne RY, White DJG, Rolles K et al: Prolonged survival of pig orthotopic heart grafts treated with Cyclosporin A. Lancet June 3, 1183–1185, 1978
10. Cannom DS, Rider AK, Stinson EB et al: Electrophysiologic studies in the denervated transplanted human heart. Am J Cardiol 36(7):859–866, 1975
11. Cannom DS, Graham AF, Harrison DC: Electrophysiological studies in the denervated transplanted human heart. Response to atrial pacing and atropine. Circ Res 32:268–278, 1973
12. Carrel A, Guthrie CC: The transplantation of veins and organs. Am Med 10:1101–1102, 1905
13. Carrel A: The surgery of blood vessels. Johns Hopkins Hosp Bull V15:18–28, 1907
14. Caves PK, Stinson EB, Billingham ME et al: Diagnosis of human cardiac allograft rejection by serial cardiac biopsy. J Thorac Cardiovasc Surg 66(3):461–466, 1973
15. Caves PK, Stinson EB, Billingham ME et al: Serial transvenous biopsy of the transplanted human heart. Lancet 1:821–826, 1974
16. Christopherson LK, Griepp RB, Stinson EB: Rehabilitation after cardiac transplantation. JAMA 236:2082–2084, 1976
17. Clark DA, Schroeder JS, Griepp RB et al: Cardiac transplantation in man: Review of first three years' experience. Am J Med 54:563–576, 1973

18. Copeland J, Wieden M, Feinberg W et al: Legionnaires' disease following cardiac transplantation. Chest 79(6):669–671, 1981

19. De Smet J, Niset G, Degre G et al: Jogging after heart transplantation. N Engl J Med 309:1521–1522, 1983

20. Dong E, Hurley EJ, Lower RR et al: Performance of the heart two years after autotransplantation. Surgery 56(1):270–274, 1964

21. Dummer JS, Hardy A, Poorsattar A et al: Early infections in kidney, heart, and liver transplant recipients on cyclosporine. Transplantation 36(3):259–267, 1983

22. Gaudiani VA, Stinson EB, Alderman E et al: Long-term survival and function after cardiac transplantation. Ann Surg 194:381–385, 1981

23. Goldberg M, Berman EF, Akman LC: Homologous transplantation of the canine heart. J Int Coll Surg 30(5):575–586, 1958

24. Goldman MH, Barnhart GR, Mohanakumar T et al: Cyclosporine in cardiac transplantation. Surg Clin North Am 65(3):637–659, 1985

25. Goodman DJ, Rossen RM, Cannom DS: Effect of digoxin in atrioventricular conduction studies in patients with and without cardiac autonomic innervation. Circulation 51:251, 1975

26. Graham WH, Childs JW, De Giorgi LS et al: The effect of local graft irradiation on rejection of canine cardiac allografts. J Thorac Cardiovasc Surg 60:730–736, 1970

27. Griepp RB, Stinson EB, Bieber CP et al: Control of graft arteriosclerosis in human heart transplant recipients. Surgery 81(3):262–269, 1977

28. Griffith BP, Hardesty RL, Bahnson HT: Powerful but limited immunosuppression for cardiac transplantation with cyclosporine and low-dose steroid. J Thorac Cardiovasc Surg 87:35–42, 1984

29. Griffith BP, Hardesty RL, Deeb GM et al: Cardiac transplantation with Cyclosporin A and prednisone. Ann Surg 196(3):324–329, 1982

30. Griffith BP, Hardesty RL, Trento A et al: Targeted blood levels of cyclosporine for cardiac transplantation. J Thorac Cardiovasc Surg 88:952–957, 1984

31. Hardy JD, Chavez CM, Kurrus FS et al: Heart transplantation in man. JAMA 188:114–122, 1964

32. Harley JB, Fauci AS: Cyclosporine modulates the human *in vitro* T-dependent antigen-induced synthesis of specific antibody. Transplant Proc 15:2315–2320, 1983

33. Hastillo A, Cowley MJ, Vetrovec G et al: Serial coronary angioplasty for atherosclerosis following cardiac transplantation. J Heart Transplant 4(2):192–195, 1985

34. Hess ML, Hastillo A, Mohanakumar T et al: Accelerated atherosclerosis in cardiac transplantation: Role of cytotoxic B-cell antibodies and hyperlipidemia. Circulation 68(II):94–101, 1983

35. Jamieson SW, Burton NA, Bieber CP et al: Survival of cardiac allografts in rats treated with Cyclosporin A. Surg Forum 30:289–291, 1979

36. Kahn DR, Carr EA, Oberman HA et al: Effect of anticoagulants on the transplanted heart. J Thorac Cardiovasc Surg 60:616–625, 1970

37. Kahn DR, Dufek JH, Hong R et al: Heart and kidney transplantation using total lymphoid irradiation and donor bone marrow in mongrel dogs. J Thorac Cardiovasc Surg 80:125–128, 1980

38. Kahn DR, Hong R, Greenberg AJ et al: Total lymphatic irradiation and donor bone marrow for human heart transplantation. Transplant Proc 13(1):215–217, 1981

39. Kahn DR, Hong R, Greenberg AJ et al: Total lymphatic irradiation and bone marrow in human heart transplantation. Ann Thorac Surg 38(2):169–171, 1984

40. Katz MR, Goldman MH, Barnhart GR et al: Pretransplant transfusions in cardiac allograft recipients. Circulation 70(4):173, 1984

41. Kawaguchi A, Goldman MH, Hoshinaga K et al: Monitoring of lymphocyte subpopulations in cyclosporine (CYA) and azathioprine (AZA) treated cardiac allograft recipients. Transplant Proc 16:1542–1543, 1984

42. Kaye MP, Elcombe SA, O'Fallon WM: The International Heart Transplant Registry—The 1984 Report. Heart Transplant 4(3):290–292, 1985

43. Kerman RH, Flechner SM, Van Buren CT et al: Immunologic monitoring of renal allograft recipients treated with cyclosporine. Transplant Proc 15:2302–2305, 1983

44. Kosek JC, Bieber C, Lower RR: Heart graft arteriosclerosis. Transplant Proc 3(1):512–514, 1971

45. Krikorian JG, Anderson JL, Bieber CP et al: Malignant neoplasms following cardiac transplantation. JAMA 240(7):639–643, 1978

46. Lanza RP, Cooper DKC, Cassidy MJG et al: Malignant neoplasms occurring after cardiac transplantation. JAMA 249(13):1746–1748, 1983

47. Losman JG, Barnard CN: Heterotopic heart transplantation: A valid alternative to orthotopic transplantation: Results, advantages, and disadvantages. J Surg Res 32(4):297–312, 1982

48. Losman JG, Levine H, Campbell CD et al: Changes in indications for heart transplantation. J Thorac Cardiovasc Surg 84:716–726, 1982

49. Lower RR, Dong E, Glazener FS: Electrocardiograms of dogs with heart homografts. Circulation 33:455–460, 1966

50. Lower RR, Dong E, Shumway NE: Long-term survival of cardiac homografts. Surgery 58:110–119, 1965

51. Lower RR, Dong E. Shumway NE: Suppression of rejection crises in the cardiac homograft. Ann Thorac Surg 1:645–649, 1965

52. Lower RR, Shumway NE: Studies on orthotopic homotransplantation of the canine hart. Surg Forum 11:18, 1960

53. Lower RR, Stofer RC, Shumway NE: Homovital transplantation of the heart. J Thorac Cardiovasc Surg 41:196–204, 1961

54. Macintosh AF, Carmichael DJ, Wren C et al: Sinus

node function in first three weeks after cardiac transplantation. Br Heart J 48:584–588, 1982

55. Marcus E, Wong SN, Luisada A: Homologous heart grafts: Transplantation of the heart in dogs. Surg Forum 2:212–217, 1951

56. Mammana RB, Petersen EA, Fuller JK et al: Pulmonary infections in cardiac transplant patients. Modes of diagnosis, complications, and effectiveness of therapy. Ann Thorac Surg 36(6):700–705, 1983

57. Mann FC, Priestly JT, Markowitz J et al: Transplantation of the intact mammalian heart. Arch Surg 26:219–224, 1933

58. Mason JW: Techniques for right and left ventricular endomyocardial biopsy. Am J Cardiol 41:887–892, 1978

59. Mason JW, Strefling A: Small vessel disease of the heart resulting in myocardial necrosis and death despite angiographically normal coronary arteries. Am J Cardiol 44:171–176, 1979

60. Mohanakumar T, Ellis TM, Mendez-Picon G et al: Monitoring human T-cell subpopulations: Effect of immunosuppressive therapy and blood transfusion on OKT4$^+$/OKT8$^+$ ratios. Transplant Proc 15(3): 1978–1979, 1983

61. Mohanty PK, Thames MD, Sowers JR et al: Effect of cardiac transplantation on reflex sympathetic activation in man. Clin Res 33(2):212A, 1985

62. Myers BD, Ross J, Newton L et al: Cyclosporine-associated chronic nephropathy. N Engl J Med 311:699–705, 1984

63. Neptune WB, Cookson BA, Bailey CP et al: Complete homologous heart transplantation. AMA Arch Surg 66:174–178, 1953

64. Newton M, Vetrovec G, Hastillo A et al: Coronary angiographic characteristics of chronic cardiac transplant rejection. Circulation 10:174, 1984

65. Noll RB, Kulkarni R: Complex visual hallucinations and cyclosporine. Arch Neurol 41:329–330, 1984

66. Novitsky D, Boniaszczuk J, Cooper DKC et al: Prediction of acute cardiac rejection using radionuclide techniques. S Afr Med J 65:5–7, 1984

67. Opelz G, Terasaki PI: Improvement of kidney-graft survival with increased numbers of blood transfusions. N Engl J Med 299:799–803, 1978

68. Oyer PE, Stinson EB, Bieber CP et al: Diagnosis and treatment of acute cardiac allograft rejection. Transplant Proc 11(1):296–303, 1979

69. Palmer DC, Tsai CC, Roodman ST et al: Heart graft arteriosclerosis. Transplantation 39(4):385–388, 1985

70. Pennington DG, Sarafian J, Swartz M: Heart transplantation in children. Heart Transplant IV(4):441–445, 1985

71. Pennock JL, Oyer PE, Reitz BA et al: Cardiac transplantation in perspective for the future: Survival, complications, rehabilitation and cost. J Thorac Cardiovasc Surg 83:168–177, 1982

72. Pennock JL, Reitz BA, Bieber CP et al: Cardiac allograft survival in cynomolgus monkeys treated with Cyclosporin-A in combination with conventional immune suppression. Transplant Proc 13(1):390–392, 1981

73. Perloff LJ, Barker CF: Variable response to donor-specific blood transfusion in the rat. Transplantation 38(2):178–182, 1984

74. Pope SE, Stinson EB, Daughters GT: Exercise response of the denervated heart in long-term cardiac transplant recipients. Am J Cardiol 46:213–218, 1980

75. Report of the Ad Hoc Committee of the Harvard Medical School: A definition of irreversible coma. JAMA 205(6):85–88, 1968

76. Ricci DR, Orlick AE, Reitz BA et al: Depressant effect of digoxin in atrioventricular conduction in man. Circulation 57:898–903, 1978

77. Romhilt DW, Doyle M, Sagar KB et al: Prevalence and significance of arrhythmias in long-term survivors of cardiac transplantation. Circulation 66(Suppl 1):219–222, 1982

78. Rosenthal JT, Shaw BW, Hardesty RL et al: Principles of multiple organ procurement from cadaver donors. Ann Surg 198(5):617–621, 1983

79. Rynasiewicz JJ, Sutherland DER, Kawahara K et al: Total lymphoid irradiation in rat heart allografts: Dose, fractionation, and combination with Cyclosporin A. Transplant Proc 13(1):452–454, 1981

80. Sagar KB, Hastillo A, Wolfgang TC et al: Left ventricular mass by M-mode echocardiography in cardiac transplant patients with acute rejection. Circulation 64(II):216–220, 1981

81. Sakakibara S, Konno S: Endomyocardial biopsy. Jap Heart J 3(6):537–543, 1962

82. Sayegh SF, Creech O, Harding JH: Transplantation of the homologous heart. Surg Forum 18:317–319, 1957

83. Schade RK, Guglielmi A, Van Thiel DH et al: Cholestasis in heart transplant recipients treated with cyclosporine. Transplant Proc 15:2757–2760, 1983

84. Schroeder JS: Hemodynamic performance of the human transplanted heart. Transplant Proc XI:304–308, 1979

85. Shaver JA, Leon DF, Gray S et al: Hemodynamic observations after cardiac transplantation. N Engl J Med 281:822–827, 1969

86. Siegl H, Ryffel B, Petric R et al: Cyclosporine, the renin–angiotension–aldosterone system and renal adverse reactions. Transplant Proc 15:2719–2725, 1983

87. Starzl TE, Hakala TR, Shaw BW et al: A flexible procedure for multiple organ procurement. Surg Gynecol Obstet 158:223–230, 1984

88. Steed DL, Brown B, Reilly JJ et al: General surigcal complications in heart and heart-lung transplantation. Surgery 98(4):739–744, 1985

89. Stinson EB, Shroeder JS, Griepp RB et al: Observations on the behavior of recipient atria after cardiac transplantation in man. Am J Cardiol 30:615–622, 1972

90. Thames M: Personal communication

91. Thomas FT, Szentpetery S, Mammana RE et al:

Long-distance transportation of human hearts for transplantation. Ann Thorac Surg 26(4):344–350, 1978

92. Thompson ME: Selection of candidates for cardiac transplantation. Heart Transplant III(1):65–69, 1983

93. Thomson JG: Production of severe atheroma in a transplanted human heart. Lancet, November, 1088–1092, 1969

94. Toledo-Pereyra LH: Multiple organ harvesting for transplantation. Surg Gynecol Obstet 158:572–576, 1984

95. Uretsky BF, Murali S, Lee A et al: Development of coronary atherosclerosis in the transplanted heart immunosuppressed with cyclosporine and prednisone. J Am Coll Cardiol 7(2A):9, 1986

96. Watson DC, Reitz BA, Baumgartner WA et al: Distant heart procurement for transplantation. Surgery 86(1):56–59, 1979

97. Watson DC, Reitz BA, Oyer PE et al: Sequential orthotopic heart transplantation in man. Transplantation 30(6):401–403, 1980

98. Webb WR, Howard HS: Cardiopulmonary transplantation. Surg Forum 8:313–317, 1957

99. Webb WR, Howard HS, Neely WA: Practical methods of homologous cardiac transplantation. J Thorac Surg 37:361–366, 1959

100. Weil R, Clarke DR, Iwaki Y et al: Hyperacute rejection of a transplanted human heart. Transplantation 32(1):71–72, 1981

101. Yusuf S, Theodoropoulos S, Dhalla N: Effect of betablockade on dynamic exercise in human heart transplant recipients. Heart Transplant IV(3):312–314, 1985

102. Zumbro GL, Shearer G, Kitchens WR et al: Mechanical assistance for biventricular failure following coronary bypass operation and heart transplantation. Heart Transplant IV(3):348–352, 1985

CHAPTER 35

Liver Transplantation

Robert D. Gordon   Shunzaburo Iwatsuki   Carlos O. Esquivel
Leonard Makowka   Andreas G. Tzakis   Satoru Todo
Thomas E. Starzl

Since the introduction of cyclosporine into clinical practice, patient survival for both adults and children has improved from less than 35% at 1 year and 20% at 5 years to approximately 70% and 60%, respectively.

The principal indications for transplantation in children have been biliary atresia, postnecrotic cirrhosis, and inborn errors of metabolism. In adults, postnecrotic cirrhosis, inborn errors of metabolism, sclerosing cholangitis, and primary liver tumors have been the most frequent reasons for liver replacement.

Although overall results have been good, most tumor patients eventually have succumbed to recurrent tumor, often within 1 year. B-virus antigen carriers transplanted for postnecrotic cirrhosis have a high incidence of recurrent hepatitis after transplantation. Transplantation of infants continues to be complicated by a high incidence of hepatic artery thrombosis.

Retransplantation for allograft rejection, technical complications, or primary graft failure has been necessary in approximately 20% of cases.

Donor organs can be safely cooled by rapid aortic infusion of cold electrolyte solutions followed by an expeditious, bloodless dissection of the liver and en bloc removal of the kidneys. This reduces the risk of warm ischemic injury during mobilization of the liver and kidneys. Routine use of a venovenous bypass during the anhepatic phase of the recipient operation has improved graft success.

Although liver transplantation across ABO blood groups is usually successful, results have been best between ABO compatible donor–recipient pairs. A positive donor-specific cytotoxic antibody crossmatch has not been shown to be a significant barrier to transplantation of the liver. Rehabilitation after liver transplantation has been excellent.

HISTORICAL NOTES

The idea of transplanting the liver apparently was conceived first by C. Stewart Welch[49] in the early 1950s. He reported research on transplanting an extra liver in a heterotopic site (such as the right paravertebral gutter) without disturbing the host liver. All of his experiments were without immunosuppression. Orthotopic liver replacement apparently was first conceived by Dr. Jack Cannon,[5] but his publication in 1956 gave no details and did not mention whether any of his animals (species unspecified) survived.

In the summer of 1958, two research programs on liver replacement were established independently, one at the Peter Bent Brigham Hospital in Boston[21] and the other at Northwestern University in Chicago.[39,40] From these first efforts, the general requirements for liver transplantation and the events of rejection in unmodified canine recipients were worked out.

Protracted survival in experimental animals after liver transplantation was achieved in Denver in 1963 using azathioprine[41] and soon after using antilymphocyte globulin (ALG).[42] A number of animals from that original work survived for years.[29] The longest survivor lived a full canine lifetime and died almost 11 years after transplantation, having been without immunosuppression for all but 4 months of this time.

Renal transplantation became a practical form of treatment almost 25 years ago with the demonstration that azathioprine and steroids were synergistic.[44] Emboldened by successes with the kidney, the first clinical efforts at liver transplantation were made in Denver[43] in March, 1963, followed by similarly unsuccessful single attempts in Boston and in Paris.[7,22] The failure of the first seven patients to survive for as long as 1 month caused a moratorium to be declared until 1967. In 1966, ALG was added to the immunosuppressive armamentarium with trials in animals and in human kidney recipients.[41,42] Finally, in 1967, the first successful liver transplantations were carried out at the University of Colorado under azathioprine, steroids, and ALG.[32] The longest survivor in the world today has survived almost 17 years post-transplant.

Through the 1970s, further successes were achieved with liver transplantation, but between one half and two thirds of the recipients died within the first postoperative year.[38] The operation was so unpredictable and unreliable that it was justifiably considered to be an experimental operation as opposed to a service. This perception was drastically changed with the introduction of the new immunosuppressive agent cyclosporine by Calne et al in 1978[3,4] and with systematic combination of this agent with prednisone.[38,45] The first reports of nearly 80% 1-year survival of liver recipients[45] when this drug was combined with low doses of steroids have been confirmed as the numbers of cases have increased in the ensuing years.[37,38]

At the same time, technical improvements have played a significant role. It became obvious that optimal biliary tract reconstruction involved anastomosis of the donor and recipient ducts over a T-tube (or stent) and that the only reasonable alternative was anastomosis of the donor duct to a defunctionalized limb of jejunum (Roux-en-Y).[38] These techniques greatly reduced bile fistulas and obstructions as well as the infectious complications that were resulting from imperfect drainage of the biliary tree. Later, the introduction of non-heparin venovenous bypasses[26] made the operation different from the high-tension procedure that it had been previously. In turn, it became possible to train younger surgeons who could take the technology to new centers for further development.

Finally, the development of techniques for multiple organ procurement proved to be a crucial final step in making liver transplantation practical.[33]

THE DECADE OF THE 1980S

During the past 5 years, there has been a dramatic increase in the transplantation of extrarenal organs.

By the end of 1985, 1787 heart, 1441 liver, 381 pancreas or islet cell, and 79 heart–lung transplantations had been performed in the United States (Fig. 35-1A). Approximately 45% of these transplants were done in 1985 (Fig. 35-1B).

The institutional resources and technical expertise required for heart transplantation are the most available, and heart transplantation programs have been proliferating faster than those for other extrarenal organs. Pancreas transplantation and heart–lung transplantation are still regarded as experimental procedures and remain limited to investigational programs in a few major university transplant centers. Liver transplantation requires both exceptional surgical expertise and institutional support. Nearly half the liver transplantations performed in the United States have been done as part of the Denver–Pittsburgh series, but there has been a significant increase in the number of programs in the last few years (Fig. 35-1C).

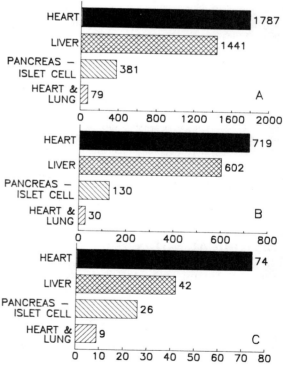

FIGURE 35-1.   (A) The total number of extrarenal organ transplants performed in the United States through December, 1985. (B) The number of extrarenal transplants performed in the United States during the calendar year 1985. (C) The number of centers that reported performing extrarenal transplants through December, 1985. (Data provided by the Office of Health Technology Assessment, U.S. Department of Health and Human Services.)

THE IMPACT OF CYCLOSPORINE

There can be no doubt that introduction of cyclosporine for clinical immunosuppression has been the most significant factor in the expansion of liver and heart transplantation.[36,37,38] For orthotopic liver transplantation, 1-year patient survival has risen from 32.9% under conventional immunosuppression with azathioprine and high-dose steroids to 69.4% with cyclosporine and low-dose steroids in the Denver–Pittsburgh series (Fig. 35-2). Only 29 (17.1%) of the 170 patients who were managed with azathioprine and steroids remain alive, but nearly all of these patients were surviving more than 10 years after transplantation and are enjoying an excellent quality of life. Of the first 500 Denver–Pittsburgh patients transplanted using cyclosporine, 340 (68.0%) of the patients are alive, including 108 patients more than 3 years after transplantation.

For both azathioprine- and cyclosporine-treated patients, the major patient mortality after liver transplantation has occurred within 6 months of transplantation (Fig. 35-2). Patient and graft loss beyond the first year after surgery has always been modest. Improved survival after liver transplantation has to a large extent depended upon effective prevention or treatment of acute rejection in the first 6 months after transplantation and the major impact of cyclosporine has been to increase graft and patient survival in this critical early period through better control of rejection (Figs. 35-2 and 35-3). Monoclonal anti-T-lymphocyte antibody (Orthoclone OKT-3, Ortho Pharmaceuticals, Raritan, NJ) has also proved highly effective in clinical trails for reversal of acute steroid-resistant cellular rejection in cyclosporine-treated patients.[9,31]

Cyclosporine is a cyclic polypeptide derived from two strains of fungi. It can be administered intravenously or orally. Since absorption of the drug is highly variable and is poor in the early postoperative period, it is customary to give the drug intravenously for the first few days after transplantation, followed by a period of combined intravenous and oral therapy with daily monitoring of trough serum or blood levels. Cyclosporine is lipid soluble, and its gastrointestinal absorption is dependent upon bile and bile salts.[48] T-tube clamping is usually followed by a significant increase in cyclosporine absorption.[1] Also, the principal route of elimination of cyclosporine is by hepatic metabolism. Drugs such as phenobarbital, phenytoin, and rifampin, which are potent inducers of hepatic enzymes, can increase cyclosporine elimination and result in reduced blood levels. Erythromycin, an inhibitor of hepatic enzymes, can increase cyclosporine blood levels. Hepatic function and bile production after liver transplantation are variable; therefore, monitoring of drug levels is essential.

In general, patients receive 2 mg/kg of cyclosporine intravenously every 8 hours immediately after transplantation. As soon as gastrointestinal function permits, oral cyclosporine, 17.5 mg/kg administered as a divided dose twice a day, is begun. Intravenous administration can be reduced to twice a day in many patients after oral therapy has begun if drug levels are adequate. Within 3 to 6 weeks of transplantation, doses of 10 mg/kg per day are often all that is required to maintain adequate drug levels. Renal excretion of cyclosporine is minimal, but the drug is nephrotoxic. Dosage may have to be reduced in patients with renal dysfunction. Cyclosporine is not removed by dialysis. In patients with severe

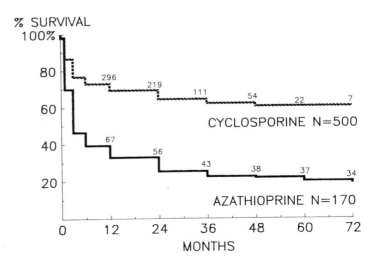

FIGURE 35-2. *Actuarial patient survival after orthotopic liver transplantation for 170 recipients treated with azathioprine (Imuran) and high-dose steroids and 500 recipients treated with cyclosporine (Sandimmune) and low-dose steroids.*

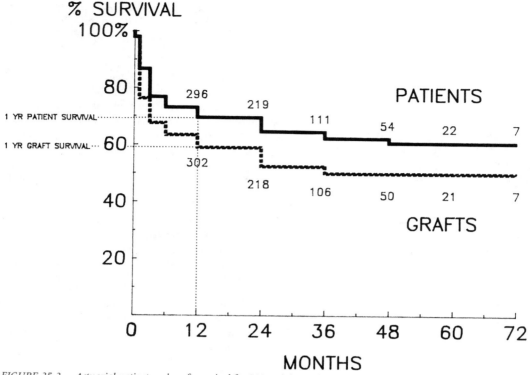

% SURVIVAL

1 YR PATIENT SURVIVAL

1 YR GRAFT SURVIVAL

PATIENTS

GRAFTS

MONTHS

296   219   111   54   22   7

302   218   106   50   21   7

FIGURE 35-3.   *Actuarial patient and graft survival for 500 recipients of 647 orthotopic liver allografts performed using cyclosporine and low-dose steroid therapy.*

renal dysfunction, a 2-week course of monoclonal antibody therapy can permit sparing of cyclosporine until renal function recovers.

Conventional bacterial infections are better tolerated with cyclosporine than with azathioprine. This may be due to the selective action of cyclosporine on T cells and to the lower doses of prednisone required with cyclosporine. Opportunistic fungal infections, *Pneumocystis carini* and *Legionella* pneumonias, and viral infections remain as significant problems.

INDICATIONS FOR TRANSPLANTATION IN ADULTS

The indications for liver transplantation in adults and children differ; therefore, it is useful to consider these groups separately. Of the 297 adults (patients over 19 years of age) in our first 50 cyclosporine-treated patients, 97 (66.3%) are living. One-year survival is 68.9%, and 5-year survival is 54.8% (Fig. 35-4A). The most common indications for liver transplantation in adults have been chronic active

hepatitis, primary biliary cirrhosis, sclerosing cholangitis, inborn errors of metabolism, and primary liver tumors (Fig. 35-5).

Transplantation for Primary Liver Cancer

The first orthotopic human liver transplantations were done for hepatic tumors that could not be treated by subtotal resection. It was hoped that this patient population would be especially favorable for transplantation, since portal hypertension and its complications are usually not present. Although early patient survival has been excellent, long-term patient survival has been poor (Fig. 35-6B) because of a high rate of tumor recurrence in these immunosuppressed patients.

Our experience with transplantation for hepatic malignancy has recently been reviewed by Iwatsuki and colleagues.[15,17] None of the 14 patients who were found to have a coincidental hepatic tumor at the time of transplantation for other diseases such as postnecrotic cirrhosis or biliary atresia have died of recurrent tumor. All of these lesions would have

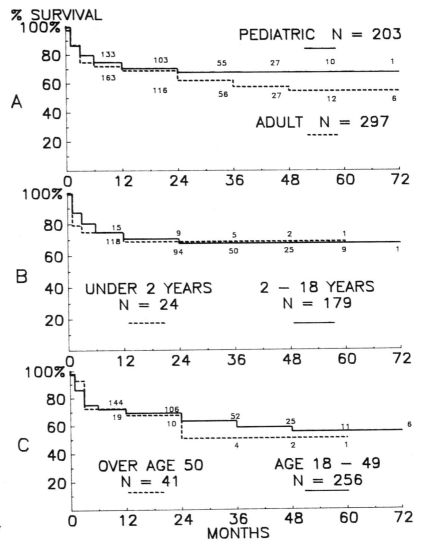

FIGURE 35-4. *(A) Actuarial patient survival for 203 pediatric and 297 adult recipients of human orthotopic liver allografts treated using cyclosporine and high-dose steroids. (B) Actuarial patient survival for 24 pediatric liver allograft recipients younger than 2 years of age compared with 179 pediatric recipients between 2 and 18 years of age at the time of transplantation. (C) Actuarial patient survival for 41 adult liver allograft recipients older than 50 years of age compared with 256 adult recipients 18 to 49 years of age at the time of transplantation.*

been suitable for subtotal hepatic resection if other diseases of the liver had not necessitated transplantation.

Forty-nine patients have been transplanted for liver tumors too extensive for conventional subtotal resection, including 21 patients transplanted using azathioprine–steroids and 28 transplanted with cyclosporine–steroids. Twenty-nine of these patients were transplanted for hepatocellular carcinomas. Thirty-two patients survived more than 3 months after surgery. Tumor has recurred in 20 patients (63%), and the liver graft is frequently the first site of recurrence. Less than half of the patients remained tumor free for at least 1 year. However, six of seven patients with fibrolamellar hepatoma re-

mained free of tumor for more than 1 year. Although there is a high ultimate recurrence rate even for this variant of hepatocellular carcinoma, palliation is longer lasting.

Conventional chemo- and radiotherapy have been used in combination with total hepatic resection and transplantation in an effort to improve survival, but results have still been poor. Of our four patients with nonfibrolamellar hepatoma treated with Adriamycin and other chemotherapeutic agents, two developed recurrence within a few months. The immunosuppression necessary to prevent graft rejection may accelerate the growth of extrahepatic nests of malignant cells unrecognizable at the time of transplantation. The high incidence

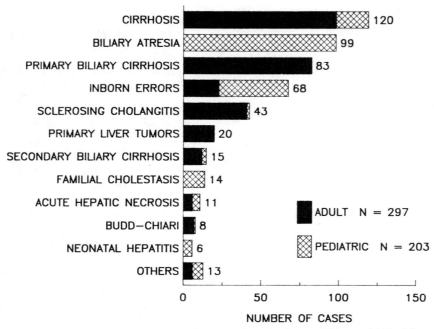

FIGURE 35-5.   *Indications for orthotopic liver transplantation in 203 children and 297 adults treated with cyclosporine and low-dose steroids.*

of recurrence in the graft suggests that these cells are able to home back to the favorable environment of the liver. Nevertheless, the high survival of patients with coincidental malignancies demonstrates that long survival after transplantation in the presence of a hepatic malignancy is possible. Even in the patients with unresectable malignancy, significant palliation can be achieved, especially in patients with less aggressive tumors such as fibrolamellar hepatoma.

Cirrhosis

Cirrhosis is the most common indication for liver replacement in adults (see Fig. 35-5). Most of these patients have chronic active hepatitis, but there are also small numbers of patients with cryptogenic cirrhosis or Laennec's cirrhosis. One-year survival after transplantation for cirrhosis in adults is 67.2%, but it drops to 50.9% at 3 years (Fig. 35-6B). Until recently, survival for cirrhotic patients over 40 years of age has been poor, but this appears to relate to the coexistence of other risk factors in these patients rather than an effect of age itself.[28] There is a significant incidence of recurrence of hepatitis in B-virus carriers. Alcoholic patients have always constituted a high-risk group, since their medical con-

dition is often poor and recidivism is a constant concern. However, we continue to offer transplantation to carefully selected candidates with Laennec's cirrhosis.

Primary Biliary Cirrhosis (PBC)

Primary biliary cirrhosis (PBC) is the second leading indication for transplantation in adults. This is an uncommon disease, most often affecting late middle-aged women. The cause is unknown but it is considered to be an autoimmune disorder. Fatigue, jaundice, pruritis, hepatomegaly, and osteoporosis ("hepatic rickets") are characteristic features of the disorder, which may progress over many years. There is no effective medical therapy, although a variety of agents, including D-penicillamine, chlorambucil, colchicine, and even cyclosporine have been tried. A sudden increase in the rate of rise of serum bilirubin, progression of osteoporosis, or complications of portal hypertension (variceal bleeding, encephalopathy, intractable ascites) are indications for transplantation. The risk of recurrence of PBC after transplantation is unknown, but the results so far are encouraging. Of the 83 patients transplanted for PBC, 58 are alive 3 months to 6 years after surgery. Actuarial survival is 68.4% at 1

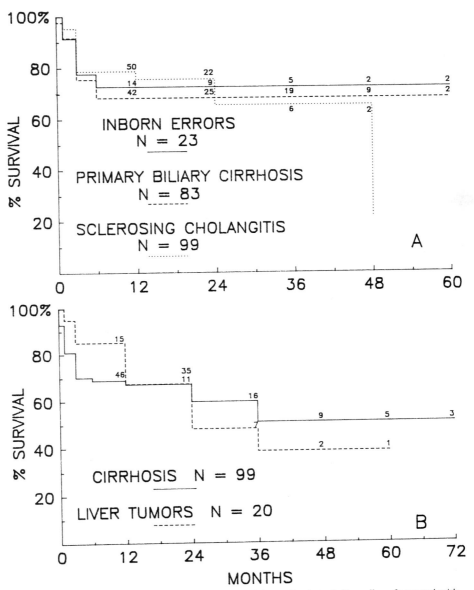

FIGURE 35-6. *Actuarial patient survival of adult recipients of orthotopic liver allografts treated with cyclosporine and low-dose steroids transplanted for (A) inborn errors of metabolism, primary biliary cirrhosis, and sclerosing cholangitis, and (B) cirrhosis (chronic active hepatitis, cryptogenic cirrhosis, or Laennec's cirrhosis) and primary liver tumors.*

and at 5 years (Fig. 35-6A). There have been no deaths and no confirmed recurrences of disease among the 42 patients surviving more than 1 year.

Sclerosing Cholangitis

Sclerosing cholangitis may occur in a primary form or in association with other diseases, especially in-

flammatory bowel disease. It is associated with an increased risk of carcinoma of the bile duct. Many of these patients have had attempts at surgical biliary diversion, which complicates transplantation and should be avoided except in patients with well-defined extrahepatic lesions. Survival after transplantation has been improving and is currently 75.7% at 1 year (Fig. 35-6A). The risk of late recurrence of disease or late development of bile duct cancer after transplantation for sclerosing cholangitis is not yet known. If proctocolectomy for associated bowel disease is indicated, it is best deferred until 3 to 6 months after liver transplantation.

Inborn Errors Off Metabolism

Twenty-three adults were transplanted for inborn errors of metabolism, including alpha$_1$-antitrypsin deficiency (11 cases), Wilson's disease (8 cases), hemochromatosis (2 cases), tyrosinemia (1 case), and cystic fibrosis (1 case). Survival in this group of patients has been good (Figs. 35-6A and 35-8) except for those patients who present in advanced stages of hepatic encephalopathy with acute hepatic decompensation from Wilson's disease. Mortality in the encephalopathic patient is 50%.

INDICATIONS FOR TRANSPLANTATION IN CHILDREN

Of the 203 children (aged 18 and younger) in the series, 143 (70.4%) are living with 1-year and 5-year actuarial survival at 70.4% and 67.7%, respectively (see Fig. 35-4A). As in adults, most of the mortality after liver transplantation in children is in the first 6 months after surgery.

Biliary Atresia

Biliary atresia is the most common indication for liver replacement in children (see Fig. 35-5). Most of these patients have had previous operations, usually portoenterostomies (Kasai procedure) and occasionally portosystemic venous shunts, often with little if any benefit. Previous surgery in the hepatic hilum makes liver transplantation much more difficult and, for most children with biliary atresia, transplantation is the only genuine hope of long-term survival. Conservative use of portoenterostomy, however, is still appropriate. There is a severe shortage of donors for small children, and a successful Kasai operation can stabilize the patient and buy valuable time. Although previous surgery is associated with an increased morbidity after liver transplantation, it has not been associated with increased mortality.[6] However, revision of Kasai operations and stoma creation are rarely of significant benefit and greatly increase the difficulty of liver transplantation. Portosystemic venous shunts should also be avoided whenever possible.

The results of liver transplantation for biliary atresia are very gratifying, and long-term survival

has been excellent.[8,16] In our first 500 transplantation with cyclosporine, 68 of 99 patients with biliary atresia are surviving 3 months to 6 years after surgery. Actuarial survival is 68.4% at 1 year and 66.7% at 5 years (Fig. 35-7). Only 4 of the 65 patients who have survived more than 1 year after transplantation for biliary atresia have died. Since only modest doses of prednisone are required with cyclosporine, growth and development in most of these children are essentially normal.[47]

Inborn Errors of Metabolism

The second most common indication for liver transplantation in children has been inborn errors of metabolism. Survival after liver transplantation for inborn errors of metabolism in children has been excellent (73.8% at 1 and 5 years, Figs. 35-7 and 35-8). Transplantation has been performed at alpha$_1$-antitrypsin deficiency (27 cases), Wilson's disease (6 cases), tyrosinemia (5 cases), glycogen storage disease (5 cases), hypercholesterolemia (1 case) and sea-blue histiocyte syndrome (1 case). Two patients (one adolescent and one adult) have been transplanted for chronic active hepatitis contracted as a result of factor VIII therapy for hemophilia, and the one survivor (the adolescent now 14 months post-transplantation) appears to have been cured of his hemophilia.[19]

Two years ago, a simultaneous heart–liver transplant was performed in Pittsburgh in a 6-year-old girl with homozygous familial hypercholesterolemia.[24,30] She had already required two coronary artery bypass operations and a mitral valve replacement for severe arteriosclerotic heart disease but was failing despite this. A heart transplant was performed, followed immediately by a liver transplant from the same donor. Although the liver appeared grossly normal, extensive studies of the child indicated that the metabolic defect responsible for her disease was a defect in hepatic-based metabolism. Now more than 2 years after the double transplantation, the child is doing well and has a sustained improvement in her lipid and cholesterol profile.[2]

OTHER INDICATIONS IN ADULTS AND CHILDREN

Most of the other pediatric liver transplantations in the Denver–Pittsburgh series have been done for cirrhosis (21 cases), familial cholestasis (14 cases), and neonatal hepatitis (giant cell hepatitis). One-year survival for these indications is over 75%.

Eight patients have been transplanted for

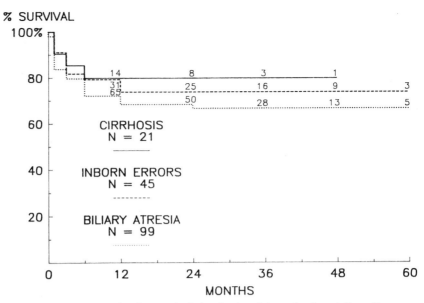

FIGURE 35-7. *Actuarial patient survival of pediatric recipients of orthotopic liver allografts treated with cyclosporine and low-dose steroids transplanted for biliary atresia, inborn errors of metabolism, or cirrhosis.*

Budd–Chiari syndrome, with four survivors, all on permanent anticoagulation. Extensive thrombectomy of the portal system, the vena cava, and iliofemoral veins may be required. Use of the venous bypass can be hazardous in this group of patients. After transplantation, these patients should be kept on permanent anticoagulation therapy.

Seven patients have been transplanted for acute hepatic necrosis. Four patients have survived, including three patients now more than 2 years since transplantation. There is a chance of survival if patients are not in deep coma at the time of surgery or have been in coma only briefly.

SELECTION AND PREPARATION OF PATIENTS FOR TRANSPLANTATION

Since liver transplantation is a complex procedure, it is often assumed that the evaluation and preparation of patients for surgery must also be complex.

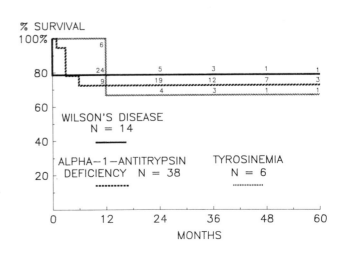

FIGURE 35-8. *Actuarial patient survival after orthotopic liver transplantation for alpha₁-antitrypsin deficiency (11 adults, 27 children), Wilson's disease (8 adults, 6 children), and tyrosinemia (1 adult, 5 children).*

In fact, the evaluation of liver transplant candidates can often be accomplished quickly and at minimal expense if the immediate needs of the patient are not confused with the research interests of the physicians. Most patients are referred to the transplant center with an established diagnosis and a poor prognosis without transplantation. A major gastrointestinal bleed, a history of repeated bouts of encephalopathy, progressive neuropathy, refractory ascites, a recent precipitous deterioration in liver function (e.g., a recent increase in the rate of rise of serum bilirubin), poor hepatic synthetic function (low serum albumin and elevated prothrombin time), rapid progression of bone disease, and severe wasting are indications for early transplantation.

Many of these patients have been needlessly explored and subjected to useless if not mutilating biliary tract operations, questionable portosystemic venous shunting, or unnecessary cholecystectomy or splenectomy. Variceal bleeding in patients awaiting transplantation is a common problem but can usually be managed by sclerotherapy. In the rare case in which a venous shunt is required, mesocaval or splenorenal shunts rather than portocaval shunts should be done. Splenectomy in patients with advanced cirrhosis and portal hypertension often results in portal vein thrombosis and may ruin the patient's chances for successful transplantation. Percutaneous needle biopsy is sufficient for tissue diagnosis in nearly all patients.

Computed tomographic (CT) scans are useful to detect the presence of tumors, with or without extrahepatic extension. Laparatomy to rule out extrahepatic metastatic disease in candidates for transplantation for primary liver cancer is best carried out at the time that the patient is taken to the operating room for transplantation. If extrahepatic spread of disease is found, a backup candidate can then be quickly substituted.

A general evaluation of pulmonary, renal, and cardiac function is appropriate to assess surgical risk and prepare the patient for surgery. Portal vein patency can be assessed by noninvasive ultrasound. We reserve invasive angiographic studies for patients whose portal vein cannot be visualized by ultrasound or in patient with previous venous shunts in whom it is important to assess the status of both the shunt and the portal vein.

The patient's weight, height, ABO blood group, and ultrasound measurements of liver size are important in donor selection. Most patients with postnecrotic cirrhosis have a small liver, whereas patients with sclerosing cholangitis and primary biliary cirrhosis usually have substantial hepatomegaly.

Liver transplantation can be successfully done across ABO blood groups and in the presence of preformed anti-donor antibody without significant risk of hyperacute rejection. Survival of grafts in patients with preformed anti-donor antibody or high panel reactive antibody (Fig. 35-9) is the same or better than survival of grafts in patients without antibody.[10] However, long-term graft survival for ABO matched grafts (Fig. 35-10) has been better than that for ABO compatible but non-identical or ABO incompatible grafts.[11] Thus, we recommend that ABO compatible donors be used except in urgent situations or for young children where donor availability is a critical problem.

The improved patient survival offered with cyclosporine has encouraged referral of better candidates and has expanded the indications for liver transplantation. For example, just a few years ago, liver transplantation was limited to patients younger than 55 years of age. However, survival of the 41 patients older than 50 years of age in our first 500 cyclosporine-treated patients has been just as good as survival for 256 patients between 18 and 49 years (see Fig. 4C). Six of the seven patients over the age of 60 years have survived, including one patient 67 years old at the time of transplantation.

Predicting which patients will succeed and which will fail based on preoperative risk factors is a difficult task. Shaw and associates[27] recently performed a retrospective analysis of 118 liver transplantations in Pittsburgh over a 4-year period to determine whether survival in the first 6 months could be predicted on the basis of preoperative condition. Variables coded on the analysis included mental status, malnutrition, ascites, previous surgery, and complications (variceal bleeding, biliary sepsis, or spontaneous bacterial peritonitis). Operative blood loss was also analyzed. The analysis produced a sigmoidal curve, with most patients on the steep slope of the curve between inflection points. Thus, it is difficult to predict early outcome based on these preoperative factors for most patients. Patients in deep coma at the time of transplantation, however, rarely survive unless their condition can be improved to the point that they are awake and off the respirator when taken to the operating room. Nevertheless, even patients in *acute* hepatic failure and coma have survived if transplanted quickly.

Given this unpredictability of survival, we continue to select patients for transplantation based on liver size, ABO blood group, and medical urgency. Only patients in deep, irreversible, subacute, or chronic coma have little chance of survival.

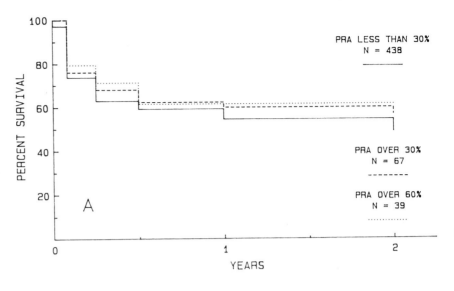

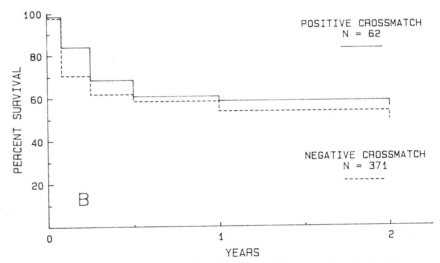

FIGURE 35-9. *(A) Actuarial graft survival after orthotopic liver transplantation in 438 pa-*
tients with a panel reactive antibody (PRA) less than 30% compared with 67 recipients with a
PRA greater than 30%, including 39 patients with a PRA greater than 60% at the time of
transplantation. (B) Actuarial graft survival after orthotopic liver transplantation for 62 recipi-
ents with a positive donor-specific antibody crossmatch compared with 371 recipients with a
negative crossmatch. There is no significant difference in graft survival based on either PRA or
antibody crossmatch. (Adapted from Gordon et al[10].)

ORGAN PROCUREMENT

The development of effective techniques for multiple organ recovery has been essential to the expansion of renal, liver, and heart transplantation.[27,33,34] An insufficient supply of brain-dead organ donors re-

mains the single greatest limiting factor in solid organ transplantation.

Public awareness of the progress in organ transplantation and the need for organ donors has resulted from media attention, professionally sponsored educational programs, and government

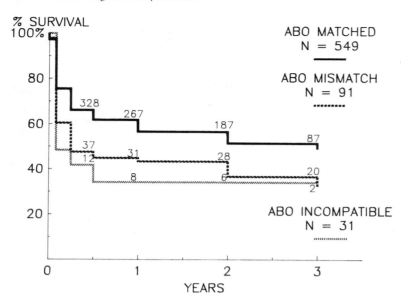

FIGURE 35-10. *Actuarial graft survival for 549 recipients of ABO identical liver allografts, 91 ABO nonidentical but compatible (mismatched) liver allografts, and 31 ABO incompatible liver allografts. Survival of ABO identical grafts is significantly better than that of ABO mismatched or incompatible grafts. (Adapted from Gordon et al[11].)*

interest. Our voluntary system of organ donation has for the most part worked well. The public's response has been highly supportive, but significant resistance to organ donation has come from physician apathy or reluctance to raise the issue of donation with potential donor families. Legislation to require hospitals to request permission for organ donation has been passed in several states in the past year and is under active consideration by many other states.

TECHNICAL CONSIDERATIONS

Donor Hepatectomy

A well-preserved, promptly functioning allograft is essential for successful liver transplantation. Techniques have been developed that permit the liver, kidneys, and thoracic viscera to be obtained from a single donor.[33,34]

In the traditional procurement technique, the abdomen and thorax are entered through a complete midline sternal splitting incision. The left lateral segment of the liver is mobilized, and the aorta is encircled just above or below the diaphragm.

Great care must be taken to identify and deal with the frequent variations in hepatic arterial supply. The gastrohepatic ligament is palpated and inspected for the presence of a branch of the left gastric artery to the liver (Fig. 35-11) which, if present, is preserved by dissection of the left gastric artery back to its origin from the celiac axis. The division of the left gastric artery to the greater curvature of the

stomach can then be safely ligated and divided. the right hepatic artery (or, rarely, the common hepatic artery) may originate from the superior mesenteric artery and lie posterior to the portal vein. This artery must be preserved in continuity with the proximal superior mesenteric artery. Special techniques have been developed for reconstruction of livers with multiple arteries (Fig. 35-11).[13]

Once the preliminary dissection is completed, cannulas are inserted in the abdominal aorta and inferior vena cava and cold Ringer's lactate is slowly infused through the portal vein cannula to cool the donor to 30°C to 32°C (Fig. 35-12). The central venous pressure and consistency of the liver are carefully monitored, and the inferior vena cava cannula is opened as needed to remove excess volume and prevent hepatic congestion. Once the liver is cool, or if the donor becomes unstable, the aorta is crossclamped at the diaphragm and cold Collins' solution is infused through the aortic and portal vein cannulas. The inferior vena cava is divided at its junction with the right atrium.

After a brief but thorough flush of the liver, the aorta is divided proximal and distal to the origin of the hepatic arterial supply taking care not to injure the renal arteries. A clamp is placed just proximal to the renal vessels to permit continued cold perfusion of the kidneys after division of the upper aorta. The diaphragm is cut leaving a wide cuff containing the suprahepatic vena cava. The infrahepatic vena cava is then mobilized and entered anteriorly just above the renal veins. The orifices of the renal veins can be seen inside the opened vena cava, which is then safely divided. The liver is taken

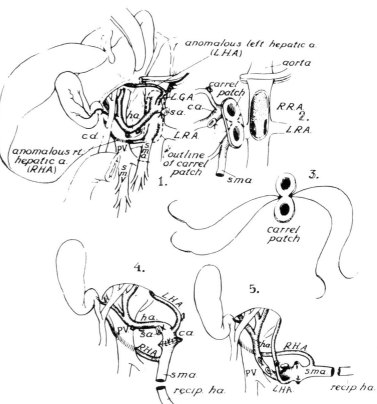

FIGURE 35-11. *Methods for reconstruction of complex donor anomaly: (1) Complex arterial supply to the liver originating from the left gastric artery (LGA), celiac axis (ca), and superior mesenteric artery (sma). (2) A patch of anterior aorta, including the origins of the celiac axis and superior mesenteric artery, is removed. The renal artery orifices are protected. (3) Folding of the aortic patch permits safe anastomosis of the celiac axis to the superior mesenteric artery. (4) The superior mesenteric artery distal to the right hepatic artery is used for anastomosis to the recipient artery (recip ha). (5) The reconstructed arterial supply of the graft may be rotated to match the orientation of the host vessel. (sa = splenic artery; LRA = left renal artery; RRA = right renal artery; PV = portal vein; smv = superior mesenteric vein; reproduced with permission from Gordon et al[13].)*

to the back table, given a final flush of Collins' solution through the portal vein, and packaged for transfer to the recipient hospital.

The kidneys can be rapidly excised en bloc and separated on the back table. The left renal vein is divided at its origin from the vena cava. The vena cava should not be split in half, but rather should be left intact attached to the right renal vein for use in providing additional length.

The aortoiliac arteries and the iliac veins are also harvested. These grafts are often necessary for reconstruction of the arterial supply and portal vein in recipients with inadequate native vessels. Iliac vein segments can also be grafted to the right renal vein to add length during transplantation of the right kidney.

The standard technique of procurement can be modified to permit rapid removal of the liver as may be necessary in an unstable donor.[34] No preliminary dissection is performed except encirclement of the proximal aorta and placement of distall aortic and vena cava cannulae. If the heart is to be taken, it is then prepared, and, when the thoracic team is ready

to arrest circulation, the proximal aorta is cross-clamped. A rapid infusion of cold Collins' solution is then begun through the aortic cannula (Fig. 35-13). The inferior vena cava is divided at its junction with the right atrium. The heart is then removed while the liver continues to flush. The intestines and portal vein will blanch within 2 to 3 minutes, and the liver will be palpably cold. In adults, 2 liters to 3 liters of flush are sufficient to cool the liver to a cryoprotective temperature of less than 28°C. Once this has been achieved, the aortic flush is slowed and the hepatic arterial supply and hilum is dissected in a bloodless field. The same care must be taken to identify and preserve arterial anomalies as with the standard technique. The liver is then excised in a manner similar to the standard method, leaving a cuff of diaphragm and the adrenal gland attached to the hepatic portion of the vena cava. In experienced hands, the donor hepatectomy can be performed in only half an hour by this method.

The final preparation of the allograft occurs on a back table in the recipient operating room. The adrenal gland and excess diaphragm are removed,

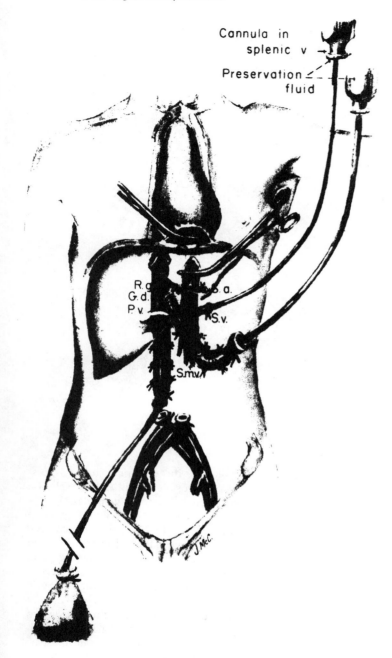

Cannula in
splenic v
Preservation
fluid

R. g.   ___. s. a.
G. d.
P. v.
S. v.

Smv.

J. McC.

FIGURE 35-12.   In situ infusion technique for combined donor hepatectomy and nephrectomy. (Rg = right gastric artery; Gd = gastroduodenal artery; Sa = splenic artery; Sv = splenic vein; Pv = portal vein; Smv = superior mesenteric vein; reproduced with permission from Starzl et al[33].)

and the vascular cuffs are prepared for anastomosis. All technical anomalies are reported to the recipient surgeon so that he may make any changes in recipient technique necessary to accommodate the graft.

The Recipient Operation

The recipient hepatectomy is often the most difficult part of the liver transplant procedure, and there is

no single best method. Individual dissection of hepatic hilar structures may be impossible because of previous surgery or because of massive formation of varices. Mobilization of the liver from the hepatic fossa may result in massive hemorrhage if the hepatic arterial and portal venous blood supply have not first been controlled.

Occlusion of the vena cava and portal vein without bypass may result in cardiovascular insta-

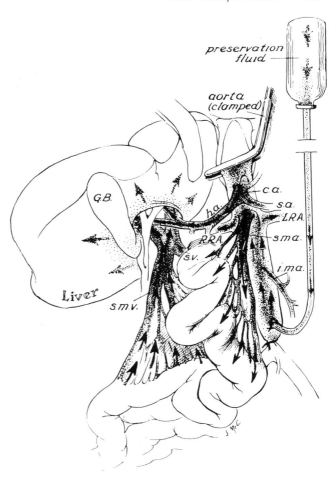

FIGURE 35-13. *Method of rapid liver cooling that does not require any preliminary dissection except for the insertion of a distal aortic cannula and cross-clamping of the aorta at the diaphragm. The infusion fluid quickly reaches the portal system through the splanchnic capillary bed, providing double inflow cooling. (GB = gallbladder, ima = inferior mesenteric artery; reproduced with permission from Starzl et al [7 in Ch. 34])*

bility, splanchnic and renal venous hypertension, and increased hemorrhage from thin-walled venous collaterals. Since 1983, we have routinely used a pump-driven venovenous bypass system without systemic heparinization during the anhepatic phase of the recipient operation. We believe that this has contributed to a significant reduction in morbidity and mortality.[26] Use of the bypass has permitted modifications in the technique of recipient hepatectomy, decreased transfusion and fluid requirements, and reduced cardiopulmonary and renal complications.[34]

When possible, the individual structures in the hepatic hilum are skeletonized, but no other dissection is necessary. Bypass is then established by placement of cannulas in the portal vein and saphenofemoral vein. Return to the superior vena cava can usually be done through a cannula in the axillary vein. If the hilar dissection is difficult, a vascular clamp is placed across all the hilar structures, which are then transected (Fig. 35-14). The

individual structures are then identified, dissected back, and the portal vein is cannulated.

Division and cannulation of the portal vein greatly facilitates mobilization of the liver from the hepatic fossa and dissection of the infrahepatic vena cava. The triangular ligaments and peritoneal reflections that make up the coronary ligament are cut, and the right lobe of the liver is elevated into the wound. The suprahepatic and infrahepatic segments of the vena cava are then encircled. If it is not possible to encircle either the upper or lower vena cava, the liver can be shelled out from above or below as shown in Figures 35-15 and 35-16.

Once the liver has been removed, use of the venovenous bypass provides time to close the raw areas created during the hepatectomy as shown in Figure 35-17. This will minimize bleeding during performance of the vascular anastomoses. Adequate vena cava cuffs and sufficient length of portal vein must have been developed before the graft is brought into the field for anastomosis.

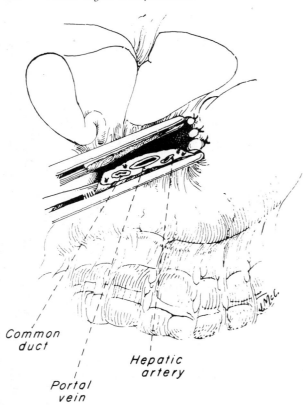

Common
duct

Portal
vein

Hepatic
artery

FIGURE 35-14.   *Mass clamping of the portal structures. This maneuver is performed if there is great difficulty in individually dissecting the structures of the portal triad. The vessels can then be dissected back from the cut ends. (Reproduced with permission from Starzl et al*[37].)

The anastomosis of the suprahepatic vena cava is performed first, followed by the infrahepatic vena cava. Near completion of the lower cava anastomosis, the liver is flushed with cold lactated Ringer's solution to remove entrapped air and concentrated potassium. The portal bypass cannula is then removed, leaving the patient on vena cava bypass while the portal vein is reconstructed. The liver is then revascularized with portal flow, and all remaining bypass cannulas are removed. After reasonable hemostasis is obtained, the hepatic artery is reconstructed.

Successful reconstruction of the portal venous and hepatic arterial circulations demands flawless technique. Failure of either anastomosis usually leads to patient death or retransplantation. A modified continuous suture technique with 6-0 or 7-0 polypropylene suture is used such that the knot is tied a significant distance from the vessel wall.[35] This permits the vessel to distend to full caliber as the suture recedes back into the vessel and redistributes itself after restoration of flow. A single interrupted suture placed where the two ends of the continuous suture meet prevents separation of the vessel at the growth factor (Fig. 35-18).

Direct anastomosis of the graft to the recipient hepatic artery is often not possible because of inadequate size, disease, or injury of the native artery. Alternative methods of reconstruction must be used in these cases.[25] Our preferred method is to use a segment of donor iliac artery that is anastomosed to the infrarenal aorta and tunneled under the pancreas and duodenum to reach the graft. Conduits of donor aorta left in continuity with the celiac axis and hepatic artery and anastomosed to the recipient infrarenal aorta have also been used in small children.

Before the biliary reconstruction is attempted, complete hemostasis should be obtained. In recent years, direct duct-to-duct reconstruction over a T-tube (Fig. 35-19A) has been our preferred method of biliary reconstruction. When this is not possible, such as in patients with disease of the extrahepatic biliary system, Roux-en-Y choledochojejunostomy over an internal stent is used (Fig. 35-19B).

POSTOPERATIVE CARE AND COMPLICATIONS

Initial Care

After surgery, initial care is similar to that for other patients undergoing a major general surgical pro-

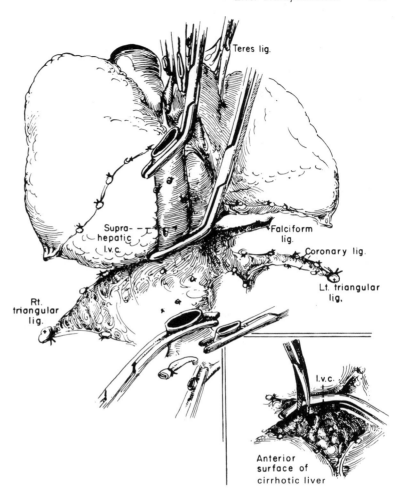

Teres lig.

Supra-
hepatic
l.v.c.

Falciform
lig.

Coronary lig.

Lt. triangular
lig.

Rt.
triangular
lig.

I.v.c.

Anterior
surface of
cirrhotic liver

FIGURE 35-15. Technique of removing the liver by peeling it out from below upward. The infrahepatic vena cava has been divided, and the liver is removed from the hepatic fossa by dissecting upward until the suprahepatic cava is reached. Inset—The suprahepatic vena cava has been crossclamped and is dissected away from the liver to increase the length of the suprahepatic cava cuff. (Reproduced with permission from Starzl et al[37].)

cedure. The patient is kept in intensive care until he or she is alert, extubated, and hemodynamically stable. Many patients are ready to return to the regular hospital floor within 48 hours after transplantation. Antibiotic prophylaxis for biliary tract organisms (*Klebsiella, Escherichia coli,* and enterococci) is begun before surgery and continued for 5 days.

Nearly all patients leave the operating room with a significant excess of fluid, and most patients will have oliguria in the first 24- to 48-hour period. Diuretics and colloid are often required. Vigorous use of crystalloid can easily result in pulmonary edema. Fresh frozen plasma (FFP) should be used with restraint, because overzealous correction of clotting parameters may contribute to postoperative hepatic artery thrombosis. We generally avoid use of FFP unless the prothrombin time is persistently over 25 seconds or there is evidence of major ongoing blood loss with abnormal clotting parameters.

It is best to give potassium as bolus when needed rather than add it to the maintenance intravenous fluids. Graft necrosis (primary nonfunction or hepatic artery thrombosis) can result in unpredictable increases in serum potassium. Children can rapidly develop low ionized calcium levels and hypo- or hyperglycemia after liver transplantation. Thus, glucose and ionized calcium levels must be monitored closely during the first 48 hours.

Mental status, prothrombin time, and urine output are important indicators of the quality of early graft function. Narcotic and other medications that may interfere with the evaluation of mental status are contraindicated. Primary graft failure occurs infrequently but is a very serious complication. The patient decompensates quickly and will show markedly abnormal liver function, coagulopathy, oliguria, and severe central nervous system (CNS) changes. Stage IV coma, alkalosis, hyperkalemia, and hypoglycemia characterize the terminal phase

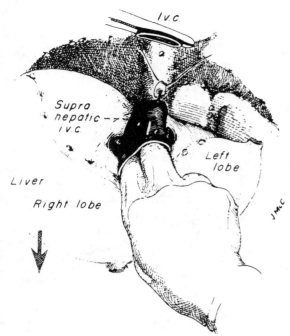

FIGURE 35-16.   *An alternative method for removal of the liver when the infrahepatic cava is difficult to crossclamp. The suprahepatic cava is divided, and fingers are thrust into the intrahepatic cava to prevent massive hemorrhage. The liver is then removed from above downward. (Reproduced with permission from Starzl et al[37].)*

of this acute hepatic decompensation. Avoid giving any potassium, give FFP every 4 to 6 hours, and keep the gastric *p*H more than 5. Urgent retransplantation is required.

Hypertension is a common problem in the postoperative patient. Hydralazine and beta-blockers (labetalol, propranolol) are first-line drugs. Minoxidil (Loniten), clonidine (Catapres), and captopril (Capoten, often preferred for children) are alternatives in patients requiring other agents. Avoid methyldopa (Aldomet), which is hepatotoxic. Intravenous nitroglycerine can be used when appropriate for patients in the intensive care unit. Sodium nitroprusside must be used with caution because of the potential for cyanide toxicity. Nifedipine (Procardia), 10 mg, administered under the tongue, is useful in an emergency.

In cases of refractory hypertension, labetalol (trandate normodyne), a beta- and alpha-adrenergic blocking drug with selective action on peripheral vascular receptors, can be given intravenously. The drug must be given by a physician with continuous blood pressure monitoring in the intensive care unit.

It is given in 20-mg doses over 2 minutes and may be repeated every 10 minutes up to a total of 300 mg or can be administered as a continuous intravenous infusion at 2 mg/min, adjusted according to the blood pressure.

Immunosuppression and Rejection

Cyclosporine therapy has been discussed previously. Patients with persistent oliguria or elevated serum creatinine require reduction of cyclosporine dosage. In cases of severe renal failure, cyclosporine is discontinued and treatment with monoclonal OKT-3 antibody is substituted for as long as 2 weeks to allow renal function to recover.

The patient is given 1 g methylprednisolone intraoperatively and then begun on a steroid taper after surgery. Adults are begun on 200 mg per day given in four divided doses and tapered 40 mg per day until a maintenance dose of 20 mg per day is reached. Children are begun at 100 mg per day and are tapered by 20 mg per day. Very small children are maintained on only 10 mg to 15 mg per day. As soon as oral intake is established, oral prednisone is substituted for the intravenous steroid.

Hyperacute rejection of the liver is a controversial entity and, if it exists, is a rare event. Acute allograft rejection usually occurs 7 to 21 days after operation but can occur at any time. Early "accelerated" rejection is occasionally seen. Liver biopsy may be required to distinguish between early rejection and ischemic injury.

Rejection is most commonly manifested by malaise, fever, graft swelling and tenderness, and diminished graft function. A rise in bilirubin and transaminases is usually seen and T-tube biliary drainage may be thin and light in color. Clinical rejection is treated initially by a 1 g IV bolus of methylprednisolone followed by a complete recycle of the postoperative steroid taper. If response is poor, biopsy and treatment with monoclonal antibody should be considered.

Monoclonal mouse anti-human thymocyte globulin (OKT-3) has been approved for clinical use by the U.S. Food and Drug Administration. It is used for the treatment of acute steroid-resistant rejection or for sparing of cyclosporine in toxic patients. It is given as a single daily dose of 5 mg IV over 5 minutes (2.5 mg in children less than 30 kg). Benadryl and Solucortef are given prior to it to reduce unpleasant reactions. Complete blood count (CBC), hematocrit, platelet count, and T cell ratios are monitored during therapy.

Chills and fever are common with the first few doses of OKT-3. Bronchospasm, hypotension, chest

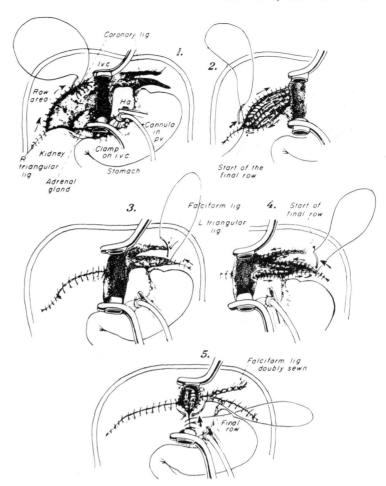

FIGURE 35-17. Elimination of the raw areas in the hepatic fossa with continuous polypropylene suturing. (Reproduced with permission from Starzl et al[37].)

pain, nausea, vomiting, and diarrhea may also occur. Pulmonary edema can occur in patients who are fluid overloaded. Acute respiratory symptoms ("anaphylactoid reactions") or anaphylaxis, manifested by joint pains, shortness of breath, and hypotension, may occur and require stopping the drug and administering epinephrine, steroids, and oxygen.

Therapy is usually continued for 10 to 14 days. Patients may develop antibodies to the mouse protein with subsequent loss of efficacy.

Post-Transplant Hepatitis

Infection is responsible for much of the morbidity and mortality after liver transplantation, and it can be difficult to distinguish rejection from postoperative viral hepatitis. Cytomegalovirus (CMV) infection of the liver is the most common troublesome offender.[12] It is diagnosed by serologic changes and/or isolation of the virus. Liver biopsy may show the typical inclusion bodies in the hepatocytes, but biopsy material should always be cultured.

CMV infection may be primary, as established by seroconversion, or be a result of reactivation of prior infection, as documented by a fourfold or greater rise in antibody titer. Many CMV infections are self-limited if immunosuppression is managed with restraint. Steroid maintenance should be reduced and cyclosporine levels kept as low as possible.

Hepatitis B virus, adenovirus, and herpes virus are other less common offenders. Hepatitis B is also often self-limited and managed by reduced immunosuppressive therapy. Herpes and adenovirus graft hepatitis have a poorer prognosis, and early retransplantation may offer the best chance of survival for patients with these infections.

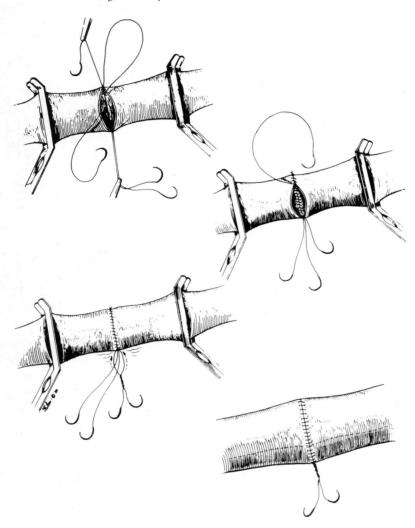

FIGURE 35-18. *(1) Intraluminal technique for sewing the back wall of the vena cava and portal vein. The hepatic artery cannot be sewn from inside but, instead, is sewn from the outside and then rotated 180° to complete the anastomosis. (2) The mate of one end suture is used to construct the other half of the circumference. (3) The two ends are tied together away from the vessel wall. The adjacent stay suture is then tied flush with the vessel wall to prevent separation. (4) Expansion and bulging of the suture line are evident as the extra polypropylene suture is taken up. (Reproduced with permission from Starzl et al[35].)*

Technical Complications

Surgical mortality (death within 30 days of operation) has significantly declined since 1980 and is currently less than 10% (Fig. 35-20). Technical complications are still responsible for a significant portion of the morbidity and mortality after liver transplantation. Our first 393 transplantations in 313 cyclosporine-treated patients were recently reviewed by Lerut and colleagues.[18] Of 393 transplantations, there were technical complications in 87 (22.1%), with 24 directly related deaths, including 52 biliary tract complications (13.2%) responsible for 5 deaths and 27 hepatic artery thromboses (6.8%) responsible for 16 deaths.

Direct duct-to-duct biliary reconstruction over a T-tube or Roux-en-Y choledochojejunostomy over

an internal stent was successful in 305 of 334 (91.3%) grafts. Failures of duct-to-duct reconstruction are best managed by conversion to Roux-en-Y choledochojejunostomy.

Hepatic arterial thrombosis is the most common technical complication requiring retransplantation and accounts for nearly 40% of the retransplantations in children (Fig. 35-21). It is the most common indication for retransplantation in children younger than 2 years of age. Despite this, survival of children younger than 2 years of age has been no different than that of older children (Fig. 35-4B).

Fever with gram-negative septicemia is almost pathognomonic of hepatic artery thrombosis, and the clinical presentation generally follows one of three patterns: acute hepatic gangrene, delayed biliary fistula, or relapsing bacteremia.[46] The ischemic

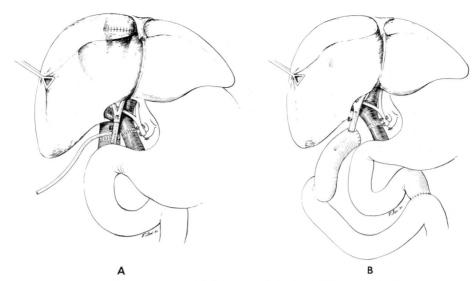

FIGURE 35-19. (A) Direct duct to duct (choledochocholedochostomy) biliary reconstruction over a T-tube that is brought out through a stab incision in the recipient bile duct contralateral to the nearby portal vein and hepatic artery anastomoses. (B) Choledochojejunostomy performed over an internal polyethelene feeding tube stent using an 18-inch Roux-en-Y limb of proximal jejunum. (Reproduced with permission from Starzl et al[38].)

injury to the biliary tree often results in intrahepatic abscess formation or biliary fistula. Doppler ultrasound studies are useful in assessing the patency of the hepatic artery.[23] If pulsations are not well visualized, an arteriogram is indicated. Ultrasound or CT scans may demonstrate abscesses in the hepatic parenchyma. A few patients, mostly small children, have survived hepatic artery thrombosis without retransplantation, but, for most patients, replacement of the graft is eventually, if not urgently, required.

RETRANSPLANTATION

Of our first 500 cyclosporine-treated patients, 147 (22.7%) have required retransplantation for allograft rejection (53.1%), technical complications (27.9%), or primary graft failure (19.0%); (Fig. 35-21). Fortunately, survival after retransplantation has also improved. Patient survival after retransplantation for loss of a first transplant, regardless of cause, is 46.4% at 1 year; for loss of a second graft, patient survival is 53.4% at 1 year (Fig. 35-22A).

For patients retransplanted for loss of a first graft to rejection, 1-year survival is 59.5%, and, for technical failures (mostly hepatic artery thrombosis), it is 43.1% (Fig. 35-22B). Primary nonfunction is a devastating complication, since the patient is in acute hepatic failure, is often septic, and is in urgent

need of another liver. One-year survival after retransplantation for primary failure of a first transplant is only 27.4% (Fig. 35-22B).

CONCLUSION

In the past 5 years, liver transplantation has been accepted as the treatment of choice for most causes of end-stage liver failure in children and adults. Many major commercial and Blue Cross medical

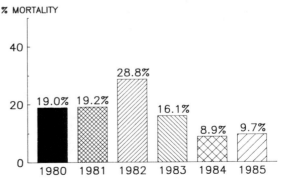

FIGURE 35-20. Surgical (30-day) patient mortality after orthotopic liver transplantation by calendar year in the Denver–Pittsburgh series.

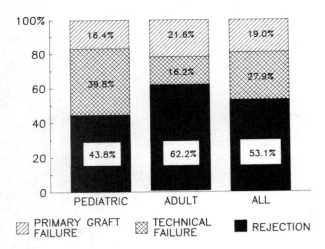

FIGURE 35-21.   *The indications for retransplanttion in 203 pediatric and 297 adult recipients of orthotopic liver allografts treated with cyclosporine and low-dose steroids.*

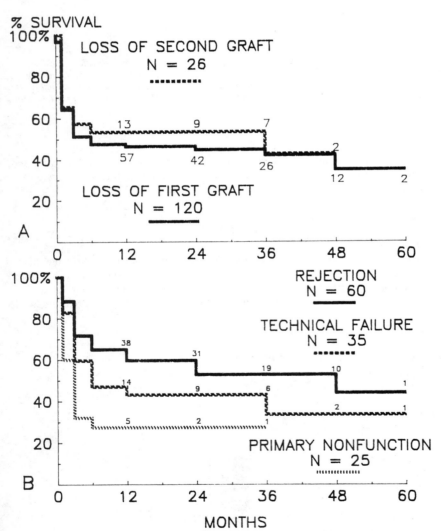

FIGURE 35-22.   *(A) Actuarial patient survival after retransplantation for loss of a first (120 cases) or second (26 cases) orthotopic liver allograft regardless of cause. (B) Actuarial patient survival after retransplantation for loss of a first orthotopic liver allograft to rejection (60 cases), technical failure (35 cases), or primary nonfunction (25 cases).*

insurance programs now provide coverage for this procedure. Most of the patients who survive the operation return to a relatively normal lifestyle within 1 year of operation. Although the immediate costs of the operation are considerable, averaging over $150,000 for medical costs and family expenses, the reward is also high. Death from liver failure is also expensive, and nothing is returned to society. Most of the patients who require liver transplantation are either children soon to enter or adults in the productive years of life. The worth to society of the advances in knowledge that have and will continue to accrue from programs in organ transplantation are incalculable.

Liver transplantation is often cited in critics as an example of "high-tech" medicine, which contributes to the escalation of health care costs. Luebs[20] has replied, "when the cost of health care in our society is attacked as being too high, one must ask "compared to what?" Is it too high compared with the cost of national drug and alcohol consumption? Is it too high compared with our nation's defense bill or our payment of interest on the national debt? . . . the true cost of health care, although taking a large portion of our nation's gross national product, is reasonable in a society concerned with suffering and the quality of life."

Organ transplantation depends upon public goodwill, since it is the public that provides both essential resources: money and organs. The public's enthusiastic support of organ donation and its charitable financial support of transplantation programs is a clear signal that the nation has not lost its traditional commitment to the relief of individual suffering.

REFERENCES

1. Andrews W, Iwatsukii S, Shaw BW Jr et al: Bile diversion and cyclosporine dosage (Letter to the editor). Transplantation 39:338, 1985
2. Bilheimer DW, Goldstein JL, Grundy SC et al: Liver transplantation provides low density lipoprotein receptors and lowers plasma cholesterol in a child with familial hypercholesterolemia. N Engl J Med 311:1658–1664, 1984
3. Calne RY, Rolles K, White DJG et al: Cyclosporin A initially as the only immunosuppressant in 34 patients of cadaveric organs; 32 kidneys, 2 pancreases, and 2 livers. Lancet 2:1033–1036, 1979
4. Calne RY, White DJH, Thiru S et al: Cyclosporin A in patients receiving renal allografts from cadaver donors. Lancet 2:1323–1327, 1978
5. Cannon JA: Transplant Bull 3:7, 1956
6. Cuervas-Mons V, Rimola A, Van Thiel DH et al: Does previous abdominal surgery alter the outcome of pediatric patients subjected to orthotopic liver transplantation? Gastroenterology 90:853–857, 1986
7. Demeirleau, Nourredine, Vignes et al: Tentative d'homogreffe hepatique (Attempted hepatic homograft). Mem Acad Chir (Paris) 90:177–179, 1964
8. Esquivel CO, Starzl TE: Liver transplantation for biliary atresia. In Glassman J (ed): Biliary Atresia. New York, McGraw-Hill, 1987
9. Fung JJ, Demetris AJ, Porter KA et al: Use of OKT-3 with cyclosporine and steroids for reversal of acute kidney and liver allograft rejection. Nephron 1986 (in press)
10. Gordon RD, Fung JJ, Markus B et al: The antibody crossmatch in liver transplantation. Surgery 100:705–715, 1986
11. Gordon RD, Iwatsuki S, Esquivel CO et al: Liver transplantation across ABO blood groups. Surgery 100:342–348, 1986
12. Gordon RD, Makowka L, Bronsther O et al: Complications of liver transplantation. In Organ Transplantation: Medical and Surgical Complications. New York, Marcel Dekker, 1986
13. Gordon RD, Shaw BW Jr, Iwatsuki S et al: A simplified technique for revascularization of liver homografts with a variant right hepatic artery from the superior mesenteric artery. Surg Gynecol Obstet 160:474–476, 1985
14. [Deleted]
15. Iwatsuki S, Gordon RD, Shaw BW Jr et al: Role of liver transplantation in cancer therapy. Ann Surg 202:401–407, 1985
16. Iwatsuki S, Shaw BW Jr, Starzl TE: Liver transplantation for biliary atresia. World J Surg 8(Suppl 1):51–56, 1984
17. Iwatsuki S, Starzl TE: Liver transplantation in the treatment of cancer. In (Ishak K, Okuda K (eds): Neoplasms of the Liver, 2nd ed. New York, Springer-Verlag, 1987
18. Lerut J, Gordon RD, Iwatsuki S et al: Biliary tract complications in human orthotopic liver transplantation. Transplantation 43:47–50, 1987
19. Lewis JH, Bontempo FA, Spero JA et al: Liver transplantation in a hemophiliac (Letter to the editor). N Engl J Med 312:1189, 1985
20. Leubs HW: Cost considerations. Semin Liver Dis 5:402–411, 1985
21. Moore FD, Wheeler HB, Demissianos HV et al: Experimental whole organ transplantation of the liver and of the spleen. Ann Surg 152:374–387, 1960
22. Moore FD, Birtch AG, Dagher F et al: Immunosuppression and vascular insufficiency in liver transplantation. Ann NY ACad Sci 102:729–738, 1964
23. Segel MC, Zajko AB, Bowen A III et al: Hepatic artery thrombosis after liver transplantation. The value of

non-invasive imaging as a screen after liver transplantation. Am J Roentgenol 146:137–141, 1987

24. Shaw BW Jr, Bahnson HT, Hardesty RL et al: Combined transplantation of the heart and liver. Ann Surg 202:667–672, 1985

25. Shaw BW Jr, Iwatsuki S, Starzl TE: Alternative methods of arterialization of the hepatic graft. Surg Gynecol Obstet 159:490–493, 1984

26. Shaw BW Jr, Martin DJ, Marquez JM et al: Venous bypass in clinical liver transplantation. Ann Surg 200(4):524–534, 1984

27. Shaw BW Jr, Rosenthal JT, Griffith BP et al: Early function of heart, liver, and kidney allografts following combined procurement. Transplant Proc 16(1):238–242, 1984

28. Shaw BW Jr, Wood RP, Gordon RD et al: Influence of selected patient variables and operative blood loss on six-month survival following liver transplantation. Semin Liver Dis 5:394–401, 1985

29. Starzl TE (with the assistance of Putnam, CW): Experience in Hepatic Transplantation. Philadelphia, WB Saunders, 1969

30. Starzl TE, Bilheimer DW, Bahnson HT et al: Heart–liver transplantation in a patient with familial hypercholesterolemia. Lancet 1:1382–1383, 1984

31. Starzl TE, Fung JJ: OKT-3 in treatment of allografts rejecting under cyclosporine-steroid therapy. Transplant Proc 4:937–941, 1986

32. Starzl TE, Groth CT, Brettschneider L et al: Orthotopic homotransplantation of the human liver. Ann Surg 168:392–415, 1968

33. Starzl TE, Hakala TR, Shaw BW Jr et al: A flexible procedure for multiple cadaveric organ procurement. Surg Gynecol Obstet 158:223–230, 1984

34. Starzl TE, Iwatsuki S, Esquivel CO et al: Refinements in the surgical technique of liver transplantation. Semin Liver Dis 5:349–356, 1985

35. Starzl TE, Iwatsuk S, Shaw BW Jr: A growth factor in fine vascular anastomoses. Surg Gynecol Obstet 159:164–165, 1984

36. Starzl TE, Iwatsuki S, Shaw BW Jr et al: Immunosuppression and other non-surgical factors in the improved results of liver transplantation. Semin Liver 5:334–343, 1985

37. Starzl TE, Iwatsuki S, Shaw BW Jr et al: Factors in the development of liver transplantation. Transplant Proc (Suppl 2):107–119, 1985

38. Starzl TE, Iwatsuki S, Van Thiel DH et al: Evolution of liver transplantation. Hepatology 2:614–636, 1982

39. Starzl TE, Kaupp HA, Brock DR et al: Reconsturctive problems in canine liver transplantation with special reference to the postoperative role of hepatic venous flow. Surg Gynecol Obstet 22:733–743, 1960

40. Starzl TE, Kaupp HA, Brock DR et al: Studies on the rejection of the transplanted homologous dog liver. Surg Gynecol obstet 112:135–144, 1961

41. Starzl TE, Marchioro TL, Porter, KA et al: Factors determining short- and long-term survival after orthotopic liver homotransplantation in the dog. Surgery 58:131–155, 1965

42. Starzl TE, Marchioro TL, Porter KA et al: The use of heterologous antilymphoid agents in canine renal and liver homotransplantation and in human renal homotransplantation. Surg Gynecol Obstet 124:301–318, 1967

43. Starzl TE, Marchioro TL, von Kaulla K et al: Homotransplantation of the liver in humans. Surg Gynecol Obstet 117:659–676, 1963

44. Starzl TE, Marchioro TL, Waddell WR: The reversal of rejection in human renal homografts with subsequent development of homograft tolerance. Surg Gynecol Obstet 117:385–395, 1963

45. Starzl TE, Weil R III, Iwatsuki S et al: The use of Cyclosporin A and prednisone in cadaver kidney transplantation. Surg Gynecol Obstet 151:17–26, 1980

46. Tzakis A, Gordon RD, Shaw BW Jr et al: Clinical presentation of hepatic artery thrombosis after liver transplantation in the cyclosporine era. Transplantation 40:667–71, 1985

47. Urbach AH, Gartner JC Jr, Malatack JJ et al: Linear growth following pediatric liver transplantation. Am J Dis Child (in press)

48. Venkataramanan R, Starzl TE, Yang S et al: Biliary excretion of cyclosporine in liver transplant patients. Transplant Proc 17:286–289, 1984

49. Welch CS: A note on transplantation of the whole liver in dogs. Transplant Bull 2:54, 1955

CHAPTER 36

Pancreas Transplantation

David E. R. Sutherland   Kay C. Moudry   John S. Najarian

Pancreas transplantation is performed to establish a normoglycemic state and to favorably influence the secondary complications of diabetes. For this reason, pancreas transplantation is restricted to patients whose complications are, or predictably will be, more serious than the potential side-effects of chronic immunosuppression.

The first pancreas transplantation in a human was performed in 1966. By April 1986, 830 cases have been recorded by the Pancreas Transplant Registry.

Either the whole pancreas or a segment can be transplanted. The three most commonly used techniques for management of the pancreatic duct and the exocrine secretions are polymer injection, enteric drainage, and urinary drainage. Polymer injection is safe but may lead to fibrosis of the gland. Enteric drainage is physiologic but results in bacterial contamination. Urinary drainage allows exocrine function to be monitored directly by measurement of urinary amylase activity and is being used with increasing frequency by direct anastomosis of the graft duodenum or pancreatic duct to the bladder. A decline in exocrine function may precede hyperglycemia as a manifestation of rejection, thus allowing earlier treatment to be instituted.

The highest graft and patient survival rates have been achieved in recipients immunosuppressed with a combination of cyclosporine and azathioprine. The technical failure rate with pancreas transplantation has been approximately 20%, but rejection is the major cause of graft loss. Diabetes mellitus appears to be an autoimmune disease resulting in a specific destruction of beta cells, and recurrence of disease in the graft has been described. In general, however, immunosuppression prevents this occurrence.

Pancreas transplantation clearly restores a normoglycemic, insulin-independent state. Limited information on the effect of pancreas transplantation on secondary complications of diabetes is beginning to emerge. Pancreas transplantation simultaneous with a kidney will prevent recurrence of diabetic nephropathy in the transplanted kidney. Improvement in neuropathy has also been described.

Pancreas graft and patient survival rates have been calculated for cases reported to the Pancreas Transplant Registry, and there has been a progressive improvement in results. For 565 cases during 1983 to 1986, the 1-year graft and patient survival rates were 41% and 78%, respectively. The results were also similar for the three most commonly used techniques, bladder drainage, polymer injection, and enteric drainage. Results were also similar for segmental and whole pancreas grafts, with 1-year function rates of 42% and 39%, respectively. Short preservation times were associated with better results than long preservation times. The 1-year graft survival rates for those who did not receive cyclosporine in the immediate post-transplant period, for those who received cyclosporine without azathioprine, and for those who received both cyclosporine and azathioprine were 38%, 40%, and 44%, respectively. Most of the pancreas grafts were transplanted in patients with end-stage diabetic nephropathy (ESDN), and the 1-year graft survival rates were higher in recipients with ESDN than in those without ESDN (44% vs 28% at 1 year). However, patient survival rates were higher in those without ESDN than in those with ESDN (84% vs 77% at 1 year).

Several institutions currently have 1-year graft survival rates between 50% and 70%. Pancreas transplants can be performed at this time in selected diabetic patients with reasonably high success rates. The limiting factors to widespread application is the need for generalized immunosuppressive therapy. Methods are needed to identify patients who will develop secondary complications.

SIGNIFICANCE AND NEED FOR PANCREAS TRANSPLANTATION

Pancreas transplantation is performed to provide physiologic insulin replacement therapy in Type I diabetes mellitus, a disease in which the beta cells within the islets of Langerhans are destroyed by an autoimmune process resulting from a complex interplay between genetic and unknown environmental factors.[29] The ultimate goal is to prevent secondary complications of diabetes.

Insulin is essential for carbohydrate metabolism, and a deficiency leads to hyperglycemia and other metabolic perturbations. Normal beta cells are programmed to release insulin by demand to maintain plasma glucose levels constantly within a very narrow range. Exogenous insulin, administered by standard parenteral techniques, cannot reliably prevent wide excursions in plasma glucose levels in diabetics.[82] Systems designed to administer insulin frequently or continuously, even with close monitoring plasma of glucose levels, do not mimic the precise control provided by functioning beta cells and carry the specific risk of hypoglycemia.[125] Thus, most diabetic patients are managed by exogenous insulin regimens that prevent or minimize the frequency of the extremes of either ketoacidosis or hypoglycemia.

The dysmetabolism of diabetes, as manifested by chronic or intermittent hyperglycemia, is thought to be responsible for the development of microvascular and other lesions that affect the eye, kidney, nerves, and other systems.[45,117] By 20 years after onset of the disease, more than 50% of persons with Type I diabetes mellitus are either blind, in renal failure, or have sensory or motor disturbances.[14,130] The incidence and severity of lesions is generally less in diabetic patients judged to have "good" as opposed to "poor" control of hyperglycemia. The lesions also develop in patients who become diabetic as a result of total pancreatectomy or disease processes that secondarily involve the islets.[117] Lesions similar to those observed in diabetic patients also occur in the animal models of primary and secondary diabetes.[65] The lesions in animals can be prevented, arrested, or reversed following restoration of normal metabolism by islet or pancreas transplantation.[92] Furthermore, kidneys transplanted from normal donors to diabetic rats[65] or humans[66] develop lesions of diabetic nephropathy. Conversely, such lesions in kidneys taken from diabetic donors will regress following transplantation to nondiabetic rat[65] or human[2] recipients.

The demographic features of diabetes mellitus in the United States are well described.[44,130] There are more than one million insulin-dependent Type I diabetic patients in the United States. The annual incidence of Type I diabetes mellitus is approximately 55 new cases per million population, or 12,000 new cases per year. The majority of the cases are in children, although all age groups are at risk. In the United States, diabetes mellitus is the fourth leading cause of death by disease, is the leading cause of new blindness, and is the cause of 25% of all cases of renal failure. Persons with diabetes are four to seven times more likely to require an amputation and twice as likely to die of heart disease than is the general population. Thus, there is great potential for pancreas transplantation to have a significant impact on the health maintenance of the diabetic population at large.

Data to show that pancreas transplantation favorably influences the course of secondary complications in diabetic patients are sparse. However, kidneys transplanted to diabetic recipients simultaneously with a pancreas have not developed the lesions of diabetic nephropathy[10] that would otherwise be expected in a high proportion of the grafts.[65] An improvement in diabetic neuropathy following pancreas transplantation has also been reported.[124] Whether or not pancreas transplants can influence existing complications is uncertain, but the results of animal experiments suggest that this might be the case if the lesions are in an early stage.[92]

It is important to realize that pancreas transplantation, unlike heart or liver transplantation, is not an immediate lifesaving measure. The objective of pancreas transplantation is to improve the quality of life and to favorably influence the secondary complications of diabetes that would otherwise take their toll several years hence. Pancreas transplantation is akin to kidney transplantation—where if the kidney fails, the patient can resume dialysis. Rejection or other causes of pancreatic graft failure should be followed by a return to exogenous insulin therapy and resumption of a lifestyle no different than that achieved pretransplant.

HISTORY OF PANCREAS TRANSPLANTATION

The discovery that the pancreas is an organ essential for carbohydrate metabolism was made by von Mering and Minkowski,[127] who, in 1890, produced fatal diabetes in dogs by total pancreatectomy. The first transplant of a pancreas was by Hedon,[47] who, in 1892, reported that free grafting of a portion of a totally resected pancreas prevented the development of diabetes in a dog.

The impetus to pursue pancreas transplantation as a treatment for diabetes was diminished by the discovery of insulin by Banting and Best[4] in 1922. Insulin was able to prevent the acute mortality from the metabolic derangements of diabetes and dramatically extended the life span of diabetes. Before the discovery of insulin, the secondary complications of diabetes were rarely seen, because most patients at risk did not live sufficiently long for their development. After the discovery of insulin, the secondary complications of diabetes became the major cause of diabetic morbidity and mortality.[117] The inability to achieve perfect metabolic control by exogenous insulin made prevention of complications difficult, and major efforts were focused on treatment of secondary complications, culminating with the application of kidney transplants for treatment of diabetic nephropathy[72] and laser procedures for treatment of diabetic retinopathy.[54] Such treatments, however, did not solve the basic problem, the dysmetabolism of diabetes experimental pancreas transplantation continued.[92]

The first successful transplants of immediately vascularized pancreatic grafts were made in dogs by Gayet and Guillaumie,[36] in 1927 and Houssay[51] in 1929. Brooks and Gifford[12] in the 1950s, DeJode and Howard[24] in the early 1960s, and Lillehei and colleagues[61] and Largarider and associates[58] from the mid 1960s to the early 1970s worked out the techniques of pancreas transplantation in large animal models that led to the first clinical attempts at pancreas transplantation and that formed the basis of current pancreas transplant research.[31,92]

The first pancreas transplant in a human was performed by Kelly and Lillehei and associates at the University of Minnesota on December 17, 1966.[53] A cadaver donor segmental (body and tail) pancreas graft, based on a vascular pedicle of the splenic artery in continuity with the celiac axis and the splenic vein in continuity with the portal vein, was transplanted to the iliac fossa of an uremic diabetic woman, and the duct of the graft was ligated. A kidney was transplanted to the opposite iliac fossa. The patient became normoglycemic and insulin-independent immediately, but she died 2 months post-transplant from a combination of rejection and sepsis. Lillehei and associates[60,61] then went on to perform a series of 13 pancreas transplants between the end of 1966 and 1973. Only one of the pancreas grafts functioned for more than 1 year.[103]

Lillehei and co-workers[61] had originally reasoned that for kidney transplants to succeed in uremic diabetic patients, the diabetic condition would have to be corrected. However, Najarian and associates,[72] in the early 1970s, showed that kidney transplantation could be performed with a success rate nearly as high in diabetic as in nondiabetic recipients. Thus, the rationale to perform pancreas transplants solely to promote kidney graft function became untenable, and kidney transplantation alone became the treatment of choice in diabetic patients.

A few other groups also performed pancreas transplants in the 1960s and early 1970s, but only a few patients survived with long-term graft function.[39] Gliedman and associates[38,39] popularized the segmental pancreas transplant technique that had been used by Kelly and Lillehei in their first case but advocated exocrine drainage into a hollow viscus, either the ureter or bowel.[39]

Of the cases done in the late 1960s and early 1970s, approximately half were whole pancreas or pancreaticoduodenal grafts and half were segmental grafts; the success rate was relatively low. The American College of Surgeons/National Institutes of Health (ACS/NIH) maintained an organ transplant registry until 1977 and received information on 57 pancreas transplants.[37] The 1-year pancreas graft function rate was only 3%, and 1-year patient survival rate was only 40% in these pioneering cases.[93]

The incentive to perform pancreas transplants was low during these years, and, in the 1970s, a surge of interest developed in islet transplantation following the report by Ballinger and Lacy[3] that islets isolated from the rat pancreas could be transplanted as free grafts to ameliorate streptozocin-induced diabetes. The development of islet isolation techniques in rodents, followed by their adaptation in large animals, led many investigators to believe that islet transplantation would supercede pancreas transplantation for clinical application.[92] However, trials of islet transplantation at the University of Minnesota in the mid- and late 1970s met with limited success (no recipients became insulin independent),[73,112,113] and a more recent trial at Washington University at St. Louis had a similar disappointing outcome.[81] Isolation of a sufficient quantity of islets from the human pancreas has been most difficult, and it remains an area of active investigation.[40]

The perception that development of islet transplantation into a clinical reality would take many years led to the resumption of pancreas transplantation at the University of Minnesota in 1978.[106] Other institutions began programs,[15,19,27,40,85,89] and, since 1978, a near doubling of pancreas transplant activity has occurred every other year (Fig. 36-1). The increase in the number of transplants has been justified as the results of pancreas transplantation have improved.

The history of clinical pancreas transplantation largely revolves around development and application of various surgical techniques for grafting. The

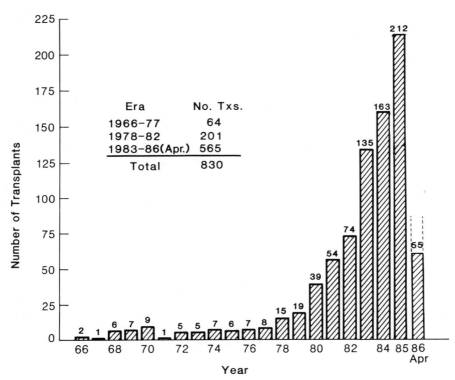

FIGURE 36-1.   *Number of pancreas transplants, by year, reported to the Registry between December 1966 and April 1986.*

first pancreas transplant was segmental with duct ligation.[53] Lillehei and colleagues[60,61] however, favored the whole pancreas transplant technique with anastomosis of the graft duodenum or a button of the papilla of Vater to the recipient bowel. Gliedman and associates[38] introduced the novel technique of anastomosis of the duct of a segmental pancreas graft to the recipient ureter in uremic diabetic patients. A modification for urinary drainage was made by Sollinger and associates[85] in which the pancreatic duct of segmental grafts or a portion of the duodenum of whole pancreas grafts was anastomosed directly to the recipient bladder.[80] Groth and colleagues[42] applied segmental pancreas transplants with anastomosis to a Roux-en-Y limb of recipient bowel in the early 1970s; this group has continued to use this basic technique with certain refinements into the 1980s.[41] In 1978, Dubernard and co-workers[27] reported on a new method of pancreas transplantation in which the duct was injected with a synthetic polymer. This technique completely avoided bacterial contamination, was safe, was soon adapted by several institutions, and has been used for more pancreas transplants than any other technique. However, even this technique is not free of complications, and fibrosis may be induced in the graft by duct injection.[9,83] A return to the original method of Lillehei and associates,[61] in which a whole pancreas transplant was used with anastomosis of the graft duodenum to the recipient bowel was resurrected in the 1980s.[90] Today, the three most popular techniques for management of the graft pancreatic duct are polymer injection, enteric drainage, and bladder drainage, all of which have relative merits and all of which can succeed.

PANCREAS RECIPIENT SELECTION AND CRITERIA FOR PANCREAS TRANSPLANTATION

Since generalized immunosuppression is necessary to prevent rejection, pancreas transplantation has been restricted to patients whose secondary complications of diabetes are, or predictably eventually would be, more serious than the potential side-effects of antirejection therapy. Ideally, pancreas transplantation should be performed before the secondary complications of diabetes are manifest. However, because of uncertainty as to which diabetic patients are prone to develop secondary complications, almost all pancreas transplants have been performed in patients who already manifest diabetic nephropathy, retinopathy, or neuropathy. Because of the uncertainty of the effects of the immunosuppression necessary to prevent rejection on these complications, most pancreas transplants have been performed in diabetic patients with end-stage diabetic nephropathy (ESDN) who are either undergoing or have had a kidney transplant and in whom immunosuppressive therapy is obligatory. As a result of such a selection process, most pancreas transplant patients have had such advanced complications that reversal or stabilization of the lesions may not be possible.

Nevertheless, nonuremic patients who do not need kidney transplants should also be considered as candidates for pancreas transplantation, particularly those with preproliferative retinopathy, who are at great risk for loss of vision,[54] or those with albuminuria, a marker of diabetic nephropathy that is otherwise inevitably progressive.[126] The largest series of pancreas transplants in non-uremic, non–kidney transplant patients is at the University of Minnesota.[95,108] The criteria for surgery in such patients is given in Table 36-1. In general, such patients have serum creatinine levels less than 2 mg/dl and have normal or nearly normal vision but with a preproliferative diabetic retinopathy.

All patients considered for pancreas transplantation should undergo an evaluation that includes the tests listed in Table 36-2. The tests are repeated at yearly or biyearly intervals after pancreas transplantation to document the degree of graft function and to assess the impact of transplantation on the course of secondary complications. A most important part of the evaluation is that of the cardiovascular system, since significant coronary artery disease may be present without angina in diabetic recipients with neuropathy. A relatively high incidence of myocardial infarctions has been reported in some series of pancreas transplants.[18] Thus, stress electrocardiograms or thallium stress tests are performed, and patients with abnormalities undergo coronary arteriograms followed by pre-pancreas transplantation angioplasty or coronary artery bypass surgery if significant and correctable lesions are detected.

Because of the side-effects of immunosuppression, pancreas transplantation has been almost exclusively limited to adult recipients over the age of 18 years and usually to those in the 20- to 40-year age group. When immunosuppressive regimen with

TABLE 36-1 Criteria for Pancreas Transplant Patients at the University of Minnesota

1. At least some evidence of secondary complications (e.g., preproliferative or background retinopathy, albuminuria).
2. Progressive complications, but not so far advanced as to be in a self-perpetuating stage independent of the metabolic state.
3. Complications that predictably are, or will be, more serious than potential side-effects of chronic immunosuppression.
4. Imperfect metabolic control on exogenous insulin.
5. Ability to pay.

TABLE 36-2 Pre- and Post-Pancreas Transplant Evaluation at the University of Minnesota

24-hour metabolic profile
Glucose tolerance tests
Urine and serum C-peptide
Stimulation with islet hormone secretogogues
Insulin withdrawal (if no history of ketosis)
Glycosylated Hb and islet cell antibodies
Neurologic evaluation
   Clinical exam, nerve conduction, autonomic tests, and quantitation of sensory loss
Opthalmologic evaluation
   Visual acuity, retinal photography, fluorescein angiography
Renal evaluation
   Serum creatinine, creatinine clearance, glomerular filtration rate, renal blood flow, sieving curve, fractional protein clearance, provocative urinary albumin excretion, kidney biopsy
Cardiovascular evaluation
   Stress EKG or thallium stress test, coronary arteriogram if stress test positive or history of angina or myocardial infarct
Camptodactyly (soft tissue) and joint evaluation
   Clinical exam, goniometry, hand prints, tracking, skin collagen quantitation
Psychiatric evaluation

fewer side-effects become available, the criteria for pancreas transplantation could be liberalized and younger patients at an earlier stage of their disease may be accepted.

Whether pancreas transplants should be performed simultaneously with or after a kidney transplant has been extensively debated.[94] Most groups prefer to perform simultaneous pancreas and kidney transplants from the same donor, since such an approach allows monitoring of the kidney for rejection, leading to earlier diagnosis and treatment of pancreas graft rejection.[28] In addition, such an approach subjects the recipient to only one operative procedure. On the other hand, if complications with the pancreas transplant occur, the complications may be more likely to lead to loss of a kidney than if a pancreas transplant occurs after a kidney transplant is well established. At this time, the most prudent course would appear to be to perform simultaneous kidney and pancreas transplants when logistically feasible. If only a kidney is available, a solitary kidney transplant with the option of later adding a pancreas is preferable to no transplants at all for a diabetic patient on dialysis.

A major consideration of recipient selection at this time is financial. Unlike kidney transplants, pancreas transplants have not been covered by Medicare or other government programs. At the University of Minnesota Hospital, the average cost of the pancreas transplant is $35,000. Patients undergoing pancreas transplantation must have insurance coverage for the procedure or pay out of pocket. At least 20 insurance companies have indicated that they will pay for pancreas transplants. Potential recipients can be admitted for a pretransplant evaluation, and the findings during the evaluation are often sufficient to convince the patient's insurance company that it will be cost-effective to pay for a pancreas transplant, which may halt the progression of secondary complications that would ultimately be even more expensive to treat.

PANCREAS DONOR SELECTION

Cadaver Pancreas Donors

Virtually any brain-dead cadaver that is suitable for use as a kidney donor is suitable for use as a pancreas donor provided that there is no history of diabetes. In addition, brain-dead cadavers that may not be acceptable as kidney donors (e.g., those with a history of benign kidney disease) may be suitable as a donor for the pancreas and other organs.

Brain-dead cadavers are often hyperglycemic owing to the administration of steroids and intravenous infusion of large amounts of dextrose-containing solutions. Such donors also often exhibit a resistance to insulin and require high doses to restore normoglycemia. Nevertheless, grafts taken from hyperglycemic cadaver donors have functioned perfectly in recipients.[49]

Hyperamylasemia is also often present in brain-dead cadavers and is usually not associated with any apparent pancreatic injury. Hyperamylasemia is a known consequence of isolated brain trauma.[49] Normal function in the recipient without the occur-

rence of pancreatitis in grafts taken from hyperamylasemic donors has been documented.[49] Thus, the only contraindication to the use of a brain-dead cadaver as a pancreas donor is a history of diabetes, intra-abdominal trauma with bacterial contamination, direct injury to the pancreas, or abnormalities of the pancreas on gross inspection.

Whole- or segmental pancreas grafts can be obtained from virtually every cadaver donor, regardless of what other organs are also procured. One should never forego obtaining a liver from a donor simply to use the pancreas; removal of both organs from the same donor is technically feasible.[96]

Related Pancreas Donors

The same rationale for use of related donors for kidney transplants also applies to use of related donors for segmental pancreas transplants.[109] A portion of the body and tail of the pancreas can be removed from a living donor, based on a vascular pedicle of the splenic vessels.[97] The spleen of the donor can survive on collateral circulation,[107] and the remainder of the body, head, the uncinate process of the pancreas is sufficient to maintain normoglycemia in the donor.[108]

Most pancreas transplants from living-related donors have been performed at the University of Minnesota. Criteria that prospective living-related donors must meet before being evaluated are listed in Table 36-3.[5]

Prospective donors undergo oral and intravenous glucose tolerance tests.[30] All glucose values

TABLE 36-3 *Criteria for Selection of Living-Related Pancreas Donors*

A. *Pre-evaluation Criteria**
   1. Recipient and donor discordant for diabetes for at least 10 years.
   2. Donor at least 10 years older than age of onset of diabetes in recipient.
   3. In cases of sibling donation, no family members other than the proband are diabetic.
B. *Post-evaluation Criteria*
   1. Normal oral glucose tolerance test (OGTT) result by criteria of Fajans and Conn and of the Natural Diabetes Data Study Group.
   2. Delta insulin > 90 µU/ml for sum of 0-, 60-, 120-, and 180-minute values during cortisone-stimulated OGTT minus sum during standard OGTT according to technique of Fajans and Conn.
   3. No islet cell antibodies.
   4. Other metabolic parameters normal (see text).

* When these demographic features pertain, donor is not statistically at higher risk to become diabetic than the general population (Barbosa J et al: Clin Invest 60:489, 1977)

during standard oral glucose tolerance tests (OGTT) must be within an arbitrarily defined normal range (fasting < 105 mg/dl, 60-minute value ≤ 185 mg/dl, 90-minute value ≤ 160 mg/dl, and 120-minute value ≤ 140 mg/dl).

An analysis of the initial related donors showed that if the serum insulin values at 0, 1, 2, and 3 hours during the preoperative cortisone-stimulated glucose tolerance test were 90 microunits greater than the sum of the values during standard glucose tolerance tests (delta insulin), almost all the donors had normal glucose tolerance tests postoperatively.[108] Thus, the criteria have now been refined so that for a person to be accepted as a donor, the delta insulin must be greater than 90 microunits (Table 36-3). A more recent unpublished analysis has shown that if the peak serum insulin values during the intravenous glucose tolerance test are greater than 100 μU/ml, the donor will also have a normal OGTT postdonation. This test could be used in lieu of the cortisone stimulation test. The mean glucose values during standard glucose tolerance tests have been 10 mg/dl to 15 mg/dl higher postoperatively than preoperatively.[109] The longest follow-up of the donor has been 6 years; the donor's glucose tolerance test results have remained normal during the entire follow-up period, with no further deviation from the base line obtained in the immediate postoperative period. The changes in glucose tolerance test results after hemipancreatectomy are of similar magnitude to those seen in creatinine clearance after uninephrectomy from a living-related kidney donation, and long-term follow-up with kidney donors has shown that deterioration does not occur.[129] Similar studies are ongoing in our pancreas donors.[110] The risk of developing diabetes in the living-related pancreas donor is small, with one occurrence of Type II diabetes in 54 donors at the University of Minnesota (< 2%). The incidence has been 0% in those with a preoperative delta insulin greater than 90 microunits.

Complications of surgery, including (1) the need for splenectomy (n = 2), (2) postoperative development of intraperitoneal sterile fluid collections (n = 3), and (3) one reoperation to religate the distal duct, have occurred in 10% of the donors. The complication rate in living-related pancreas donors has been similar to that in living-related kidney donors.[109,129]

Living-related donor pancreas grafts have a decreased propensity to be rejected.[108,109] For technically successful transplants, the functional survival rate was 73% for pancreas allografts from living-related donors and 32% from those of cadaveric donors.[105] In another subgroup, those receiving a pancreas graft from a related donor of a previous kidney, the 1-year functional survival rate has been 100% for technically successful grafts, and no rejections have been seen in this situation.[108] Although most pancreas transplants will be from cadaver donors, the option of using related donors should be considered when family members are highly motivated. This option is particularly attractive when the recipient has a high percentage of HLA antibodies (PRA) but has a negative crossmatch against a living relative.

TECHNIQUE OF PANCREAS DONOR OPERATION

The entire pancreas (whole pancreas with or without the duodenum) or the tail and body alone (segmental graft) can be transplanted. For transplants from living-related donors, the segmental technique is obligatory, whereas in cadaver donors, either whole-pancreas or segmental grafts can be procured. For a cadaver donor from whom the liver is also obtained, procurement of a segmental graft is simpler than procurement of the whole-pancreas graft, because the head of the pancreas and the liver are supplied with vessels that have a common origin. However, with appropriate vascular reconstructive techniques, an equitable division of the blood supply to the liver and pancreas can be made so that the whole pancreas and liver can be procured. However, many groups still prefer to transplant segmental grafts; thus, both operations, segmental and whole organ pancreatectomy, are described.

Segmental Pancreas Donation

The pertinent anatomy of a segmental pancreas transplant donor is shown in Figure 36-2. The arterial blood supply to the tail and most of the body of the pancreas is derived from the splenic artery, which has its origin from the celiac axis. The dorsal and transverse pancreatic arteries ramify with the branches of the superior mesenteric artery through the neck of the pancreas, but, occasionally, the origin of these branches is directly from the superior mesenteric artery, which, if unrecognized, can lead to devascularization of the tail of the pancreas during hemipancreatectomy for segmental transplantation.

The venous drainage of the tail and most of body of the pancreas is the splenic vein, which discharges into the portal vein. The narrowest portion of the pancreas is overlying the portal vein. It is in this area where a plane between the dorsal surface

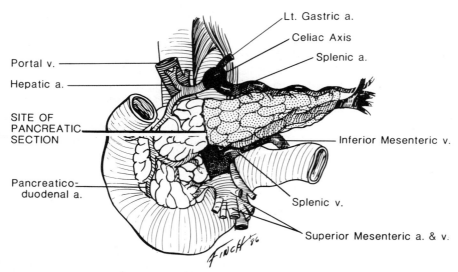

FIGURE 36-2.   *Pertinent pancreatic anatomy in segmental graft donor. The pancreas is transected at its neck where it crosses the ventral through the portal vein. The blood supply to the pancreatic tail is from the splenic artery off the celiac axis.*

of the pancreas and the portal vein is developed and where the pancreas can be transected. The length of vessels that can be obtained depends upon whether the segmental graft is procured from a cadaver or a related donor, and, in the case of a cadaver donor, whether or not a liver is also procured.

Segmental Pancreatectomy Without Liver Procurement

In non-liver donors, the proximal splenic artery does not have to be dissected. Rather, the celiac artery is identified, the left gastric and hepatic arteries are ligated and divided at their origin, and the splenic artery alone remains in continuity with the celiac. Likewise, the termination of the splenic vein into the portal vein does not have to be isolated. Tributaries to the portal vein, including the coronary vein and the short vessels from the pancreatic head, are ligated, as is the superior mesenteric vein, leaving the portal vein in continuity from its junction with the splenic vein to the hilum of the liver. The distal pancreas is now completely free except for the vascular pedicle (Fig. 36-3). The final maneuvers for removal from the donor include detachment of the celiac axis encompassed within a Carrel patch of the aorta and transection of the portal vein in the hilum of the liver (Fig. 36-4). A segmental pancreas graft can be removed either before or after the heart and kidneys or after removal of the heart and simultaneously with removal of the kidneys en bloc following in situ perfusion.

Segmental Pancreatectomy With Procurement of the Liver From the Donor

When the liver is also procured from a segmental pancreas graft donor, the celiac axis is usually retained in continuity with the donor hepatic artery so that it is available for arterial anastomosis in the liver recipient. In this situation, the pancreas has to be removed, with only the donor splenic artery available for arterial anastomosis in the pancreas recipient. Thus, the splenic artery has to be isolated and divided at its origin from the celiac axis. Likewise, when a liver is procured, the usual practice is to leave the portal vein intact and in continuity with the liver. The splenic vein is isolated at its termination in the portal vein where it is transected. If the pancreas segment is procured with a vascular pedicle consisting solely of the splenic artery and vein, it can be removed prior to the other organs and without any jeopardy whatsoever to the liver. An isolated pancreatic segment following removal from a cadaver liver donor is similar to the segment shown in Figure 36-4, except that only the splenic artery and vein remain with the graft.

Related Donor Segmental Pancreatectomy

The technique for excision of the body and tail of the pancreas from a living donor is similar to that described for segmental pancreatectomy in a cadaver donor in which the liver is also procured (Fig. 36-5A) and is well illustrated elsewhere.[97] In living

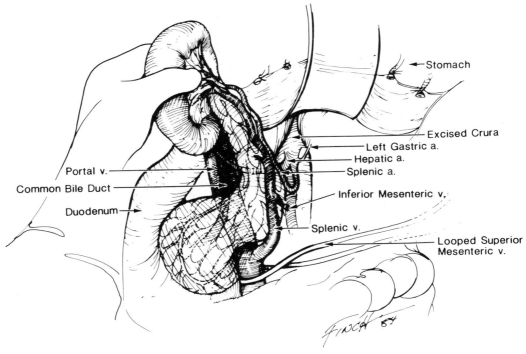

FIGURE 36-3. *Mobilization of tail of pancreas from a cadaveric donor. The short gastric and gastroepiploic vessels and inferior mesenteric vein are divided, following which the pancreatic tail can be lifted from its bed to the level of the superior mesenteric vessels.*

donors, the superior mesenteric and portal vein remain intact and the splenic vein stump is oversewn. The splenic artery and vein are ligated and divided near the hilum of the spleen, with preservation of the collateral circulation to the spleen from the short gastric and left gastroepiploic vessels. The pancreas is divided over the portal vein. The splenic artery is isolated at its origin from the celiac axis and the splenic vein at its termination into the portal vein. The stumps of the splenic vessels are oversewn on

the donor, as is the pancreatic duct and the cut surface of the proximal pancreas. Fifty percent of the pancreas remains in the recipient, a quantity sufficient to maintain a normoglycemic state.[109]

Other Considerations in Segmental Pancreatectomy

With living-related hemipancreas donation, a functioning spleen should be retained in the donor. However, for cadaver segmental pancreas transplan-

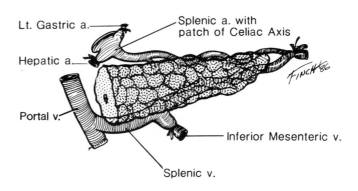

FIGURE 36-4. *Pancreatic segment following removal from a non–liver donor in which the splenic vessels are maintained in continuity with the celiac artery and portal vein.*

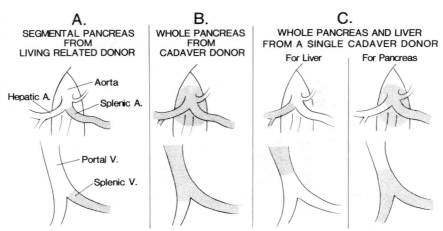

A.
SEGMENTAL PANCREAS FROM LIVING RELATED DONOR

B.
WHOLE PANCREAS FROM CADAVER DONOR

C.
WHOLE PANCREAS AND LIVER FROM A SINGLE CADAVER DONOR
For Liver   For Pancreas

Aorta
Hepatic A.   Splenic A.

Portal V.
Splenic V.

FIGURE 36-5.   *Options for management of the blood vessels to the pancreas. (A) With a seg-mental pancreas graft from either a living-related or a cadaveric liver donor, the splentic artery and splenic vein only are retained with the pancras graft. (B) If a liver is not procured from a cadaveric donor, all collateral vessels to the pancreas can be retained and a patch of aorta encom-passing the celiac and superior mesenteric arteries procured along with the entire portal vein. (C) When a whole pancreas and liver are both procured from a cadaveric donor, the hepatic artery and portal vein must be retained with the liver. If only the hepatic artery is used for anastomoses in the liver recipient, the splenic artery is used for anastomoses in the liver recipient, the splenic artery can be retained in continuity with the celiac artery, and a Carrel patch to include the latter as well as the superior mesenteric artery can be fashioned; alternatively, the celiac artery can be retained in continuity with the hepatic artery for the liver, and the splenic artery and superior mesenteric artery with the pancreas. In either event, the short portal vein segment retained with the pancreas is lengthened with an iliac vein extension graft.*

tation, the spleen can be included with the graft.[55,86] The rationale for its inclusion is to increase the blood flow in the splenic vessels and thus decrease the probability of vascular thrombosis. Inclusion of the spleen carries the risk of graft-versus-host disease[22,23]; thus, most groups no longer include the spleen with the pancreas.

Another maneuver to increase the flow rate in the splenic vessels is the creation of a distal fistula between the graft splenic artery and vein.[16] How-ever, the incidence of thrombosis has not been dif-ferent from segmental transplants with or without atrioventricular (A-V) fistulae.[96]

Whole-Pancreas or Pancreaticoduodenal Procurement from Cadaver Donors

Whole-pancreas transplantation from cadaver donors is preferred in the United States,[19,70,87,90,98,101,111] although segmental pan-creas transplants are used by most European cen-ters.[11,13,26,57,123] Whole-pancreas grafts have a higher blood flow, which may reduce the propensity for thrombosis, present more options for drainage of the exocrine secretions, and provide an islet mass that is normal and approximately double that of

segmental grafts. Some of these considerations are largely theoretical, since the islet mass of a segmen-tal graft is sufficient to maintain normoglycemia.[108] The thrombosis and graft survival rate for segmental and whole-organ grafts has been similar.[114]

Procurement of the whole pancreas is no more complicated than procurement of a segmental graft in a cadaver donor from whom a liver is not ob-tained. Whole-pancreas grafts can be procured with the duodenum either left intact, or trimmed to a patch encompassing the papillae of the ducts of San-torini and Wirsung, or with the duodenum com-pletely separated from the pancreas.

Procurement of a whole pancreas includes the basic maneuvers described for mobilization of the tail and body of the pancreas as depicted in Figure 36-3 except that the neck of the pancreas does not have to be isolated. In addition, the duodenum and head of the pancreas are mobilized to the ligament of Treitz. The ligament is also divided from the left side so that the jejunum and duodenum are freed in continuity posterior to the course of the proximal superior mesenteric artery.

The other maneuvers required for whole-pan-creas donation can be performed in a variety of sequences, depending upon the organs to be removed and the particular anatomy encountered. It is expeditious to completely abolish the lesser sac by division of the hepato-, duodeno-, gastro-, and splenocolic ligaments along with ligation and division of the gastroepiploic vessels and the midcolic vessels inferior to the pancreas. These maneuvers allow the entire transverse colon, including the hepatic and splenic flexures to be reflected into the pelvis. Whole-pancreas grafts can be procured from cadavers who are donors of any organ, but the maneuvers to isolate the vascular supply will differ depending upon whether or not a liver is procured (see Fig. 36-5).

Whole-Organ Pancreatectomy Without Liver Procurement

If a liver is not procured, the pancreas and duodenum can be removed with the entire blood supply to the pancreas left intact, including the splenic and heptic-gastroduodenal-superior-pancreaticoduodenal arcade off the celias axis and the transverse pancreatic and inferior pancreaticoduodenal arcade off the superior mesenteric artery, as well as the corresponding pancreatic veins that drain into the portal vein (Fig. 36-6). The portal lymphatic vessels, common hepatic artery, and bile duct are divided and ligated in the liver hilum; the only structure remaining intact in the portal hepatis is the portal vein. The celiax axis and superior mesenteric artery are isolated at their origins from the aorta.

At this point, the pancreas is tethered only by its vascular supply, the duodenum, and the small bowel mesentery, including the superior mesenteric vessels inferior to the pancreas. If the pancreas is procured with the entire duodenum, it is now ready for excision. It can also be excised at this point even if the intent is to transplant the pancreas with only a patch or without the duodenum, provided that the pancreaticoduodenal separation is performed ex vivo after flushing and cooling. Alternatively, this separation may be carried out in situ as previously described.

Any other organs to be transplanted should also be mobilized and prepared for removal. The superior mesenteric artery and vein and encompassing lym-

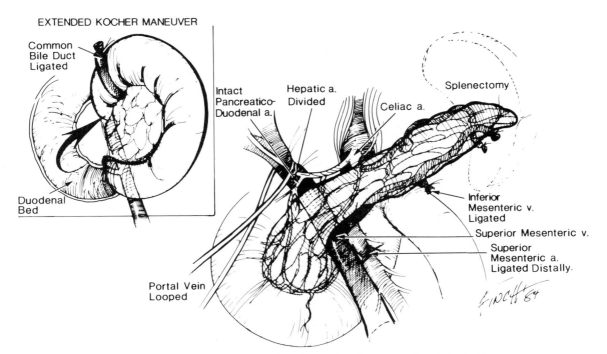

FIGURE 36-6. *Whole pancreas procurement in the non–liver donor. The entire pancreas is mobilized with division of the ligament of Treitz via an extended Kocher maneuver. The entire blood supply to the pancreas remains intact, including the hepatic-superior pancreaticoduodenal arterial arcade. In a liver donor, the gastroduodenal artery is ligated and divided, and the superior pancreaticoduodenal artery is fed by the inferior pancreaticoduodenal artery, so the entire length of the common and proper hepatic arteries can remain with the liver.*

phatic vessels in the small bowel mesentery are ligated and divided caudad to the duodenum and distal to the origin of the inferior pancreaticoduodenal vessels. If desired, the distal aorta is cannulated for in situ flushing of the kidney and pancreas with cold organ preservation solution. Alternatively, the organs can be rapidly excised and flushed ex vivo. In either event, the kidneys are excised with the aorta and vena cava, taking care to divide the aorta just below the origin of the superior mesenteric artery and above the origin of the right and left renal arteries. The aorta is also divided proximal to the origin of the celiac axis, so a Carrel patch encompassing the celiac and mesenteric arteries can be fashioned ex vivo. The portal vein is also divided, and the pancreas graft is removed. The sequence of the maneuvers depends in part upon several considerations, such as how much duodenum is retained with the graft and whether a heart is also considered. For example, when a heart is procured, if the suprahepatic portion of the vena cava is clamped, it is necessary to either transect the portal vein or drain the inferior vena cava to prevent venous congestion within the pancreas. Pertinent considerations as to how much duodenum is retained with the pancreas graft follow.

1. *Whole-pancreas procurement with retention of a duodenal segment (pancreaticoduodenal graft).* During the dissection, the duodenal lumen should be irrigated with antimicrobial solution through a nasogastric tube. When a pancreaticoduodenal graft is procured (Fig. 36-7), no further dissection between the pancreas and duodenum other than that previously described as necessary. Using a gastrointestinal stapling device, the proximal and distal portions of the duodenum are divided, leaving that portion of the duodenum most intimate with the pancreas attached to the graft. Early division of the prox-

imal duodenum facilitates the dissection within the portahepatis. Following excision of the graft, a lateral duodenotomy can be made to empty the duodenum of its contents and to instill cold preservation solution.

2. *Retention of a duodenal patch only with a whole-pancreas graft.* If a whole-pancreas graft with a duodenal patch encompassing the papilla of Vater and the duct of Santorini is procured, the small branches of the pancreaticoduodenal vascular arcade to the duodenum are meticulously isolated and ligated, while the branches to the pancreas are preserved. This dissection can be performed in situ or ex vivo after pancreaticoduodenectomy as previously described. Following separation of the majority of the duodenum and pancreas, the duodenum is excised leaving only a patch encompassing the papilla of Vater and the duct of Santorini, as illustrated elsewhere.[96,98] With careful dissection, the blood supply to the head of the pancreas and the duodenal patch will remain completely intact.

3. *Whole-pancreas procurement without the duodenum.* Procurement of the whole pancreas without the duodenum is generally done only if the duct injection technique is used. In this situation, the dissection separating the pancreas and the duodenum includes not only the vessels to the duodenum but also the pancreatic ducts, as illustrated elsewhere.[96,98] The pancreas and duodenum can be separated ex vivo following excision of the pancreas and duodenum as previously described, but there are advantages to performing the dissection in situ. The duodenum does not have to be divided, thus eliminating the possibility of enteric bacterial contamination, and in situ dissection also allows certain identification and ligation of the duodenal branches from the pancreatic duodenal vascular arcade.

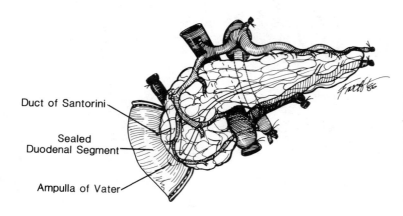

Duct of Santorini

Sealed
Duodenal Segment

Ampulla of Vater

FIGURE 36-7. *Isolated pancreaticoduodenal grafts from a cadaveric donor. The first portion of the duodenum has been stapled distal to the pylorus but proximal to the entry of the duct of Santorini, and the second portion of the duodenum has been stapled and divided distal to the ampulla of Vater at a point where the duodenum is easily separable from the pancreas.*

Whole-Organ Pancreatectomy with Procurement of the Liver from the Donor

The main technical considerations when both the whole pancreas and liver are removed from a multiorgan cadaver donor is preservation of the arterial blood supply to both organs and preservation of an adequate length of portal vein with the liver. If only the donor common hepatic artery is used for the arterial anastomosis of the liver graft, a full arterial blood supply to the pancreas can be retained. However, usually the entire hepatic artery (common hepatic and hepatic proper in continuity) are needed for the liver; thus, the gastroduodenal artery (which in turn gives rise to the superior pancreaticoduodenal artery) must be ligated and divided at its origin from the hepatic artery. This can be done, because the superior pancreaticoduodenal artery is in continuity with the inferior pancreaticoduodenal artery; the latter has its origin from the superior mesenteric artery, and the latter is retained with the pancreatic graft. It is possible to retain the celiac axis with the pancreatic segment if the hepatic artery

proper itself is used for vascular anastomosis in the liver recipient. However, it is also usually desirable to retain the celiac axis with the liver, and, in this situation, the splenic artery must be divided at its origin from the celiac axis. The splenic artery and superior mesenteric artery can then either be anastomosed to the recipient iliac vessels separately, or, as has been practiced at the University of Minnesota, the splenic artery can be anastomosed to the graft superior mesenteric artery, allowing a single anastomosis of a patch of aorta encompassing the graft superior mesenteric artery in the recipient.[96]

When the liver is procured, the portal vein is divided just proximal to the termination of the splenic vein into the portal vein. A segment of donor iliac vein is then procured and anastomosed ex vivo to the portal vein stump of the pancreas graft. In this way, a sufficiently long venous conduit from the graft is available for anastomosis in the recipient. The specific maneuvers necessary for procurement of both a whole pancreas and liver graft from a cadaver donor are illustrated in Figure 36-8.

It is best to adapt a flexible policy (as has been

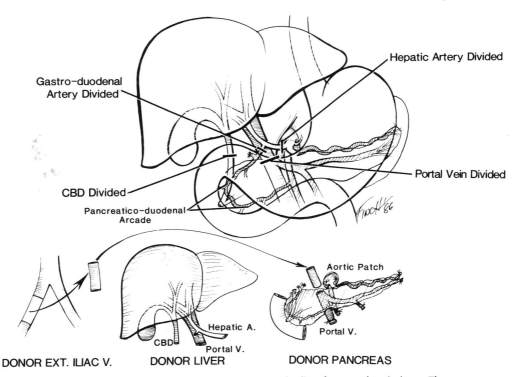

FIGURE 36-8. *Maneuvers for removal of a whole pancreas and a liver from a cadaveric donor. The gastro-duodenal artery must be divided so the common and proper hepatic arteries can remain in continuity and be retained with the liver. The portal vein is divided just superior to the entrance of the splenic vein, and then the pancreatic portion is lengthened by an iliac vein graft. The celiac and superior mesenteric arteries can remain with the pancreas to be encompassed by a Carrel patch, or the celiac artery can remain with the liver and the donor splenic artery anastomosed directly to the superior mesenteric artery feeding the pancreas.*

advocated by Starzl and colleagues[90] for multiple organ donor procurement in general), making allowances for anatomical variations that may be encountered during the procurement procedure. For example, if the right hepatic artery originates from the superior mesenteric artery, procurement of the whole pancreas can either be abandoned and a segment can be procured, or some other provision can be made. In most instances, however, it should be possible to procure all organs from all donors.

Preservation of the Pancreas

Most groups have preserved pancreas grafts by cold storage in the intracellular electrolyte solution used for kidney preservation and make an effort to transplant the pancreas within 6 hours of procurement. The failure rate is higher with longer than with shorter storage times (see later section on results).

Solutions superior to the intracellular electrolyte solutions for organ preservation have been developed.[32] A silica gel filtered (SGF) plasma solution made hyperosmolar by addition of glucose and hyperkalemic by addition of potassium chloride was uniformly successful in preserving canine pancreas grafts for 48 hours in experiments by Florack and associates.[33] A non–plasma-based colloid solution containing hydroxyethyl starch and raffinose as the osmotic agent was shown by Wahlberg and coworkers[128] to preserve canine pancreas for up to 72 hours. Equally good results were obtained by Heise and associates[48] when SGF was made hyperosmolar by mannitol rather than by glucose.

Modified hyperosmolar silica gel–filtered plasma solutions have been used for cold storage of

human pancreases with adequate function of pancreas grafts stored for 12 to 24 hours.[1] Of 20 grafts stored for 6 to 12 hours, 19 functioned, as did 18 of 19 stored for 12 to 24 hours, for a primary nonfunction rate of only 5%. The composition of the solution used for pancreas preservation at the University of Minnesota is given in Table 36-4. After removal of the human pancreas from the donor, the arteries to the graft are flushed at a low pressure with a volume of preservation solution just sufficient to clear the venous effluent (50 ml–100 ml). The pancreas is then immersed in the same solution (approximately 400 ml) and stored at 4°C until the time of transplantation.

TECHNIQUE OF PANCREAS RECIPIENT OPERATION

A variety of techniques have been used for both segmental and whole-organ pancreas transplantation. The most important variations revolve around the methods for management of the pancreatic duct and the exocrine secretions. Duct drainage can be external or into the peritoneal cavity, but usually a hollow viscus is used. The graft can be placed solely in the retroperitoneum or placed intraperitoneally to take advantage of the capacity of the peritoneum to absorb peripancreatic secretions.

Segmental Pancreas Transplantation

Revascularization of Segmental Pancreas Transplants

Most segmental pancreas transplants have been revascularized using the iliac vessels of the recipient for anastomosis to the celiac (or splenic) artery and portal (or splenic) vein of the graft. If no kidneys are transplanted, the right iliac vessels are generally used; if a kidney has been transplanted, the side opposite the kidney is usually used.

A procured cadaveric segmental graft in which the celiac axis and portal vein are retained with the pancreas is easily revascularized by end-to-side anastomoses to the common iliac vessels of the recipient, as illustrated in Figure 36-9. In recipients of segmental grafts from living-related donors, or from cadaver donors, in which the celiac axis and portal vein remain in the donor or were retained with the donor liver, the recipient hypogastric artery can be used for end-to-end anastomosis to the short proximal splenic artery of the graft, as illustrated elsewhere.[96,99]

Other options for revascularization of segmen-

TABLE 36-4 Pancreas Preservation Solution Used at the University of Minnesota

INGREDIENTS AND ADDITIVES	CONCENTRATION/ LITER
Silica gel–filtered plasma (SGF) (base solution)	45 g protein* (17 g albumin)
Human albumin	47 g*
Mannitol	7.5 g
Sodium	135 mmol
Potassium	40 mmol
Magnesium	4 mmol
Phosphate	122 mg
Calcium	60 mg
Chloride	99 mmol
Ampicillin	500 mg
Solu-medrol	500 mg
Osmolarity	410 mOsm

* Total protein concentration is 92 g/liter, and final albumin concentration is 64 g/liter.

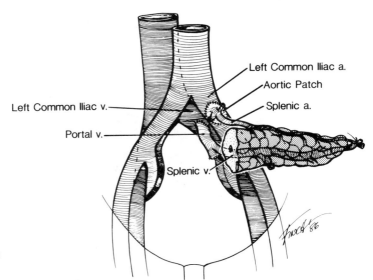

Left Common Iliac v.

Portal v.

Splenic v.

Left Common Iliac a.

Aortic Patch

Splenic a.

FIGURE 36-9. *Technique for revascularization in the recipient of a segmental pancreatic graft from a cadaveric non–liver donor. The celiac axis (on a Carrel patch) and portal vein of the graft are anastomosed to the iliac vessels of the recipient.*

tal grafts include end-to-side anastomosis of the graft splenic vessels to the splenic vessels of the recipient, as described by Calne,[13] or end-to-end anastomosis of the graft splenic artery and vein to the inferior mesenteric artery and vein of the recipient (Fig. 36-10).[102] These alternative methods drain the graft venous effluent into the portal circulation of the recipient, but a metabolic advantage of such an arrangement has not been shown.

Duct Management Techniques for Segmental Pancreas Grafts

Several methods have been used for management of the duct and exocrine secretions of segmental grafts, including duct ligation,[53] duct injection with synthetic polymers,[27] anastomosis to recipient bowel,[41] and anastomosis to the urinary system of the recipient.[38,85] Free drainage into the peritoneal cavity[106] and duct ligation have largely been abandoned but duct injection or anastomosis to the recipient's bowel or urinary system are in common use.

Duct-Injection With Synthetic Polymers. Segmental pancreas transplantation with injection of a synthetic polymer into the pancreatic duct has been used for more clinical cases than any other technique (Fig. 36-10). A variety of polymers hae been used, including neoprene,[11,26] prolamine,[57] polyisoprene,[67] cyanoacrylate,[119] and silicone rubber.[104] No differences in graft survival rates can specifically be attributed to the type of polymer used.[114] The polymers suppress endocrine function, probably by

direct toxic effects on the acinar cells, and block residual secretions.

Fibrosis in the graft is produced by polymer injection.[9,83] Whether or not fibrosis leads to islet dysfunction is uncertain, and injected grafts have functioned normally for several years.[75,108]

Some groups have delayed injection of the pancreatic duct until several weeks after transplantation.[8,91] With this method, the catheter is left in the duct and is brought externally through the abdominal wall. Approximately 3 weeks after transplantation, the polymer is injected into the gland and the catheter is withdrawn.

Enteric Drainage of Segmental Grafts. *Intestinal Drainage.* Drainage into the small intestine is the most physiologic of all the pancreas transplant duct management techniques and is the second most commonly used technique. A Roux-en-Y limb of recipient small intestine is created. Following revascularization of the pancreas graft, direct anastomosis of the pancreatic duct on the cut surface of the pancreas can be made to the intestinal mucosa. More commonly, however, the cut surface of the pancreas is intussuscepted into the end of the Roux-en-Y limb (Fig. 36-11). The duct is stented with a catheter, which is secured with an absorbable suture. Eventually, the suture holding the catheter will dissolve, and the catheter will pass through the intestine. An alternative,[40] is to bring the catheter through the intestine and the abdominal wall, facilitating diversion and allowing external collection of the pancreatic graft secretions in the catheter (Fig.

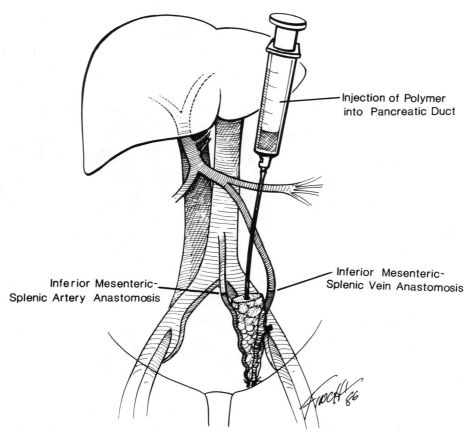

Injection of Polymer
into Pancreatic Duct

Inferior Mesenteric-
Splenic Artery Anastomosis

Inferior Mesenteric-
Splenic Vein Anastomosis

FIGURE 36-10.   *Injection of a synthetic polymer into the duct of a segmental pancreas graft following revascularization. Approximately 4 ml to 6 ml of the polymer is injected, followed by ligation of the duct. In this particular case, revascularization was to the recipient inferior mesenteric vessels.*

36-11). This technique also allows for direct monitoring of the graft exocrine function.[120] The external catheter is removed, usually at 3 to 4 weeks posttransplant.

Gastric Drainage.   Calne[13] devised a method for drainage of the graft excretion secretions directly into the stomach following placement of a segmental graft in a paratopic position with end-to-side anastomosis of the graft vessels to the splenic artery and vein of the recipient as illustrated elsewhere.[96] The number of cases performed with gastric drainage is small, but the outcome has been similar to that of intestinal-drained segmental pancreas grafts.[114,122]

Urinary Drainage of Segmental Pancreas Graft Secretions.   The main advantage of the urinary drainage technique is the provision of a direct

method for measurement of exocrine function. A decrease in urinary amylase secretion may precede a rise in plasma glucose secondary to a rejection episode, leading to earlier diagnosis and treatment.[76]

Pancreticoductoureterostomy.   A drawback to this method is the need for a nephrectomy, making it inapplicable to patients other than those with end-stage renal failure. The complication rate with this technique has been relatively high; it has essentially been abandoned.

Segmental Pancreaticocystostomy.   The exocrine secretions of segmental grafts can be drained directly into the bladder.[85] Although most groups using the bladder drainage methods now transplant whole-pancreas grafts,[74,76] a few groups have persisted in combining segmental transplantation with bladder drainage.[114] During revascularization, the graft is

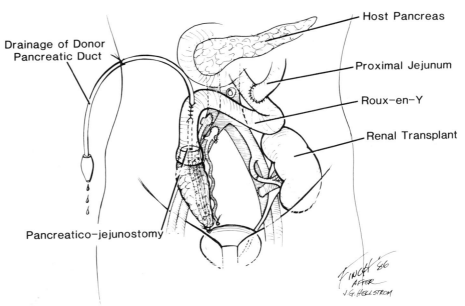

Host Pancreas

Proximal Jejunum

Roux-en-Y

Renal Transplant

Drainage of Donor
Pancreatic Duct

Pancreatico-jejunostomy

FIGURE 36-11. *Enteric drainage of a segmental pancreas graft to a roux-en-Y limb of the recipient jejunum. Temporary external drainage of the pancreatic secretions to the catheter brought to the roux-en-Y loop and the abdominal wall is illustrated, as practiced by the Stockholm group.*

oriented such that the neck of the pancreas is projected directly toward the bladder. A direct mucosal-to-mucosal anastomosis of the graft duct to the bladder can be made over a stent. Alternatively, the cut surface of the pancreas can be intussuscepted into the bladder as a pancreaticocystostomy. The success rate with segmental and whole-organ grafts has been approximately equal.[114]

Whole-Pancreas or Pancreaticoduodenal Transplantation

Whole pancreas transplantation can be performed with either a suprainguinal, retroperitoneal approach or through a midline intraperitoneal incision. Even if the retroperitoneal approach is used, following revascularization, the peritoneum is usually opened to facilitate the absorption of perigraft secretion. The orientation of the whole-pancreas graft depends upon the method for management of the pancreatic duct and the exocrine secretions. For example, with enteric drainage, the head of the pancreas and the duodenum can project transversely or cephalad. If the bladder drainage techniqe is used, the graft is oriented so that the head and duodenum project caudad, directly into the pelvis and bladder. The same basic techniques for management of the

duct exocrine secretions are used for both whole-pancreas and segmental pancreas transplantation.

Revascularization of Whole-Organ Grafts

The revascularization technique is similar for whole-organ grafts whether or not the duodenum or portion thereof is included with the pancreas. The graft portal vein (or in the case of pancreas grafts obtained from liver donors, a donor iliac vein extension graft conduit) is anastomosed end-to-side to the recipient iliac vein or vena cava. A Carrel patch of graft donor aorta encompassing both the celiac axis and superior mesenteric arteries or, in cases in which the graft has been obtained from a liver donor in whom the celiac axis was retained with the liver, encompassing only the superior mesenteric artery to which the donor splenic artery has been joined, is anastomosed end-to-side to the recipient common or external iliac artery. These anastomoses are facilitated by full mobilization of the recipient iliac vessels, including ligation and division of the hypogastric veins. If the left iliac vessels are used, with an intraperitoneal approach, the vessels can be isolated in their proximal portion medial to the sigmoid colon, thus facilitating complete intraperitoneal placement of the graft and avoiding entrapment of perigraft pancreatic secretions within the retroperitoneum lateral and posterior to the sigmoid colon.

The initial maneuvers for revascularization of whole-pancreas grafts are illustrated elsewhere.[96,99]

Techniques for Management of the Exocrine Secretions of Pancreas or Pancreaticoduodenal Grafts

The basic methods described for management of the exocrine secretions of segmental grafts are applicable for whole-pancreas grafts. Again, simple ligation or open duct intraperitoneal drainage have largely been abandoned, but duct injection, enteric drainage, and urinary drainage continue to be used, with the latter becoming increasingly popular.

Whole-Pancreas Transplantation With Duct Injection. Following revascularization of a whole pancreas graft, the papilla of Vater or the duct of Wirsung is directly cannulated, injected with 6 ml to 10 ml of the desired polymer, and ligated as illustrated elsewhere.[96,99] The duct of Santorini can also be injected separately, but, unless there is pancreatic division, this maneuver is probably unnecessary, and the duct of Santorini can simply be ligated. If the ligation of the duct of Santorini is deferred until the duct of Wirsung has been injected, the confluence of the two ducts can be ascertained, because the polymer will enter the proximal duct of Santo-

rini by retrograde flow from the duct of Wirsung and will egress at the minor papilla.

Enteric Drainage of Pancreaticoduodenal Grafts or Whole-Pancreas Grafts with a Duodenal Patch. Enteric drainage of whole-pancreaticoduodenal transplants can be accomplished by side-to-side anastomosis of the graft duodenum to the recipient bowel. The anastomosis can be made directly to an intact loop of the recipient intestine.[19,90] Alternatively, the duodenum can be anastomosed side-to-side to a Roux-en-Y limb of recipient jejunum, as illustrated in Figure 36-12. If only a duodenal patch is used, anastomosis to a Roux-en-Y limb can also be accomplished by direct anastomosis of the duodenal patch to a small enterotomy on the side of the distal limb of the Roux, as illustrated in the insert in Figure 36-12.

Urinary Drainage of Pancreaticoduodenal Grafts or Whole-Pancreas Grafts with a Duodenal Patch. _Ureteral Drainage of Whole-Pancreas Grafts._ Two approaches have been used for ureteral drainage of whole-pancreas grafts: a flank approach, and intraperitoneal approach. The recipient's ureter is divided (sacrificing the kidney) on the side of the transplant, and an anastomosis is carried out directly between a small patch of duodenum encom-

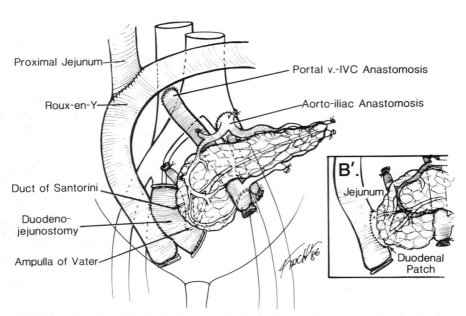

FIGURE 36-12. _Enteric drainage of a pancreaticoduodenal or whole-pancreas graft with a duodenal patch (insert). The side-to-side anastomosis is made between the graft duodenum and the roux-en-Y limb of the recipient jejunum. Alternatively, a patch of graft duodenum is anastomosed to the recipient bowel._

passing the papilla of Vater and the ureter or kidney pelvis. Only a few whole-pancreas transplants with ureteral drainage have been performed, and the graft survival rate has been statisticaly significantly lower with the ureteral than with the bladder drainage technique.[114]

Bladder Drainage of Pancreatioduodenal or Whole-Pancreas Grafts With a Duodenal Patch.   Bladder drainage of pancreaticoduodenal or whole-pancreas grafts with a patch of duodenum has become the most popular technique for pancreas transplantation in the United States. The technique as originally described by Solinger and colleagues[85,87,88] entails two incisions in the bladder with anastomosis of a patch of duodenum encompassing the papilla of Vater and the duct of Santorini to the posterior wall of the bladder through anterior cystotomy (Fig. 36-13). More recently, the duodenocytostomy has been made directly without a counter incision.[87]

A variation on the bladder drainage technique is to transplant a whole pancreaticoduodenal graft with side-to-side anastomosis of the duodenum to the bladder.[74] With this technique, the side of the duodenum is anatomosed directly to the posterior wall of the dome of the bladder, using a two-layer anastomotic technique (Fig. 36-14). There have been no leaks in a series of 20 consecutive transplants by this method at the University of Minnesota.[110] If pancreas transplant is performed simultaneously with a kidney, an extra vesicle ureteroneocystostomy is also easily accomplished following completion of the duodenal system (Fig. 36-14). The duodenum in essence constitutes a bladder diverticulum, but there has been no apparent increased incidence of urinary tract infection or other problems with this technique, and it appears to have been adopted by most transplant groups using bladder drainage in the United States.

PATIENT MANAGEMENT OF PANCREAS TRANSPLANT RECIPIENTS

Except in cases in which there is pancreatic exocrine insufficiency, the sole purpose of pancreas transplantation is to provide beta cells. Thus, 98% of the graft consists of accessory or unnecessary tissue, the exocrine pancreas, a potential source of complications that are not seen with transplants of other organs. On the other hand, the immunosuppression necessary to prevent rejection is similar to that of other organs, but monitoring for rejection is based on functional parameters peculiar to the pancreas.

General Postoperative Management of Pancreas Transplant Recipients

In part, the postoperative management of pancreas transplant recipients depends upon the technique

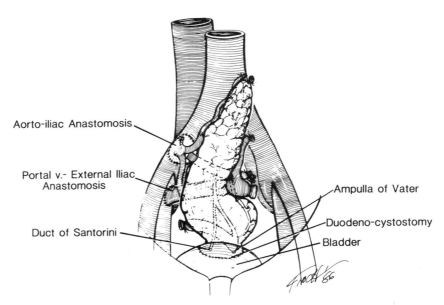

Aorto-iliac Anastomosis

Portal v.- External Iliac Anastomosis

Duct of Santorini

Ampulla of Vater

Duodeno-cystostomy

Bladder

FIGURE 36-13.   *Whole-pancreas transplantation with bladder drainge. A duodenal patch encompassing the duct of Santorini and ampulla of Vater is anastomosed directly to the dome of the bladder.*

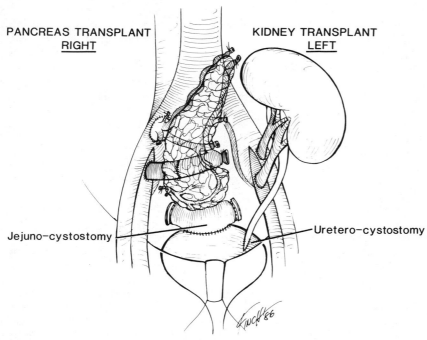

PANCREAS TRANSPLANT
RIGHT

KIDNEY TRANSPLANT
LEFT

Jejuno–cystostomy

Uretero–cystostomy

FIGURE 36-14.   *Pancreaticoduodenal transplantation with bladder drainage. A side-to-side anastomosis of the duodenal segment is made to the dome of the bladder. If a kidney is also transplanted, a ureteral neocystostomy can be accomplished at the site away from the duodeno-cystostomy. In this particular example, the whole-pancreas graft was obtained from a liver donor.*

used for duct management; specific recommendations have been made by the various groups practicing one or another of the specific techniques, such as duct injection,[25,27] enteric drainage,[121] or urinary drainage.[71,74,76,87]

When transplants are placed intraperitoneally, patients are treated with nasogastric suction and intravenous fluids during the first few postoperative days until bowel function returns. Feeding is a stimulus to pancreatic exocrine secretion, but once normal bowel function has been established, oral alimentation can be initiated. While the patients are on intravenous fluids, plasma glucose levels may fluctuate, and insulin is administered to maintain plasma glucose levels less than 150 mg/dl. The drawback to using insulin during this period is the inability to accurately monitor graft endocrine function. Our practice is to administer insulin in the early post-transplant period, because chronic hyperglycemia is detrimental to islet cells.[125] Once oral alimentation is initiated, however, no insulin is given unless there is loss of graft function.

Sollinger and co-workers,[87] using the duodenal patch technique, recommended leaving the Foley catheter in place for at least 2 weeks. However,

using the whole-pancreaticoduodenal technique with a segment of duodenum attached to the graft and a side-to-side duodenocystostomy, we have removed the catheters at 4 to 7 days postoperatively without any anastomotic leaks in 20 consecutive cases.[110]

Because of the propensity for vascular thrombosis in pancreas transplants (12%), many transplant groups anticoagulate the recipients.[19,121] Our approach is to administer low–molecular weight dextran (Rheomacrodex), 20 ml/hr intravenously, until the patients can take oral medication. The patients than receive dipyridamole and aspirin, and the Rheomacrodex is discontinued.

Immunosuppression in Pancreas Transplant Recipients

In the precyclosporine era the basic regimen was azathioprine and prednisone with or without use of an antilymphocyte globulin (ALG) preparation.[104] Cyclosporine was first used in pancreas transplant recipients by Calne and White,[15] and this drug is now used by almost all groups performing pancreas transplants.[114] Some groups give azathioprine and

TABLE 36-5 *Current Immunosuppressive Protocol for Non-Uremic, Non–Kidney Transplant Recipients of Pancreas Grafts at the University of Minnesota*

CYCLOSPORINE

Preoperative oral dose of 14 mg/kg

Immediate postoperative continuous intravenous infusion of 0.125 mg/kg/hr, adjusted to keep blood level approximately 300 ng/ml and serum creatinine concentration ≤ 150% of preoperative concentration

Convert to oral cyclosporine when enteral alimentation begins (usually 2–7 days post-transplant) at a dose of 8 mg/kg/day in divided doses (b.i.d.), adjusted to keep whole-blood levels at approximately 200 ng/ml

AZATHIOPRINE

5 mg/kg/day tapered to 2.5 mg/kg/day by 1 week and adjusted to maintain white blood count > 4000 cells/min[3]

PREDNISONE

1 mg/kg/day tapered to 0.5 mg/kg/day by 1 month, to 0.25 mg/kg/day by 6 months, and to 0.15 mg/kg/day by 1 year

ANTILYMPHOBLAST GLOBULIN (MINNESOTA ALG)

20 mg/kg/day intravenously for seven doses beginning at the end of the first post-transplant week

prednisone initially and either add cyclosporine later[121] or substitute cyclosporine for azathioprine.[19] Our own approach has been to give all three drugs (cyclosporine, azathioprine, and prednisone) initially and continually as long as the recipient has a functioning graft[105] (Table 36-5). Administration of ALG is delayed to reduce the risk of infection in the immediate postoperative period from any enteric bacterial contamination that may have occurred at the time of transplantation. The immunosuppressive protocol was designed for the highly immunocompetent non-uremic patients without renal allografts.[105] For recipients of simultaneous pancreas and renal grafts, cyclosporine is not given until the renal graft is functioning. Recipients of pancreas grafts from a related donor of a previous kidney as simply maintained on their current immunosuppressive regimens.[109]

Rejection episodes are treated by a temporary increase in prednisone or with anti-OKT3 monoclonal antibody or with ALG. An increase in prednisone as well as administration of ALG or anti-OKT3 may be used, depending upon the severity of the rejection episodes. Administration of OKT3 or ALG alone has the advantage of avoiding a further increase in plasma glucose from steroids. A flexible policy toward treatment of rejection episodes, depending upon individual circumstances of the recipient, should be used.[110]

Biochemical Monitoring of Pancreas Graft Function

The most important parameter to monitor in a pancreas transplant recipient is plasma glucose levels. A functioning graft will maintain plasma glucose levels less than 200 mg/dl in the absence of exogenous insulin, and usually plasma glucose levels are entirely within the normal range. In the immediate post-transplant period, high–plasma glucose levels or the need for exogenous insulin may signal graft thrombosis. If an insulin-independent state is established, an increase in plasma glucose levels above base line levels may indicate a decrease in loss of graft function from rejection or thrombosis. In some patients, steroids or other drugs such as thiazides or beta-blockers, may result in mild increases in plasma glucose levels, mimicking rejection.

Base line plasma glucose levels should be established in all patients by performing a metabolic profile prior to discharge from the hospital. The patients then monitor plasma glucose levels at home using commercially available glucometers.

Whether hyperglycemia is a consequence of total or of partial loss of graft function can be distinguished by measurement of serum C-peptide levels. C-peptide rather than insulin is measured because most recipients have circulating antibodies to insulin for at least the first 2 months after transplant owing to a prior immune response to heterologous insulin injection. In addition, if hyperglycemia occurs, insulin may be administered.

Serum amylase levels are usually elevated in the immediate post-transplant period but eventually return to normal. A precipitous decline may indicate deterioration of graft function. On the other hand, a precipitous rise followed by an immediate drop may also be an indication of rejection. If such is the case, a rise in plasma glucose would soon follow. Changes in serum amylase levels are difficult to interpret.

In recipients of a kidney transplant from the same donor as the pancreas, serum creatinine levels are important to monitor for possible renal allograft rejection. A rise in serum creatinine level as a manifestation of rejection will, in general, occur before a rise in plasma glucose as a manifestation of pancreas rejection.[34] Thus, in recipients of both a kidney and a pancreas graft from the same donor, rejection of the pancreas can be treated earlier in its course than in recipients of pancreas graft alone.

In patients in whom the pancreas graft exocrine secretions have been drained into the urinary system, the exocrine function of the graft can be monitored by measurement of urine amylase levels.[76,87] A decrease in urine amylase activity will precede a rise in plasma glucose levels during a rejection episode.[77] With a fully functioning graft, urinary amylase activity will generally range between 10,000 and 100,000 units per liter. Because urine amylase concentration will vary according to urine volume, urine amylase activity per hour is measured by performing time collections. With a fully functioning graft, urine amylase activity usually ranges between 1,000 and 8,000 units/hour. A base line is established on each patient, and, generally, the day-to-day variation is no more than 25%. A decline of urine amylase activity of more than 25% is suggestive of rejection, and a decline of 50% is virtually diagnostic. With severe rejection, urinary amylase activity will fall to less than 1,000 units/hour and with loss of function to pretransplant levels (< 100 units/hr). After discharge from the hospital, daily monitor of urinary amylase is impractical; thus, patients are instructed in *p*H monitoring of the urine. Because of the excretion of bicarbonate from the pancreas, urine *p*H levels are generally greater than 7. A post-transplant base line is established, and a decline in *p*H to less than 7 is an indication to obtain a urinary amylase level. A decline in urine amylase activity associated with a moderate rise in plasma glucose levels should be considered rejection and should lead to treatment. Severe or advancing rejection will lead to severe hyperglycemia, and the objective should be to treat rejection before this stage is reached.

Post-Pancreas Transplant Problems and a Clinical Approach to Such Problems in Pancreas Graft Recipients

A variety of problems in addition to hyperglycemia, including fever, abdominal pain, ascites, and development of an intra-abdominal mass, can occur in pancreas transplant patients.

Hyperglycemia

An increase in plasma glucose levels signifies graft dysfunction. In the immediate post-transplant periods, hyperglycemia is usually not caused by rejection but by some technical problem. If insulin is required during the first few post-transplant days, thrombosis should be confirmed by a technetium flow study, and if no uptake is visualized, an arteriogram should be performed. A thrombosed graft should be removed.

If there is blood flow to the graft in the presence of hyperglycemia, graft dysfunction could be secondary to early rejection or to preservation injury; graft function may improve with time, and insulin can be temporarily administered.

Infection

Fever should be investigated by blood and urine cultures, and intravenous lines should be changed. Positive blood cultures usually signify an abscess unless the fever disappears after the intravenous lines are changed. Intra-abdominal abscess is also heralded by pain. Diagnostic studies conclude with sonography and computed tomography (CT) scans.[21,29,59,64] Sterile collections can be treated by aspiration alone, but, if pus is encountered or subsequent cultures grow bacteria, percutaneous drainage by itself has usually not been successful.[50] Operative drainage is the most effective treatment. Unless the infection is minor, the best treatment is graft removal and cessation of immunosuppression.

When cytomegalovirus (CMV) or other herpes infections occur, immunosuppression is reduced until the syndrome resolves. In severe cases, hyperimmune globulin can be administered. Nonviral opportunistic infections will also occur, but some may be prevented. Sulfa-containing drugs should be given indefinitely to all patients. With such prophylactic treatment, infections such as Nocardia or those caused by *Pneumocystis carinii* do not occur.

Recurrence of Disease (Diabetes) Versus Rejection in a Transplanted Pancreas

Most cases of Type I diabetes mellitus appear to be due to an autoimmune process that results in insulitis and specific destruction of beta cells.[29] Pancreas transplantation restores beta cells and can provoke a secondary immmune response to beta cell antigen independent of the rejection process. Fortunately, the immunosuppression given to prevent rejection will usually also prevent insulitis and recurrence of disease. However, a few recipients of related donor pancreas transplants who were given low-dose cyclosporine alone or no immunosuppression (identical twin donors) had recurrence of diabetes with insulitis and selective beta cell destruction on graft biopsies.[84,116] Such a process mimics rejection in that hyperglycemia occurs, although other signs of rejection are absent. Nevertheless, rejection can be manifested by hyperglycemia alone; thus, with living-related recipients on low-dose immunosuppression, a distinction might not be possible without a graft biopsy. With the immunosuppressive regimen of cyclosporine, azathioprine, and prednisone (triple therapy), recurrence of disease has not occurred, even with related donors.[110]

Pancreas Graft Biopsies

When duct management has been by polymer injection or by enteric drainage and when there is not a kidney allograft from the same donor, a diagnosis of rejection may be uncertain. Thus, some patients may require a biopsy of the graft.[100] This requires a laparotomy, but, in some patients with hyperglycemia, rejection is not seen. The most important feature of rejection is vasculitis.[83] When rejection was not seen on graft biopsy, graft dysfunction has generally resolved. In some cases, hyperglycemia was due to drug toxicity (e.g., steroids, thiazides, or beta-blockers).[43] Since converting to the urinary drainage technique, the use of biopsy has declined; however, a biopsy may still be instructive in selected cases.

RESULTS OF PANCREAS TRANSPLANTATION

Metabolic Effect of a Functioning Pancreas Transplant

A fully functioning pancreas graft establishes an insulin-independent normoglycemic state in recipients, with plasma glucose levels usually ranging between 80 mg/dl and 120 mg/dl in the fasting state and between 100 mg/dl and 180 mg/dl in the nonfasting state. OGTT and intravenous glucose tolerance test results are also usually normal or nearly normal in most patients.[108] An example of a metabolic profile in a patient with a functioning graft is illustrated in Figure 36-15. Post-transplantation, the patient is insulin-independent and consistently normoglycemic. The mean glucose values during metabolic profiles and during OGTT in 18 patients with functioning pancreas grafts studied at 1 year post-transplant show normal values.[111]

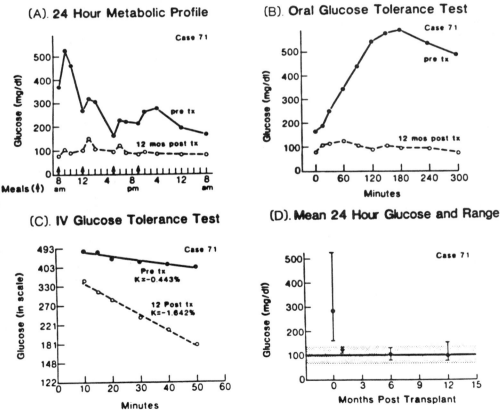

FIGURE 36-15. Results of metabolic profiles (A &D) and oral (B) and intravenous (C) glucose tolerance tests before (on insulin) and 1 year (off insulin) after a segmental pancreas transplant with enteric drainage of the pancreatic duct and systemic drainage of the graft venous effluent. Results after transplantation are entirely normal. (From Sutherland et al: Pancreas transplantation from related donors. Transplantation 38:625–633, 1984.)

Glycosolated hemaglobin levels, serum C-peptide, and urine C-peptides are also normal in pancreas transplant recipients with functioning grafts.[19,115] In general, the response of the pancreas graft to various secretagogues[75] is normal. For example, insulin response to arginine has been documented.

In the few patients in whom portal venous drainage has been established, the results of the metabolic studies have not been significantly better than in those with systemically drained grafts.[14,35,102]

Normal metabolism is sustained in pancreas transplant recipients as long as they have a functioning graft. Such a situation is virtually impossible to obtain with exogenous insulin regimens in Type I diabetic patients.[82]

Effect of Pancreas Transplantation on Secondary Complications of Diabetes

Limited information is available on the effect of pancreas transplantation on the secondary complications of diabetes. Recurrence of renal disease is not seen in renal allografts placed simultaneously with a pancreas transplant as a long as the pancreas graft functions.[10] Recurrence of diabetic nephropathy is seen in kidneys transplanted alone in diabetic recipients.[66] This observation is not surprising, because if diabetic nephropathy was seen in kidneys transplanted to recipients maintained in the normoglycemic state by a pancreas transplant, all theories as to the pathogenesis of diabetic nephropathy would have to be revised.

The light microscopic lesions of diabetic nephropathy in kidneys transplanted some years prior to a pancreas transplant have regressed following restoration of a normoglyemic state.[108] It is not known whether or not diabetic nephropathy in the native kidneys of pancreas transplant recipients regresses.

An effect of pancreas transplantation on diabetic retinopathy is also difficult to document, although an improvement in visual acuity and regression or stabilization of vascular proliferative processes in the retina have been described after combined kidney and pancreas transplants by the Munich group.[52] Most recipients of pancreas transplants have advanced retinopathy, and the disease at this point may be self-perpetuating. The incidence of progression of retinopathy has been similar during the first year after pancreas transplantation in patients with either failed or successful grafts.[78]

Subjective improvement in neuropathy is common with functioning grafts. Objective documentation of regression of neuropathy by nerve conduction tests or quantitative studies of autonomic neuropathy may have occurred in preliminary observations.[124]

The success rate of pancreas transplantation has improved, and it is anticipated that long-term observations will establish what effect pancreas transplantation has on secondary complications.

Pancreas Grafts and Patient Survival According to Pancreas Transplant Registry Data

The ACS/NIH Registry maintained an Organ Transplant Registry until June 30, 1977, and received information on 57 pancreas transplants in 55 patients.[37] In 1980, a new international Pancreas and Islet Transplant Registry was founded,[93] and the information in the ACS/NIH Registry was transferred to the new international registry. Information collected in the Registry on more than 1000 cases includes demographic data on the donor and recipient, type of transplant and method of duct management, length of preservation time, type of immunosuppression, duration of graft function, and cause of graft failure, the results of an actuarial analysis of all reported cases (Fig. 36-1) are summarized in the following sections.

Overall Results of Pancreas Transplantation Between 1966 and 1986

Between December 1966, and April 1986, 830 pancreas transplants in 775 diabetic patients, performed in 79 institutions, were reported to the Registry. Cadaver donors were the source of 778 transplants (726 primary, 48 secondary, and 4 tertiary grafts), and living-related donors were the source of 52 grafts (49 primary, 3 secondary).

Two hundred fifty-three patients had fully functioning grafts (insulin-independent) from 1 month to 7.8 years post-transplant. Twenty-three patients had partially functioning grafts (receiving small doses of insulin, but with C-peptide levels above a pretransplant base line). One hundred seventy-nine grafts have fully functioned (recipients insulin-independent) for more than 1 year, including 132 grafts in recipients who were listed as insulin-independent as of April 1986.

The overall patient survival, graft function, and insulin-independent rates for all cases are depicted in Figure 36-16. The 1-year patient survival rate was 73%, and the overall 1-year graft function (full and partial) rate was 34%. The 1-year insulin-independent rate (full graft function) was 32%). All subsequent figures and graft function will refer only

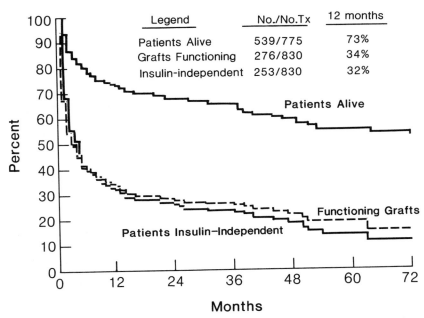

FIGURE 36-16. *Patient survival rates after primary transplantation and graft functional survival (full and partial) and insulin independent (full function) rates for all cases reported to the Registry between December 1966 and April 1986.*

to those in which the recipients were insulin independent, that is, had full function.

Of the 830 transplants, 227 (27%) failed for technical reasons. Two hundred fifty-nine technically successful grafts functioned before subsequently failing because of rejection or undetermined causes (31%). Ninety-one recipients died with functioning grafts (11%). The 250 grafts listed as having full function represent 30% of the total number of transplants.

Fifty-one patients underwent a second pancreas transplant after the first transplant failed; and four of these patients received a third transplant after a second graft failed. The functional survival rate of retransplants is 23% at 1 year, insignificantly less ($p > 0.1$) than that of primary transplant cases. Retransplantation has been safe, with a 1-year patient survival rate of 82%, as opposed to 73% for primary cases ($p > 0.1$).

An analysis of graft survival rates according to duct management techniques showed that the 1-year actuarial function rates were 47% for bladder drainage (n = 113), 33% for enteric drainage (n = 302), 32% for duct injection (n = 325), 19% for open duct intraperitoneal drainage (n = 31), 14% for ureteral drainage (n = 30), and 0% for duct ligation (n = 20). There were no statistically significant dif-

ferences in the results between the first three techniques, but the differences between the last three techniques and the first three techniques just listed were almost statistically significant ($p < 0.08$). Graft survival rates have been similar for whole (n = 227) and segmental (n = 623) pancreas transplants (33% vs 32% at 1 year).

The graft survival rate was significantly higher ($p < 0.01$) for pancreases stored less than 6 hours than those stored at least 6 hours (38% vs 30% at 1 year). This difference could be attributed to the significantly ($p < 0.05$) higher technical failure rate in those stored at least 6 hours (36%) than in those stored less than 6 hours (25%).

Graft survival rates were significantly higher ($p < 0.001$) in those who initially received cyclosporine (n = 522) than in those who did not (n = 283; 40% vs 21% at 1 year). When the analysis was restricted to only technically successful cases, the same relative differences were seen, with a 1-year actuarial graft function rate of 54% in recipients initially treated with cyclosporine (n = 383), and 29% in those who were not (n = 203). Graft survival rates in recipients who initially received cyclosporine were about the same as those in recipients who also initially received azathioprine (n = 199) and in those who did not (n = 323) (43% vs 38%). If the same analysis was performed only in recipients of technically successful grafts, however, the difference would be statistically significant (60% vs 51%).

Pancreas graft functional survival rates were significantly higher ($p < 0.001$) in those with ESDN (n = 650) than in those without ESDN (n = 180; 36% vs 21% at 1 year). Pancreas graft survival was about the same with simultaneous or prior kidney transplantation.

In patients who received a pancreas transplant after a kidney transplant, the 1-year graft survival rate was 52% for those who received the pancreas and the kidney from the same donor (n = 17), and 28% for those who received the pancreas from a different donor(n = 28), a difference that reflects the fact that all "same donors" were living relatives.

Most recipients of pancreas transplants have had ESDN, and 622 of the 770 patients in the Registry received kidney transplants (80%), either simultaneously with (n = 472) or before (n = 143) a pancreas transplant. The functional survival rate of kidneys transplanted before a pancreas (93% at 1 year) was higher than that of those transplanted simultaneously with a pancreas (57% at 1 year), simply because these patients had to survive and the kidneys had to function in order for a subsequent pancreas transplant to be performed. The Registry does not have data to determine whether or not the survival rate of kidneys transplanted with a pancreas is different than that achieved with kidney transplants alone in a similar diabetic population. However, the kidney graft functional survival rate for those transplanted simultaneously with a pancreas are similar to those reported for diabetic recipients of kidney grafts alone in an analysis of those cases reported to the UCLA Kidney Transplant Registry for the years 1978 to 1985 (53% at 1 year for 1233 cadaver cases).[118]

Results of Pancreas Transplantation by Era

The results of pancreas transplantation have progressively improved. The pancreas graft functional survival rates in the three eras, 1966 to 1977, 1978 to 1982, and 1983 to 1986, were 3%, 20%, and 41%, respectively, at 1 year (Fig. 36-17A). Patient survival rates have also improved, being 40%, 72%, and 78%, respectively (Fig. 36-17B). Current results (1983–1986) are summarized in the following subsection and represent the minimal standards for pancreas transplantation today.

Results for 1983–1986 Cases According to Multiple Variables.   Between January 1983, and April 1986, 565 pancreas transplants in 526 patients performed at 63 institutions were reported to the Registry. When analyzed (1986), 413 of the recipients (79%) were alive, and 234 patients (45%) had a fully functioning graft (insulin-independent), including 114 that were more than 1 year post-transplant. One hundred fifty-five of the grafts failed for technical reasons. Thirty-nine patients (7%) died with technically successful functioning grafts, and 136 grafts (24%) that were technically successful functioned before failing as a result of rejection or undetermined causes. The results of pancreas transplantation and a variety of subcategories are summarized in the following paragraphs.

Results of Retransplantation.   At 1 year, graft survival rates were 30% for retransplant cases and 42% for primary cases, whereas the corresponding patient survival rates for primary transplantation were 91% and 71%, respectively, statistically insignificant differences (Fig. 36-18). The results indicate that retransplantation is safe and can be performed with a success rate that is similar to that expected in primary transplantation.

Results According to Technique for Management for the Pancreatic Duct and the Exocrine Secretions.   For 1983–1986 cases, almost all pancreas transplants had been managed by either polymer injection, enteric drainage, or urinary drainage. Ureter drainage (n = 19) or bladder drainage (n = 111) was associated with a 1-year graft survival rate of 16% or 47%, respectively. In regard to enteric drainage, the stomach (n = 22) or jejunum (n = 201) were associated with similar graft survival rates ($\geq$ 40% at 1 year; Fig. 36-19). With duct injection (n = 188), the 1-year graft survival rate was 44%, and there were no differences according to the type of polymer used. Thus, the functional survival rates for graft management by the three most common techniques, bladder drainage, enteric drainage, and polymer injection do not significantly differ from one another (> 40% at 1 year in each group; Fig. 36-20A). Patient survival rates also do not differ significantly between the three major duct management categories (Fig. 36-20B).

Results of Segmental Versus Whole-Pancreas Transplants.   During 1983–1986, there were 193 whole- and 372 segmental pancreas grafts; the functional survival rates (39% vs 42% at 1 year) were similar (Fig. 36-21A). Whole- or segmental graft survival rates were not significantly different for enteric drainage and duct injection. Bladder-drained grafts had functional survival rates that were significantly higher for whole than for segmental grafts (Fig. 36-21B–D).

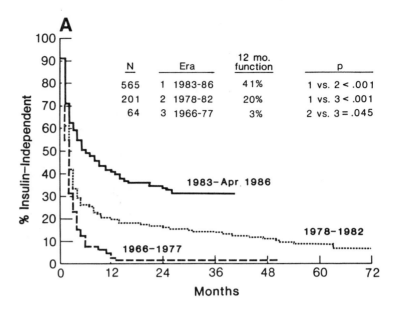

N	Era	12 mo. function	p
565	1 1983-86	41%	1 vs. 2 < .001
201	2 1978-82	20%	1 vs. 3 < .001
64	3 1966-77	3%	2 vs. 3 = .045

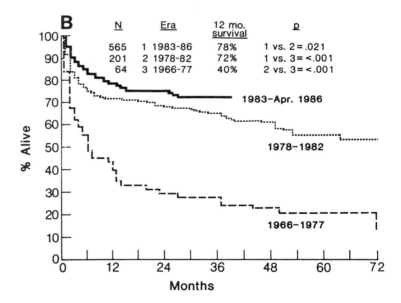

N	Era	12 mo. survival	p
565	1 1983-86	78%	1 vs. 2 = .021
201	2 1978-82	72%	1 vs. 3 = <.001
64	3 1966-77	40%	2 vs. 3 = <.001

FIGURE 36-17. *(A) Insulin independent rates and (B) patient survival rates for all pancreas transplant cases reported to the Registry by era for 1966–1977, 1978–1982, and 1983–April 1986.*

Results According to Duration of Graft Preservation. The graft survival rate was significantly higher for pancreases stored less than 6 hours than for those stored more than 6 hours (45% vs 34% at 1 year; Fig. 36-22). The difference correlated with a significantly higher ($p < 0.05$) technical failure rate (as defined by loss of graft function within the first 3 days) for grafts stored at least 6 hours (56 of 151, 37%) than for those stored less than 6 hours (82 of 346, 24%). Advances in preservation have been made,[1,33] and a recent analysis suggests that the results with longer storage times are improving.[114]

Results According to Immunosuppression Modality in the Recipients. For purposes of this Registry analysis, the various immunosuppressive regimens were classified according to the immunosuppressive drugs administered in the immediate post-transplant period and not according to the maintenance regimen. For all cases, the 1-year graft survival rate was 42% in patients initially treated with cyclosporine (n=446) and 38% in patients who did not receive cyclosporine in the immediate post-transplant period (n = 106). In recipients of technically successful grafts only, the corresponding 1-year graft survival

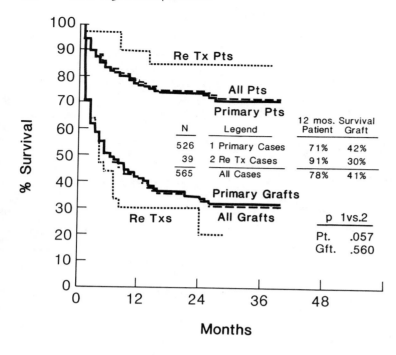

FIGURE 36-18. *Insulin independent (graft survival) and recipient (patient) survival rates for primary transplants, retransplants, and all transplant cases reported to the Registry from 1983–April 1986.*

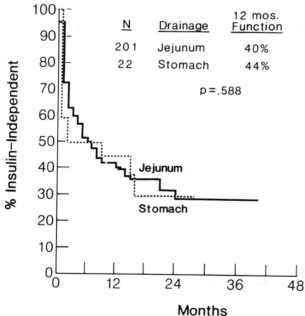

FIGURE 36-19. *Insulin independent rates for 1983–1986 pancreas transplant recipients of enteric drained grafts according to whether drainage was into the jejunum (PJ) or stomach.*

rates were 58% (n=324) and 53% (n=75) (p = 0.027).

The results were also analyzed according to whether or not the recipients received azathioprine in the immediate post-transplant period (Fig. 36-23). In an analysis of all (Fig. 36-23A) and for technically successful cases (Fig. 36-23B) the graft survival rates were slightly higher in cyclosporine-treated patients who also received azathioprine than in those who received cyclosporine without azathioprine.

The combination of cyclosporine and azathio-

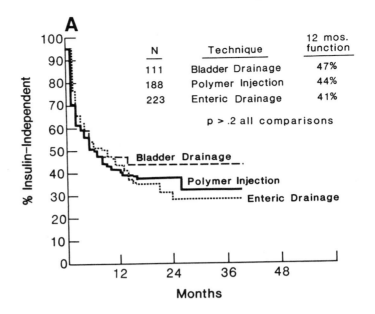

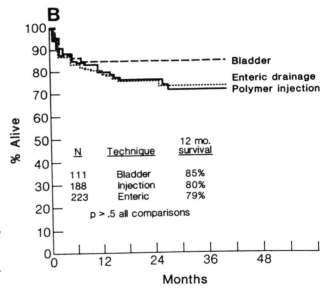

FIGURE 36-20. *(A) Insulin independent rates and (B) patient survival rates for 1983–1986 pancreas transplants according to the most commonly used duct management techniques: bladder drainage, polymer injection, or enteric drainage.*

prine, usually also given with prednisone (triple therapy), was not associated with a penalty in terms of patient survival (Fig. 36-23C and D). The cyclosporine–azathioprine (with or without prednisone) group had a patient survival rate significantly higher than that in the other immunosuppressive groups (86% at 1 year vs 77% in the cyclosporine-treated patients not given azathioprine and 71% in those given azathioprine but not cyclosporine in the immediate post-transplant period). It appears that the

combination of cyclosporine and azathioprine is a safe and effective immunosuppressive regimen.

Results According to the Presence or Absence of ESDN in the Recipients. The pancreas graft survival rate was higher in recipients *with* ESDN than in those *without* ESDN (44% vs 28% at 1 year; Fig. 36-24A). Conversely, patient survival rates for all cases were higher in those without ESDN than in those with ESDN (84% vs 77% at 1 year; Fig. 36-24B). The

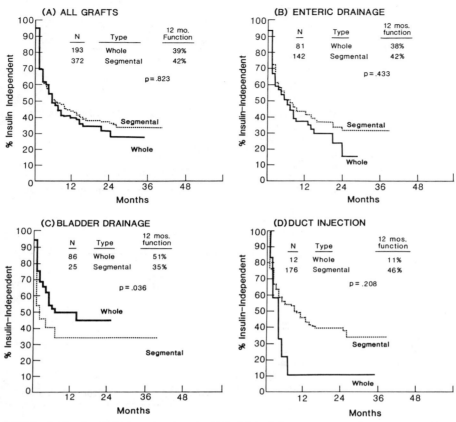

FIGURE 36-21.   *Insulin independent rates for 1983–1986 whole-versus segmental pancreas transplant cases for (A) all grafts, (B) enteric-drained grafts, (C) bladder-drained grafts, and (D) duct-injected grafts.*

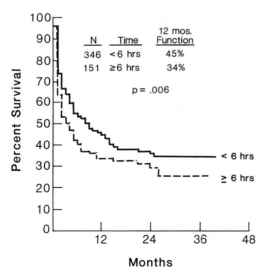

FIGURE 36-22.   *Insulin independent rates for 1983–1986 cadaveric pancreas transplants according to duration of graft preservation prior to transplantation.*

actuarial functional survival rate for pancreas grafts transplanted simultaneously with kidney grafts was higher than that of pancreas grafts transplanted after kidney grafts (46% vs 38% at 1 year), but the differences were not significant (Fig. 36-25A).

Patient survival rates (Fig. 36-25B) were higher at 1 year in recipients of pancreas transplants after a kidney transplant than in recipients of simultaneous pancreas and kidney transplants, but the overall survival rate curves were not significantly different between these two groups (Fig. 36-25B). The highest patient survival rate and graft survival rate (60%) was seen in the small subgroup of eight patients who received a pancreas after a previous kidney from a related donor.

Results of Kidney Transplants in Pancreas Transplant Recipients.   Primary renal allograft functional survival rates in 444 recipients of pancreas transplants during the 1983–1986 period were 71% at 1 year. This calculation was made on all patients with

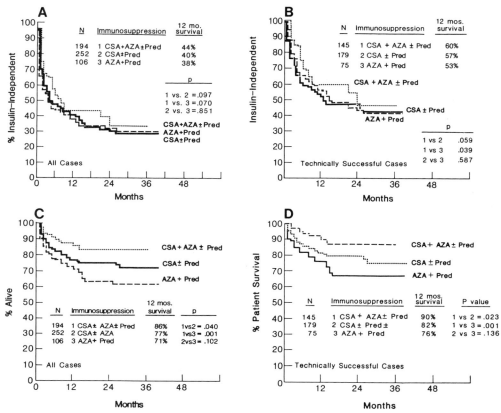

FIGURE 36-23. Insulin independent rates for (A) all and for (B) technically successful 1983–1986 pancreas transplant cases, with corresponding patient survival rates for (C) all and (D) technically successful cases according to the initial immunosuppressive regimen given the recipient. CSA plus AZA ± prednisone includes 6 who did not receive prednisone, of which 5 were technically successful. CSA ± prednisone includes 29 who did not receive prednisone, of which 20 were technically successful.

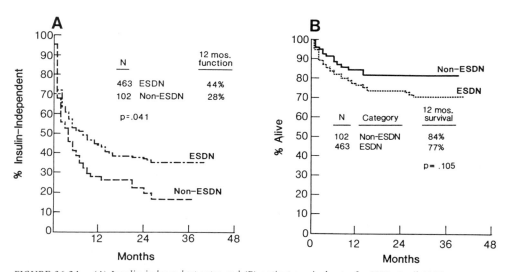

FIGURE 36-24. (A) Insulin independent rates and (B) patient survival rates for 1983–April 1986 pancreas transplant recipients with or without end-stage diabetic nephropathy (ESDN).

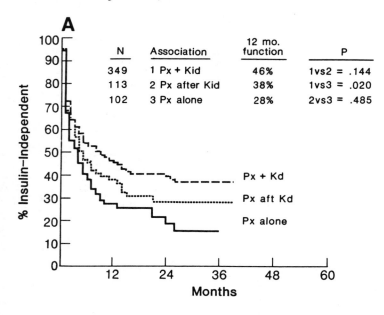

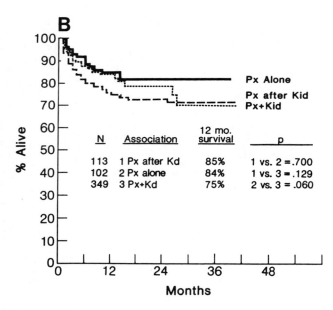

FIGURE 36-25.   *(A) Insulin independent rates and (B) patient survival rates for 1983–April 1986 pancreas transplant cases according to association with or without kidney transplants.*

ESDN, combining those who had a kidney transplant prior to a pancreas transplant with those who received a pancreas transplant simultaneously with a kidney transplant. The 1-year renal allograft functional survival rate following pancreas transplantation in patients who received a kidney transplant before a pancreas transplant was 95% (Fig. 36-26); the kidney graft survival rate is high, because such patients had to survive with a functioning kidney in order to receive the pancreas transplant, most of

which were performed more than 1 year after the kidney transplant. For recipients of simultaneous kidney and pancreas transplants, the 1-year renal graft function rate was 63%; however, after 1 year, the function survival rate curve paralleled that for kidneys transplanted prior to a pancreas. The 63% 1-year renal allograft survival rate for kidneys placed simultaneously with a pancreas for the 1983–1986 period is similar to that of 65% for 264 cyclosporine-treated and 56% for 291 non-cyclos-

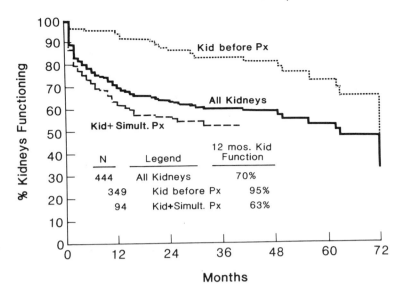

FIGURE 36-26. *Renal graft functional survival rates in 1983–April 1986 recipients of pancreas transplants for all kidneys and according to the timing of kidney transplant relative to the pancreas.*

porine-treated diabetic recipients of renal allografts alone reported to the UCLA kidney transplant registry for 1983–1985 cases.[17]

Results Reported in the Literature from the Currently Active Institutions with the Largest Experiences. The general trend for improvement in pancreas transplant results as documented in the Registry is reflected in the reports from individual institutions. Often, medical centers with significant experience will report results much better than those reported by the Registry.

Beginning in 1984, the University of Minnesota transplant group[76] began to use the bladder drainage technique in some cases and have gradually converted to using this technique now for practically all cadaver recipients.[110] This change has been associated with an improvement in graft survival rates.[77] This group also began to use a triple or quadruple regimen in 1983,[108] consisting of cyclosporine, azathioprine, and prednisone with or without ALG; this protocol has also been gradually refined with a concomitant improvement in graft survival rates.[105] This same group has also used living-related donors for pancreas transplants and has been able to assess the differences in rejection rates according to donor source.[109]

From January 1, 1983, through the first 9 months of 1986, 99 pancreas transplants were performed at the University of Minnesota, with an overall 1-year patient survival rate of 88% and a graft survival rate of 40%. There were 70 cadaver donor transplants, and 29 living-related donor transplants, with 1-year graft survival rates of 35%

and 48%, respectively. When technically successful grafts were analyzed, the 1-year graft survival rates for 42 enteric- and 17 bladder-drained grafts were 64% and 100%, respectively. For technically successful cases only in patients who were non-uremic (no kidney transplant), the 1-year graft survival rates for 32 enteric- and 13 bladder-drained grafts were 57% and 100%, respectively. These results suggest that there is an advantage for monitoring rejection with the bladder-drained grafts.

The same trends for the entire series since 1983 are also seen in a separate analysis of the 1985–1986 cases at the University of Minnesota. For 59 transplants, the 1-year patient survival rate was 91%, and the 1-year graft survival rate was 43%. Of 44 cadaver and 15 living-related donor grafts, the 1-year patient survival rates were 39% and 53%, respectively. Again, a striking advantage for bladder drainage was seen, with a 1-year graft survival rate for 26 enteric- and 13 bladder-drained grafts being 36% and 100%, respectively. Rejection has been particularly difficult to diagnose and treat in non-uremic patients. However, the triple therapy regimen has been associated with a high patient survival rate and an improved graft survival rate.

The University of Wisconsin with the next largest series, has used exclusively the bladder drainage technique, with a gradual shift from segmental to whole-pancreas transplants and an evolution of a quadruple immunosuppressive regimen.[88] In the overall series for 1983–1986, the 1-year graft survival rate was 62%, and the 1-year patient survival rate was 91%.[96] The best results were in the latest series of 28 patients; 18 patients received a pancreas transplant after kidney transplant, and 10 patients had a simultaneous kidney and pancreas transplant.[88] For the combined groups, the 1-year patient survival rate was 96%, and the 1-year graft survival rate was 74%. Rejection losses are infrequent, and this outcome may reflect the ability to monitor for rejection episodes by urine amylase measurements.

The University of Iowa has the third largest series of pancreas transplants in the United States,[18] including 46 cases for 1983–1986, with an overall 1-year pancreas graft survival rate of 46%, and a patient survival rate of 76%.[96] The University of Iowa has used the whole-pancreaticoduodenal transplant method, with enteric drainage initially,[19] but with bladder drainage in the most recent cases.[18] Results of 29 pancreases transplanted simultaneously with kidneys from March 1984, to May 1986, showed a 1-year pancreas graft survival rate of 57%, a kidney graft survival rate of 68%, and a patient survival rate of 78%.[18] Corry and associates[18] have stressed the importance of careful screening for cardiac disease prior to accepting the diabetic patients for pancreas transplantation.

Unlike the United States, where almost all groups are now using the bladder drainage technique for cadaver pancreas transplants, in Europe, either duct injection or enteric drainage are used by most centers. At the University of Munich, all grafts are placed simultaneously with a kidney graft[57] and all transplants have been segmental grafts injected with prolamine. In a recent analysis of 1983–1986 Munich cases, the 1-year pancreas graft function rate for all cases (n = 53) was 56%, and, for 49 pancreases transplanted simultaneously with the kidney, it was 59%.[96]

Huddinge Hospital in Stockholm is one of the pioneering institutes in the field of pancreas transplantation.[42] This group has used the segmental method and has used enteric drainage for most grafts.[41] The best results were in the subgroup of 37 patients who received segmental grafts drained into a Roux-en-Y loop of intestine simultaneously with the kidney transplant, with a 1-year pancreas graft function rate of 52%. In 28 consecutive combined renal and pancreas transplants with enteric exocrine drainage performed between June 1984, and May 1986, the 1-year actuarial survival rates were 69% for the pancreas grafts, 67% for the kidney grafts, and 90% for the patients.

Herriot Hospital in Lyon is another pioneering institute in pancreas transplantation.[27] Until recently, this institution used exclusively the segmental technique with duct injection, and most recipients of pancreas grafts received simultaneous kidney transplants.[26] For 1983–1986, the overall 1-year

graft and patient survival rates for 42 cases were 55% and 73%, respectively. In one of the most recent reports from the Lyon series,[25] the several changes in protocol that have contributed to a progressive improvement in results were described. Of 27 patients treated initially with azathioprine followed by conversion to cyclosporine, the pancreas graft survival rate at 1 year was 51%, and of six patients treated with cyclosporine and azathioprine from the onset, it was 60%.

The University of Oslo[11] reported 39 cases for 1983–1986, with an overall 1-year graft and patient survival rate of 55% and 91%, respectively.[96] The Oslo group has used exclusively the segmental tecnique with duct injection with neoprene, and almost all pancreas grafts have been placed simultaneously with a kidney graft in pancreas graft recipients. The most recent published report from the University of Oslo described 19 cases, with 1-year pancreas and kidney graft survival rates of 60% and 77%, respectively, in doubly transplanted patients.[11]

DISCUSSION

The application of pancreas transplantation for the treatment of diabetes has increased as the success rate has improved. Pancreas transplantation can clearly restore normal metabolism, and long-term graft function (up to 8 years) has been documented in several patients.[96] Currently, 1-year graft function rates of more than 40% are being achieved worldwide, and several institutions are reporting graft survival rates in selected patients of more than 60%. Patient survival rates have also improved; overall they are 80% at 1 year. Again, several institutions have patients survival rates in excess of 90%. Thus, pancreas transplantation has the potential to have the same impact on the treatment of diabetes as kidney transplantation has had on the treatment of end-stage renal disease (ESRD). Significant information related to the nature of diabetes mellitus, such as etiology or its association with microvascular and other complications, may also be forthcoming from observations in pancreas transplant recipients.[6]

It is clear that segmental grafts can sustain normal metabolism.[75,108,132] The theoretical advantages to whole-pancreas grafts are an increased blood flow and an increased islet mass that may provide greater reserve if rejection episodes occur. Both segmental and whole-pancreas grafts can be taken from cadaver donors whether or not a liver is procured;

thus, it would seem best to take a whole pancreas whenever possible.[96]

The three-duct management techniques used most frequently (polymer injection, intestinal drainage, and bladder drainage) have been associated with equivalent graft survival rates. Also, there were no significant differences in graft survival rates for whole- versus segmental pancreas transplants. The Registry data could be interpreted to mean that the debates about technique are moot. However, the merits of each approach must still be considered, and the data are rapidly changing.

Duct injection has been associated with a low complication rate.[96] This advantage has not been associated with a higher long-term graft survival rate than that of the duct drainage techniques, indicating that some grafts indeed may fail because of polymer-induced damage.[9,83] The duct injection technique does not usually allow for monitoring graft exocrine function. Thus, long-term monitoring of graft function must depend solely upon endocrine function or on the function of a simultaneously transplanted kidney.

Enteric drainage is physiologic and will preserve the architectural integrity of the graft, but, again, monitoring of exocrine function is difficult except in the immediately postoperative period if a catheter from the duct has been brought externally.[41,62] For long-term monitoring of pancreas graft function, only endocrine responses can be assessed. Again, the only other parameter that could be used for early diagnosis of rejection would be assessment of function of a simultaneously transplanted kidney from the same donor.[28]

The advantage of the urinary drainage technique is the ability to directly monitor exocrine function, which has been shown in animal studies and in preliminary observations in humans to decrease prior to hyperglycemia during rejection episodes.[76,85] Theoretically, earlier treatment of rejection should result in higher graft survival rates. The major advantage of the bladder drainage technique may not become apparent until a large series of transplants has been accumulated in patients without ESRD who have not also received a kidney from the same donor. The only large series of pancreas transplants in non-uremic, non–kidney transplant recipients is at the University of Minnesota, and the graft survival rates have been higher in those who received transplants by the bladder drainage technique than in those by the enteric drainage technique.[77,110] This supports the thesis that being able to monitor exocrine function for evidence of early rejection will lead to a higher graft survival rate. This thesis is further strengthened by observations

in patients who receive pancreas transplants after a kidney transplant from a different donor, where the grafted kidney cannot be used for monitoring for rejection of the pancreas. The University of Wisconsin has a large number of transplants in this category, again with high graft survival rates.[88]

In the Registry, preservation times of less than 6 hours have been associated with graft survival rates higher than those for pancreases stored longer than this time. However, most of the grafts have been preserved in simple electrolyte solutions designed for the kidney. A hyperosmolar silica gel filter plasma has been used with reliable preservation for up to 24 hours for human pancreases.[1] Although every effort should be made to shorten the preservation time as much as possible, if the preservation limits can be expanded, the logistics of pancreas transplantation will be greatly simplified, and expansions of its application facilitated as become appropriate.

Rejection is still the most frequent cause of graft failure. The use of cyclosporine has been associated with an improvement in pancreas graft functional survival, but not the the level reported for kidney transplants.[15] Recently, cyclosporine has been combined with azathioprine (with or without prednisone). In the Registry data[114] and in reports of individual institutions,[88,105] this regimen has been more effective in preventing rejection than other regimens. Combination therapy also appears safe, since patient survival rates are higher for cyclosporine–azathioprine-treated recipients than those associated with other regimens.[114] Nevertheless, none of the immunosuppressive regimens currently used are entirely satisfactory. Because the side-effects of immunosuppression can be more serious than the complications of diabetes in some patients, pancreas transplantation will not be generally applicable until even less toxic antirejection regimens are devised.

No strictly defined criteria can be applied to the selection of patients to undergo pancreas transplantation. The potential benefit is rather limited in those with advanced complications, yet the majority of pancreas transplants to date have been performed in patients with ESRD. According to the Registry, pancreas graft survival rates are higher in patients who had simultaneous kidney transplants than in non-uremic, non–kidney transplant recipients of pancreas grafts alone or in the recipient of a pancreas graft after a kidney graft.[114] One possible explanation is that it is easier to diagnosis rejection of the pancreas, leading to earlier treatment in those who receive a kidney from the same donor as the pancreas because of the relative ease by which the kidney can be monitored. On the other hand, the patient survival rates are higher in recipients of pancreas transplants alone, and the number of patients in this category is gradually increasing as results improve. It is in such a group that the potential benefit is the greatest.

Nevertheless, generalized immunosuppression is necessary to prevent rejection. Therefore, pancreas transplantation is currently restricted to patients whose secondary complications of diabetes are, or predictably will be, more serious than the potential side-effects of antirejection therapy. Patients who have either had a kidney transplant or are obligated to immunosuppressive therapy meet this criteria. However, many non-uremic, non-kidney transplant patients are also in this category, such as those with preproliferative retinopathy who are great risk for loss of vision,[54] or those with albuminuria and thus have early, but inevitably progressive, diabetic nephropathy.[126]

For maximal therapeutic benefit, pancreas transplants should be performed in very early stage of disease. Because of the need at this point for generalized immunosuppression, the patients selected must clearly be difficult to manage for the metabolic standpoint or be at high risk for secondary complications when subjected to conventional (exogenous insulin) treatment of diabetes. Methods to identify such patients are needed.[69] High plasma levels of inactive renin are associated with microvascular complications in diabetic patients.[63] High levels of insulin-like growth factor I are also seen in patients who do have accelerated progression of diabetic retinopathy.[68] Diabetic children with stiff joints have a high incidence of subsequent microvascular complications.[79] Diabetics who have impaired counterregulatory mechanisms are at high risk for hypoglycemic reactions while on an insulin pump or other intensified insulin therapy regimens, and such patients can be identified by measurement of adrenergic and other responses to stress.[131] Persons with such characteristics are those who are most likely to benefit from a pancreas transplant. At current levels or organ procurement, a sufficient number of pancreas should be available for this select group of diabetics.[7]

When immunosuppressive therapy is improved to the point at which side-effects are minimal, many more diabetics could be considered for pancreas transplantation, and donor procurement will have to be increased. However, at this time, procurement should not be a problem. More than 7000 kidney transplants are currently being done each year in the United States.[46] The yearly incidence of Type I diabetes mellitus in the United States is estimated at approximately 12,000 new cases per year, and fewer than half the patients with the disease develop serious complications.[130] Thus, the current kidney transplant rate is similar to the incidence of complication-prone Type I diabetes. Only a small proportion of the potential donors are currently used as a source of organs,[7] but it should be possible to increase the procurement rate; each donor could give the pancreas as well as other organs for transplantation.

For pancreas transplantation, the major question still revolves around whether or not the procedure can favorably influence the course of secondary complications. Preliminary observations in a few pancreas transplant recipients suggest that development of lesions in kidneys can be halted[10] and that neuropathy may also improve,[124] but definitive answers to these questions may not be forthcoming until advances in immunosuppressive and improvement in results justify transplantation soon after the onset of disease, allowing for longitudinal observations in a large number of patients.

In conclusion, pancreas transplantation can effectively treat Type I diabetes mellitus in humans. Islet transplants have been successful in animals, but, at this time, pancreas transplantation is the only practical method of total endocrine replacement therapy in diabetic humans. Pancreas transplantation could potentially be applied on as large a scale as kidney transplantation. As future advances in immunosuppression occur, pancreas transplantation could eventually be routinely performed at a stage sufficiently early to prevent the development of diabetic nephropathy and other lesions and could supercede kidney transplants and other procedures in the management of complication-prone diabetic patients.

REFERENCES

1. Abouna GM, Sutherland DER, Florack G et al: Function of transplanted human pancreatic allografts after preservation in cold storage for 6–26 hours. Transplantation 43(5):630–635, 1987
2. Abouna GM, Al-Adnani MSA, Kremer GM et al: Reversal of diabetic nephropathy in human cadaveric kidneys after transplantation into nondiabetic recipients. Lancet 2:1274–1276, 1983
3. Ballinger WF, Lacy PE: Transplantation of intact pancreatic islets in rats. Surgery 72:175, 1972
4. Banting FG, Best GH: The internal secretion of the pancreas. J Lab Clin Med 7:251, 1922

5. Barbosa J, King R, Goetz FC, et al: Histocompatibility antigens (HLA) in families with juvenile insulin dependent diabetes mellitus. J Clin Invest 60:989–999, 1977

6. Barker CF, Naji A, Perloff LJ et al: Invited commentary: An overview of pancreas transplantation—Biologic aspects. Surgery 92:113, 1982

7. Bart KJ, Macon EJ, Whittier FC et al: Cadaveric kidneys for transplantation. A paradox of shortage in the face of plenty. Transplantation 31:374, 1981

8. Baumgartner D, Bruhlmann W, Largarider F: Technique and timing of pancreatic duct occlusion with prolamine in recipients of simultaneous renal and intraoperative segmental pancreas Allotransplants. Transplant Proc 16:1134–1135, 1986

9. Blanc-Brunat N, Dubernard JM, Touraine JL et al: Pathology of the pancreas after intraductal neoprene injection in dogs and diabetic patients treated by pancreatic transplantation. Diabetologia 25:97, 1983

10. Bohman SO, Tyden G, Wilezek A: Prevention of kidney graft diabetic nephropathy by pancreas transplantation in man. Diabetes 34:306, 1985

11. Brekke IR, Dyrbekk D, Jakobsen A: Combined pancreas and kidney transplantation for diabetic nephropathy. Transplant Proc 18:1125–1126, 1986

12. Brooks JR, Gifford GH: Pancreatic homotransplantation. Transplant Bull 6:100–103, 1959

13. Calne RY: Paratopic segmental pancreas grafting: A technique with portal venous drainage. Lancet 1:595–597, 1984

14. Calne RY, Brons IGM: Observations on paratopic segmental pancreatic grafting with splenic venous drainage. Transplant Proc 17:340, 1985

15. Calne RY, White DJG: The use of cyclosporine in clinical organ grafting. Ann Surg 196:330, 1982

16. Calne RY, McMaster P, Rolles K et al: Technical observations in segmental pancreas transplantation: Observations on blood flow. Transplant Proc 12 (Suppl 2):51–57, 1980

17. Cats S, Gallon J: Effect of original disease on kidney transplant outcome. In Terasaki PI (ed): Clinical Kidney Transplantation—1985, p 35. Los Angeles, University of California at Los Angeles Press, 1985

18. Corry RJ, Nghiem DD, Schanbacher B: Critical analysis of mortality and graft loss following simultaneous renal-pancreaticoduodenal transplantation. Transplant Proc 19:2305–2306, 1987

19. Corry RJ, Nghiem DD, Schulak JA et al: Surgical Treatment of diabetic nephropathy with simultaneous pancreatic duodenal and renal transplantation. Surg Cynecol Obstet 162:547–555, 1986

20. Crass JR, Feinberg SB, Sutherland DER et al: Radiology of human segmental pancreatic transplantation. Gastroenterol Radiol 7:153–158, 1982

21. Crass JR, Sutherland DER, Feinberg SB: Sonography of the segmental human pancreatic transplantation. J Clin Ultrasound 10:149–152, 1982

22. DaFoe DC, Campbell DA, Marks WH et al: Karyotypic chimerism and rejection in a pancreaticoduodenal splenic transplant. Transplantation 40:572–574, 1985

23. Deierhoi MH, Sollinger HW, Bozdec MJ et al: Lethal graft versus host disease in a recipient of a pancreas–spleen transplant. Transplantation 41:544–546, 1986

24. DeJode LR, Howard JM: Studies in pancreaticoduodenal homotransplantation. Surg Gynecol Obstet 114:553–558, 1962

25. Dubernard JM, Faure JL, Gelet A et al: Simultaneous pancreas and kidney transplantation: Long-term results and technical discussion. Transplant Proc 19:2285–2287, 1987

26. Dubernard JM, Monti LD, Faure JL et al: Report on 63 pancreas and kidney transplants in uremic diabetic patients. Transplant Proc 18:1111–1113, 1986

27. Dubernard JM, Traeger J, Neyra P et al: A new method of preparation of segmental pancreatic grafts for transplantation: Trials in dogs and in man. Surgery 84:633, 1978

28. Dubernard JM, Traeger J, Touraine L et al: Patterns of renal and pancreatic rejection in double-grafted patients. Transplantation Proc 13:305, 1981

29. Eisenbarth GS: Type I diabetes mellitus: A chronic autoimmune disease. N Engl J Med 314:1360–1368, 1986

30. Fajans S, Conn JW: An approach to the prediction of diabetes mellitus by modification of the glucose tolerance test with cortisone. Diabetes 3:296–304, 1954

31. Florack G, Sutherland DER, Cavallini M et al: Technical aspects of segmental pancreatic autotransplantation in dogs. Am J Surg 146:565, 1983

32. Florack G, Sutherland DER, Heil J et al: Preservation of canine segmental pancreatic autografts. Cold storage vs pulsatile machine perfusion. J Surg Res 34:493–504, 1983

33. Florack G, Sutherland DER, Heil J et al: Long term preservation of segmental pancreas autografts. Surgery 92:260–269, 1982

34. Florack G, Sutherland DER, Sibley RK et al: Combined kidney and segmental pancreas allotransplantation in dogs. Transplant Proc 17:374–377, 1985

35. Florack G, Sutherland DER, Squifflet JP et al: Effect of graft denervation, systemic drainage and reduction of beta cell mass on insulin levels after heterotopic pancreas transplantation in Dogs. Surg Forum 33:351–353, 1982

36. Gayet R, Guillaumie M: Laregulation de la secretion interne pancreatique par un processus normorler dermontree par des plantation de pancreas. CR Soc Biol 97:1613, 1927

37. Gerrish EW: Final Newsletter, American College of Surgeons/National Institutes of Health Organ Transplant Registry, June 30, 1977

38. Gliedman ML, Gold M, Whittaker J et al: Clinical segmental pancreatic transplantation with ureter–pancreatic duct anastomosis for exocrine drainage. Surgery 74:171–180, 1973

39. Gliedman ML, Tellis VA,, Soberman R et al: Long-term effects on pancreatic transplant function in patients with advanced juvenile onset diabetes. Diabetes Care 1:1–9, 1978

40. Gray DWR, Morris PJ: Prospects for pancreatic islet transplantation. World J Surg 10:410–421, 1986

41. Groth CG, Collste H, Lundgren G et al: Successful outcome of segmental human pancreatic transplantation with enteric exocrine diversion after modifications in technique. Lancet 2:522–524, 1982

42. Groth CG, Lundgren G, Arner P et al: Rejection of isolated pancreatic allografts in patients with diabetes. Surg Gynecol Obstet 143:933–940, 1976

43. Gunnarson R, Klintmalm G, Lundgren G et al: Deterioration in glucose metabolism in pancreatic transplant recipients after conversion from azathioprine to cyclosporine. Transplant Proc 16:709–712, 1984

44. Harris MJ, Hanaman RF (eds): Diabetes in America. Bethesda, Maryland, NIH Publication 85-1468, 1985

45. Harrisen KF, Dahl-Jorgenson K, Lauritzen J et al: Diabetic control and microvascular complications: The near normoglycemic experience. Diabetologia 10:677–684, 1986

46. Health Care Financing Administration (HCFA) Office of Special Programs. End-Stage Renal Disease Program Medical Information System, Facility Survey Tables, Department of Health and Human Services, USA, HCFA. January 1–December 31, 1985

47. Hedon E: Sur la consommation du sucre ches le chien apres l'extirpadon de pancreas. Arch Physiol Norm Pathol 5:154, 1893

48. Heise J, Sutherland DER, Heil J: Comparison of two colloid osmotic solutions for 72 hours preservation of pancreatic segments in a dog. Autotransplant Model (in press)

49. Hesse UJ, Najarian JS, Sutherland DER: Amylase activity and pancreas transplants. Lancet 2:726, 1985

50. Hesse UJ, Sutherland DER, Simmons RL et al: Intraabdominal infections in pancreas transplant recipients. Ann Surg 203:2,153–162, 1986

51. Houssay BA: Technique de la greffe pancreaticoduodenale au con. CR Soc Biol (Paris) 100:138–140, 1929

52. Kampik A, Ulberg M: Is proliferative diabetic retinopathy an indication for pancreatic transplantation. Transplant Proc 18:62–63, 1986

53. Kelly WD, Lillehei RC, Merkel FK et al: Allotransplantation of the pancreas and duodenum along with the kidney in diabetic nephropathy. Surgery 61:827, 1967

54. Klein BEK, Davis MD, Segal D et al: Diabetic retinopathy: Assessment of severity and progression. Ophthalmology 91:10–17, 1984

55. Koostra G, von Hooff JP, Jorning PJG et al: A new variant for whole pancreas grafting. Transplant Proc 19:2314–2318, 1987

56. Lafferty KJ: Pancreatic islet transplantation—experimental experience and clinical potential. West J Med 143:853–857, 1985

57. Land W, Landgraf R, Illner WD et al: Improved results in combined segmental pancreatic and renal transplantation in diabetic patients under cyclosporine therapy. Transplant Proc 17:317, 1985

58. Largarider F, Lyons GW, Hidalgo F et al: Orthopathic allotransplantation of the pancreas. Am J Surg 113:70–76, 1967

59. Letourneau JG, Maile CW, Sutherland DER et al: Ultrasound and computerized tomography in the evaluation of pancreatic transplantation. Radiol Clin North Am 25:345–355, 1987

60. Lillehei RC, Ruiz JO, Acquino C et al: Transplantation of the pancreas. Acta Endocrinol 83 (Suppl 205):303, 1976

61. Lillehei RC, Simmons RL, Najarian JS et al: Pancreaticoduodenal allotransplantation: Experimental and clinical experience. Ann Surg 172:405–436, 1970

62. Liu T, Sutherland DER, Heil J et al: Beneficial effects of establishing pancreatic duct drainage into a hollow organ (bladder, jejunum, or stomach) compared to free intraperitoneal drainage of duct-injection. Transplantation Proc 17:366–371, 1985

63. Luetscher JA, Kraemer FS, Wilson DM et al: Increased plasma inactive renin: A marker to microvascular disease. N Engl J Med 312:1412, 1985

64. Maile CW, Crass JR, Frick MP et al: Computerized tomography of pancreas transplants. Invest Radiol 20:557–562, 1985

65. Mauer SM, Steffes MW, Brown DM: Studies of diabetic nephropathy in animals and man. Diabetes 25:850–857, 1976

66. Mauer SM, Steffes MW, Connett J et al: Development of lesions in the glomerular basement membrane and mesangium after transplantation of normal kidneys to diabetic patients. Diabetes 32:948–952, 1983

67. McMaster P, Michael J, Adu D et al: Experience in human segmental pancreas transplantation. World J Surg 8:253, 1984

68. Merimee TJ, Zapf J, Froesch ER: Insulin-like growth factors. Studies in diabetes with and without retinopathy. N Engl J Med 309:527, 1983

69. Mogenson CE, Christiansen CK: Predicting diabetes nephropathy in insulin-dependent diabetic patients. N Engl J Med 311:89–93, 1984

70. Munda R, First MR, Weiss et al: Synchronous pancreatic and renal allografts with urinary tract drainage of the pancreas. Transplant Proc 19:2343–2344, 1987

71. Munda R, Tom WW, First MR: Pancreatic allograft exocrine urinary tract diversion: Pathophysiology. Transplantation 42: Dec, 1986 (in press)

72. Najarian JS, Kjellstrand CM, Simmons RL et al: Renal transplantation for diabetic glomerulosclerosis. Ann Sur 178:477–485, 1973

73. Najarian JS, Sutherland DER, Matas AJ et al: Human islet transplantation: A preliminary experience. Transplant Proc 9:233–236, 1977

74. Nghiem DD, Gowana TA, Corry RJ: Metabolic effects of urinary diversion of exocrine secretions in pancreatic transplantation. Transplantation 43:70–73, 1987

75. Pozza G, Traeger J, Dubernard JM et al: Endocrine

responses of Type I (insulin-dependent) diabetic patients following successful pancreas transplantation. Diabetologia 24:244, 1983

76. Prieto M, Sutherland DER, Fernandez-Cruz L et al: Experimental and clinical experience with urinary amylase monitoring for early diagnosis of rejection in pancreas transplantation. Transplantation 43:71–79, 1987

77. Prieto M, Sutherland DER, Fernandez-Cruz L et al: Diagnosis of rejection in pancreas transplantation. Transplant Proc 19:2348–2349, 1987

78. Ramsay RC, Goetz FC, Sutherland DER et al: Diabetic retinopathy following pancreas transplantation for insulin dependent diabetes mellitus: A prospective study. Transplant Proc 18:1774, 1986

79. Rosenbloom AL, Silverstein JH, Lezotte DC et al: Limited joint mobility in childhood diabetes mellitus indicates increased risk for microvascular disease. N Engl J Med 305:191, 1981

80. Rynasiewicz JJ, Sutherland DER, Fergguson RM et al: Cyclosporin A for immunosuppression: Observations in rat heart, pancreas and islet allograft models and in human renal and pancreas transplantation. Diabetes 31 (Suppl 4):92–108, 1982

81. Scharp DW, Lacy PE: Human islet isolation and transplantation. Diabetes 34 (Suppl 1):5A, 1985

82. Service FJ, Molnar GD, Rosevar JW et al: Mean amplitude of glycemic excursions, a measure of diabetes instability. Diabetes 19:644–655, 1970

83. Sibley RK, Sutherland DER: Pancreas transplantation: A immunohistological and histopathologic examination of 92 grafts. Am J Pathol (in press)

84. Sibley RK, Sutherland DER, Goetz FC et al: Recurrent diabetes mellitus in the pancreas iso- and allograft. A light and electron microscopic and immunohistochemical analysis of four cases. Lab Invest 53:132–144, 1985

85. Sollinger HW, Cook K, Kamps D et al: Clinical and experimental experience with pancreaticocystostomy for exocrine pancreatic drainage in pancreas transplantation. Transplant Proc 16:749, 1984

86. Sollinger H, Kalayoglu M, Hoffman RM et al: Results of segmental and pancreaticosplenic transplantation with pancreaticocystostomy. Transplant Proc 17:360–362, 1985

87. Sollinger H, Kalayoglu M, Hoffman RM et al: Experience with whole pancreas transplantation and pancreaticoduodenocystostomy. Transplant Proc 18:1759–1761, 1986

88. Sollinger HW, Kalayoglu M, Hoffman RM: Quadruple immunosuppressive therapy in whole pancreas transplantation. Transplant Proc 19:2297–2299, 1987

89. Starzl TE, Hakali TR, Show BW et al: A flexible procedure for multiple cadaveric organ procurement. Surg Gynecol Obstet 158:223–230, 1984

90. Starzl TE, Iwatsuki S, Shaw BW: Pancreaticoduodenal transplantation in humans. Surg Gynecol Obstet 159:265, 1984

91. Steiner E, Klima J, Niederwieser D et al: Monitoring of the pancreatic allograft by analysis of exocrine secretion. Transplant Proc 19:2336–2338, 1987

92. Sutherland DER: Pancreas and Islet transplantation. I. Experimental studies. Diabetologia 20:161–185, 1981

93. Sutherland DER: International Human Pancreas and Islet Transplant Registry. Transplant Proc 12 (No 4, Suppl 2):229, 1980

94. Sutherland DER: Selected issues of importance in clinical pancreas transplantation. Transplant Proc 16:661, 1984

95. Sutherland DER: Transplantation in nonuremic diabetic patients. Transplant Proc 18:1747–1749, 1986

96. Sutherland DER: Pancreas transplantation. Curr Probl Surg (in press)

97. Sutherland DER, Ascher NL: Distal donation from a living relative. In Najarian JS et al (eds): Manual of Vascular Access, Organ Donation and Transplantation, Chapter 11, pp 144–152. New York, Springer-Verlag, 1984

98. Sutherland DER, Ascher NL: Whole pancreas donation from a cadaver. In Simmons RL et al: (eds): Manual of Vascular Access, Organ Donation, and Transplantation, Chapter 10, pp 105–143. New York, Springer-Verlag, 1984

99. Sutherland DER, Ascher NL, Najarian JS: Pancreas transplantation. In Simmons RL et al (eds): Manual of Vascular Access, Organ Donation, and Transplantation, Chapter 17, pp 237–254. New York, Springer-Verlag, 1984

100. Sutherland DER, Casanova D, Sibley RK: Role of pancreas graft biopsies in the diagnosis and treatment of rejection after pancreas transplantation. Transplant Proc 19:2329–2331, 1987

101. Sutherland DER, Elick BA, Najarian JS: Maximization of islet mass in pancreas grafts by near total or total whole organ excision without duodenum from cadaver donors. Transplant Proc 16:111, 1984

102. Sutherland DER, Goetz FC, Abouna GM et al: Use of recipient mesenteric vessels for revascularization of segmental pancreas transplants. Transplant Proc 19:2300–2304, 1987

103. Sutherland DER, Goetz FC, Carpenter AM et al: Pancreaticoduodenal grafts: Clinical and pathological observations in uremic versus nonuremic recipients. In Touraine JL et al (eds): Transplantation and Clinical Immunology, Vol X, pp 90–195, Amsterdam, Excerpta Medica, 1979

104. Sutherland DER, Goetz FC, Elick BA et al: Experience with 49 segmental pancreas transplants in 45 diabetic patients. Transplantation 34:330, 1982

105. Sutherland DER, Goetz FC, Najarian JS: Improved pancreas graft survival rates by use of multiple drug combination immunotherapy. Transplant Proc 18:1770–1773, 1986

106. Sutherland DER, Goetz FC, Najarian JS: Intraperitoneal transplantation of immediately vascularized segmental pancreatic grafts without duct ligation: A clinical trial. Transplantation 28:485, 1979

107. Sutherland DER, Goetz FC, Najarian JS: Living related donor segmental pancreatectomy for transplantation. Transplant Proc 12 (No 4, Suppl 2):33–39, 1980

108. Sutherland DER, Goetz FC, Najarian JS: 100 pancreas transplants at a single institution. Ann Surg 200:414, 1984

109. Sutherland DER, Goetz FC, Najarian JS: Pancreas transplants from related donors. Transplantation 38:625, 1984

110. Sutherland DER, Goetz FC, Najarian JS: Pancreas transplant donor and recipient selection, management and outcome. Transplant Proc (in press)

111. Sutherland DER, Kendall DM, Najarian JS: One institution's experience with pancreas transplantation. West J Med 143:838–844, 1985

112. Sutherland DER, Matas AJ, Goetz FC et al: Transplantation of dispersed pancreatic islet tissue in humans: Autografts and Allografts. Diabetes 29 (Suppl 1):34, 1980

113. Sutherland DER, Matas AJ, Najarian JS: Pancreatic islet cell transplantation. Surg Clin North Am 58:365–382, 1978

114. Sutherland DER, Moudry KC: Pancreas Transplant Registry Report–1986. Clin Transplant 1:3–17, 1987

115. Sutherland DER, Najarian JS, Greenberg BZ et al: Hormonal and metabolic effects of an endocrine graft: Vascularized segmental transplantation on the pancreas in insulin-independent patients. Ann Intern Med 95:537, 1981

116. Sutherland DER, Sibley RK, Zu X-Z et al: Twin-to-twin pancreas transplantation reversal and reenactment of the pathogenesis of Type I diabetes. Trans Assoc Am Physicians XCVII:80–87, 1984

117. Tchobroutsky G: Relation of diabetes control to development of microvascular complications. Diabetologia 15:143, 1978

118. Terasaki PI, Toyotome A, Mickey MR: Patient, graft and functional survival rates. In Terasaki PI (ed): Clinical Transplantation—1985, pp 1–26. Los Angeles, University of California at Los Angeles Press, 1985

119. Toledo-Pereyra LH: Pancreas transplantation. Surg Gynecol Obstet 157:49, 1983

120. Tyden G, Brattstrom G, Haggmark A: Studies on the exocrine secretion of human segmental pancreatic grafts. Surg Gynecol Obstet 164:404–408, 1987

121. Tyden G, Brattstrom C, Lundgren G et al: Improved results in pancreatic transplantation by avoiding non-immunological graft failures. Transplantation 43:674–676, 1987

122. Tyden G, Lundgren G, Ostman J et al: Grafted pancreas with portal venous drainage. Lancet 1:964–966, 1984

123. Tyden G, Wilczek H, Lundgren G et al: Experience with 21 intraperitoneal segmental pancreatic transplants with enteric or gastric exocrine diversion in humans. Transplant Proc 17:331–335, 1985

124. Tzakis AG, Carrol PB, Makowaka L et al: Effect of pancreatic transplantation on diabetic complications in adults. J Surg Res (in press)

125. Ungar RH: Meticulous control of diabetes: Benefits, risks and precautions. Diabetes 31:479, 1982

126. Viberti GC, Hill RD, Jarre HRJ et al: Microalbuminuria as a predictor of clinical diabetic nephropathy. Lancet 1:1430–1432, 1982

127. von Mering J, Minkowski O: Diabetes mellitus after pancreas extirpation. Arch Exp Pathol Pharmakol 26:371–387, 1889

128. Wahlberg JA, Lowe R, Landegaard L et al: 72-Hour preservation of the canine pancreas. Transplantation 43:5–8, 1987

129. Weiland D, Sutherland DER, Chavers B et al: Information on 628 living related kidney donors at a single institution, with long-term follow-up in 472 cases. Transplant Proc 16:5–7, 1984

130. West KM: Epidemiology of Diabetes and It's Vascular Lesions. New York, Elsevier, 1978

131. White N, Skor DA, Cryer PE et al: Identification for Type I diabetic patients at increased risk for hypoglycemia during intensive therapy. N Engl J Med 308:485, 1983

132. Wilczek H, Gunnarsson R, Felig P et al: Normalization of hepatic glucose regulation following heteroptic pancreatic transplantation in humans. Transplant Proc 17:315, 1985

CHAPTER 37

Transplantation of Pancreatic Islets

Clyde F. Barker   Ali Naji   James F. Markmann

The vascular complications of diabetes appear to be due to failure of conventional insulin therapy to sufficiently approximate normoglycemia. Since there is no pancreatic exocrine deficiency in diabetes, effective transplantation and control of blood glucose could be accomplished by implantation of isolated islets. Islets transplanted in rodents from genetically identical donors have been demonstrated to permanently reverse diabetes. However, allogeneic islets appear to be especially vulnerable to rejection.

Immunosuppressive agents such as azathioprine, Cytoxan, and cyclosporine have in general been minimally effective for islet allografts, as have adrenal corticosteroids. The results with antilymphocyte serum (ALS) are better, but, unless ALS is combined with other methods such as minimizing histocompatibility or allograft antigen manipulation, even this potent immunosuppressive agent is less effective for islets than for other allografts.

Success has been reported for islet allografts in immunologically privileged sites such as the anterior chamber of the eye, the cerebral cortex, and the testicle. The clinical impracticality of these sites is unfortunate.

It is possible that the sensitization that follows islet transplantation is caused by graft elements other than the endocrine cells, that is, vascular, exocrine, and passenger leukocytes. These cells may be removed from the graft by pretransplant tissue culture or by treatment of grafts with anti-donor antibody or ultraviolet irradiation. Islets treated by these methods have been found not to provoke an immune response, although they may serve as targets of rejection.

It may also be necessary to contend with another biological barrier to successful transplantation, that is, autoimmune destruction of transplanted islets by diabetes. Pretransplant tissue culture may overcome this type of immune damage of islet just as it does rejection. Despite the lack of success with human islet allografts, both the technical problems of isolating human islets and the immunologic problems are probably solvable.

Of great interest to the 5% of the population afflicted with insulin-dependent diabetes and to physicians caring for them is the recent demonstration that pancreatic transplantation can totally normalize carbohydrate metabolism in human diabetics.[125] Whether this therapy can also prevent or reverse the vascular complications commonly seen in diabetics treated with insulin remains to be shown, but it seems likely in view of evidence that optimal control of blood sugar by insulin therapy minimizes complications.[67,127] The results of vascularized pancreas transplantation have improved in recent years, but the operation and necessary immunosuppression continue to carry a significant morbidity and mortality. Since many of the problems encountered have been related either to surgical technique or to the exocrine portion of the transplanted pancreas, simple implantation of purified isolated islets of Langerhans is an attractive alternative. In this chapter, the following questions are discussed, some of which should be answered prior to extensive clinical application of islet transplantation. Do the usual rules of histocompatibility prevail, or are islets immunologically privileged, as has been claimed for some endocrine tissue? Would fetal islets have advantages over adult islets, such as diminished antigenicity and capability for growth? Can islets be stored, and, if so, would this decrease their immunogenicity? If rejection were prevented, would transplanted beta cells be destroyed by the original disease process, leading to recurrence of diabetes? In this chapter, the outcome of clinical islet transplantation is reviewed, but since most of the available information pertinent to these questions has been provided by experimental studies in animals, these will be described first and in greatest detail.

EXPERIMENTAL ISLET TRANSPLANTATION

Techniques of Islet Preparation

In the development of islet isolation techniques and the initial successful islet transplants, rodents were the experimental animals used, because, in these species, the soft consistency of the pancreas facilitates enzymatic digestion and separation of islets from exocrine tissue. Several types of prepared pancreas have been transplanted as free grafts, including (1) mechanically fragmented pancreas; (2) enzymatically dispersed pancreas; (3) isolated islets (selectively removed from finely dispersed pancreas); and (4) fetal or neonatal pancreas either whole, fragmented or digested.

Pancreatic Fragments.   Beginning in 1893, sporadic unsuccessful attempts were made to reverse diabetes in animals and humans by implants of pancreatic fragments.[22] In these experiments, the pancreas was mechanically disrupted, sliced, or chopped but not digested. Only within the last few years has success been reported with such a technique, and then only when very large amounts of finely minced fetal pancreas (20 to 30 donors) were used.[137] Thus, fragmentation alone appears to be an inefficient method for pancreas transplant preparation, and further effort to separate islets from acinar tissue is preferable.

Dispersed Pancreas.   Since the initial reports of partial reversal of diabetes in 1972 by Ballinger and Lacy[7] and complete reversal in 1973 by Reckard and Barker,[95] dispersed pancreas has been successfully transplanted by many investigators. This technique involves mechanical preparation of small fragments of pancreas, which are then digested with collagenase or other enzymes while being agitated to dislodge islets from the acinar tissue. Alternatively, enzymes may be inoculated into the duct of the intact pancreas, which is then agitated to facilitate disintegration and islet separation. The digested tissue is then washed to remove the enzymes, but no separation of exocrine and endocrine elements is attempted. All techniques that have been devised to remove acinar tissue result in substantial islet loss, usually to the extent that multiple donors are needed for a successful transplant.[65] Minimizing islet losses by accepting impurity of a dispersed pancreas preparation is probably essential for autotransplants in which, by definition, only one donor is available. However, the large amount of enzymatically active acinar tissue content in dispersed pancreas is a major disadvantage. Acinar tissue may be tolerated in some implant sites such as the peritoneal cavity because of the large absorptive surface of the canine spleen, which is very tough. However, injection of dispersed adult pancreas into a closed space such as intramuscular or subcutaneous tissues may cause enzymatic digestion of the islets and the entire transplant site, with disastrous results. Inoculation of impure dispersed pancreas into the portal vein has also been reported to cause portal hypertension, venous occlusion, and disseminated intravascular coagulation.[119,120]

Isolated Islets.   This exacting technique is the most appealing on theoretical grounds and also the one that has most commonly led to successful transplantation.[55] From preparations of dispersed pancreas, individual islets are separated from acinar, ductal, and vascular components, either with a pipette under low-power magnification or by centrifugation of the preparation through density gradients of Ficoll. Although this method results in very significant islet loss (up to 95%), it is capable of yielding 150 to 450 intact islets from a single rat pancreas. Since it is necessary for successful transplantation to transplant 600 to 1500 islets, 2 to 6 donors may be required. Agents that decrease enzymatic content of acinar cells (pilocarpine) or that cause acinar atrophy (DL-ethionine) or acinar destruction (antiacinar cell antibody) may be useful in minimizing the acinar content of islet preparations.[61,90,103,135] Another variation uses a filtration device in which the pancreatic tissue is placed for digestion.[106] Islets that become separated from the pancreas early in the process are filtered out, thus protecting them from excessive digestion while further digestion of the remaining pancreatic tissue is continued to free additional islets.[103] Modification and improvement of techniques have recently been reported to increase islet yield sufficiently to allow reversal of diabetes by transplantation of islets from a single donor, but multiple donors are still required by most workers for each successful transplant.[21,36]

Fetal and Neonatal Pancreas. The ratio of endocrine to exocrine tissue is high in fetal and neonatal pancreases compared with that in adult pancreas.[66] Immature pancreatic tissue also has the advantage that it can be dispersed by minimal enzymatic digestion, avoiding the islet damage that results from prolonged digestion. However, a disadvantage of digested fetal or neonatal pancreas, which has about 11% of the islet mass of the adult pancreas, is the need for large numbers of donors for reversal of diabetes, sometimes as many as 20 or 30.[133] However, because of the capacity for islet growth, small numbers of whole fetal pancreas (usually four), if implanted as a free graft under the kidney capsule, will eventually reverse diabetes over several weeks.[18]

Technique and Site of Islet Implantation

Theoretically, endocrine grafts implanted anywhere should be capable of satisfactory function. However, for islet grafts, the transplant site has been a crucial consideration, and success has been achieved in only a few transplant sites. An "ideal" transplant site should have the following characteristics: (1) sufficient vascularity for graft "take"; (2) superficial location accessible for simple inoculation of islets and for biopsy to evaluate viability or rejection; (3) an expansile nature to accommodate the large volume of an impure dispersed pancreas preparation; (4) resistance to damage by enzymatic impurities; (5) expendability, so that tissue damage by enzymatic activity or excision of the graft and transplant site is acceptable; (6) portal venous drainage, so that insulin from the transplanted islets goes directly to the liver in the usual physiologic manner; (7) if possible, the characteristics of an "immunologically privileged site," to minimize rejection. Unfortunately, no known transplant site has all of these characteristics.

Peritoneal Cavity. The peritoneal cavity is accessible for islet inoculation and is large enough to accommodate a sizable volume of nonpurified dispersed pancreas. Its absorptive surface is relatively resistant to damage by enzymatically active acinar tissue. Pancreatic fragments that adhere to the peritoneal surface become well vascularized, but others may float free, decreasing the percentage of islets that eventually "take." Other disadvantages of this site are its lack of accessibility or expendability for excision of infected grafts, the nonportal nature of the venous drainage, and the lack of immunologically privileged status. Despite these disadvantages, this site was the one first used successfully for amelioration of diabetes.[7,95] It is acceptable in rats or mice but would be the site of choice only for impure dispersed pancreas, since, in this case, the tolerance of the peritoneal surface for enzymatic activity becomes a crucial consideration. However, the site is inefficient, and more islets are needed here than if the intraportal route is used.[99] The intraperitoneal site has not been used extensively in large animals or in humans.

Portal Vein. Inoculation of islets to this unique transplant site was first described by Kemp and colleagues,[46] who hypothesized that insulin secreted by islets within the portal outflow tract might prove particularly effective because it would reach the liver directly. The observation that only 300 to 600 isolated rat islets (prepared from three to six donors) inoculated intraportally cured diabetes, whereas as many as 800 to 2400 islets from 4 to 12 donors transplanted intraperitoneally were less effective, also demonstrated the efficiency of this site.[99] Inoculated islets lodge in the terminal portal venules and, even before neovascularization takes place, are nourished by and secrete insulin into the blood, reversing diabetes within 24 hours (Fig. 37-1A and B). Neovascularization of islets occurs within a few days, and "take" has been estimated at greater than 50%.[94] An important attribute of the liver as a transplant site is its double blood supply, which allows the complete occlusion of the portal venules caused by embolized islets to be tolerated without infarcting the transplant site, which remains nourished by hepatic arterial blood. Intra-arterial transplantation of islets to areas not provided with a double blood supply (e.g., the spleen) results in infarction of the transplant site and failure of the graft.

If nonpurified dispersed pancreas is inoculated intraportally, the activated enzymes and bulkiness of the transplanted tissue may lead to occlusion of major portal venous channels, causing portal hypertension, hepatic damage, hypotension, and disseminated intravascular coagulation.[69] These complications are especially severe in the dog, although they have also been encountered in rats and humans. Another potentially serious risk of intraportal transplants is dissemination of contaminating microorganisms. Finally, the intraportal transplant site is not easily accessible, and inoculation has usually been done intraoperatively, although we have used a transcutaneous, transhepatic approach to the hu-

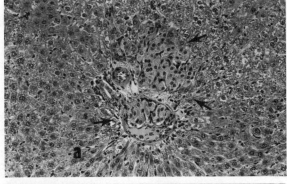
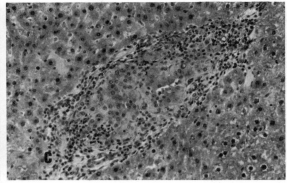
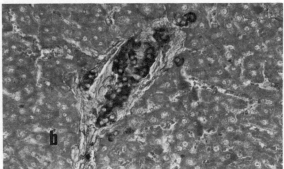

FIGURE 37-1.   (a) Histologic picture of an intraportally inoculated islet isograft that has lodged in a portal venule. Migration of some cells has taken place through adjacent hepatocytes hematoxylin and eosin; (arrows).
(b) Well-established intraportal islet graft showing well-granulated beta cells stained for insulin with Aldehyde Fuchin stain.
(c) Liver biopsy at the time of the recurrence of diabetes in a spontaneously diabetic BB rat tolerant of WF antigens that remained normoglycemia for only 12 days following successful intraportal transplantation of Wistar Furth islets. Islets reveal heavy mononuclaer infiltration (insulitis) suggestive of recurrence of the original autoimmune disease since rejection cannot take place because of immunologic tolerance.

man portal system in human islet autotransplantation.[13]

Despite these multiple disadvantages, the intraportal transplant site has proved effective more often than any other site, and it should probably be considered the islet transplant site of choice in most instances, especially if it is possible to use a highly purified nontoxic islet preparation.

Spleen.   The spleen has several potential advantages as a transplant site: excellent vascularity, portal venous drainage, and relative expendability (compared with the liver or kidney). However, the spleen is neither safely nor easily accessible for the nonoperative implantation of islets. In the dog, this organ is expansile enough to accept large volumes of impure dissociated pancreas and is quite resistant to damage. In this species, intrasplenic autotransplantation of nonpurified islets can prevent diabetes after total pancreatectomy.[52,53,71,96] Favorable results have also been noted in other species, such as the rat and the mouse, but the risk of significant splenic injury is higher.[28] Although the site has also been used in humans, splenic rupture is to be feared.

Intravenous.   Most islets inoculated into peripheral veins lodge in the lung and have been reported to correct hyperglycemia in rats.[113] However, because of the serious consequences that could occur from wide dissemination of infected islets and because large numbers of islets are needed for successful intravenous transplants, this site is not worth of serious consideration.

Superficial Sites (Intramuscular, Subcutaneous).
These sites are ideally accessible and expendable. Although it would be predicted that vascularity is adequate for islet "take," even transient function of islets transplanted to these sites has rarely occurred.[51,137] Another serious drawback is the susceptibility of these sites to enzymatic digestion if impure preparations are used. In the few instances of success in these sites, islet preparations of minimal enzymatic activity were used, suggesting the possibility that autodigestion of the transplanted islets might be the usual cause of failure.

Omentum.   A novel islet transplantation site is the peritoneal-omental pouch constructed in rats by encasing the omentum in a pouch of parietal peritoneum; it is reported to sustain long-term function of islet isografts.[141] Advantages of this site are that (1) insulin secreted by the islets is released into the portal venous system, and (2) the grafts could be retrieved easily if required.

Kidney Capsule. Although this site appears to have none of the characteristics of an ideal transplant site other than good vascularity, it is effective for implants of whole-fetal pancreas, which become rapidly vascularized and reverse hyperglycemia of diabetic rats.[18] Although the site is too small to accommodate a large volume of impure dissociated pancreas grafts, it is suitable for inoculation of pure islet preparations.[100] There is some evidence that this site may be more preferable than the liver from an immunologic standpoint.[138]

Characteristics of Rejection of Islet Allografts

Despite the known immunologically privileged status of certain endocrine tissues (e.g., parathyroid, ovary, thyroid), which, for unknown reasons, are partially exempt from rejection, early islet allograft experiments indicated just the opposite for islets.[60,74,93]

The first technical success in transplanting allogeneic islets was followed by rejection within only a few days.[95] Cessation of insulin secretion was accompanied by the classic histologic picture—infiltration of the graft by mononuclear cells and by the appearance of specific cytotoxic alloantibody.[30,31,108] Attempts to exclude acinar elements by "hand picking" islets failed to improve survival, appearing to confirm that endocrine tissue itself was capable of provoking rejection and was highly vulnerable to it. In addition, it was found that conventional immunosuppression was less effective in prolonging survival of islet allografts than those of skin or other endocrine tissues.[142] Vascularized pancreas allografts also survived longer than isolated islets, in that pancreas allografts transplanted across major histocompatibility barriers survive about as long in rats as those of kidney or heart (7–12 days), whereas major histocompatibility complex (MHC)-compatible heart and pancreas grafts survived for many weeks, compared with much shorter islet allograft survival.[92] These findings, in conjunction with the demonstration that isolated islet allografts in other species (dogs and baboons) are also rejected within a few days, provide convincing evidence that in unmodified hosts, isolated islet allografts fare worse than vascularized organ transplants.[70,122]

The explanation for the anomalously short-lived survival of allogeneic islets is obscure but possibly depends on the generic vulnerability to humoral immunity exhibited by dissociated cellular grafts (a factor known to prejudice the survival of other dissociated cellular grafts such as bone marrow). Naji and colleagues[75,77,91] examined the vulnerability of islet allografts to humoral factors, using long-standing healthy islet allografts in immunologically tolerant rat hosts as targets. Administration of alloantiserum specific for the donor strain rapidly destroyed well-established adult islet allografts, while similarly established allografts of skin, parathyroid, and vascularized or fetal pancreas did not succumb. Other researchers have confirmed the sensitivity of islets to antibody using a rat-to-mouse xenograft model.[20,30] For whatever reason, the results of all experimental allogeneic islet transplants (except those using methods that decrease islet immunogenicity) indicate that free grafts of isolated adult islets are unusually susceptible to immune damage.

Methods for Avoiding Rejection

Strategies to prevent rejection include (1) histocompatibility matching; (2) modification of the recipient's immune system (e.g., immunosuppression or induction of specific unresponsiveness); (3) use of weakly immunogeneic tissue (e.g., fetal) or modification of donor tissue to decrease immunogenicity; and (4) protection of the allograft by implantation in a privileged site.

Histocompatibility Matching. The validity of this method of prolonging survival of allografts is most convincingly demonstrated by the outcome of MHC-identical human sibling kidney transplants, which is vastly superior to that possible with MHC-incompatible donors. Experimentally, "matching" has also proved effective in nonimmunosuppressed animals for extending survival of endocrine allografts (i.e., parathyroid, thyroid, and ovary), which may enjoy permanent survival if donor and recipient are MHC compatible, whereas MHC incompatible grafts are rejected promptly.[10,74,93] However, the initial assessment of histocompatibility matching of islet allografts suggested that it was of little benefit.[8,98] In rats, islets transplanted across MHC-incompatible barriers by portal vein inoculation were rejected in 3 to 5 days, whereas MHC-compatible islets did not survive much longer (7.8 days).[14] Also, in mice, H-2 compatible allogeneic islets survive no more than a week, only a few days longer than H-2 incompatible allogeneic islets.[29,76] Indeed, transplanted islets are rejected even when donor and recipients are members of the same inbred strain and differ only with respect to the weak sex-determined H–Y antigen, results that generate little optimism for the usefulness of histocompatibility matching. In all these instances, islet preparations heavily contaminated with acinar tissue were used. However, somewhat different results have recently been obtained with highly purified islets obtained by Percoll/Ficoll gradient centrifugation and "hand picking." The increased purity appears to lengthen survival of islet allografts, especially those transplanted across weak histocompatibility barriers. In some instances, very prolonged survival of MHC-compatible islet allografts has been observed (e.g., in WF to BB rats, 50% graft survival at 100 days; and, in WF to WAG rats, 75% survival at 100 days).[140] It has also been found that in certain mouse strains, H-2-matched fetal pancreatic grafts are likely to fare much better than H-2-incompatible grafts, although these experiments are not comparable to those with adult islets, since the fetal grafts were cultured (a process that alters immunogenicity).[34] Interestingly, although MHC-matching is beneficial in delaying rejection of pure islets, it may be associated with a greater likelihood of autoimmune damage to islets.[140]

Modification of the Recipient's Immune System

Nonspecific Immunosuppression. Nonspecific immunosuppressive agents that have been used to prolong islet allograft function include pharmacologic agents and antilymphocyte serum (ALS). The results with the former have been quite disappointing. Cyclophosphamide prolongs (DAxLewis)F$_1$ islet survival in Lewis rats only to 6.8 days, compared with an islet survival in controls of 4.2 days.[27,72] Using azathioprine, allograft survival could not be extended beyond 25 days in the rat.[64] Corticosteroids, a mainstay of clinical immunosuppression, have proved to be of no benefit in delaying the onset of rejection of islet allografts nor in reversing islet rejection in rats when used in high doses similar to those useful for aborting ongoing rejection episodes in human renal allograft recipients.[84,107] In dogs, high-dose steroids were actually detrimental to islet function, perhaps not surprising in view of the known diabetogenic effect of these agents.[122]

Disappointingly, the new pharmacologic immunosuppressive agent cyclosporine, which has been so successful in prolonging survival of renal, heart, and liver allografts, appears to be considerably less effective for pancreas and isolated islet allografts.[38,102] In addition to being nephrotoxic and hepatotoxic, this agent has been reported to have a detrimental effect on glucose metabolism. In rats, 50 mg/kg of cyclosporine (a large but not significantly nephrotoxic dose in this species) induces severe degeneration of beta cells and causes hypoinsulinemia and hyperglycemia.[41,45] Cyclosporine has an inhibiting effect on mouse islet cell replication that is evident in the cells of isografted islets and in those of the native pancreas.[49] Deterioration of islet

transplant function after cyclosporine has also been noted in other species, including dogs, although it was found that the major toxicity of the drug for canine islet autografts occurred during the early post-transplant period, suggesting that the adverse effect was on revascularization of the graft. In human pancreas recipients, a consistent deterioration of allograft function was noted when immunosuppression was changed from azathioprine to cyclosporine. Whether the detrimental effect reflects direct beta cell toxicity, inhibition of protein synthesis, or induction of insulin resistance is not clear.[40] Whatever the reason, present indications are that cyclosporine will be less effective for pancreas and islet transplants than for other allografts.

ALS, another relatively nonspecific immunosuppressive agent, prolongs the function of islet allografts with substantially greater success than pharmacologic agents, including cyclosporine.[98] In rats, rejection of intraperitoneal islets can be delayed from a control of 8.5 days to 30.5 days by a 5-day course of ALS treatment. The efficacy of this agent in extending allograft survival has been confirmed. For instance, prolonged survival of Lewis rat islets in Fischer recipients has been obtained for 200 days with ALS therapy; and, in the closely related DA to ACI rat combination, even a short course of ALS is followed by function of islets in some recipients for 150 days.[37,143] In the latter study, long-term islet recipients were found to accept DA skin grafts, indicating that the islets in conjunction with ALS could induce a state of specific immunologic unresponsiveness, a finding confirmed by Zitron and associates[144] who used cultured islets and postulated that suppressor cells are involved. Even islet xenograft survival can sometimes be accomplished with ALS in rat-to-mouse transplants.[20,30,56]

Although, because of species differences, the effect of immunosuppressive protocols in animals should not be expected to generate data directly applicable to clinical transplantation, important general principles learned from the laboratory are applicable and allow the following predictions: (1) once technical success is achieved, currently available immunosuppression should allow prolonged function of islet allografts and possibly even of xenografts in concordant species; and (2) identical immunosuppressive protocols are less effective in prolonging survival of islets than of vascularized whole-organ grafts (kidney, heart, pancreas) unless some method of decreasing islet allograft immunogenicity is also used.[83,92]

Induction of Donor-Specific Unresponsiveness. The effectiveness of inducing donor-specific unresponsiveness for islets has been demonstrated in experimental animals and suggests eventual clinical feasibility. Immunologic tolerance is a form of unresponsiveness induced by neonatal inoculation of recipients with lymphohematopoietic cells of the prospective donor strain. Tolerance allows permanent engraftment of all types of allografts, including islets, but, unfortunately, the method is practical only in rodents, which, unlike man and most other species, are immunologically quite immature at birth. However, further examination of the model of experimental tolerance may be useful in defining the specific properties of islets that are responsible for their anomalously rapid rejection.

Enhancement is a form of immunologic unresponsiveness dependent upon "blocking antibody." It may be induced by administration of donor antigen and/or anti-donor antibody and is an effective method of promoting survival of experimental *vascularized* organ transplants (including pancreas), although it is generally ineffective for free grafts such as skin or isolated islet allografts.[83,87,97] In fact, it has been noted that the same enhancing protocols that promote very long survival of vascularized heart or pancreas allografts in rats actually prejudice the survival of transplanted islets, perhaps because islets are susceptible to the cytotoxic properties of antibody.[92] Also, when donor whole blood was administered to prospective mouse islet allograft recipients, accelerated rejection was seen instead of enhancement. However, immunization with whole blood that had first been treated with anti-Ia antibody and complement (to remove leukocytes such as B-lymphocytes and macrophages) did prevent islet rejection.[54] In an analogous study in rats, prolonged islet allograft survival was achieved in recipients preimmunized with donor whole blood that had been irradiated with ultraviolet light, a procedure that allegedly inactivates the Ia (Class II) antigen–bearing leukocytes (which include cells with known antigen-presenting capability, such as macrophages).[57] Markmann and colleagues[63] investigated the survival of islet allografts in rats pretreated with donor-type blood from which virtually all leukocytes (whether bearing Class I or II antigens or both) were mechanically removed. Since erythrocytes in the rat, unlike humans, express MHC antigens (but only Class I MHC antigens), these experiments determined the effect of pretransplant exposure of recipients to donor MHC Class I antigens in the absence of Class II antigen–bearing cells. The exposure of hosts to pure donor erythrocytes did not prolong survival of subsequent islet allografts unless the islets were cultured prior to transplantation. However, cultured islets, which contain no Class II expressing cells, did survive permanently when transplanted to rats immunized with purified

donor erythrocytes. The experiments of these three investigators support the hypothesis that selective immunization to Class I MHC antigens may be a particularly effective form of enhancement; this may be especially true if the graft contains only Class I antigens.

Use of Weakly Immunogenic Donor Tissue. Strategies by which islets might be transplanted to recipients in a weakly immunogenic or nonimmunogenic state include the use of fetal or neonatal tissue and the use of grafts that have been manipulated prior to transplantation to modify their cellular composition or immunogenicity.

Fetal tissue has less predilection for rejection than does adult tissue. In rats and mice, fetal or neonatal skin allografts may have permanent survival even though adult skin allografts are always rejected promptly.[136] The possibility of a similar immunologic advantage for fetal pancreas was examined by Spence and colleagues,[114,115] who found that transplantation of fetal pancreas allografts under the kidney capsule of diabetic rats was followed by destruction of the pancreas by a mononuclear infiltrate within only 4 days. However, fetal pancreas may enjoy a slight immunologic advantage over adult tissue, since, in tolerant hosts, established fetal pancreas grafts are less vulnerable than adult islets to adoptively transferred immunity.[91] Other experiments using a variety of forms of cultured immature pancreas also confirm the generality that islets transplanted by this method are likely to have extended survival compared with adult tissue allografts.[62,111,112]

Another method aimed at diminishing immunogenicity is alteration of donor tissue prior to transplantation. Several such methods have recently been demonstrated to improve islet allograft survival in rodents (Fig. 37-2).[17,24,58] As previously noted, unmodified allogeneic islets elicit both cellular and humoral immune responses and usually undergo an anomalously rapid rejection. However, it is also known that the transplantation of a small number of allogeneic leukocytes will provoke a similar strong immune response.[117] Thus, it might be difficult to distinguish the immunization that follows islet transplantation from that which might actually be caused by "passenger leukocytes" contained in the transplanted islets.

There is, in fact, some evidence that the endocrine cells in islets are themselves deficient in histocompatibility antigens. H-2 antigens could not be found on the surface of beta cells of dissociated islets with an immunoferritin-labeling technique, although H-2 antigens were present on pancreatic acinar, ductal, and capillary endothelial cells.[88] Class

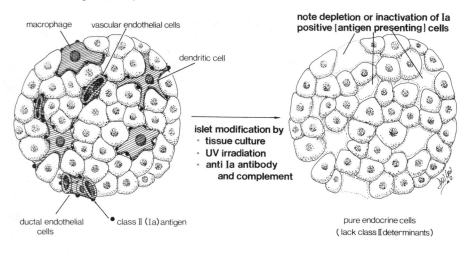

FIGURE 37-2.   *Schematic diagram of a single isolated islet composed of both endocrine and non-endocrine cellular components. Several methods are indicated that alter immunogenicity of donor islet prior to transplantation. Generally these techniques alter the antigenic make-up of the lymphoid "passenger leukocytes" or vascular endothelial cells.*

I antigens have been detected on islet cells but without evidence of Class II antigens.[6,23] It is generally accepted that cells expressing MHC Class II antigens such as macrophages and dendritic cells are the relevant ones in presenting transplantation antigens or inciting an immune response.[116] Thus, Class II antigens (or the cells expressing them) may be the sole stimulators of immune responses, although cells expressing Class I antigens serve as excellent targets for immune reactivity. This could explain the success of Lacy[54] and Bowen and co-workers[17] in extending islet allograft survival by a pretransplant period of tissue culture. This is because Class II expressing passenger leukocytes, especially those of the macrophage series, are particularly susceptible to destruction by prolonged culture if there is high O_2 tension in the culture medium.[89] This may also be true of nonlymphoid cell types expressing Class II antigens, such as vascular or ductal endothelium, while pancreatic beta cells should, it is hoped, survive in tissue culture. Islets treated by tissue culture might therefore confront their allogeneic hosts only with Class I antigens, having been deleted of all the cells expressing Class II determinants and (more importantly) all cells capable of presenting antigen and inciting an immune response. Thus, the transplanted islet cells might thrive because they escape the notice of the host's immune system. However, because of their continued expression of Class I an-

tigens, transplanted islets would remain targets for rejection if stimulation by antigen-presenting cells of the donor strain took place at some other time, either before or after the islet transplant.

Unfortunately, it has been noted that under prolonged culture conditions at high-oxygen tension, islet cells as well as passenger leukocytes are likely to be damaged.[54,126] Other details of culture conditions may also be important (e.g., temperature), and further work is necessary before ideal conditions can be defined.[139] Nevertheless, it is now finally established that islet allograft survival can be prolonged by pretransplant culture, especially if temporary immunosuppression is used.

Another method aimed at eliminating the graft of antigen-presenting cells is treatment with donor-specific antibody. In the mouse, Faustman and associates[24] reported prolonged survival of noncultured islet allografts after pretreating islets with anti-Class II antibody and complement to delete the antigen-presenting population of passenger leukocytes. Subsequently, prolonged mouse islet allograft survival following pretransplant treatment of islets with a mouse antidendritic cell monoclonal antibody and complement was reported.[25] These experiments lend further support to the contention that of Class II MHC expressing passenger leukocytes, the dendritic cell has the predominant role in initiation of graft rejection. Unfortunately, attempts to apply these techniques in rat islets experiments have been less encouraging. Pretransplant treatment of rat islets with anti-Ia antibody alone resulted in no increase in survival unless combined with cyclosporine immunosuppression.[128] Even in the mouse, other investigators have had difficulty in reproducing Faustman's results, making it apparent that this is an exacting method.[35]

An analogous strategy is the treatment of donor islet allografts with ultraviolet irradiation prior to their transplantation. Stimulated by the observations that ultraviolet (UV) irradiation abrogated the stimulatory capability of leukocytes for in vitro mixed lymphocyte reaction (MLR), Hardy and coworkers[43] found that UV irradiated Lewis donor islets transplanted to nonimmunosuppressed ACI recipients survived for 80 days.[47] Rather than destroying the Class II-expressing antigen-presenting cells, this method appears to inactivate them. Further refinements of the method are necessary before clinical application, because endocrine cells are also somewhat susceptible to UV damage. Also unfortunate is the finding that attempts to transpose these extremely provocative results to other species or even other rat strains have thus far met with little success.[43]

Further confounding interpretation of the aforementioned inconsistencies is the result of studies indicating a possible role of MHC-restriction in transplantation immunity.[15] Following tissue culture in high-oxygen tension conditions, islet allograft survival in diabetic mice was prolonged only if donor and recipient were MHC-incompatible. A proposed explanation of this unexpected finding is that cultured endocrine grafts usually fare better than noncultured grafts because their antigen-presenting cells fail to survive the culture conditions. However, if, after culture, the graft is transplanted to MHC-compatible hosts, the antigen-presenting function can be assumed by the MHC-compatible host macrophages, whereas in more disparate hosts, MHC-restriction precludes this.[140]

Immunologically Privileged Sites

Allografts of several endocrine tissues have been transplanted to immunologically privileged sites with great success, and it is probable that this approach might also be useful for islets if technical considerations allow implantation.[12]

Anterior Chamber of the Eye. A variety of malignant and benign tissue allografts, including pancreatic fragments, have been successfully grafted to this classic privileged site, although reversal of diabetes was not accomplished by the latter.[19] Protection of foreign grafts in this site probably depends upon the absence of lymphatic drainage.[9,12] Some anterior chamber allografts are rejected because they become vascularized by contact with the iris, allowing passenger leukocytes to escape or peripheral sensitization to occur. Survival of allografts is almost always precluded in presensitized hosts. From a practical standpoint, the anterior chamber may be too small to accommodate enough islets to reverse diabetes, even if the risk of impairing vision by such an implant were acceptable.

Brain. Allografts of tumors and endocrine tissues implanted in the brain often survive indefinitely, apparently avoiding rejection because of the lack of a conventional lymphatic drainage. The transplantation of allogeneic isolated islets and dissociated islet cells to the brain of streptozotocin-induced diabetic rats reversed diabetes for as long as 170 days.[131] It is questionable whether the risk of using this site in humans could ever be justified. Interestingly, transplanted syngeneic islets into the cerebral ventricles of rats had long-term functional success, whereas allogeneic islets were rejected, presumably because contact with meninges was not avoided and lymphatic communication with the host caused sensitization.[68]

Testicle. The testicle, unlike other privileged sites, has a rich lymphatic drainage, and its privileged status (long established for thyroid and parathyroid allografts) may depend upon high local concentrations of male steroid hormones or the peculiar blood testis barrier known to exist around seminiferous tubules.[12] Histologic evidence of intratesticular islet allograft survival for up to 90 days, but not reversal of the diabetic state, has been reported in guinea pigs.[26] Also, long-term reversal of diabetes in rats by intratesticular implantation of a rat insulinoma in syngeneic hosts has been achieved.[1] Other investigators have also found that intratesticular xenografts and allografts, respectively, survived for prolonged intervals in the intratesticular site.[16,109] The latter investigators made the interesting observation that only when the testicle was relocated to the abdominal cavity was there sufficient insulin production by implanted islets to reverse diabetes, apparently indicating the importance of the temperature for islet function but decreasing the possible usefulness of this transplant site for clinical use.

Muscle and Subcutaneous Tissue. Skeletal muscle, which is poor in lymphatics, has some of the properties of a privileged transplant site. Barker and Billingham[9,11] found that grafting allogeneic skin to large open muscle beds isolated from contact with edges of surrounding host skin approximately doubled their usual survival. Naji and Barker[74] noted that when rat parathyroid allografts were implanted in muscle, they often survived for more than 100 days, especially if there was major locus histocompatibility of donor and recipient, whereas parathyroid allografts in sites of normal lymphatic vascularity were rejected promptly. This superficial and readily accessible site deserves to be further evaluated as a possible site for isolated islet grafts, but, as previously noted, even syngeneic intramuscular islet grafts have usually failed for obscure reasons.

There is also evidence that subcutaneous fat may be a partially privileged site, as shown for skin allografts, although this has not been shown for isolated islets.[42] A similar fatty site, the cleared mammary fat pad, extends the survival of allogeneic islet grafts in the mouse.[86]

Kidney Capsule. The kidney capsule is not a true privileged site, and allografts of skin and parathyroid implanted here are rejected promptly. However, it appears that at least in rats, survival of purified allogeneic isolated islets is likely to be prolonged in this site compared with those embolized to the liver by the portal vein; MHC-incompatible kidney subcapsular islets survive 8.4 days, compared with 4.0 days for intraportal islets.[100]

Even more dramatic results were recently obtained using spontaneously diabetic BB rat recipients and finding that while all intraportal grafts were rapidly rejected (WF in 12.7 days, and Lew in 4.7 days), three of five WF grafts and four of five Lewis grafts survived indefinitely when transplanted beneath the renal capsule.[138] Islet damage in these spontaneously diabetic rats can occur either from rejection or autoimmune insulitis, but, in either case, it was prevented by transplantation to the renal subcapsule. This site has also been advocated in dogs, although these experiments using non purified pancreas require confirmation.[130]

Artificial Privileged Sites

Surgically Constructed Privileged Sites. The common denominator for most immunologically privileged sites appears to be an abnormality in lymphatic drainage. The most convincing evidence of the critical nature of an intact lymphatic circulation from the graft bed to regional lymph nodes was provided by the experiments of Barker and Billingham,[9] who surgically created islands of skin and muscle on the trunk of guinea pigs, separated from contact with surrounding skin by plastic chambers glued to the body wall. Nourishment of the islands was provided by a neurovascular bundle left intact in the surgical procedure but shown by dye injections to contain no lymphatics. Skin allografts transplanted to these alymphatic sites failed to sensitize their hosts and enjoyed prolonged survival, a finding confirmed in rats by Tilney and Gowans.[129] The model has been used successfully with tumor allografts and would be promising for islets if technical problems were overcome with regard to islet "take" in subcutaneous tissue and muscle.[32]

Millipore Diffusion Chambers. Artificial devices were first used to prevent allograft rejection using chambers made of semipermeable material having a pore size of 0.1 μm to 0.8 μm, which served several functions: (1) to prevent escape of antigenic particles or cells; (2) to exclude immunized host cells or antigen-sensitive cells of host origin, thus preventing peripheral sensitization; and (3) to admit nutrient-containing fluids to support the grafted tissue or egress of hormones secreted by the graft.[5] Antibody and complement penetrate such chambers with difficulty (depending upon the pore size), but, if this does occur, allogeneic or xenogeneic tissues may be destroyed, probably accounting for the failure of porcine islet xenografts transplanted in diffusion chambers.[101]

Prolonged success of islet allograft survival in Millipore chambers was reported by early workers in the field. Although islets recovered 10 weeks after transplantation were found to be viable as evidenced by their in vitro secretion of insulin when stimulated by glucose, the very small amount of islet tissue used in these experiments invites skepticism that the implant was actually responsible for the reported reversal of diabetes.[33,118]

The most difficult problem in maintaining survival of transplants in Millipore chambers is that host fibrin and adhesions eventually clog the pores and interfere with diffusion of nutrients. A variant of the Millipore chamber has been used in an attempt to obviate this problem by allowing continuous circulation of rapidly moving blood past the membrane. Knazek and associates[48] reported culturing islet cells on the outer surface of artificial capillaries while culture medium circulates inside the lumen of the capillary. The material constituting the "capillary wall" of the hollow fiber capillaries consists of a thin retentive skin surrounded by an outer macroporous spongy layer on which cells are seeded. The membrane has pores large enough to admit glucose or insulin but not cells or antibody.

The implantation of such chambers into the aorta of diabetic rats allows blood to circulate through the lumen of the hollow fibers, with isolated islets growing on the macroporous outside layer of the membranes.[132] Blood glucose levels returned toward normal, and serum insulin was significantly increased. However, clotting of blood or bleeding from excessive heparinization limited the function of the system to 13 hours, indicating that major obstacles would need to be solved before this method could be attempted clinically.

Biologically Compatible Capsules. Possibly more promising is the incorporation of isolated islets into biocompatible spherical capsules 100 μm to 500 μm in diameter, using alginate polylysine membranes.[59] Microencapsulated islets have remained morphologically and functionally intact for up to 15 weeks in culture. Encapsulated islets transplanted intraperitoneally in diabetic rats were capable of reversing hyperglycemia, but, after 2 to 3 weeks, recurrence of diabetes occurred, apparently because the polymer used to form the capsule was not totally compatible, and the resultant inflammatory reaction eventually culminated in its disintegration. However, O'Shea and Sun[85] recently reported that implantation of microencapsulated xenogeneic rat islets in diabetic mice allowed normoglycemic for 100 days, encouraging hopes for eventual clinical applications of this technique.

Recurrence of Autoimmune Diabetes in Transplanted Islets

Implicit in the emerging consensus that Type I diabetes mellitus is a disease of autoimmune etiology, is the question of whether autoimmunity in a naturally diabetic host might destroy transplanted islets, even if rejection could be avoided.[79] The outcome of islet and pancreas transplantation has been thoroughly studied mainly in animals in which diabetes was artificially induced by a beta cell toxin such as streptozotocin. To study the effect of spontaneous diabetes, Naji and associates[80–82] selected BB rats, an outbred strain in which about 50% of individual members develop a form of spontaneous diabetes similar to human insulin-dependent diabetes. In order to distinguish rejection from autoimmune damage, two approaches were used: (1) comparison of the results of islet allografts in rats of the BB stock which had either developed diabetes spontaneously or had it induced by streptozotocin; and (2) determining the outcome of islet transplantation in diabetic BB rats in which rejection was avoided by immunologic tolerance.[78] In these experiments, the rapid failure of islet grafts in spontaneous BB diabetics, whereas grafts across the same weak histocompatibility barrier in artificially induced diabetics had prolonged survival, is difficult to explain on any basis other than vulnerability of transplanted islets to autoimmune destruction. However, since rejection theoretically could have contributed to the failure of these allografts, islet transplantation was performed in BB recipients in which immunologic tolerance precluded rejection.

Diabetes-prone BB rats were rendered tolerant by neonatal inoculation of donor strain bone marrow cells from Wistar Furth (WF) rats. BB rats tolerant of WF antigens that had failed to develop diabetes by 150 days of age were rendered artificially diabetic with streptozotocin and transplanted with WF islets. This resulted in permanent normoglycemia, confirming that rejection of allogeneic islets could be avoided by the induction of tolerance. However, in other BB rats also tolerant of WF antigens but *spontaneously* diabetic, transplantation of isolated islets from WF donors, initially normalizing blood glucose, was always followed by recurrent diabetes and insulitis within a few days (Fig. 37-1c). In these tolerant hosts, since the transplanted islet failure could not be attributed to rejection, autoimmune damage must have been responsible.

These two experiments collectively appear to provide conclusive evidence that the original disease process can destroy the transplanted islets. It has since been noted in several instances of human identical twin pancreatic transplants that initially successful transplants failed almost surely from recurrent autoimmune insulitis.[110] Immunosuppression appears to be useful in avoiding pancreas failure in twins.

On theoretical grounds, it seems likely that recurrence of autoimmune diabetes might be influenced by MHC restriction, and this has proved to be the case for glomerulonephritis, which is more likely to recur in transplanted human kidneys if HLA-identical donors are used.[73] Evidence in support of this possible cause of islet failure was recently obtained in BB rats.[140] Cultured and noncultured islets from MHC-compatible WF donors were promptly destroyed (after 12.7 and 13.4 days, respectively) in spontaneously diabetic BB rats, whereas cultured MHC-incompatible Lewis islets survived permanently. Thus, although there is general agreement that minimizing donor–recipient disparity favorably influences the outcome of allografts by reducing the impact of rejection, it may, on the other hand, increase the chances of recurrent autoimmunity. The balance of these two threats to graft survival may be particularly complex with respect to islet and/or pancreas allografts compared with other organ grafts for several reasons. First, Type I diabetics carry HLA/DR3 and HLA/DR4 alleles, which, in all probability, are linked to the susceptibility gene(s) for the disease. Second, the destruction of the target organ (pancreatic beta cells) in insulin-independent diabetes could result from an abnormal autoantigen, which, in diabetes, is expressed on the surface of beta cells.[79]

CLINICAL RESULTS OF ISLET TRANSPLANTATION

Islet Allografts

Since 1924, sporadic attempts have been made to reverse human diabetes with allografts of pancreatic fragments.[44] Until the mid 1970s, lack of understanding of technical problems in obtaining from the donor sufficient numbers of viable islets or appreciation of the need for immunosuppression of the recipient precluded any chance of success. Following development of islet isolation techniques and the demonstration in 1973 that experimental diabetes in animals could be cured by islet transplantation, a flurry of attempts at clinical application took place. Since then, information on 166 islet transplants had been collected by Sutherland's Pancreas Transplant Registry through 1984.[121] Most of the isolation techniques and transplant sites described in this chapter for experimental transplants were tried. The largest well-studied series (18 transplants in 13 patients) was performed at the University of Minnesota in diabetics who were previous recipients of successful kidney transplants.[124] In none of these patients was it possible to discontinue insulin therapy for more than 4 days, and there was no instance of long-term islet function. Other reports of islet transplantation have, for the most part, documented similar failures. In a few instances, diabetes was thought to have been favorably influenced, but evidence of this was always incomplete. Kolb and Largaiader[50] reported that 9 months after an intrasplenic islet transplant, insulin therapy was stopped for the remainder of the patient's life (11 months), but autopsy did not confirm the presence of transplanted islets. In one of nine diabetic patients transplanted by Groth and colleagues,[39] marginal function of transplanted islets for 4 months was confirmed by small amounts of C-peptide in the blood, although insulin could never be withdrawn. Insulin requirements were reported to be reduced in one of six patients transplanted in Berlin and in several patients who received fetal pancreas transplants in China and Russia. Valente and associates[134] reported that in 3 of 24 patients who received transplanted pancreatic fragments, insulin therapy was withdrawn. Thus, of a combined series of 166 patients, in only 4 was it reported that insulin was temporarily withdrawn. Considerable reservation remains about the results in these cases, because confirmation of transplant function by C-peptide assays or histology was not obtained, and pretransplant withdrawal of insulin therapy had presumably not been attempted in these patients to substantiate that they were indeed insulin-dependent. In most of these cases, very impure islet preparations were used and were transplanted to a variety of sites.

The closest approximations to isolated islet preparations have been used recently by Alejandro and colleagues[4] and Alderson and associates.[2] Alejandro and co-workers[3] described perfecting a reasonably purified islet preparation in dogs, using antiacinar antibody and, in this species, has reported successful transplantation using only one donor. In three patients, islet allografts were performed with a similarly purified islet preparation; at least a temporary decrease in insulin requirements was found.[4]

A recent carefully studied series of six clinical islet allografts performed by Scharp and colleagues[104] probably represents the current state of the art. Using more than 180 pancreases procured from local and distant centers from heart beating cadavers, they evolved an islet isolation technique based on digestion, filtration, and elutriation, which yielded a preparation of 20% of the islet tissue known to be present in the entire pancreas (compared with about 5% achieved in the earlier Minnesota trials).[105] Their patients, all of whom were diabetic successful renal allograft recipients already on immunosuppression, received an average of 240,000 islets, inoculated into the spleen. Three of the six had definite allograft function documented by the presence of C-peptide in the blood and decreased insulin requirements. However, evidence of allograft function lasted no longer than a few weeks prior to probable islet rejection in these patients, in whom there was no significant increase in immunosuppression. Further technical improvements have since been made by the St. Louis group, who now believe that their islet yield has been increased to 60% to 80% in some instances.[2] Viability of their human isolated islets has been substantiated by in vitro glucose challenge.

In summary, convincing documentation that diabetes has actually been completely reversed for a meaningful period of time has not been shown in a single human islet allograft recipient. Nevertheless, it appears that substantial progress in human islet isolation techniques has recently occurred, and adequate islet tissue may soon be available to test whether current immunosuppression can safely prevent islet rejection. If not, animal experiments indicate that further improvements in purification of islets may eventually allow techniques for pretransplant modification of islet tissue to be used to diminish immunogenicity and allow successful transplantation, possibly even without immunosuppression.

Islet Autotransplant

Islet autotransplantation has been used by several investigators in an attempt to prevent the diabetes that usually follows total or near-total pancreatectomy.[121,123] This technique should not be considered in cases of malignant disease, since tumor might be implanted, and it would rarely be necessary for pancreatic trauma, since only 10% of a pancreatic remnant is needed to prevent diabetes. Thus, the indication for autotransplantation exists only in patients undergoing pancreatectomy for the unrelenting pain of chronic pancreatitis. Seventy-nine such patients were reported to the islet registry as of 1984.[121] Many of these transplants were done by groups that had previous experience with islet allotransplantation, using the same technique. The transplant site was the portal vein in most instances. Knowing the poor results of islet allotransplanta-

tion, one might have predicted little success with this procedure. In fact, about half of the patients were reported to be insulin-independent after the transplant, perhaps suggesting that rejection plays a very significant part in the unsuccessful allograft experience. In several of the autograft patients, a total pancreatectomy had been done, proving that the transplanted islets were responsible for preventing diabetes. But, in most instances, the unresected pancreatic remnant (roughly estimated as 5%, but no doubt exceeding this in some instances) is likely to be providing some of the insulin and is partly or totally responsible for insulin independence.

Pancreatic autotransplantation is not without significant risks, and at least three patients have died as a result.[69,124] Infusion of nonpurified, enzymatically active, dispersed pancreas into the portal vein can lead to portal hypertension, systemic hypotension, portal vein occlusion, and disseminated intravascular coagulation. Thus, islet autotransplantation will probably continue to carry significant risk until human islet isolation procedures are perfected and sufficient numbers of very pure islets can be extracted from a single pancreas to prevent diabetes.

Also disquieting is the possibility of late failure of initially successful islet autografts. In a substantial proportion of patients who initially appear to have functioning islet autografts (and are off insulin), the onset of diabetes has occurred after several months.[124]

REFERENCES

1. Akimaru GM, Stuhmiller GM, Seigler HF: Autotransplantation of insulinoma into the testis of diabetic rats. Transplantation 32:227, 1981
2. Alderson D, Ineteman NM, Scharp DW: The isolation of purified human islets of Langerhans. Diabetes 35:81(A), 1986
3. Alejandro R, Cutfield R, Shienvold FL et al: Successful long-term survival of pancreatic islet allografts in spontaneous or pancreatectomy-induced diabetes in dogs. Cyclosporine-induced immune unresponsiveness. Diabetes 34:825, 1985
4. Alejandro R, Russell E, Kyriakides G et al: Islet cell transplantation in patients with type I diabetes mellitus. Diabetes 35:139(A), 1986
5. Algiere GH, Weaver JM, Prehn RT: Growth of cells in vivo in diffusion chambers. I: Survival of homografts in immunizing mice. J Natl Cancer Inst 15:493, 1954
6. Baekkeskov S, Kanatsuna T, Klareskog L et al: Expression of major histocompatibility antigens in pancreatic islet cells. Proc Natl Acad Sci USA 78:6456, 1981

7. Ballinger WF, Lacy PE: Transplantation of intact pancreatic islets in rats. Surgery 72:175, 1972
8. Barker CF: Transplantation of islets of Langerhans and the histocompatibility of endocrine tissue. Diabetes 24:766, 1975
9. Barker CF, Billingham RE: The role of the lymphatic system in the rejection of skin homografts. J Exp Med 128:197, 1968
10. Barker CF, Billingham RE: Comparison of fates of Ag-B locus compatible homografts of the skin and heart in inbred rats. Nature 225:851, 1970
11. Barker CF, Billingham RE: Analysis of local anatomic factors that influence the survival time of pure epidermal and full thickness homografts in guinea pigs. Ann Surg 176:597, 1972
12. Barker CF, Billingham RE: Immunologically privileged sites. Adv Immunol 25:1, 1977
13. Barker CF, Naji A: Pancreatic and islet cell transplantation. In Howard JM, Jordan GL, Reber HA (eds): Surgical Diseases of the Pancreas, p 912. Philadelphia, Lea & Febiger, 1987
14. Barker CF, Naji A, Silvers WK: Immunological prob-

lems in islet transplantation. Diabetes 29:86, 1980

15. Bartlett ST, Naji A, Silvers WK et al: Influence of culturing on the functioning of major-histocompatibility-complex-compatible and incompatible islet grafts in diabetic mice. Transplantation 36(Suppl 6):687, 1983

16. Bobzien B, Yasunami Y, Majercik M et al: Intratesticular transplants of islet xenografts (rat to mouse). Diabetes 32:213, 1983

17. Bowen KM, Andrus L, Lafferty KJ: Successful allotransplantation of mouse pancreatic islets to non-immunosuppressed recipients. Diabetes 29(Suppl 1):98, 1980

18. Brown J, Clark WF, Molnan G et al: Fetal pancreas transplantation for reversal of streptozotocin-induced diabetes in rats. Diabetes 25:56, 1976

19. Browning H, Resnik P: Homologous and heterologous transplantation of pancreatic tissue in normal and diabetic mice. Yale J Biol Med 24:141, 1951

20. Delmonico FL, Chase CM, Russell PS: Transplantation of rat islets of Langerhans into diabetic mice. Transplant Proc 9:367, 1977

21. Dibelius A, Konigsberger H, Walter P et al: Prolonged reversal of diabetes in the rat by transplantation of allogeneic islets from a single donor and cyclosporine treatment. Transplantation 41:426, 1986

22. Downing R: Historical review of pancreatic islet transplantation. World J Surg 8:137, 1984

23. Faustman D, Hauptfeld V, Davie M et al: Murine pancreatic beta cells express H-2 and H-2D but not Ia antigens. J Exp Med 151:1563, 1980

24. Faustman D, Hauptfeld V, Lacy PE et al: Prolongation of islet allograft survival by pretreatment of islets with antibody directed at Ia determinants. Proc Natl Acad Sci 78:5156, 1981

25. Faustman DL, Steinman RM, Gebel HM et al: Prevention of mouse islet allograft rejection by elimination of intraislet dendritic cells. Transplant Proc 17(No 1):420, 1985

26. Ferguson J, Scothorne RJ: Extended survival of pancreatic islet allografts in the testes of guinea pigs. J Anat 124:1, 1977

27. Finch DRA, Morris PJ: The effect of increasing islet numbers on survival of pancreatic islet allografts in immunosuppressed diabetic rats. Transplantation 23:104, 1977

28. Finch DRA, Wise PH, Morris PJ: Successful intrasplenic transplantation of syngeneic and allogeneic isolated pancreatic islets. Diabetologia 13(3):195, 1977

29. Frangipane LG, Barker CF, Silvers WK: Importance of weak histocompatibility factors in survival of pancreatic islet transplants. Surg Forum 28:294, 1977

30. Frangipane LG, Poole TW, Barker CF: Vulnerability of allogeneic and xenogeneic islets to alloantisera. Transplant Proc 9:371, 1977

31. Franklin WA, Schulak JA, Reckard CR: The fate of transplanted pancreatic islets in the rat. Am J Pathol 94:85, 1979

32. Futrell JW, Albright NL, Myers GH Jr: Prevention of

33. Gates RJ, Hunt MI, Smith R et al: Return to normal of blood glucose plasma insulin and weight gain in New Zealand obese mice after implantation of islets of Langerhans. Lancet II:567, 1972

34. Georgiou HM, Mandel TE: Pancreatic islet transplantation across partial major histocompatibility complex barriers. Transplant Proc XVII (Suppl 2):1723, 1985

35. Gores PF, Sutherland DER, Platt JL et al: Elimination of Ia-positive cells does not influence islet allograft survival of the renal subcapsular position. Surg Forum 36:326, 1986

36. Gotoh M, Maki T, Kiyoizumi T: An improved method for isolation of mouse pancreatic islets. Transplantation 40(4):437, 1985

37. Gray BN, Watkins E: Prolonged relief from diabetes after syngeneic or allogeneic transplantation of isolated pancreatic islets in rats. Surg Forum 15:382, 1974

38. Gray DWR, Morris PF: Cyclosporine and pancreas transplantation. World J Surg 8:230, 1985

39. Groth CG, Andersson A, Bjorken C et al: Attempts at transplantation of fetal pancreas to diabetic patients. Transplant Proc 12(Suppl 2):208, 1980

40. Gunnarsson R, Klintmalm G, Lundgren G et al: Deterioration in glucose metabolism in pancreatic transplant recipients after conversion from azathioprine to cyclosporine. Transplant Proc XVI(Suppl 3):709, 1984

41. Hahn HJ, Laube F, Lucke S et al: Toxic effects of cyclosporine on the endocrine pancreas of Wistar rats. Transplantation 41:44, 1986

42. Hamilton MS, Billingham RE: Privileged status of the subcutaneous site for skin allografts in rats. Transplantation 28:199, 1979

43. Hardy MA, Reemtsma K, Lau HT: Induction of indefinite rat islet allograft survival with direct UV irradiation and peritransplant cyclosporine. Transplant Proc 17(No 1):423, 1985

44. Hegre, OD, Lazarow A: Islet cell transplantation. In Volk BW, Wellman, KF (eds): The Diabetic Pancreas, p 517. New York, Plenum Press, 1977

45. Helmchen U, Schmidt WE, Siegel EG et al: Morphological and functional changes of pancreatic B cells in Cyclosporin A-treated rats. Diabetologia 27:416, 1984

46. Kemp CB, Knight MJ, Scharp DW et al: Effect of transplantation site on the results of pancreatic islets in diabetic rats. Diabetologia 9:486, 1973

47. Kindahl-Kiessling K, Safwenberg J: Inability of UV irradiated lymphocytes to stimulate allogeneic cells in mixed lymphocyte culture. Int Arch Allergy 41:670, 1971

48. Knazek RA, Gullino PM, Kohler PO et al: Cell culture on artificial capillaries: An approach to tissue growth in vitro. Science 178:65, 1972

49. Kojima Y, Sandler A, Andersson A: Cyclosporine in-

tumor growth in an "immunologically privileged site" by adoptive transfer of tumor-specific transplantation immunity. J Surg Res 12:62, 1972

hibits mouse islet cell replication. Transplant Proc XVII:37, 1986

50. Kolb E, Largaiader F: Transplantation of pancreatic microfragments in patients with juvenile diabetes. In Bretzol R, Federlin K, Schatz H (eds): Proceedings of 1980 Giessen Workshops on Islet Transplantation Culture and Cryopreservation. Stuttgart, Thieme, 1981

51. Kramp RC, Congdon CC, Smith LH: Isogeneic and allogeneic transplantation of duct-ligated pancreas in streptozotocin diabetic mice. Eur J Clin Invest 5:249, 1975

52. Kretschmer GJ, Sutherland DER, Matas AJ et al: Autotransplantation of pancreatic islets without separation of exocrine and endocrine tissue in totally pancreatectomized dogs. Surgery 82:74, 1977

53. Kretschmer GJ, Sutherland DER, Matas AJ et al: The dispersed pancreas: Transplantation without islet purification in totally pancreatectomized dogs. Diabetologia 13:495, 1977

54. Lacy PE: Experimental immunoalteration. World J Surg 8:198, 1984

55. Lacy PE, Kostianovsky M: Method for the isolation of intact islets of Langerhans from the rat pancreas. Diabetes 16:35, 1967

56. Lacy PE, Davie JM, Finke EH: Prolongation of islet xenograft survival without continuous immunosuppression. Science 209:174, 1980

57. Lau H, Reemtsma K, Hardy MA: Pancreatic islet allograft prolongation by donor-specific blood transfusion treated with ultraviolet irradiation. Science 221:754, 1983

58. Lau H, Reemtsma K, Hardy MA: Prolongation of rat islet allograft survival by direct ultraviolet irradiation of the graft. Science 223:607, 1984

59. Lim F, Sun AM: Microencapsulated islets as bioartificial endocrine pancreas. Science 210:908, 1980

60. Linder OEA: Comparisons between survival of grafted skin, ovaries and tumors in mice across histocompatibility of different strengths. J Natl Cancer Inst 27:351, 1961

61. Long JA, Adair WF, Scharp DW: An immunological approach to islet cell purification. J Cell Biol 95:4061, 1982

62. Mandel TE: Transplantation of organ-culture fetal panacreas: Experimental studies and potential clinical application in diabetes mellitus. World J Surg 8:158, 1984

63. Markmann JF, Silvers WK, Barker CF et al: Influence of donor-specific erythrocyte transfusion on the survival of rat islet allografts. Transplant Proc XVII(1):1101, 1985

64. Marquet RL, Heysteck GA: The effect of immunosuppressive treatment on the survival of allogeneic islets of Langerhans in rats. Transplantation 20:428, 1975

65. Matas, AJ, Sutherland, DER, Steffes MW et al: Short-term culture of adult pancreas fragments for purification and transplantation of islets of Langerhans. Surgery 80:183, 1976

66. Matas AJ, Sutherland DER, Steffes MW et al: Islet transplantation using neonatal rat pancreata: Quantitative studies. J Surg Res 20:143, 1976

67. Mauer SM, Sutherland DER, Steffes MW et al: Pancreatic islet transplantation: Effects on the glomerular lesions of experimental diabetes in the rat. Diabetes 23:748, 1974

68. McEvoy RC, Leung PE: Transplantation of fetal rat islets into the cerebral ventricles of alloxan-diabetic rats. Amelioration of diabetes by syngeneic but not allogeneic islets. Diabetes 32:852, 1983

69. Mehigan DG, Ball WR, Zuidema GD et al: Disseminated intravascular coagulation and portal hypertension following pancreatic islet autotransplantation. Ann Surg 191:287, 1980

70. Mieng CJ, Smit JA: Autotransplantation of pancreatic tissue in totally pancreatectomized baboons. S Afr J Surg 16:19, 1978

71. Mirkovich V, Campiche M: Intrasplenic allotransplantation of canine pancreatic tissues. Maintenance of normoglycemia after total pancreatectomy. Eur Surg Res 9:173, 1977

72. Morris PJ, Finch DR, Garvey JF et al: Suppression of rejection of allogeneic islet tissue in the rat. Diabetes 29:107, 1980

73. Morzycka, M. Croker BP, Seigler HF et al: Evaluation of recurrent glomerulonephritis in kidney allografts. Am J Med 72:588, 1982

74. Naji A, Barker CF: The influence of histocompatibility and transplant site on parathyroid allograft survival. J Surg Res 20:261, 1976

75. Naji A, Barker CF: Relative vulnerability of isolated pancreatic islets. Parathyroid and skin allografts to cellular and humoral immunity. Transplant Proc 11:560, 1979

76. Naji A, Frangipane LG, Barker CF et al: The survival of H–Y incompatible endocrine grafts in mice and rats. Transplantation 31:145, 1981

77. Naji A, Reckard CR, Ziegler MM et al: Vulnerability of pancreatic islets to immune cells and serum. Surg Forum 26:459, 1975

78. Naji A, Silvers WK, Barker CF: Islet transplantation in spontaneously diabetic rats. Transplant Proc 13:826, 1981

79. Naji A, Silvers WK, Barker CF: Autoimmunity and type I (insulin-independent) diabetes mellitus. Transplantation 36:355, 1983

80. Naji A, Silvers WK, Bellgrau et al: Prevention of diabetes in rats by bone marrow transplantation. Ann Surg 194:328, 1981

81. Naji A, Silvers WK, Plotkin SA et al: Successful islet transplantation in spontaneous diabetes. Surgery 86(No 2):218, 1979

82. Nakkooda AF, Like AA, Chappel CI et al: The spontaneously diabetic Wistar rat: Metabolic and morphologic studies. Diabetes 26:100, 1979

83. Nash JR, Peters M, Bell PRF: Comparative survival of pancreatic islets, heart, kidney and skin allografts in rats with and without enhancement. Transplantation 24:70, 1977

84. Nelken D, Morse SI, Beyer MM et al: Prolonged survival of allotransplanted islet of Langerhans cells in the rat. Transplantation 22:74, 1976

85. O'Shea GM, Sun AM: Encapsulation of rat islets of Langerhans prolongs xenograft survival in diabetic mice. Diabetes 35(Suppl 1):325(A), 1986

86. Outzen HC, Leiter EH: Transplantation of pancreatic islets into cleared mammary fat pads. Transplantation 32:101, 1981

87. Panijananond P, Monaco AP: Enhancement of pancreatic islet allograft survival with ALS and donor bone marrow. Surg Forum 379, 1974

88. Parr EL: The absence of H-2 antigens from mouse pancreatic beta cells demonstrated by immunoferatin labelling. J Exp Med 150:1, 1979

89. Parr EL, Bowen KM, Lafferty KJ: Cellular changes in cultured mouse thyroid glands and islets of Langerhans. Transplantation 30:135, 1980

90. Payne WD, Sutherland DER, Matas AJ et al: DL-ethionine treatment of adult pancreatic donors: Amelioration of diabetes in multiple recipients with tissue from a single donor. Ann Surg 189:248, 1979

91. Perloff LJ, Naji A, Barker CF: Islet sensitivity to humoral antibody. Surg Forum 32:390, 1981

92. Perloff LJ, Naji A, Silvers WK et al: Whole pancreas vs isolated islet transplants: An immunological comparison. Surgery 88:222, 1980

93. Perloff LJ, Utiger RD, Barker CF: The thyroid graft: Influence of histocompatibility and transplant site on survival. Ann Surg 188:186, 1978

94. Pipeleers–Marichal M, Pipeleers DG, Cutler J et al: Metabolic and morphologic studies in intraportal transplanted rats. Diabetes 25:1041, 1976

95. Reckard CR, Barker CF: Transplantation of isolated pancreatic islets across strong and weak histocompatibility barriers. Transplant Proc 5:761, 1973

96. Reckard CR, Franklin W, Schulack JA: Intrasplenic vs intraportal pancreatic islet transplants: Quantitative, qualitative and immunological aspects. Trans Am Soc Artif Intern Organs 24:232, 1978

97. Reckard CR, Stuart FF, Schulak JA: Immunologic comparisons of isolated pancreatic islets and whole organ allografts. Transplant Proc 11:563, 1979

98. Reckard CR, Ziegler MM, Barker CF: Physiological and immunological consequences of transplanting isolated pancreatic islets. Surgery 74:91, 1973

99. Reckard CR, Ziegler MM, Naji A et al: Physiological immunological status of long functioning transplanted pancreatic islets in the rat. Surg Forum 25:374, 1974

100. Reece–Smith H, DuToit DF, McShane P et al: Prolonged survival of pancreatic islet allografts transplanted beneath the renal capsule. Transplantation 31:305, 1981

101. Reemtsma K: Experimental islet cell grafting: A transplantation model. Transplant Proc 2:513, 1970

102. Rynasiewicz JJ, Sutherland DER, Kowahara K et al: Cyclosporin A: Prolongation of segmental pancreatic and islet allograft function in rats. Transplant Proc 12:270, 1980

103. Scharp DW: Isolation and transplantation of islet tissue. World J Surg 8:143, 1984

104. Scharp DW, Lacy PE, Santiago JV et al: Clinical islet transplantation: A report of six allografts and one autograft. (in press)

105. Scharp DW, Lacy PE, Alderson D et al: The procurement and distribution of cadaver human pancreas for islet isolation and transplantation. National Diabetes Research Interchange Proceedings of the Second Int'l Conference: The use of human tissues and organs for research and transplant, p 61, October 2–4, 1985

106. Scharp DW, Murphy JJ, Newton WT et al: Transplantation of islets of Langerhans of diabetic Rhesus monkeys. Surgery 77:100–105, 1975

107. Schulak JA, Franklin W, Reckard CR: Morphological and functional changes following intraportal islet allograft rejection: Irreversibility with steroid pulse therapy. Surg Forum 28:296, 1977

108. Schulak JA, Reckard CR: Experimental transplantation of pancreatic islet allografts. J Surg Res 25:562–571, 1978

109. Selawry HP, Whittington: Extended allograft survival of islets grafted into intra-abdominally placed testis. Diabetes 33:405–406, 1984

110. Sibley RK, Sutherland DER, Goetz F et al: Recurrent diabetes mellitus in the pancreas iso- and allograft. Lab Invest 53:132, 1985

111. Simeonovic CJ, Agostino M, Lafferty KJ: Control of diabetes: Comparative immunogenecity and function of fetal pancreas and isolated islets. Transplant Proc XVI(No 4):1064–1065, 1984

112. Simeonovic CJ, Wilson JD, Hegre OD et al: Reversal of diabetes by proislet isotransplantation. Transplant Proc XVII(Suppl 2):1728–1730, 1985

113. Slijepcevic M, Heline K, Federlin K: Islet transplantation in experimental diabetes in the rat. II. Studies in allogeneic streptozotocin treated rats. Horm Metab Res 7:456–461, 1975

114. Spence RK, Perloff LJ, Barker CF: The role of the implant site in rat fetal pancreas transplantation. Trans Am Soc Artif Intern Organs 23:352–357, 1977

115. Spence RK, Perloff LJ, Barker CF: Fetal pancreas in treatment of experimental diabetes in rats. Transplant Proc 11:533–536, 1979

116. Steinman RM, Witmer MD: Lymphoid dendritic cells are potent stimulators of the primary mixed leukocyte reaction in mice. Proc Natl Acad Sci USA 75:5132, 1978

117. Steinmuller D: Immunization with skin isografts taken from tolerant mice. Science 158:127–129, 1967

118. Strautz RL: Studies of hereditary-obese mice (ob/ob) after implantation of pancreatic islets in Millipore filter capsules. Diabetologia 6:306–312, 1970

119. Sutherland DER: Pancreas and islet transplantation. I. Experimental studies. Diabetologia 20:161–185, 1981

120. Sutherland DER: Pancreas and islet transplantation. II. Clinical trials. Diabetologia 20:435–450, 1981

121. Sutherland DER, Kendall D: Clinical pancreas and islet transplant registry report. Transplant Proc XVII(No 1):307–311, 1985

122. Sutherland DER, Kretschmer GJ, Matas AJ et al: Experience with auto and allotransplantation of pancreatic fragments to the spleen of totally pancreatectomized dogs. Trans Am Soc Intern Organs 23:723, 1977

123. Sutherland DER, Matas AJ, Goetz FC et al: Transplantation of dispersed pancreatic tissue in humans: Autografts and allografts. Diabetes 29(Suppl 1):10–18, 1980

124. Sutherland DER, Najarian JS: Pancreas and islet transplantation. In Brooks JR Jr (ed): Surgery of the Pancreas, pp 334–469. Philadelphia, WB Saunders, 1983

125. Sutherland DER, Najarian JS, Greenberg BZ et al: Hormonal and metabolic effects of an endocrine graft: Vascularized segmental transplantation of the pancreas in insulin-dependent patients. Ann Intern Med 95:537, 1981

126. Talmage DW: Effect of oxygen, temperature, and time of culture on the survival of mouse thyroid and pancreas allografts. Diabetes 29(Suppl 1):105–106, 1979

127. Tchobroutrky G: Relation of diabetic control to development of microvascular complications. Diabetologia 15:143–152, 1978

128. Terasaka R, Lacy PE, Hauptfeld V et al: The effect of Cyclosporin A, low-temperature culture, and anti-Ia antibodies on prevention of rejection of rat islet allografts. Diabetes 35:83–88, 1985

129. Tilney NL, Gowans JL: The sensitization of rats by allografts transplanted to alymphatic pedicles of skin. J Exp Med 133:951–962, 1971

130. Toldeo-Pereyra LH, Bandlien KO, Gordon DA et al: Renal subcapsular islet cell transplantation. Diabetes 33:910–914, 1984

131. Tze WJ, Tai J: Successful intracerebral allotransplantation of purified pancreatic endocrine cells in diabetes rat. Diabetes 32:1185–1187, 1983

132. Tze WJ, Wong FC, Chen LM et al: Implantable artificial endocrine pancreas unit used to restore normoglycemia in the diabetic rat. Nature 264:466–467, 1976

133. Usadel KH, Schwedes U, Lenacker U et al: Development of isologous transplants of cell suspensions of the fetal pancreas in the rat. Acta Endocrinol (Copenh) 84(Suppl 205):97, 1974

134. Valente U, Ferro M, Barocci S et al: Report of clinical cases of human fetal pancreas transplantation. Transplant Proc 12(Suppl)2:213–217, 1980

135. Vrobova H, Theodorosa NA, Tyhurst M et al: Transplantation of islets of Langerhans from pilocarpine-treated rats: A method of enhancing islet yield. Transplantation 28:433–435, 1979

136. Wachtel SS, Silvers WK: The role of passenger leukocytes in the anomalous survival of neonatal skin grafts in mice. J Exp Med 135:388–404, 1972

137. Weber CJ, Hardy MA, Pi-Sunyer FX et al: Tissue culture preservation and intramuscular transplantation of pancreatic islets. Surgery 84:166–174, 1978

138. Woehrle M, Markmann JF, Armstrong J et al: Subrenal capsule islet grafts are protected from rejection and autoimmune damage. Transplant Proc 19:925–927, 1987

139. Woehrle M, Markmann JF, Silvers WK et al: Effect of temperature of pretransplant culture on islet allografts in BB rats. Transplant Proc 18(6):1845–1847, 1986

140. Woehrle M, Markmann JF, Silvers WK et al: Transplantation of cultured pancreatic islets to BB rats. Surgery 100(2):334–340, 1986

141. Yasunami Y, Lacy PE, Finke EH: A new site for islet transplantation—a peritoneal-omental pouch. Transplantation 36(2):181–182, 1983

142. Ziegler MM, Reckard CR, Barker CF: Long-term metabolic and immunological considerations in transplantation of pancreatic islets. J Surg Res 16:575–581, 1974

143. Ziegler MM, Reckard CR, Naji A et al: Extended function of isolated pancreatic islet isografts and allografts. Transplant Proc 7:743–745, 1975

144. Zitron IM, Ono J, Lacy PE et al: Active suppression in the maintenance of pancreatic islet allografts. Transplantation 32:156–158, 1981

CHAPTER 38

Heart–Lung Transplantation

William H. Frist   Stuart W. Jamieson

Potential recipients typically have advanced pulmonary disease, incapacitating symptoms, and functional disability not amenable to conventional medical or surgical therapy. Potential donors are younger than 35 years of age and must manifest no evidence of cardiac or pulmonary disease.

The most challenging technical aspect of the operation is excision of the recipient heart and lungs. Maintenance of the integrity of the phrenic, vagus, and recurrent laryngeal nerves and meticulous attention to hemostasis of the mediastinal and collateral circulation are essential. Implantation of the heart and lungs is performed with sequential tracheal, right atrial, and aortic anastomoses.

Postoperative care demands rapid diuresis and optimization of function of the denervated lungs. Suppression of the immune response is achieved with cyclosporine, azathioprine, and steroids, the latter withheld for the first 2 weeks after surgery to optimize healing.

Rejection of the heart and lungs may occur asynchronously, and each must be monitored independently, the former with percutaneous transvenous endomyocardial biopsy, and the latter with chest radiographs, arterial book gases, body temperature, and white blood cell count.

The current actuarial 1-year survival for all centers combined is 58%. Thirty-one combined heart–lung transplants have been performed at Stanford, with the longest survivor almost 5 years after transplantation. In this series, actuarial survival predicts a 1-year survival of 62%, and a 3-year survival of 54%. Although still early in its evolutionary history, combined heart–lung transplantation offers the first effective treatment for what until recently has been considered untreatable disease.

In March 1981, the first successful combined heart–lung transplantation was performed in a 45-year-old woman with primary pulmonary hypertension at Stanford University Medical Center. The initiation of a clinical heart–lung program at Stanford was prompted by the refinement of surgical and immunosuppressant techniques in the laboratory in primates and by the encouraging recent experience with cyclosporine.[21] This drug was investigated in the Stanford laboratories in 1978 and used in the clinical cardiac transplantation program in 1980.[12,20] By January 1986, more than 100 patients throughout the world had undergone cardiopulmonary transplantation. One third of these transplants have been performed at Stanford, the other major programs being those at Pittsburgh and Harefield Hospital in England.

The selection criteria for the recipient and donor, the intricacies of the operation, the unique features of postoperative care, and the concept of pulmonary rejection have all undergone revision as clinical experience has been gained. In this chapter, we review the current state of cardiopulmonary transplantation, including preoperative selection, operative technique, postoperative care, results, current problems, and future directions.

HISTORICAL BACKGROUND

Although attempts to transplant the heart and lungs into the neck were made as early as 1907,[5] the earliest successful investigations of combined heart–lung transplantation were those of Demikhov,[10] who, in the late 1940s and early 1950s, attached the donor dog's heart and lungs in parallel with the recipient's organs, later excluding the recipient's heart and lung. Demikhov achieved survival of more than 5 days in 2 of 67 animals, with most deaths attributed to bronchopneumonia in the lower lobes, thrombosis of blood vessels at the anastomotic sites, and an abnormal respiratory pattern generated by denervation of the lungs. These remarkable investigations, performed without the benefits of hypothermia or cardiopulmonary bypass, demonstrated the technical feasibility of combined heart and lung transplantation.

Other early studies were also performed in dogs. In 1953, survival for 6 hours in dogs who underwent heart–lung transplantation using circulatory arrest and central cooling was achieved.[19] Four years later, others increased the survival to 22 hours.[25] In these investigations, the airway anastomoses were performed at the bronchial level. In 1961, 6-day survival was achieved using the simplified (and currently clinically applied) technique of tracheal rather than bronchial anastomosis.[17] Denervation of the lungs with consequent disruption of the respiratory pattern appeared to be the common underlying fatal phenomenon in all these early investigations.

Within several years, however, an important species difference in respiratory function following loss of pulmonary innervation was reported.[11,18] Primates, unlike the dog and other species, were able to maintain a normal respiratory pattern in spite of pulmonary denervation. Spontaneous respiration, apparently regulated by the midbrain, is preserved. Subsequently, in 1972, with autotransplantation in baboons, 2-year survival in 5 of 25 animals was reported.[6,7] The first long-term survivors after cardiopulmonary allografting in primates were reported by the Stanford group in 1980.[21] In this series of experiments, 27 monkeys underwent heart–lung transplantation, with postoperative cyclosporine immunosuppression, and most survived for several months. One of these monkeys remains alive today, 6 years after transplantation of the heart and lungs, and is the longest living recipient of such transplantation. These pioneering experimental investigations underscored the technical feasibility of cardiopulmonary transplantation and demonstrated long-term survival.

The early clinical experience of cardiopulmonary transplantation was disappointing. In 1968, Cooley and associates[9] attempted the first such procedure in a 2-month-old infant with a complete atrioventricular canal defect; the patient died 14 hours after surgery. A year later, Lillehei[16] performed the second procedure in a 43-year-old patient with emphysema and pulmonary hypertension; the patient died 8 days later of pneumonia. A third operation was performed in Cape Town on a 49-year-old patient with chronic obstructive disease, bronchiectasis, and cor pulmonale. The patient developed necrosis of the bronchial anastomoses and died on the twenty-third day.[1]

The first successful transplantation, performed at Stanford University Medical Center, was not carried out until a decade later. During this time, significant advances had been made in the field of clinical orthotopic heart transplantation, including the endomyocardial biopsy technique for the diagnosis of rejection, techniques for monitoring immunologic status, and the introduction of rabbit anti-thymocyte globulin.[2,3,8] The final stage for embarking on a clinical cardiopulmonary transplant program was set with the emergence of cyclosporine as a powerful immunosuppressant agent, which permitted the deletion of perioperative steroids, thereby improving the likelihood for tracheal anastomotic healing.[4]

In March 1981, the clinical program in combined heart–lung transplantation at Stanford was initiated, and, since that time, more than 30 such transplants have been performed at this center.

THE RECIPIENT

Indications for Transplantation

Indications for heart–lung transplantation and the criteria for recipient selection vary from center to center, although uniformly the recipient has advanced pulmonary disease, incapacitating symptoms, and functional disability not amenable to conventional medical or surgical therapy. At Stanford, transplantation has been specifically restricted to two groups of patients with end-stage pulmonary vascular disease: (1) those with primary (idiopathic) pulmonary hypertension, and (2) those with congenital heart disease and Eisenmenger's syndrome (secondary pulmonary hypertension). Several factors suggest that patients with these disease entities are those most likely to benefit from the procedure. The patients are usually young, and the tracheobronchial tree is generally sterile. In both conditions, the lung and the heart are damaged to some degree, and other organs are generally only secondarily (and reversibly) involved. In addition, the likelihood of recurrence of the original disease in the transplanted organs is small.

There are, however, a variety of other disorders that might be considered indications for transplantation, including end-stage chronic obstructive pulmonary disease, cystic fibrosis, fibrosing alveolitis, pulmonary fibrosis secondary to irradiation or medicines, and idiopathic pulmonary fibrosis. In addition to primary pulmonary hypertension and Eisenmenger's syndrome, patients with cystic fibrosis, eosinophilic granuloma of the lung, and emphysema have received transplants. However, patients with chronic debilitating diseases of the lung should be considered less than ideal candidates because of frequently associated malnutrition or distortion of thoracic anatomy or both.

Selection of the Recipient

General criteria for prospective recipients are consistent with those applied to orthotopic cardiac transplantation. Elderly and severely debilitated patients are not suitable candidates. In-depth psychosocial evaluation should identify features that may limit or preclude rehabilitation after transplantation, especially with regard to compliance to a strict, lifelong medical regimen.

Contraindications include previous cardiac or thoracic surgery (because of the increased risk of intraoperative hemorrhage), insulin-dependent diabetes, active infection, or any systemic disease that might independently limit survival, such as malignancy. The associated renal and hepatic toxicity of cyclosporine dictate that patients with a bilirubin of more than 3.5 mg/dl or a significantly diminished creatinine clearance should not be considered for surgery.

Within these rather rigid criteria, there exists latitude for acceptance, depending upon the absolute supply of donors compared with the number of optimal candidates.

SELECTION OF THE DONOR

The principal limitation to expanding heart–lung transplantation is the scarcity of donors. Although, at Stanford, all cardiac donors are initially considered as potential heart–lung donors, fewer than 10% qualify because of associated pulmonary morbidity. Brain death is frequently associated with factors that adversely affect the respiratory system, including neurogenic pulmonary edema, thoracic trauma, aspiration of gastric contents, and pulmonary infection, the latter often a product of inadequate pulmonary toilet during prolonged ventilation. Currently, at Stanford, potential donors must be younger than 35 years of age and have no history of pre-existing cardiac or pulmonary disease. ABO blood group compatibility and a negative lymphocyte crossmatch (lack of cytotoxic effect of recipient's serum on donor lymphocytes) are required.

The chest roentgenogram must be clear, with no evidence of pulmonary contusion or infection. The donor's weight and height must be reasonably matched with those of the recipient. Mismatch of donor lung and recipient thoracic cavity size may cause compression of pulmonary parenchyma, atelectasis, and arteriovenous shunting, all of which might contribute to infection in the immunocompromised host. Available cultures and the appearance of the sputum must confirm no evidence of ongoing infection. The potential donor must demonstrate adequate gas exchange and pulmonary compliance, with an ability to maintain a PaO_2 of more than a 100 mm Hg on 40% inspired oxygen, with peak inspiratory pressures of less than 30 mm Hg at normal tidal volumes.

Cardiac assessment involves a normal electrocardiogram (ECG) and myocardial function sufficient to maintain adequate systemic perfusion without high-dose inotropic support at a central venous pressure of less than 12 mm Hg. Physical examination should reveal no murmurs or gallops, and a chest roentgenogram should demonstrate a normal cardiac silhouette. Intraoperative inspection must reveal normal contractility, absence of thrills, and no palpable coronary lesions.

Careful donor management is critical to the overall success of the procedure. In addition to the usual guidelines of donor management for orthotopic heart transplantation, critical and aggressive attention from the outset must be directed toward protection of the lungs from infection, atelectasis, gastric aspiration, and the complication of neurogenic pulmonary edema.

OPERATIVE TECHNIQUE

The Donor Operation

Until recently, preservation of explanted lungs for periods of more than an hour was unreliable, and the donor and recipient operations were performed at the same center. The donor procedure does not require cardiopulmonary bypass, although the Harefield group have recently used this as a method of cooling the heart and lungs so as to allow long-distance transport.

After excision of all thymic tissue and complete pericardiectomy, including both phrenic nerves, the descending aorta, the innominate artery, and superior and inferior venae cavae are mobilized, and the azygos vein is divided. The trachea is dissected in a limited fashion, with care taken to preserve the peritracheal vascular and lymphatic tissue in the supracarinal region. Important collaterals that contribute to healing of the tracheal anastomosis lie in the areolar tissue between the left atrium and carina.

The donor is heparinized. The superior vena cava is doubly ligated and divided, the inferior vena cava is divided, the aorta is crossclamped, and the tip of the left atrial appendage is amputated to decompress the left side of the heart. Cold hyperkalemic cardioplegia is infused into the aortic root, and 1.5 liters of cold modified Collins' solution (high osmolality and high potassium) are infused into the pulmonary artery at a pressure of 20 mm Hg during gentle ventilation (with unwarmed room air) to promote adequate distribution. Cold topical saline is applied to the heart.

The aorta is divided at the level of the innominate artery, and the trachea is clamped as high as possible and divided above the clamp. The heart and lungs are removed en bloc by dividing the posterior pleural reflections and pulmonary ligaments and then placed into cold Ringer's solution and transported to the recipient operating room for implantation.

Recipient Operation

Excision of the Recipient Organs

The most challenging technical aspect of cardiopulmonary transplantation is excision of the recipient heart and lungs. Although it is possible to remove the heart and lungs en bloc, visualization of the nerves and vessels is markedly improved by excising first the heart and then each lung separately.[13] Maintenance of the integrity of the phrenic, vagus, and recurrent laryngeal nerves is vital to the preservation of adequate ventilatory mechanics postoperatively in the denervated lung, return of satisfactory gastrointestinal function, and protection of the airway from aspiration. Meticulous attention to hemostatic control of the mediastinal and bronchial collateral circulation, usually large and friable in patients with Eisenmenger's syndrome, is also essential.

After median sternotomy and pericardiotomy, thymic fat is excised, and the left and right pleural cavities are entered through the anterior pleuropericardial reflections. Accessible adhesions are divided with the electrocautery prior to heparinization. The aorta is cannulated adjacent to the innominate artery, and the superior and inferior venae cavae are each cannulated through the sinus venosus aspect of the right atrium. Total cardiopulmonary bypass and systemic cooling are initiated.

The heart is excised in a fashion similar to orthotopic heart transplantation, with the aorta transected at its sinus ridge, the pulmonary artery at its midpoint, and the atria at the atrioventricular junction. A cuff of right atrium is preserved for anastomosis to the donor heart.

Bilateral longitudinal incisions are made in the pleuropericardium parallel to the phrenic nerves, such that a broad ribbon of pericardium containing each nerve and its blood supply is preserved (Fig. 38-1). The left atrium is divided longitudinally through the oblique sinus, so that the right and left pulmonary veins are separated. The left pulmonary veins and atrial segment can then be drawn out beneath the pericardial ribbon, although care must be taken in this dissection to preserve the vagus nerves, lying immediately posterior. Division of the pulmonary ligament, pulmonary artery, and left main bronchus now allows removal of the left lung. A similar technique is used on the right. The remaining structures to be removed are the right and left main bronchi and the remnants of the pulmonary artery. A rim of pulmonary artery at the level of the ductus is left undisturbed to avoid possible recurrent laryngeal nerve injury. The remaining stumps of the right and left bronchi are removed after transection of the trachea just above the carina.

Dissection in the region of the trachea is minimized to preserve local blood supply and to avoid disturbance of the vagus nerve plexus adjacent to the esophagus. After evisceration of the organs, absolute hemostasis of the hilar regions and posterior mediastinum must be achieved because of the inaccessibility of these regions after implantation of the donor organs.

Implantation

Implantation is achieved by sequential tracheal, right atrial, and aortic anastomoses[7] each constructed with continuous polypropylene sutures (Figs. 38-2–38-4). The donor trachea is trimmed to within one or two cartilages above the carina, and the entire heart–lung specimen is positioned in the chest cavity, with the right lung passed beneath the recipient right atrial cuff and phrenic nerve pedicle, and the left lung passed beneath the left phrenic nerve pedicle. A curvilinear incision, which extends from the posterolateral aspect of the inferior vena caval orifice to the base of the right atrial appendage, is made to avoid the region of the sinoatrial node. Myocardial protection is enhanced by continuous topical application of cold saline.

After construction of the three anastomoses, ventilation is begun with 40% oxygen, routine deairing maneuvers are performed, the crossclamp is removed, and the heart is resuscitated. After re-

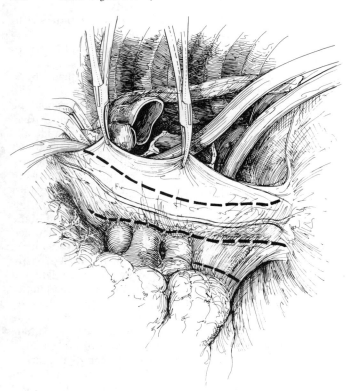

FIGURE 38-1.   *The pericardium is incised 3 cm anterior and 3 cm posterior to the right phrenic nerve. The phrenic nerve on the right lies closer to the hilum than that on the left. (Reproduced with permission from Jamieson SW: Transplantation. In Jamieson SW, Shumway NE (eds): Operative Surgery—Volume on Cardiac Surgery. Stoneham, MA, Butterworth Publishers, 1986.)*

warming, cardiopulmonary bypass is discontinued, and an isoproterenol infusion is titrated to maintain a heart rate of 100 beats per minute. Drainage tubes are placed in the pericardial and pleural cavities, and the chest is closed.

Operative Techniques

The intricacies of operative technique have been continually refined as experience has been gained with the procedure. Early in the Stanford experience, three patients sustained injuries to nerves in the mediastinum. Modifications in surgical technique, including retention of the rim of pulmonary artery in the region of the left recurrent laryngeal nerve, construction of broad ribbons of pericardium containing the phrenic nerves, and minimization of overall dissection, all substantially reduce the likelihood of injury.

Postoperative bleeding, a major cause of morbidity in most programs, may be minimized by insistence on absolute hemostasis of the posterior mediastinum before implantation of the heart–lung block and exclusion of potential recipients who have undergone previous major intrathoracic procedures.

IMMEDIATE POSTOPERATIVE CARE AND IMMUNOSUPPRESSION

After arrival in the intensive care unit, the patients are isolated, and strict sterile precautions are taken. Otherwise, they are generally treated in a fashion similar to other cardiac surgical patients. Initially ventilated with a volume ventilator, patients are maintained on the lowest possible concentration of inspired oxygen to maintain a PaO_2 of 80 mm Hg to 100 mm Hg and are commonly extubated on the first postoperative day. Secretions are mobilized from the tracheobronchial tree by postural percussion physiotherapy and frequent coughing and deep-breathing exercises. The entire heart and lung block is without any type of neural connection; the direct bronchial-arterial blood supply and lymphatic drainage has also been interrupted. The loss of these connections causes surprisingly little functional disruption. Patients resume spontaneous and rhythmic breathing immediately postoperatively.

Chest radiographs are obtained at least daily for the first 2 weeks. Prophylactic broad-spectrum antibiotics are continued for 48 hours or until mediastinal and pleural tubes have been removed. Low-dose isoproterenol is maintained after surgery

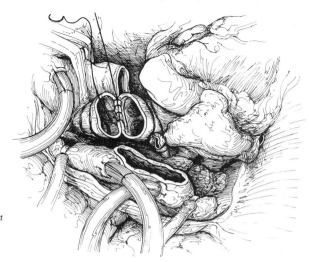

FIGURE 38-2. *The tracheal anastomosis is constructed immediately above the carina. (Reproduced with permission from Jamieson SW: Transplantation. In Jamieson SW, Shumway NE (eds): Operative Surgery—Volume on Cardiac Surgery. Stoneham, MA, Butterworth Publishers, 1986.)*

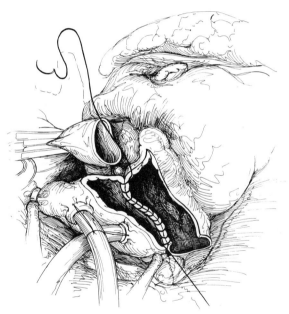

FIGURE 38-3. *After the tracheal anastomosis, the atrial anastomosis is performed. On the posterior aspect, all remnants of the left atrium and the intra-atrial groove are included in the suture line. (Reproduced with permission from Jamieson SW: Transplantation. In Jamieson SW, Shumway NE (eds): Operative Surgery—Volume on Cardiac Surgery. Stoneham, MA, Butterworth Publishers, 1986.)*

until the patient's heart rate is stabilized and cardiac output is satisfactory. In an effort to avert pulmonary edema, patients are rapidly diuresed to below preoperative weight.

Suppression of the immune response after cardiopulmonary transplantation is required indefinitely. Acute rejection episodes occur almost invar-

iably, with the highest frequency during the first 2 months. The use of cyclosporine and azathioprine as immunosuppressants permits avoidance of steroids during the first 2 post-transplant weeks, thereby promoting tissue healing, especially that of the tracheal anastomosis. Cyclosporine (18 mg/kg) is administered preoperatively and continued postoperatively in two divided doses (18 mg/kg/day initially), with dosages adjusted to maintain trough serum levels of 150 ng/ml to 200 ng/ml.

Methylprednisolone (500 mg) is given after discontinuation of cardiopulmonary bypass and (125 mg) is given every 8 hours for three doses. Steroids are then discontinued for a 2-week period, after which prednisone is initiated at 0.2 mg/kg/day. Azathioprine is administered at 1.5 mg/kg/day or adjusted to maintain a total white blood cell count of 3000 to 5000 cells/mm^2. Rabbit anti-thymocyte globulin (ATG) is given intramuscularly for the first 3 days to reduce the circulating thymic-derived lymphocyte population (as measured by the e-Rosette test) to less than 5%. Periodic surveillance cultures of blood, urine, and sputum are obtained. Postoperative fever or any suggestion of a pulmonary infiltrate demands aggressive evaluation, including transtracheal aspiration for stains and culture/sensitivities, to differentiate between infection, implantation response, and rejection.

POSTOPERATIVE COMPLICATIONS

Rejection

Although it was initially thought that significant pulmonary rejection would not occur without biopsy evidence of cardiac rejection, it is now clear

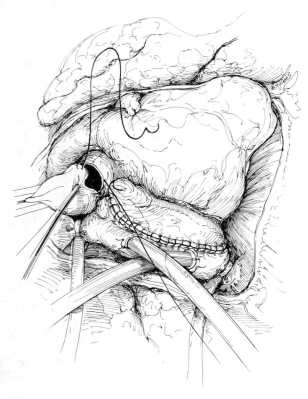

FIGURE 38-4. *The aortic anastomosis is performed with a single 4-0 polypropylene suture. (Reproduced with permission from Jamieson SW: Transplantation. In Jamieson SW, Shumway NE (eds): Operative Surgery—Volume on Cardiac Surgery. Stoneham, MA, Butterworth Publishers, 1986.)*

that the heart and lungs present two immunologically distinct axes, each subject to rejection.[15,22]

Percutaneous transvenous endomyocardial biopsy, the mainstay of the diagnosis of cardiac graft rejection, is performed routinely on a weekly basis for approximately 3 weeks or until two negative biopsies have been obtained. Cardiac rejection episodes during the first month are treated with methylprednisolone (1000 mg daily) for 3 days; after 1 month, rejection can be adequately treated with augmented oral steroids.

The ability to biopsy repetitively and safely the transplanted heart and thereby establish a definitive diagnosis of rejection has no parallel for the lungs. Thus, the true incidence of rejection of the lung in transplanted patients is not known. There are currently no clnically reliable techniques to document pulmonary rejection, and the diagnosis is made principally on clinical grounds. Differentiation from the implantation response and infection is vital. Manifestations of rejection include worsening infiltrate on chest radiograph, deteriorating arterial blood gases, low-grade fever, and elevated white blood cell count. Episodes of acute pulmonary rejection are treated with methylprednisolone (1000 mg daily) and rabbit ATG for 3 days.

As with cardiac transplantation, the frequency of rejection episodes is highest within the first 2 months after transplantation. Although slightly different immunosuppressive regimens are used for cardiac and cardiopulmonary transplantation, at Stanford, fewer rejection episodes have been observed in cardiopulmonary patients.

Implantation Response

The *implantation* response, a transient phenomenon that occurs most commonly between 4 and 21 days after transplantation, is a reversible defect in pulmonary gas exchange, loss of pulmonary compliance, and elevation of pulmonary vascular resistance coupled with roentgenographic interstitial edema.[14,23] This syndrome, initially termed the *reimplantation* response, is a phenomenon peculiar to the transplantation of pulmonary tissue, whether unilateral or combined with the cardiac graft.[24]

Typically, a patient will be extubated 24 to 48 hours after transplantation, and the chest roentgenogram will be clear. With the implantation response, the patient will become febrile and tachypneic, and a diffuse pulmonary infiltrate develops on chest radiograph. It is associated with a ventilation–perfusion mismatch and a marked fall in arterial Pao_2 and rise in Pco_2.

It is likely that the etiology is multifactorial, with lymphatic interruption, ischemia, denervation, and surgical trauma all contributing to the syndrome. It is important to differentiate this transient phenomenon, which has been observed in more than 80% of the patients in the Stanford series, from pulmonary infection and rejection because treatment for each is different yet vital to patient survival. In anticipation of this response, all patients are diuresed in the early postoperative period, with the goal of maintaining patient weight 2 kg to 3 kg below preoperative level. The syndrome lasts an average of 7 days and responds to chest physiotherapy and diuresis. Occasionally, endotracheal intubation and ventilation with positive airway pressure have been necessary for a short period of time while lung function recovers.

OUTPATIENT CARE

Patients are discharged after 4 to 8 weeks of hospitalization and are initially evaluated on a twice-weekly outpatient basis. The frequency of clinic visits decreases over time, and, ultimately, patients return home. Routine monitoring includes frequent chest radiographs, serial pulmonary function evaluation, and periodic endomyocardial biopsy. Patients return annually to Stanford for invasive cardiac evaluation and pulmonary evaluation. Immunosuppression is maintained indefinitely. Long-term survivors continue to sustain the risks of cardiac or pulmonary rejection, infectious complications associated with chronic immunosuppression, progressive restrictive or obstructive disease of the lung, and development of graft atherosclerosis. Therefore, they must remain under close medical supervision.

RESULTS

The international experience with heart—lung transplantation, as reported by the Registry of the International Society for Heart Transplantation, is shown in Table 38-1. The average age for these recipients was 31 years (range 8 months to 51 years). The 1-year and 2-year survival rates are 58% and 56%, respectively. The combined perioperative (30-day) mortality rate reported by all centers is 28%, although currently experienced centers report a much lower rate. Cause of death was infection in 71%, ventricular failure in 13%, acute rejection in 10%,

TABLE 38-1 *International Experience with Heart—Lung Transplants*

YEAR	NUMBER OF TRANSPLANTS
1981	5
1982	7
1983	16
1984	32
1985	47
1986	85
Total	192

Source: Registry of International Society for Heart Transplantation

and cardiac arrest in 6%. Current 1-year survival has improved to 68%.

Results at Stanford

As of March 1986, 31 combined heart—lung transplants had been performed in 30 recipients at Stanford (Table 38-2). Of these recipients, 15 presented with congenital heart disease and Eisenmenger's syndrome, 14 suffered from primary pulmonary hypertension, 1 had a cardiomyopathy and secondary pulmonary hypertension, and 1 had pulmonary hypertension as a result of repeated pulmonary emboli (diagnosed at operation). There were 12 women and 19 men, and the patients ranged in age from 22 to 46 years.

There have been 10 early deaths, defined as deaths within the initial hospitalization. Previous chest surgery or major pulmonary adhesions (as in the patient with repeated pulmonary emboli) is a substantial risk factor; 6 of the early deaths have been associated with bleeding from pulmonary adhesions. There have been 5 late deaths: the third patient in the series died from complications of appendicitis 44 months after transplantation, and 1 patient died 3 years after transplantation from progressive severe respiratory dysfunction before a second donor could be found. The other late death not previously reported was the nineteenth patient, who sustained severe pulmonary rejection on the third week postoperatively without evidence of cardiac rejection. Although he required reintubation, he survived this episode and made a good initial recovery. Shortly after discharge, he suffered progressive dyspnea related to respiratory obstructive disease, which could not be reversed with augmented immunotherapy. Repeated courses of steroid therapy eventually led to superinfection with cytomegalovirus (CMV) and pneumocystis, and he died 11 months after transplantation.

The remaining 15 recipients are alive. Total fol-

TABLE 38-2   Patient Data and Follow-Up

NO.	AGE (YR)	AGE OF DONOR	DIAGNOSIS	FOLLOW-UP (MONTHS)	OUTCOME
1.	46	15	pph	59	Alive
2.	39	21	E	57	Alive (re-tx at 37 months)
3.	28	22	E	0	Died 4 days
4.	40	19	E	44	Died 44 months
5.	37	30	pph	50	Alive
6.	26	15	pph	0	Died 23 days
7.	22	27	E	0	Died at operation
8.	40	23	E	39	Alive
9.	22	18	E	37	Died 37 months
10.	27	22	E	14	Died 14 months
11.	38	17	E	37	Alive
12.	32	32	E	15	Died 15 months
13.	33	21	pph	32	Alive
14.	28	15	pph	0	Died 15 days
15.	42	20	E	1	Died 23 days
16.	22	26	pph	27	Alive
17.	37	18	pph	26	Alive
18.	33	16	pph	22	Alive
19.	40	19	E	11	Died 11 months
20.	42	14	h-l tx	20	Alive
21.	20	21	pph	19	Alive
22.	31	25	pph	18	Alive
23.	37	20	E	0	Died 10 days
24.	34	25	E	0	Died 1 day
25.	43	18	pph	10	Alive
26.	24	23	pph	10	Alive
27.	29	18	PE	0	Died 13 days
28.	32	21	pph	7	Alive
29.	37	22	CM	0	Died 8 days
30.	30	27	E	0	Died 28 days
31.	25	17	pph	0	Alive

Abbreviations: M = male; F = female; pph = primary pulmonary hypertension; E = Eisenmenger's syndrome; h-l tx = heart–lung transplant (reoperation); PE = pulmonary embolus; CM = cardiomyopathy

low-up is now 556 patient-months, with the longest survivor now almost 5 years after transplantation. Actuarial survival predicts a 1-year survival rate of 62% ± 9.0% (± SEM), and a 2- and 3-year survival rate of 54% ± 9.5% for all patients. Comparable survival figures for simple cardiac transplantation recipients at this center over the same time period are 83% ± 3.0%, 74% ± 3.8%, and 69% ± 4.3%, respectively (Fig. 38-5).

Late Complications at Stanford

Systemic hypertension, as for the cardiac transplant patients, is universal, although it is usually well controlled with a conventional regimen of diuretics and vasodilators. Similarly, cyclosporine nephrotoxicity has been universal and has required withdrawal of cyclosporine in two patients.

The patient who required retransplantation after 3 years remains well and fully active.

Seven patients (including the patient who was retransplanted) have experienced late symptoms, having initially recovered well with normal or near-normal respiratory function. As previously described, these changes include progressive dyspnea with or without chronic bronchitis and recurrent pulmonary infections. The characteristic histologic change at biopsy or autopsy is the appearance of bronchiolitis obliterans, with pulmonary vascular intimal thickening and bronchiectasis. At autopsy, diffuse coronary graft atherosclerosis accompanies these findings.

It is likely that rejection is the major cause of this late pathology. However, in three of the patients, there has been a distinct temporal link to CMV infection. It is still unclear as to whether this is coincidence, causal, or concomitant. The long-term complications are by no means invariable, however, and the remaining survivors are well and enjoy normal activity. The Pittsburgh group have also encountered the long-term impairment of function seen in some patients later after transplantation.

STANFORD TRANSPLANTATION

SURVIVAL STATISTICS

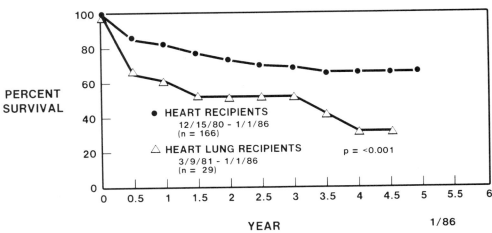

FIGURE 38-5. *Actuarial survival of heart–lung recipients and of heart recipients at Stanford, 1980–1986.*

CONCLUSION

Patients with terminal pulmonary disease, most notably primary pulmonary hypertension and Eisenmenger's syndrome, suffer a progressive and ultimately fatal illness. Although still early in its evolutionary history, combined heart–lung transplantation offers the first effective treatment for what until recently has been considered untreatable disease. The actuarial survival rate at Stanford is 62% at 1 year, and 54% at 3 years. Continued improvement in perioperative and late survival may be anticipated with refinement of patient selection and advances in diagnosing and monitoring pulmonary rejection.

Persistent clinical effort based on a rational approach and a thorough investigational background has led to the current understanding of the selection of patients, the intricacies of the operation, and the complex unique postoperative problems. Long-term complications such as obliterative bronchiolitis of the lungs and proliferative atherosclerosis of the heart are challenges that remain and must be aggressively addressed.

REFERENCES

1. Barnard CN, Cooper DKC: Clinical transplantation of the heart: A review of 13 years' personal experience. J Royal Soc Med 74:670–674, 1981
2. Bieber CP, Griepp RB, Oyer PE et al: Use of rabbit antithymocyte globulin in cardiac transplantation: Relationship of serum clearance rates to clinical outcome. Transplantation 22:478, 1976
3. Bieber CP, Griepp RB, Oyer PE et al: Relationship of rabbit ATG serum clearance rates to circulatory T-cell levels, rejection onset, and survival in cardiac transplantation. Transplant Proc 9:1031–1036, 1977
4. Borel JF, Feurer C, Gubler HU et al: Biological effects of Cyclosporin A: A new antilymphocytic agent. Agents Actions 6:468–475, 1976
5. Carrel A: The surgery of blood vessels. Bull John Hopkins Hosp 18:18, 1907
6. Castaneda AR, Arnar O, Schmidt-Habelman P et al: Cardiopulmonary autotransplantation in primates. J Cardiovasc Surg 37:523–531, 1972
7. Castaneda AR, Zamora R, Schmidt-Habelman P et al: Cardiopulmonary autotransplantation in primates (baboons). Late functional results. Surgery 72:1064–1070, 1972
8. Caves PK, Stinson EB, Billingham ME et al: Percutaneous transvenous endomyocardial biopsy in human heart recipients. Ann Thorac Surg 16:325, 1973
9. Cooley DA, Bloodwell RD, Hallman GL et al: Organ transplantation for advanced cardiopulmonary disease. Ann Thorac Surg 8:30–42, 1969
10. Demikhov VP: Some essential points of the techniques of transplantation of the heart, lungs and other organs. In Basil Haigh (trans): Experimental Transplantation

of Vital Organs Chapter II, pp 29–48. Medgiz State Press for Medical Literature in Moscow, Moscow, 1960, New York, Consultants Bureau, 1962

11. Haglin J, Telander RL, Muzzall RE et al: Comparison of lung autotransplantation in the primate and dog. Surg Forum 14:196–199, 1963

12. Jamieson SW, Burton NA, Bieber CP et al: Cardiac allograft survival in rats treated with Cyclosporin A. Surg Forum 30:289–291, 1979

13. Jamieson SW, Stinson EB, Oyer PE et al: Operative technique for heart–lung transplantation. J Thorac Cardiovasc Surg 87:930–935, 1984

14. Jamieson SW, Stinson EB, Oyer PE et al: Heart–lung transplantation for irreversible pulmonary hypertension. Ann Thorac Surg 38:554–562, 1984

15. Jamieson SW: The current status of heart and heart–lung transplantation. Transplant Proc 17:199–203, 1985

16. Lillehei CW: In discussion of Wildevuur CRH, Benfield JR: A review of 23 human lung transplantations by 20 surgeons. Ann Thorac Surg 9:489–515, 1970

17. Lower RR, Stofer RC, Hurley EJ et al: Complete homograft replacement of the heart and both lungs. Surgery 50:842–845, 1961

18. Nakae S, Webb WR, Theodorides T et al: Respiratory function following cardiopulmonary denervation in dog, cat, and monkey. Surg Gynecol Obstet 125:1285–1292, 1967

19. Neptune WB, Cookson BA, Bailey CP et al: Complete homologous heart transplantation. Arch Surg 66:174–178, 1953

20. Oyer PE, Stinson EB, Jamieson SW et al: One-year experience with Cyclosporin A in clinical heart transplantation. Heart Transplant 1:285–290, 1982

21. Reitz BA, Burton NA, Jamieson SW et al: Heart and lung transplantation: Auto- and allotransplantation in primates with extended survival. J Thorac Cardiovasc Surg 80:360–372, 1980

22. Scott WC, Haverich A, Billingham ME et al: Lethal lung rejection without significant cardiac rejection in primate heart–lung allotransplantation. Heart Transplant 4:33–39, 1984

23. Siegelman SS, Sinha SB, Veith FJ: Pulmonary reimplantation response. Ann Surg 177:30–36, 1973

24. Veith FJ, Montefusco C, Kamholz SL et al: Lung transplantation. Heart Transplant 2:155–164, 1983

25. Webb WR, Howard HS: Cardiopulmonary transplantation. Surg Forum 8:313–317, 1957

CHAPTER 39

Transplantation of Endocrine Tissue

Hans W. Sollinger   Debra A. Hullett   Robert B. Love

The goal of endocrine transplantation research is to develop methods of allotransplantation without immunosuppressive therapy. Therefore, many laboratories have focused their attention on developing techniques for modulating endocrine tissue immunogenicity.

Endocrine allograft survival has been prolonged with extended organ culture, culture in an atmosphere of 95% O_2 with 5% CO_2, ultraviolet (UV) irradiation of the donor tissue, treatment with antilymphocyte serum (ALS) or monoclonal antibodies to Class II molecules and complement, and interim hosting in the nude mouse.

Although isolated, cultured islets have been successfully transplanted across allogeneic barriers in animal systems, no long-term reversals of hyperglycemia have been noted in human trials. Initial experimental results with human fetal pancreas culture and transplantation showing tissue differentiation and maturation in the nude mouse indicate that this tissue is functionally suitable for human transplantation.

Thyroid and parathyroid transplantation in selected patients is a viable alternative to chronic supplement therapy. Using the interim host system, patients with long-standing hypoparathyroidism have been successfully transplanted without immunosuppressive therapy.

Endocrine tissue transplantation in many instances represents an alternative to chronic replacement therapy. In particular, insulin therapy for diabetes mellitus is not sufficient to prevent disease-related complications. The potential significance of whole-organ pancreas and islet of Langerhans transplantation has attracted considerable attention and provides an attractive alternative to conventional therapy. Clinical indication for parathyroid transplantation is well defined.[37] Autotransplantation is appropriate for generalized parathyroid hyperplasia and severe secondary hyperparathyroidism. Allotransplantation, although more involved since systemic immunosuppression may be required, is indicated in cases of congenital parathyroid absence (DiGeorge's syndrome) or iatrogenic hypoparathyroidism, which is not controllable with replacement therapy. Autotransplantation of adrenal cortical tissue has been used following adrenalectomy for treatment of Cushing's disease.

Current methods of endocrine transplantation require the use of immunosuppressive therapy. Although the benefits of a pancreas transplant may outweigh the risks of immunosuppressive therapy, the benefit of thyroid, parathyroid, and adrenal transplants do not. Therefore, many laboratories have focused their attention on developing techniques for modulating the immunogenicity of endocrine tissues.

THE PASSENGER LEUKOCYTE CONCEPT

Rejection of transplanted foreign tissues is the result of immune response by the host to non-self cell surface antigens presented on the transplanted tissue.[13,19] Graft rejection was originally proposed to proceed through the ability of nucleated cells, expressing donor antigens, to be passively transported to the regional draining lymph node, where they activated the rejection response.[30,41] These stimulatory cells were termed **passenger leukocytes.**[6] Lymphocyte activation was shown not to occur in the regional draining lymph node when Strober and Gowans[48] demonstrated effective sensitization of P1 rat lymphocytes by in vivo or in vitro perfusion through a (P1 × P2) F1 kidney. Steinmuller[44,45] proposed an active role for passenger leukocytes in triggering allograft rejection when he showed that allogeneic lymphocytes present within a skin graft conferred immunologic reactivity upon a syngeneic naive recipient. Further support for an active role of passenger leukocytes in generating an allograft response came from studies of graft-versus-host reactivity[6] and from the ability of donor peritoneal exudate cells to induce rejection of cultured thyroid grafts.[50] Two findings suggest that allograft pretreatment to remove passenger leukocytes can prevent or delay graft rejection. First, blood cell removal from graft tissue prior to transplantation successfully prolongs allograft survival.[20] Second, in vitro culture of donor tissue prior to transplantation also prolongs allograft survival.[21,28,32] Ultraviolet (UV) irradiation,[16] culture in the presence of deoxyguanosine,[35] and the use of the nude mouse interim host system[43] will also prolong allografted endocrine tissue. The passenger leukocyte model of allograft rejection has been reviewed.[25]

MECHANISM OF ALLOGRAFT REJECTION

The role of passenger leukocytes in generating an allograft response does not reside solely in passive antigen delivery to alloreactive T cells. Mitomycin C–treated allogeneic lymphocytes, rendered metabolically inactive but still expressing antigen, inoculated subcutaneously into a recipient, generated a barely detectable immune response in the regional draining lymph node.[38] This result suggested that alloantigen recognition alone could not account for T cell activation and led to the hypothesis that two signals were required for T cell activation.[1,24,42] One signal is provided by the binding of alloantigen to the T cell receptor and the second signal, co-stimulator activity, is provided by a metabolically active stimulating cell (antigen-presenting cell). In the case of direct activation, alloantigen and co-stimulator activity reside within the same cell.

The T cell receptor for nominal antigen recognizes antigen in the context of major histocompatibility complex (MHC)-encoded self Class I and Class II cell surface molecules. Alloantigen recognition is thought to arise from the resemblance of alloantigen to self plus nominal antigen.[5] Alternatively, alloantigen may be processed by the antigen-presenting cell and presented to the T cell receptor in a context or self Class II molecules.

Research to improve allograft survival has focused on attempts to remove passenger leukocytes, the source of co-stimulator activity. Prolongation of endocrine allograft survival has been achieved with extended organ culture, culture in an atmosphere of 95% O_2 with 5% CO_2 and 25 PSI,[26] UV irradiation of donor tissue,[16] treatment with antilymphocyte serum (ALS)[14] or monoclonal antibodies to Class II molecules and complement,[8] and interim hosting in the nude mouse.[43]

TRANSPLANTATION OF PANCREATIC TISSUES

The most active research in endocrine tissue transplantation is concerned with developing alternatives to traditional whole-organ pancreas transplantation in diabetic patients. To effect a cure for the diabetic patients, one must eliminate the problems associated with donor exocrine pancreas while preserving islet functional integrity as well as decreasing tissue immunogenicity. There are two major experimental branches in this regard; islet isolation and transplantation, and human fetal pancreas culture and transplantation. Using these approaches, a number of investigators have shown prolongation of pancreatic graft survival without the use of immunosuppression.

Over the last 10 years, much interest has focused on islet and beta cell isolation, culture techniques, and transplantation. There are various methods of handling islet tissue, and these have been discussed in detail in another section of this text. These procedures are designed to decrease tissue immunogenicity while preserving cellular insulin production. Several conclusions can be made from the research in this area. First, islet isolation techniques are extremely tedious and technically difficult. Second, islet culture can be performed with good tissue survival using special media and growth conditions. However, there is little evidence to suggest that the tissue will function adequately after manipulation and transplantation. Third, isolated islet tissue is difficult to transplant. The procedure requires a large volume of cells in the form of a suspension that is difficult to manipulate. Currently, investigators are advocating an intrasplenic or intraportal route for tissue placement. More research is needed to further delineate this problem. Finally, although islets can be isolated and reconstituted into neoislets that resemble normal islets histologically, there is no evidence that neoislets will function normally in the new microenvironment.

Other investigations are primarily concerned with intact fetal pancreas transplantation and developing techniques for modulating immunogenicity. Tissue culture, interim hosting, and treatment with specific monoclonal antibodies have been used.[7,8,12,21,22,29,32,43] Transplantation of intact fetal tissue has the theoretical advantage of closely approximating the islet microenvironment and could result in better endocrine function.[3,39,51] Although recent studies have shown apparent immunologic privilege in some endocrine tissue transplantation, such as thyroid,[34] these results are not seen with fresh allogeneic islet tissue transplantation.[2] Therefore, it is necessary to develop techniques for immune modulation of donor pancreatic tissue.

To date, there are no clinical cures using either human islet or human fetal pancreatic tissue. The amount of tissue required to effect a cure is uncertain. The problem of tissue function in a new and different microenvironment may be compounded by the maturity of the fetal tissue transplanted.

TRANSPLANTATION OF THYROID AND PARATHYROID TISSUES

Thyroid and parathyroid tissue transplantation has been used extensively to elucidate the mechanisms of allograft rejection. Early experiments using parathyroid tissue transplantation indicated that thyroid tissue was highly immunogeneic and that immunosuppressive therapy or immunologic manipulation of the donor tissue was necessary to achieve graft survival.[31,53] Successful transplantation of parathyroid allografts has been achieved after treatment of the recipient with immunosuppressive therapy, including antilymphocyte globulin (ALG), prednisone, and azathioprine.[53] Naji and Barker[31] followed parathyroid allograft rejection in rats while examining the role of histocompatibility differences and transplantation site on allograft rejection. Several methods of immunologic manipulation of the donor tissue prior to transplantation have been pursued.

Allogeneic parathyroid survival in dogs after tissue culture has been accomplished and suggests that tissue culture changes the antigen composition of the allograft.[47] Others have suggested that short periods of in vitro culture prolong parathyroid graft survival.[9,10,18] For instance, Lafferty and associates[22] demonstrated that 26-day cultured Balb/c thyroids transplanted to CBA recipients maintained their function for greater than 100 days. Further, cyclophosphamide treatment (300 mg/kg) of donor mice 2 and 4 days prior to graft harvest significantly reduced the in vitro culture period required to achieve thyroid allograft survival.[23] We have demonstrated that organ culture was effective in making possible

successful xenotransplantation of closely related species, such as rat and mouse. La Rosa and Talmage[26] demonstrated that thyroid culture in 95% O_2, 5% CO_2 pressurized to 23 PSI significantly prolonged allograft survival.

In contrast to the consistent prolonged survival of thyroid allografts after culture, parathyroid culture does not consistently prolong graft survival. Gough and Finnimore[14] were unable to demonstrate parathyroid allograft survival after 3 weeks of culture and treatment with donor-specific ALS. We have found that it is extremely difficult to obtain reproducible viability of cultured parathyroid tissue. In an attempt to reproducibly preserve tissue viability while reducing the passenger lymphocyte content, several investigators have used the nude mouse interim host system.[40,43] BALB/c thyroids irradiated with 1000 rads and maintained in the BALB/c interim host for 4 weeks survived indefinitely when transplanted to CBA recipients.[43] We have used the interim host system for human parathyroid transplantation in two patients with long-standing hypoparathyroidism.[43] Donor tissue was irradiated with 1000 rads and immediately transplanted beneath the kidney capsule of Balb/c nude mice. After 16 to 19 days of interim hosting, parathyroid tissue was retransplanted into the brachioradialis muscle of the patient's left forearm. One patient has been completely removed from calcium and vitamin D therapy, the other is receiving approximately one third of the initial calcium dose. Parathyroid hormone levels have risen with a difference between the left and right antecubital area in both patients. These results suggest that in vitro culture and/or interim hosting of thyroid and parathyroid tissue will prolong allograft survival and allow transplantation without immunosuppression therapy.

Organ culture success in abrogating thyroid allograft rejection has led to the use of this system in elucidating rejection mechanisms.[42] LaRosa and Talmage[27] have investigated the role of minor antigens in graft rejection. They proposed that in cultured allografts with minor-plus-MHC antigenic deficiencies, minor antigens are shed from the graft, processed by recipient antigen presenting cells, and induce a delayed-type hypersensitivity (DTH) response. The localized DTH response would produce sufficient lymphokines to activate cytotoxic T cells against the donor alloantigens of the Class I type and subsequently mediate graft rejection. This hypothesis would account for the observed synergism of rejection observed in minor-plus-MHC antigenic differences. Silvers and colleagues[40] have postulated that MHC-restricted cytotoxic T cells are generated directly against minor antigens presented by recipient antigen-presenting cells. These authors have proposed that cultured thyroid allografts will be more likely to survive in MHC-incompatible recipients. MHC-compatible minor antigen-mismatched allografts survival is not prolonged by culture, suggesting a different mechanism of rejection.

Cultured thyroid allograft rejection has been used to study the cells responsible for graft rejection. Warner and Pemburg have shown that cultured thyroid allografts can be rejected after transfer of sensitized LyT 2[+] T cells but not L3T4[+] T cells.[52] The confusion over which T cells mediate allograft rejection may be explained by the ability of L3T4[+] T cells to stimulate cytotoxic T cell differentiation and provide IL-2.[46]

TRANSPLANTATION OF ADRENAL CORTICAL AND OVARIAN TISSUES

Adrenal cortical tissue autotransplantation has largely been used in animal models to elucidate the mechanisms of endocrine regulation.[36] In humans, adrenal autotransplantation following adrenalectomy for treatment of Cushing's disease has met with limited success. The degree of autotransplant survival is highly variable. Adrenal implants showing marginal survival on early biopsy often continue to grow to produce recurrent Cushing's syndrome.[15] Allotransplantation of adrenal cortical tissue has not been studied.

Ovarian tissue survives and maintains endocrine function when transplanted across minor histocompatibility barriers.[4,11] Jacobs[17] has shown significant prolongation of allograft survival after in vitro culture for 8 to 12 days. Ovarian autotransplants have been used to determine age-related changes in the ovary and uterus.[33] Nance and coworkers[33] have shown alterations in the endocrine control mechanism of rats bearing ovarian grafts.

REFERENCES

1. Bach FH, Bach ML, Sondel PM: Differential function of major histocompatibility complex antigens in T-lymphocyte activation. Nature 259:273, 1976
2. Barker CF, Silvers WK: Immunologic problems in islet transplantation. Diabetes (Suppl 1) 29:86, 1980
3. Brown J, Heininger D, Kurel J et al: Islet cells grow after transplantation of fetal pancreas and control of diabetes. Diabetes 30:9–13, 1981
4. Camilleri AP, Micallef T, Ellul J et al: Homograft transplantation of the ovary. Transplantation 22:308, 1976
5. Cohn M: The T cell receptor mediating restrictive recognition of antigen. Cell 33:657, 1983
6. Elkins WL, Guttmann RD: Pathogens of a local graft versus host reaction. Immunogenicity of circulating host leukocytes. Science 159:1250, 1968
7. Faustman DL, Hauptfield V, Lacy P et al: Prolongation of murine islet allograft survival by pretreatment of islets with antibody directed to Ia determinants. Proc Natl Acad Sci USA 81:5156, 1981
8. Faustman DL, Steinman RM, Gebel HW et al: Prevention of mouse islet allograft rejection by elimination of intraislet dendritic cells. Transplant Proc 17:420, 1985
9. Feind CR, Weber CJ, Derenoncourt F et al: Survival and allotransplantation of cultured human parathyroids. Transplant proc 11:1011, 1979
10. Gaillard PJ: Preservation and autotransplantation of normal tissues. Gaillard PJ: Growth, differentiation and function of explants of some endocrine glands Symp Soc Exp Biol 2:139–144, 1948
11. Goldman MB: Immunogenetic factors in the survival of ovarian transplants. Transplantation 17:518, 1974
12. Gores PE, Sutherland DER, Platt JL et al: Elimination of Ia-positive cells does not influence islet allograft survival in the renal subcapsular position. Surg Forum 36:326, 1985
13. Gorner PA: The genetic and antigenic basis of tumor transplantation. J Pathol Bacteriol 44:691, 1937
14. Gough IR, Finnimore M: Rat parathyroid transplantation. Allograft pre-treatment with organ culture and anti-lymphocyte serum. Transplantation 29:149, 1980
15. Hardy JD, Moore DO, Langford HG: Late follow-up of 17 adrenalectomy patients with emphasis on eight with adrenal autotransplants. Ann Surg 201:595, 1985
16. Hardy MA, Reemtsma K, Lau HT: Induction of indefinite rat islet allograft survival with direct ultraviolet irradiation and peritransplant cyclosporine transplant. Transplant Proc 17:423, 1985
17. Jacobs BB: Ovarian allograft survival. Prolongation after passage in vitro. Transplantation 18:454, 1974
18. Jordan GL: An experience with parathyroid homotransplantation. Adv Surg 2:199, 1966
19. Kaliss N, Kardutsch AA: Acceptance of homografts by mice injected with antiserum. I. Activity of serum fractions. Proc Soc Exp Biol Med 91:118, 1956
20. Lafferty KJ, Jones MAS: Reaction of the graft versus host (GVH) type. Aust J Exp Biol Med Sci 47:17, 1969
21. Lafferty KJ, Cooley MA, Woolnough J et al: Thyroid allograft immunogenicity is reduced after a period in organ culture. Science 188:259, 1975
22. Lafferty KJ, Bootes A, Dart G et al: Effect of organ culture in the survival of thyroid allografts in mice. Transplantation 22:138, 1976
23. Lafferty KJ, Bootes A, Killoy AA et al: Mechanism of

thyroid autograft rejection. Aust Exp Biol Med Sci 54:573–586, 1976

24. Lafferty KJ, Andris L, Prowse SJ: Role of lymphohine and antigen in the control of specific T cell responses. Immunol Rev 51:279, 1980

25. Lafferty KJ, Prowse SJ, Simeonovic CJ: Immunobiology of tissue transplantation: A return to the passenger leukocyte concept. Ann Rev Immunol 1:143, 1983

26. LaRosa FG, Talmage DW: The failure of a major histocompatibility antigen to stimulate a thyroid allograft reactivation after culture in oxygen. J Exp Med 157:898, 1983

27. LaRosa FG, Talmage DW: Synergism between minor and major histocompatibility antigens in the rejection of cultured allografts. Transplantation 39:480, 1985

28. Lueker DC, Sharpton TR: Survival of ovarian allograft following maintenance in culture. Transplantation 18:457, 1974

29. Mandel TE, Koulmanda M: Effect of culture conditions on fetal mouse pancreas in vitro and after transplantation in syngeneic and allogeneic recipients. Diabetes 34:1082, 1985

30. Medawar PB: The immunology of transplantation. Harvey Lect 52:144, 1956–57

31. Naji A, Barker CF: The influence of histocompatibility and transplant site on parathryoid allograft survival. J Surg Res 20:261–267, 1976

32. Naji A, Silvers WK, Barker CF: Effect of culture in 95% O$_2$ of parathryoid allografts. Surg Forum 30:109, 1979

33. Nance DN, Moser WH, Wilkinson M: Neuroendocrine control of ovarian autografts. Endocr Res Commun 9:185, 1982

34. Perloff LJ, Barker CF: The thyroid graft: Influence of histocompatibility and transplant site on survival. Ann Surg 188:186, 1978

35. Ready AR, Jenkinson EJ, Kingston R et al: Successful transplantation across major histocompatibility barrier of deoxyguanosine-treated embryonic thymus expressing class II antigens. Nature 310:231, 1984

36. Saxe AW, Connors M: Autotransplantation of adrenal cortical tissue: A rodent model. Surgery 98:995, 1985

37. Schwartz SI, Shires GT, Spencer FC et al: Principles of Surgery, 4th ed. New York, McGraw-Hill, 1984

38. Scollay RG, Lafferty KJ, Poskitt DC: Allogeneic stimulation modulates the strength of transplantation antigen. Transplantation 18:6, 1974

39. Shizura J, Trager D, Merrell RC: Structure, function, and immune properties of reassociated islet cells. Diabetes 34:1082, 1985

40. Silvers WK, Bartlett ST, Chen HD et al: Major histocompatibility complex restriction and transplantation immunity. A possible solution to the allograft problem. Transplantation 87:28, 1984

41. Snell GD: Enhancement and inhibition of the growth of tumor homotransplants by pretreatment of the hosts with various preparations of normal and tumor tissue. J Natl Cancer Inst 13:719, 1952

42. Sollinger HW, Bach FH: Collaboration between *in vivo* responses to LD and SD antigens of major histocompatibility complex. Nature 259:487, 1976

43. Sollinger HW, Mack E, Cook K et al: Allotransplantation of human parathyroid tissue without immunosuppression. Transplantation 36:6, 1983

44. Steinmuller D: Immunization with skin allografts taken from tolerant mice. Science 158:127, 1967

45. Steinmuller D: Passenger leukocytes and the immunogenicity of skin allografts. J Invest Dermatol 75:107, 1980

46. Steinmuller D: Which T cells mediate allograft rejection? Transplantation 40:229, 1985

47. Stone HB, Owings JC, Gey GO: Living grafts of endocrine glands. Am J Surg 24:386–395, 1934

48. Strober S, Gowans JL: The role of lymphocytes in the sensitization of rats to renal homografts. J Exp Med 122:347, 1965

49. Summerlin WT, Broutbar C, Foanes RB et al: Acceptance of phenotypically differing cultured shin in man and mice. Transplant Poc 5:707, 1973

50. Talmage DW, Dart G, Radovich J et al: Activation of transplant immunity. Effect of donor leukocytes on thyroid allograft rejection. Science 191:358, 1976

51. Tuch BE, Ng ABP, Jones A et al: Maturation of the response of human fetal pancreatic explants to glucose. Diabetologia 28:28–31, 1985

52. Warren HS, Pemburg RG: Rejection of cultured thyroid allografts by the transfer of sensitized LyT 2$^+$ T cells. Transplantation 41:421, 1986

53. Wells SA, Burdick JF, Christiansen CL et al: Long-term survival of dogs transplanted with parathyroid glands and autografts and as allografts in immunosuppressed hosts. Transplant Proc 5:769–771, 1973

CHAPTER 40

Bone Marrow Transplantation

E. Donnall Thomas   Mukund Sargur

Bone marrow transplantation provides a means for curative correction of a number of lethal congenital and acquired disorders of the hematopoietic and lymphoid systems.

The initial successful marrow transplants were carried out with identical twins. Most experience is derived from allogeneic marrow transplants from HLA-identical sibling donors. Successful allogeneic marrow transplants have also been carried out using other family members, with one-HLA haplotype being genetically identical with the patient and the other haplotype being phenotypically partially identical. Recently, successful transplants have been carried out using unrelated donors phenotypically HLA-identical with the patients. Successful transplants have been carried out in patients younger than 1 year to almost 60 years of age, with the best results in patients younger than 30 years.

Marrow transplantation is the treatment of choice for severe combined immunologic deficiency, severe aplastic anemia, and genetically determined disorders of the marrow. Marrow transplantation offers the only hope of cure for patients with acute leukemia once relapse has occurred or for those with chronic myelogenous leukemia in the blastic phase. For patients younger than 30 years with acute nonlymphocytic leukemia in first remission, marrow grafting is the treatment of choice. For patients between ages 30 and 50 years, the choice between combination chemotherapy or marrow transplantation may be considered debatable, but, if these patients are treated with combination chemotherapy, marrow grafting is the treatment of choice when relapse occurs. For chronic myelogenous leukemia, marrow transplantation offers the only hope of cure. The risk of early death from the complications of marrow grafting must be weighed against the benefit of long-term survival and cure. *

HISTORY

In the 1950s, it was shown in rodent, canine, and human models that intravenous infusion of bone marrow cells protected against otherwise lethal exposure to total body irradiation. By the use of immunologic and cytogenetic markers, it was shown that the regenerating marrow was of donor origin. In the late 1950s, marrow transplantation was undertaken for patients with leukemia who had failed conventional therapy. Since very little was known about tissue typing at that time, the only successful transplants were those cases in which the patients had an identical twin. During the 1960s, studies in rodent models provided an understanding of the genetic factors governing the success or failure of a bone marrow transplant, and studies in the canine model demonstrated that long-term, healthy chimeras could be achieved in an outbred species. At the end of the 1960s, the increasing knowledge of human histocompatibility typing and the ability to provide supportive care for the patient without bone marrow function set the stage for the "modern" era of human bone marrow transplantation.*

Bone marrow transplantation as a treatment for patients with acute or chronic leukemias, malignant lymphomas, severe aplastic anemia, thalassemia major, congenital immunologic deficiency diseases, or inborn errors of metabolism has met with increasing success in the past two decades.[8] Clinical trials of human marrow transplantation followed observations in experimental animals that showed a decreased incidence of graft-versus-host disease (GVHD) and an increased recipient survival when

* (For a full review, see Thomas ED, Starb R, Clift RA et al: Bone-marrow transplantation. N Engl J Med 292:832–843, 895–902, 1975.)

the donor and recipient were identical at the major histocompatibility complex (MHC). Advances in the knowledge of human histocompatibility typing made it possible to select sibling donor–recipient pairs genetically identical for human leukocyte antigens (HLA) determined by a series of loci, the MHC, or chromosome 6 of humans. The immune system is sufficiently intact in patients other than those with severe combined immunodeficiency disease (SCID) to reject an allogeneic marrow transplant. Therefore, preparative chemoradiotherapy or chemotherapy alone is needed to immunosuppress the recipient so that a graft will be accepted, to eliminate the existing abnormal marrow elements, and to create space in the microenvironment for the donor marrow to develop. Damage to marrow stem cells can be ignored, since the donor marrow will restore marrow function, and anticancer therapy can be given prior to marrow transplantation in doses limited only by toxicity to organ systems other than marrow.

HISTOCOMPATIBILITY AND DONOR SELECTION

Human marrow transplantation has stressed the use of histocompatible donor marrow as determined by serologic typing for the alleles of HLA-A, -B, -C, -DR, and -D loci and nonreactive mixed lymphocyte cultures (MLC). Obviously, identical twins with identity at all genetic loci are an ideal source of donor marrow. Allogeneic transplantation has been accomplished between HLA-identical siblings who inherited the same haplotype of chromosome 6 from each parent but are dissimilar for other genetic loci. The chance of HLA-identity for a patient with a sibling is one in four. In our experience, about 40% of young patients will have an HLA-identical donor because there is more than one normal sibling in the family. In countries in which the tendency is to have very small families, it is more difficult to find a matched sibling.

Because most patients have neither a twin nor an HLA-identical sibling, recent efforts have focused on identifying acceptable selection criteria for partially matched parent–offspring or sibling pairs and with phenotypically HLA-identical unrelated donors.[3] Donor banks are being established to search for matched unrelated donors, thereby increasing the number of patients who could benefit from transplantation.

ABO blood group incompatibility between donor and recipient is not a major problem.[4] Isohemagglutinins against the donor's blood group need to

be removed by plasma exchange or extracorporeal perfusion over affinity columns designed to deplete the patient's plasma of isohemagglutinins. To avoid hemolysis of donor erythrocytes, transplantation of marrow that is depleted of erythrocytes is also effective. The donor must be in good health, and the donor, or an appropriate advocate of the donor, must be capable of giving informed consent for the marrow donation. Major complications in marrow donors have been rare, but the potential risks of anesthesia are of concern.[5]

PREPARATIVE REGIMEN FOR THE RECIPIENT

The type of conditioning regimen used to prepare recipients for marrow transplantation is determined by the underlying disease and by previous therapy. Organ functions and previous chemoradiotoxicity to various organs should be assessed, and additional insult by conditioning regimens should be avoided if possible. As in all critical care situations, good vascular access (double-lumen right atrial catheter) is essential for administration of blood products, parenteral nutrition, antibiotics, and blood drawing. Allogeneic transplantation can be performed in children with SCID without immunosuppression. Patients with severe aplastic anemia require immunosuppression to prevent rejection.[12,14] Children with nonmalignant disorders associated with active bone marrows (such as Wiskott-Aldrich syndrome and thalassemia major) receive chemotherapy to provide immunosuppression and to eradicate the affected marrow.[9,10] Patients with hematologic malignancies and lymphoma require both immunosuppression and chemoradiotherapy to destroy the tumor cells and allow engraftment.[20]

Specific preparative regimens for aplastic anemia include cyclophosphamide at 50 mg/kg on each of 4 successive days, followed 36 hours later by marrow transplantation. Other regimens include cyclophosphamide (120 mg/kg–200 mg/kg) with 3 to 10 Gy total body irradiation, with or without partial lung shielding, thoracoabdominal irradiation, or total lymphoid irradiation.

Patients with genetically determined nonmalignant disorders have been conditioned with cyclophosphamide (200 mg/kg), used with either busulfan (3.5 mg/kg/day, p.o., for 4 days) or dimethyl busulfan (5 mg/kg IV).[18] These regimens provide immunosuppression and marrow eradication. The combination of procarbazine, anti-thymocyte globulin, and total body irradiation has also been used successfully in patients with Wiskott-Aldrich syndrome.[10]

Patients with leukemia or other hematologic malignancies require larger doses of chemoradiotherapy to eliminate the malignant cells. With the notable exception of the conditioning regimen consisting of busulfan (4 mg/kg/day for 4 days) and cyclophosphamide (50 mg/kg per day for 4 days) described by the Johns Hopkins group,[13] most transplant teams use total body irradiation as a principal element in their conditioning regimens.

The initial preparative regimen at Seattle consisted of cyclophosphamide (60 mg/kg/day for 2 days), followed 3 days later by 10 Gy as a single exposure from opposing radioactive cobalt (^{60}Co) sources given at a rate of 5 to 8 cGy/min.[20] More recently, 12 Gy to 15.75 Gy midline dose at 6 to 7 cGy/min in six to seven fractions have been given to reduce radiation toxicity and increase leukemic cell kill.

Several marrow transplant teams are exploring new regimens using hyperfractionated total body irradiation with or without chemotherapy with high-dose cytosine arabinoside, VP16 or VM26.[8] These manipulations of the preparative regimens are directed at reducing acute and delayed toxicity while optimizing the destruction of leukemic cells.

BONE MARROW HARVEST AND INFUSION

Marrow aspiration is similar to diagnostic aspirations except that 150 to 200 aspirates are performed under general or spinal anesthesia in the operating room.[19] From 10 ml/kg to 15 ml/kg body weight is obtained from the posterior iliac crests and, if necessary, from anterior iliac crests and sternum. The heparinized marrow is screened through a series of increasingly finer mesh screens and given intravenously to the recipient. The infused marrow stem cells grow almost exclusively in the marrow cavities. Proof of engraftment is obtained by rising peripheral counts (which occurs in 2–4 weeks), by cytogenetics, and by isoenzyme and restriction enzyme fragment length polymorphisms that distinguish donor from host cells.

SUPPORTIVE CARE DURING POST-TRANSPLANT PERIOD

The conditioning regimens ablate the hematopoietic and lymphopoietic systems, leading to profound immunodeficiency and pancytopenia. Therefore, the recipient is at increased risk of bleeding and infection. Nearly all patients are transfusion-dependent for several weeks. During this period, the hematocrit is maintained between 25% and 30%, and the platelet count is maintained at a minimum of 20,000/mm³ by transfusion. Other supportive measures include a protective environment (laminar air flow rooms), prophylactic antibiotics, and hyperalimentation.

Owing to severe impairment of all immunologic parameters, marrow graft recipients are prone to life-threatening infections with bacterial, fungal, and viral infections.[7] Although the absolute number of peripheral blood cells usually returns to near normal within 4 to 6 weeks, immune functions do not return to normal in uncomplicated patients for several months. Fungal infections are common, necessitating the frequent use of amphotericin B. Approximately half of all allogeneic transplant patients develop self-limiting infections with herpes simplex or varicella-zoster viruses. Acyclovir is useful in shortening the course of these infections. The most serious infections are the interstitial pneumonias, which occur between 1 and 3 months after marrow grafting. Currently, 60% of interstitial pneumonias are due to cytomegalovirus (CMV), with 85% mortality. Attempts at preventing or treating CMV pneumonia have been frustrating. Prophylaxis using CMV immune plasma or hyperimmune globulin has been of some value. Recently, an acyclic nucleoside structurally related to acyclovir but with increased activity against CMV in vitro, called DHPG (9-2-hydroxy-1-[hydromethyl]ethoxymethyl guanine), has been introduced into clinical trials. It is the first antiviral agent showing activity against CMV in vivo, and it is being evaluated in the earlier management of serious infections in the immunocompromised host. The other 40% of interstitial pneumonias are not caused by identifiable infectious agents, but they may be the consequence of cumulative toxicity to the lung by chemotherapy and irradiation. High-dose steroids (at 16 mg/kg) have occasionally produced responses.

IMMUNOLOGIC RECONSTITUTION

Return to normal immune function is dependent upon appropriate proliferation, maturation, and differentiation of cells of donor origin.[21] Studies have shown that all marrow graft recipients have profound impairment of most immune functions during the first 4 to 5 months after grafting regardless of underlying disease, type of preparative regimen, source of marrow (syngeneic, allogeneic, or autologous), and postgrafting immunosuppression (methotrexate or cyclosporine). Healthy recipients return to normal or near normal in a year. Patients who develop chronic GVHD have delayed immune recovery, leaving them at increased risk for life-threatening infections.

GRAFT-VERSUS-HOST DISEASE (GVHD)

Acute

Pathophysiology, Incidence and Immunologic Events

About half the recipients of genotypically HLA-identical sibling marrow develop acute GVHD, which, theoretically, is due to disparities of "minor" histocompatibility antigens.[20] The immunocompetent T-lymphocytes in the marrow inoculum recognize these minor host antigens, become sensitized, proliferate, and attack host tissue, producing the clinical syndrome of GVHD. The principal target organs are the skin, gut, and the liver. The clinical manifestations range from mild transient skin rashes, impairment of liver function tests, and gastrointestinal disturbances (nausea, vomiting, and diarrhea) to severe life-threatening involvement with loss of skin, liver failure, bloody diarrhea, and depressed immune function. Approximately 5% to 10% of transplanted patients die of acute GVHD; 50% of those die of infection.

With donor–recipient pairs that are partially matched for HLA, the incidence and severity of acute GVHD appears to increase with increasing antigenic disparity.[3] However, survival of recipients of partially matched marrow is determined primarily by the type and stage of disease.

Prevention and Treatment

A variety of immunosuppressive agents have been used pre- or post-grafting to prevent the development of acute GVHD. Methotrexate and cyclosporine were compared in a randomized prospective study, showing no difference in the incidence of GVHD or survival. A combination of anti-thymocyte globulin (ATG), methotrexate, and prednisone decreased the incidence of acute GVHD but did not improve overall survival. Recently, a prospective randomized study showed significant reduction of acute GVHD and improvement in survival from the combination of a short course of methotrexate with a long course of cyclosporine.[14a]

More recent approaches have been directed at elimination of T cells from the marrow inoculum by incubating the marrow with ATG, with monoclonal antibodies to T cells, or by lectin agglutinin sedimentation or sheep erythrocyte rosetting.[8] The major problem associated with T cell–depleted marrow has been graft failure.[6] Drugs such as prednisone, cyclosporine, ATG, and anti-T monoclonal antibodies have been used to treat established GVHD, with a 35% to 50% response.

Chronic

Chronic GVHD occurs in 35% to 45% of patients receiving HLA-identical marrow transplants any time from 100 days to 15 months after grafting.[15] Chronic GVHD is more likely to occur in older patients and in patients who had developed acute GVHD. The clinical picture resembles autoimmune diseases, with involvement of the skin and sometimes the liver and/or the gut. This analogy is supported by the findings of circulating autoantibodies and immunoglobulin and complement deposits at the dermal-epidermal junction. Left untreated, fewer than one fifth of patients survive without major disabilities. Two thirds of patients will respond completely to prednisone and/or azathioprine.

Late Complications

Late complications are primarily due to the effects of chemoradiotherapy and the problems related to chronic GVHD. Sterility is likely in almost all patients. Cataracts occur in 1 to 3 years in approximately 80% of patients given single exposure total body irradiation and 25% of patients given fractionated total body irradiation. Restrictive and obstructive chronic pulmonary disease occurs in 10% to 15% of patients who develop chronic GVHD. There may be an increased risk of secondary malignancy after high doses of irradiation. Studies of growth and development show that most children with aplastic anemia who were prepared by cyclophosphamide alone have normal growth. Those with leukemia, almost all of whom had received prior chemotherapy and prophylactic cranial irradiation, receiving cyclophosphamide and total body irradiation before grafting have delayed growth and development.[11]

Graft-Versus-Leukemia Effect.   Residual leukemic cells persisting after ablative chemoradiotherapy may be destroyed by donor lymphocytes reacting against non-HLA antigens on the surface of leukemic cells ("graft-versus-leukemia effect"). Retrospective analyses of the clinical data showed a reduced incidence of leukemic relapse in patients with GVHD compared with those without GVHD. In recipients transplanted for leukemia in relapse or in second remission who survived at least 150 days, 50% were alive at 2 years for those who had Grade II to Grade IV acute GVHD compared with 25% for those who had Grade 0 to Grade I acute GVHD. Ongoing clinical trials in patients transplanted in relapse are directed at manipulating GVHD for its apparent antileukemic effects.

Nature of Recurrent Leukemia. The recurrence of leukemia post-transplant is still a major complication.[8,16] As indicated by genetic markers, the majority of leukemic relapses occur in the host cells, reflecting a failure to eradicate all the original leukemic cells. However, in eight cases, the leukemic relapse occurred in donor-type cells (about 5% of recurrences).

There are several possible explanations for leukemic relapse occurring in donor cells. Perhaps the simplest explanation would be that leukemia is a disease of "regulation," so that any cells in the abnormal environment would become leukemic. A second explanation would involve the possibility of cell fusion between donor and host cells followed by a loss of chromosomal material or "diploidization." A third possibility would be that the immunodepression in the marrow graft recipient leads to a breakdown in immune surveillance defenses against malignant cell clones that might develop spontaneously in the regenerating engrafted tissue. It is possible that transfection of an oncogene from DNA of degenerating host leukemic cells to the DNA of developing donor cells occurs. Fortunately, this type of recurrence is rare, but advances in technology to distinguish cell surface antigens, cytogenetic markers, and DNA restriction fragment length polymorphisms may shed more light on the phenomenon.

CLINICAL RESULTS OF MARROW TRANSPLANTATION

Genetic Diseases

Marrow transplantation is the treatment of choice in SCID, with better than 60% long-term survivors.[9] These patients are immunodeficient because of their disease and do not require further immunosuppression for successful engraftment. Patients with Wiskott-Aldrich syndrome and X-linked immunodeficiency with a triad of eczema, thrombocytopenia, and recurrent infections have hypercellular marrows and require cyclophosphamide and busulfan or irradiation to permit full replacement of the diseased marrow.

Patients with Fanconi's anemia are unusually sensitive to preparative regimens, which may be the result of impaired mechanisms of somatic cell repair manifested by in vitro chromosomal fragmentation after exposure to irradiation or alkylating agents. Reducing the dose of cyclophosphamide and/or other agents in the preparative regimen has been associated with increased success in this disease.

Other genetic diseases in which marrow grafts have been performed with varying degrees of success include infantile agranulocytosis, chronic granulomatous disease, osteopetrosis, ataxia telangiectasia, Blackfan-Diamond anemia, congenital red cell aplasia, cartilage-hair hypoplasia, neutrophil actin deficiency, neutrophil membrane GP-180 deficiency, mucopolysaccaridosis, Gaucher's disease, and paroxysmal nocturnal hemoglobinuria.[10]

Thalassemia major, a frequent disorder in many countries, is an anemia resulting from genetic defects in hemoglobin synthesis. Conventional management includes transfusions and chelation therapy to prevent iron overload. Although patients may live one or more decades, the treatment is expensive and compromises one's life-style. Marrow grafting from a suitable donor has now been carried out after preparation with dimethyl busulfan or busulfan and cyclophosphamide in approximately 100 patients. About 15% of the recipients died of transplant complications, and 5% of the surviving patients have chronic GVHD. Ten percent have had their own marrow regenerate and again have thalassemia major. About 70% appear to be cured of the disease and are leading normal lives. Thus, the risk of early death or cure by transplantation must be weighed against the problems and expense of transfusions and chelation over a period of many years.[18]

Severe Aplastic Anemia

Bone marrow transplantation from an HLA-identical sibling is very effective treatment for severe aplastic anemia, and it is the treatment of choice for patients younger than 40 years.[14] Graft rejection occurred in 36% of the first 82 multiply transfused patients transplanted prior to 1975 in Seattle. Graft rejection is due to sensitization of the patients to "minor" histocompatibility antigens of their donors through multiple blood transfusions. Early transplantation, prior to the administration of multiple blood products, minimizes the problem of graft rejection, and sustained hematopoietic engraftment has been the rule in untransfused patients. Administration of additional donor buffy coat cells helps to prevent graft rejection in transfused patients. Figure 40-1 compares the probability of survival in aplastic anemia patients for untransfused, transfused, and transfused patients who received donor buffy coat cells. The present emphasis for physicians

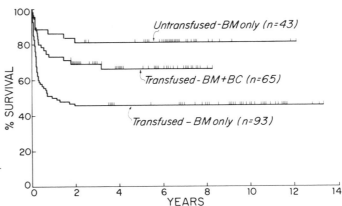

FIGURE 40-1. Kaplan–Meier product limit estimates for survival of patients with severe aplastic anemia given a marrow transplant from an HLA identical sibling. The recipients were prepared with cyclophosphamide. Sixty-five patients were given additional donor buffy coat cells. All patients received intermittent methotrexate in the first 100 days after grafting.

referring patients for transplantation is to avoid all transfusions if possible. If transfusion is required, family members should not be used until tissue typing can be completed to determine whether or not the patient has a suitable marrow donor.

Some transplant teams have modified the preparative regimen to include some form of total body irradiation. Although rejection rates declined, the overall survival was not improved, largely because of an increase in complications from GVHD and interstitial pneumonia. For instance, cyclophosphamide combined with total lymphoid irradiation results in 73% survival at 5 years after grafting.

For patients without donors and who do not undergo transplantation, ATG is of benefit. As many as 60% of approximately 150 patients have responded, and 40% of these patients are long-term survivors. Patients over the age of 40 years are generally considered to be "poor-risk" candidates for transplantation. ATG may be used as first-line therapy for these patients, even if they have an HLA-identical sibling. Marrow grafting could then be undertaken if ATG treatment is unsuccessful, but there is considerable risk of death during the 8 to 12 weeks of therapy and observation needed to evaluate response to ATG.

Acute Leukemia

Acute leukemia is now responsive to systemic chemotherapy, so that with present-day induction regimens, 60% to 90% of patients can be put into remission. However, depending upon the type of acute leukemia, the likelihood of cure ranges from 50% to 0%. Patients who relapse are destined to die of the disease, even though additional remissions can be achieved. Thus, marrow transplant teams are exploring various regimens for patients with acute leukemia in relapse or in remission designed to improved the likelihood of cure.

Transplantation for Acute Leukemia in Relapse Using HLA-Identical Sibling Donors

Initially, it was unethical to transplant patients with acute leukemia until they had failed conventional chemotherapy. Ten end-stage patients underwent marrow transplant after preparation with total body irradiation only, and 100 end-stage patients were prepared with cyclophosphamide and total body irradiation.[16] There were many early deaths from advanced disease, infection, GVHD, and recurrence of leukemia. However, 12 patients (3 with chronic GVHD) survived 9 to 14 years without recurrence of leukemia, indicating that some end-stage patients can be cured. Several marrow transplant teams, using newer chemotherapy and/or radiation regimens, are reporting initial results indicating 20% to 60% survival of patients transplanted in relapse.[8]

Transplantation in Acute Lymphoblastic Leukemia (ALL) in Remission Using HLA-Identical Sibling Donors

Encouraged by the initial success with patients in relapse, earlier transplantaton seemed indicated for patients with ALL.[16] Chemotherapy alone may result in the cure of up to 50% of patients with ALL. However, once relapse occurs, the prognosis is very poor, and a trial of transplanting during the second or a subsequent remission was evaluated. Several reports now reflect a disease-free survival of 25% to 35% at 5 years with this approach. Relapse remains the main obstacle, with approximately 60% of those transplanted destined to relapse in the absence of other causes of death. New regimens are exploring monoclonal antibodies directed against leukemic cells and the use of interferon after marrow grafting.

Transplantation for Acute Nonlymphoblastic Leukemia (ANL) in Remission Using HLA-Identical Sibling Donors

Patients with ANL who achieve an initial remission have a poor prognosis, and median survival in most series is 12 to 24 months, with a 5-year survival of approximately 20%. In an initial series of 22 patients transplanted for ANL, during the first remission, about half are alive in remission 7 to 10 years later (Fig. 40-2).[11,16] About half of these patients had chronic GVHD, but four have recovered and are off treatment. The one patient with active chronic GVHD has a performance score of 90% on the Karnofsky scale, and the other 11 score 100%. Other transplant centers are reporting comparable or even better results, although with a shorter follow-up time.

Marrow Transplantation for Chronic Myelogenous Leukemia (CML)

The results of marrow transplantation for CML in blast crisis are similar to those obtained in patients with acute leukemia in relapse.[17] Disease-free long-term survival following marrow transplantation is approximately 20%. Cytogenetics on the marrow cells of these patients do not show the Philadelphia chromosomes, indicating that the leukemic clone has been eliminated resulting in cure of the disease.

Marrow transplantation in the chronic phase of CML promised to improve survival and cure. The initial trial began with 12 patients with chronic-phase CML who had cytogenetically normal identical twin marrow donors. These patients were prepared with dimethyl busulfan (5 mg/kg IV), cyclophosphamide (60 mg/kg × 2) and 10 Gy total body irradiation as a single dose. All 12 patients had complete remissions associated with disappearance of the Philadelphia chromosome. Of the 12 patients 8 survive in remission without evidence of the Philadelphia chromosome 6 to 10 years later; the remaining either died or relapsed. These results encouraged clinical trials at multiple centers using HLA-identical sibling donor–recipient combinations for the treatment of CML in chronic phase. Figure 40-3 shows the survival after marrow grafting of patients with CML according to the stage of the disease. Reported long-term survivals are 47% to 80%, with absence of the Philadelphia chromosome indicating cure. The longest disease-free survivors are now 6 years postgrafting, and continued follow-up will be necessary for full evaluation.[17]

Non-Hodgkin's Lymphoma

The results of allogeneic bone marrow transplantation for non-Hodgkin's lymphoma, although limited, have been encouraging.[1,2] Eight patients with disseminated non-Hodgkin's lymphoma who failed conventional chemotherapy were given grafts from healthy monozygous twins after conditioning with high-dose chemoradiotherapy. Three patients died from interstitial pneumonia. One relapsed at 10 months, was retreated with chemotherapy, and is alive more than 7 years after grafting. Half of the patients are alive in remission 2 to 12 years after grafting. However, in another series, 20 patients with disseminated disease after failure of conventional chemoradiotherapy were transplanted with allogeneic marrow, and only 4 are alive in complete remission up to 2 years post-transplant.

Other Malignancies

Allogeneic bone marrow transplantation has been

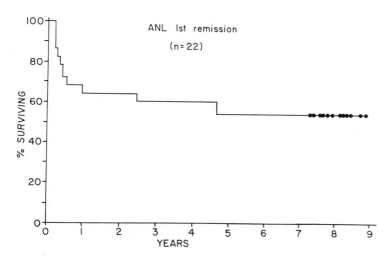

FIGURE 40-2. *Kaplan–Meier product limit estimates for survival after marrow grafting for 22 patients transplanted for acute nonlymphoblastic leukemia in first remission. The dots indicate living patients.*

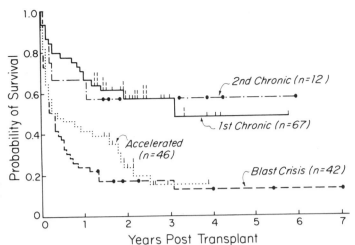

FIGURE 40-3. *Kaplan–Meier product limit estimates for survival following marrow transplantation for patients with chronic myelogenous leukemia given allogeneic grafts in first chronic phase, second chronic phase, accelerated phase, or blastic phase. The tick marks and dots indicate surviving patients. (Thomas ED, Clift RA, Fefer A et al: Marrow transplantation for the treatment of chronic myelogenous leukemia. Ann Intern Med 104:155–163, 1986)*

TABLE 40-1   *Marrow Transplantation for Hematologic Diseases; Summary of Current Results*

DISEASE/STATUS AT TIME OF TRANSPLANT	5-YEAR DISEASE-FREE FRACTION (APPROXIMATE)	LONGEST DISEASE-FREE SURVIVOR (YR)
MALIGNANT		
Acute lymphoblastic leukemia—remission	0.30	9
Acute lymphoblastic leukemia—relapse	0.15	14
Acute myelogenous leukemia—remission	0.60	10
Acute myelogenous leukemia—relapse	0.15	14
Chronic myelogenous leukemia—chronic phase	0.60	10
Chronic myelogenous leukemia—blastic phase	0.10	9
NONMALIGNANT		
Severe combined immunodeficiency disease	0.60	16
Aplastic anemia—multiply transfused	0.65	14
Aplastic anemia—untransfused	0.85	10
Thalassemia major	0.75	5

successful using conditioning regimens of cyclophosphamide and total body irradiation for treatment of patients with Hodgkin's disease, multiple myeloma, myelofibrosis, preleukemia, and hairy cell leukemia. Several pilot studies are evaluating marrow transplantation for radiosensitive solid tumors in pediatric and adult populations. Marrow grafting for ovarian carcinoma, testicular carcinoma, and small cell lung cancer after failure of conventional therapy has not been successful.

SUMMARY AND OUTLOOK FOR THE FUTURE

Marrow transplantation has evolved from and experimental treatment used only in terminally ill patients to being the preferred treatment for several diseases if a suitable donor is available (Table 40-1). Marrow grafting for aplastic anemia is generally successful if performed early in the course of the disease. Marrow grafting for patients with acute leukemia who have relapsed once, whether or not a subsequent remission has been achieved, is the only approach that offers long-term survival, with 10% to 30% cures. Although still controversial, it appears that marrow grafting is the treatment of choice for patients with ANL in first remission and for patients with CML in chronic phase, since approximately 50% to 70% of these patients are surviving in complete remission and are cured. Marrow grafting is the only effective treatment for patients with immunologic deficiency diseases. It offers a probability of cure for the majority of patients with a genetic disorder of hematopoiesis. It is being actively explored in patients with lymphoma, Hodgkin's disease, multiple myeloma, small cell lung cancer, breast cancer, testicular cancer, and ovarian cancer.

To extend marrow transplantation to larger numbers of patients, partially matched family members who share one-HLA-haplotype genetically with the patient are being used as donors. More than 200 patients have been transplanted from such donors, and the overall results appear to reflect the type and stage of the disease more than the type and match of donor.

Five years ago, the Seattle team reported a successful transplant for a patient with leukemia using an unrelated donor. This illustrated the feasibility of using unrelated donors. Data banks with information on unrelated donors are being established in England, Canada, and the United States to determine the feasibility and usefulness of phenotypically matched unrelated donors.

REFERENCES

1. Appelbaum FR, Sullivan KM, Thomas ED et al: Allogeneic marrow transplantation in the treatment of MOPP-resistant Hodgkin's disease. J Clin Oncol 3:1490–1494, 1985

2. Appelbaum FR, Thomas ED: Review of the use of marrow transplantation in the treatment of non-Hodgkin's lymphoma. J Clin Oncol 1:440–447, 1983

3. Beatty PG, Clift RA, Mickelson EM et al: Marrow transplantation from related donors other than HLA-identical siblings. N Engl J Med 313:765–771, 1985

4. Bensinger WI, Buckner CD, Thomas ED et al: ABO-incompatible marrow transplants. Transplantation 33:427–429, 1982

5. Buckner CD, Clift RA, Sanders JE et al: Marrow harvesting from normal donors. Blood 64:630–634, 1984

6. Martin PJ, Hansen JA, Buckner CD et al: Effects of in vitro depletion of T cells in HLA-identical allogeneic marrow grafts. Blood 66:664–672, 1985

7. Meyers JD, Thomas ED: Infection complicating bone marrow transplantation. In Rubin RH, Young LS (eds): Clinical Approach to Infection in the Immunocompromised Host, Chapter 20. New York, Plenum press, (in press)

8. O'Reilly RJ: Allogeneic bone marrow transplantation: Current status and future directions. Blood 62:941–964, 1983

9. O'Reilly RJ, Brochstein J, Dinsmore R et al: Marrow transplantation for congenital disorders. Semin Hematol 21:188–221, 1984

10. Rappeport JM, Smith BR, Parkman R et al: Application of bone marrow transplantation in genetic diseases. Clin Haematol 12:755–773, 1983

11. Sanders JE, Thomas ED, Buckner CD et al: Marrow transplantation for children in first remission of acute nonlymphoblastic leukemia: An update. Blood 66:460–462, 1985

12. Santos GW, Sensenbrenner LL, Anderson PN et al: HLA-identical marrow transplants in aplastic anemia, acute leukemia, and lymphosarcoma employing cyclophosphamide. Transplant Proc 8:607–610, 1976

13. Santos GW, Tutschka PJ, Brookmeyer R et al: Marrow transplantation for acute nonlymphocytic leukemia after treatment with busulfan and cyclophosphamide. N Engl J Med 309:1347–1358, 1983

14. Storb R, Thomas ED, Buckner CD et al: Marrow transplantation for aplastic anemia. Semin Hematol 21:27–35, 1984

14a.Storb R, Deeg HJ, Whitehead J et al: Methotrexate and cyclosporine compared with cyclosporine alone for prophylaxis of acute graft versus host disease after marrow transplantation for leukemia. N Engl J Med 314:729–735, 1986

15. Sullivan KM, Shulman HM, Storb R et al: Chronic graft-versus-host disease in 52 patients: Adverse natural course and successful treatment with combination immunosuppression. Blood 57:267–276, 1981

16. Thomas ED: Marrow transplantation for malignant diseases (Karnofsky Memorial Lecture). J Clin Oncol 1:517–531, 1983

17. Thomas ED, Clift RA, Fefer A et al: Marrow transplantation for the treatment of chronic myelogenous leukemia. Ann Intern Med 104:155–163, 1986

18. Thomas ED, Sanders JE, Buckner CD et al: Marrow transplantation for thalassemia. Ann NY Acad Sci 445:417–427, 1985

19. Thomas ED, Storb R: Technique for human marrow grafting. Blood 36:507–515, 1970

20. Thomas ED, Storb R, Clift RA et al: Bone-marrow transplantation. N Engl J Med 292:832–843, 895–902, 1975

21. Witherspoon RP, Deeg HJ, Lum LG et al: Immunologic recovery in human marrow graft recipients given cyclosporine or methotrexate for the prevention of graft-versus-host disease. Transplantation 37:456–461, 1984

CHAPTER 41

Bone Transplantation

Gary E. Friedlaender

Bone grafts are required for a wide variety of reconstructive procedures related to congenital, traumatic, degenerative, and neoplastic disorders. The acquisition of autogenous tissue is associated with potential morbidity, and their supply is limited. An increasing interest in limb-sparing tumor resections has focused attention on the use of osteochondral allografts.

Bone graft incorporation involves both graft-derived and host-derived contributions. The recipient bed provides for the ingrowth of new blood vessels that bring with them primitive mesenchymal cells capable of differentiating into bone resorbing and bone-forming populations. The graft acts passively as a template (osteoconduction) as well as actively inducing the host response to occur (osteoinduction); both these properties are independent of viable cellular contributions from the graft. It is possible, therefore, to recover graft material many hours following death and preserve these tissues for later use. Immune responses to bone allografts can be monitored, and the magnitude of immunogenicity is influenced by approaches to graft preservation. Correlation to sensitization and biologic fate remains unclear.

Bone banking methodology consistent with safety for recipients and predictable biological properties has been established. Grafts can be acquired under sterile conditions or can be secondarily sterilized by chemical or physical means and then subjected to a long-term preservation technique such as deep-freezing or freeze-drying.

Clinical applications of osteochondral allografts are associated with success comparable to autografts. Of most significance, graft incorporation provides a repair based ingrowth of host bone, and this regenerated skeletal tissue gets stronger with time. Synthetic implants, on the other hand, gradually wear and fatigue and are, therefore, less well suited for younger and more active persons.

HISTORY AND INTRODUCTION

Bone transplantation specifically and limb transplantation more generally have captured the interest of scientists and the imagination of the public throughout recorded history. This theme appears in ancient medical records, mythology, and even Biblical references but is most dramatically illustrated by the purported exploits of Cosmas and Damian.[3,18] These patron saints of medicine are credited with the transplantation of a lower extremity from a Moor to replace the diseased limb of a parishioner during the 4th century. Jobi Meekren, a Dutch surgeon, apparently used dog cranium to repair the skull wound of a soldier during the 17th century but was forced to remove the graft prematurely, under threat of excommunication.[3]

The foundation for our contemporary approach to bone transplantation was provided by the investigations of Ollier,[24] pertaining to the osteogenic properties of bone and periosteum in the mid 1800s, and by the clinical use of bone allografts in children reported by Macewen[20] in 1881. Although the innovative use of massive bone allografts described by Lexer[19] between 1908 and 1925 was only partially successful, it provided the necessary incentive for Parrish,[26] Ottolenghi,[25] and Volkov and Imamaliev[36] to pursue the clinical development of limb-sparing tumor resections followed by osteochondral allograft reconstruction beginning in the 1950s. This approach has been further refined by the work of Mankin and associates,[22] and is described in more detail below.

At present, more than 100,000 autogenous bone grafts are used annually in the United States to support reconstructive approaches addressing a wide variety of skeletal disorders. These autografts represent the maximal available biological potential, circumvent concern for transfer of disease from donor to recipient, and are histocompatible by definition. Despite clear advantages, the acquisition of osteochondral autografts requires sacrifice of normal structures as well as the potential morbidity associated with an additional surgical procedure and site that may include wound infection, substantial blood loss, increased postoperative discomfort, and fracture of weakened bone. Of even greater pragmatic significance, autogenous bone is available in limited size, shape, and quantity. For these reasons, allogeneic and even xenogeneic bone grafts have been used with increasing frequency over the past century and continue to support innovative approaches to reconstructive challenges.[13]

Credible use of osteochondral allografts, or other biologic substitutes for bone, must be predicted upon efficacy and safety. It must be demonstrated that the graft material is biological useful and predictable, that potential transfer of disease from donor to recipient can be minimized, if not eliminated, and that consequences of histocompatibility differences are of no practical concern. These issues can be met satisfactorily by nonvascularized osteochondral allografts preserved by deep-freezing or freeze-drying (lyophilization), using rigorous banking methodology, and transplanting with attention to appropriate surgical principles.

GRAFT BIOLOGY

Autografts

Bone graft incorporation is an interactive process between transferred osteogenic tissue and the host bed into which it is placed. A portion of the reparative response is vested in the graft, while other definable aspects of the process are provided by the recipient site.

Following implantation, bone grafts are enveloped in a hematoma that gradually transforms into a fibrovascular response over the next 1 to 2 weeks. Only those cells at or very near the surface of bone trabeculae can survive by diffusion. The remainder of cells undergo necrosis unless the vascular supply to that segment is immediately re-established by surgical anastomosis analogous to solid organ transplantation. Unlike organs, graft cell viability is not crucial to success of the transplant. However, there does appear to be a favorable role for viable graft-derived cells, related either to their direct osteogenic potential or as a source of humoral mediators or mitogens for repair and homeostasis. Consequently, the relatively few cells that survive fresh autograft

transplantation provide a momentum to or amplification of biological events leading to graft incorporation that is absent from allografts and may account for much of the observed differences in speed and completeness of repair.

The next phase of bone graft incorporation is revascularization, followed by recruitment of osteogenic cells responsible for repair.

As previously mentioned, both the graft and the recipient site play distinct but complementary and indispensable roles in the biological process. The graft functions passively as a scaffold or template onto which new bone is formed (osteoconduction), and protein(s) residing in the matrix actively stimulate the host response leading to osteogenesis (osteoinduction).[35] Aside from the limited but important role of the few residual viable graft-derived cells, these conductive and inductive properties are independent of graft cell viability.

Bone incorporation does, however, require active cellular responses emanating from the host bed. The recipient site provides ingrowth of blood vessels that are accompanied by multipotential mesenchymal cells able to differentiate into the bone-resorbing (osteoclastic) and bone-forming (osteoblastic) populations responsible for graft incorporation and remodeling. Cancellous bone is repaired more rapidly and completely than cortical tissue, but, in either case, incorporation leads to formation of physiologically and biomechanically competent bone of host origin.[5,17]

The systemic and local control mechanisms responsible for osteogenesis, whether for purposes of homeostasis or repair, are only superficially understood and represent an area of intense investigation. Improved knowledge of graft biology will provide an opportunity to manipulate and enhance the reliability and quality of bone incorporation. Similarly, factors that interfere with graft repair can be identified, and attention to these events may also favorably impact upon end results. For example, circumstances that adversely affect the recipient bed or the circulating pool of recruitable osteogenic cells will detract from the bone graft incorporation process. Of particular relevance in cases of skeletal reconstruction following limb-sparing tumor resections are the local consequences of irradiation and the systemic influence chemotherapy.[15] Radiation therapy causes fibrosis of its target tissue sufficient to interfere with revascularization efforts and also injures the metabolic and replicative potential of local multipotential cells such that recruitment from distant sites by way of the circulation is required. As pointed out, however, delivery of these osteogenic cells to the graft is hampered by radiation-induced soft tissue scarring. Chemotherapy results in both local and systemic depletion of required precursor cells. The inflammatory exudate associated with infection may also interfere with delivery of host-derived contributions to graft incorporation sufficient to preclude a satisfactory result.

Each of these adverse circumstances can be addressed, at least in part, by the use of grafts immediately revascularized by (micro) vascular anastomosis following tissue transfer. Vascularized bone does not undergo necrosis or the slow but cellularly intense process of repair. Instead, it maintains graft cell viability, continues in an uninterrupted fashion the ongoing remodeling characteristic of homeostasis, and unites to the host skeleton by the relatively rapid process of fracture healing.[37] Bone grafts available on a vascular pedicle are confined to autogenous tissues from a small number of sites, such as a fibula, rib, and iliac crest.

Allografts

The biology of bone allograft repair is analogous to autograft incorporation, particularly if the graft has been preserved by deep-freezing or freeze-drying, except that allogeneic bone requires longer periods of time to repair and is less completely replaced or remodeled.[5,6,16] This probably reflects the lack of viable graft-derived osteogenic cells and greater dependence upon host cell contributions. As is the case with autografts, allogeneic bone is both osteoconductive and osteoinductive, provided that this letter characteristic has not been destroyed by preservation techniques. The usefulness of osseous and osteochondral allografts has been repeatedly confirmed in numerous animal models and in various clinical circumstances.[5,6,13,17,22,31,32]

IMMUNOLOGIC CONSIDERATIONS

Studies pertaining to the immunogenicity of osteochondral allografts and xenografts reflect idiosyncrasies of the model chosen for evaluation, the nature of assay methodology used, and the specific target antigen identified.

Bone is composed of mineral, collagen, matrix, and cells. The hydroxyapatite crystal (mineral phase of bone) is not antigenic, and collagen is, at best, a weak immunogen. Matrix components, particularly proteoglycan subunits and link protein, have been shown to evoke immune responses in allogeneic and xenogeneic systems, whereas other matrix components, including hyaluronic acid and the glycosaminoglycans associated with the core protein, appear nonreactive.[11,28,29] The major source of sensitization in bone grafts resides with the heterogeneous cell populations reflecting osteogenic, chondrogenic, fibrous, fatty, neuronal, hematopoietic, and vascular components intrinsic to skeletal tissue. These diverse cells share surface antigens associated with the major histocompatibility complex (MHC), and antibodies to both Class I and Class II MHC antigens have been demonstrated in numerous animals models and in humans following graft implantation.[8]

The magnitude of anti-MHC responses varies with different animal models in relation to such factors as orthotopic versus heterotopic implantation sites, cortical versus cancellous bone, segmental versus particulate tissues, dose, timing, route, and preservation techniques applied to the graft material. Similarly, assay techniques have varied over the past 30 years, beginning with histologic evaluation of surrounding cellular infiltrates, regional lymph node responses, skin graft rejection patterns, and numerous in vivo and in vitro assay techniques of increasing sophistication.[6,8]

Although some differences exist, most studies confirm the immunogenicity of fresh osteochondral allografts, the reduction in sensitization following deep-freezing of the implant, and further compromise of responses subsequent to freeze-drying.[8,14] The limited data available from clinical investigations closely reflect animal-derived information.[9]

Despite the monitored presence of immune responses, the significance of osteochondral allograft immunogenicity, particularly in humans, remains unanswered. In a recent multi-institution study, presensitization to DR antigen or lack of any detectable sensitization following transplantation were both circumstances associated with favorable radiographic and clinical results. Development of antibodies against Class I antigens was a less reliable prognostic indicator but appeared most compatible with intermediate biological results.[10] These preliminary observations require scrutiny and confirmation based on additional experience. Further correlation of immune responses with graft histology as well as noninvasive parameters of biological status will be required to accurately establish the significance of bone graft immunogenicity.

DONOR SELECTION AND MANAGEMENT

Banking methodology addresses aspects of donor selection, tissue recovery, preservation and storage, and recordkeeping. This sequence of events must be used to comprehensively screen prospective donors for potentially harmful diseases and provide biologically useful grafts of predictable mechanical properties. Guidelines and standards have been developed by the American Association of Tissue Banks to ensure that these goals are achieved.[1,13,34]

Donor Selection

Donor selection criteria are based on careful review of the past medical history and circumstances surrounding death in the case of cadaver donors. Contraindications to donation include the presence of local infection in the bone to be recovered or systemic sepsis; a history of hepatitis, venereal disease, or acquired immunodeficiency syndrome (AIDS); metabolic bone disease; malignancy; or the presence of toxic substances in potentially harmful amounts. Appropriate laboratory tests and an autopsy help confirm the clinical impressions.

Because cell viability is not crucial to bone graft success, tissue can be recovered up to 12 to 24 hours following death, including cessation of circulatory function, provided that the donor is maintained in a refrigerated environment during the period of ischemia. Donor age constraints reflect potential clinical applications. Bone with open epiphyses (prior to skeletal maturity) are not suitable for segmental replacement, because the growth plate may slip during the incorporation process. When transplanted portions of bone do not include the physis or are used in particulate form, young donors are acceptable. Older persons are susceptible to osteoporosis and loss of mechanical strength, and this may affect the appropriateness of bone from these donors for certain applications that depend upon physical properties. Otherwise, age per se is not an issue with respect to bone donation.

Tissue Recovery

Virtually any bone with potential clinical application can be obtained from cadaver sources following ante mortum consent from the individual or post mortum authorization from the next of kin. Allografts can be acquired in a sterile environment using standard operating room technique, with sufficient bacteriologic cultures accomplished to document freedom from contamination; this is the author's preference. It is also feasible to recover bone in a clean but nonsterile manner, but this requires an effective method of secondary sterilization. Both high-dose irradiation and ethylene oxide have been used effectively for this purpose in the past.[4,30] Potential disadvantages of the required megarad doses of irradiation include structural changes, apparent loss of inductive properties, and the lack of assurance that all potential contaminants have been eliminated (particularly viruses).

Preservation and Storage

Bone can be stored for prolonged periods of time by deep-freezing. Temperatures in the $-70°C$ to $-80°C$ range ensure substantial retardation of the autolysis that would otherwise occur even at $-20°C$,[7] but specific shelf lives have never been determined for bone stored under various low-temperature conditions. Freeze-drying used in conjunction with other preservation approaches, particularly demineralization, has generally been efficacious for providing osteoinductive graft material. Mechanical integrity, however, is altered by lyophilization, and this change in properties must be compatible with intended clinical application.[27]

Cartilage, in contrast to bone, requires survival of existing chondrocytes, and this necessitates use of a cryoprotectant agent (dimethyl sulfoxide or glycerol) prior to deep-freezing. Articular cell viability in the range of 40% to 50% can be achieved by this approach, and this appears consistent with clinical success.[33]

Grafts are packaged in a sterile fashion and can be stored frozen or, in the case of freeze-dried bone, in evacuated containers at room temperature for future applications. Recordkeeping is an indispensible part of bone banking and must be meticulous.

RECIPIENT APPLICATIONS

Bone allografts have been used for a wide variety of reconstructive procedures associated with congenital, traumatic, degenerative, and neoplastic disorders of the skeleton.[13] This growing experience has been encouraging, such that clinical outcome now closely approximates results obtained using fresh autogenous bone graft in most, if not all, circumstances. There is, for example, no difference in the rate at which benign cystic defects of long bones respond to curettage and packing with bone graft whether autogenous or allogeneic sources are used.[32] Similar patterns have been documented with anterior cervical fusions[31] and arthrodesis for scoliosis.[2] Clinical success with bone allografts in these circumstances approximates 90%, the same that can be anticipated with autografts.

The application of massive osteochondral allografts in support of reconstruction of substantial skeletal deficits following severe trauma or limb-sparing tumor ablation has been most exciting and rewarding (Fig. 41-1).[12,22] In the case of skeletal malignancy, this approach requires removal of large portions of tumor-bearing long bones (especially the distal femur, proximal humerus, and proximal tibia), and a portion of the articular surface may often be included in the resection specimen (Figs. 41-2 and 41-3). The use of large osteochondral allografts in musculoskeletal oncology was introduced in the United States by Parrish,[26] and this experience has been expanded more recently by Mankin, whose large series of more than 300 cases has been most carefully reviewed and provides a benchmark of data.[12,22,23] To date, evaluation of success has been based on clinical function and x-ray criteria, with little opportunity to directly monitor biological function. This noninvasive approach suggests that 75% to 80% of patients have achieved a satisfactory (excellent or good) result, meaning return to work and nonathletic activities with little or no discomfort and without the need for crutches or braces on a routine basis. The success of segmental bone grafts that do not include articular surfaces (joints) is even better, with predictable satisfactory results in 90% to 95% of cases. Just as important, the success rate does not deteriorate after the first 2 years of follow-up, based on more than 10 years of observations.

Alternative reconstructive procedures for extensive bony deficits may include amputation, joint fusion, or, perhaps, custom-made synthetic implants. Each of these approaches has specific disadvantages as well as advantages. For example, synthetic prostheses have been excellent options for restoring function of the hip and, more recently, the knee joint when compromised by degenerative disease in a sedentary and elderly population. This approach provides rapid return to activity. However, long-term fixation to the skeleton, wear, and implant fatigue continue to limit durability, especially for younger and more active persons. Allografts require a significant investment in time while incorporating into the skeleton, but, when successful, these transplants are replaced by regenerated host bone capable of responding to physiologic stress and, in fact, get stronger over time. The relatively high rate of unsatisfactory results associated with massive osteochondral allografts remains a concern. Reasons for failure include the occurrence of infection, nonunion at the osteosynthesis site (junction of the allograft and host skeleton), fracture of the segment during the reparative process, and instability at the joint.[21] Infection is most devastating and has been better controlled in recent years by careful patient selection, specifically by avoiding circum-

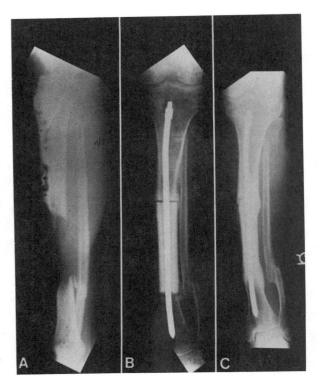

FIGURE 41-1. Replacement of the tibial shaft by a bone allograft following traumatic loss of a similar segment. (A) The deficit of the middle third of the tibia. (B) The bone allograft in place shortly after transplantation. (C) The grafted segment well on the way to incorporation 23 months later.

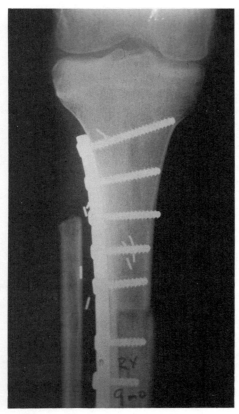

FIGURE 41-2.   Allograft relacement of the proximal tibia 9 months following resection of a low-graft bone tumor. (Courtesy of HJ Mankin)

stances in which irradiation or other injuries to the necessary soft tissue coverage may exist. Chemotherapy likewise compromises the repair potential[15] and represents a relative contraindication to this biological reconstructive approach. When complications can be avoided, the clinical success rate for osteochondral allografts is over 95%.

THE FUTURE

The future for bone and cartilage transplantation is bright and will continue to grown in terms of numbers, scope, and innovation. Better understanding of mechanisms controlling the biology and isolation of osteogenic "mitogens" or growth factors (bone morphogenic proteins) will contribute to favorable and predictable results. Continued careful attention to bone banking procedures will ensure maximal availability of graft material with minimal risk of disease transferred inadvertently to recipients. An opportunity to better understand and correlate the nature of immune responses, biology, and clinical success will further enhance our ability to repair and reconstruct deficits of the skeleton and set a stage for limb transplantation. This latter circumstance will be preceded by development of approaches to clinically efficacious revascularized bone allografts (an extension of current experience with autografts) and, of course, a substantial improvement in our understanding of nerve regeneration.

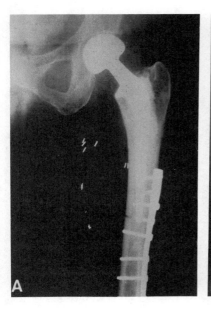

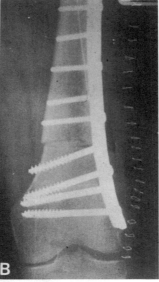

FIGURE 41-3.   Allograft replacement of the proximal three fourths of the femur combined with prosthetic replacement of the hip joints following limb-sparing tumor resection. (A) The immediate postoperative appearance of the proximal half of the allograft with a prosthetic femoral component cemented into the transplant. (B) The distal half of the same segment, including the osteosynthesis site where graft (on top) joins the remaining host femur just above the flare of the metaphysis.

REFERENCES

1. American Association of Tissue Bank Guidelines for the Banking of Musculoskeletal Tissues. Newsletter Am Assoc Tissue Banks 3:12, 1979
2. Aurori BF, Weiderman RJ, Lowell HA et al: Pseudarthrosis after spinal fusion for scoliosis: A comparison of autogeneic and allogeneic bone grafts. Clin Orthop 199:153, 1985
3. Bick EM: Source Book of Orthopaedics, p 243. New York, Hafner, 1968
4. Bright, RW, Smarsh JD, Gambill VM: Sterilization of human bone by irradiation. In Friedlaender GE, Mankin HJ, Sell KW (eds): Osteochondral Allografts: Biology, Banking and Clinical Applications, p 223. Boston, Little, Brown and Co, 1983
5. Burchardt H: The biology of bone graft repair. Clin Orthop 174:28, 1983
6. Burwell RG: The fate of bone grafts. Recent Adv Orthop 6:115, 1969
7. Ehrlich MG, Lorenz J, Tomford W et al: Collagenase activity in banked bone. Transact Orthop Res Soc 8:166, 1983
8. Friedlaender GE: Immune responses to osteochondral allografts: Current knowledge and future directions. Clin Orthop 174:58, 1983
9. Friedlaender GE: Immune responses to preserved bone allografts in humans. In Friedlaender GE, Mankin HJ, Sell KW (eds): Osteochondral Allografts: Biology, Banking and Clinical Applications, p 159. Boston, Little, Brown and Co, 1983
10. Friedlaender GE: Morphologic and immunologic responses to bone allografts in humans: A preliminary report. In Enneking WF (ed): International Symposium on Limb-Preservation Surgery, New York, Churchill Livingstone
11. Friedlaender GE, Ladenbaure-Bellis IM, Chrisman OD: Immunogenicity of xenogeneic cartilage matrix components in a rabbit model. Yale J Biol Med 56:211, 1983
12. Friedlaender GE, Mankin HJ: Transplantation of osteochondral allografts. Ann Rev Med 35:311, 1984
13. Friedlaender GE, Mankin HJ, Sell KW: Osteochondral Allografts: Biology, Banking and Clinical Applications. Boston, Little, Brown and Co, 1983
14. Friedlaender GE, Strong DM, Sell KW: Studies on the antigenicity of bone. I. Freeze-dried and deep-frozen allografts in rabbits. J Bone Joint Surg 858A:854, 1976
15. Friedlaender GE, Tross RB, Doganis AC et al: Effects of chemotherapy on bone. I. Short-term methotrexate and doxorubicin (Adriamycin) treatment in a rat model. J Bone Joint Surg 66A:602, 1984
16. Heiple KG, Chase SW, Herndon CH: A comparative study of the healing process following different types of bone transplantation. J Bone Joint Surg 45A:1593, 1963
17. Heiple KG, Goldberg VM, Powell AE et al: Biology of cancellous bone graft repair. In Friedlaender GE, Mankin HJ, Sell KW (eds): Banking, Biology and Clinical Applications of Osteochondral Allografts, p 37. Boston, Little, Brown and Co, 1983
18. Kahan BD: Cosmas and Damion in the 20th century. N Engl J Med 305:280, 1981
19. Lexer E: Joint transplantation and arthroplasty. Surg Gynecol Obstet 40:782, 1925
20. Macewen W: Observations concerning transplantation of bone: Illustrated by a case of inter-human osseous transplantation, whereby over two-thirds of the shaft of a humerus was restored. Proc R Soc Lond 32:232, 1881
21. Mankin HJ: Complications of allograft surgery. In Friedlaender GE, Mankin HJ, Sell KW (eds): Osteochondral Allografts: Biology, Banking and Clinical Applications, p 259. Boston, Little, Brown and Co, 1983
22. Mankin HJ, Doppelt SH, Sullivan TR et al: Osteoarticular and intracalary allograft transplantation in the management of malignant tumors of bone. Cancer 50:613, 1982
23. Mankin HJ, Gebhardt MC, Tomford WW: The use of frozen cadaveric osteoarticular allografts in the treatment of benign and malignant tumors about the knee. In Enneking WF (ed): International Symposium on Limb-Preservation Surgery. New York, Churchill Livingstone
24. Ollier L: Traite experimental et clinique de la regeneration des os et de la production artificielle de tissu osseux. Paris, Victor Masson et fils, 1867
25. Ottolenghi CE: Massive osteo and osteoarticular bone grafts: Techniques and results of 62 cases. Clin Orthop 87:156, 1972
26. Parrish FF: Allograft replacement or part of the end of a long bone following excision of a tumor: Report of twenty-one cases. J Bone Joint Surg 55A:1, 1973
27. Pelker RR, Friedlaender GE, Markham T: Biomechanical properties of preserved allografts. Clin Orthop 174:54, 1983
28. Poole R, Reiner A, Choi H et al: Immunological studies of proteoglycan subunit from bovine and human cartilages. Transact Orthop Res Soc 4:55, 1979
29. Poole AR, Reiner A, Tang LH et al: Immunological studies of link protein from bovine nasal cartilage. Transact Orthop Res Soc 4:56, 1979
30. Prolo DJ, Oklund SA: Sterilization of bone by chemicals. In Friedlaender GE, Mankin HJ, Sell KW (eds): Osteochondral Allografts: Biology, Banking and Clincal Applications, p 233. Boston, Little, Brown and Co, 1983
31. Schneider JR, Bright RW: Anterior cervical fusion using preserved bone allografts. Transplant Proc 8(Suppl 1):73, 1976
32. Spence KF Jr, Bright RW, Fitzgerald SP et L: Solitary unicameral bone cyst: Treated with freeze-dried crushed cortical bone allograft: A Review. J Bone Joint Surg 58A:636, 1976

33. Tomford WW, Duff GP, Mankin HJ: Experimental freeze-preservation of chondrocytes. Clin Orthop 197:11, 1985

34. Tomford WW, Friedlaender GE: 1983 bone banking procedures. Clin Orthop 174:15, 1983

35. Urist MR, Silverman BG, Buring K et al: The bone induction principle. Clin Orthop 53:243, 1967

36. Volkov MV, Imamaliev AS: Use of allogenous articular bone implants as substitutes for autotransplants in adult patients. Clin Orthop 114:192, 1976

37. Weiland AJ, Moore JR, Daniel RK: Vascularized bone autografts: Experience with 41 cases. Clin Orthop 174:87, 1983

CHAPTER 42

Corneal Transplantation

Richard S. Smith

HISTORY

Transplantation of the human cornea ranks as the oldest technique of transplantation of a human organ. The concept was discussed in the early part of the 19th century and was first accomplished with successful visual improvement by von Hippel in 1877. He also demonstrated that only homotransplantation would result in a clear graft. In the early part of the 20th century, Elschnig developed the technique to a point of clinical usefulness. Widespread use of keratoplasty did not appear until the late 1940s, when finer suture materials, surgical microscopes, and delicate instrumentation became widely available. Over the ensuing years, there was rapid development of surgical techniques and postoperative management. Penetrating keratoplasty is now the most frequent form of organ transplantation.

TYPES OF KERATOPLASTY

Lamellar keratoplasty was the most commonly used technique early in the history of corneal transplantation. In this procedure, the anterior two thirds of the donor cornea is placed in a bed from which a corresponding portion of the recipient cornea has been removed. The advantage of this technique is that it can be performed without entering the eye, thereby decreasing the surgical risks of intraocular infection. It was also believed that lamellar keratoplasty was less likely to induce an immune response. The current principal value of lamellar keratoplasty is in patch grafting. Corneal perforation may occur from trauma, corneal ulcers, or melting of the corneal stoma from a variety of causes. The consequent loss of substance prevents primary closure. A lamellar patch of corneal donor material may be fashioned to cover the defect and seal the perforation. This procedure may preserve the integrity of the eye and permit a later penetrating keratoplasty for visual purposes.

It is not a feasible procedure for patients with full thickness corneal disease or for indications in which dysfunction of the corneal endothelium is the primary pathology. Although lamellar keratoplasty is still used, penetrating keratoplasty, in which the full-thickness cornea is transplanted, is the most common operation and the one that will be discussed in detail in this chapter.

Because the normal human cornea is an avascular structure, many of the problems associated with other types of organ transplantation are avoided. It has been shown that the turnover of corneal protein is very slow and that lateral diffusion to the vessels at the corneoscleral junction occurs in only minimal amounts. In addition, there is usually a 2-mm to 4-mm margin of the recipient's own tissue that separates the graft from the host vessels. Because of these factors, the host immune system has limited access to the foreign protein of the donor. Immune corneal rejection occurs, but in only 5% to 10% of cases. Systemic immunosuppression is not used routinely with corneal transplants. Topical corticosteroids (1% prednisolone acetate) are almost always sufficient to avoid graft rejection or to treat an acute episode. Problems are encountered principally in those patients with vascularized corneas or in instances of multiple grafts in the same eye. Here, the possibility of a graft–host immune reaction is greatly enhanced. In such cases, systemic immunosuppression may play a role, and tissue typing may improve the chance for graft survival.

PATIENT SELECTION

Normal vision is possible only when the cornea is clear. The collagen of the normal cornea is highly organized at the ultrastructural level. Any scar or deposit that disturbs this organization results in scattering of light and visual distortion. Many corneal conditions are indications for penetrating keratoplasty, including trauma, post-infectious scarring, congenital corneal abnormalities, metabolic diseases, and degenerations. The prognosis for visual success varies with the surgical indications. Situations in which the peripheral cornea is clear and avascular have the best visual prognosis. Examples of good prognosis cases include central avascular scars or degenerative changes limited to the central cornea. In such instances, the prognosis for a visually successful graft exceeds 90%.

Once corneal vascularization has occurred, the immune system has access to the donor tissue and the possibility of rejection is enhanced many times. The issue of histocompatibility testing has been raised with respect to keratoplasty, but, thus far, the experimental evidence is far from strong. There may be some indication to use HLA matching in grafting of vascularized corneas.[5] ABO compatibility testing is not useful in keratoplasty.

DONOR SELECTION AND PRESERVATION

The age of a corneal donor may range from 1 to 80 years, but most surgeons prefer corneas between 5 and 50 years of age. Younger donors often have corneas that are too thin for transplantation, and older persons have a lesser population of endothelial cells. The monolayer of endothelial cells on the posterior corneal surface is vital for proper function of the cornea. In the preferred donor age range, the endothelial cell count is between 2000 mm^2 and 3000/mm^2. Because these cells do not undergo mitosis in the adult human eye, the surgeon is limited by what is available in the donor tissue. Prospective donor tissue may be examined in the eye bank laboratory to determine the endothelial cell density.[2,4] If the cell count is below normal, there is a strong possibility of primary donor failure, soon after transplantation.

The corneal endothelium is important, because it is necessary for maintenance of corneal dehydration, which, in turn, is necessary for maintenance of corneal transparency. The endothelium is a relatively tight anatomic barrier to diffusion of fluid and electrolytes from the aqueous humor. Failure of endothelial function results in progressive leakage of fluid into the corneal stroma. As fluid accumulates, the cornea loses its transparency and vision is compromised.

As with other organ transplants, there are a number of reasons for rejection of prospective donor tissue, including serum hepatitis, syphilis, lymphoma, leukemia, acquired immunodeficiency syndrome (AIDS), and potential slow virus infections. With regard to the latter, both rabies and Jakob-Creutzfeldt disease have been transmitted to corneal recipients. Screening for AIDS is a particular problem in corneal transplantation, since most donor material comes from cadaver sources, making acquisition of adequate blood samples for testing difficult. Since November 1985, all corneal donor tissue in the United States has been routinely screened for HTLV-III. This is necessary because the virus has been detected in tears.

Corneal surgeons are fortunate in that their donor material can be taken after death, within 4 to 12 hours. Initially, corneas were used within 48 hours of enucleation and preserved solely by refrigeration. Currently, the most common form of preservation is in a modified tissue culture medium. In this technique, the cornea and a rim of sclera are removed from the donor eye and placed in the solution under refrigeration. This method is helpful in preserving the health of the corneal endothelium and also allows the donor material to be used for a period of 72 to 96 hours after enucleation. Additionally, corneas may be frozen, using cryoprotectant solutions, and used up to 18 months after enucleation. In a new technique, known as organ culture, corneas are preserved in a tissue culture solution under scrupulous aseptic control at 37°C for as long as 3 weeks. These techniques offer the corneal surgeon several options and usually permit surgery to take place on a scheduled basis.

TECHNICAL ASPECTS

Both donor and recipient corneas are cut with a calibrated trephine and then sutured in place with monofilament synthetic sutures. Most corneal surgeons use either 10-0 or 11-0 monofilament nylon sutures, which necessitate surgery under the operating microscope with fine microsurgical instrumentation (Fig. 42-1). Great care must be taken to achieve exact alignment of the various anatomic structures of the cornea. Failure to do so can produce wound leakage, irregular astigmatism, and ingrowth of fibrous tissue, which can lead to ultimate failure of the graft. Patients who have coexisting corneal conditions and cataracts may undergo a triple procedure in which the cataract is removed, an intraocular lens is inserted, and a graft is done, all at the same time. This saves the patient a second procedure and also reduces the risk of damage to

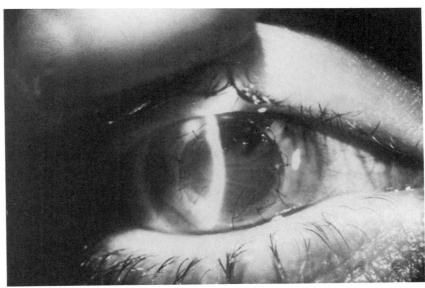

FIGURE 42-1.   *Corneal graft, 5 days postoperative. The cornea is slightly edematous, which is normal at this stage. The central 7.5-mm diameter graft is held in place by interrupted 11-0 monofilament nylon sutures.*

the graft if the cataract removal is done at a later time.

POSTOPERATIVE MANAGEMENT

Frequent and careful observation of the patient during the wound-healing process is essential. Although some investigators have suggested systemic immunosuppressive treatment, a routine graft is usually handled with topical corticosteroids as the only agent. Because of the potential danger of infection, prophylactic postoperative antibiotics are frequently used. Depending upon the surgical technique, sutures may remain indefinitely or may be removed when the wound is healed (Fig. 42-2). The healing period for corneas is prolonged, and sutures may stay in for several months before the wound is secure.

COMPLICATIONS

A variety of complications may occur after keratoplasty.[3] If the donor material is unsatisfactory, a primary donor failure may occur, with graft opacification within a few days. This is most often due to unhealthy donor endothelium. An immunologic

graft rejection may occur any time after keratoplasty but is not often observed before 8 weeks.[1] With increasing postoperative time, the risk of rejection decreases, but never completely disappears. Graft rejection episodes have been seen as late as 20 years after surgery. These are usually handled successfully with topical corticosteroids but may lead to graft failure if not recognized and treated promptly and with appropriate medication. All grafts undergo a certain amount of endothelial cell loss. A low endothelial cell count may be compatible with a clear graft, but obviously leaves the patient in a more precarious position.

Careful surgical technique is critical for success. Most important is precise alignment of the edges of donor and host corneas. Unpublished studies from our ocular pathology laboratory suggest that graft failure is frequently due to poor surgical alignment. As with other forms of transplantation, infection may also occur with keratoplasty. It is an established fact that topical corticosteroids enhance the chances of infection, which can permanently alter graft clarity. Nevertheless, steroids are essential, especially in the early postoperative period to avoid graft rejection. Vascularization may be pre-existing or may develop after keratoplasty. Such an event may promote immune rejection or scarring and distortion of the graft.

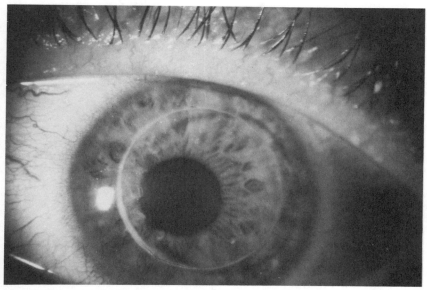

FIGURE 42-2.   *A well-healed corneal graft, 1 year after surgery. The patient's vision is 20/20. A faint white scar demarcates the margins of the graft.*

NEW FRONTIERS

Even though keratoplasty is a highly successful procedure for restoring vision, there are many patients in whom it fails. In recent years, there has been extensive basic science research into the possibility of transplanting healthy tissue-cultured endothelial cells. This has been successfully accomplished in experimental animals. If the laboratory results can be transferred to humans, this technique might be used to treat situations in which endothelial cell loss is the primary pathology.

Corneal vascularization remains a major cause of graft failure. The recent biochemical characterization of angiogenin may offer an experimental tool by which to test inhibitors of angiogenesis. If the mechanism of corneal vascularization could be understood and controlled, the success of keratoplasty in situations such as alkali burns could be greatly enhanced.

An additional refractory problem in keratoplasty is how to deal with patients with severe primary or secondary tear deficiency, such as occurs following Stevens-Johnson syndrome, chemical burns of the cornea, or ocular pemphigus. These patients frequently have severe corneal vascularization, are extremely prone to infection, and show very poor wound healing. Although the idea was tried more than one hundred years ago, implanta-tion of a plastic cornea to restore vision is a concept currently undergoing intense study. Many problems still exist with regard to tissue/plastic interactions, and success in this area has yet to be seen in a consistent fashion.

SUMMARY

Successful transplantation of the human cornea has now been performed for more than one hundred years. The modern era of corneal grafting dates from the post-war era, when operating microscopes, fine sutures, and delicate microsurgical instrumentation became available. the development of an understanding of the immune system has played a major role in increased graft success, although the role of tissue typing in keratoplasty remains uncertain.

Modern techniques of keratoplasty utilize full-thickness corneal replacement with utilization of cadaver tissue. The donor material may be preserved in a variety of ways, including fresh refrigerated, tissue culture media, cryopreservation, and organ culture. Donor material is rejected if there is a history of serum hepatitis, syphilis, leukemia, lymphoma, AIDS, or slow virus infection.

Postoperative management of potential immune reactions is usually handled with topical corticosteroids. Systemic immunosuppression is necessary only in unusual cases of multiple failed grafts. Immune reactions to the donor tissue occur in no more than 5% to 10% of cases but may occur many years after surgery. More common causes of graft failure are secondary infections and errors in surgical technique in which there is poor graft–host tissue alignment. If corneal vascularization occurs, the possibility of an immune rejection is enhanced.

REFERENCES

1. Alldredge OC, Krachmer JH: Clinical types of corneal transplant rejection. Arch Ophthalmol 99:599, 1981
2. Bourne WM, Kaufman HE: The endothelium of clear corneal transplants. Arch Ophthalmol 94:1370, 1976
3. DeVoe AG: Complications of keratoplasty. Am J Ophthalmol 79:907, 1975
4. Neubauer L, Smith RS, Leibowitz HM, et al: Endothelial findings in cryopreserved corneal transplants. Ann Ophthalmol 16:980, 1984
5. Vannas S. Karjailainen K, Ruusvaara P et al: HLA-compatible donor cornea for prevention of allograft reaction. Graefes Arch Clin Exp Ophthalmol 198:217, 1976

CHAPTER 43

Skin Transplantation

Arnold Luterman   P. William Curreri

Skin provides the outer barrier to microbial invasion and helps to internally maintain heat and water. When destroyed, it has limited regenerative ability, and "replacement" coverage is often required.

Allograft "takes" in the same way as autograft. Skin banks cryopreserve donor skin obviating problems or short self life. The major source is cadaver donors. Rejection is inevitable after "take" has occurred. This may be delayed by careful crossmatching and ABO blood types or by immunosuppression with antilymphocytic serum (ALS). Allograft is used for immediate coverage of superficial burns, as a test material prior to autografting, to cover granulating areas between crops of autografts in large burns, and as an immediate cover following major excision.

Amniotic membranes are allotissues readily available and easy to prepare, used in the same way as cutaneous allograft, with similar disadvantages.

Porcine xenografts are the major type of xenograft tissue used as a biological dressing. Viable xenografts may "take" but reject very quickly. They are commonly used in all situations in wound treatment like allograft except in the specific circumstance in which "take" for prolonged coverage is required.

A synthetic skin system includes autologous tissue membranes (cultured epidermal cells) and composite grafts (fibroblast-seeded collagen).

Synthetic bilaminate membranes, which are totally synthetic membranes, have not gained wide use.

Collagen synthetic composite membranes include biobrane and artificial skin. Preliminary results are encouraging.

Skin is a compound organ with a limited ability to regenerate itself. The skin provides the outer envelope to the body and serves as a selective barrier for water, heat, and bacteria. When skin loss occurs, the body's normal healing process attempts to restore surface continuity. The biological process involves the formation of scar tissue with all its morbid, functional, and cosmetic consequences. the process of scar formation progressing to wound closure is slow, and, in the interim, the open wound provides a portal for egress of fluid and heat and for entrance of microbial invaders. Transplantation of tissues or synthetic materials to close these defects becomes a priority of treatment, because the morbidity of an open wound varies directly with its size and the length of time that it remains open.

Burn injuries are the most common injuries that produce an urgent requirement for massive skin replacement. The burn wound is an open wound despite the presence of necrotic tissue (eschar). Vir-

tually all modalities of skin transplantation with biological and synthetic materials are used in treating burn patients. In this chapter, we discuss currently available methods to close these wounds and the advantages and disadvantages of each. This field is rapidly changing, and new techniques and materials are constantly appearing. The purpose of this chapter is to introduce the reader to the avenues of research that are currently being pursued and the broad categories of techniques that are clinically available.

AUTOGRAFTS

Skin grafts may be classified into split-thickness (partial thickness) or full-thickness grafts, depending upon the amount of dermis present. Partial thickness grafts have the distinct advantage over full-thickness grafts in that the donor site can spon-

TABLE 43-1   *Microscopic Events in the Creation of Split-Thickness Skin Graft Circulation**

TIME POST-GRAFT	
0–6 hr	Survival of graft dependent on plasmatic circulation alone
6–12 hr	Graft and host vessels form communications at interface
12–24 hr	Host vessels grow into graft
24–48 hr	Graft–host vascular communications established
48–72 hr	Active circulation into graft established
72 hr–8 days	Development of mature complex of capillaries, arterioles, and venules

Modified from Moncrief JA: Grafting. In Artz CP, Moncrief JA, Pruitt BA (eds): Burns—A Team Approach. Philadelphia, WB Saunders, 1979

taneously regenerate and restore itself, allowing for reharvesting of further tissue. Full-thickness grafts are generally used only when small defects need resurfacing. Successful transfer of a skin graft ("take") depends upon the rapid and complete revascularization of the graft from the recipient bed, adequate fixation of the graft, absence of collections of blood or serum beneath the graft, and absence of infection. For the first few hours following transfer of a split-thickness skin graft, survival is dependent upon plasmatic circulation and absorption alone (Table 43-1). Graft and host vessels form communications by 12 hours. Active blood flow into the graft usually occurs by 2 to 3 days. The development of a mature complex of capillaries, arteries, and vessels occurs by 6 to 8 days after transplantation.[63] The clinical vascularization of a skin graft occurs primarily through the direct anastomoses of vessels within the graft to underlying host vessels, reinforced later by ingrowth of new host vessels into the graft.

The thicker the skin graft, the more durable it will be at its recipient site. The thinner the skin graft, the more likely it is to survive on its recipient bed. This is due to an enhanced ability to survive the phase of plasmatic absorption and delay in definitive vascularization when compared with thicker grafts. In general, in large wounds, split-thickness skin grafts are preferred, because the increased "take" guarantees faster closure. The donor site for a thin split-thickness skin graft re-epithelializes more rapidly than for a thick graft. The donor site for a full-thickness graft will not re-epithelialize at all; therefore, it must be closed primarily or allowed to granulate, scar, and contract to achieve closure. Donor site of 0.014 inches in depth may be reharvested at 15- to 16-day intervals,[23,43] although with thinner grafts, even shorter intervals are possible.

Although it has traditionally been accepted that the absolute thickness of the graft determined the amount of contracture, it is now known that the contracture is also a function of the underlying donor bed.[40,51] The earlier that a wound is grafted, the smaller the amount of contracture observed.

Split-thickness skin grafts are either applied as sheets or meshed graft prior to placement on recipient sites. Pinch grafts or stamp grafts, once popular, are no longer used in burn centers. The most commonly used device to mesh the grafts is a Tanner mesher.[58] The split-thickness skin graft is passed through this device, and, in the process, small slits are cut in the full thickness of the graft in a pattern that allows for expansion of the graft in a 1 1/2:1, 3:1, or 6:1 ratio, in an accordian-like fashion. Spread of epidermal cells from the margins of the fenestrated grafts results in rapid closing of the interstices of the mesh, thereby achieving wound closure. This technique is particularly valuable in patients in whom donor skin is limited. Mesh grafts must be kept moist and have firm dressings applied in order to achieve good "take."[25] If exposed to air too soon after grafting, the exposed recipient bed (through the holes of mesh) will desiccate and delay healing.

As mesh grafts heal, the mesh pattern may persist for varying periods of time, often permanently. Therefore, in cosmetically critical areas such as the face, sheet grafts are preferred. Similarly, because bulky moist occlusive dressings are not required for sheet grafts, they are the preferred graft for functionally critical areas such as the hands, where dressings will delay the onset of physical therapy.

When skin grafting is required, particularly in the massively burned patient, a planned approach to the multiple procedures that may be required is created using the following general guidelines.

1. The donor areas must be assessed for availability and thickness. In general, the skin of the medial portions of the thighs and calves, medial portion of the upper arm, the volar surface of the forearm, and the anterior trunk is relatively thin skin. The anterolateral and posteriolateral aspects of the thighs, the lateral aspects of the calves, the lateral and dorsal aspects of the upper extremities, the lumbar area of the back, and the buttocks are sites of intermediate thickness skin, whereas the back, and the buttocks are sites of intermediate thickness skin, whereas the back, the back of the neck, and the scalp sites of very thick skin.

2. Donor sites should not be created below the elbow or knee unless a lifesaving measure

owing to unfavorable functional and cosmetic results.

3. Donor sites may need to be reharvested. The thinner the split-thickness skin graft, the faster reharvesting can be accomplished.[28]

4. Priority areas for coverage consist of face and neck, axillae, elbows, hands, knees, and feet. These anatomic areas are always addressed first, once survival is ensured, because of their cosmetic and functional importance.

The maturation process of a split-thickness skin graft takes months to years. The earlier a wound is closed, the less the scar tissue buildup in the bed and resultant contracture.[43] Reappearance of the many functional elements of the skin occurs at varying times following grafting. Spotty hyperpigmentation often occurs, so avoidance of sunlight for 12 to 18 months is required. Reinnervation occurs by the ingrowth of nerves from the depth of the recipient bed and not by ingrowth from the margins; however, abnormal sensation inevitably results in the grafted area. for excellent sensation, flaps rather than split-thickness skin grafts are required.[46] Hypersensitivity to heat or cold is the rule with split-thickness skin grafts because of changes in nerve supply to the vessels. With time, as the graft bed fully matures, a soft pliable graft is the rule unless heavy scarring has supervened.

ALLOGRAFTS

The first recorded cutaneous allograft was performed in 1869 at the Charite Hospital in Paris by Reverdin.[45] Small grafts were taken from the arm of this French surgeon to treat a patient with extensive burns. Over the ensuing 20 years, clinical trials gave conflicting results, with claims by some of long-term host acceptance of allograft, while others claimed graft loss 5 to 8 weeks following application.[8,15,19,24,30] In 1881, Gindner[24] reported the use of cadaver allograft in treating a patient with a severe burn. He noted a 75% immediate graft take. In 1930, Loeb[35] conclusively demonstrated that an allograft would ultimately reject. Medawar[42] performed extensive experiments in the 1940s which finally elucidated the mechanisms of allograft rejection. Following his work, allografts were reserved for lifesaving circumstances when sufficient autografts were not available. During the next four decades, numerous reports of allograft use as a lifesaving measure in extensive burns have appeared.[2,10,11,26,39]

Today, allograft use is a major component in burn treatment, particularly in the salvage of massive injuries. Early excision of burned tissue in massive injuries has improved survival from previously fatal injuries.[9,12] The techniques and supportive measures required for the excision of burned tissue have developed rapidly; however, closure of the open wound has remained a problem. In theory, allograft satisfies the four major principles of the care of open wounds: (1) prevent infection, (2) preserve deeper tissues, (3) provide timely closure, and (4) maintain function and relieve pain. Thus, allografts have become the biological material of choice to treat open wounds when an autograft is unavailable because of limited donor sites.

The major limitations to allograft use have been limited availability, cost, potential risks of transferring disease from donor to host, and ultimate rejection of the material by the host.

Over the past 15 years, major advances have been made in correcting some of these problems; however, the results from use of allograft remain unpredictable in individual patients.

Limited Availability

There are potentially three sources of allografts: amputated limbs, live donors, and cadaver donors. Amputated limbs are of limited use. Large quantities of skin are generally not available from these limbs because of the pathologic process that led to the amputation. Live donors have also presented a number of major problems. If sufficient amounts of skin are to be obtained, the donor must be hospitalized (cost of hospitalization), placed at risk (infection, blood loss, anesthesia), and possibly permanently scarred (hypertrophic scarring in donor sites). Despite these factors, live donors have occasionally been used, particularly the parents of burned children or in twins.[12]

The availability of cadaver donors has made this the preferred allograft source. Postmortem skin remains viable for 3 to 4 hours without refrigeration and up to 16 hours if early refrigeration of the body occurs.[18] When cryopreserved, these allografts have the same properties as those obtained from live donors.

If careful selection of donors is undertaken, the risk of transmitting disease from donor to recipient is rare. Postmortem blood tests are used to rule out hepatitis or treponemal infection. Multiple bacteriologic cultures are taken throughout the processing procedure to detect contamination.

Skin banks have developed across the country. In 1979, a survey of 20 such banks by May and DeClement[41] found that 868 cadaver donors were procured. The skin donation rate was found to be unrelated to the population base but, instead, was correlated with the number of skin procurement personnel. The yield was substantially increased if a medical examiner source existed that yielded one half of all donors. The cost of the skin was indirectly related to the number of donors.

When a donor is identified and consent from next of kin is obtained, the body is taken to a clean area (usually an operating room), and the areas of the body to be used are surgically prepped and draped. The skin once removed is cryopreserved using a controlled-rate freezing protocol ($-1°C$ per minute to $-40°C$, then $-10°C$ per minute to $-100°C$, then quickly cooled to $-196°C$) and stored in liquid nitrogen at $-196°C$.[38] Most skin banks that have developed in the United States currently use a set of guidelines prepared by the American Association of Tissue Banks,[57] which outline criteria for donor selection, collection and processing procedures, and storage of the allograft. In general, donors with malignancy, systemic microbial infection, diffuse dermatitis, treponemal antibody in their serum, or history of viral hepatitis or jaundice are excluded. Collection is recommended within 18 hours of death, and cryoprotection and cryopreservation to maintain viability are suggested.

With the standardization of the skin banking facilities, viable safe allografts are now available from many banks.

Clinical Studies

The use of allografts to provide wound coverage following excision in massive burn injuries is limited by the ultimate rejection of the material. This necessitates frequent removal and replacement of the material and inconsistent results. In 1975, 11 children with massive third-degree burn injuries (70% body surface area or greater) underwent major excision at the Shriner's Institute in Boston.[12] These wounds were covered with allograft, and immunosuppression was achieved with anti-thymocyte globulin (ATG). Seven children survived and were capable of returning to normal productive lives. The most compatible family member as determined by tissue typing was chosen as the donor. Of the 11 children, 9 received allografts from their mother or father. Allograft survival was maintained for 30 to 50 days before surgical removal was performed and autograft closure was completed. Other centers also report similar scattered reports of children who survived their injury with the use of this technique.[20] To date, these results have not been obtained in adults.

Allograft use requires that it be changed before rejection occurs; otherwise, immunosuppression must be used to delay this rejection. Five days after an allograft is applied, a round cell infiltrate can be identified in the tissue deep to the graft, which is suggestive of early rejection. If allowed to progress, this rejection reaction produces severe systemic toxic symptoms in already debilitated patients and results in a granulating wound that is ill prepared for grafting and susceptible to invasive sepsis.[55]

Although it has been shown that HLA and ABO closely matched skin allografts will survive longer than poorly matched skin,[5,16,27] most of the viable allografts available in the United States are not being tissue typed. The major reason is one of supply and demand. Allografts are also used for other aspects of burn care and are not recovered for the specific situation in which "take" is required. The major uses of allografts are summarized in Table 43-2. Only in indication Number 5 is "take" essential, and this constitutes a small proportion of the use of this material.

If all available allografts were used solely for situations in which "take" was essential, theoretically, it would be possible to select a panel of donors from skin bank stores (previously typed) that would most likely be able to provide prolonged "take."

In a computer analysis study performed to determine the required pool size in order to match HLA-B and HLA-DR between donor and recipient using recurrence relationships, it was shown that with 1000 donors, there was a 91% probability of a three-antigen match, whereas with 10,000 donors, there was a 42% chance of a four-antigen match.[36] Unfortunately, economic constraints do not allow for restriction of use of allografts for this sole indication. The cooperative effort required nationwide to create this static-type donor pool resource is not available; thus alternate approaches to the problem have been pursued.

Glutaraldehyde is a bifunctional reagent capable of reacting rapidly in aqueous solutions with the E-amino group of lysine and with the alpha-amino

TABLE 43-2   Homograft Use

1. Immediate coverage of superficial second-degree burns
2. Débridement of "untidy" wounds after eschar separation
3. "Test" material prior to autografting
4. Coverage of granulation tissue between "crops" of autograft in large burns
5. Immediate coverage following excision

groups of amino acids. These properties make it an efficient reagent for the crosslinking of proteins.[4,49] In theory, glutaraldehyde could directly and covalently bind to the histocompatibility antigen molecules or in their close vicinity. These antigens would therefore be masked and become inaccessible to the immune apparatus of the recipient.[53]

Despite some encouraging preliminary results in both animals and humans, the practice of pretreating allografts with glutaraldehyde has not become widespread.[54] Glutaraldehyde treatment kills the allograft and converts it to a biological dressing. True "take" with vascularization of the graft is not seen.[29] Allografts so treated may adhere temporarily to a graft bed but are of limited value as transplants when prolonged coverage is required. Similarly, pretreatment of the grafts with corticoids, thalidomide, urethran, radiation, or electrophosesis have been assessed and abandoned.[29] To date, no effective method is available to alter the antigenicity of the allograft material without destroying its viability and converting it to a biological dressing. The material may then adhere temporarily to the wound bed; however, it will not "take," achieve vascularization, or effectively close the wound for prolonged periods of time.

AMNIOTIC MEMBRANES

Amniotic membrane was used as an allograft tissue as early as 1912 by Sabella.[52] The material is readily available from the delivery room and is inexpensive to prepare.[50] True biological union with host-to-graft vascular connection is uncertain,[17] and the material is very thin and breaks down easily. Because of these limitations, amnion has had limited use in the treatment of burn patients.

XENOGRAFTS

It is only natural that over the years, scientists have attempted the transplantation of animal skin to humans. At different times, the skins of lizards, chickens, pigeons, dogs, guinea pigs, rats, rabbits, cats, frogs, pigs, and cows were used as the source.[47] The most common species currently used to provide xenografts for burn treatment is the pig. Porcine cutaneous xenografts decrease the rate of bacterial growth in the underlying wound but not as effectively as cutaneous allografts.[32] Porcine xenografts also adhere to wound beds but, again, not as well as allografts. The graft-to-host union is produced by fibrovascular ingrowth of granulation tissue into the dermis of the graft, and vessel-to-vessel connection

between host and graft does not occur as it does with cutaneous allografts.[56] There is no evidence of revascularization of the graft nor evidence of host sensitization after sloughing 7 to 10 days later.[3] There are some reports of true "take" of porcine xenografts, but rejection occurs rapidly.[59] Even with immunosuppression, this response cannot be delayed despite continued retention of allografts in these same patients.[20] This emphasizes the limited use of xenografts in achieving long-term coverage of wounds.

When porcine xenografts are used as wound dressings, care must be taken not to apply them to heavily contaminated wounds. Marked subgraft bacterial proliferation may occur, which may convert partial thickness injuries to full-thickness injuries. In the case of full-thickness injuries, the infection may become invasive, with involvement of local unburned tissue and may even produce systemic dissemination. In general, biological dressings should not be applied to deep partial-thickness burns prior to removal of the superficial debris, to full-thickness burns prior to eschar separation or removal, or to any wound with a bacterial population density of more than 10^5 organisms per gram of tissue as determined by semiquantitative biopsy of the burn wound.

Porcine xenografts are commonly used in burn centers despite these limitations. When applied to clean partial-thickness wounds, they exert the same effect on water vapor loss as do allografts[31] and promote epithelialization like allografts when compared with the rate of epithelialization under topical antibacterials.[14] Viability per se is not the critical factor in the function of a biological dressing when permanent "take" is not required. As such, currently available preparations are processed to prolong shelflife and are not viable.

Porcine xenografts are far cheaper than allografts. A variety of commercial preparations exist so that storage is no longer an issue. Pigskin is the most commonly used biological dressing in burn treatment and is used in all cases in which a biological dressing is required except for the single circumstance when true vascularization of the graft for prolonged coverage is required.[37] In this circumstance, an allograft or one of the newer artificial skin systems must be used.

SYNTHETIC SKIN SYSTEMS

No discussion of skin transplantation is complete without a review of the current status of artificial skin. In the past 20 years, there has been a proliferation of new synthetic materials to substitute for skin. When faced with a failing organ or devitalized tissue, physicians have historically first searched the animal kingdom or other humans for a replacement. With time, technology has provided a synthetic to replace the biological material. In general, these synthetics are more durable and free of the problems of rejection. They can be mass produced, have an indefinite shelf life, and, eventually, become inexpensive. Joints, heart valves, and blood vessels now have suitable synthetic replacements.

Most of the current research in skin transplantation, particularly in burns, is focused on the development of an artificial skin. To date, major advances have been made in a number of new materials and, currently, are undergoing clinical evaluations.[13] A clinically effective skin substitute must have certain properties (Table 43-3). The new materials are either bilaminate membranes that are a composite of heterologous biodegradable tissue and synthetic material, bilaminate membranes that are totally synthetic and biologically inert, or membranes composed of autologous tissue that either persist or are gradually replaced by host tissue.

Although each system offers both advantages and disadvantages, none, as yet, fulfills all the requirements of the ideal "artificial" skin. Many offer such benefit that they are currently preferred over allografts as the skin substitute of choice to close massive open wounds.

Autologous Tissue Membranes

The tissue culture growth of autologous components of skin is now possible. Single cell suspensions of epidermal cells obtained from the prospective recipient can be grown into sheets in vitro. These multilayered sheets of epidermal cells have a lower layer of cells morphologically similar to the basal cells of normal epidermis.[21] When reimplanted in humans, sheets of epidermal cells have produced less than optimal results. The resultant epidermis lacks rete pegs as late as 6 months following application. The resultant graft remains thinner than normal and often develops traumatic fissures. It is subject to desiccation and totally lacks a normal dermis. The fibrous structure of the skin is reconstituted by granulation tissue deep to these sheets of epidermal cells and matures into scar tissue.[44]

Recently, "a living skin equivalent" has been proposed, which consists of a composite consisting of a fibroblast-seeded collagen fibrillar lattice upon which dissociated epidermal cells are cultured and proliferate.[7] The addition of fibroblasts to a solution of Type I collagen causes the collagen to form a fibrillar lattice that subsequently decreases in volume and increases in consistency. The composite,

TABLE 43-3 Essential Properties of Skin Substitutes

1. Non antigenic
2. Tissue compatible
3. Non-toxic
4. Water-vapor transmission similar to normal skin
5. Bacterial barrier
6. Rapid and sustained adherence to wound surface
7. Inner surface stricture which allows for ingrowth of fibrovascular tissue
8. Flexible, pliable and elastic to allow for conformation to irregular wound surfaces and permit underlying body tissue movement
9. Strong enough to resist fragmentation
10. Deeper layers which will sustain tissue ingrowth must be biodegradable
11. Low Cost
12. Indefinite shelf life
13. Easily stored

Modified from Pruitt BA, Levine NS: Characteristics and uses of biologic dressings and skin substitutes. Arch Surg 119:312, 1984

when applied to full-thickness wounds (following excision), rapidly vascularizes. The composite graft can persist as long as 10 months, with considerable remodeling of the dermal component occurring. Radioactive-labeled fibroblasts in the composite persist for up to 5 weeks. The dermal component of the graft serves as a scaffold for replacement by host tissue. By 10 weeks following application, the graft dermis thins to approximately half the thickness of the adjacent host dermis.[6] Epidermal hypertrophy has been observed, the histologic sections show tongues of host epidermis invading the periphery of such composite grafts, which may represent replacement of the graft epidermis by scar epithelium of the host.

The major limitation to the clinical use of this material is the time required to produce the composite graft. To create a 100 sq cm composite graft from a 1 sq cm biopsy specimen takes 20 to 26 days. Patients with massive burn injuries must be excised earlier than 3 weeks, because, by that time, colonization of the wounds like bacteria inevitably has occurred. Excision with closure is usually performed during the first week post burn; hence, this technique of creating the composite graft of autogenous tissue is of little value.

Totally Synthetic Bilaminate Membranes

Another path of development has been to find a totally synthetic biologically inert bilaminate membrane. The composition of the inner layer that appeared to be most promising was a nylon stocking fragment.[33] This material was found to be superior to a variety of other membranes with which it was compared when assessed for tissue compatibility, lack of fragmentation, and retention of foreign bodies at the time of membrane removal. The material was flexible and elastic and conformed to irregular wound surfaces. This material was more in keeping with a wound dressing and has not been widely accepted.

Collagen-Synthetic Composite Membranes

Two materials are not available that fall into this category of skin replacements. The first to be available is a bilaminate membrane. The outer layer is an ultrathin sheet of silicone rubber that is mechanically bound to a fine-kit flexible nylon fabric. Type 1 porcine collagen is covalently bonded to the fabric to provide an inner layer into which granulation can grow. The material is sold under the name Biobrane. It is extremely elastic, easily draped over even the most difficult contours, and permits full range of motion of grafted body parts.

The material is best suited for application to clean wounds such as donor sites or after excision, because adhesion is severely impaired if bacterial colonization has occurred.[22] This material, when applied to clean wounds, appears to be as effective an allograft in providing long-term wound stability. The use of Biobrane is particularly useful on donor sites and as an overlay graft on widely meshed 6:1 or greater autograft if it is peeled off before the fifth postoperative day. If it is retained beyond the fifth day, it may interfere with re-epithelialization.[34] This overlay technique has also been described with allografts, with favorable results.[1] The ultimate cosmetic appearance of this technique is acceptable, and this type of approach offers significant advantages for grafting of extensively burned patients with limited donor sites.

The second of the bilaminate membranes is now undergoing extensive clinical evaluation and appears to show great promise. In developing this material, the concept of nonreactivity to tissue was abandoned, and, instead, an attempt was made to design a material with biochemical, mechanical, and physiochemical properties intended to optimize physical and chemical properties, such as surface energy, elasticity, energy of fracture, and moisture permeability. In addition, the material was designed to induce the migration of normal fibroblasts and vessels into the material. The artificial material would act as a template for the synthesis of a new dermal matrix while controlling the rate of implant biodegradation in order to maintain the physical

and biological properties of skin necessary for physiologic wound closure. This nonantigenic membrane would act as biodegradable scaffolding inducing the syntheses of a "neodermis."

Reconstitution of a neodermis restores structural integrity of the skin with a fibrous structure with the same characteristics as normal dermis, not scar. From a functional and cosmetic point of view, this line of thinking must be viewed as a major breakthrough in advancing this field.

Artificial skin was developed and tested by John F. Burke, Ioannis V. Yannas, William C. Quinby, and associates and is currently undergoing a multi-institutional evaluation prior to being commercially available. The material is a bilayer membrane made of a distinct epidermal and dermal portion.[60] The function of each portion physiologically resembles its counterpart in normal skin. The raw material used to manufacture the dermal portion is a preparation of bovine hide collagen and chondroitin-6-sulfate obtained from shark collagen. Physiochemical, biochemical, and mechanical properties are controlled by the content of chondroitin-6-sulfate, methods of crosslinking, crosslink density, and mean pore size.[61] The epidermal portion of the artificial skin consists of a homogeneous layer of medical grade Silastic that is approximately $1/10$ mm thick. This material controls water flux from the dermis, making it approximately equal to that of normal skin. It also protects the wound from mechanical trauma and microbial invasion. The composite can be stored in 70% isopropyl alcohol or can be freeze-dried for storage.

The material itself, when applied firmly, adheres to the wound bed, and early vascularization of the dermal component is evident within 3 to 5 days. Whenever donor sites are available, the Silastic is removed and the neodermis is covered with thin epidermal autografts (0.1 mm thick). Progressive host tissue invasion and replacement of the dermal analog occurs slowly over the ensuing months. Pore size is critical to the successful function of the dermal analog, because a pore size smaller than that of normal dermis retards cellular invasion and leads to the development of thick fibrous tissue. No inflammatory or immunologic reactions occur as the biodegradation occurs.

Once adherent, the artificial skin effects closes the wound. The Silastic can remain in place for weeks following its application. A true "take" of this material occurs without fear of rejection. The thin epidermal grafts, when applied, rapidly mature, and the final result is a smooth homogenous appearance identical to normal skin. No evidence of hypertrophic scarring or contracture occurs. The use of this material produces a final healed area that is softer and more elastic and pliable than areas in which the excised wounds are closed by immediate application of meshed autograft skin. The major problems in the use of this material have been premature separation of the Silastic epidermis and scar formation at seam lines between sheets of artificial skin.

In vitro seeding of the dermal analog with dissociated autologous basal cells has been attempted in animal models. Rapid basal cell proliferation occurs with the formation of sheets of keratinized epidermis at the laminar interface of the composite within 14 days of application to a wound.[62] This technique may prove to be useful in the second step in which epidermal grafts are required to replace the Silastic.

CONCLUSION

Skin transplantation is required when skin is destroyed. If donor areas are not available in adequate quantities, substitutes are essential. The open wounds rapidly deplete the host and are a ready portal for microbial invasion. Xenografts are dressings, and application to wounds achieves only short-term closure. Allografts ''take'' and effectively close the wound; however, rejection ultimately occurs. Synthetic materials currently offer the best promise for achieving all the requirements of skin replacement, particularly the bilaminar membrane, which allows for formation of a true neodermis. Not only can it effectively restore the physical and biochemical functions of the skin, but it also creates a cosmetic result that to date has not been obtainable by any other technique.

To the burn patient, transplantation of skin or its substitutes is essential first and foremost for survival, but also for cosmetic and functional rehabilitation. As new techniques and materials are developed, the prognosis for the patient who has suffered massive skin loss will continue to improve, making this one of the most dynamic and exciting new arenas for research and development.

REFERENCES

1. Alexander JW, MacMillan BG, Law E et al: Treatment of severe burns with widely meshed skin autograft and meshed skin allograft overlay. Trauma 21:433, 1981
2. Artz CP, Recker JM, Sako Y et al: Postmortem skin homografts in the treatment of extensive burns. Arch Surg 71:682, 1955
3. Artz CP, Rittenbury MS, Yarbrough DR: An appraisal of allografts and xenografts as biological dressings for wounds and burns. Ann Surg 175:934, 1972
4. Avrameas S, Ternynck T: The cross-linking of proteins with glutaraldehyde and its use for the preparation of immunoabsorbents. Immunochemistry 6:53, 1969
5. Batchelor JR, Hatchett M: HL-A matching in treatment of burned patients with skin allografts. Lancet 1:581, 1970
6. Bell E, Ehrlich HP, Buttle DJ et al: Living tissue formed in vitro and accepted as skin equivalent tissue of full thickness. Science 211:1052, 1981
7. Bell E, Ehrlich HP, Sher S et al: Development and use of a living skin equivalent. Plast Reconstr Surg 67:386, 1981
8. Blair VP, Brown JB: The use and uses of large splitskin grafts of intermediate thickness. Surg Gynecol Obstet 49:82, 1929
9. Bondoc CC, Burke JF: Clinical experience with viable frozen human skin and a frozen skin bank. Ann Surg 174:371, 1971
10. Brown JB, Fryer MP: Postmortem homografts to reduce mortality in extensive burns: Early biological closure and savings of patients for permanent healing. Use in mass casualties and in national disaster. JAMA 156:1163, 1954
11. Brown JB, Fryer MP, Randall PL et al: Postmortem homografts as biological dressings for extensive burns and débrided areas: Immediate and preserved homografts as life-saving procedures. Ann Surg 138:618, 1953
12. Burke JF, Quinby WC, Bodoc CC et al: Immunosuppression and temporary skin transplantation in the treatment of massive third degree burns. Ann Surg 182:183, 1975
13. Burke JF, Yannas IV, Quinby WC et al: Successful use of a physiologically acceptable artificial skin in the treatment of extensive burn injury. Ann Surg 194;413, 1981
14. Burleson R, Eiseman E: Effect of skin dressings and topical antibiotics on healing of partial thickness skin wounds in rats. Surg Gynecol Obstet 136:158, 1973
15. Carrel A: The preservation of tissues and its application in surgery. JAMA 59:523, 1912
16. Cepellini R et al: Survival of test skin groups in man: Effects in genetic relationship and blood group incompatibility. Ann NY Acad Sci 129:421, 1966
17. Colocho G, Graham WB III, Greene AE et al: Human amniotic membrane as a physiologic wound dressing. Arch Surg 109:370, 1974
18. Dago G: Survival and utilization of cadaver skin. Plast Reconstr Surg 10:10, 1952
19. Davis JS: Skin transplantation. John Hopkins Hosp Reports 15:307, 1910
20. Diethelm AG, Dimick AR, Shaw JF et al: Treatment

of the severely burned child with skin transplantation modified by immunosuppression therapy. Ann Surg 180:814, 1974

21. Eisenger M, Morden M, Raaf JH et al: Wound coverage by a sheet of epidermal cells grown in vitro from dispersed single cell preparations. Surgery 88:287, 1980

22. Frank DH, Wachtel T, Frank HA et al: Comparison of Biobrane, porcine and human allograft as biologic dressings for burn wounds. J Burn Care Rehab 4:186, 1983

23. Gilman T, Penn J, Bronks D et al: A reexamination of certain aspects of the histogenesis of healing cutaneous wounds. Br J Surg 43:141, 1955

24. Gindner JH: Skin grafting with grafts taken from the dead patient. Med Rec NY 20:119, 1890

25. Hagstrom NS Jr et al: the importance of occlusive dressings in the treatment of mesh skin grafts. Plast Reconstr Surg 38:137, 1966

26. Haynes BW Jr: Skin homografts: A life saving measure in severely burned children. J Trauma 3:217, 1963

27. Higuchi D, Sei Y, Takivchi I: Influence of histocompatibility antigens on skin homograft survival in an extensively burned patient. J Dermatol 8:47, 1981

28. Hinshaw JR, Miller ER: Histology of healing split thickness, full thickness autogenous skin grafts and donor sites. Arch Surg 91:658, 1965

29. Im HM, Simmons RL: Mechanism for the prolonged survival of glutaraldehyde-treated skin allografts. Transplantation 14:527, 1972

30. Ivanova SS: The transplantation of skin from dead body to granulating surface. Ann Surg 12:354, 1890

31. Lamke LO, Nillsson GE, Reithner HS: The evaporative water loss from burns and the water-vapor permeability of grafts and artificial membranes used in the treatment of burns. Burns 3:159, 1978

32. Levine NS, Lindberg RA, Salisbury RE et al: Comparison of coarse mesh gauge with biologic dressings on granulating wounds. Am J Surg 131:727, 1974

33. Levine NS, Salisbury RE, Peterson HD:: Continued evaluation of split-thickness cutaneous xenograft and synthetic materials as temporary biologic wound covers for burned soldiers. Annual Research Progress Report. Fort Sam Houston, Texas, U.S. Army Institute of Surgical Research, Brooke Army Medical Center Section 40, June 1984

34. Lin SD, Robb BS, Nathan P: A comparison of 1P-758 and Biobrane in rats as temporary protective dressings on widely expanded meshed autografts. J Burn Care Rehab 3:220, 1982

35. Loeb L: Transplantation and individuality. Physiol Rev 10:547, 1930

36. Luterman A, Braun D, Kraft E et al: Skin banking, transplantation with tissue typing: What size donor pool is required? Am Burn Assoc Proc 13:1981

37. Luterman A, Kraft E, Bookless S: Biologic dressings: An appraisal of current practices. J Burn Care Rehab 1:18, 1980

38. Luterman A, Kraft E, Kirchner S: What's new in skin banking? Hosp Physician 16:51, 1980

39. MacMillan BG: Homograft skin: A valuable adjunct to the treatment of thermal burns. J Trauma 2:130, 1962

40. Madden JW: Plastic Surgery ACS Bulletin p 12, Nov–Dec, 1973

41. May SR, DeClement FA: Skin banking Part I: Procurement of transplantable cadaveric allograft skin for burn wound coverage. J Burn Care Rehab 2:7, 1981

42. Medawar PB: Notes of the problems of skin homografts. Bull War Med 4:1, 1943

43. Moncrief JA: Grafting. In Artz CP, Moncrief JA, Pruitt BA (eds): Burns—A Team Approach. Philadelphia, WB Saunders, 1979

44. O'Connor NE, Mulliken JB, Banks-Schlegel S et al: Grafting of burns with cultured epithelium prepared from autologous epidermal cells. Lancet 1:75, 1981

45. Palmer JF: The origin of skin grafting—a reminiscence. Med Magazine London 15:477, 1906

46. Porten B: Grafted skin observations on innervation and other qualities. Acta Chir Scand Suppl 257:1, 1960

47. Pruitt BA, Curreri PW: The use of homograft and heterograft skin. In Polk HC, Stone HH (eds): Contemporary Burn Management. Boston, Little, Brown and Co, 1971

48. Pruitt BA, Levine NS: Characteristics and uses of biologic dressings and skin substitutes. Arch Surg 119:312, 1984

49. Richards FM, Knowles JR: Glutuaraldehyde as a protein cross-linking reagent. J Mol Biol 37:231, 1968

50. Robson MC, Krizek TJ, Koss N et al: Amniotic membranes as a temporary wound dressing. Surg Gynecol Obstet 136:904, 1973

51. Rudolph R: Skin graft preparation and wound contraction. Surg Forum 26:560, 1975

52. Sabella N: Use of fetal membranes in skin grafting. Med Rec NY 83:478, 1913

53. Schechter I: Prolonged survival of glutaraldehyde-treated skin homografts. Proc Natl Acad Sci USA 68, 1590, 1971

54. Schechter I: Prolonged retention of glutaraldehyde treated skin allografts and xenografts. Ann Surg 182:699, 1975

55. Shuck JM: Biologic dressings. In Artz CP, Moncreif JA, Pruitt BA (eds): Burns—A Team Approach, Philadelphia, WB Saunders, 1979.

56. Silverstern P, Curreri PW, Muster AM: Evaluation of fresh viable porcine cutaneous xenografts as a temporary wound cover. Annual Research Progress Report. Sam Houston, Texas, U.S. Army Surgical Research Unit, Brooke Army Medical Center, Section 51, June 30, 1971

57. Standards Committee of the Skin Council of the American Association of Tissue Banks: Guidelines for the banking of skin tissues. Am Assoc Tissue Banks Newsletter 3(1):5, 1979

58. Tanner JC, Vandeput J, Olley JF: The mesh skin graft. Plast Reconstr Surg 34:287, 1964

59. Wood M, Hale HW: The use of pigskin in the treatment of thermal burns. Am J Surg 124:720, 1972

60. Yannas IV, Burke JF: Design of an artificial skin. I.

Basic design principles. J Biomed Mater Res 14:65, 1980

61. Yannas IV, Burke JF, Gordon PL et al: Design of an artificial skin. II. Control of chemical composition. J Biomed Mater Res 14:107, 1980

62. Yannas IV, Burke JF, Orgill DP et al: Wound tissue can utilize a polymeric template to synthesize a functional extension of skin. Science 215;174, 1982

63. Zarem HA: Transplantation of the skin. In Krizek TJ, Hoopes JE (eds): Symposium on Basic Science in Plastic Surgery. St Louis, The CV Mosby Co, 1976

CHAPTER 44

Small Bowel Transplantation

Zane Cohen   Ramses Wassef   Richard Silverman

There has been a great increase in the number of patients undergoing major small bowel resections. An alternative to total parenteral nutrition (TPN) and the complications of the short bowel syndrome is small interstitial transplantation.

Allotransplantation of the small intestine without immunosuppression invariably results in death of the recipient from small bowel rejection. In addition to rejection, the large lymphoid mass transplanted with the intestine included in the mesentery predisposes the recipient to graft-versus-host disease. Attempts at overcoming rejection and graft-versus-host disease with conventional immunosuppressive regimens have proved significantly more difficult than for other organ transplants. Survival has been shown to be increased with low-dose graft irradiation alone and with lymphadectomy of the donor small intestine.

Cycylosporine alone or in combination with steroids has prolonged survival in both the dog and pig and has also prevented the rejection response in a unidirectional rat intestinal transplantation model. Factors that have hindered successful small intestinal transplantation have been (1) the immunologic reactions of rejection, (2) graft-versus-host disease, (3) the very high technical failure rate of 40% to 60% following intestinal transplantation in large animal models, and (4) inadequate preservation. The optimal route of venous drainage is still uncertain.

In view of the success of home parenteral nutrition, it is difficult to define candidates for intestinal transplantation. Long-term survivors in large animal models have been few, and, at the present time, there have been eight documented published reports of small intestinal transplantation in humans. None have been successful, with the longest survivor being 76 days with no useful function of the allograft.

At the moment, there are few patients who should be deemed suitable candidates for this experimental procedure.

Patients undergoing major resections of their small intestine secondary to small bowel infarction owing to (1) vascular thrombosis, (2) embolus of the superior mesenteric artery, (3) volvulus, or (4) multiple resections for extensive Crohn's disease may become unable to absorb nutrients.[37] Oral feeding will cause diarrhea and steatorrhea because of the rapid transit of nutrients through the small bowel. In addition to insufficient protein and caloric intake and the risk of dehydration, patients suffering from the crippling short bowel syndrome inevitably develop vitamin and mineral deficiencies that require parenteral correction. These patients become dependent upon parenteral nutritional support, which must provide glucose, amino acids, electrolytes, vitamins, trace minerals, and lipids. Long-term parenteral alimentation has proved lifesaving in some patients with massive small intestinal resections. In some cases, this therapy has been administered outside the hospital under the supervision of specialized centers offering home total parenteral nutrition (TPN). This undoubtedly leads to an improvement in the lifestyle of these patients, freeing them from the confines of the hospital and allowing most of them to resume an active life at home or at work. However, these patients still face several major problems.

Although long-term survivors in excess of 10 years on home TPN programs have been reported, the nutritional management of these patients still requires close monitoring owing to the nonphysiologic route of alimentation.[16] Metabolic complications include deficiency states such as hyponatremia, hypokalemia, hypophosphatemia, and magnesium and calcium disorders.[10] In addition, long-term venous access can be associated with catheter complications at the time of insertion and, later, sepsis, thrombosis, and embolism. Psychosocial limitations resulting from either the inability to eat or the dependency on an external means for survival are common. Patients and their relatives must understand feeding schedules and follow aseptic technique in handling the catheters and the intravenous (IV) solutions. Some patients feel overwhelmed by the complexity of such programs and are thus unable to benefit maximally from this therapy. Finally, the cost of such a program approximates $45,000 per patient per year for the IV solutions alone. The additional expenses of catheters, dressings, repeated hospitalizations, and frequent biochemical and hematologic assays often make such care prohibitively expensive on a long-term basis.

HISTORY

In 1959, experimental small intestinal transplantation was attempted by Lillehei and co-workers.[20] Their interest in this concept was a natural sequela of their work on the relationship between irreversible shock and intestinal ischemia. It was quickly realized, however, that this model could have great implications in the treatment of patients suffering from the short bowel syndrome.

The initial surgical technique for canine small intestinal transplantation and for bowel preservation was developed by this group. This technique consisted of dividing the mesentery of the proximal and distal small bowel and exposing the superior mesenteric artery and vein. After dividing the duodenum and terminal ileum, both superior mesenteric artery and superior mesenteric vein were divided between clamps (Figs. 44-1 and 44-2). Cooling of the graft by a cold saline solution (4°C) through the superior mesenteric artery or by placing the bowel in a sterile bag and immersing it in cold saline preserved the bowel for periods of 4 to 5 hours. Preservation by hypothermia and hyperbaric oxygenation were also successful for up to 48 hours.[24] The vessels were reconstructed by anastomosing to the host superior mesenteric artery and vein, respectively. Continuity of the bowel was restored by a proximal and distal anastomosis. Initial experiments with autotransplants in dogs yielded indefinite survival. Although diarrhea and steatorrhea occurred immediately following surgery, the stools became normal within a few weeks. Injection of dye into a lymph duct of the small bowel mesentery subsequently demonstrated prompt regrowth of the lymphatics, with the dye quickly appearing in the thoracic duct.[13] This lymphatic regeneration was completed within 4 weeks of autotransplantation.[18]

However, allotransplantation of the small intestine without immunosuppression invariably resulted in the death of the recipient, usually by the eighth postoperative day.[12] Death was originally attributed solely to graft-versus-host disease because of the relatively normal growth and histologic appearance of the bowel. Hypertrophy of the mesenteric lymph nodes in the allograft further substantiated this hypothesis.[25] Later experiments disclosed, however, that both graft rejection and graft-versus-host disease occurred in small intestinal allotransplantation. The length of the graft and, thus, the amount of lymphoid tissue transplanted determined the dominant reaction, with short intestinal segments showing prompt and definite rejection, and long segments causing mainly graft-versus-host disease.[22] However, the predominant reaction in animals in whom a total intestinal transplant has been performed seems to be allograft rejection.

Attempts at overcoming rejection and graft-versus-host disease with conventional immunosuppressive regimens proved more difficult than for the kidney or the heart.[15] Antilymphocyte serum (ALS), prednisone, azathioprine, and several other immunosuppressive drugs were administered alone or in combination to allotransplanted dogs. Survival could be increased only to a mean of 25 days.[29] Low-dose graft irradiation alone was shown to prolong survival in a canine small bowel allograft model to a mean of 28 days.[34] In contrast, irradiation of the graft with a higher dose of 150 rads resulted in death of the recipient animals at a mean of 9.2 days, apparently from allograft rejection. It was postulated that a balance was struck between the allograft rejection reaction and graft-versus-host disease in the low-dose radiation group, resulting in prolonged survival.

A better understanding of the intricate interactions between graft and host in small intestinal transplantation was provided by Monchik and Russel[26] in their study of small intestinal transplantation using inbred strains of rats and their Fl hybrid offspring. Fl hybrids are the products of matings between rats from two different isogeneic strains. In accordance with mendelian principles, the hybrids possess all the histocompatibility genes and antigens present in each of the parental strains. Consequently, Fl hybrid cells do not recognize parental tissue as antigenetically dissimilar. Thus, unilateral reactions of rejection (Fl graft in a parental recipient) and graft-versus-host disease (parental graft in an Fl recipient) could be separated and studied. These genetic combinations had previously been used to circumvent allograft rejection and allow

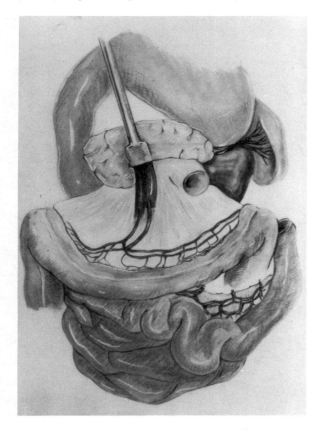

FIGURE 44-1.   Harvesting the small bowel. Note dissection to base of middle colic vessels beneath pancreas.

graft-versus-host reactions to occur.[3] Their technique consisted of harvesting the small bowel and mesentery from the distal duodenum to the terminal ileum along with the attached portal vein and superior mesenteric artery with an aortic cuff. The resected specimen was cooled by immersion in a crushed ice–saline solution. The recipient was prepared by isolating the inferior vena cava and the aorta. The graft was then revascularized in a heterotopic position by microvascular anastomosis between the graft's aortic cuff with the recipient aorta and the graft's portal vein with the recipient's inferior vena cava. The ends of the graft were exteriorized and sutured to the abdominal wall was a duodenostomy and ileostomy, respectively. With heterotopic small bowel transplantation, the rejection or graft-versus-host reactions that occurred in the appropriate Fl parental donor–recipient combination uniformly proved fatal in 9 to 17 days. However, graft-versus-host disease could be eliminated by total donor irradiation, with 700 rads producing indefinite survival in recipients. This provided a strong demonstration of the importance of graft-versus-host disease in small bowel transplantation.

RECENT ADVANCES OF SMALL INTESTINE TRANSPLANTATION

The major advance in organ transplantation during the last decade has been the utilization of the immunosuppressive agent Cyclosporin A (CsA), introduced in 1974 by Borel and associates.[4] This led to a flurry of clinical trials in kidney and later in liver and other organ transplantations in humans. Because of cyclosporine's initial success with other organ transplants and because of its effect against graft-versus-host disease, it rekindled interest in small intestinal transplantation.

Cyclosporine has been used experimentally in three major animal models, including the dog, the pig, and the rat.

Large Animal Models of Small Intestinal Transplantation

Our group has studied total orthotopic small intestinal transplantation in unmatched mongrel dogs treated with cyclosporine as the sole immunosuppressant.[7] The success of small bowel transplanta-

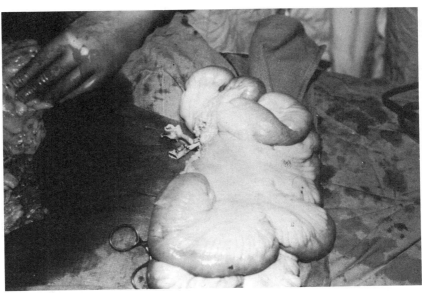

FIGURE 44-2. *The entire small bowel harvested on a cuff of aorta and the superior mesenteric vein.*

tion in dogs without cyclosporine, oral cyclosporine (25 mg/kg), or parenteral CsA was 12, 34, or 104 days of survival, respectively; survival in excess of 400 days was observed in the parenteral group. Diliz-Perez and colleagues[9] recently reported prolonged survival in dogs following total small intestinal transplantation using a combination of cyclosporine and steroids as immunosuppressants 4 of 12 survived more than 4 months, and 2 of 12 survived more than 500 days). This length of survival had never been reported previously in an experimental model. However, the majority of animals in all prior series died of early technical failures and survived for fewer than 50 days. It is an important observation that cyclosporine given to dogs orally with incontinuity transplants can provide prolonged survival, but the overall survival does not approach the survival of animals treated with parenteral cyclosporine. This may reflect poor initial absorption of CsA; therefore, cyclosporine in human trials should be given parenterally to ensure adequate immunosuppression. Other groups, using a variety of immunosuppression protocols, have also reported prolonged survival in pigs and dogs with small bowel allografts.[1,30,31]

One of the problems in small intestinal transplantation is diagnosing rejection and monitoring the effect of rejection on allograft function. Our laboratory has evaluated a method for histologic monitoring of the allografted bowel by exteriorizing two isolated segments of the graft as blind pouches, thus rendering the graft easily accessible for serial biopsies.[23] This technique was first used by Fortner and associates[11] to monitor the histology of the allografted bowel in a human trial of intestinal transplantation. The histologic sequence of rejection as well as the effect of cyclosporine therapy on the appearance and progression of rejection were recently documented. In the presence of rejection, as documented by graft histology from isolated pouch biopsies, the peak absorption of ^{14}C-labeled glucose from these blind-ended pouches is significantly delayed, and absolute absorption is sharply reduced[27]; with normal histology, there is normal absorption of ^{14}C-labeled glucose from the mucosa of these isolated pouches.

Cyclosporine alone or in combination with steroids occasionally provides prolonged survival following large animal small intestinal transplantation; however, survival is inconsistent.

Small Animal Models of Intestinal Transplantation

When the graft-versus-host reaction is eliminated by using the appropriate Fl hybrid graft into parental strain, cyclosporine treatment for 7 days prevents rejection indefinitely, with uniform graft survival in these rodents of greater than 100 days.[17] In addition, morphologic and functional defects associated with rejection were partially prevented as measured by the intestinal epithelial potential difference and resistance. Similarly, when rejection is eliminated by a parental graft into Fl hybrid, prolonged administration of cyclosporine delays the onset of fatal graft-versus-host disease until cyclosporine is discontinued.

A considerable body of evidence implicates the lymphoid tissue within the transplanted intestine as the cause of graft-versus-host disease following small bowel transplantation. Irradiation of the donor graft or lymphadenectomy of the accompanying lymph nodes prior to transplant will prevent graft-versus-host disease. In addition, cyclosporine given for 14 days in a unilateral graft-versus-host reaction in the rat will produce survival of greater than 120 days in 71% of inbred rats treated in this way.[8]

Graft-versus-host reaction in intestinal transplantation seems to be heavily dependent upon a functional T cell population. Intestine from Lewis "B rats" made deficient of T cells by thymectomy, irradiation, and reconstitution with syngeneic T cell–depleted bone marrow failed to cause graft-versus-host disease in Fl recipients. Reconstitution of these "B rats" with T cells before transplantation restored the graft-versus-host disease response. Although an Fl rat model can separate the rejection from the graft-versus-host response, this model and approach cannot be duplicated in large animal work nor in the human clinical situation in which a bidirectional immunologic response is anticipated. It appears that when both reactions are operating, the rejection reaction will supercede the graft-versus-host response.

TECHNICAL CONSIDERATIONS IN SMALL BOWEL TRANSPLANTATION

Technical problems in small bowel transplantation in the dog and pig have been significant. There is an extremely high incidence (40%–60%) of early arterial and/or venous thrombosis. Survival of less than 5 days is usually due to technical failures. The cause of the high incidence of thrombosis is unknown, because a technical problem with the anastomosis is rarely identified.[30] A low flow state possibly aggravated by inadequate bowel preservation may predispose it to thrombosis. There has been very little new information on preservation of the small bowel since the observation of Toledo-Pereyra and associates[36] approximately 10 years ago. Pulsatile perfusion of the small intestine allowed successful transplantation after 24 hours and was thought to be superior to cold storage in Collins'

solution. This technique, however, has not gained wide acceptance. More recently, there has been interest in cryopreservation of the small intestine, particularly free fetal intestinal transplants. With cyclosporine, cryopreserved free allogenic fetal grafts are capable of growth.[14] This concept provides successful intestinal transplantation. At the present time, no conclusive data exist on long-term immunologic nutritional or metabolic consequences of systemic rather than portal venous drainage of the small bowel except in questionable models of portal hypertension.[19,33] Most investigators prefer to use systemic venous drainage for technical ease. this approach would most likely reflect the clinical condition in which the portal vein may be thrombosed or unavailable for anastomosis.

PATIENT SELECTION

In view of the success of home TPN, it is difficult to define candidates for intestinal transplantation. Long-term survivors in large animal models, while present, have been few. The absorptive capacity of the surviving allografts has never completely returned to normal. This makes it difficult to determine how much of the small intestine to transplant. The general goal of intestinal transplantation would be to avoid the use of home TPN. This can only be done if the graft functions relatively normally and is capable of maintaining the nutritional status of the patient. To date, long-term experimental intestinal allografts have not been able to accomplish this function. Therefore, because the required amount of transplanted intestine is uncertain, the appropriateness of a larger segment of intestine from a cadaveric transplant or a shorter segment from a living-related transplant is extremely difficult to determine, both scientifically and ethically.

HUMAN SMALL BOWEL TRANSPLANTATION

Despite the rather poor experimental results documented in the past 25 years, seven attempts at human small intestinal transplantation were performed and summarized by Kirkman.[30] Five of these failed within 7 days, presumably for technical reasons, and, in only one case was graft survival sufficiently long to minimally contribute to the patient's nutritional status. All seven patients died because of bowel necrosis or sepsis possibly related to graft rejection (Table 44-1).

There have been two recent reports on human

TABLE 44-1   Results of Human Trials

SURGEON	DATE	TRANSPLANTED	SEGMENT TRANSPLANTED	OUTCOME
Detterling[35]	1964	Mother to child	Ileum	Died—hours
Detterling	1964	Cadaver to child	Small bowel	Removed—Day 2
Lillehei[21]	1967	Cadaver to adult	Jejunum, ileum, right colon	Died—hour
Okumura[32]	1968	Cadaver to adult	Jejunum, ileum, right colon	Died—12 days
Olivier[28]	1969	Cadaver to adult	Small intestine, right colon	Died—26 days
Alican[2]	1971	Mother to child	Ileal segment	Removed—Day 7
Fortner		Sister to sister*	Ileal segment	See text

* HLA-identical

small bowel transplantation. Starzl and co-workers[34] reported transplantation of a pancreaticoduodenal segment in humans in which two patients also received long jejunal segments in the composite graft. Despite cyclosporine and steroids, cramps, watery diarrhea, and severe hypoalbuminemia required reoperation and removal of the jejunum and distal duodenum; both showed inflammatory changes in the mucosa with patchy epithelial regeneration. Whether this intestinal injury resulted in a protein losing enteropathy caused by rejection, ischemia, or other factors could not be definitely determined.

In 1985, a 26-year-old blood group A patient underwent small bowel transplantation.[6] The patient had had a prior extended subtotal colectomy, followed within a year by total removal of the small bowel because of desmoid tumor of the mesentery. Because of great difficulty in managing this patient with TPN, a small bowel transplant from an O blood type cadaver donor was performed. The ends of the intestine were exteriorized; the SMA was anastomosed to the aorta; and the superior mesenteric vein was anastomosed to the inferior vena cava, with a total ischemic time of under 90 minutes.

Immunosuppression with parenteral cyclosporine and steroids was instituted. Daily biopsies of the graft did not show any significant changes during the first week post transplantation. However, a moderately severe hemolytic episode was noted on Day 5 due to anti-A antibodies formed by the graft lymphocytes. On the ninth postoperative day, the patient became deeply comatose. A laparatomy on the tenth postoperative day demonstrated a graft that appeared grossly normal. Nevertheless, the graft was removed, and the immunosuppression discontinued, she died on the eleventh postoperative day. Histologic examination of the graft showed a moderate mononuclear infiltration; however, the gross architecture of the graft remained normal. The autopsy demonstrated a brain infarction in the area of the thalami, possibly explaining her comatose state. The exact cause of this brain infarction remains unknown.

Thus, there have been approximately 10 attempts at intestinal transplantation without success, but the clinical need and experimental results suggest a future role for intestinal transplantation

There are some encouraging accomplishments in small bowel transplantation. Long-term survival in large animals has been reported. The understanding of the rejection process of the small bowel is increasing, and monitoring of the immunologic status of the graft is possible. Cyclosporine has improved the clinical courses of such transplants. Nevertheless, small intestine transplantation is highly experimental and should be currently attempted only in those rare cases in which TPN is impossible or absolutely refused by the patient. There is little question that the results, similar to the evolution of transplantation of the kidney, heart, liver, and pancreas will improve. The improvement will await (1) a better understanding of the causes of early graft necrosis, (2) improved preservation techniques, (3) minimizing graft-versus-host reactions, and (4) possibly successful immunomodulation of the recipient. These problems will be solved and await the intelligent and persistent investigator.

REFERENCES

1. Aeder MI, Payne WD, Jeng LB et al: Use of cyclosporine for small intestinal allotransplantation in dogs. Surg Forum 35:387, 1984

2. Alican F, Hardy J, Cayirli M et al: Intestinal transplantation: Laboratory experience and report of a clinical case. Am J Surg 121:150, 1971

3. Billingham RE: Reactions of grafts against their hosts. Science 130:947, 1959

4. Borel JF, Feurer C, Magnee C et al: Effects of the new antilymphocyte peptide Cyclosporin A in animals. Immunology 32:1017, 1977

5. Cohen Z, MacGregor AB, Moore KTH et al: Canine small bowel transplantation: a study of the immunological responses. Arch Surg 111:248, 1976

6. Cohen Z, Silverman RE, Wassef R et al: Small intestinal transplantation using Cyclosporine A (CsA). Transplantation 42(6):613–621, 1986

7. Craddock GN, Nordgren S, Reznick RK et al: Small bowel transplantation in the dog using Cyclosporine. Transplantation 35:284, 1983

8. Deltz E, Muller-Hermelink HK, Ulrichs K et al: Development of graft versus host reaction in various target organs after small bowel intestine transplantation. Transplant Proc 13:1215, 1981

9. Diliz-Perez HS, McClure J, Bedetti C et al: Successful small bowel transplantation in dogs with Cyclosporine and prednisone. Transplantation 37:127, 1984

10. Fisher JE: Nutritional support in the seriously ill patient. Curr Probl Surg 17(9):466–532, 1980

11. Fortner JG, Sichuk G, Litwin SD et al: Immunologiical responses to an intestinal allograft with HLA identical donor-recipient. Transplantation 14:531, 1972

12. Goot B, Lillehei RC, Miller FA: Homografts of the small bowel. Surg Forum 10:193, 1959

13. Goot B, Lillehei RC, Miller FA: Mesenteric lymphatic regeneration after autografts of small bowel in dogs. Surgery 48:571, 1960

14. Guttman FM, Nguyen LT, Laberge JM et al: Fetal rat intestinal transplantation cryopreservation and Cyclosporine A. J Pediatr Surg (in press)

15. Hardy Ma, Quint J, State: Effect of antilymphocyte serum and other immunosuppressive agents on canine jejunal allografts. Ann Surg 171:51, 1970

16. Kennedy G, Jeejeebhoy KN: Home total parenteral nutrition. In JeeJeebhoy KN (ed): Total parenteral Nutrition in the Hospital and at Home. Boca Ratan, Fl, CRC Press, Inc, 1983

17. Kirkman RL, Lear, PA, Tilney NL: Small intestinal transplantation in the rat—immunology and function. Surgery 96:280, 1984

18. Kocandrle V, Houttuin E, Prohaska JV: Regeneration of the lymphatics after autotransplantation and homotransplantation of the entire small intestine. Surg Gynecol Obstet 122:587, 1966

19. Lee KKW, Schraut WH: Structure and function of orthotopic small bowel allografts in rats treated with Cyclosporine. Am J Surg 151:55, 1986

20. Lillehei RC, Goott B, Miller FA: The physiological response of the small bowel of the dog to ischemia including prolonged in vitro preservation of the bowel with successful replacement and survival. Ann Surg 150:543, 1959

21. Lillehei RC, Idezuki Y, Feemster JA et al: Transplantation of stomach, intestine and pancreas: Experimental and clinical observations. Surgery 62:721, 1967

22. Lillehei RC, Manax WG, Lyons GW et al: Transplantation of gastrointestinal organs, including small intestine and stomach. Gastroenterology 51:936, 1966

23. Lossing A, Mordgren S, Cohen Z et al: Histologic monitoring of rejection in small intestinal transplantation. Transplant Proc 14:643, 1982

24. Manax WG, Bloch JH, Eyal Z et al: Experimental preservation of the small bowel. Am J Surg 109:26, 1965

25. Manax WG, Lyons GW, Lillehei RC: Transplantation of the small bowel and stomach. Adv Surg 2:371, 1966

26. Monchik GJ, Russel PS: Transplantation of small bowel in the rat: Technical and immunological considerations. Surgery 70:693, 1971

27. Nordgren S, Cohen Z, Mackenzie R et al: Functional monitors of rejection in small intestinal transplants. Am J Surg 147:152, 1984

28. Olivier C, Rettori R, Olivier Ch et al: Un ca de transplantation orthotopique du jejuno-ileon et du colon droit et transverse. Presse med 77:1275, 1969

29. Preston WF, Macalalad F, Wachowski TJ et al: Survival of homografts of the intestine with and without imunosuppression. Surgery 60:1203, 1966

30. Pritchard TJ, Kirkman RL: Small bowel transplanatation. World J Surg 9:860, 1985

31. Ricour C, Revillon Y, Arnaud-Battandier JF et al: Successful small bowel allografts in piglets using Cyclosporine. Trsnplant Proc 15:3019, 1983

32. Ruiz JO, Lillehei RC: Intestinal transplantation. Surg Clin North Am 52:175, 1972

33. Schraut WH, Rosemurgy AS, Riddell RM: Prolongation of intestinal allograft survival without immunosuppressive drug therapy. J Surg Res 34:597, 1983

34. Starzl TE, Iwatzuki S, Shaw BW et al: Pancreaticoduodenal transplantation in humans. Surg Gynecol Obstet 159:265, 1984

35. Stauffer U: Der gegenwartge stand der dunndarmstransplantation. Paediatr-Paedol (Suppl) 3:59, 1975

36. Toledo-Pereyra LH, Simmons JRL, Najarian JS: Two to three day intestinal preservation utilizing hypothermic pulsatile perfusion. Ann Surg 179:454, 1974

37. Trier JS: The short bowel syndrome. In Sleisenger MH, Fordtran JS (eds): Gastrointestinal Disease. Pathophysiology, Diagnosis, Management. Philadelphia, W.B. Saunders, 1981

CHAPTER 45

Lung Transplantation

Cheryl M. Montefusco   Frank J. Veith

The problems that limit success in lung transplantation have been identified, and complete or partial solutions to them have been achieved. Transplanted lungs need not have a fixed, high vascular resistance after operation. Poor healing of the bronchial anastomosis has also been a frequent clinical occurrence. Newer methods of telescoping the donor bronchus into the recipient bronchial stump and of revascularizing and reinforcing the anastomosis and the use of cyclosporine immunosuppression have solved this problem.

The patterns of rejection that can occur have been defined and correlated with the use of various immunosuppressive regimens. Methods that can detect impending rejection episodes and, in many recipients, prevent or control rejection entirely have been developed. In very recent work, tolerance to experimental lung allografts has been achieved in some animal models.

The clinical problem of extreme scarcity of donor lungs can be ameliorated by methods that will provide good preservation of donor lungs, thus increasing their availability, and by the widespread adoption of surgical techniques of organ retrieval that permit donor lung excision after removal of the heart. To date, there have been no long-term successful lung transplants. However, the clinical successes that have been achieved in both single lung transplantation and in en bloc transplantation of the heart and both lungs suggest that these procedures can be effective therapeutic modalities.

Over the past 20 years, many advances in surgical methods, transplant immunology, donor organ procurement and preservation techniques, and post-surgical care regimens have greatly influenced the field of lung transplantation. Many of the problems that precluded success in early clinical attempts have now been completely or partially resolved, and, today, patients who have received some form of lung transplant have reasonable expectations for long-term survival and improved quality of life. Despite these recent successes, however, several problems continue to prevent widespread application of lung transplantation for relief of end-stage pulmonary disease. In this chapter, we will summarize progress in lung transplantation to date and review the problems still under active investigation.

PREFERRED METHODS OF LUNG TRANSPLANTATION

Heart–Lung Transplants

Combined autotransplants of the heart and both lungs have been performed successfully in baboons.

Late physiologic studies revealed essentially normal cardiopulmonary function up to 2 years after operation.[6] However, 5 of the 14 patients in the Stanford group of long-term heart–lung transplant survivors have developed obstructive airway disease of varying degrees of severity, with no tendency for spontaneous improvement of flow rates.[4] Despite these late complications, 10 of the 14 surviving patients continue to lead a relatively normal life.

Lung allograft rejection in cyclosporine-treated animals can produce subtle vascular changes that increase pulmonary vascular resistance.[30,46] Although such changes do not occur universally and can be reversed with appropriate glucocorticosteroid treatment, they can occur in the absence of any other roentgenographic or ventilatory abnormality.[30,46] These changes may, therefore, be difficult to detect, and, if left untreated, this form of rejection (Fig. 45-1) may cause irreversibly increased pulmonary vascular resistance.

The recent success with combined transplantation of the heart and both lungs suggests that this procedure may be optimal for any patient who requires a lung transplant. Since 1981, 19 patients

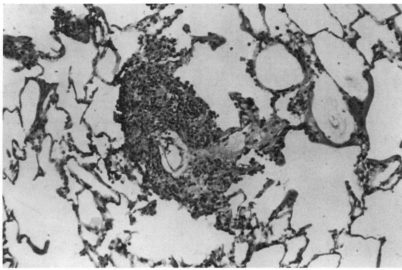

FIGURE 45-1.   *Hematoxylin and eosin stain of a section of allografted lung taken from a dog that was immunosuppressed with cyclosporine. The perivascular cuffing is prominent while the alveoli are normal. Increased vascular resistance was present.*

have undergone heart–lung transplantation at Stanford University, with 14 long-term survivors.[4] This remarkable achievement highlights the advantages of combined transplantation of the heart and both lungs, that is, relative technical simplicity, secure healing of the tracheal anastomosis, and elimination of all diseased lung tissue, and the maximal amount of functioning pulmonary parenchyma is provided. Clearly, this is the procedure of choice for patients with terminal heart and lung disease and in those with end-stage cardiac disease accompanied by severe pulmonary vascular disease. However, the optimal unit of lung tissue necessary for amelioration of terminal acute or chronic lung disease that is *not* accompanied by advanced cardiac disease or severe infection remains questionable. In these patients, single lung transplantation may be better than the heart–lung procedure for several reasons.

First, the improved immunonsuppression provided by cyclosporine has helped to eliminate some of the complications previously observed with bronchial anastomotic healing in single lung transplant recipients. This has certainly been demonstrated in our laboratory studies[30,46] and in two patients who received single lung transplants.[18,19] Other surgical advances, such as wrapping the bronchial anastomosis with an omental or intercostal pedicle, have also proved helpful.[25,29]

Second, a single lung transplant that is free of significant functional impairment is effective in the treatment of bilateral chronic lung diseases.[12,45,50,52]

Third, any procedure involving simultaneous transplantation of both lungs requires a donor with two healthy lungs—a relatively rare circumstance.

Fourth, in some cases of acute but very severe pulmonary insufficiency, it may be advisable to leave one lung in place so that it might ultimately recover.

Fifth, as improvements are made in techniques for the earlier and more accurate diagnosis of lung allograft rejection,[10,11,30,46] it would be inadvisable to replace a normal heart with a transplant in those patients with only end-stage lung disease.

Finally, separate procurement from a single donor, preservation and transplantation of the heart and two single lungs, or the bilateral lung bloc is now technically feasible[3] and may provide better overall utilization of this scarce resource.

Single Lung Transplants

End-stage pulmonary disease is usually accompanied by advanced pulmonary vascular disease. Therefore, any single lung transplant must carry most of the pulmonary blood flow at pressures that are tolerable to the right ventricle. A properly constructed vascular anastomosis[50] in a single lung transplant can provide total pulmonary function with normal pulmonary artery pressures.[47,49,50,52] Although these findings were disputed initially, they have now been substantiated in dogs and baboons by several investigators.[1,9,13,17,55]

TABLE 45-1   *Human Single Lung Transplants (1980-Present)*

CASE NUMBER AND TRANSPLANT TEAM	DATE	INDICATION FOR TRANSPLANT	DURATION OF SURVIVAL	CAUSE OF DEATH/GRAFT FAILURE
1. F.J. Veith	3/10/82	Interstitial fibrosis; chronic ARDS*	14 days	Respiratory insufficiency; renal failure; rejection
2. J.D. Cooper[†]	8/29/82 9/15/82	Toxic pneumonitis (paraquat)	88 days	Bilateral bronchopneumonia; trachea-innominate artery fistula; cerebrovascular accident
3. F.J. Veith[‡]	9/24/82	Toxic pneumonitis (paraquat)	49 days	Bronchopleural fistula of right pneumonectomy stump; pseudomonas empyema; right hemothrax
4. J.D. Cooper	11/7/83	Interstitial fibrosis	Continues to survive	—
5. F.J. Veith	12/22/83	Interstitial fibrosis; chronic ARDS*	16 days	Bilateral ARDS*
6. J.D. Cooper	11/30/84	Intersitial fibrosis	Continues to survive	—

* Adult respiratory distress syndrome
[†] Toronto Lung Transplant Group: J Thorac Cardiovasc Surg 89:734–742, 1985
[‡] Kamholz SL et al: NY State J Med 84:82–84, 1984

Experience with four patients demonstrated that transplantation of a single lung can immediately relieve some forms of severe pulmonary hypertension and that a single lung can carry the entire cardiac output at easily tolerable pulmonary artery pressures (Table 45-1).[12,19,45] Although the vascular resistance of transplanted lungs with greatly increased cardiac outputs (e.g., in strenuous exercise) is not known, the finding that animals could survive transplantation of one lung and immediate ligation of the opposite pulmonary artery, and the observation that patients without pulmonary function in their remaining lung could survive solely on the function of their single lung transplant,[8,12,18,19] prove conclusively that one transplanted lung can provide total respiratory and vascular pulmonary function at all times after its insertion.

DONOR LUNG PROCUREMENT

Human donor lungs suitable for transplantation are scarce.[26] In the past 3 years, we have had more than 50 potential recipients (Table 45-2) but have been able to perform only three lung transplants. Many of the remaining transplant candidates died before a suitable lung donor could be identified. This occurred despite the fact that more than 10 potential kidney donors are identified in our region annually.

Human donor lungs are much more difficult to obtain than other human donor organs for several reasons. First, even short periods of ischemia of a donor lung cause significant transient malfunction after transplantation.[42] Donor lung ischemic damage must, therefore, be minimized, and this is best accomplished when the donor and recipient are located in the same institution. Achieving such proximity requires a level of cooperation that is sometimes impossible to obtain from the donor's family and from other physicians. Second, pulmonary edema and pneumonia are common in prospective donors.[26] Third, the size of the donor lung, its hilar structures, and, particularly, its bronchus must approximate those of the recipient.[49]

Selection of Lung Donors

Potential lung donors must be younger than 50 years of age and must have blood type compatibility with the recipient. The size of the donor hilar structures must approximate those of the recipient. Ideally, the recipient should be free of persisting antibodies to donor lymphocytes, although this ideal may not always be possible to evaluate because of logistic considerations, and experiences with heart and liver transplants indicate that the historical presence of such antibodies does not always preclude success. At least one of the donor's lungs must be free of infiltrates visible on chest roentgenogram. Tracheobronchial secretions must be nonpurulent and relatively free of organisms demonstrable with Gram's stain. The donor must have an arterial oxygen tension over 250 mm Hg with an F_{IO_2} of 1.0.[28]

Even in those circumstances in which all of the aforementioned criteria are satisfied, donor lungs are excluded from further consideration for trans-

TABLE 45-2   *Single Lung Transplant Recipient Criteria*

Indications for Single Lung Transplantation

End-stage pulmonary disease, including:

1. Pulmonary interstitial fibrosis of all types
2. Emphysema (including alpha-l-antitrypsin deficiency)
3. Chronic obstructive pulmonary disease
4. Adult respiratory distress syndrome (ARDS)
5. Age less than 60 years

Exclusive Criteria (Risk Factors)

1. Age greater than 60 years
2. Morbid obesity or cachexia
3. Significant prior chest surgery
4. Extensive pleural disease
5. Malignant disease
6. Active or recurrent infection
7. Significant psychiatric disorder or psychopathology
8. Coagulopathy
9. Bronchiectasis (particularly with recurrent infection)
10. Cardiac functional abnormalities
11. Liver and renal functional abnormalities
12. Active gastric and/or colonic ulcerative disease
13. Presence of circulating immune complexes

plantation if the donor has sustained bilateral penetrating chest trauma or has a history of lung disease, regular intravenous drug abuse, or malignant disease.[28] Of course, as with most other organ donations, the lung donor must meet acceptable criteria for brain death yet retain circulatory integrity before and during lung retrieval surgery.[27]

Surgical Methods of Donor Lung Retrieval

We have evaluated the following alternatives for donor lung retrieval:

1. Left or right pneumonectomy by lateral thoracotomy. This technique leaves on otherwise intact, heart-beating cadaver available for donation of other organs, including the heart.
2. En bloc retrieval of the heart and both lungs by median sternotomy with subsequent ex vivo separation and transplantation of these organs into different recipients.[3] This alternative is also used for retrieval of the heart–lung bloc.
3. Retrieval of the heart followed by retrieval of the left or right lungs by median sternotomy.
4. Retrieval of the heart followed by retrieval of the bilateral lung bloc by median sternotomy.

If the organs below the diaphragm are procured, a midline celiotomy is performed simultaneously, and cannulation of the infrarenal aorta and inferior vena cava is performed for in situ organ perfusion and cooling with the supraceliac aorta crossclamped while the hear and lungs are procured. Whenever possible, alternative number 3 in the preceding paragraph should be used, because the heart is procured first using this technique. While the abdominal organs are being cooled in situ, the lung or lungs are removed after in situ perfusion. Removal of the heart and left lung requires approximately 15 to 20 minutes. If consent was not obtained for heart donation, alternative number 1 may be used for removal of the lung. With this technique, the patient may be turned for procuring of the kidneys and liver in the standard fashion, that is, performing the dissection while the circulation continues to be maintained.

The heart and both lungs can be removed so that all three organs are suitable for separate transplantation.[3] This is accomplished by fashioning a slightly smaller left atrial cuff on the heart. To do this, the left atrial wall must be divided to provide three suitable cuffs. Standard cardiac procurement methods divide the left atrium through the orifice of the pulmonary veins, leaving insufficient donor left atrium for single lung transplantation (Fig. 45-2A and B).[2,5,38,42] We have demonstrated in human cadaver heart–lung bloc dissections that there is 1.5 cm to 3.0 cm of left atrial wall between the left inferior pulmonary vein and the coronary sinus, and 3.0 cm to 6.0 cm of left atrial wall between the right inferior pulmonary vein and the coronary sinus. With appropriate division of the left atrium to provide an atrial cuff for the left lung transplant, more than 0.7 cm of left atrial wall remains on the heart above the coronary sinus (Fig. 45-3A). This is an adequate left atrial cuff for heart transplantation. After removal of the right lung from the heart, the remaining atrial cuff on the heart extended at least 2.0 cm above the coronary sinus (Fig. 45-3B). Creation of a left atrial cuff for the right lung may require dissection into Sundergard's groove. This occasionally includes a small portion of the superior limbus of the interatrial septum. The left atrial cuffs harvested with lung specimens in our human cadaver studies measured at least 3.5 cm × 5.5 cm in diameter and were entirely suitable for transplantation (Fig. 45-4A and B).

PRESERVATION

The scarcity of donor lungs would be partially ameliorated by the development of methods that permitted a lung to be procured in one institution, preserved for 24 hours or more, and transported to

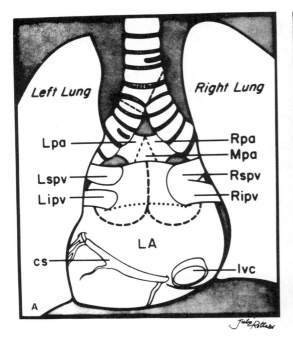
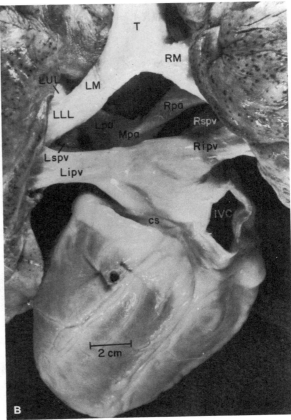

FIGURE 45-2.   *(A) Diagram of the posterior aspect of the left atrium, pulmonary arteries, and lower airway. Dashed lines (- - -) indicate sites of division of left and right mainstem bronchi, left and right pulmonary arteries, and atrial cuffs for left and right pulmonary veins when harvesting the heart and two lungs all suitable for separate transplantation. Adequate left atrial tissue remains on the heart to form a cuff suitable for transplantation of this organ. The dotted line (· · ·) indicates the line of division made between the right and left inferior pulmonary veins when the heart alone is harvested by standard methods. This leaves insufficient tissue to facilitate single lung transplantation. (abbreviations: T = trachea; LM = left mainstem bronchus; LUL = left upper lobe bronchus; LLL = left lower lobe bronchus; RM = right mainstem bronchus; RUL = right upper lobe bronchus; BI = bronchus intermedius; LPA = left pulmonary artery; RPA = right pulmonary artery; MPA = distal main pulmonary artery; LSPV = left superior pulmonary vein; RSPV = right superior pulmonary vein; LIPV = left inferior pulmonary vein; RIPV = right inferior pulmonary vein; LA = left atrium; RA = right atrium; CS = coronary sinus)*
(B) Posterior aspect of a human cadaver heart–lung bloc. Mediastinal tissues and pericadial reflections have been dissected from the specimen. Note that the left inferior pulmonary vein is in closer proximity to the coronary sinus than is the right inferior pulmonary vein.

another institution for transplantation. If such methods did not add to the ischemic damage of the transplant procedure, they would permit donor procurement almost anywhere in the world. Until recently, such a system did not exist, and it has been found that lungs are more difficult to preserve without functional impairment than are other organs.[42]

In the last several years, methods have been developed that permit donor lungs to be preserved up to 24 hours, transported, and then transplanted.[42] These methods include flushing the inflated lung against outflow resistance with a cold (4°C) hypertonic hyperkalemic solution. After the pulmonary vessels are clamped, the lung is immersed in this solution for storage. Transportation at 4°C is accomplished using a solid/liquid mixture of an organic chemical, l-hexadecene. When lungs thus preserved were allografted into immunosup-

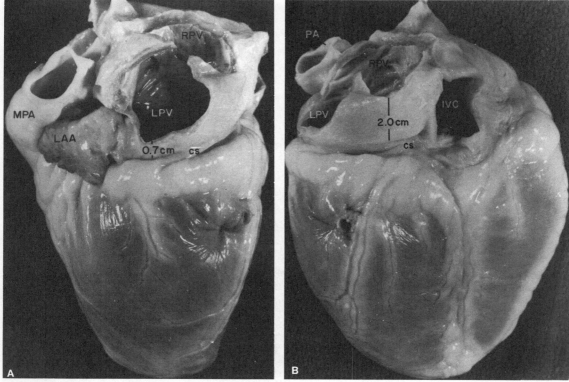

FIGURE 45-3.   *(A) The site of excision of the left lung (LPV) with its required atrial cuff leaves at least 0.7 cm of left atrium on the heart in this particular specimen. The distal main pulmonary artery (MPA) remaining with the heart is adequate for pulmonary artery anastomosis. (B) Because the left inferior pulmonary vein lies closer to the coronary sinus than the right inferior pulmonary vein, excision of the right lung with a left atrial cuff (RPV) suitable for single lung transplantation leaves a broader band of atrium on the heart at this site compared with the left pulmonary vein excision site. In this specimen, a minimum of 2.0 cm of left atrium remains on the heart after removal of the right pulmonary veins.*

pressed dogs and followed by immediate right pulmonary artery ligation, the function of the preserved transplant was excellent, proving equal to that of nonpreserved transplanted lungs.[42] These preservation techniques have also been used successfully in canine lung autografts and in lung allografts harvested after cardiac arrest.[7,23] The preserved autotransplants have been able to provide continuous total pulmonary function up to 4 years after operation.[31,47]

Some modifications of donor technique are required to suit the surgical method of donor lung retrieval used.[23,47] Use of these or similar methods will allow maximal utilization of organ donors and will permit appropriate therapeutic lung, heart, or heart–lung transplantation for patients with a variety of disease processes.

THE REIMPLANTATION RESPONSE

This is defined as the morphologic, roentgenographic, and functional changes that occur in a lung transplant in the early postoperative period as the result of surgical trauma, ischemia, denervation, lymphatic interruption, and other injurious processes (exclusive of rejection) that are unavoidable aspects of the transplant operation. Although the reimplantation response occurs in lung allografts, it can only be examined experimentally in lung autografts in which manifestations of rejection cannot occur.

Several experimental studies have shown that the reimplantation response consists of alveolar edema that is evident on histologic examination and alveolar infiltrates that may be seen on plain chest

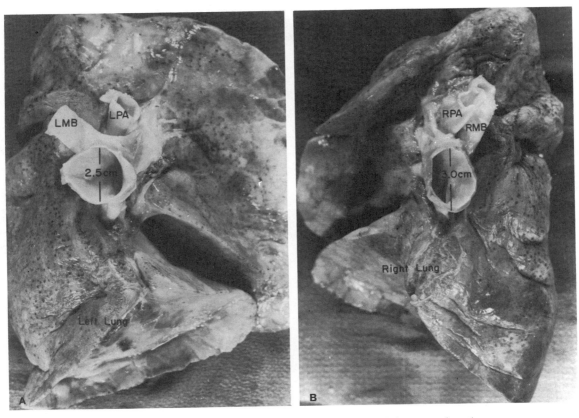

FIGURE 45-4.   Excised left (A) and right (B) lungs are anatomically suitable for single lung transplantation. Note the adequate left atrial cuffs on both organs for pulmonary venous anastomosis.

roentgenograms. In animal models, these changes seem to reach their peak within 3 days after transplantation and then gradually regress over the next 3 weeks.[36] Functionally, the reimplantation response produces a temporary impairment of ventilation/perfusion ratio in the transplanted lung, although there may also be some transient impairment of blood flow.[39]

The reimplantation response is not unique to single lung transplantation and has been noted regularly in experimental and clinical heart–lung transplants.[16,33,35] In addition to the contributing factors already mentioned, intercurrent rejection, expanded blood volume, or overhydration will act synergistically to exacerbate the functional defects produced by the reimplantation response. Therefore, vigorous diuresis and, if necessary, ultrafiltration hemodialysis should be used to remove excess fluid in any instance of pulmonary insufficiency. Percutaneous transvenous endomyocardial biopsy should be used to detect any component of rejection, so that the

correct diagnosis may be made and effective treatment instituted. Cardiac rejection is a reliable guide to pulmonary rejection in combined heart–lung transplants in the early post-transplant period.[34] More recent data in long-term heart–lung transplantation in primates indicates that the observed pulmonary histologic abnormalities may be the result of chronic rejection not accompanied by any evidence of chronic rejection in the heart.[15]

TRACHEAL OR BRONCHIAL ANASTOMOTIC COMPLICATIONS

Before cyclosporine was available, complications resulting from defective healing of the bronchial anastomosis were a major problem in single lung transplantation. These complications have included anastomotic disruption with air leakage, infection, bleeding, and stenosis or mucosal necrosis with aspiration pneumonia. In the 38 patients who received lung transplants prior to January 1981, these complications contributed directly to the deaths of most recipients who survived 10 days or more after operation.[48]

Bronchial anastomotic complications have generally been attributed to ischemia of the transplanted bronchus, which derives nutrition solely by retrograde perfusion from pulmonary artery collateral vessels. On this basis, some investigators have advocated direct revascularization of the transplant bronchial arterial circulation by implanting a button of donor aorta containing the origin of these vessels into the recipient aorta;[14,24] this is a difficult procedure that greatly adds to the complexity of the transplant operation. Accordingly, we and others have tried to minimize bronchial problems by means of simpler operative techniques, such as shortening the donor bronchial stump, reinforcing the anastomosis with surrounding vascularized tissue,[22] and using an intussuscepting anastomotic method.[32,40,49] These techniques have helped to prevent bronchial problems in experimental models but were not entirely successful in human lung transplant recipients. Defective healing of the bronchial anastomosis sometimes became manifest many weeks after operation.[45] This late occurrence suggests that the pathogenesis of the poor healing observed is more complex than had been previously thought and that it may also be partially caused by rejection, high-dose corticosteroids, and size discrepancy between donor and recipient bronchi.

The feasibility and the effects of wrapping an ischemic canine bronchial anastomosis with a pedicled intercostal muscle flap have been evaluated.[25] The pedicles adhere strongly and provide early neovascularity as well as mechanical support to the bronchial anastomosis. These technical improvements, as well as the better control of rejection and the decreased need for corticosteroids brought about by cyclosporine, have resulted in secure bronchial healing in both canine and human lung transplant recipients.[18,19]

LUNG ALLOGRAFT REJECTION

Diagnosis, Prevention, and Treatment

If a lung is allotransplanted without immunosuppressive treatment, it undergoes rapid rejection with destruction of all its component parts, loss of ventilatory and vascular function, and thrombosis of its blood vessels. The recipient usually dies within 10 days.[41] Standard immunosuppression with azathioprine, corticosteroids, and ALS modifies and attenuates the rejection process, but fewer than 10% of allografted lungs treated this way will function well beyond a month.[21,51,54] Cyclosporine immunosuppression completely prevents lung allograft rejection in an occasional recipient, attenuates it to a far greater extent than does standard immunosuppression in most recipients, and often modifies it, when it does occur, to produce a milder, more easily and completely reversible form of lung allograft rejection.[18,30,,33,46] Although some manifestations of rejection occur in most animals and patients receiving lung transplants with cyclosporine immunosuppression, with appropriate treatment, the function of the lung allograft can be preserved in the majority of recipients.[18,46] Thus, for the first time, cyclosporine has made therapeutic lung transplantation a real possibility.

Manifestations

Three distinct patterns of lung allograft rejection have been defined.[46,53] The first of these is the **classic** form, in which perivascular cuffs of round cells are prominent, along with alveolar exudates containing desquamated pneumocytes and a mixture of inflammatory cells (Fig. 45-5). Physiologically, this **classic rejection** is associated with decreased transplant ventilation and perfusion that occur concomitantly.[43] This form of rejection is always observed in nonimmunosuppressed recipients. It also occurs in some animals treated with standard immunosuppression and in a few treated with cyclosporine.[46,53]

The second form of rejection, termed atypical or **alveolar rejection,** is observed in some animals and in patients receiving standard immunosuppressive agents.[43,53] This form of rejection is characterized by the presence of fibrinous alveolar exudates with a relative paucity of round cells and no perivascular cuffing (Fig. 45-6). Radiographically and functionally, alveolar rejection is associated with transplant opacification and decreased ventilation without a corresponding reduction in blood flow.[43] This atypical, alveolar form of rejection, which was never observed in autografts, can produce serious ventilation/perfusion imbalances and respiratory insufficiency of the type that has caused the deaths of several emphysematous human lung transplant recipients who were treated with aziathoprine, corticosteroids, and antilymphocyte globulin (ALG).[37,56] Other factors such as ventilation/perfusion mismatching secondary to the presence of an emphysematous lung in parallel with a transplant were thought to be more important. On this basis, double lung transplantation, with or without the heart, was considered essential if lung transplantation was to

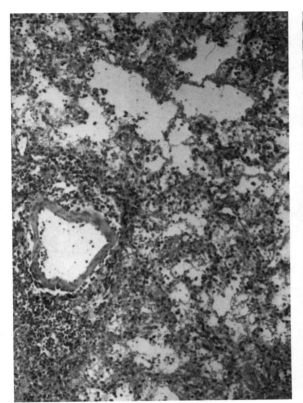

FIGURE 45-5.   *Hematoxylin and eosin stain of a section of allografted lung taken from a dog that was not immunosuppressed. Rejection occurred within 6 days and was manifested histologically by the occurrence of perivascular cuffs of round cells with the simultaneous appearance of cellular alveolar exudates.*

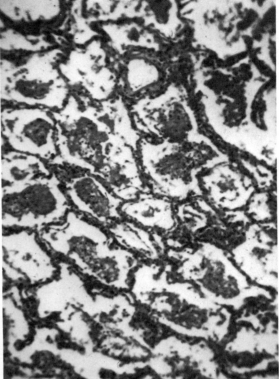

FIGURE 45-6.   *Hematoxylin and eosin stain of a section of allografted lung taken from a patient who was immunosuppressed with azathioprine, prednisone, and antilymphocyte serum. This form of rejection is characterized histologically by the presence of fibrinous alveolar exudates without concomitant perivascular cuffing.*

be performed in emphysematous recipients. However, subsequent experience has not supported this requirement. Rejection, often in the atypical or alveolar form, seems to have been a very important cause of the poor transplant function that has contributed to the disappointing results of clinical single lung transplantation.[43] When rejection is prevented, a single functioning lung transplant is sufficient to provide adequate pulmonary function, as it did for our emphysematous patient who survived for 6 months after receiving a single lung transplant.[45] When this patient's allograft was not rejecting, he was greatly improved clinically and had normal arterial oxygen and carbon dioxide tensions with minimal ventilation/perfusion imbalances.[45]

The third form of lung allograft rejection, which as been observed only in recipients treated with cyclosporine, involves primarily and predominantly the small and medium-sized blood vessels. This **vascular form of rejection** is manifested by perivascular cuffs of round cells with alveoli and interstitial

areas that are relatively normal. Vascular resistance is increased, and blood flow is decreased to the allografted lung.[30,46] Results of plain chest roentgenogram and ventilation scans may be completely normal, although, in the later stages, some abnormalities caused by alveolar involvement may appear.

Although typical examples of these forms of rejection are frequently observed, they represent three points on a spectrum. Many allografted lungs develop mixed forms of rejection, often with some degree of superimposed fibrosis.[21,30,43] Moreover, superimposed infection is often observed with allograft rejection. This has been prominent, particularly in recipients receiving high doses of standard immunosuppressive agents.[21,43]

Diagnosis

Early and accurate diagnosis of rejection is necessary for optimal treatment. Until 1981, rejection in lung allografts was best diagnosed by the rapid appearance of an infiltrate seen on plain chest roentgenograms that was accompanied by fever, leukocytosis, a decrease in arterial oxygen tension, and, importantly, no change in the sputum bacteria as evaluated with serial Gram's stain examination.[45] Better methods are needed for rapid and reliable differentiation among rejection, pneumonia, and the reimplantation response, because the latter two processes can produce changes that mimic those of rejection. In the laboratory, transthoracic needle biopsy has proved helpful in this regard, but transbronchial biopsy has not.[20]

In cyclosporine-treated recipients of heart–lung allografts, early lung rejection does not seem to occur without concurrent rejection of the heart, so transvenous endomyocardial biopsy has permitted early and accurate diagnosis of rejection of heart–lung grafts.[34] However, recent observations cast doubt on these conclusions. Comparable diagnosis of lung allograft rejection has also been possible by examining the returns of alveolar lavages in cyclosporine-treated canine single lung recipients.[30,46] The lectin-dependent cell-mediated cytotoxicity assay[11,12] has been particularly useful in the early diagnosis of lung rejection, even before any roentgenographic abnormalities or evidence of decreased blood flow appeared.

Treatment

In canine lung allograft recipients receiving standard immunosuppression, rejection crises can be reversed up to 40% of the time by administration of large, IV bolus doses of methylprednisolone.[44] Both the occurrence and the reversal of rejection in this model were well documented by roentgenographic and histologic evidence. However, in cyclosporine-treated recipients, the reversal of lung allograft rejection by increased doses of corticosteroids is much more effective. In a canine lung allograft model, 28 or 38 (74%) rejection episodes were reversed rapidly and completely with increased corticosteroid doses.[18] Many of these animals continue to have normal allograft function, although some lose function from chronic or recurrent infection.[18]

Clinically, the occurrence and reversal of rejection need not be followed by permanent loss of pulmonary function. In two of our patients, one immunosuppressed with cyclosporine and the other treated with standard agents, excellent allograft function and near-normal structure were observed following the reversal of multiple rejection episodes (Fig. 45-7).[18,19,45] Reitz and colleagues[34] report sim-

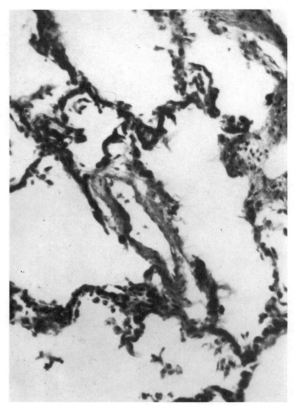

FIGURE 45-7.   Postmortem section of the transplanted lung of a patient who received cyclosporine and survived 7 weeks after operation. Four rejection episodes were successfully reversed with boluses of methylprednisolone. The patient succumbed to a bronchopleural fistula at the site of a contralateral pneumonectomy. The left, transplanted lung was functioning well at the time of death and was mainly normal histologically.

ilar successful treatment of six rejection episodes that occurred in four of their patients who had received heart–lung allografts and who were immunosuppressed with cyclosporine and a low-dose combination of other agents.

The optimal immunosuppressive regimen, using cyclosporine alone or in combination with other agents, awaits definition. Cyclosporine with initial (first 14 days after operation) azathioprine is the best immunosuppressive regimen for canine single lung transplant recipients at this time.[18] Clinically, the Stanford group recommends an immunosuppressive protocol for heart–lung allograft recipients that consists of cyclosporine with an initial course of rabbit anti-thymocyte globulin (ATG). Azathioprine is given for the first 2 weeks and then replaced with prednisone.[16]

REFERENCES

1. Alican F, Cayirili M, Isin E et al: Left lung reimplantation with immediate right pulmonary artery ligation. Ann Surg 174:34, 1971
2. Baumgartner WA, Reitz BA, Oyer PE et al:: Cardiac homotransplantaion. Curr Probl Surg 16:1, 1979
3. Brodman RF, Veith FJ, Goldsmith J et al: Multiple organ procurement from one donor. Heart Transplant 4:254, 1985
4. Burke CM, Theodore J, Dawkins KD et al: Post-transplant obliterative bronchiolitis and other late sequelae in human heart–lung transplantation. Chest 86:824, 1984
5. Cabrol C, Gandjbakhch I, Pavie A et al: Heart and heart–lung transplantation: Techniques and safeguards. Heart Transplant 3:110, 1984
6. Castaneda AR, Zamora, R, Schmidt-Haberman P et al: Cardiopulmonary autotransplantation in primates (baboons): Late functional results. Surgery 72:1064, 1972
7. Crane R, Torres M, Hagstrom JWC et al: Twenty-four hour preservation and transplantation of the lung without functional impairment. Surg Forum 26:111, 1975
8. Derom F, Barbier F, Ringoir S et al: Ten-month survival after lung homotransplantation in man. J Thorac Cardiovasc Surg 61:835, 1971
9. Ebert PA, Hudson BH: Pulmonary hemodynamics following lung autotransplantation: Studies in unanesthetized dogs with the opposite pulmonary artery ligated. J Thorac Cardiovasc Surg 62:188, 1971
10. Emeson EE, Norin AJ, Veith FJ et al: Cytotoxic T cells in rejecting canine lung allografts. Am Rev Respir Dis 125:59, 1982
11. Emeson EE, Norin AJ, Veith FJ: Lectin-dependent cell-mediated cytotoxicity: A new and simple method to quantitate cytotoxic T cell activity in dogs. Transplantation 33:365, 1982
12. Fell SC, Mollenkopf FP, Montefusco CM et al: Revascularization of ischemic bronchial anastomoses by an intercostal pedicle flap. J Thorac Cardiovasc Surg 90:172, 1985
13. Haglin JJ, Arnar O: Pulmonary function in the baboon with lung reimplantation and subsequent contralateral pneumonectomy: Four year follow-up. In The Baboon in Medical Research, Vol 2, p 77. Austin, Texas, University of Texas Press, 1968
14. Haglin JJ, Ruiz E: Histologic studies of human transplantation. In Widlevuur C (ed): Morphology In Lung Transplantation, pp 13–22. Basel, Switzerland, S. Karger, 1973
15. Haverich A, Dawkins KD, Baldwin JC et al: Long-term cardiac and pulmonary histology in primates following combined heart and lung transplantation. Transplantation 39:356, 1985
16. Jamieson SW, Reitz BA, Oyer PE et al: Combined heart and lung transplantation. Lancet 1:1130, 1983
17. Joseph WL, Morton DL: Immediate function with survival following left lung autotransplantation and contralateral pulmonary artery ligation in the baboon. J Thorac Cardiovasc Surg 60:859, 1970
18. Kamholz SL, Veith FJ, Mollenkopf FP et al: Single lung transplantation with cyclosporine immunosuppression. J Thorac Cardiovasc Surg 86:537, 1983
19. Kamholz SL, Veith FJ, Mollenkopf FP et al: Single lung transplantation in paraquat intoxication. NY State J Med 84:82, 1984
20. Koerner SK, Hagstrom JWC, Veith FJ: Transbronchial biopsy for the diagnosis of lung transplant rejection: Comparison with needle and open biopsy techniques in canine lung allografts. Am Rev Respir Dis 114:575, 1976
21. Kondo Y, Cockrell JV, Kuwaharo O et al: Histopathology of one-stage bilateral lung allografts. Ann Surg 180:753, 1974
22. Lima O, Goldberg M, Peters WJ et al: Bronchial omentopexy in canine lung transplantation. J Thorac Cardiovasc Surg 83, 418, 1982
23. Merav AD, Crane R, Pinsker KL et al: Preservation, transportation and transplantation of lungs obtained after death. Surg Forum 28:195, 1977
24. Mills, NL, Boyd AD, Gheranpong C: The significance of bronchial circulation in lung transplantation. J Thorac Cardiovasc Surg 60, 866, 1970
25. Mollenkopf FP, Fell SC, Torres M et al: Intercostal pedicle flap for improved bronchial anastomatic healing. Surg Forum 34:119, 1983
26. Montefusco CM, Mollenkopf FP, Kamholz SL et al: Maintenance protocol for potential organ donors in multiple organ procurement. Hosp Physician 20:9, 1984
27. Montefusco CM, Veith FJ: Maintenance of potential organ donors for multiple organ procurement. In Kamholz SL (ed): Pulmonary Aspects of Neurologic Illness: Diagnosis and Treatment. New York, Spectrum Publications, in press
28. Montefusco CM, Veith FJ: Organ selection and preservation for transplantation. Part I: Cornea, kidney, heart and lung. Hosp Physician 21:98, 1985
29. Morgan E, Lima O, Goldberg M et al: Successful revascularization of totally ischemic bronchial autografts with omental pedicle flaps in dogs. J Thorac Cardiovasc Surg 84:204, 1982
30. Norin AJ, Emeson EE, Kamholz SL et al: Cyclosporin A as the initial immunosuppressive agent for canine lung transplantation: Short and long term assessment of rejection phenomena. Transplantation 34:372, 1982
31. Pinsker KL, Kamholz SL, Montefusco CM et al: Long-term functional adequacy of canine lung autografts after 24-hour preservation. Transplantation 13:715, 1981
32. Pinsker KL, Koerner SK, Kamholz SL et al: The effect of donor bronchial length on healing: A canine model to evaluate bronchial anastomotic problems in lung transplantation. J Thorac Cardiovasc Surg 77:669, 1979

33. Reitz BA, Burton NA, Jamieson SW: Heart and lung transplantation: Auto and allo transplantation in primates with extended survival. J Thorac Cardiovasc Surg 80:360, 1980

34. Reitz BA, Gaudiani VA, Hunt SA et al: Diagnosis and treatment of allograft rejection in heart-lung transplant recipients. J Thorac Cardiovasc Surg 85:354, 1983

35. Reitz BA, Wallwork JL, Hunt SA et al: Heart–lung transplantation: Successful therapy for patients with pulmonary vascular disease. N Engl J Med 306:557, 1982

36. Siegelman SS, Sinha SBP, Veith FJ: Pulmonary reimplantation response. Ann Surg 117:30, 1973

37. Stevens PM, Johnson PC, Bell RL et al: Regional ventilation and perfusion after lung transplantation in patients with emphysema. N Engl J Med 282:245, 1970

38. Stinson EB, Dong E, Iben AB et al: Cardiac transplantation in man. III. Surgical aspects. Am J Surg 118:182, 1969

39. Streider DJ, Barnes BA, Aronow S et al: Xenon 133 study of ventilation and perfusion in normal and transplanted dog lungs. J Appl Physiol 23:359, 1967

40. Trummer MJ, Berg P: Lung Transplantation, pp 10–21. Springfield, IL, Charles C Thomas, 1968

41. Veith FJ, Blumenstock DA: Lung transplantation. J Surg Res 11:13, 1971

42. Veith FJ, Crane R, Torres M et al: Effective preservation and transportation of lung transplants. J Thorac Cardiovasc Surg 72:97, 1976

43. Veith FJ, Hagstrom JWC, Anderson WR: Alveolar manifestations of rejection: An important cause of the poor results with human lung transplantation. Ann Surg 175:336, 1972

44. Veith FJ, Koerner SK, Siegelman SS et al: Diagnosis and reversal of rejection in experimental and clinical lung allografts. Ann Thorac Surg 16:172, 1973

45. Veith FJ, Koerner SK, Siegelman SS et al: Single lung transplantation in experimental and human emphysema. Ann Surg 178, 473, 1973

46. Veith FJ, Norin AJ, Montefusco CM et al: Cyclosporin A in experimental lung transplantation. Transplantation 32:474, 1981

47. Veith FJ, Montefusco CM: Long-term fate of lung autografts charged with providing total pulmonary function. II. Hemodynamic, functional and angiographic studies. Ann Surg 190:654, 1979

48. Veith FJ, Montefusco CM: Lung transplantation. In Glenn WL, Baue AE, Geha AS et al (eds): Thoracic and Cardiovascular Surgery, pp 326–337. Norwalk, CN, Appleton-Century-Crofts, 1983

49. Veith FJ, Richards K: Improved technique for canine lung transplantation. Ann Surg 171:553, 1973

50. Veith FJ, Richards K: Mechanism and prevention of fixed high vascular resistance in autografted and allografted lungs. Science 163:699, 1969

51. Veith FJ, Richards K, Lalezari P: Protracted survival after homotransplantation of the lung and simultaneous contralateral pulmonary artery ligation. J Thorac Cardiovasc Surg 58:829, 1969

52. Veith FJ, Siegelman S, Dougherty JC: Long-term survival after lung transplantation and immediate contralateral pulmonary artery ligation. Surg Gynecol Obstet 133:425, 1971

53. Veith FJ, Sinha SBP, Dougherty JC et al: Nature and evolution of lung allograft rejection with and without immunosuppression. J Thorac Cardiovasc Surg 63:509, 1972

54. Veith FJ, Sinha SBP, Siegelman SS et al: Single lung transplantation with immediate ligation of the opposite pulmonary artery in the dog. A model for assessing the functional adequacy of transplanted lungs. In Harmison LT (ed): Research Animals In Medicine, p 437. DHEW Publication No.: (NIH) 72-333, 1973

55. Wagner OA, Edmunds LH, Heilbron DC: Vascular pressure-flow relationship in denervated and reimplanted lungs of dogs. Surgery 75:91, 1974

56. Wildevuur CRH, Benfield JR: A review of 23 human lung transplantations by 20 surgeons. Ann Thorac Surg 9:489, 1972

PART FIVE

Artificial Organ Replacement

CHAPTER 46

The Artificial Heart and Mechanical Assistance Prior to Heart Transplantation

Mark M. Levinson   Jack G. Copeland

A large segment of our population displays myocardial dysfunction not amenable to surgical or medical therapy, making cardiac replacement the definitive form of treatment. Improved criteria for patient selection and the introduction of anti-thymocyte globulin (ATG) and cyclosporine have improved graft survival. Endomyocardial biopsy allows a more specific diagnosis of rejection and appropriately directed therapy. The 1-year survival rate has gradually improved from 20% in 1968 to close to 85% with current protocols.

Because limitations on donor organs have meant that between 20% and 40% of waiting patients die each year before a suitable donor cannot be located, a variety of mechanical circulatory assist devices have been developed to maintain hemodynamic stability until a donor heart can be found. Three basic devices are in use today: (1) the intra-aortic counterpulsation balloon (IABP), (2) ventricular assist devices (VADs), and (3) the total artificial heart (TAH). Successful temporary application of each category of device followed by explantation and transplantation has now been achieved in man.

The techniques of cardiac transplantation were developed in the late 1950s by Drs. Shumway, Lower, Hardy, and others.[32,37,41,42,44,60,62] In their laboratories, the scientific basis for cardiac replacement with a donor organ was established. Very few modifications have been made since the basic surgical technique was published in 1960.[42] An initial human case was attempted by Hardy and associates[32] in 1964. A 68-year-old man received the heart of a 98-pound chimpanzee when a prospective human donor was not thought to be brain dead and the recipient was near death. Cardiac function in the donor heart was restored, but the graft was too small to support the circulation, and it failed approximately 1 hour following cardiopulmonary bypass.

In December 1967, Dr. Christian Barnard[3] of Cape Town, South Africa, performed the first human-to-human allograft transplantation in a 58-year-old man with ischemic heart disease. Although this patient only survived 18 days, he provided dramatic proof that the concept of cardiac replacement was valid. The excitement generated by this successful case stimulated profuse activity in transplantation during 1968. Unfortunately, the promise of successful cardiac replacement appeared to dwindle as most patients expired within the first few weeks or months. By mid 1969, 146 cases were reported with only 34 survivors.[29] The American Medical Association cautioned against overspread of this new technique to centers without adequate preparation and commitment.[54]

When the initial excitement waned, diligent pursuit of success continued at only a few centers, most notably Stanford University Hospital under the direction of Dr. Norman Shumway. Gradually improving survival rates were obtained as the many pitfalls were identified and solutions were found.[9,20,30,31,47,48] Improvement in patient selection and the introduction of anti-thymocyte globulin (ATG) as an immunosuppressive agent started the initial upswing in results. One of the most important breakthroughs was the adaptation of endomyocardial biopsy to cardiac transplantation by Dr. Phillip Caves and colleagues.[7] This technique provided direct histologic evidence of rejection prior to irreversible myocardial damage and hemodynamic compromise. Antirejection therapy could be directed in a more specific fashion with a correspondent lessening of complications. With these improvements, the 1-year survival rate rose from only 20% in 1968 to almost 70% by 1976.[33]

Another major milestone was marked in 1976, when Jean Borel and co-workers[4] described the effects of Cyclosporin A, a cyclic polypeptide with profound immunosuppressive properties. In human cardiac transplantation, this agent has been found useful in decreasing the severity and acuity of rejection episodes, sparing the use of large doses of steroids, decreasing the frequency of infections, lowering the overall morbidity/mortality, and decreasing the cost of cardiac transplantation.[13,31,33,47,48,59] With improving safety and effectiveness demonstrated, the application of cardiac transplantation has broadened to a larger potential recipient population, as well as to multiple centers interested in performing this operation. The total number of cardiac transplants has once again risen exponentially. There are now more than 60 centers in the United States that have transplanted at least one patient and perhaps 140 centers expressing interest in starting a program in the next 2 years. Whereas only 36 transplants were performed in 1979, more than 500 were performed in 1985 (Fig. 46-1).[22]

HISTORY

Although the 1-year survival following cardiac transplantation is now approximately 70% to 80% in major centers, it is impossible to universally apply this operation to the enlarging groups of potential recipients. It is estimated that only 2,000 to 3,000 potential organ donors exist in the United States per year.[22,23] Of these, less than half (700–800) meet the selection criteria for cardiac donation.[22] The National Heart Transplantation Study completed in 1984 projected a maximal number of cardiac transplants at 700 per year by 1990.[22] The estimated need for cardiac replacement, however, is between 15,000 and 75,000 people per year.[22]

With donor shortages, it is estimated that 20% to 40% of transplant candidates awaiting a donor organ will expire before one becomes available. Currently, the average wait for a donor heart in our hospital is 36 days. In addition, because some donor organs cannot be used because of poor timing, wrong location, incompatible blood group, and inappropriate size differential,[21] there is a great stimulus to perfect an interim mechanical support program analogous to renal dialysis. This "bridge-to-transplantation" would allow preservation of life in the near-death cardiac transplant candidate until a donor could be found.

The idea of a mechanical circulatory assist device is not a new one. The application to human patients, however, has had to wait for many developments in the technology of organic polymers, electronics, and mechanical engineering. Initial laboratory investigations in the late 1800s and early 1900s demonstrated that hydraulic pumps could propel fluids similar to cardiac action. In 1953, a primitive artificial heart was devised in preparation for pharmacologic experiments in cats and dogs.[27,28] During that same year, primitive circulatory perfusion experiments were performed in a dog with a centrifugal pump.[2]

The development of clinically useful blood pumps began with the description of the roller pump in the early 1930s.[16,57] Continuing experiments by Gibbon[25,26] culminated in the development of the heart–lung machine with vertical screen oxygenator suitable for the performance of intracardiac operations. Following introduction of this cardiopulmonary bypass (CPB) circuit into clinical practice in 1954, there are now more than 200,000 CPB procedures performed each year in the United States.

The next breakthrough in mechanical support was the invention of the intra-aortic counterpulsation balloon pump (IABP).[43] The concept of counterpulsation was first described by Clauss and associates[10] in 1961 and was used successfully in the early 1960s by Lefemine and colleagues.[38] Six years later, the first clinical experience with IABP in patients with cardiogenic shock was reported.[34] Subsequently, the use has expanded, and approximately 10,000 patients per year in the United States have benefited from this device, mainly for support of the failing left ventricle in ischemic heart disease.

The development of a partial or total artificial heart (TAH) has been pursued along with these other developments. The first attempt to completely replace the heart of an experimental animal with a mechanical device was performed in 1937 by Demikhov,[18] a cardiac surgeon in the Soviet Union, and the first effort in the United States was performed at the Cleveland Clinic in 1957 by Akutsu

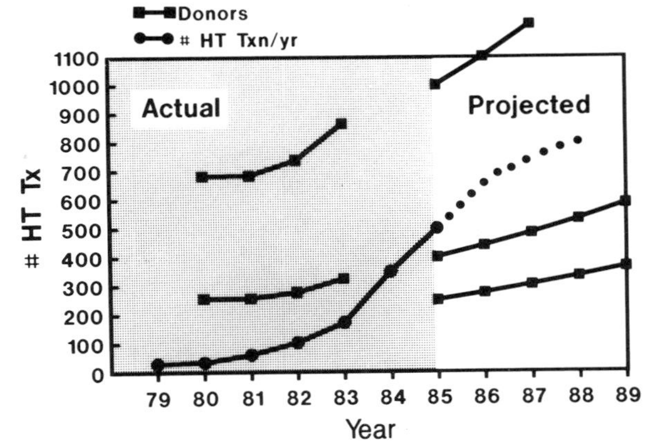

FIGURE 46-1   Heart transplantation activity in the United States: Results of the National Heart Transplantation Study by Evans et al. There has been a marked rise in transplant activity that is rapidly approaching the maximal number of potential heart donors. (Minimal, average, and maximal numbers of cardiac donors per year is illustrated by separate plots. The actual numbers of donors in the years 1980 to 1983 are given as maximum and minimum depending on variations in selection criteria from center to center).

and Kolff.[1] After relocating at the University of Utah, Salt Lake City, Kolff and associates continued the pursuit of a mechanical heart. Under his direction, Robert Jarvik, a mechanical engineer, developed the Jarvik-7, which was first implanted into animals in 1979.[35] Separately, the Texas Heart Institute kept alive its interest in this field. Two total artificial heart devices, the Liotta heart[11] and the Akutsu heart,[12] were developed there and later implanted into human patients. Under the direction of William S. Pierce, M.D., Pennsylvania State University at Hershey has maintained a developmental program in artificial devices leading to the successful use of both assist devices and the total artificial heart.[50,52] Currently, there are multiple centers throughout the world (Paris, Vienna, Berlin, Tokyo, Osaka) where new engineering and design ideas for artificial hearts and assist devices are being tested.

The feasibility of temporary mechanical replacement of the failing heart followed by successful transplantation has now been demonstrated in both animals and man. Cortesini and co-workers[15] reported four surviving calves in 1977 following TAH implantation and subsequent transplantation. At this time, the Jarvik-3 device was used. In 1981, Olsen and associates[45,46] reported several short-term and one long-term survival in calves following removal of a Jarvik-5 TAH and transplantation from a twin sibling. This ingenious experimental model in twins did not require immunosuppression. Their work has verified the concept that the native heart can be excised and replaced by an artificial device followed later by transplantation. In addition, Chiang and colleagues[8] verified the durability of such implants. In 1984, they reported calves surviving up to 268 days and sheep surviving up to 297 days on the Jarvik-7 device. Subsequent fatigue testing of this blood pump has shown durability in vitro

for up to 5 years. These data confirm the feasibility of temporary TAH use and imply that success in humans will be a matter of eliminating complications as experience develops.

MECHANICAL ASSIST AND REPLACEMENT DEVICES

The major categories of devices currently available for circulatory support include the IABP, ventricular assist devices (VADs), and the TAH. Temporary support of end-stage cardiac patients has been successful to date with each type of device. However, there are considerable differences, advantages, and disadvantages to each system.

Intra-Aortic Balloon Pump (IABP)

The single greatest application of the IABP is in the support of the failing left ventricle following cardiac surgery; other indications include unstable angina and cardiogenic shock.[24,34] Counterpulsation is designed to augment coronary blood flow while reducing afterload, thus decreasing oxygen supply/demand mismatch in ischemic heart disease. This technique may not be useful to stabilize patients who have other forms of cardiac disease. Afterload reduction by the IABP is moderate in low output hypotensive patients, and the device does not reduce preload as do other types of assist devices. In low cardiac output situations in which death is imminent, the IABP may be inadequate. Appropriate timing with the ECG or arterial pulse wave is essential to its function. This device cannot pump blood that has not already exited the aortic valve; thus, the actual increase in cardiac output is usually on the order of only 10%, or less than 800 ml/min.[24,50]

TABLE 46-1   Intra-Aortic Balloon Pump

ADVANTAGES	DISADVANTAGES
1. Relatively available and inexpensive	1. ECG triggered (usually) needs high-quality ECG signal and tracks poorly during arrythmias
2. Famliarity of staff to concepts and equipment	2. Limited increase in CO ($\leq$ 10%)
3. Reliability	3. Diastolic augmentation of coronary blood flow may be ineffective in absence of coronary obstruction
4. Patients not totally dependent upon device should drive system require change	4. Failure to insert (12%)
5. No special secondary equipment required	5. Thromboembolic complications
6. Anticoagulation not absolutely necessary (desirable for long-term use [>48 hours])	6. Vascular complications
7. Percutaneous technique[52] greatly increases ease of placement	7. Infection at insertion site
	8. Thrombocytopenia
	9. Mesenteric infarction

This limited augmentation of the cardiac output by the IABP is a distinct disadvantage (Table 46-1).

Ventricular Assist Devices

These units are designed to pump blood in parallel to the failing cardiac chamber. This means that the device drains oxygenated blood from the left atrium or ventricle and returns it under pressure to the aorta. Initially, roller or centrifugal pumps used for CPB have been adapted for this use. For longer durations of pumping, centrifugal pumps (Fig. 46-2) have proved simpler and safer, thus enjoying wider use. However, the non-pulsatile nature of centrifugal pumping is deleterious to organ perfusion over long periods of time.

Several forms of pulsatile assist devices have been developed. Although not intended for use in cardiopulmonary bypass, these devices appear to be better than nonpulsatile systems in supporting the failing ventricle. Most current designs are powered by compressed air, because this energy source is the easiest and simplest to work with in initial design phases. Currently, the only device approved by the FDA for temporary use is the Pierce-Donachy pneumatic VAD (Fig. 46-3A and B). The Novacor, Inc MK22D[53] electrically actuated LVAD (Fig. 46-4) has been implanted for temporary use in two patients prior to transplantation. Several other designs are being developed but have not yet been used in patients.

Total Artificial Heart (TAH)

Finally, TAHs are designed for complete replacement of ventricular function and are attached to the atrial and vascular remnants left after excision of the native ventricles. The blood pumps are implanted in the patient's mediastinum and connected to their power source by transthoracic pneumatic drive lines. Three basic types of pneumatic TAH blood pumps are currently being used (Fig. 46-5). The earliest model, a sac pump, is designed around a single monolayer of organic polymer formed into a round or ovoid sac. The sac, in turn, is encased in a hard plastic or metal housing and is compressed by surrounding pressurized gas. Filling of the sac may be controlled by passive or active means (i.e., negative pressure). With improvements in molding techniques, the diaphragm pump evolved.[36] A semi-ridged or ridged housing with an inner coating of blood contacting polymer is mounted on a flexible membrane that separates the blood chamber from the pressurized gas chamber. Techniques to mold the housing and flexible diaphragm as a single unit have decreased the thrombogenicity and increased the versatility of this type of blood pump.[36] Finally, pusher plate pumps utilize a moveable plate that compresses a blood sac, expelling blood through the outflow port. At least one model of pneumatically actuated pusher plate TAH has been tested in animals.[56]

Biocompatible organic polymers are essential to the design of all these devices. A surface that is minimally thrombogenic but withstands multiple flexion cycles is a major challenge to design. Many materials have been discarded because of their mechanical or thrombogenic characteristics. Currently, the most effective and widespread organic polymers in use are the family of compounds known as segmented polyurethanes. Initially developed by Boretos and Pierce[5] in the 1960s, these compounds have been widely applied because they have desirable molding characteristics, resistance to flexing stresses, and relative blood compatibility. Additives such as polydimethylsiloxane, the chemical backbone of "silicone rubber," has improved the blood contacting properties of solution cast films of segmented polyurethanes. Avcothane 51, a segmented polyether polyurethane, also retains many desirable

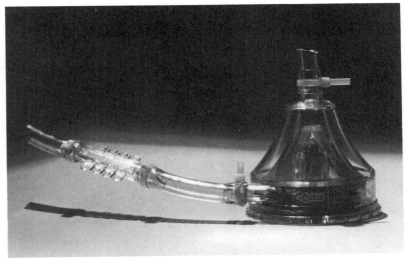

FIGURE 46-2.   *Biomedicus Centrifugal Blood Pump. This pump is currently used for temporary nonpulsatile bypass of either left, right, or both ventricles (drive unit not shown).*

properties and is commonly used in experimental circulatory assist devices.[52]

CANDIDATE GROUPS

Potential for Future Transplantation

Selecting patients for circulatory support with the intent to perform transplantation should closely follow the guidelines set forth for selection of candidates for cardiac transplantation.[14,30,55] Failure to follow these guidelines could possibly create the untenable situation of a patient who is both unweanable from mechanical support and nontransplantable. As is possible, alternative therapies must be constantly entertained for those who are excluded by the established criteria for transplantation. Table 46-2 summarizes the exclusion criteria accepted by most active transplant centers.

The target group for use of *interim* mechanical support with potential for transplantation consists of patients with severe end-stage left ventricular failure, often with associated right ventricular failure. In our experience, the majority of these patients can be stabilized with inotropes, afterload reduction, and antiarrythmics. Table 46-3 lists categories of patients who are likely to be refractory to these therapies at the end-stages of their disease and be candidates for mechanical circulatory support followed by transplantation. Most suffer from either idiopathic or ischemic cardiomyopathy. In addition, some patients who fail to wean from CPB and meet the criteria for transplantation can be included.

Hopefully, some of these patients can be preselected based on their cardiac lesion and myocardial reserve so that the possibility of dependence upon bypass and use of interim mechanical circulatory support followed by staged transplantation can be anticipated. This option could then be discussed with the patient and family preoperatively. Recently, it has been our policy to discuss with patients who have high-risk operative lesions and limited myocardial reserve the possibility of placement of one of several types of circulatory assist devices before undertaking conventional reparative operations.

In addition to the aforementioned patients, those affected by persistent low cardiac output following cardiac surgery or rapidly declining postopertive courses might also be considered in the candidate group if they meet the transplant criteria. Also, patients who are transplanted but subsequently developed fulminant rejection unresponsive to aggressive therapy may develop cardiogenic shock with impending death in a matter of hours. Retransplantation for the irreversibly injured cardiac allograft is possible if the patient can be adequately supported in the interim. Other causes of acute myocardial failure following transplantation that may induce near-fatal complications that could also serve as an indication for mechanical support include ischemic injury to the donor heart during transport, preservation problems, and undetected positive serologic crossmatch with hyperacute rejection.

In the future, a potentially large group of patients with acute myocardial infarctions may be can-

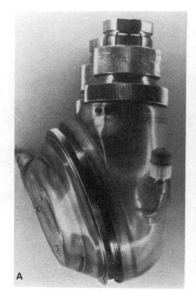
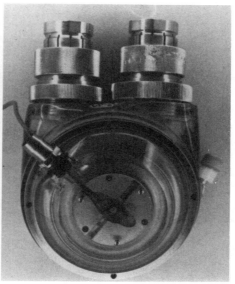

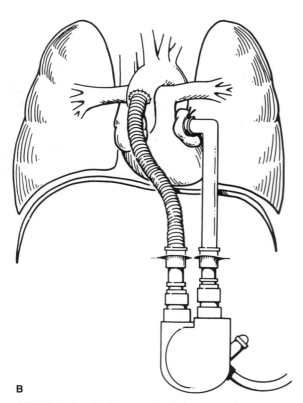

FIGURE 46-3.   (A) Photographs of Pierce–Donachy Ventricular Assist Device (VAD). (Courtesy of the Journal of Heart Transplantation) (B) Schematic of Pierce–Donachy VAD inserted to support failing left ventricle (left atrium-to-aorta).

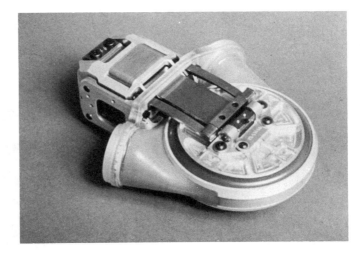

FIGURE 46-4. The Novacor MK22D electrically actuated VAD. This device was designed for permanent support of the failing left ventricle. Recently, two patients have been implanted on a temporary basis prior to transplantation. (Photo courtesy of Peer Portner, Ph.D., Novacor Corporation, Oakland, California)

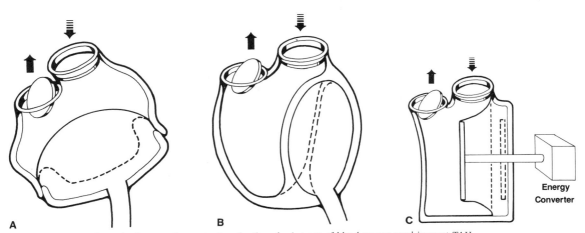

FIGURE 46-5. Schematic diagram demonstrating the three basic types of blood pumps used in most TAH and VAD designs. (A) Diaphragm type; (B) sac type; (C) pusher plate type.

didates for bridge-to-transplantation with artificial devices. Currently, the acute cardiogenic shock patient has a mortality of 30% to 50% in the first postinfarction week. It is extremely difficult, however, to determine which of these patients will recover enough function to avoid the need for cardiac replacement.

Because of the limited human experience, there are currently no standardized guidelines for application of the TAH as a temporary support device. We have formulated tentative guidelines to allow us to optimally utilize available alternatives. All candidates should have end-stage cardiac failure with either acute cardiogenic shock or a prognosis for survival of less than 48 hours; thus, all conventional therapy must have failed. All candidates must meet the acceptance criteria for cardiac transplantation and an emergency search for a donor heart must have been unsuccessful. If appropriate, a condensed pretransplant evaluation should be undertaken to include assessment of the function of major body systems (e.g., pulmonary, renal, hepatic, neurologic, coagulation). In addition, investigation of the emotional and financial resources of the patient and family contribute to the decision about transplantability. In the absence of contraindications, acceptance as an active transplant candidate implies that the patient would also be a candidate for interim mechanical support if hemodynamic deterioration becomes unmanageable.

TABLE 46-2   Contraindications to Heart Transplant (1986)

1. Age: > 55 (? 60)
2. Pulmonary hypertension: (PVR ≥ 8 Woods units)
3. Active infection
4. Irreversible hepatic dysfunction
5. Irreversible renal dysfunction
6. History of malignancy
7. Life-limiting systemic diseases
8. Insulin-dependent diabetes mellitus?
9. Symptomatic severe peripheral or cerebral vascular disease
10. Active peptic ulcer disease
11. Prohibitive psychosocial handicaps

TABLE 46-3   Possible Candidates for TAH-Bridge

TRANSPLANTABLE PATIENTS WITH:

1. Idiopathic cardiomyopathy
   a. Acutely deteriorated
2. Ischemic cardiomyopathy
   a. Acutely deteriorated
   b. Superimposed acute M.I.
   c. Life-threatening arrythmias
3. Failure to wean from CPB
   a. Despite pharmacologic Rx
   b. IABP first
   c. LVAD first ?
4. Post pump refractory low C.O.
5. Acute MI—cardiogenic shock
   a. Failure of IABP
6. Acute myocarditis
7. Acute failure of donor heart
   a. Ischemic injury
   b. Hyperacute rejection
   c. Positive crossmatch

CPB = cardiopulmonary bypass; IABP = Intra-aortic balloon pump; LVAD = left ventricular assist device

Rapid Loss of Cardiac Function

The next major criterion for consideration of interim TAH is evidence of rapid deterioration of cardiac function. In those patients thought to have a reversible injury, temporary VAD support may be better suited, whereas in those with irreversible left or biventricular failure, TAH and eventual transplantation should be considered. As previously mentioned, approximately 20% to 40% of accepted transplant candidates deteriorate and expire before a suitable organ donor is found. This constitutes the most immediate group under consideration for interim TAH support. It is common for medical intervention to temporarily stabilize such patients while an intensive donor search is undertaken. Often, a donor organ can be located, and the preferred procedure, orthotopic transplantation, can be performed. Patients with idiopathic cardiomyopathy often respond to Dobutamine in moderate to high doses (10 µg/kg/min to 30 µ/kg/min). In addition, gentle volume loading and low doses of alpha or mixed alpha-beta vasopressors (e.g., epinephrine, dopamine, norepinephrine) often serve to stabilize patients for days or weeks with minimal complications.

It is not uncommon for such patients to be on high doses of diuretics and to develop dehydration during their initial evaluation period, with subsequent hypotension or symptoms of low cardiac output and diminished perfusion. Cautious use of fluids to support filling pressures without inducing pulmonary edema is occasionally helpful. Although pulmonary artery catheters are a popular means of assessing fluid status and cardiac output, they may be associated with an unnecessary risk of septicemia in all but the sickest of these patients. Any fever from invasive monitoring lines removes the patient from active consideration for transplantation until the source of the fever can be determined and treated. With the extreme shortage of organ donors, the optimal time for transplantation may bypass a febrile patient with disastrous results.

Experience has shown that impending death may be predicted in part by clinical findings. Multiple organ failure and/or acidosis despite near-normal cardiac outputs implies inadequate organ perfusion and impending death. Vasoconstriction, air hunger, extreme weakness, postural hypotension, systolic pressure less than 90 mm Hg combined with a pulse pressure less than 20 mm Hg, and a waxing-waning state of consciousness or delirium are often seen. Pharmacologic therapy may temporarily abate these findings for several days or weeks. However, tachyphylaxis or recurrence of symptoms, particularly episodic hypotension, dizziness, and arrythmias is common. Foreboding re-entry ventricular arrythmias are notoriously unresponsive to lidocaine and other standard antiarrythmics in the end stages of cardiomyopathy. At this point, strong consideration for mechanical support should be given before a terminal event occurs.

The National Association of Transplant Coordinators (NATCO) and the United Network of Organ Sharing (UNOS) have made available a 24-hour per day urgent procurement classification to deal with these situations. NATCO has designated four classifications of potential cardiac recipients based on their hemodynamic status. The highest priority, status 9, is used to notify this network of a less than 48-hour prognosis. If an intensive donor search fails and hemodynamic stabilization begins to deteriorate, preparations for interim mechanical circulatory support should be initiated.

CLINICAL APPLICATION OF ASSIST DEVICES

Most hospitals with active cardiac catheterization laboratories and cardiopulmonary bypass facilities also have the technology to provide intra-aortic balloon counterpulsation. This form of mechanical support is undoubtedly the easiest and simplest to establish, least expensive, most widely available, and best understood. In addition, the simplicity of insertion of the IABP has been markedly improved by the development of the percutaneous transfemoral technique.

Intra-Aortic Balloon

In 1980, Bregman and associates[6] reported a needle-guidewire-dilator technique for IABP insertion. Previously, a femoral arterial cut-down was required. With the percutaneous technique, a tightly wrapped 40-ml balloon can be passed over a guidewire into the descending aorta up to the level of the subclavian artery origin. The unwrapped balloon is connected to a driving console, which is synchronized to either the ECG or arterial pulse wave of the patient. A safety chamber with "slave" balloon is incorporated between the console and the patient. Compressed air inflates the slave balloon, which transfers the energy to the carbon dioxide–filled intra-aortic balloon. Carbon dioxide is readily soluble in blood and provides a measure of safety against air embolism in case there is a structural failure of the intra-arterial portion.

During native systole, the balloon is rapidly deflated, creating a sudden drop in arterial pressure and afterload. This reduces the resistance to left ventricular ejection and reduces myocardial work. During native diastole, the balloon is inflated in synchrony to the timing of aortic valve closure. This increases pressure in the arterial tree at the moment of maximal coronary artery blood flow. In this way, the IABP reduces myocardial oxygen demand while increasing supply. Counterpulsation has proved to be extremely helpful in a larger number of patients with ischemic events such as unstable angina, acute myocardial infarction, and cardiogenic shock. In addition, since the IABP increases mean arterial blood pressure, it has also found a place in stabilizing some hypotensive pretransplant patients.

The intra-aortic balloon has several disadvantages, however, which are summarized in Table 46-1. More than 10% of patients develop a balloon-related complication, the most common being arterial thrombosis or embolization in the ipsilateral extremity. Occasionally, amputation is the end result. Arterial laceration, arterial dissection, dislodgement of atherosclerotic emboli, and perforation of the iliac artery or descending aorta are also potential complications. Bowel ischemia and mesenteric embolization may also occur.[61] In a large series, 4% of patients developed major complications and 7% minor complications such as superficial bleeding, superficial infection, or thrombocytopenia.[61] Insertion is not possible in 12% of patients in whom the attempt is made.[61] Counterpulstion is often ineffective in patients with normal coronary arteries. The balloon will augment diastolic coronary flow but remains dependent upon the native cardiac outut displaced through the aortic valve for its effects. Afterload reduction is moderate in low output hypotensive patients, but the device does not provide preload reduction as will VADs. Augmentation of cardiac output is at best between 5% and 10%, whereas reduction in myocardial oxygen consumption and increased oxygen delivery remain the major potential benefits.[24,50]

Ventricular Assist Devices— Nonpulsatile

Centrifugal and roller pumps have been designed primarily for CPB. Their adaptation for mechanical circulatory support of the failing left ventricle is a natural extension of their performance of this task. However, their minimally pulsatile or nonpulsatile characteristics fail to duplicate the physiology of the normal circulation. In addition, peak pump flow through the small aortic cannulas commonly used with this technique may be inadequate, especially for long periods of time. High-flow velocities across these catheters have been associated with hemolysis, platelet activation, and increased bleeding compications. These systems seem best suited for patients who fail to wean from CPB. In this situation, the aortic cannula can be converted to an infusion line, and the system can be completed by a drainage catheter inserted into the left atrium. With appropriate connections, these catheters can be brought out transthoracically and connected to the extracorporeal pumps. Because commercially available centrifugal pumps are not exceptionally expensive or difficult to use by trained perfusionists, this technology has disseminated rapidly and is well within the range of any currently practicing cardiac surgical team.

The currently available centrifugal pumps are

easy to prime in an emergency situation. Removal of air from centrifugal pumps has been less critical than with roller pumps because small air bubbles are often trapped in the vortex of the pump. However, the initial suggestion that these devices do not pump air at all has proved to be untrue, since large boluses of air can occasionally be transmitted to the arterial line. In addition, heat generated by friction as well as the high-speed motor (2,000 to 5,000 RPM) can induce denaturization of serum proteins. Small blood coagulum can form on the plastic cones or the base plate of the pumping chamber. Improvements in pump design have lessened, but not totally eliminated, this potential for thrombus formation. It is recommended that the pump head be changed every 24 hours in order to diminish the risk of embolization or pump dysfunction from thrombosis.[17] It is, of course, a disadvantage to break the sterility of the system for daily pump head changes; septicemia has been a major problem in this group of patients.[17] Disadvantages of this technique include bleeding complications, which are extremely common, particularly at cannulation sites and suture lines.

Ventricular Assist Devices—Pulsatile

Superior physiologic control, myocardial decompression, and elimination of myocardial work are provided by pulsatile VADs. These pneumatic pumps provide approximately 65 ml of stroke volume per cycle. To obtain this flow, they drain the pulmonary venous return and thus decompress the left heart. Various cannulation techniques have been attempted to obtain adequate inflow and complication-free outflow. Oxygenated blood can be obtained from either the right superior pulmonary vein, the left atrial appendage, the left atrial free wall, or the left ventricular apex. A specially designed outflow cannula attached to a Dacron graft is also provided; it is sewn to the ascending aorta using side-biting clamp techniques (Fig. 46-3B). This large-bore outflow does not generate significant pressure gradients across the cannula during systole.

An alternative for inflow is the use of a left ventricular apex cannula. This technique decompresses the left ventricle better and provides higher flows than the atrial cannulation technique. It is undesirable to place a ventricular apical cannula in a patient with a small left ventricle or in a patient with potentially recoverable myocardial injury such as low output syndrome after conventional surgery. Bridge-to-transplant patients with dilated myopathy are probably more suitable for apex cannulation. Although the ventricular cannula gives more complete decompression, thrombi may form around the cannula tip in the left ventricle.

There are other disadvantages of the ventricular assist systems (Table 46-4). All extracorporeal devices with transcutaneous cannulas provide a continuous risk of ascending infection spreading into the mediastinum during the implant period.

The reliance on a single left-sided device (LVAD) is unsuccessful in approximately 20% to 30% of candidates.[49] In the presence of pulmonary hypertension, pulmonary edema, or severe right heart failure, inadequate filling of the left-sided pump may prevent its support of the circulation. Inotropic therapy (Isuprel) and prostaglandin E1 infusion have been used successfully to restore function of the right heart and pulmonary circulation. If this fails, a right-sided VAD may be required.

Total Artificial Heart (TAH)

The temporary use of TAH devices offers several theoretical advantages over extracorporeal assistance. Because the entire heart is removed, control of the circulation lies with the device and not the patients' failing cardiovascular system. Unlike the diseased native heart, TAH devices have almost no limitation in the ability to eject blood during systole. Their only limitation is the inefficiency of diastolic filling, which can be overcome by various design and driving adjustments. This total control over the cardiovascular system has permitted patients to recover from the multiorgan damage of end-stage heart failure, be removed from ventilators, and even begin ambulation and oral nutrition again prior to undergoing the rigors of heart transplantation.

Current units have demonstrated long-term reliability and freedom from sudden mechanical failure. Valuable diagnostic and hemodynamic data are generated electronically by feedback circuitry in the drive systems. Thus, with cardiac outputs available continuously, freedom to control the hemodynamics of the recipient is always available. In addition, acute pulmonary vascular resistance changes and right ventricle failure are no longer limiting factors in pump performance as they are in LVAD systems.

The use of temporary TAH devices in humans is still in its early phase; however, disadvantages are already apparent. Owing to their unusual shape and size, TAHs fit poorly in the human pericardial space. Obstruction of systemic or pulmonary venous return can occur if there is insufficient room or improper placement of the device. Bleeding complications have been common but will probably be manageable with more surgical experience. The risk of embolism, particularly stroke, has been high in the first

TABLE 46-4   *Advantages and Disadvantages of Temporary Left Ventricular Assist Devices*

ADVANTAGES	DISADVANTAGES
1. Readily implantable	1. Bleeding complications are common
2. Native heart remains in place	2. Removal can be technically difficult
3. Patient not totally device dependent	3. Large transcutaneous cannulation stomas
4. Low rate of embolic complications	4. Thrombosis around atrial or ventricular cannulas
5. No absolute need for anticoagulation	5. Large cannulas, difficult to position without inflow obstruction
6. Can relieve ventricular arrythmias	6. Left-sided pump efficiency dependent upon performance of right heart and low pulmonary vascular resistance
7. May be used despite arrythmias	7. BVAD may be required
	8. Patent foramen ovale leads to right-to-left shunting and cyanosis with LVADs
	9. Fusion of aortic valve leaflets if periodic native ejection is absent
	10. Inadequate myocardial recovery may prolong implant
	11. May not totally decompress LVEDP
	12. Cannulas may compress coronary or mammary artery grafts

BVAD = biventricular assist device

TABLE 46-5   *Selection of Anticoagulants for Short-Term TAH Recipients: Advantages and Disadvantages*

	MECHANISM	DURATION	IV/PO	ACUTELY "REVERSIBLE"	EASE OF TITRATION	RISK OF BLEEDING AT TX*
Heparin	Antithrombotic	30 min	IV	Yes	Yes	Minimal
Warfarin	Antithrombotic	3–5 days	PO	No	None	Moderate
ASA	Antiplatelet	7–10 days	PO	No	None	High
Dipyridamole	Antiplatelet	6–8 hr	PO	No	None	Minimal
Sulfinpyrazone	Antiplatelet	18 hr	PO	No	None	?
Dextran 40	Antiplatelet	6–12 hr	IV	No	Minimal	Minimal

* TX = transplantation

several recipients of the Jarvik-7 TAH.[39] Attempts to prevent this with anticoagulants (Table 46-5) have not been effective and have led to worsened bleeding complications. Advances in anticoagulant therapy and improvement in device design offer great hope for reduction in thromboembolic complications. However, drive line infection, total dependence on the artificial heart, and complexity of the procedure are other major disadvantages.

Enthusiasm for the Jarvik-7 in patients awaiting transplantation has been tempered by the concern for stroke. The initial human trials of the Jarvik-7 have disclosed a relatively high incidence of cerebral thromboembolism. This particular complication appears to be the most serious current drawback related to the design.[39] Explanted Jarvik-7 devices have shown that anatomic crevices created during the formation of the blood pump, particu-

larly around the inflow and outflow valves and the quick connectors, provide a nidus for thrombus formation.[39] These connections and the methods of valve mounting in the Penn State heart are different, but, currently, human experience is limited to only two patients. With more human experience, the cause and associated aggravating factors precipitating stroke are being identified. In addition, it is anticipated that elimination of crevices and areas of stasis in future designs will decrease the threat of thromboembolism.

Other important complications of the TAH seen in some patients include lymphocytopenia, granulocytopenia, thrombocytopenia, thrombocytosis, renal insufficiency and renal failure, hemolysis, respiratory failure, mechanical failure (valve fracture), and invasive line complications (valve obstruction, valve regurgitation, bacteremia).

Continuing developmental work and animal implantation has led to improvements in the technology of pneumatic total artificial hearts. Several promising designs have reached the phase of pre-clinical trials. In 1980, approval for implantation of the Jarvik-7 TAH was granted by the FDA for use in patients who fail to wean from cardiopulmonary bypass. Shortly thereafter, Phase I clinical investigation (restricted to 7 patients) was granted for the implantation of this device as a "permanent" cardiac replacement. The first patient survived for 112 days.[19] This landmark case provided the dramatic proof that mechanical cardiac replacement can succeed in humans for extended periods of time. Subsequently, four other patients have had "permanent" implantations, with three long-term (greater than 30 days) survivors.

In the spring of 1985, FDA approval for the temporary use of the Jarvik-7 and the Penn State pneumatic artificial hearts was granted to investigators in several centers. Initial experience has shown promise in eliminating some of the problems associated with VAD systems.

CLINICAL EXPERIENCE

Currently, the surgical experience of staged cardiac transplantation consists of isolated case reports from many different centers. As an overview, Table 46-6 demonstrates the details of the 15 initial cases. The calendar years 1985 to 1987 showed a dramatic resurgence in interest in all devices, particularly the TAH. For the purposes of this chapter, an account of the first few TAH cases is warranted not only for historic value but also to illustrate the complexity of the entire field of bridging-to-transplantation with mechanical devices. The first human case of the TAH in staged cardiac transplantation was performed at the Texas Heart Institute in April 1969.[11] The device was designed by Dr. Domingo Liotta and manufactured in cooperation with the Cullen Research Laboratories of the Texas Heart Institute. The pump was comprised of a diaphragm-type reciprocating design constructed of Silastic impregnated fibers of Dacron polyester. The blood contacting surface was lined with a reticular Dacron fabric to induce formation of a pseudointima and to reduce potential embolism. One-way flow was obtained with Wada-Cutter hingeless tilting disk valves (Fig. 46-6). Great vessel conduits were made from woven Dacron grafts, and the atrial connections were cuffs of Silastic-embedded Dacron fabric.

The patient failed to wean from CPB following resection of a large ventricular aneurysm. Support of the circulation by the Liotta TAH was uneventful for 64 hours, following which orthotopic cardiac transplantation was performed. However, the patient expired 32 hours later from severe *Pseudomonas* pneumonia. Complications during implant were primarily related to poor renal function, hemolysis, and leukocyte destruction, probably secondary to the fabric lining of the blood contacting surface.[11]

The second patient was implanted with the Akutsu III pneumatic TAH in July 1981 (Fig. 46-7).[12] Because of a cardiac arrest in the intensive care unit (ICU) following triple coronary bypass, an emergency placement of the Akutsu heart was undertaken, with a CPB time of 100 minutes. The major difficulty was a size discrepancy between the device and the thoracic cavity, causing compression of the left pulmonary veins and unilteral pulmonary edema. The sternum could not be closed, and pump outputs were only 3.5 to 4 liters/min. Cardiac transplantation was performed after 39 hours of TAH support, but the patient expired from gram-negative and *Candida* septicemia and multiorgan failure. The Akutsu Series III TAH appeared to perform with less trauma to the cellular blood elements than did the Liotta heart. The blood contacting surface was a seamless smooth layer of Avcothane, and Bjork-Shiley convexo-concave disk valves were used in the inflow and outflow positions (Fig. 46-7).

The third human case was performed at the University Medical Center in Tucson, Arizona, by Drs. J. G. Copeland and Cecil Vaughn in March, 1985. The patient had severe coronary artery disease, a history of two massive myocardial infarctions, and was an acceptable transplant candidate. The immediate performance of the donor heart was suboptimal, and the patient was returned to surgery and placed on CPB while receiving open cardiac massage. When a second cardiac donor could not be located after 4 hours of CPB, the Phoenix pneumatic TAH (Fig. 46-8b) was implanted, and the patient was removed from bypass after a total of 7 1/2 hours.[40,58] Because this device was designed for calf experiments, it was too large for the human pericardial space, and the sternum could not be closed. Retransplantation was performed, but the second donor heart had difficulty maintaining perfusion against the newly increased pulmonary vascular resistance; the patient died on the second day following transplantation from pulmonary edema and sepsis.[40,58] The TAH device used in this case (Fig. 46-9) was molded from Biomer (a segmented polyurethane); St. Jude bileaflet tilting disk valves were used in the inflow and outflow positions. The atrial connector was a plastic stent in which the inflow valves were mounted. This in turn was de-

TABLE 46-6   Registry of Temporary TAH Prior to Transplantation

#	PATIENT	AGE	SEX	DIAGNOSIS	DATE	IMPLANT #DAYS/ HOURS	OUTCOME	SURGEON/ CENTER	DEVICE
1	HK	47	M	IHD	4/4/69	64 hr	Died/ sepsis	DA Cooley Texas Heart Inst	Liotta
2	WM	36	M	IHD	7/23/81	54 hr	Died/ sepsis	DA Cooley Texas Heart Inst	Akutsu III
3	TC	33	M	IHD	3/4/85	12 hr	Died	JG Copeland C Vaughn, Univ Med Ctr, Tucson	Phoenix
4	MD	25	M	ICM	8/29/85	9 days	Alive	JG Copeland Univ Med Ctr, Tucson	Jarvik-7
5	AM	44	M	IHD	10/18/85	12 days	Died	WS Pierce Hershey Med Ctr	Penn State
6	TG	47	M	ICM	10/24/85	4 days	Alive	B Griffiths Univ of Pittsburgh	Jarvik-7
7	ML	40	F	VCM	12/18/85	45 days	Died	L Joyce Abbott-NW, Minn	Jarvik-7 70 ml
8	BC	40	F	VCM	2/3/86	4 days	Rejected reimplant	JG Copeland Univ Med Ctr, Tucson	Jarvik-7 70 ml
9	JB	39	M	IHD	2/3/86	12 days	Alive	B Griffiths Univ of Pittsburgh	Jarvik-7
10	HK	41	M	IHD	2/3/86	31 days	Alive	OH Frazier DA Cooley Texas Heart Inst	Jarvik-7
11	BC	40	F	AR	2/9/86	Ongoing	Alive	JG Copeland Univ Med Ctr, Tucson	Jarvik-7 70 ml
12	UP	26	M	VHD	3/6/86	1 day	Died	F Unger Landeskranken anstalten, Salzburg, Austria	Unger
13	HH	39	M	IHD	3/7/86	4 days	Died	E Burcherl West End Clinic, West Berlin	Berlin
14	RC	48	M	AR	3/17/86	Ongoing	Alive	WS Pierce Hershey Med Ctr	Penn State
15	GB	43	M	ICM	3/23/86	18 days	Died	B Griffiths Univ of Pittsburgh	Jarvik-7

IHD = ischemic heart disease; ICM = idiopathic cardiomyopathy; VCM = viral cardiomyopathy; AR = acute rejection; VHD = valvular heart disease

signed to fit inside the residual atrioventricular (A-V) groove after resection of the A-V valve. Transannular horizontal mattress sutures were used to support and guide the atrial connector into the A-V groove, and the atrium was gathered around the connector with a pursestring suture (Fig. 46-10).[58] Conventional woven Dacron conduits to the great vessels fitted with quick connectors completed the connections. Hemodynamic stability was excellent, and there were no mechanical failures during this 12-hour implant period. No anticoagulants were given.

The fourth patient implanted with a Jarvik-7 TAH in August, 1985 by the same group had severe

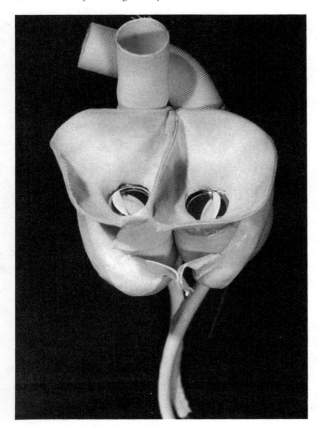

FIGURE 46-6.   *The Liotta heart. The first human recipient of a TAH was implanted with this device on April 4, 1969 by Dr. Denton A. Cooley at the Texas Heart Institute. The patient was a 47-year-old man who could not be weaned from cardiopulmonary bypass following resection of a left ventricular aneurysm.*

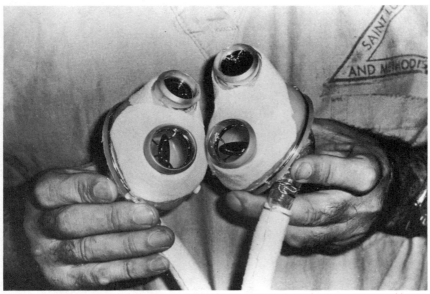

FIGURE 46-7.   *The Akutsu III TAH implanted by Dr. Denton A. Cooley into a 36-year-old man with ischemic heart disease on July 23, 1981.*

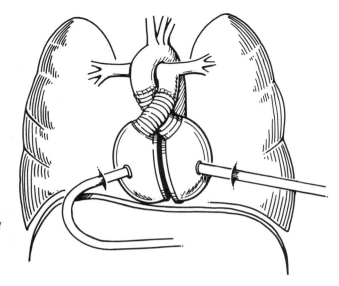

FIGURE 46-8.   Final orientation of the Phoenix TAH designed and built by Kevin Cheng, D.D.S. and implanted by Dr. Jack Copeland and Dr. Cecil Vaughn into a 33-year-old man with a failed donor heart on March 6, 1985.

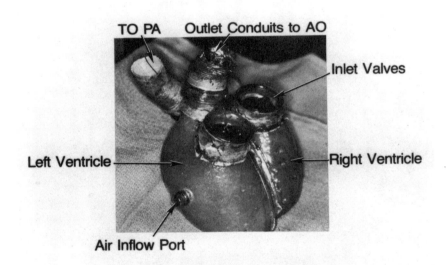

FIGURE 46-9.   The explanted Phoenix TAH from the human case described in Fig. 46-8. All four valves are St. Jude bileaflet tilting disc prothesis.

end-stage idiopathic cardiomyopthy with rapidly deteriorating hemodynamics. After a period of severe hypotension associated with severe unresponsive ventricular arrhythmias and an unsuccessful donor search, a Jarvik-7 was implanted (Fig. 46-11). During the implant period, severe pulmonary edema occurred, mandating 4 days of mechanical ventilation. On the seventh postimplant day, a cerebral embolic event occurred, and, although all deficits eventually cleared, this event prompted urgent consideration for transplantation.[39] Following explanation of the device on the ninth day and cardiac transplantation, the patient was discharged from the hospital 68 days following transplantation with no neurologic deficits and fully ambulatory;[40] the patient continues to enjoy a normal lifestyle post-transplant and has returned to full-time employment.

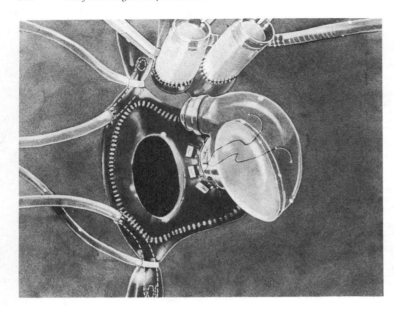

FIGURE 46-10.   *Implantation technique of the Phoenix Heart using pledgetted horizontal mattress sutures in the A-V valve annulus of the failed donor heart. Aortic and pulmonary dacron grafts are illustrated already sewn in place. (Drawing courtesy of Dr. Cecil Vaughn and St. Luke's Medical Center, Phoenix, Arizona).*

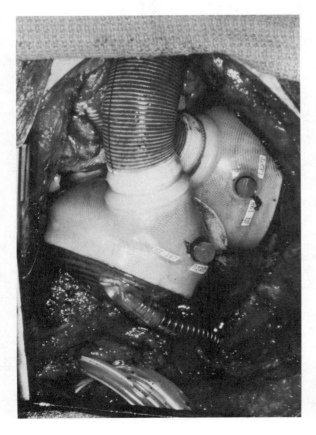

FIGURE 46-11.   *Jarvik-7 TAH implanted by Dr. Jack Copeland, Tucson, Arizona into a 25-year-old man with rapidly deteriorating idiopathic cardiomyopathy. This patient was the first human survivor of bridge-to-transplantation with a total artificial heart.*

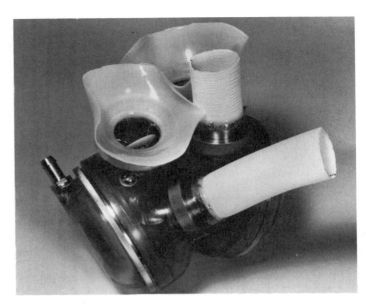

FIGURE 46-12. *The Pennsylvania State TAH designed, built, and implanted on October 18, 1985 by Dr. William S. Pierce and associates at the Milton S. Hershey Medical Center. The patient was a 44-year-old man with severe ischemic cardiomyopathy.*

The fifth TAH-bridge patient had severe ischemic cardiomyopathy and was supported with an IABP but continued to deteriorate. The pneumatic Penn State TAH (Fig. 46-12) was implanted in October 1985 and performed well during the ensuing 11 days; there was no evidence of embolic events. Immediately post-transplantation, he developed severe pancreatitis and a disseminated fungal infection and expired.[51]

Shortly after implantation of the Penn State heart, a Jarvik-7 was implanted as a bridge-to-transplantation at the University of Pittsburgh Hospital in a patient with end-stage idiopathic cardiomyopathy who failed to stabilize with inotropic and IABP support. Mediastinal exploration for bleeding took place shortly following the artificial heart implantation. Otherwise, the patient was free of complications during the implant and post-transplant period. After 4 1/2 days, the TAH was replaced with a human donor heart, and the patient left the hospital 2 weeks later, clinically well.

CONCLUSIONS

Clinical activity in mechanical assistance has blossomed in the 1980s. Simultaneously, several devices finally progressed from developmental stages to initial clinical trials. At the same time, experience with cyclosporine has shown a marked reduction in morbidity (particularly infections) and better long-term survival than previous steroid/azathioprine protocols. These improvements in heart transplantation have stimulated greater numbers of referrals as well as a proliferation of transplant centers. However, competition among centers for fixed donor resources keeps getting worse. There remains an attrition rate of 20% to 40% in potential recipients during the waiting period. The application of mechanical assistance or TAH replacement of the failing heart has now proved to be an important means of preventing this attrition. Although results were initially poor, progress in this area has been extremely rapid.

The first human to survive a bridge-to-transplantation with an artificial heart was implanted with a Jarvik-7 on August 29, 1985, by Jack Copeland. In the 20 months following this historic case, 53 more implants in 51 patients took place. Of these patients, 27 are alive. In just over 1 year, attempts were made with six different TAH designs. This kind of technology was once restricted to a few dedicated research centers; now there are fully equipped TAH implant teams in nine American and six European cities, with many more scheduled to begin soon. The whole field of circulatory support has benefited by the clarification of the unique problems such as stroke, coagulopathy, and infections seen in these complex patients. As experience grows and improvements occur, the TAH and related devices will surely assume a major role in transplantation, if not in all cardiovascular medicine.

REFERENCES

1. Akutsu T, Kolff WJ: Permanent substitutes for valves and hearts. Trans Am Soc Artif Intern Organs 4:230, 1958

2. Barcroft H: Observations on the pumping action of the heart. J Physiol 78:186–195, 1933

3. Barnard CN: The operation, a human cardiac transplant: An interim report of a successful operation performed at Groote Schuur Hospital, Cape Town. SAfr Med J 41:1271–1274, 1967

4. Borel JF, Feurer C, Gubler HV et al: Biological effects of Cyclosporin A: A new antilymphocytic agent. Agents Actions, 6(4):468–475, 1976

5. Boretos JW, Pierce WS: Segmented polyurethanes: a new elastomer for biomedical application. Science 158:1481–1482, 1967

6. Bregman D, Casarella WJ: Percutaneous intra-aortic balloon pumping: Initial clinical experience. Ann Thorac Surg 29:153–155, 1980

7. Caves PK, Stinson EB, Graham AF et al: Percutaneous transvenous endomyocardial biosy. JAMA 225(3):288–291, 1973

8. Chiang BY, Olsen DB, Dries D et al: An analysis of animals surviving over 100 days on the total artificial heart. In Progress in Artificial Organs, Vol 1, pp 211–216. IVth Congress of ISAO, Kyoto, Japan Nov 1983. Atsumi K, Naekawa M, Ota K (eds): ISAO press #204 Cleveland 1984

9. Clark DA, Schroeder JS, Griepp RB et al: Cardiac transplantation in man, review of first three years experience. Am J Med 54:563–576, 1973

10. Clauss RH, Birtwell WC, Abertal G et al: Assisted circulation I. The arterial counter pulsator. J Thorac Cardiovasc Surg 41:447, 1961

11. Cooley DA, Liotta D, Hallman GL et al: Orthotopic cardiac prosthesis for two-staged cardiac replacement. Am J Cardiol 24:723–730, 1969

12. Cooley DA, Akutsu T, Norman JC et al: Total artificial heart in two-staged cardiac transplantation. Cardiovasc Dis Bull Texas Heart Inst 8(3)305–319, 1981

13. Copeland JG, Emery RW, Levinson MM et al: Cyclosporine; an immunosuppressive panacea? Thorac Cardiovasc Surg 91(1):26–39, 1986

14. Copeland JG, Solomon NW: Recipient selection for cardiac transplantation. Ariz Med XXXVII(11):758–760, 1980

15. Cortesini R, Cucchiara G, Famulari et al: Perspectives on heart substitution: Temporary implantation of artificial heart followed by heart allograft. Transplant Proc IX No. 1:305–307, 1977

16. DeBakey M: A simple continuous-flow blood transfusion instrument. New Orleans M&SJ 87:386–389, 1934

17. Dembitsky WP, Daily PO, Raney AA et al: Temporary extracorporeal support of the right ventricle. J Thorac Cardiovasc Surg 91:518–525, 1986

18. Demikhov VP: In Haigh B (ed): Experimental Transplantation of Vital Organs, Chapter 5, pp 212–213. Moscow, Translation-Medqiz, 1969

19. DeVries WC, Anderson JL, Joyce LD et al: Clinical use of the total artificial heart. N Engl J Med 310(5):273–278, 1984

20. Dong E Jr, Shumway NE: Current results of human heart transplantation. World J Surg 1:157–164, 1977

21. Emery RW, Cork RC, Levinson MM et al: The cardiac donor: A six year experience. Ann Thorac Surg 41(4):356–362, 1986

22. Evans RW, Manninen DL, Overcast TO et al: The National Heart Transplantation Study: Final Report, Seattle, Washington: Batelle Human Affairs Research Centers, 1984, Tables 19–7, 19–8, 30–2, 10–5

23. Evans RW: The heart transplantation dilemma. Issues in Science and Technology, pp 91–101, Spring 1986

24. Frazier OH, Painvin GA, Urrutia CO et al: Medical circulatory support: Clinical experience at the Texas Heart Institute. Heart Transplant 2(4):299–306, 1983

25. Gibbon JH Jr: The maintenance of life during experimental occlusion of the pulmonary artery followed by survival. Surg Gynecol Obstet 69:602, 1939

26. Gibbon JH Jr: Application of a mechanical heart and lung apparatus to cardiac surgery. Minn Med 37:171, 1954

27. Gibbs OS: An artificial heart. J Pharmacol Exp Ther 38:197–215, 1930

28. Gibbs OS: An artificual heart for dogs. J Pharmacol Exp Ther 49:181–186, 1933

29. Haller JD, Cerruti MM: Heart transplantation in man: Compilation of cases II January 23, 1964–June 22, 1969. Am J Cardiol 24:554–563, 1965

30. Hallman GL, Leachman RD, Leatherman LL et al: Factors influencing survival after human heart transplantation. Ann Surg 170(4):593–602, 1969

31. Hardesty RL, Griffith BP, Debski RF et al: Experience with cyclosporine in cardiac transplantation. Transplant Proc XV No. 4 Suppl 1:2553–2558, 1983

32. Hardy JD, Chavez CM, Kurrus FD et al: Heart transplantation in man. Developmental studies and report of a case. JAMA 188(13):1132–1140, 1964

33. Jamieson SW, Oyer P, Baldwin J et al: Heart transplantation for end-stage ischemic heart disease: The Stanford experience. Heart Transplant 3(3):224–227, 1984

34. Kantrowitz A, Tjonneland S, Freed PS et al: Initial clinical experience with intraaortic balloon pumping in cardiogenic shock. JAMA 203:113–118, 1968

35. Kolff WJ, Lawson J: Perspectives of the total artificial heart. Transplant Proc, XI No. 1:317–324, 1979

36. Kolff WJ: Artificial organs—forty years and beyond. Trans Am Soc Artif Intern Organs XXIX 6–27, 1983

37. Kondo Y, Gradel F, Kantrowitz A: Homo transplantation of the heart in puppies under profound hypothermia: Long survival without immunosuppressive treatment. Ann Surg 162:837, 1965

38. Lefemine AA, Low HB, Cohen ML et al: Assisted circulation III. The effect of synchronized arterial counter pulsation on myocardial oxygen consump-

tions and coronary flow. Am Heart J 64:789–795, 1962

39. Levinson MM, Smith RG, Cork RC et al: Thromboembolic complications of the Jarvik-7 total artificial heart: Case report. Artif Organs 10(3):236–244, 1986

40. Levinson MM, Smith RG, Cork R et al: Clinical problems associated with the total artificial heart as a bridge to transplantation. Artif Organs The W.J. Kolff Festschrift (in press)

41. Lower RR, Shumway NE: Studies on orthotopic homo transplantation of the canine heart. Surg Forum 11:18–19, 1960

42. Lower RR, Stoffer RC, Shumway NE: Homovital transplantation of the heart. J Thorac Cardiovasc Surg 41:196, 1961

43. Moulopoulos SD, Topaz S, Kolff WJ: Diastolic balloon pumping (with carbon dioxide) in the aorta: A mechanical assistance of the failing circulation. Am Heart J 63:669–675, 1962

44. Neptune WB et al: Complete homologous heart transplantation. Arch Surg (Chicago) 66:174, 1953

45. Olsen DB, DeVries WC, Oyer PE et al: Artificial heart implantation, later cardiac transplantation in the calf. Trans Am Soc Artif Intern Organs XXVII 132–136, 1981

46. Olsen DB, Gaykowski R, Blaylock RC et al: Twin calves, total artificial heart, cardiac transplantation. Artif Organs 7(1):74–77, 1983

47. Oyer PE, Stinson EB, Jamieson SW et al: Cyclosporine in cardiac transplantation: A 2 1/2 year follow-up. Transplant Proc XV No. 4 Suppl 1:2546–2552, 1983

48. Oyer PE, Stinson EB, Jamieson SW et al: One year experience with cyclosporine A in clinical heart transplantation. Heart Transplant 1(4):285–290, 1982

49. Pennington DG, Merjavy JP, Swartz MT et al: The importance of biventricular failure in patients with postoperative cardiogenic shock. Ann Thorac Surg 39(1):16–26, 1985

50. Pennock JL, Wisman CB, Pierce WS: Mechanical support of the circulation prior to cardiac transplantation. Heart Transplant 1(4):299–305, 1982

51. Personal communication: Richenbacker W, Pierce WS: Milton S. Hershey Medical Center

52. Pierce WS, Myers JL, Donachy JH et al: Approaches to the artificial heart. Surgery 90(2):137–148, 1981

53. Portner PM, Oyer PE, Jassawalla JS et al: An implantable permanent left ventricular assist system for man. Trans Am Soc Artif Intern Organs Vol XXIV:98–103, 1978

54. Statement on heart transplantation. JAMA 207(9):1704–1705, 1969

55. Thompson ME: Selection of candidates for cardiac transplantation. Heart Transplant 3(1):65–69, 1983

56. Tomita K, Harasaki H, Takatani S et al: Total artificial hearts: physiological and technical limitations. Heart Transplant 1(2):163–171, 1982

57. Van Allen CM: A pump for clinical and laboratory purposes which employs the milking principle. JAMA 98:1805–1806, 1932

58. Vaughn CC, Copeland JG, Cheng K et al: Interim heart replacement with a mechanical device; an adjunct to management of allograft rejection. J Heart Transplant 4(5):502–505, 1985

59. Wallwork J, Cory-Pierce R, English TA: Cyclosporine for cardiac transplantation: UK trial. Transplant Proc XV No. 4 Suppl 1:2559–2566, 1983

60. Webb WR et al: Practical methods of homologous cardiac transplantation. J Thorac Surg 37:361, 1959

61. Weintraub RM, Thurer RL: the intra-aortic balloon pump—a ten year experience. Heart Transplant 3(1):8–15, 1983

62. Willman VL et al: Autotransplantation of the canine heart. Surg Gynecol Obstet 115:299, 1962

Replacement of Pancreatic Function Through the Use of Mechanical or Electronic Devices

Louis Vignati   Steven V. Edelman

In order to mimic normal pancreatic B cell function, an artificial pancreas should consist of a glucose sensor capable of detecting small changes of plasma glucose concentrations, calculate and rapidly deliver insulin to insulin-sensitive tissues in appropriate amounts, and be safe and reliable over a long period of time with minimal professional or patient input. Electromechanical devices have been either "closed loop," containing a glucose sensor, which provides feedback to the unit to adjust insulin infusion rate, or "open loop," where the device has a programmed finite basal infusion rate and additional insulin is infused to accommodate meals at the discretion of the patient.

The most promising sensors are based on the oxidation of glucose or by electrocatalytic conversion. In both systems, reaction products generate electrical current proportional to glucose concentration. In vivo studies with existing sensors have been limited because of the short life span that makes them unsuitable for intracorporeal implantation.

In vivo experience with open loop implantable infusion devices is more extensive and has successfully maintained euglycemia for periods of 1 to 30 months.

Despite differential insulin levels, no difference in regulation of glucose disposal or production can be demonstrated when peripheral or portal insulin delivery routes are compared.

Bioincompatibility of materials for the glucose sensor and insulin preparations remains a major obstacle to development of an artificial pancreas. Tissue reaction around the sensor results in prolongation of the response time for insulin release and loss of glycemic control. Insulin stored in reservoirs at body temperature tends to aggregate with subsequent occlusion of catheters.

External and internal open loop devices to control diabetes have been successful and provide evidence that more sophisticated implantable devices may benefit the diabetic patient.

Despite 64 years of therapeutic insulin use, restitution of physiologic plasma insulin levels are not achievable. Conventional subcutaneously administered insulin does not mimic the rapid modulation of insulin produced by the beta cell. Normally, the beta cell instantaneously increases or decreases insulin release and production proportional to the ambient-glucose concentration. In addition, because of its anatomical location, the beta cell delivers insulin directly to the liver, an organ that is exquisitely sensitive to small changes of insulin concentration.

Controversy continues as to whether restoration of the dynamic balance of insulin and glucose in insulin-dependent diabetes mellitus (IDDM) will prevent the long-term complications of the disease. Although there is considerable evidence to support this, a prospective study may not be feasible until normal insulin secretory dynamics can be restored.

Although effective, multiple daily insulin injections or continuous subcutaneous insulin infusion (CSII) are unable to consistently achieve normoglycemia over a long period of time.

The cost and complexity of transplantation of the whole pancreas and the failure of islet transplants has resulted in an effort to produce an artificial beta cell, with the following properties: (1) capable of detecting small changes in blood glucose levels, (2) rapid delivery of insulin to insulin-sensitive tissues in appropriate amounts, and (3) safe and reliable over a long period of time with minimal professional or patient input.

Most work has been done using electromechanical devices, either "closed loop," containing a glucose sensor, which provides feedback to the unit to adjust insulin infusion rate, or "open loop," where the device has a programmed finite basal infusion rate and additional insulin to accommodate meals is infused at the discretion of the patient or physician.

Albisser and associates[1] provided early evidence that such a device was capable of achieving near normoglycemia in the diabetic state. However, because of the technical difficulties in providing reliable glucose sensors, biocompatible insulin preparations, and units of sufficient size and reliability, a clinically useful device is not yet available.

GLUCOSE SENSORS

The lack of an implantable glucose sensor has been a major roadblock to closing the loop in a functioning artificial pancreas. An ideal glucose sensor would be totally implantable, able to distinguish minute changes of glucose concentration over long periods of time, and made of materials that are biocompatible with body tissues. The most promising sensors under development have involved some form of glucose oxidation reaction, either enzymatically on or by use of a catalyst. Other sensors developed have depended upon displacement of measurable reactants by glucose (affinity sensor) or measurement of physical properties of glucose such as optical rotation.

Electroenzymatic Sensor

The electroenzymatic sensor is based on the polarographic measurement of hydrogen peroxide generated by glucose oxidase held between two membranes.[10] An outer membrane allows diffusion of glucose, which interacts with glucose oxidase to produce hydrogen peroxide. The resultant product diffuses across the second inner cellulose acetate membrane to the electrode surface, where an electrical current is generated. The inner membrane is impermeable to other interfering plasma substrates that might stimulate electrical currents such as ascorbate or urate. The electrical current generated is proportional to the glucose concentration and increases linearly with glucose concentrations up to 1000 mg/dl in diluted samples. Unfortunately, in undiluted samples of blood or plasma, the response is nonlinear above 100 mg/dl. Although this sensor was developed for a possible in vivo intravascular or tissue implant usage, it has found considerable use in the extracorporeal closed loop system (Biostator). The Biostator continuously withdraws blood, which is diluted, so that the response of the sensor is linear over the entire physiologic range. A number of various refinements of this basic sensor have been outlined, many of them resulting in improved enzyme stability and membrane diffusion characteristics. These have included covalent binding of the glucose oxidase to collagen[64] or addition of outer hydrophobic layers of albumin and nylon to allow selective diffusion of oxygen,[66] one of the substrates needed for the glucose oxidation. Assurance of adequate oxygen diffusion allows for a more linear reliable response to glucose concentration.

Information with regard to sensor response time and reliability is based on in vitro data. However, accuracy of blood glucose readings up to 7 days in dogs has been achieved with implantation of a sensor in the intravascular or intersittial space.[23,50]

A number of difficulties remain with enzymatic sensors, including the ability to recalibrate the sensor while implanted, variability of available oxygen in the different body components, time delay between changes in actual blood glucose concentration and the ability of the sensor to generate an electrical current, life span of the enzymatic membrane, and the ability to immobilize glucose oxidase on a membrane.[17,35]

Electrocatalytic Sensor

A second sensor based on oxidation of glucose is referred to as an electrocatalytic sensor.[22,27,28,40] In this model, the glucose reacts at a platinum catalyst electrode that generates a current based on the following potential equation:

$$C_6H_{12}O_6 \rightarrow C_6H_{10}O_6 + 2H + 2e-$$

Although this has been a reliable sensor in vitro and in animal experiments, further development is needed to prolong the life span of the electrode and screen out competing coreactants present in biolog-ical tissues.

Fluorescein Sensor

The affinity with which glucose binds to concana-valin A has been used to create a glucose sensor.[51] In this model, fluorescein-labeled dextran is com-petitively displaced from concanavalin A, and the resulting fluorescence is measured by an optical fi-ber system. This model has provided high selectivity and sensitivity depending upon the choice of the binding protein and the competitive ligands or bind-ing sites. The system has been miniaturized and placed in a 27-gauge needle, which may be placed subcutaneously. The model does not depend upon diffusion of glucose across membranes and therefore minimizes response time.

Other Sensors

All body tissues, to some degree, equilibrate with regard to glucose concentration.[68] A number of novel approaches to continuous glucose measure-ments in different body compartments have been made.

A noninvasive scleral contact lens has been de-veloped using a miniaturized electro-optic unit to estimate the aqueous humor glucose concentra-tion.[33,39] Potentially, it could be used in conjunction with a telemetric component to transfer information to a computerized insulin pump located elsewhere on the patient. In this model, the electro-optic unit correlates aqueous humor glucose concentration by optical rotation determinations. Although this model has given statistically indistinguishable re-sults from simultaneous blood glucose assays in animals, major difficulties arise because other inter-fering biochemical materials in aqueous humor con-tribute significantly to the optical rotation.[16]

Sites of Implantation

Most investigators have concentrated on extravas-cular implantation of glucose sensors, because the intravascular space has proved to be a hostile en-vironment with increased potential for infection, embolization, thrombosis, and hemorrhage. Poten-tial extravascular sites have included interstitial tis-sue and intramuscular, intraperitoneal, intrapleural, and intrapericardial sites. It is important that in any site chosen, there be adequate perfusion and micro-convection currents so that an implanted glucose sensor would closely reflect any changes in concen-tration of glucose.[66]

Production materials and the shape of the unit also play a role in the durability and reliability of any sensor. Histologic studies suggest that a flat disc or smooth-surfaced implant, such as that seen with Teflon-coated pacemakers and silicone breast prostheses, are nonreactive and invoke less of an inflammatory response. The stimulation of fibro-blasts or giant cells around an irregularly surfaced implant would create a relatively impermeable bar-rier between the implant and the vascular system. It has been suggested that a porous sponge-like ma-terial around an implant might incite a chronic in-flammatory response and generation of vascular granulation tissue that might act as a successful in-terface between the sensor and the surrounding sub-cutaneous tissue.[69]

IMPLANTABLE OPEN LOOP SYSTEMS

Despite the lack of reliable glucose sensors, inves-tigation has proceeded with the development of in-sulin infusers suitable for implantation. The devices consist basically of an insulin reservoir and pumping device designed to give a continuous basal infusion of insulin, with or without additional capability to increase insulin flow rates to accommodate meals. These implantable devices have a major advantage of allowing long-term access to central venous or portal venous routes for insulin delivery with min-imal chance of infection. In addition, any implant-able device would be protected from environmental traumas.

As of September 1984, 35 investigators had used 159 implanted devices in 142 patients. All the devices except for 10 were constant rate infusion, without the capability for supplemental infusion for meals. Of the insulin infusion, 51% was intrave-nous, and the remainder was intraperitoneal.[22]

The majority of the reported patients have used an Infusaid pump. This is a hollow titanium disc, separated into two chambers by a titanium bellows. A volatile liquid in equilibrium with its vapor phase in the outer chamber produces sufficient vapor pres-sure to propel the infusate from the inner chamber at a constant rate of flow into a vein or other desired location. Flow rate is controlled by a capillary flow restrictor. The pump is implanted in the supraclav-icular fossa and is filled transcutaneously through a self-sealing port. Implantation of an infusaid pump, modified to provide supplementary insulin infusion in addition to the basal infusion rate to dogs, nor-malized glycemic excursions in response to intra-venous glucose and mixed meals.[4,7] Although in-sulin levels are not reported, the normalization of glucose was at the expense of hyperinsulinemia, as evidenced by the preprandial hypoglycemia. Encouraged by this work, Buchwald and associates[7] used this system in Type II insulin–requiring diabetics. Despite the use of an open loop system without capacity to supplement the basal infusion with additional insulin, glucose control was maintained at a level significantly lower than that achieved in the same patients by intermittent subcutaneous insulin or CSII. In a follow-up study with a nonprogrammable infusaid pump, Kritz and colleagues[24] were able to control insulin-dependent diabetes, although, for larger nutrient challenges, additional supplemental insulin had to be given by subcutaneous injection, demonstrating that an insulin-dependent patient could benefit by an implantable pump that lacked supplemental insulin infusion rates.

A second, more conventional, device used is an electromechanical device developed by the Siemans Company (Siemans AG, Erlangen Germany),[18] which consists of two components, a pump and an external device. The external component using carrier frequency is able to program the pump mechanism to specific basal infusion rates, as well as higher demand rates for meals. The external device is also capable of monitoring pump functions, such as insulin reserve. Irsigler and co-workers,[19] using the Siemans two-part device were able to achieve glycemic control over a 6-month period of time. This device was implanted over the facia of the external oblique abdominal muscle, with placement of the delivery catheter intraperitoneally in the left hypogastrum.

A third, but similar, device has the internal component divided into a reservoir, rotary solenoid pump, and separate energy source.[55] An external programmer permits alteration of the basal infusion rate and monitors pump function. Schade and associates,[49] using a separate remotely programmable device and intraperitoneal delivery of insulin, were able to achieve improvement in euglycemia in an insulin-dependent diabetic.

This success with implantable devices has been reconfirmed in larger series, with treatment of both Type I and Type II patients[9,45,45a] using implanted devices for up to 30 months. The use of these implantable pumps, however, has not been without technical difficulties, in particular stability of the insulin preparations at body temperature.

External Open Loop Insulin Systems

Open loop external insulin infusion pumps were introduced clinically several years ago, with the goal of improving the conventional means of treating insulin-dependent diabetes mellitus (IDDM).[61] At the present time, several thousand diabetics are currently using one of the 13 different models in the United States. The basic system consists of an external device that pumps insulin through a thin plastic tube connected to a 25- to 27-gauge needle (Fig. 47-1). The needle is implanted subcutaneously by the patient in almost any area where usual injections are taken (triceps area of the arm, abdomen, thigh, and upper outer quadrant of the buttocks) and held in place by tape or adhesive material. The needle site is changed every 24 to 48 hours.

Most insulin pumps have two infusion rates. A preprogrammed basal rate (usually programmed between 0.5 to 1.5 units/hour), given as small pulses of 0.1 units spaced evenly throughout a 24-hour period. This basal rate is designed to prevent hepatic glucose output in the fasting state without causing hypoglycemia. The newer insulin pumps have the ability to deliver multiple basal rates in order to accommodate the variability of basal insulin secretions needed to maintain normoglycemia.

The second basal infusion rate, which is patient initiated, consists of a larger premeal insulin dose (usually 5–15 units), given 30 minutes before eating. This method allows more physiologic plasma insulin levels and improved glucose control and may allow a more flexible lifestyle, in terms of meals and exercise. Continuous subcutaneous insulin infusion (CSII) has been shown to improve glucose and glycohemoglobin levels for extended periods of time.[34] In addition to the effect on carbohydrate metabolism, there is improvement in triglyceride, cholesterol, and free fatty acid levels,[59] mineral metabolism by decreasing urinary calcium and phosphate losses,[14] motor nerve conduction velocity,[37] somatomedin C levels, and abnormal coagulation factors found in the diabetic. CSII therapy also lowers the exercise-induced microalbuminuria[67] and exercise-induced release of counterregulatory hormones such as epinephrine, glucagon, and growth hormone.[54,60] CSII has been extensively used in the management of pregnant diabetics, since improved metabolic control throughout the pregnancy minimizes the incidence of congenital anomalies and perinatal mortality and morbidity.[21,44]

Some of the problems encountered with these pumps are (1) small abscesses or areas of inflammation at the needle implantation site (one reported case of subacute endocarditis); (2) mechanical failure (low batteries, kinked or defective tubing, and insulin aggregation and clogging), resulting in hyperglycemia or, potentially, ketoacidosis; (3) patient fatigue of wearing the pump; (4) initial weight gain

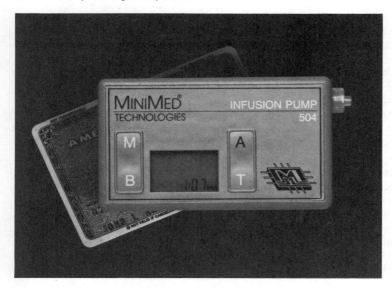

FIGURE 47-1.   *Electromechanical pump utilized for continuous subcutaneous delivery of insulin infusion (CSII, photographed larger than lifesize).*

seen in some patients; and (5) although patients experience fewer hypoglycemic reactions, the recognition may be diminished secondary to lower levels of counterregulatory hormones.[30,54]

The Center for Disease Control in Atlanta has intensively investigated 35 deaths occurring in diabetics while using CSII and concluded that there was no association with excess mortality compared with specific death rates for conventionally treated patients with Type I diabetes.[62] The ideal patient for CSII is a Type I diabetic of almost any age who is motivated, compliant, educated about diabetes, yet not prone to unrecognized hypoglycemia reactions or recurrent skin infections.

CLOSED LOOP SYSTEM

Because of the lack of prolonged reliability of glucose sensors, the closed loop systems have remained extracorporeal. The majority of studies with closed loop systems have used the Biostator (Life Sciences Div, Ames Company, Elkhart, Indiana). This device consists of an electroenzymatic glucose oxidase sensor, which monitors continuously withdrawn blood from the patient, an on-line computer, and a multichannel roller infusion pump. The lag time for glucose analysis is less than 60 seconds; insulin and/or glucose infusion is based on actual glucose concentrations and the rate of change of glucose concentrations. This second component for determination of insulin infusion ensures early prandial

infusion of insulin, which is needed to achieve optimal plasma glucose control.[20] The device is relatively large and requires two intravenous access lines, which limits the patient's mobility, although Schichiri and colleagues[50] reported treatment of IDDM with a portable closed loop device.

The Biostator is capable, using the appropriate parameters for each patient, of restoring a euglycemic state in the insulin-dependent diabetic and establishing physiologic patterns of plasma insulin levels.[41] The Biostator has functioned primarily as a research tool and as a standard of comparison for open loop systems of insulin infusion. The clinical use has been limited to determination of insulin requirements for IDDM,[26] control of glycemia during surgery,[52] facilitation of resection of insulinomas,[25] and management of the diabetic during labor and delivery.[70]

The Biostator overestimates the insulin required in the ambulatory diabetic treated with subcutaneous insulin.* At present, it is not clear whether the hyperinsulinism resulting from the closed loop intravenous infusion is a result of the route of delivery or rate of delivery of insulin as determined by the present algorithm. In addition, the clinical use is limited by the size of the device and the personnel intensive effort required to operate it, as well as the need for frequent recalibration.

* Unpublished data.

UNRESOLVED ISSUES WITH ARTIFICIAL PANCREAS

Insulin Aggregation

Early investigators using both portable and implantable insulin delivery systems were frustrated by the interruption of insulin infusion and subsequent hyperglycemia owing to occlusion of the delivery catheter. This was particularly true with indwelling intravenous catheters left in place for months. The problem occurs with CSII but does not represent as serious a problem because of the frequency and ease of catheter changes. As demonstrated by a number of investigators and reviewed by Lougheed and associates[32] and Feingold and colleagues,[11] the occlusions are the result of aggregation of insulin into polymers and soluble denatured forms, which accumulate at the surface of the narrowing catheter. Factors that affect the extent and rapidity of aggregation include the presence of metal ions, purity of insulin, *p*H, temperature, agitation of insulin solution, and reservoir composition.

Aggregation of insulin can be minimized by manipulation of the insulin formulations. Manipulatin of the *p*H is particularly important, as change of *p*H of the insulin solution toward the isoelectric point within the reservoir or during transit along the infusion catheter can lead to aggregation of the insulin. The insulin solution can be stabilized by addition of bicarbonate[46] or autologous serum-containing bicarbonate.[2,31] After a number of trials of various buffers and chelating agents, Buchwald and co-workers[6] stabilized the insulin by diluting with glycerol; however, the high osmotic solution limits the infusion to a central venous route. Additional methods have used surface active agents containing polypropylene glycol polymer to prevent aggregation.[19]

Insulin Infusion Route

Another question facing the development of an artificial pancreas is the question of the most appropriate site of insulin delivery. There are four potential sites for insulin delivery from an extracorporeal or implanted artificial pancreas: interstitial or subcutaneous, systemic venous, portal venous, or intraperitoneal. Physiologically, the liver is the central organ in regulating supply of glucose to insulin-dependent and independent tissue. At meals, hepatic glucose uptake increases dramaticaly and hepatic gluconeogenesis decreases, thereby modifying post-meal plasma glycemic excursions. These changes in hepatic activity are mediated by a prompt rise in portal insulin concentrations.[42] Peripheral levels of insulin are also regulated by hepatic extraction,[12] since 40% to 60%, depending upon the portal insulin concentration, of portal insulin is extracted by the liver. Therefore, the insulin delivered by portal vein could theoretically dampen post-meal glucose fluctuations while minimizing the risk of intraprandial or fasting hypoglycemia.[57]

Intravenous routes of delivery, either peripherally or by central venous line, provide rapid distribution of infused insulin and the potential for variation of plasma insulin profiles. However, these routes of delivery are subject to phlebitis and thrombosis.[53] Current studies comparing portal vein infusion to systemic intravenous infusion show no difference in glucose disposal or appearance rates in response to a glucose load or mixed meal.[13,43] Given the technical difficulties of direct portal vein infusion, it appears to offer no advantage over the intravenous route. The experience with whole-organ pancreas transplantation in which insulin delivery is by way of the systemic circulation supports this conclusion.

Intraperitoneal insulin is a feasible route for insulin delivery, particularly from implantable devices. The liver will be exposed to high concentrations of insulin in comparison to peripheral tissues, since insulin readily crosses the peritoneal membrane to capillaries draining into the portal vein, particularly if the catheter is placed high in the peritoneal cavity. Intraperitoneal delivery of insulin using implanted or extracorporeal devices provide glycemic control equal to that achieved with intravenous insulin and superior to subcutaneously delivered insulin.[15,19] Absorption of intraperitoneal insulin is rapid, achieving peak peripheral plasma insulin levels 15 to 30 minutes post infusion, depending upon the concentration of insulin and the duration of infusions.[51,47,48]

The subcutaneous route, although having the advantage of ease of access, has been associated with local irritation or frequent mechanical failures.[38]

BIOARTIFICIAL PANCREAS AND OTHER NOVEL APPROACHES

A major difficulty to date with pancreatic transplants or beta cell implantations has been transplant rejection. Attempts have been made to prevent host-cytotoxic cells from destroying implanted islet cell tissue by creating a mechanical barrier between the tissue and the cytotoxic cells. This barrier has taken the form of semipermeable membranes, which allow diffusion of glucose and insulin but prevent passage of large molecular weight substances and cytotoxic cells. Early studies using islets sandwiched between membranes were disappointing because of delay of diffusion across the membrane of either glucose or insulin. This resulted in prolonged responsiveness of the islet to glucose changes.

Improvement of responsiveness to ambient glucose levels is achieved by cultivating cells on the outside of capillary tubes and subsequently enclosed in an outer jacket. This device placed in a vascular shunt[3,3a,8,58,65] was successful in achieving euglycemia in experimental animals, but prolonged use was limited by thrombus formation within the capillary units.[65] Other methods of encapsulation of beta cells within capillary tubes and then planted interperitoneally have been successful in maintaining euglycemia for up to 12 months. Optimal therapy with these devices has depended upon the available mass of the insulin-producing tissue, source and insulin secretion capacity of such tissue, diffusion time of the insulin through the semipermeable membrane.[63]

In order to optimize kinetics of insulin release, there must be minimal distance for diffusion of glucose or insulin. To approach this problem, individual islets have been encapsulated with semipermeable materials. Islets encapsulated in alginate polylysinealginate have been implanted to the intraperitoneal space of streptozocin diabetic rats, with subsequent control of the diabetes for up to 1 year.[29,36]

A more novel implantable device designed to deliver insulin in a physiologic way consists of implanted pellets containing glycosylated insulin bound to concanavalin A. The insulin thus bound is competitively displaced by glucose, thereby producing a biochemical artificial pancreas.[5,56]

REPLACEMENT OF PANCREATIC FUNCTION

The development of electromechanical devices to replace normal pancreatic function is conceptually easy but has been technically difficult to achieve. Although preliminary animal and human clinical trials are promising, long-term reliability of these devices have limited their utilization.

Future advances in the formulation of insulin, development of reliable sensors, and improved understanding of physiologic insulin secretory patterns will result in clinically useful devices. Whether the development of such devices will precede successful transplantation of biologic tissue in the form of micro- or macroencapsulated islets or segmental pancreatic transplants cannot be foreseen at this time. Once appropriate devices are available for clinical use, there will be a need for prospective trials to evaluate the efficiency of such devices and their potential for prevention of chronic diabetic complications.

REFERENCES

1. Albisser AM, Leibel TG, Eward TG et al: An artificial endocrine pancreas. Diabetes 23:389–396, 1974
2. Albisser AM, Lougheed W, Perlman K et al: Non-aggregating insulin solutions for long term glucose control in experimental and human diabetes. Diabetes 29:241–243, 1980
3. Altman JJ, Houlbert D, Chollier A et al: Encapsulated human islet transplants in diabetic rats. Trans Am Soc Artif Intern Organs 30:382–384, 1984
3a. Altman JJ, Houlbert D, Callard P et al: Long term plasma glucose normalization in experimental diabetic rats with macroencapsulated implants of benign human insulinomas. Diabetes 35:625–633, 1986
4. Blackshear PJ, Rohde TD, Grotting JC et al: Control of blood glucose in experimental diabetes by means of a totally implantable insulin infusion device. Diabetes 28:634–639, 1979
5. Brownlee M, Cerami A: a glucose-controlled insulin delivery system: Semi-synthetic insulin bound to lectin. Science 206:1190–1192, 1979
6. Buchwald H, Rohde TD, Dorman FD et al: A totally implantable device: Laboratory and clinical experience using a model with single flow rate and new design for modulated insulin infusion. Diabetes Care 3:351–358, 1980
7. Buchwald H, Varco RL, Rupp WM et al: Treatment of a type II diabetic by a totally implantable insulin infusion device. Lancet 1233–1235, 1981
8. Chick W, Perna JJ, Lauris V et al: Artificial pancreas using living B cells: Effect on glucose homeostasis in diabetic rats. Science 197:780–782, 1977
9. Chute EP, Rupp WM, Rohde TD et al: Continuous single rate long term insulin infusion using a totally implantable pump. Trans Am Soc Artif Intern Organs 30:387–398, 1984
10. Clark LC, Duggan CA: Implanted electroenzymatic glucose sensors. Diabetes Care 5:174–180, 1982
11. Feingold, Jenkins AB, Kraegen WW: Affect of contact material on vibration-induced insulin aggregation. Diabetologia 27:373–378, 1984

12. Field JB, Rojdmark S, Harding P et al: Role of liver in insulin physiology. Diabetes Care 3:255–260, 1980
13. Fischer U, Rizza RA, Hall LD et al: Comparison of peripheral and portal venous insulin administration on postprandial metabolic responses in alloxan-diabetic dogs. Diabetes 3:579–584, 1982
14. Gerfner JM, Tamborlane WV, Honst RL et al: Mineral changes accompanying treatment with a portable subcutaneous insulin infusion system. J Clin Endocrinol Met 50:862–866, 1980
15. Gooch BR, Abumrad NN, Robinson RP et al: Near normalization of metabolism of IDDM: Comparison of continuous subcutaneous versus intraperitoneal insulin delivery. Horm Metab Res (Suppl) 1:190–194, 1984
16. Gough DA: The composition and optical rotary dispension of bovine aqueous humor. Diabetes Care 5:266–270, 1982
17. Guilbault GG: Enzymatic glucose electrodes. Diabetes Care 5:181–183, 1982
18. Hepp KD, Renner R, Piwernetz K et al: Control of insulin dependent diabetes with portable miniaturized infusion systems. Diabetes Care 3:309–313, 1980
19. Irsigler K, Kritz H, Hagmüller G et al: Long term continuous intraperitoneal infusion with an implanted remote controlled insulin infusion device. Diabetes 30:1072–1075, 1981
20. Kerner W, Thum CH, Tamasjun GY et al: Attempts at perfect normalization of glucose tolerance test of severe diabetics by artificial B cell. Horm Metab Res 8:256–261, 1976
21. Kitzmiller JL, Younger D, Hare JW et al: Continuous subcutaneous insulin therapy during early pregnancy. Obstet Gynecol 66:606–611, 1985
22. Knatterud G, Fisher M: Report from international study group on implantable insulin delivery devices. Diabetes Care 8(3):308, 1985
23. Kondo T, Ito K, Ohkura K et al: A miniature glucose sensor, implantable in the blood stream. Diabetes Care 5:218–221, 1982
24. Kritz H, Hagmüller G, Lovett R et al: Implanted constant basal rate insulin infusion devices for type I diabetic patients. Diabetologia 25:78–81, 1983
25. Kudlow JE, Albisser AM, Angel A et al: Insulinoma resection facilitated by the artificial endocrine pancreas. Diabetes 27:774–777, 1978
26. Lambert AE, Buysschaert M, Marchand E et al: Determination of insulin requirements in brittle diabetic patients by the artificial pancreas. Diabetes 27:825–833, 1978
27. Lerner H, Soeldner JS, Cotton CK et al: Measurement of glucose concentration in the presence of coreactants with a platinum electrode. Diabetes Care 5:229–237. 1982
28. Lewandowski, Szczepanska-Sadowska E, Krzymien J et al: Amperometric glucose sensor: Short-term, in vivo test. Diabetes Care 5:238–244, 1982
29. Lim F, Sun AM: Microencapsulated islets as bioartificial endocrine pancreas. Science 210:908–909, 1980
30. Lock DR, Rigg LA: Hypoglycemia coma associated with subcutaneous insulin infusion by portable pump. Diabetes Care 4:389–391, 1981
31. Lougheed WD, Fischer U, Perlman K et al: A physiologic solvent for crystalline insulin. Diabetologia 20:51–53, 1981
32. Lougheed WD, Woulfe-Flanagan H, Clement JR et al: Insulin aggregation in artificial delivery systems. Diabetologia 19:1–9, 1980
33. March WF, Rabinovitch B, Adams RL: Noninvasive glucose monitoring of the aqueous humor of the eye: Part II. Animal studies and the scleral lens. Diabetes Care 5:259–265, 1982
34. Mecklenburg RS, Benson EA, Benson JW et al: Long term metabolic control with insulin pump therapy. N Engl J Med 313:465–468, 1985
35. Oberhardt JB, Fogt EJ, Clemens AH: Glucose sensor characteristics for miniaturized closed-loop insulin delivery: A step towards implantation. Diabetes Care 5:213–217, 1982
36. Oshea GM, Goosen MFA, Sun AM: Prolonged survival of transplanted islets of Langerhan's encapsulated in a biocompatible membrane. Biochem Biophys Acta 804:133–136, 1984
37. Pietri A, Ehle AL, Raskin P: Changes in nerve conduction velocity after six weeks of glucoregulation with portable insulin infusion pumps. Diabetes 29:668–671, 1980
38. Pietri A, Raskin P: Cutaneous complications of chronic continuous subcutaneous insulin infusion therapy. Diabetes Care 4:624–626, 1981
39. Rabinovitch B, March WF, Adams RL: Noninvasive glucose monitoring of the aqueous humor of the eye: Part I. Measurement of very small optical rotation. Diabetes Care 5:254–258, 1982
40. Richter GJ, Luft G, Gebhardt V: Development and present status of an electrocatalytic glucose sensor. Diabetes Care 5:224–228, 1982
41. Rizza RA, Gerich JE, Haymond MW et al: Control of blood sugar in insulin dependent diabetes: Comparison of artificial endocrine pancreas, continuous subcutaneous insulin infusion, and intensified conventional insulin therapy. N Engl J Med 303:1313–1318, 1980
42. Rizza RA, Mandarino LJ, Gerich JE: Dose response characteristics for the effects of insulin on glucose production, glucose utilization and overall glucose metabolism in man: Determination using sequential infusion in conjunction with glucose clamp technique. Am J Physiol 3:E630–639, 1981
43. Rizza RA, Westland RE, Hall LD et al: Effect of peripheral versus portal venous administration of insulin on postprandial hyperglycemia and glucose turnover in alloxan-diabetic dogs. Mayo Clin Proc 56:434–438, 1981
44. Rudolf MCJ, Coustan DR, Sherwin RS et al: Efficacy of the insulin pump in the home treatment of pregnant diabetics. Diabetes 30:891–895, 1981
45. Rupp WH, Barbosa JJ, Blackshear PJ et al: The use of inplantable insulin pump in the treatment of type II diabetes. N Engl J Med 307:265–270, 1982

45a. Saudek CD, Pitt HA, Dempsey RE et al: The programable implantable medication system: The first human implantations. Diabetes 36:77a, 1987

46. Schade DS, Easton PR, Carlson GA et al: Future therapy of insulin dependent diabetic patients—The implantable insulin delivery system. Diabetes Care 4:319–374, 1981

47. Schade DS, Eaton PR, Davis T et al: The kinetics of peritoneal insulin absorption. Metabolism 30:149–155, 1981

48. Schade DS, Eaton PR, Friedman NM et al: Intraperitoneal delivery of insulin by portable microinfusion pump. Metabolism 29:699–702, 1980

49. Schade DS, Eaton PR, Friedman NM et al: Five day programmed intraperitoneal insulin delivery in insulin dependent diabetic men. J Clin Endocrinol Metab 52:1165–1169, 981

50. Schichiri M, Kawamori R, Halkui N et al: The development of a wearable-type artificial endocrine pancreas and its usefulness in glycemic control of human diabetes mellitus. Biomed Biochem Acta 435:561–568, 1984

51. Schultz JS, Mansouri S, Goldstein IJ: Affinity sensor: A new technique for developing implantable sensors for glucose and other metabolites. Diabetes Care 5:245–253, 1982

52. Schwartz SS, Horwitz DL, Zehfus B et al: Use of a glucose controlled insulin infusion system (artificial beta cell) to control diabetes during surgery. Diabetologia 16:157–164, 1979

53. Selam JL, Slingemeyer A: Long term ambulatory peritoneal insulin infusion of brittle diabetes mellitus compard with IV and subcutaneous routes. Diabetes Care 6(2):105–111, 1983

54. Simonson DC, Tamborlane WV, Defronzo RA et al: Intensive insulin therapy reduces counterregulatory hormone responses to hypoglycemia in patients with type I diabetes. Ann Intern Med 103:184–190, 1985

55. Spencer WJ, Bair RE, Carlson GA et al: Some engineering aspects of insulin delivery systems. Diabetes Care 3:345–350, 1980

56. Stephen RL, Kim SW, Jacobsen SC: Potential novel methods for insulin administration: II. Self regulating internal drug delivery systems. Biomed Biochem Acta 43, 5:559–560, 1984

57. Stevenson RW, Parsons JA, Alberti KG: Insulin infusion into the portal and peripheral circulation of unanesthetized dogs. Clin Endocrinol 8:335–347, 1978

58. Sun AM, Parisus W, Healy GM et al: The use in diabetic rats and mnkeys of artificial capillary units containing cultured islets of Langerhan. Diabetes 26:1136–1139, 1977

59. Tamborlane WV, Genel M, Sherwin RS et al: Restoration of normal lipid and amino acid metabolism in diabetic patients treated with a portable insulin infusion pump. Lancet 1:1258–1261, 1979

60. Tamborlane WV, Sherwin RS, Kovisto V et al: Normalization of the growth hormone and catecholamine response to exercise in juvenile-onset diabetic subjects treated with a portable insulin infusion pump. Diabetes 28:785–788, 1979

61. Tamborlane WV, Sherwin RS, Genel M et al: Reduction to normal of plasma glucose in juvenile diabetes by subcutaneous administration of insulin with a portable infusion pump. N Engl J Med 300:573–578, 1979

62. Teutch SM, Herman WH, Whyer DM et al: Mortality among diabetic patients using continuous subcutaneous insulin infusion pumps. N Engl J Med 310:361–368, 1984

63. Theodorou NA, Howell SL: an assessment of diffusion chambers for use in pancreatic islet cell transplantation. Transplantation 27(5):350–352, 1979

64. Thevenot DR, Sternberg, Coulet P: A glucose electrode using high-stability glucose-oxidase collagen membranes. Diabetes Care 5:203–206, 1982

65. Tze, WJ, Tai J, Wong FC et al: Studies with implantable artificial capillary units containing rat islets on diabetic dogs. Diabetologia 19:541–545, 1980

66. Updike SL, Shults M, Ekman B: Implanting the glucose enzyme electrode: Problems, progress and alternative solutions. Diabetes Care 5:207–212, 1982

67. Viberti B, Pickup JC, Bilous RW et al: Correction of exercise-induced microalbuminuria in insulin-dependent diabetes after three weeks of subcutaneous insulin infusion. Diabetes 30:813–823, 1981

68. Wingard LB, Chung CL, Wolfson SK et al: Potentiometric measurement of glucose concentration with an immobilized glucose oxidase/catalase electrode. Diabetes Care 5:199–202, 1982

69. Woodward SC: How fibroblasts and giant cells encapsulate implants: Considerations on the design of glucose sensors. Diabetes Care 5:278–281, 1982

70. Younger MD, Vlachokosta F, Kitzmiller J et al: Marked decrease in insulin requirements in diabetics during labor and delivery. Diabetes 29:119, 1980

PART SIX

Special Topics in Transplantation

CHAPTER 48

Ethics in Organ Transplantation

Roberta G. Simmons   Linda Abress

Medical advances in organ transplantation over the past twenty years have not brought resolution to the ethical debates that were generated. Three areas include (1) whether the level of patient rehabilitation justifies the expense of transplantation; (2) whether patient selection is equitable; and (3) ethical issues of live and cadaver donation.

The majority of living donors have a positive attitude toward their decision. Among relatives, the decision to donate a kidney appears to be most frequently an instantaneous rather than a deliberative one, and independent information-seeking is low, even in cases of deliberation. Evasion and postponement of decision making is evidenced among a few donors and among a sizeable minority of relatives who fail to volunteer to donate. Similar studies of living unrelated donors should be conducted, given the increase in the use of such donors who are emotionally close to the recipient but genetically unrelated.

Medical successes in organ transplantation over the past 25 years have been spectacular. Nevertheless, many of the ethical ramifications that were originally present[77] still remain at issue. Whereas some problems seem less urgent, others have emerged to replace them. Basically, there have been three foci of concern: (1) Is the level of rehabilitation substantial enough for different types of patients to justify these extremely expensive treatments?[8,35,38,39,54] (2) Does the health care delivery system ensure equitable treatment for all patients?[21,29,32,63*] (3) Are donors (living as well as cadaver) being treated in ways that satisfy high ethical standards?[17,20,77,80]

Very recently, the ethical issues of organ transplantation have received increased attention in the press, in the government, and in professional societies. In the United States, The Federal Task Force on Organ Transplantation was created by Public Law 98-507, "The National Organ Transplant Act," signed by President Reagan, October 19, 1984. The general charge of this task force is to examine medical, legal, ethical, economic, and social issues presented by human organ procurement and transplant. Also, awareness of the abuses in the procurement, distribution, and use of human organs for transplants has prompted professional organizations such as The Council of the Transplantation Society[17] and The American Society of Transplant Surgeons (see Appendix) to adopt positions and develop guidelines and resolutions directed to the problems and controversies. The controversies have also received a great deal of public press. Recently, the Pittsburgh Press published a five-part series entitled "The Challenge of a Miracle: Selling the Gift," which received wide attention and was the basis of a recent episode of ABC's "20/20."

In this chapter, many of these issues and controversies will be discussed, and it is hoped that this discussion will shed light on the debates that exist within government, the medical community, and society in general. Our own work[40,74–77] has dealt extensively with ethical issues related to patient rehabilitation, equity of health care delivery, and donor use, primarily in regard to kidney transplantation. In this chapter, the relevant literature as well as an analysis from our own work, particularly in regard to the decision making of the living-related kidney donor, will be reviewed.

* A Report of the Standards Committee on Organ Procurement of the ASTS: Prioritization of candidates for extra-renal transplants. 1985

PATIENT REHABILITATION IN GENERAL

The findings cited in Chapter 33 (Rehabilitation After Kidney Transplantation) indicate that quality of life as perceived by the patient is quite high 1 year after a successful transplant compared with rehabilitation on alternative therapies for end-stage renal disease (ESRD). Furthermore, new immunosuppression regimens appear to be associated with improvements in life quality. The ethical question of whether federal dollars are well allocated to ESRD is addressed by these data.

Clearly, one benefit of transplantation is life extension. In terms of survival, Evans[22] notes the following:

... it is estimated that 80 percent of all heart transplant recipients will live one year, 50 percent will live 5 years, and more than 25 percent will live 10 years or longer. About 50 percent of liver transplant recipients also will live five years or longer. (p. 7)

However, given limits on resources, these high-cost therapies need to be evaluated in more rigorous ways than assessing the ability of an organ transplant to prolong life. Life quality as well as life extension is important. The work on quality of life and rehabilitation of kidney patients is substantial (see Chapter 33). There is less information on quality of life of patients who have received other types of organ transplants. However, heart transplant patients have a lower overall quality of life than do kidney transplant patients.[24] The ability for liver transplant patients to achieve a satisfactory quality of life has also been questioned.[58]

Other related ethical issues also remain of concern. These issues deal with the attempt to place a value on the quality of life, that is, to determine whether the quality of life is high enough generally for transplant patients to substantiate the enormous amounts of federal money being spent. They also include more specific issues such as equitable health care delivery, organ supply, and sale of organs.

For the physician, ethical ambiguity is focused primarily around two domains: (1) selection of patients in a way as to ensure equity, and (2) the use of organs from related and unrelated living donors.

SELECTION OF PATIENTS

Originally, the shortage of money and facilities meant that many patients with ESRD had to be denied treatment. The criteria to be used in condemning kidney patients to certain death were unclear and controversial. Whether centers should use factors such as apparent psychological strength, social worth, social class, intelligence level, or predicted ability to cooperate with the treatment regimen were significant matters of controversy.[77] With the government now paying for the treatment of kidney disease, and facilities therefore expanding, few patients need to worry about being turned away, and many of these arguments have become moot for this therapy.[17,65] For transplantation of other organs and for future new technologies, such issues still remain highly relevant, however.[5,50,64]

The expansion of facilities for kidney transplantation and dialysis has made treatment available for high-risk groups who would not otherwise have been eligible for treatment—the elderly, diabetics, and those with other physical diseases.[78] The question still remains whether such an expensive treatment should be allocated to those for whom life quality is likely to be severely compromised.[77] If elderly patients on dialysis become senile and incapable of caring for themselves or if physically ill patients are severely restricted by other diseases, is the maintenance of physical existence contraindicated?[59,90] Physicians and policy advocates alike are concerned that if the federal cost of this program skyrockets because of such patients, this and other future catastrophic disease programs will be threatened.

The most pronounced difference between the treatment of chronic kidney disease in Great Britain and the United States is that virtually every afflicted patient in the United States is treated, whereas many patients in Great Britain are not.[1,51] Many centers in Great Britain turn away diabetic patients, older patients, and other high-risk persons whose medical problems make them less likely to react favorably to dialysis or transplantation. However, these types of patients are treated in large numbers elsewhere.[1,23,51,78]

There are three alternatives for such high-risk patients, all of which have their proponents: (1) not to accept them for treatment, (2) to accept them but withdraw treatment if quality of life becomes exceedingly poor, or (3) to accept and treat them as long as they can maintain life. The entire issue of removing a patient from treatment, either at his own suggestion or that of the physician, has been difficult to resolve.[59]

The patient at high physical risk is not the only person who poses selection problems for transplantation of kidneys and other organs. Should patients apparently at psychological risk prior to treatment be accepted for treatment? What policy should apply to social deviants? Should the patients who have revealed a strong tendency to violate medical orders be allowed these expensive therapies? On the basis of a dying person's behavior, can a psychologist or psychiatrist predict his reaction to a medical regimen that will restore him to partial or full health? James F. Childress, a medical ethicist and a member of the Federal Task Force on Organ Transplantation, suggests that organ transplantation be based on medical utility rather than social utility. However, he notes that it is possible to transform judgments of social utility into judgments of medical utility. For example, rehabilitation is affected by the availability and commitment of family and friends. Thus, the presence of this type of social support could be considered as a criterion for selection for transplantation.*

Basically, selection issues are tied to resources, namely available organs and funding. Nationally, we are developing the perception that we have reached the limits of our resources.[66] Although changes may not be made in the ESRD program, other transplant programs may develop different allocation procedures in the face of scarcity.[66] For example, the current practices for patient selection in heart transplantation use medical criteria and psychosocial criteria such as requiring that a patient has a strong "will to live," a "stable or rewarding family or vocational environment to return to after the transplant," and no history of "alcoholism, job instability, or antisocial behavior."[56] The concern of a current article by Merrikin and Overcast[56] was that patient selection for heart transplantation may be in violation of the Rehabilitation Act of 1973, which prohibits discrimination against the handicapped in any program receiving federal funds.

Thus, questions have been raised as to whether it is appropriate to exclude high-risk patients, elderly patients, and less psychologically stable patients from transplantation. Another question that has received less attention involves the transplantation of newborns and other infants.[6] The effects of such early transplantation and of long-term immunosuppression remain to be evaluated, although studies of somewhat older children who have received kidney transplants indicate favorable quality of life for the majority.[43,44]

Another controversy that has arisen over patient selection concerns the transplantation of foreign nationals.[3] The issue is that wealthy foreign nationals will absorb resources provided, in part, by federal dollars. On the other hand, questions can be raised about the ethics of denying treatment based on nationality. The debate has focused on whether foreign nations should be denied access to waiting lists, whether they should be treated only if suitable Americans are unavailable, or whether quotas should be established. According to the current draft of the guidelines for organ donation from The American Society of Transplant Surgeons, a consensus has been reached that U.S. citizens or persons residing in the United States on a permanent basis should be preferentially transplanted, and foreign nationals will be transplanted using a quota as a guideline. (See Appendix for The American Society of Transplant Surgeons guidelines.)

USE OF ORGAN DONORS

The ethical issues concerning the use of organ donors have proved even more ambiguous than those concerned with selection of patients. In this section, we will discuss (1) the current controversial issues of the sale and exportation of organs, (2) alternative laws to enhance the cadaver donor supply, and (3) the issues involved in the use of living donors, both related and unrelated. Highlighted in this section is our empirical study of the donor decision-making process.

The Sale of Organs

The question of the sale of organs has become a recent controversial issue.[57,60] The National Organ Transplant Act (passed by the U.S. Congress in 1984) bans the sale or purchase of organs. Similarly, both the Council of the Transplantation Society[17] and the American Society of Transplant Surgeons (see Appendix) strongly renounce the sale of organs. Both organizations maintain that offending members of either society be expelled. However, there is evidence that organs are being sold in many countries[69] and that foreign nationals from such countries attempt to convince transplant centers that a potential, compensated donor is their relative. Some believe that organ sales make sense from a utilitarian perspective, with the donor able to save the recipient's life, as well as provide financially for his or her family.[7] For an extended discussion of this controversy, see a special section of *Progress in Clinical and Biological Research.*[62]

The two main policy arguments summarized by Annas[4] in favor of allowing living donors to sell their nonvital organs are: (1) It could increase the supply, and (2) individuals should have the liberty to use and dispose of their bodies as they see fit. Annas[4] argues that if the major issue is supply, there

* See Childress JF: The scarcity of human organs for transplantation: Charity, justice, and public policy. Presented at a Colloquium, The Wilson Center, July 9, 1985

should be increased efforts to make the present procurement methods more efficient in order to avoid all the problems and controversy of this radical alternative. The individual liberty argument appears more compelling, but there are many examples of ways in which the government prevents persons from placing themselves at risk (e.g., limits on third trimester abortions, occupational health and safety laws, seat belt laws).[4]

The arguments against the sale of organs are numerous. First, there is the concern that the product will be less dependable[17,34] and that poor-quality kidneys could be sold more cheaply than good-quality ones. Second, there is the problem of deciding what a kidney is worth[34,61] or, stated another way, "the pricing of a priceless gift."[4] Third, a market in body parts is an unsavory idea.[5,16] From a legal perspective according to Annas,[4] the major argument against permitting a competent adult to sell his or her nonvital organs is that ". . . . sale is an act of such desperation that *voluntary* consent is impossible." As an example, consider the following letter. This letter was sent to one of the major American transplant centers in August 1985, from a Mexican citizen:

Permit me to address you with the finest attention you deserve, and to divert you for a little while from your many occupations in order to explain to you the following case: When I encounter a desperate economy, I decided to sell a kidney and wish to go to trouble so that I am a useful intermediary in order to be able to sell it.

The amount that I request for the kidney is the following: $60,000 which I wish that you send $5,000 for expenses, . . . (translated from Spanish)

This letter paints the dangers quite well; low-income persons would be the ones to sell their kidneys with the well-to-do person ending up with better access to organs despite the use of public moneys in funding transplantation. In some cases, poor and powerless persons would be under direct pressure. And, in some instances, a network of "middle men" might emerge to capture some of the profit: Flaherty and Schneider[30] report a case of a loan shark from Tokyo who allowed his debtors to pay him with their kidneys.

Fourth, a weakening of altruism might occur. Voluntary gifts from cadaver donors might decrease if organ sales were encouraged. Like Annas,[4] several commentators,[15,16,92] suggest greater efforts to make the present procurement mechanism of cadaver organs more efficient so that the ethically problematic sale of organs can be avoided. It has been estimated that each day, 10 U.S. families donate a family member's organs for transplantation.[70] Still, the waiting lists for cadaver organs have been very long in the past few years.

Organ Exportation

Closely connected to the issue of organ sales is the problem of organ exportation. Flaherty and Schneider[31] report that kidneys are being exported from the United States to private hospitals for private patients while U.S. citizens continue to wait for available organs. The American Society of Transplant Surgeons guidelines now suggest that there be verifiable evidence that an attempt has been made to place these organs in the United States. While such action encourages equitable access to organs regardless of financial background, it raises the issue of protectionism and nationalism versus an open international exchange.

Laws to Enhance Cadaver Donor Supply

Aside from the allocation of cadaver kidneys, the problem of retrieving kidneys from brain-dead patients has raised substantial ethical concerns over the years.[10,41,86,87,93] With time, the ethical and legal problems associated with brain death seem to be less distressing for transplant physicians than the issues involving living donors.[41] As long as families give consent for the use of cadaver donors, there appears to be relatively little controversy. Greater difficulty arises over the ethical issue of "opting out" laws that would entitle governments to remove organs unless families objected or unless the person carried a refusal card.[11,49,85,88]

"Presumed consent" policies specify, as previously noted, that consent for retrieval of organs is presumed unless the patient or family explicitly opt out.[53,84,85] (Other terms that have been used are "opting out"[85] or "contracting out."[84]) Strong and Strong[85] report that 13 countries have presumed consent laws, but, in 6 of the 13, families are notified before proceeding with the organ donation. A recent survey by Stuart and associates[87] indicated that countries with presumed consent laws seem to have an increased organ supply, although sizeable waiting lists for kidney transplants still exist.

Those who argue against opting out and presumed consent laws suggest that they involve "diminished voluntarism" on the part of donors.[85,98] Manninen and Evans[49] conducted a survey of a representative sample of the American population concerning attitudes and behaviors regarding organ donation and found that only 7% of those questioned supported the presumed consent idea. In the United States, it is doubtful whether such a law could be instituted because of constitutional questions.[84] The issue of paying "just compenstion" to the next of kin for nonconsensual removal requires deciding whether or not cadaver organs are property in the traditional sense. The free exercise of religion can be a reason for nonparticipation in organ donation.[84] However, as previously noted, the main ethical dilemma in opting-out stems from the notion that voluntary donation is more desirable than presumptive donation.[84]

Another policy recently initiated in the United States does not compromise voluntarism. This policy was originally suggested by Caplan[13] as a method of dealing with the organ shortage problem and involves "required (professional) request." When the attending physician pronounces a suitable patient brain dead and determines that medical intervention should cease, the hospital personnel are required to ask about organ donation. In the past few years, some investigators have noted that the single largest barrier to increasing the number of organs donated is the failure of physicians to approach families of patients with the issue.[91] As Simmons and associates[77] describe, the possibility of donation is unlikely to occur to the grieving family members themselves because of their emotional state. In fact, studies of actual cadaver donor families indicate that the local physician who cares for the potential cadaver donor is usually the one who first raises the issue of donation.[77] However, the option of donation may not even occur to the caretaking physician; or it may be emotionally difficult to approach the grieving family; or the local physician may not be well enough acquainted with a transplant center for referral to be psychologically easy.[77] Both Skelley[79] and Matas and colleagues[53] have discussed the many barriers that seem to prevent hospital personnel from obtaining consent for cadaver donation, such as unfamiliarity with procedure and the transplant center, lack of clear delineation of responsibility for referral, uncertainty as to the extent of care that the brain-dead donor should receive prior to donation because of the transplant, and lack of compensation for local staff time.

Within the last year, however, these barriers have been reduced. Fifteen states have enacted "required request" or routine inquiry laws.[48] The results have been even more successful than were anticipated. Notably, organ transplant officials from the first three states to pass the law reported that donations increased immediately after the bills took effect.[48] Caplan[13] also suggests that beyond mandating the required request policy through legislation, it could be made a part of the criteria for accreditation of hospitals.

Living Donors

The shortage of cadaver kidneys could also be reduced if living relatives were given more encouragement to donate.[79,80] Nationally, the 3-year graft survival has been 67% if the kidney comes from a living-related donor, as opposed to 45% if the kidney comes from a cadaver.[45] At the same time, at the University of Minnesota, the 3-year graft survival for all age patients transplanted from 1977 to 1980 has been 76% if the kidney comes from a living-related donor and 55% if the kidney comes from a cadaver. Recent results with living-related donors are even better with the use of either donor-specific transfusions or cyclosporine in HLA-identical donors.

Support for living-related donation has rested largely on the clinical evidence that these transplants are more successful, even though this conclusion has been challenged.[83] However, Najarian and co-workers[89] have also emphasized the importance of related donation in reducing organ shortage:

We would continue to use living-related donors even if the results of cadaveric and living-related donor transplantation were equivalent, otherwise end-stage renal disease patients would be denied transplantation because of the shortage of cadaver kidneys.

In fact, centers vary dramatically in their willingness to use kidneys from related donors: Only 9% of the kidneys transplanted in Europe[46] are from related donors, in contrast to 25% in the United States[36] and 46% at the University of Minnesota. In cases in which the donor is living, the issue is especially difficult for many physicians. Transplantation has placed physicians in an unusual position, where they may cause harm to one person to save the life of another. The reluctance to use related donors at many centers is in part due to a fear of harm to the donor (see below), but also in part due to a widespread feeling that family members are unable to make such a decision willingly, that they will respond to family pressure and later regret their sacrifice.[80,83]

According to Caplan,[12] informed consent includes three aspects: (1) competency to decide, (2) freedom of choice, and (3) adequate knowledge. Competency refers to age and mental capability. Freedom of choice refers to the absence of coercion. A number of factors can contribute to coercion, such as fear, the power of authority, embarrassment, and suddenness. Although adequate or sufficient knowledge is difficult to quantify, Caplan[12] emphasizes the following:

Full and complete disclosure of reasonable risks and benefits, disclosure of possible alternative sources for getting the tissue and comprehension of the information would seem necessary.

There is controversy over the question of whether a family member can really give informed consent or whether the sense of obligation or coercion by other family members is so strong that an informed decision is never really made.[55,77]

Transplant centers also ponder the risks involved in living-related donation. For some surgeons, the fact that there has been an occasional death of a living donor does not make such donation inappropriate. In the words of one surgeon whose center had experienced no related donor deaths:[20]

... when you then look at these situations of people waiting for a cadaver kidney and weigh the salvage against the potential loss of a donor or possibly a serious accident to the donor, well, I think you have a reasonable trade off. And that is the reason why it does not bother me. It concerns me that someday someone may die in our program, but weighing that against the fact that there are patients who are living well because of a living related donor transplant is, I think, far away from any considerations that I can see to make it obsolete.

On the other hand, another transplant surgeon states "we have come close to disaster" with the 15 or 16 living-related donors who have died.[20] In general, a recent study by the Spitals[81] concludes that living-related donors are the preferred source of kidneys at many U.S. transplant centers.

There is controversy not only over whether living relatives should be selected at all but also to what extent the physicians should make the decision in regard to a specific relative. For example, in a case reported by Fox and Swazey,[33] the "gatekeeping" physician refused to allow a willing donor to proceed because his wife was opposed; the donor was told that he was medically ineligible, although this was not the fact. Different centers vary in the placement of the onus of responsibility, with some placing greater emphasis on the physicians and surgeons responsible for the patient care, whereas others allow the potential donor more voice.[77]

At one extreme, the Spitals argue that the competent donor should have a greater voice than he or she has now in his or her suitability for donation and should be able, in fact, to "accept small or unknown added risk."[77,81] In cases in which there is a small or unknown risk, they believe that the donor is better qualified than the physician to make the decision.[80]

Given the continuing uncertainty over the psychological reaction of living-related donors, we now address some of our own empirical work in this area.

The Donor's Reaction and Decision Making

Specifically in terms of the ethics of living-related donation, it is important to consider both the psychological reaction of the donor after the transplant and the decision-making process that a potential donor experiences prior to the transplant. Rather than simply speculating on the donor's psychology, it is necessary to study actual reactions. For that reason, we have investigated the actual social-psychological experiences of a cohort of living-related donors.

To investigate donor decision making, we followed all families presenting for kidney transplantation at the University of Minnesota between 1970 and 1972, beginning with the donor search and continuing to long-term follow-up 5 to 9 years later. These studies of decision making involved 205 families and 114 related donors. All family members possible were interviewed in depth repeatedly during the donor search—a total of more than 900 relatives. Interviews were transcribed, and material was coded or classified into categories by two independent coders. Reliability between the two coders for the material to be presented was satisfactory.[77] In addition to the in-depth studies, we also attempted to administer quantitative surveys to all related donors from 1970 to 1973 at four points in time: (1) prior to transplantation, (2) 5 days after transplantation, (3) 1 year after transplantation, and (4) 5 to 9 years after transplantation. One hundred and fifty donors (90% consent rate) participated in this quantitative aspect of the study.[71]

The Reaction to Altruism. A question at issue is the extent to which altruism, or help-giving behavior without expectation of external reward, is really possible and the nature of the psychological consequences of altruism. Altruism in both the theoretical and lay literature has "fallen into disrepute."[27,28] According to exchange and reinforcement theory, persons "give" to others to obtain certain rewards for themselves.[37] "Merely" saving the life of a loved one is not regarded as strong enough motivation for sacrificing an important body organ at the risk to one's own life. The search is for other rewards that the donor expects to receive or the negative consequences he expects to avoid. The emphasis is on the disillusion and regret that the donor will feel when rewards do not match the sacrifice.

Our quantitative and qualitative data from the historical transplant group and their living-related donors (1970–1973) suggest, however, that altruistic behavior is intrinsically rewarding for great numbers of donors whose self-images and levels of happiness rise after the donation.[71] Because of their ability to undergo self-sacrifice to benefit another person, a high proportion of donors in our studies feel that they have become better and more worthwhile persons with a greater appreciation of life.[73] The entire experience of having rescued a close relative from death is frequently regarded as a peak life experience; and the donors perceive themselves as, consequently, more in touch with truly important values. In fact, the successful weathering of a major family and individual crisis appears to have had a positive impact on most donors—an impact that persists as long as 5 to 9 years after the sacrifice was made.[40,71,72] The typical donors appear to be especially close to the recipient, both prior to and many years after the transplant. Studies from other donor series support this positive view for the majority of donors.[9,26,52]

Although most donors appear to react positively, our findings do not eliminate situational pressures, guilt, family pressure, low self-esteem, or other less-positive forces as operative in motivating some donors. Nor are negative reactions unknown after donation, especially when the explicit reward of family gratitude is absent. Donors who may have been motivated originally by guilt or a need to benefit their self-image are among those more likely to react negatively after the gift is given. "Black sheep" donors who have had major problems with the family in the past and donors who start out with low self-images and low levels of happiness are less likely to be happy with the donation a year later. Substantial regret over donation occurs in a few cases and more frequently when the donation is unsuccessful.[72] Severe negative reaction, particularly over the short term, in a few donors has also been reported by others.[2,19,25,67]

The Donor Decision-Making Process.

Organ donation is an example of a decision made under stress with few established norms to guide the decision-maker. It is an irreversible major life decision with high stakes in which probabilities of success or failure are known. Given this particular type of decision, what was found about the perceived process of decision making? How do these findings affect the ethical evaluation of living-related donation?

To most persons as well as to many decision theorists, decision making implies a period of deliberation followed by a conscious choice of one alternative. Although this decision is one of the most important decisions that persons might ever have to resolve, the majority of potential donors did not perceive that they had made a deliberative choice. The term *decision making* did not seem to fit many people's perception of their decision process, despite the fact that the transplant occurred and they either volunteered or did not volunteer to donate a kidney. The majority of donors and a sizeable proportion of nondonors perceived that their choice to donate or not was an instantaneous one, made at the time that they first heard of the donor need, without any period of conscious deliberation.[77]

For a few donors and a sizeable proportion of nondonors, an interesting pattern of decision postponement, evasion, and stepwise decision making was noted.[77] The *nondonors* evaded the issue; when another volunteer emerged or the patient received a cadaver kidney, they seemed to perceive that events precluding their own donation had occurred before they had thought it was time to make their own difficult choice. The *donors* in this category also postponed deciding whether to donate but agreed to take the first steps toward donation to find out whether they were eligible. If they were ineligible after the first step of the blood test or the second step of the extensive physical work-up, they never had to make a final decision. However, if they were still eligible after proceeding so far into the process, they found that others' expectations had locked them into donation without their ever having finally resolved the issue in their own minds.

Although a *deliberative* pattern of decision making is not the most common mode, it does occur for a sizeable minority of both donors and nondonors who weigh the pros and cons and arrive at a conscious choice. Yet, even in this group, independent information seeking was limited, despite the importance of the decision. About 40% of the "deliberative" donors relied on the transplant physician for information; many sought no new information other than that provided by the family prior to the blood test; and about one third of the "deliberative" nondonors sought no information. The deliberation that did occur frequently involved weighing competing obligations to the patient, on the one hand, and to one's own spouse and children, on the other.

We suggest that the more important the decision, especially in an emotionally charged area, the more uncomfortable the deliberative mode will make many persons. Where the potential costs of both alternatives are very high, thinking about these costs and taking responsibility for the resultant choice is uncomfortable. If persons feel that their obligations in one direction are overwhelming or if they believe that they have become "locked into" one alternative by the course of events, they may more easily be able to justify a course of action.

Thus, whereas both The Council of The Transplantation Society[17] and the American Society of Transplant Surgeons (see Appendix) have emphasized in policy guidelines and editorials the necessity for proper informed consent for living-related donors, it should be recognized that decision making and informed consent are complex processes. Although it is easy to insist on absence of coercion, the questions of adequate deliberation and information are more difficult to resolve.[77]

Living, Genetically Unrelated Donors

One method of alleviating the kidney shortage and avoiding many of the cadaver problems would be to use living volunteers unrelated to the organ recipient (e.g., from husband to wife). However, the lack of clear norms governing such a situation has discouraged many centers from tapping this source.

More than a decade ago, prisoners who volunteered were used as unrelated kidney donors.[18] The practice was discontinued on the grounds that "the use of penal volunteers, however equitably handled in a local situation, would inevitably lead to abuse if accepted as a reasonable precedent and applied broadly."[82]

In the past, most other centers have refrained from using unrelated living donors because of ethical considerations of this type and because of the failure of such kidneys to function any better than cadaver kidneys. However, the University of California Hospitals in San Francisco at one point did use living, genetically unrelated volunteers. Sadler and associates[68] studied the psychiatric aspects of such a donation process. In one year, three public appeals for volunteer donors generated calls from 200 persons; 22 became serious volunteers. Careful screening indicated that 18 of these volunteers were without psychological problems and that most were middle-class stable citizens, married, with children. No social and psychological complications were noted in the donors.

For a long time, however, the use of living-unrelated donors failed to emerge as a viable option owing to the increased availability of dialysis and the belief that a well-matched cadaveric transplant was equally beneficial to the recipient without incurring any harm to a living donor.[47] More recently, though, attitudes toward living-unrelated donation are changing. The primary contributing factor to the current expansion of living-unrelated donors is the shortage of cadaveric organs and the improved results with living-unrelated donors.[17, 47] The Council of the Transplantation Society[17] recently thought it necessary to address the issue of living-unrelated donors. The result was a set of guidelines that set forth fairly strict criteria as to the use of such donors. These guidelines can be summarized as follows:

1. Such donors should be used for situations in which an alternate satisfactory donor cannot promptly be found.
2. Motives should be altruistic, not self-serving or for profit, and no solicitation for profit is acceptable.
3. Motivation should be evaluated by a physician independent of the recipient and of the transplant team, and an independent donor advocate should be assigned.
4. Unrelated donors should be of legal age.
5. The same criteria apply to the selection of living-unrelated and living-related donors.
6. Informed consent without pressure should be secured.
7. No payment is allowed other than for loss of work earnings or for expenses.
8. All procedures must be performed in institutions with recognized transplant teams.
9. Living-unrelated donors should be "emotionally related."

In terms of results, it appears that some centers are able to achieve success rates with living-unrelated donors that are markedly better than with cadaveric transplants. Psychosocial benefits are also likely to accrue to the donor as well as the recipient, further justifying the procedure. As stated by the Council of the Transplantation Society:[17]

With the assurance of relative success, it does not seem unreasonable that in selected instances, donation from unrelated persons, particularly a spouse or individual with a close relationship and intense interest in the welfare of the recipient should be permitted.

Although guidelines specify the use of "emotionally related" donors,[17] this policy has its drawbacks. Once again, informed consent is seriously questioned because of the strength of the emotional relationship.[42] For instance, the spouse might feel a sense of obligation or undue pressure to donate as a result of his or her role. On the other hand, the principle of family benefit, which states that the loss of a family member may be more damaging than the loss of a kidney, can be argued.[42] (See the Appendix for a similar set of guidelines from the *American Society of Transplant Surgeons.*)

SUMMARY

The projected figure for total ESRD benefit payments by Medicare in 1989 is expected to exceed 3 billion 200 million dollars. Transplantation and related services have become a very large public investment. Ethical questions persist owing to the potential for abuses in terms of patient selection, distribution of organs, and donation from cadavers as well as from living relatives and living nonrelated persons. In particular, the public, as well as the transplant professional, have been made aware of abuses that stem primarily from organ shortages. In order to mitigate the incidence of improprieties, national law and professional societies have established guidelines for the attainment and distribution of organs.

Studies of the psychological reactions of living-related donors point to positive effects among most persons, although a few negative consequences have been observed. Among relatives, the process of deciding to donate a kidney appears to be most frequently an instantaneous rather than a deliberative one, and independent information seeking is low, even in cases of deliberation. Actual studies of donor decision making are clearly important to the issue of "informed consent." The evaluation of use of living-unrelated donors should also rely on careful investigation of their decision-making processes and reactions.

APPENDIX

Draft of Guidelines for Organ Donation and Transplantation From the American Society of Transplant Surgeons
2/24/86

The past several years have seen a growth and spread of transplantation that is due both to the improvement of transplantation results and to the application of transplantation techniques to other organs. Because of this, there has been an accentuation of certain ethical issues that the American Society of Transplant Surgeons feels must be publicly addressed. These issues are in part secondary to the basic problem of the overall shortage of organs for transplantation, and the potential for profit, however, altruistically utilized, on the part of medical centers, physicians and potential organ donors. It seems, therefore, appropriate and necessary that the American Society of Transplant Surgeons make public its position on such issues.

1. The supply of transplantable organs is a national resource, and procurement is almost exclusively fiscally supported through federal funding. Therefore, the distribution and assignment of organs to patients must be made by medical criteria and cannot be influenced by other considerations, such as political influence, monetary exchange, or center favoritism.

2. There must be no shipment of transplantable organs to foreign countries by an organ procurement organization or individual unless there is verifiable evidence that a concerted attempt has been made to place these organs somewhere in the United States. Such evidence must include the referral of the organ to a national center for organ distribution if regional patients are not available for its utilization.

3. The active recruitment or encouragement of foreign nationals for the sole purpose of transplantation in the United States is inappropriate and unacceptable to the American Society of Transplant Surgeons.

4. Organs made available for transplantation in the United States should be preferentially transplanted into U.S. citizens, individuals residing permanently in the United States, and foreign nationals under specifically defined conditions. The transplantation of any organ into individuals who come to the United States for the expressed purpose of receiving a transplant is acceptable for humanitarian reasons providing such transplantations constitute a very small percentage of organs transplanted at a given center. This percentage must not exceed on average 5% per year of the organs transplanted at any single center. Foreign nationals who are on the transplant waiting list of a U.S. center must reflect the religious, ethnic, and economic profile of their country of origin. The patient or the responsible financing agency must be charged for transplantation services on the same basis as U.S. citizens.

5. The use of living-related donors is currently acceptable because of the shortage of cadaver organs and because current long-term results with living-related donors are better than with cadaver organs. The utilization of living-related donors must ensure (a) proper informed consent with adequate documentation, (b) assurance of proper donor psychological and medical follow-up, (c) absence of financial profit by the donor, and (d) no known coercion of the donor or his family.

6. The use of living-nonrelated donors is accept-

able only under specifically defined circumstances, which include a well-documented "emotional relationship" between donor and recipient and a medical situation necessitating prompt transplantation. Where living-nonrelated donors are used, there must be clearly documented informed consent, lack of monetary exchange in excess of reasonable donor costs, and an assurance of proper donor medical and psychological follow-up. Because at this time the overall clinical results and benefits of using living-nonrelated donors are still unknown, such transplantation must be conducted with the approval of the respective center's Committee on Human Experimentation or a similar group. The American Society of Transplant Surgeons, while recognizing the occasional appropriateness of living-nonrelated donor utilization and the current justification for the use of living-related donors, is committed to the goal of there being an adequate supply of cadaveric organs with a graft success equivalent to that of living-related donors, thus, ultimately eliminating the need to use healthy living donors.

7. The Ethics Committee of the American Society of Transplant Surgeons will review complaints against individual surgeons and/or centers regarding alleged breaches of ethical practice. The Ethics Committee will present its findings to the Council of the American Society of Transplant Surgeons who will decide upon appropriate disciplinary action, which may include censure by or expulsion from the American Society of Transplant Surgeons if violations of ethical practice are confirmed. The governing board of the facility used by the offending member for the purpose of transplantation will be notified in writing if such disciplinary action is taken.

REFERENCES

1. Aaron HJ, Schwartz WB: The painful prescription: Rationing hospital care. Washington DC, The Brookings Institution, 1984
2. Abram HS, Buchanan DC: Organ transplantation: Psychological effects on donors and recipients. Med Times 88:23d, 1978
3. Anast D: Congressional hearings on 'transplantation into nonimmigrant aliens.' Contemp Dial 5(1):18, 1984
4. Annas GJ: Life, liberty, and the pursuit of organ sales. The Hastings Center Report 14:22, 1984
5. Annas GJ: The prostitute, the playboy, and the poet: Rationing schemes for organ transplantation. Am J Public Health 75(2):187, 1985
6. Associated Press: Baby shows no sign of rejecting heart. Minneapolis Star and Tribune V(69):3A, June 12, 1986
7. Bach DL: Markets in kidneys. Lancet 2(8411):1102, 1984
8. Blagg CR: After ten years of the Medicare End-Stage Renal Disease Program. Am J Kidney Dis 3(1):1, 1983
9. Brown CJ, Sussman M: A transplant donor follow-up study. Dial Transplant 11:897, 1982
10. Byrne PA, O'Reilly S, Quay PM: Brain death—An opposing view. JAMA 242:1985, 1979
11. Calne RY: What has happened to charity? Br Med J 284:998, 1982
12. Caplan AL: The right to privacy when lives are at stake. In Basson MD, Lipson RE, Ganos DL (eds): Troubling Problems in Medical Ethics: The Third Volume in a Series on Ethics, Humanism, and Medicine. Progress in Clinical and Biological Research 76:245–255. 1981
13. Caplan AL: Ethical and policy issues in the procurement of cadaver organs for transplantation. N Engl J Med 311(5):981, 1984
14. [Deleted]
15. Caplan AL, Siegler M: Risks, paternalism and the gift of life. Arch Intern Med 145:1188, 1985
16. Carpenter CB, Ettenger RB, Strom TB: 'Free-market' approach to organ donation. N Engl J Med 310:395, 1984
17. The Council of the Transplantation Society: Commercialism in transplantation: The problems and some guidelines for practice. Lancet 2(8457):715, 1985
18. Crosbie S: The administrator in the organ replacement program. Proceedings of the First International Symposium on Organ Transplantation in Human Beings. Hanover, NH, Sanadoz Pharmaceuticals, 1970
19. Eklund B, Ahonen J, Lindfors O et al: The living donor in renal transplantation. Transplant Proc XIV:68, 1982
20. Ethical aspects in renal transplantation. Kidney Int 23(Suppl 14):S-90, 1983
21. Evans RW: Health care technology and the inevitability of resource allocation and rationing decisions, Part II. JAMA 249:2208, 1983
22. Evans RW: Transplant coverage: A public policy dilemma. Business Health 3(5):5, 1986
23. Evans RW, Manninen DL, Hart LG et al: The national kidney dialysis and kidney transplantation study: Selected findings Part III. Contemp Dial Nephrol 6(11):41, 1985
24. Evans RW, Manninen DL, Maier A et al: The quality of life of kidney and heart transplant recipients. Transplant Proc XVII:1579, 1985
25. Ewald J, Aurell M, Brynger H et al: The living donor in renal transplantation: A study of physical and men-

tal morbidity and functional aspects. Scand J Urol Nephrol 38(Suppl):59, 1976

26. Fellner CH: Renal transplantation and the living donor: Decision and consequences. Psychother Psychosom 27:139, 1976/77

27. Fellner CH, Marshall JR: Twelve kidney donors. JAMA 206:2703, 1968

28. Fellner CH, Marshall JR: Kidney Donors: The myth of informed consent. Am J Psychiatr 126:1245, 1970

29. Flaherty MP, Schneider A: Richest, not sickest, often get help. The Pittsburgh Press 102(132):November 3, 1985

30. Flaherty MP, Schneider A: Sale of organs for transplant reaches U.S. The Pittsburgh Press 102(133):November 4, 1985

31. Flaherty MP, Schneider A: U.S. kidneys sent overseas as Americans wait. The Pittsburgh Press 102(135):November 6, 1985

32. Fox RC: Exclusion from dialysis: A sociologic and legal perspective. Kidney Int 19:739, 1981

33. Fox RC, Swazey JP: The Courage to Fail: A Social View of Organ Transplants and Dialysis. Chicago, University of Chicago Press, 1974

34. Green PJ: Paying for organs from living donors. Lancet 2(8448):214, 1985

35. Guttmann RD: Medical progress. Renal transplantation (Part 2). N Engl J Med 301:1038, 1979

36. Health Care Financing Administration: End-stage renal disease program medical information system, facility survey tables. Department of Health Services, USA, HCFA, January–December 31, 1984

37. Homans GC: Social Behavior: Its Elementary Forms, Rev ed. New York, Harcourt, 1963

38. Johnson JP, McCauley CR, Copley JB: The quality of life of hemodialysis and transplant patients. Kidney Int 22:286, 1982

39. Kalman TP, Wilson PG, Kalman CM: Psychiatric morbidity in long-term renal transplant recipients and patients undergoing hemodialysis: A comparative study. JAMA 250:55, 1983

40. Kamstra-Hennen L, Beebe J, Stumm S et al: Ethical evaluation of related donation: The donor after five years. Transplant Proc 13:60, 1981

41. Kaste M, Palo J: Criteria of brain death and removal of cadaveric organs. Ann Clin Res 13:313, 1981

42. Kelley, JT: Legal aspects of hemodialysis and human organ transplantation. Dial Transplant 7:506, 1978

43. Klein SD, Simmons RG: Chronic disease and childhood development: Kidney disease and transplantation. In Simmons RG (ed): Research in Community and Mental Health, Vol 1, p 21. Greenwich, CT: JAI Press, 1979

44. Klein SD, Simmons RG, Anderson CR: Chronic kidney disease and transplantation in childhood and adolescence. In Blum R (ed): Chronic Illness and Disabilities in Childhood and Adolescence. New York, Grune & Stratton, 1984

45. Krakauer H, Grauman JS, McMullan MR et al: The recent U.S. experience in the treatment of end-stage renal disease by dialysis and transplantation. N Engl J Med 308:1558, 1983

46. Kramer P, Broyer M, Brunner FP et al: Combined report on regular dialysis and transplantation in Europe, XIV, 1983. Proc Eur Dial Transplant Assoc 21:2, 1985

47. Levey AS, Hou S, Bush HL Jr: Kidney transplantation from unrelated living donors: Time to reclaim a discarded opportunity. N Engl J Med 314(14):914, 1986

48. Malcolm AH: Human-organ transplants gain with new state laws. New York Times CXXXV(46,792):1, June 1, 1986

49. Manninen DL, Evans RW: Public attitudes and behavior regarding organ donation. JAMA 253(21):3111, 1985

50. Marsden C: Ethical issues in a heart transplant program. Heart Lung 14(5):495, 1985

51. Marine SK, Simmons RG: Policies regarding treatment of end stage renal disease in the United States and United Kingdom. Int Technol Assess Health Care 2(2):253, 1986

52. Marshall JR, Fellner CH: Kidney donors revisited. Am J Psychiatr 134:575, 1977

53. Matas AJ, Arras J, Muyskens J et al: A proposal for cadaver organ procurement: Routine removal with right of informed refusal. J Health Politics, Policy, Law 10(2):231, 1985

54. Matthews DE: Beyond survival. Dial Transplant 9:657, 1980

55. Meisel A, Roth LH: What we do and do not know about informed consent. JAMA 246(21):2473, 1981

56. Merrikin KJ, Overcast TD: Patient selection for heart transplantation: When is a discriminating choice discrimination? J Health, Policy, Law 10(1):7, 1985

57. Morris PJ: Presidential address: Transplantation Society, 1984. Transplant Proc 17:615, 1985

58. Najarian JS, Ascher NL: Liver transplantation. N Engl J Med 311(18):1179, 1984

59. Neu S, Kjellstrand CM: Stopping long-term dialysis: An empirical study of withdrawal of life-supporting treatment. N Engl J Med 314(1):14, 1986

60. Novello AC, Sundwall DN: Current organ transplantation legislation: An update. Transplant Proc 17:1585, 1985

61. Porter S: Organ transplants. Part two: Questions and controversy. Ohio State Med J 80(1):33, 1984

62. Progress in Clinical and Biological Research: Ethics, Humanism and Medicine, MD Basson (ed). 38:127–146, 1980

63. Relman A, Rennie D: Treatment of end-stage renal disease: Free but not equal. N Engl J Med 303:996, 1980

64. Report of the Massachusetts Task Force on Organ Transplantation: Law Med and Health Care 13(1):8, 1985

65. Rettig RA: The policy debate on patient care financing for victims of end-stage renal disease. Law Contemp Prob 40:196, 1976

66. Rettig RA, Marks E: The Federal government and social planning for end-stage renal disease: Past, present, and future. A Rand Note. Prepared for The Na-

tional Center for Health Services Research, Published by The Rand Corporation, February 1983

67. Ringden O, Friman L, Lundgren G et al: Living related kidney donors: Complications and long-term renal function. Transplantation 25(4):221, 1978

68. Sadler AM Jr, Sadler BL, Stason EB: Transplantation and the law: Progress toward uniformity. N Engl J Med 282(13):717, 1970

69. Schneider A, Flaherty MP: Abuses blamed on kidney shortage. The Pittsburgh Press 102(137):November 8, 1985

70. Schneider A, Flaherty MP: Neglect and greed infect transplant system. The Pittsburgh Press 102(132): November 3, 1985

71. Simmons RG: Long-term reactions of renal recipients and donors. In NB Levy (ed): Psychonephrology 2. New York, Plenum, 1983

72. Simmons RG, Anderson CR: Related donors and recipients five to nine years posttransplant. Transplant Proc XIV:9, 1982

73. Simmons RG, Anderson CR: Social-psychological problems in living donor transplantation. Transplant Clin Immunol 16:47, 1985

74. Simmons RG, Anderson C, Kamstra L: Comparison of quality of life of patients on continuous ambulatory peritoneal dialysis, hemodialysis, and after transplantation. Am J Kidney Dis 4:253, 1984

75. Simmons RG, Anderson CR, Kamstra LK et al: Quality of life and alternate end-stage renal disease therapies. Transplant Proc 17:1577, 1985

76. Simmons RG, Crosnier J: Ethical and social considerations in transplantation. Transplant Proc 13:1281, 1981

77. Simmons RG, Marine SK, Simmons RL: Gift of Life: The Effect of Organ Transplantation on Individual Family, and Societal Dynamics. New Brunswick, NJ, Transaction, 1987

78. Simmons RG, Marine SK: The regulations of high cost technology medicine: The case of dialysis and transplantation in the United Kingdom. J Health Soc Behav 25:320, 1984

79. Skelley L: Practical issues in obtaining organs for transplantation. Law, Med Health Care 13(1):35, 1985

80. Spital A, Spital M: Donor's choice or Hobson's choice? Arch Intern Med 145:1297, 1985

81. Spital A, Spital M, Spital R: The living donor: Alive and well. Arch Intern Med 146:1993, 1986

82. Starzl TE: In discussion on JE Murray, Organ transplantation: The practical possibilities. In Wolstenholme GEW, O'Connor M (eds): Ethics in Medical Progress: With Special Reference to Transplantation. Ciba Foundation Symposium. Boston, Little, Brown, 1966

83. Starzl TE: Will live organ donations no longer be justified? The Hastings Center Report 15:5, 1985

84. Steinbrook RL: Kidneys for transplantation. J Health Politics, Policy, Law 6(3):504, 1981

85. Strong M, Strong C: The shortage of organs for transplantation. ANNA J 12(4):239, 1985

86. Stuart FP: Need, supply, and legal issues related to organ transplantation in the United States. Transplant Proc XVI:87, 1984

87. Stuart FP, Veith FJ, Cranford RE: Brain death laws and patterns of consent to remove organs for transplantation from cadavers in the United States and 28 other countries. Transplantation 31:238, 1981

88. Surman OS: Toward greater donor organ availability for transplantation. N Engl J Med 312(5):318, 1985

89. Weiland D, Sutherland DER, Chavers B et al: Information on 628 living-related kidney donors at a single institution, with long-term follow-up in 472 cases. Transplant Proc XVI:5, 1984

90. Westlie L, Umen A, Nestrud S et al: Mortality, morbidity, and life satisfaction in the very old dialysis patient. Trans Am Soc Artif Intern Organs 30:21, 1984

91. White JK: Update. Health Affairs 4(4):109, 1985

92. Williams GM, Feree D, Bollinger RR et al: Renal transplant wastage: An international problem. Transplant Proc XVII:1594, 1985

93. Youngner SJ, Allen M, Bartlett ET et al: Psychosocial and ethical implications of organ retrieval. New Engl J Med 13:321, 1985

CHAPTER 49

Legal Aspects of Transplantation

Thomas D. Overcast

The material in this chapter addresses legal issues that affect transplant providers (including health care facilities), organ and tissue donors, and transplant recipients.

The two broad topics in the law that affect transplant practitioners are malpractice and antitrust law. Some issues are unique to transplantation, including the required scope of consent for organ donation and the liability of the physician for failure to refer potential candidates to transplant programs. Other areas of litigation include cases arising from the transplantation of defective organs or tissues, negligence in the conduct of transplant itself, and questions over the appropriate standard of follow-up care and rehabilitation.

Antitrust law will come into increasing prominence as the "business" of medicine and that of transplantation takes shape in response to newly imposed financial incentives in health care. In transplant practice, as techniques are more widely recognized as accepted practice, competitive forces in the marketplace will force providers (both physicians and facilities) to undertake activities that will increase their productivity and economic efficiency. Chief among these will be the formation of new forms of health care delivery, exclusive staffing arrangements within existing facilities, and the imposition of specialty certification standards for transplant practitioners. Because of their potential for illegal anticompetitive effects, these and other activities will be closely scrutinized by the courts, often at the insistence of competitors who feel themselves to be at a competitive disadvantage. However, the distinct trend of recent antitrust cases in health care suggests that a variety of activities aimed at increasing efficiency and productivity can be legitimately undertaken if they are carefully developed and implemented within the constraints of the antitrust law.

Legal issues that arise out of the Uniform Anatomical Gift Act and its state-enacted counterparts include problems with physician compliance with consent procedures both for donors and next of kin. These problems and the increasing demand for transplantable organs have led to the consideration of alternatives, including a market system for organs, and required request laws that force transplant and organ procurement personnel to request consent for donation.

It has been a mere 2 years since the publication of the final report of the National Heart Transplantation Study.[6] Yet the pace of events in transplantation research and practice is such that the study seems tarnished with age, even though it is widely recognized as the standard against which other efforts at medical technology assessment must be measured. Not only have the number of transplant procedures continued apace, but new areas of transplantation have begun to receive increased public attention (e.g., neonatal cardiac transplantation). In addition, new transplant centers are emerging where before there were only a few.[23] The last few years have also been witness to the emergence of artificial hearts, both as permanent cardiac replacement devices and as what have been called "bridges to transplant." In addition to these scientific and practice advances, there has been a continuing series of political and governmental activities that have affected the transplant community.[27] Major federal legislation has been passed, and a federal task force on transplantation only recently concluded its activities. Throughout this period, the media have regularly reminded the public both of the enormous benefits of transplantation technology and of its potentially serious down-side risks. Thus, in the view of many, the verdict is still not in regarding widespread public or professional acceptance of transplantation as a safe and efficacious procedure for general use.

Although the general area of transplantation is still in a state of considerable flux, the fundamental legal issues that must be confronted remain much the same, and many of the legal dilemmas remain to be resolved. In this chapter, we review the major legal questions that surround the transplant provider, the transplant recipient, and the organ donor. We describe what currently exists in the body of law relating to transplantation, and, where appropriate, conclusions about the current state of the law will be highlighted. Where such conclusions are not warranted, trends will be identified and their implications briefly discussed.

Finally, the advent and recent use of artificial organs (most notably, cardiac assist devices and totally implantable artificial hearts) raises a host of legal and ethical questions that are more properly the subject of an entire chapter or book. However, because of the important effect that such replacement devices have on issues in transplantation, the legal implications of their development and use are discussed at appropriate points in the text.

THE TRANSPLANT PROVIDER

A dramatic change has occurred in medical research and development over the last 50 years. At one time, major developments in medicine were primarily associated with advances in the control of infections and infectious diseases. However, medical technology has now come to dominate the public's perceptions of medical innovation and progress.[10] Because of its high visibility, and some would argue, its high cost, transplantation has become a focal point for policy debates about medical technology.[12]

Physician Liability and the Transplant Patient. If hospital risk managers and attorneys in institutions with transplant programs were asked, most would agree that potential and actual transplant recipients are not likely to bring malpractice suits against their transplant centers or the health care providers involved in their care.[24] Some of the reasons are related to social factors—transplant providers and recipients and their families develop a close relationship that contrasts markedly with the impersonal nature of other areas of highly technological medical practice. Other reasons are traceable to the more practical difficulties of proving a case of mal-

practice and obtaining a sizable recovery in court. In areas of medical practice that have not yet completely evolved a set of standard procedures and are occupied by a relatively small number of providers, it is extremely difficult to define a standard of good practice against which to measure the care provided and the techniques used by a transplant team.

Transplantation practice has already given rise to a number of liability claims. Standard malpractice cases have involved claims that (1) transplantation was contraindicated,[15] (2) the transplant failed owing to faulty surgical technique, (3) known side-effects were not recognized and treated, (4) anesthesia was not properly administered, or (5) the transplant center did not exercise due care in its choice of transplant professionals. Because it involves introducing another's tissue into the recipient, with the accompanying requirement of immunosuppression and tissue typing, transplantation also involves a more unusual set of liability issues. The potential for liability is illustrated by a case in which a patient died after receiving a second heart transplant that was necessary to replace the first, which had been mismatched for blood type. Although no lawsuit may arise out of this episode, it is the kind of circumstance that will ultimately engender malpractice against individual transplant physicians and against the health care facilities in which they practice.

Finally, a recent case[11] illustrates liability issues that cut across the areas of transplantation and artificial hearts. Haskell Karp was referred for treatment of severe cardiac disease, ultimately opting for a "wedge procedure." However, the consent form stated that if death appeared imminent, Karp's heart could be removed and a mechanical substitute used until a suitable donor heart could be found. Karp's heart did fail, and the first artificial heart to be used in a human was transplanted. The patient survived for 64 hours after the implantation. The wife later filed suit (which she eventually lost), alleging that neither she nor her husband had been told about the number of animals on which the artificial heart had been tested nor the results of those tests, or of the serious risk of injury involved in the use of the artificial heart, or that it was an experimental device and procedure. She also contended that the surgeon had failed to tell her husband that another surgeon had stated that Karp was not a good candidate for surgery. The Fifth Circuit Court of Appeals ruled that a claim of failure to obtain informed consent could not be established because of the lack of evidence of any causal connection between the lack of informed consent and the harm caused to the patient, since there was no evidence that the use of the mechanical heart had caused the patient's death and no evidence that the patient would not have consented to the procedure even if the risks had been disclosed.

Failure to Refer.   In addition to the problems of informed consent such as those described in *Karp v. Cooley,* transplantation and other forms of high level medical technology involve a unique question of potential liability for the medical practitioner: Can a physician be held liable for failure to advise a potential transplant recipient of the existence of the procedure as a viable treatment alternative and for failure to refer such a patient for evaluation? The answer to this question is "perhaps."

As a general rule of law, physicians have an affirmative duty to inform their patients of alternative forms of treatment, and the failure to disclose a standard treatment alternative is generally held to be negligence.[21] The physician has a duty to inform the patient of alternatives, even though the referring physician is not competent to render any or all of the other forms of treatment. In typical cases of failure to inform, malpractice liability is based on the failure of the physician to keep up-to-date with advances in the medical profession. For example, one reason that physicians may fail to refer patients for transplantation is that the physicians are simply not aware of the latest advances in transplant practice.

Keep in mind, however, that the situation with respect to transplantation differs considerably from the normal circumstances of medical practice. Despite steady increases in survival and success rates for nearly all forms of organ and tissue transplantation, the procedures are still considered by many to be outside the realm of normal medical practice. In addition, in contrast to many other forms of medical treatment, the scarcity of resources surrounding transplantation may play an important role in determining a physician's potential liability for failure to inform a patient of the transplant alternative. Finally, the often limited availability of donor organs and tissues means that there is no guarantee that the person who is otherwise medically suitable for a transplant will be able to undergo the procedure.

These elements, particularly the latter two, may significantly influence the decision of a court or a jury on the question of whether a physician, in fact, had a duty to inform a patient of the transplant alternative. Failure to prove that the transplant could have been obtained, even if the physician had informed the patient of it, may also be a factor in determining whether the physician's failure to inform actually "caused" any injury to the patient.

Because of the physician's perception (and, in fact, the reality) that the likelihood of acceptance of any patient into the pool of potential recipients for many types of transplantation is relatively small, and the probability that the patient will actually receive a transplant is even smaller, even the physician who believes in the value of the procedure may be reluctant to advise a patient of the possibility of transplantation.

These and other legal issues that confront the provider of transplant services also appear in the context of the development and diffusion of artificial organ technology. This can be seen by the potential problems that evolved from after-the-fact questions about the legitimacy of the informed consent process used with the first recipient of the Jarvik-7 artificial heart. Critics and analysts went through the consent forms line-by-line identifying deficiencies that they argued vitiated any consent that might have originally been given. Chief among the criticisms was that the degree of detailed information was such that no one, particularly a sick patient, could have been expected to fully understand the consent form to the degree necessary to give legally sufficient "informed consent" to the implantation of the artificial heart.

An adjunct of this criticism was the question of whether anyone in the same position, where life itself was hanging in the balance, could be expected to give truly informed consent. This argument is based on the assumption that patients in immediate jeopardy of loss of life really have no choice at all and are, in fact, coerced into taking the treatment that is available. This was the essence of the argument that was used to prohibit the use of prison inmates in medical research—their situation was inherently coercive; thus, they could not give voluntary, informed consent. Parenthetically, the debate over the issue of consent has recently been fueled by speculations on the part of family members of some artificial heart recipients that, had they known in advance of the recipients' present outcomes, consent would not have been as readily given or as easily obtained from the recipients.

In any event, the consent protocols of the Utah group (and subsequently, the other locations where artificial heart implants have been performed) have been substantially revised. As experience with this procedure accumulates, the consent process and the substance of the consent obtained will change in response to medical advances and patient experiences.

In addition to questions about informed consent, artificial heart technology raises unique questions with respect to the liability of product developers and the physicians who use those products. Because there has been so little litigation experience directly related to artificial heart technology, little can be said other than speculation. However, when the cases do arise, they will clearly break new ground in defining the roles and responsibilities of physicians and health care facilities and will more clearly define the rights and expectations that patients have in medical technologies such as transplantation.

Transplant Providers and Antitrust Laws.   While the application of state and federal antitrust laws in the health care area is a relatively new phenomenon, these laws have been used to limit the ability of health care providers and insurers to control and coordinate the delivery and financing of transplantation. The antitrust laws are based on the belief that competition in all economic spheres will result in the most efficient allocation of resources, will best determine the cost of goods and services, and will most effectively promote technologic and economic progress in our society. Any business practice that interferes with a potential or current market participant's ability to compete on the merits (price, quality, and service) of a product or service is subject to antitrust challenge. The increased emphasis on competition in health care has caused providers and insurers to carefully assess their activities with an eye to potential antitrust liability.[25] Among the practices that have been the subject of considerable antitrust activity are exclusive staffing arrangements, explicit market division,[4,18] and specialty certification.[9] As an emerging, highly visible area of medical practice, transplantation will incur its share of antitrust litigation.

The application of antitrust laws to health care activities is a very complicated area of law that is still the subject of considerable debate and litigation. The increased focus on competition and market forces in health care has spawned new forms of health care delivery (i.e., HMOs, PPOs, IPAs, and a veritable alphabet soup of new delivery systems). In addition, the recent introduction of prospective payment by the federal government (and its likely adoption by private health insurers and the states) has triggered what can only be called a revolution in the delivery of health care services by individual physicians and health care facilities, and in their financing by federal and state governments, private insurers, and health care consumers. These factors have resulted in a premium being placed on cost-consciousness and innovation in the delivery.[8] As with any other newly created "industry," it is in-

evitable that business practices and activities in transplantation will collide with the antitrust laws. And physicians and health care facilities will have to carefully examine new business arrangements for their antitrust implications.

LEGAL IMPLICATIONS OF ORGAN PROCUREMENT

The organ procurement process presents a number of important and only partially resolved legal questions regarding the responsibilities and potential liability of transplant and organ procurement physicians and facilities.

"Good Faith" Immunity.   How far does the Uniform Anatomical Gift Act's (UAGA) grant of "good faith" immunity for physicians extend? There is only one reported case in which a court has considered the tort liability of a physician or hospital in connection with the organ or tissue transplant procedures performed upon a donor who had been declared dead prior to removal of his or her organs or tissues. The court held that Section 79(c) of the UAGA immunized the physicians, insofar as they had acted in good faith, from liability for conduct occurring *after* the donor's death but did not apply to treatment received by the donor prior to death. In *Williams v. Hoffman* (1974), a treating physician informed the husband of a patient that the patient had died and obtained the husband's consent to remove her kidneys for transplantation. More than 2 days later, after a mortician reported that he could not locate the body, the husband learned that his wife's body had been kept functioning through life support techniques and that she had not been officially pronounced dead. He attempted to contact the physician to stop removal of the kidneys only to discover that, even as he acted, his wife had been declared dead and her kidneys removed. The suit that he filed alleged assault and battery, negligence, willful and intentional mutilation of a corpse, negligent mutilation of a corpse, and negligence in communicating an erroneous and premature announcement of his wife's death.

Thus far, no cases have been reported alleging that transplant physicians have acted in bad faith and thus are not immune under Section 7(c) of the UAGA. Generally, however, the "good faith" standard of care connotes a state of mind on the part of the physician involving honesty of purpose, freedom from intent to defraud, and faithfulness to his or her duty. In a transplant setting, this translates into good intentions and honest exercise of the physician's best judgment about the needs of the patient. Bad faith, by way of contrast, is evidenced by actual or constructive fraud, intent to mislead or deceive another, or neglect or refusal to fulfill some duty or contractual obligation (*Williams v. Hoffman,* 1974).

The question of whether a transplant provider has acted in "good faith" will always be one of fact, which must be determined on a case-by-case basis. However, the persons involved in obtaining consent for donation and the physician who removes organs and tissues should carefully observe the procedures for valid donation that are spelled out in the UAGA. Adherence to its letter and spirit is the best preventive approach.

Living Donors. Litigation involving organ donation from living donors has generated a great deal of legal and ethical debate. The courts have had to wrestle with the difficult question of when, and under what conditions, relatives may legally consent to organ removal from mentally incompetent persons or children, an especially difficult question when the transplant procedure may save the life of another family member. The direction of the courts may be discerned from the following brief descriptions of cases that have been decided in this area:

Strunk v. Strunk[31]: Under a court order, a mentally incompetent adult was allowed to donate a kidney to his brother, in part because of the strong familial relationship that had been established between the brothers and the perceived psychological harm that might be suffered by the incompetent brother if the recipient were to die.

Little v. Little[14]: The court authorized removal of a kidney from a 14-year-old with Down's syndrome for transplantation into a brother.

Lausier v. Pescinski[13]: The court would not allow removal of a kidney from a mentally incompetent adult where he would gain no psychological benefit from the donation.

At least one court (*Hart v. Brown*[7]) has ruled that children without a mental disability have the capacity to consent to organ donation. In addition, courts have addressed the issue of whether a donor may recover damages for organ removal, claiming that the donation was necessitated by the negligent treatment of the donee. For example, the plaintiff in *Sirianni v. Anna*[28] was a mother who volunteered to permit one of her kidneys to be transplanted into the body of her adult son after the defendant surgeons had negligently removed the son's kidneys. The court ruled that the mother could not recover from the surgeons for the resulting impairment to her health resulting from the loss of one kidney.

Similarly, in *Moore v. Shah,*[19] the court ruled that the kidney donor (a son) had no cause of action for the negligent diagnosis and treatment of the donee/father. Because there have been so few cases, the trend of the law is not yet established, and decisions turn heavily on the facts of individual cases and the predilections of the judges. However, the courts are clearly very protective of the rights of organ donors regardless of their competency.

Determination of Death. One of the most difficult medicolegal problems in transplant practice has been determining the moment of the donor's death. The UAGA leaves the determination of the time of death to the attending or certifying physician and makes no attempt to define the uncertain point in time when life ceases. The issue is critical for unpaired organs and other vital tissues—to delay the declaration of death runs the risk of damaging the tissue, which can be fatal to the recipient. On the other hand, if the donor is not legally dead at the time that the organs or tissues are taken, the physician may be open to charges of wrongful death or even homicide.

The potential for legal action in this area has been exacerbated by the fact that "legal" and "clinical" definitions of death are not always the same. For example, in *Tucker v. Lower,*[32] the brother of an organ donor brought suit against a transplant surgeon, alleging in part that the donor's heart and kidneys had been removed before the donor was legally dead. As evidence that the donor was not dead, he pointed to the fact that his brother's heart was still beating at the time that death was declared. At the time of the case, Virginia had not yet adopted a standard of death based on discontinuance of brain function. The judge refused to grant the physician summary dismissal and sent the case to the jury, which found for the surgeon. The Virginia Medical Society later supported a statute (eventually adopted in Virginia) that recognized cessation of brain function as one ground for declaration of death.

The legal and medical uncertainties produced by the gap between the varied legal definitions of death and advances in medicine have resulted in some legal movement toward adoption of "brain death" as the legal standard of death. Legislators in more than half the states have enacted laws that permit reliance on brain-related criteria for determining death. In addition, the courts in several states have judicially recognized brain-death standards in the absence of statutory recognition (*State v. Fierro,*[29]; *Commonwealth v. Goldston,*[3]; *New York*

City Health & Hospital Corporation v. Sulsona,[20]). However, the standards adopted in the various states are not uniform. At least six varying standards exist, many of which have been criticized as unworkable or outmoded.

In recognition of this problem, the President's Commission for the Study of Ethical Problems in Medicine and Biomedical and Behavioral Research[26] devoted a substantial amount of its time to the issues. The Commission ultimately concluded that the necessary changes in the state and federal laws and the long-term goal of uniformity would best be served by the following definition of death.

An individual who has sustained either (1) irreversible cessation of circulatory and respiratory functions, or (2) has irreversible cessation of all functions of the entire brain, including the brain stem, is dead. A determination of death must be made in accordance with accepted medical standards.

The proposed statute recognizes that the traditional means to determine death will continue to be applied in the overwhelming majority of cases. But in those cases where artificial means of support require direct evaluation of the functions of the brain, the statute would recognize the use of accepted medical procedures.

Medical Examiners and Coroners. A large number of organ and tissue donors are victims of traumatic injuries, usually to the head. These injuries often occur under violent or suspicious circumstances in which a police investigation or autopsy may be considered. Under normal circumstances, the time delay inherent in these processes rules out the use of the victim's organs and tissues for transplantation because of rapid tissue deterioration. However, organ removal prior to investigation by the medical examiner or coroner's office may lead to questions about whether evidence relating to the causes of circumstances of death has been destroyed. This need not be the case, for example, the Dade County, Florida Medical Examiner has established a formal program of cooperation with transplant programs, and in Texas, cooperation is mandated by state law (Texas Code Art. 49.29(6) 1977).

In general, cooperation with the medical examiner or coroner in cases of potential organ donation (and the local prosecutor in suspected criminal cases) will avoid legal difficulties. Although permission of the prosecutor for organ removal is not legally required in most states, it avoids potential charges of interference with criminal law enforcement through destruction of evidence. Prosecuting attorneys will generally grant permission for organ or tissue removal when they are assured that donation will not compromise any necessary testimony regarding the cause of the donor's death.

The Source and Supply of Donor Organs. Reference to any major daily newspaper over the last several years would reveal a continuing series of stories relating the struggle of a family to find a donor organ for a relative or loved one. Many of these stories had happy endings, but, tragically, many did not, and the depth of the tragedy is compounded by considering the number of families whose stories never made the headlines. Advances in transplant technology and the diffusion of the procedure throughout the medical community are driving the demand for transplantable organs and tissues beyond the capacity of the current system to supply them. Continued reliance on the ad hoc pleas of individual families and the individual donations of organs and tissues, coupled with an uncoordinated organ procurement system in many communities and medical facilities, results in a system that simply does not meet the current needs of the transplant community. Just as surely, reliance on this system will not meet the ever-increasing needs that are just over the medical horizon.

In theory, and by virtue of its drafters' explicit intentions, the UAGA (and its state-enacted counterparts) should provide an adequate vehicle for organ procurement. In practice, however, reliance on donations has remained an unsatisfactory solution to a very pressing problem. There is considerable evidence that important provisions of the UAGA are largely ignored by organ procurement personnel.[22] For example, although the UAGA specifically recognizes donor documentation (i.e., a signed donor card) as sufficient legal evidence of an individual's intent to donate his or her organs (and, as previously noted, extends blanket immunity to physicians and other medical personnel acting in "good faith" in procuring an organ), the majority of medical institutions do not permit organ removal without the express consent of the potential donor's next of kin. This requirement often means that the donation is never made, either because the next of kin are never approached for their consent or, when approached, they refuse.

Evidence also suggests that the medical community believes that the provisions of the UAGA do not provide them with sufficient protection from legal action initiated by aggrieved next of kin. The important question, however, is whether stronger legal protections are needed to reduce physicians fears of liability and, if so, what protections would have to be given in order to bring their practices into line with the theory of the UAGA. A strong argument can be made that additional legal protections are not needed in order to encourage organ donation under the Act. Instead, it is clear that fundamental changes in people's attitudes are necessary to trigger long-term and stable increases in the number of transplantable organs and tissues made available through donation.

Recent Developments in Organ Procurement. In response to the continued shortage of organs and tissues, a number of different proposals have been offered as alternatives to continued reliance on the present system of donation. Proposals have been made to establish a market system in transplantable organs, with serious business proposals being offered by a physician in Maryland and, most recently, a Texas entrepreneur. Such proposals have been roundly condemned by legal commentators and ethicists, and perhaps made illegal by a provision in the recently enacted federal Organ Transplantation Act.

Taking another approach to the problem, a number of states have passed what are called "required request" laws, which require medical personnel to request consent for organ donation from patients (and sometimes, next of kin) admitted to health care facilities (the specific provisions of these laws vary somewhat from state to state). These laws were enacted to address the problem of the failure of physicians and organ procurement personnel to even ask patients and next of kin for an organ donation, resulting in what was seen as a shameful loss of a valuable and lifesaving resource. Although consent for a donation is certainly not guaranteed by these laws, at least it will be sought. It is too early to determine whether required request will have an appreciable effect on the number of organs and tissues donated, although these is every reason to believe that the number of such donations will increase.

In summary, any proposal to go beyond donation in organ and tissue procurement, such as a market system or compulsory removal, will inevitably raise complex legal questions that will have to be resolved either legislatively or through the courts. However, the important issues in organ and tissue donation and procurement do not involve fundamentally difficult legal issues. Rather, proponents of alternatives to donation will have to deal with the very important ethical and moral issues that surround such alternatives. Defending the legal validity of any alternative is a relatively minor technical problem, requiring careful legal research and skilled legislative drafting. The more significant undertaking will be to reconcile strongly held attitudes and beliefs and sociocultural sentiment with the implementation of alternatives to donation.

DISCRIMINATION IN PATIENT SELECTION FOR TRANSPLANTATION

Although many of the medical aspects of transplantation differ between transplant centers and physicians, the process of patient selection remains relatively constant and is usually based on a generally accepted set of medical and often psychosocial selection criteria.[2] From a legal perspective, the psychosocial criteria are more important than medical criteria in assessing the degree to which patient selection may present legal problems for the transplant practitioner. The assumption underlying the utilization of these psychosocial criteria is that they reflect on the transplant patient's overall viability, that is, the patient must have a strong "will to live," the familial and social support structure necessary to help him or her endure the stress and tension resulting from the transplant procedure (which was the basis of the recent controversy over the neonatal heart transplant case at Loma Linda Hospital in California), and the need for a considerable change in lifestyle following treatment and rehabilitation. The question here is whether patient selection processes that incorporate psychosocial selection criteria unlawfully discriminate against protected groups and whether transplant practitioners might be liable for using such selection criteria. Because this is a very complicated area of the law, the following material only briefly outlines the potential nature of the problem and summarizes the general conclusions that can be drawn on the basis of the available cases and laws regarding discrimination against the handicapped, against ethnic or racial groups, or against potential transplant recipients based on their age.

Handicap. Patient selection can discriminate against the handicapped in a number of ways, both subtle and obvious. For example, a handicapping condition may: (1) be erroneously judged to be a medical contraindication to transplantation, (2) be seen as a contributing factor to the development of post-transplant complications, resulting in a bias against selection for a new or emerging medical technology such as transplantation, (3) be inaccurately perceived as a limit on the ability of the handicapped patient to follow prescribed medical and rehabilitation procedures after the transplant, and (4) be reflected in selection criteria based on unfounded assumptions or stereotypes about the psychosocial capabilities of the handicapped.[17]

Because of the uncertainties in this area of law, it is particularly troublesome for transplant providers. The best that can be said is that although patient selection decisions must be made, regardless of whether they are based on medical suitability, a lottery, or some other means, such choices must meet the requirements of the laws prohibiting discrimination against the handicapped (Section 504 of the Rehabilitation Act) or run the risk of being challenged.[5]

Race, Color, or National Origin. It is difficult to define the parameters of the problem of racial or ethnic discrimination in patient selection for transplantation, although the results of the National Heart Transplantation Study showed that heart transplant recipients were overwhelmingly young, Caucasian and middle class. In general, there is abundant evidence demonstrating that racial minorities do not have equal access to health care facilities or services. In light of the particular need for selectivity in many forms of transplantation, the problem of unequal access will be exacerbated as the different forms of transplantation become more frequently used. However, the important question is whether the disparity in access results from unlawful discrimination or from some other secondary cause.

As is the case with other areas of discrimination, there is little specific guidance that can be given regarding the vulnerability of patient selection practices to charges of discrimination based on race or ethnicity. However, the trend of recent cases suggests that charges of discrimination will only be upheld by the courts when there is clear evidence of *intent* to discriminate against a particular group. In the absence of a patent and overt record of discrimination, it is difficult to prove that a transplant program or provider intended to discriminate through the imposition of racially neutral selection criteria, even though the effect of the selection process is to differentially enroll racial or ethnic minorities.

Age. Although not an explicit psychosocial criteria for all forms of transplantation, age is explicitly recognized as a "strongly adverse" selection factor for heart transplantation when the patient is older than 50 years of age (46 Federal Register 7073, January 22, 1981). Age is widely recognized as an important determinant of treatment outcome in a wide variety of other medical settings. The assumption underlying the age criterion is that increasing age reduces the individual's capacity to withstand the complications and rigors of the transplant procedure and the post-transplant recovery and rehabilitation regimen. The use of a strict age criterion falls within the legal purview of the Age Discrimination Act of 1975.

In spite of the lack of cases interpreting the Age Discrimination Act, a number of conclusions can be made about its potential application to the use of age as a patient selection criterion for transplantation. First, age discrimination is not viewed with the same degree of alarm as are other forms of discrimination. Thus, the use of age distinctions in patient selection will be the subject of far fewer legally imposed restrictions. If there is an empirically strong relationship between advancing age and treatment outcome, such that age can be clearly demonstrated to be a strongly adverse factor in transplant patient survival or outcome, the provisions of the Age Discrimination Act will not apply.

Many of the legal issues and quandries that surround patient selection for transplantation come up again in regard to the implantation of artificial hearts and the use of other mechanical devices.[1,34] As with other areas on the cutting edge of medical developments, recent events surrounding the development and use of artificial hearts have unfolded at an unprecedented rate.[30] One of the dominant themes from the very beginning—the selection of the first patient by the Utah group—has been the issue of patient selection and the degree to which selection guidelines have met both the needs of the patients and those of the researchers and implant teams. In fact, there were early reports in the media of a lawsuit filed by a person who had been turned down by the Utah group for implantation of the Jarvik-7. His contention was that he satisfactorily met the requirements that had been established for the first artificial heart recipient. Although there was some reported controversy over his contention, in fact, although he may have been an acceptable candidate under the established criteria, apparently he was not the *best* candidate. As far as can be discovered, the lawsuit did not progress far beyond its first appearance in the press.

These early controversies over patient selection for the artificial heart mirror in many respects those that were first reported regarding selection for kidney dialysis and other scarce medical resources. The questions centered on the suitability of recipients, both medically and socially; whether appropriate rationing decisions were being made; whether candidates were chosen too soon or too late (the implication being that if chosen too soon, they were being experimented upon and, if chosen too late, were too sick to adequately demonstrate the remedial effects of the treatment); and, finally, whether patients were adequately informed of the risks of the procedure and whether, in the face of an otherwise terminal condition, the concept of a voluntary, informed consent made any sense to begin with.

The legal issues regarding discrimination in patient selection that have been covered here have not yet come into play with regard to artificial hearts for many of the same reasons that they have not arisen in other areas of transplantation—because many of the procedures have not yet entered the mainstream of medical practice and, to a certain extent, remain experimental, where greater latitude is allowed in order to accomplish the goals of a research program. However, only two conditions must be satisfied to ensure that issues regarding discrimination will play an important role in shaping how both transplantation and artificial heart technologies are widely used. These conditions are: (1) the continued development and diffusion of more successful transplant and artificial heart procedures, to the point that they become generally accepted as appropriate therapeutic tools, and (2) the continued scarcity of resources necessary to support the widespread use of such procedures, forcing transplant physicians and institutions to use ever more restrictive selection criteria—perhaps going so far as to base access to the procedures on the ability of individual patients to pay the cost of the treatment.[16] These conditions guarantee that patient selection criteria for organ and tissue transplantation will be challenged on the basis that they discriminate against particular groups.

RECENT DEVELOPMENTS IN TRANSPLANT LAW

In addition to the material discussed above, there have been recent developments in the laws affecting transplantation that deserve special mention. These developments include the passage of some important federal legislation and the publication of the results of several major federally initiated studies addressing issues in transplantation.[4a]

Federal Laws

The National Organ Transplant Act (P.L. 98-507, October 19, 1984) is surely the most important piece of federal legislation affecting transplantation. Although its enactment is not now so recent, the content of its major provisions warrant emphasis. Title I established the Task Force on Organ Procurement and Transplantation and delineated the Task Force's responsibilities, which were to (1) conduct comprehensive examinations of the medical, legal, ethical, economic, and social issues presented by human organ procurement and transplantation, (2) assess immunosuppressive medications used to prevent organ rejection in transplant patients, and (3) prepare a report on a long list of issues relating to organ procurement and transplantation. The outcome of the Task Force's activities is described in greater detail below. Title II related to organ transplants and contained provisions relating to (1) assistance for organ procurement organizations, (2) the establishment of an organ procurement and transplantation network, and (3) the development and maintenance of a scientific registry of organ transplant recipients. Title II was the source of considerable controversy because of the failure of the Reagan administration to authorize funds for the specific activities enumerated there. Only recently have such funds been forthcoming. Title III specifically prohibits any person from knowingly acquiring, receiving or otherwise transferring any human organ for valuable consideration for use in human transplantation if the transfer affects interstate commerce. Finally, Title IV authorized a conference to study the feasibility of establishing a national registry of voluntary bone marrow donors.

The Consolidated Omnibus Budget Reconciliation Act of 1985 (COBRA) (P.L. 99-272, April 7, 1986) contained two important provisions relating to transplantation. Section 9217 documented a "sense of the Senate" resolution regarding liver transplants. After listing a set of findings, the Senate recommended that (1) a liver transplant not be considered an experimental procedure for Medicare beneficiaries solely because a potential recipient is over 18 years of age, (2) liver transplants be covered under Medicare when reasonable and medically necessary, and (3) limiting criteria be placed on coverage, including those relating to the patient's condition, the disease state, and the institution providing the care, so as to ensure the highest quality of medical care demonstrated to be consistent with successful treatment outcomes. Note that this language represents only the sense of the Senate, and the directives it contains are not binding.

Section 9507 of the COBRA related to the denial of federal payments for organ transplants unless such transplants are conducted under written standards. The section provides that Medicare payments will not be made "for organ transplant procedures unless a State plan provides for written standards respecting the coverage of such procedures and unless such standards provide that

(A) similarly situated individuals are treated alike; and
(B) any restriction, on the facilities or practitioners which

may provide such procedures, is consistent with accessibility of high quality care to individuals for the procedures under the state plan.

This provision was intended to ensure that state plans adequately address the issue of equity of access to organ transplant procedures, an issue that was noted above as a source of continuing controversy.

Even though its provisions do not take effect until October 1, 1987, the Omnibus Budget Reconciliation Act of 1986 (OBRA) (P.L. 99-509, October 21, 1986) provided perhaps the strongest impetus to effective hospital participation in organ procurement and the establishment of coherent standards for cooperation among organ procurement agencies. Section 1138.(a)(1) established a new hospital condition of participation for the Medicare program. To participate in the Medicare system, a hospital must establish written protocols for the identification of potential organ donors. And such protocols must (1) ensure that families of potential organ donors are made aware of the option of organ or tissue donation and their option to decline, (2) encourage discretion and sensitivity with respect to the circumstances, views, and beliefs of families of potential organ donors, and (3) require that an acceptable organ procurement agency be notified of potential organ donors. In addition, if a hospital performs organ transplants, the hospital must be a member of and abide by the rules and regulations of the Organ Procurement and Transplantation Network established pursuant to Section 372 of the Public Health Service Act. These requirements are generally consistent with the "required request" laws that have been enacted in many states,[4a] but adds teeth to the provisions by making them conditions of participation in Medicare programs.

Section 1138.(b)(1) similarly attaches a number of important conditions to reimbursement of procurement costs to organ procurement agencies. In addition, the Section specifies that only one organ procurement organization will be designated for each service area described in Section 371(b)(1)(E) of the Public Health Service Act.

Finally, OBRA amended the Medicare law to provide reimbursement for immunosuppressive drugs for Medicare-qualified transplant recipients. Specifically, Medicare will pay for "immunosuppressive drugs furnished, to an individual who receives an organ transplant for which payment is made under this title (Medicare), within 1 year after the date of the transplant procedure." This provisions quite effectively gives with one hand (payment for immunosuppressive drugs), while taking away

with the other (only for a 1-year period following the transplant).

On October 17, 1986, HCFA published its proposed notice, *Medicare Program; Criteria for Medicare Coverage of Heart Transplants* in the *Federal Register.* The final rules did not differ substantively from those first proposed. The regulations cover (1) criteria for facilities (including patient selection, patient management, commitment, facility plans, experience and surivial rates, maintenance of data, organ procurement, and laboratory services), (2) the process for review and approval of facilities, (3) the application procedure, and (4) detailed guidelines for patient selection criteria. Under these rules the application of the University of Washington heart transplant program was recently rejected on the basis of an insufficient number of procedures.

Reports

Three major reports addressing some of the most timely and pressing issues in transplantation have been recently completed and released. Although this chapter cannot do justice to the full scope of those reports, their contents bear directly on legal aspects of transplantation and their findings are briefly summarized here.

Under the authority of the National Organ Transplant Act, the Task Force on Organ Transplantation issued its *Report to the Secretary and the Congress on Immunosuppressive Therapies* in October of 1985. Two major considerations drove the deliberations of the Task Force with regard to immunosuppressive therapies. The first was the promise held out by the increasing use of cyclosporine. The second was the general issue of patient access to immunosuppressives, including the effect of patient ability to pay for such drugs on access to transplantation. These led to three major findings by the Task Force:

1. *Efficacy of cyclosporine:* Cyclosporine was viewed as representing a major breakthrough in organ transplantation, resulting in increased patient and graft survival rates, decreased hospital stays, and fewer episodes of infection and rejection.

2. *Cost–benefit:* As a result of the reduced rate of complications and shorter length of hospital stay, cyclosporine has a favorable impact on the cost of cadaveric renal transplants, even though it is more expensive than conventional immunosuppressive therapies in the 6-month post-transplant period. The Task Force concluded that, over the long run, the use of cyclosporine was at least cost neutral with the added benefit of fewer patient complications.

3. *Patient problems:* The Task Force concluded that there were two major categories of patient problems: (1) approximately 25% of the transplant population does not have private insurance coverage or coverage by a state Medicaid or other state program. This inability to pay for necessary immunosuppressive drugs, particularly cyclosporine, results in non-medically indicated changes in drug regimens that have adverse impacts on the long-term success of the transplant; and (2) there was evidence that inability to pay for immunosuppressive drugs was a factor in the initial selection of patients for transplantation.

Based on these findings, the Task Force recommended that any federal funding for immunosuppressive drugs be limited to assisting only financially needy Medicare-eligible transplant patients.

Organ Transplantation: Issues and Recommendations, the second major Report of the Task Force on Organ Transplantation, was issued in April 1986. It clearly contained the most sweeping analysis of technical and policy issues in organ procurement and transplantation yet to be done. Based on these analyses, the Report included a lengthy set of specific recommendations for changes in the system of organ procurement and transplantation. Although the recommendations are too detailed to reproduce here, they generally fall under the following categories:

1. *Organ and tissue donation and procurement:* The gap between the need for organs and tissues and the supply of donors is a serious problem common to all programs in organ transplantation and tissue banking and transplantation.
2. *Organ sharing:* A unified national system of organ sharing encompassing a patient registry and coordination of organ allocation and distribution will go far in ensuring equity and fairness in the allocation of organs.
3. *Equitable access to organ transplantation:* Although existing patient selection mechanisms are generally fair, they (a) must be systematized at each center and throughout the nation and (b) must be based solely on objective medical criteria that are applied fairly and open to public examination.
4. *Diffusion of organ transplantation technology:* Recognizing that the issue of designating transplant centers for reimbursement purposes is a difficult one, the Task Force adopted the commonly held principle that the volume of surgical procedures performed is positively associated with outcomes and inversely associated with cost.

Although not without considerable controversy and the publication of a minority opinion, the Task Force recommended that a minimum volume criterion be enforced, together with other criteria defining the minimal requirements for both institutional and professional support and outcome of transplantation procedures.

5. *Research in organ transplantation:* Research on all aspects of transplantation, including the social, ethical, economic, and legal considerations, should be encouraged, and funding for it increased. The free flow of transplant-related research should be facilitated and coordinated by an interinstitutional council on transplantation.
6. *Advisory board on organ transplantation:* A National organ transplantation advisory board should be authorized and funded to review, evaluate and advise with regard to the implementation of the recommendations of the Task Force on Organ Transplantation, to serve in an advisory capacity to the Office of Organ Transplantation and to other transplant-related activities of the Department of Health and Human Services.

The recommendations of the Task Force are consistent with a number of activities that were already in progress in Congress, the states, and individual transplant programs. However, the Task Force recommendations served as a focal point for national consideration of these issues and as an impetus for continuing developments in federal and state governments and the private sector.

The Access of Foreign Nations to U.S. Cadaver Organs, issued by the Region I office of the Department of Health and Human Services in August, 1986, addressed the problem of nonresident aliens coming to the U.S. to receive transplants and the practice of exporting cadaver kidneys from the U.S. to other countries. It is estimated that 300 foreign nationals received cadaveric kidney transplants in the U.S. in 1985 (5.2% of total cadaver-donor transplants) and that 200 to 250 kidneys were exported from the U.S. Based on these findings, the report recommended that

1. The Health Care Financing Administration (HCFA) undertake efforts to help ensure that cadaver kidneys not be offered to foreign nationals unless it has been determined that no suitable U.S. recipient can be found.
2. HCFA undertake efforts to help ensure that kidneys are not exported to other countries unless it has been determined that no suitable U.S. recipient can be found.

3. When kidneys are sent to other countries, HCFA should prohibit Medicare reimbursement for any of the acquisition costs of those organs.

Implementing these recommendations would allow an estimated 500 additional Medicare beneficiaries to receive cadaveric transplants at a substantial cost saving to the Medicare system.

SOME CONCLUDING THOUGHTS

There are several points that should be emphasized about the preceding discussions. First, this chapter has not covered all the potential legal issues that may confront the transplant practitioner or the transplant facility.

Second, the legal issues discussed here have been presented in their barest skeletal form. As painful as it may be, transplant physicians must deal every day in an arena that is bounded on all sides by the operation of the law. The reader is cautioned that the material in this chapter is not intended to provide the type of legal advice necessary to safely structure transplant practice.

Third, when the issues that have been discussed here are finally resolved, as they surely will be, the impact on the broader health care system will be minimal. The outcome of the necessary adjustments will, on the whole, result in a better health care system—access will be more equal, resources will be better allocated, and information will be more widely available.

Finally, on a more somber note, there is a disturbing series of developments of which all involved in the health care system are painfully aware. I refer to the continuing introduction of market principles and competition into the health care system and the emergence of a giant health care industry dominated by large vertically and horizontally integrated health care corporations.

One cannot pretend to know the nature of the legal issues that will arise out of these disputes, but, when this chapter is rewritten for the third or fourth edition of this book, it will undoubtedly have to be authored by a corporate or tax attorney, because the business and financial complexities of transplant practice will be far beyond the ken of a simple health care lawyer.

REFERENCES

1. Caplan AL: The artificial heart. The Hastings Center Report 12:22–24, 1982
2. Christopherson LK: Heart transplants. The Hastings Center Report 12:18, 1982
3. *Commonwealth v. Goldston,* 373 Mass. 249,366 N.E.2d 744, *cert. denied,* 434 U.S. 1039 (1978)
4. Copeland JG, Stinson EB: Human heart transplantation. Curr Probl Cardiol 4:1–51, 1979
4a. Cover BM, Overcast TD (eds): *Organ Procurement and Transplantation Manual: Laws, Regulations and guidelines.* Owings Mills, MD, Rynd Communications, 1987
5. Crane K: Section 504 of the Rehabilitation Act of 1973: Is it authority for federal intervention in the area of medical decision-making? Capital University Law Review 13:645–683, 1984
6. Evans RW, Manninen DL, Overcast TD et al: The National Heart Transplantation Study: Final Report. Seattle, WA, Battelle Human Affairs Research Centers, 1984
7. *Hart v. Brown,* 289 A.2d 386 (Conn. 1972)
8. Havighurst CC: Competition in health services. Vanderbilt Law Review 34:1117–1195, 1981
9. Herbsleb J, Sales BD, Overcast TD: Challenging licensure and certification. Am Psychol 40:1165–1178, 1985
10. Iglehart J: The cost and regulation of medical technology: Future policy directions. Milbank Memorial Fund Quarterly 25–79, 1977
11. *Karp v. Cooley,* 349 F. Supp. 827 (S.D. Tex. 1972), *aff'd,* 493 F.2d 408 (5th Cir. 1974)
12. Knox RA: Heart transplants: To pay or not to pay. Science 209:570–572, 574–575, 1980
13. *Lausier v. Pescinski,* 226 N.W.2d 180 (Wis. 1975)
14. *Little v. Little,* 576 S.W.2d 493 (Tex. Civ. Ct. App. 1979)
15. *McDermott v. Manhattan Eye, Ear & Throat Hospital,* 26 App. Div.2d 519, 270 N.Y.S.2d 955, *aff'd without op.,* 18 N.Y.2d 970, 278 N.Y.S.2d 200, 224 N.E.2d 717 (1966)
16. Merrikin KJ, Overcast TD: Governmental regulation of heart transplantation and the right to privacy. J Contemp Law 11:481–514, 1985
17. Merrikin KJ, Overcast TD: Patient selection for heart transplantation: When is a discriminating choice discrimination? J Health Politics, Policy, Law 10:7–32, 1985
18. Moore FD: How much cardiac transplantation—and where? Heart Transplant 1:254–256, 1982
19. *Moore v. Shah,* 458 N.Y.S.2d 33 (1982)
20. *New York City Health & Hospital Corp. v. Sulsona,* 81 Misc.2d 1002, 367 N.Y.S.2d 686 (Sup. Ct. 1975)
21. Note: The evolution of the doctrine of informed consent. Georgia Law Review 12:581–612, 1978
22. Overcast TD, Evans RW, Bowen LE et al: Problems in the identification of potential organ donors: Misconceptions and fallacies associated with donor cards. J Am Med Assoc 251:1559–1562, 1985
23. Overcast TD, Evans RW: Technology assessment, pub-

lic policy and transplantation: A restrained appraisal of the Massachusetts Task Force Approach. Law, Med Health Care 13:106–111, 1985

24. Overcast TD, Merrikin KJ, Evans RW: Malpractice issues in heart transplantation. Am J Law Med 10:363–395, 1985

25. Overcast TD, Sales BD, Pollard MR: Applying antitrust law to the professions: Implications for psychology. Am Psychol 37:517–525, 1982

26. President's Commission for the Study of Ethical Problems in Medicine and Biomedical and Behavioral Research. Defining Death: Medical, Legal and Ethical Issues in the Determination of Death. Washington, D.C.: U.S. Government Printing Office, 1981

27. Rettig R: The changing federal role in medical technology. Technol Rev 34:34–41, 1980

28. *Sirianni v. Anna,* 55 Misc.2d 553, 285 N.Y.S.2d 709 (1967)

29. *State v. Fierro,* 124 Ariz. 182, 603 P.2d 74 (1979)

30. Strauss MJ: The political history of the artificial heart. N Engl J Med 310:332–336, 1984

31. *Strunk v. Strunk,* 445 S.W.2d 145 (Ky. 1969)

32. *Tucker v. Lower,* No. 2831 (Richmond, VA L. & Equity Ct., May 23, 1972)

33. *Williams v. Hoffman,* 223 N.W.2d 844, 76 A.L.R. 880 (Wis. 1984)

34. Woolley FR: Ethical issues in the implantation of the total artificial heart. N Engl J Med 310:292–296, 1984

Index

Page numbers followed by an *f* refer to figures; those with a *t* refer to tables.

ABO blood groups, 22, 223–229
  and bone marrow transplantation, 609
  historical aspects of, 223–224
  incompatability in transplantations, 224–229, 231–233, 365
    and administration of synthetic trisaccharide A or B, 232–233
    animal models for, 233
    donor-specific platelet transfusions in, 224–225
    immunosuppressive agents in, 225
    plasmapheresis in, 225
    role of HLA antigens in, 228
    splenectomy in, 225, 226t–227t
  and liver transplantation, 520, 522f
  pretransplant matching of donor and recipient, 380
  studies in patients awaiting transplants, 224, 229, 232
Acetate in dialysate, effects of, 240
Acyclovir, in herpes simplex virus infection, 453–454, 610
Adenine nucleotide metabolism, hypothermic perfusion affecting, 301–302, 302f
Adenosine triphosphate-magnesium chloride, and cyclosporine-induced nephrotoxicity, 26
Adrenal cortical tissue transplantation, 606
Age range
  in heart transplantation, 495–496
  in kidney transplantation, 264
    in childhood, 350–351
    and tumor development, 439
  in liver transplantation, 520
  for organ donors, 275, 291, 324t
  in pancreas transplantation, 539
  and patient selection for transplants, 264, 710
AIDS
  in donors of organs, 277, 447–448
  risks of
    in corneal transplantation, 626
    in hemodialysis, 240

  in peritoneal dialysis, 242
  in pretransplant transfusions, 154–155
  in renal transplants, 269
Air embolism, in hemodialysis, 240
Alkylating agents, immunosuppressive, 121t, 122–123
Allogenotopes, 167, 172
Allograft rejection, 53–62. *See also* Rejection of grafts
Allopurinol
  interaction with azathioprine, 122
  and organ preservation, 20
Alport's syndrome recurrence in renal allograft, 267
Amniotic membranes, as allograft tissue, 634
Amylase activity in urine, in pancreas transplant recipients, 556
Amyloidosis
  and patient selection for kidney transplantation, 264
  recurrence in renal allograft, 267
Anemia, aplastic, bone marrow transplantation in, 609, 612–613, 615t
Anesthesia in multiple organ procurement, 323–324
Antacid therapy, pretransplant, 364, 465
Antibodies. *See also* Immunoglobulins
  affinity for antigens, 51
  cold, 197, 205
  receptors for, rearrangement of genetic components in, 42, 43f
  role in graft rejection, 57–58
  valency of, 51
Antigen
  active presentation of, 54, 55f
  antibody affinity for, 51
  complex with antibody, 51
  passive presentation of, 54, 55f
  processing by B cells, 52, 53f
Antigen-presenting cell, 38, 39f, 72, 73
  costimulator activity of, 44–45
  and T-cell activation, 44

Antiglobulin crossmatch test, 203–204
Antilymphocyte serum
  administration of, 85
  bone marrow cell infusions with
    in dogs, 110–112
    in humans, 113–114
    in mice, 102–110
    in primates, 112–113
  corticosteroids with, 86, 129
  cyclosporine with, 89–90
  and graft survival, 85–87
  in heart–lung transplantation, 597
  in heart transplantation, 502
  and herpes simplex virus infection, 453
  in lung transplantation, 656
  mechanism of action, 85
  in pancreas transplantation, 555, 555t
  in pancreatic islet grafts, 580
  in pediatric renal transplantation, 254
  peripheral blood lymphocytes with, 109
  platelets with, 109
  production of, 84–85
  radiation of graft with, 141
  splenocyte infusions with, 108
  toxicity of, 90–91
  in treatment of graft rejection, 87–89, 373
    high-dose steroids with, 87–88
    as sole treatment, 89
    in steroid-resistant cases, 88–89
Antimetabolites, immunosuppressive, 121t, 121–122
Antithymocyte globulin. *See* Antilymphocyte serum
α_1-Antitrypsin deficiency, liver transplantation in, 518, 519f
Arterial steal syndrome, as vascular access problem in dialysis, 255
Artificial support of organ function
  heart and circulatory support devices in, 661–677
  historical aspects of, 9–10
  legal aspects of, 705